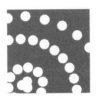

Regional Anesthesia and Analgesia

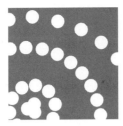

Regional Anesthesia and Analgesia

David L. Brown, M.D.

Associate Professor of Anesthesiology,
Mayo Medical School;
Consultant, Department of Anesthesiology,
Mayo Clinic and Mayo Foundation,
Rochester, Minnesota

Illustrated by
David A. Factor, M.S.

Mayo Clinic and Mayo Foundation,
Rochester, Minnesota

W.B. SAUNDERS COMPANY
A Division of Harcourt Brace & Company
Philadelphia   London   Toronto   Montreal   Sydney   Tokyo

W.B. SAUNDERS COMPANY
A Division of Harcourt Brace & Company

The Curtis Center
Independence Square West
Philadelphia, Pennsylvania 19106

Library of Congress Cataloging-in-Publication Data

Regional anesthesia and analgesia / [edited by] David L. Brown;
[illustrated by] David A. Factor. — 1st ed.

p. cm.

ISBN 0–7216–5654–4

1. Conduction anesthesia.   2. Analgesia.   I. Brown, David L.
  (David Lee). [DNLM: 1. Anesthesia, Conduction.
  2. Analgesia.   WO 300 R3351 1996]

RD84.R4225   1996

617.9′64—dc20

DNLM/DLC   95–21513

REGIONAL ANESTHESIA AND ANALGESIA   ISBN 0–7216–5654–4

Printed in the United States of America.

Last digit is the print number: 9   8   7   6   5   4   3   2   1

Dedication of this book to:

*Enthusiasts of regional anesthesia and the
patients benefiting from this interest*

Contributors

Stephen E. Abram, M.D.
Professor, Department of Anesthesiology, Medical
College of Wisconsin, Milwaukee, Wisconsin
Pharmacology of Pain Control

Alison Albrecht, M.D.
Fellow in Anesthesiology, Mayo Graduate School of
Medicine, Rochester, Minnesota
Orthopedics

Douglas R. Bacon, M.D., M.A.
Assistant Vice Chairman for Education, Department of
Anesthesiology, State University of New York at
Buffalo; Chief, Department of Anesthesiology,
Veterans Administration Medical Center, Buffalo, New
York
Regional Anesthesia and Chronic Pain Therapy: A History

David L. Brown, M.D.
Associate Professor of Anesthesiology, Mayo Medical
School; Consultant, Department of Anesthesiology,
Mayo Clinic and Mayo Foundation, Rochester,
Minnesota
Observations on Regional Anesthesia

Daniel B. Carr, M.D.
Salstonstall Professor of Pain Research, Professor,
Departments of Anesthesia and Medicine; Vice-Chair
for Research, Department of Anesthesia, New England
Medical Center, Boston, Massachusetts
The Stress Response and Regional Anesthesia

M. Soledad Cepeda, M.D.
Assistant Professor, Department of Anesthesia,
Javeriana University School of Medicine; Chief, Pain
Clinic, Department of Anesthesia, San Ignacio
Hospital, Bogota, Colombia
The Stress Response and Regional Anesthesia

David H. Chestnut, M.D.
Alfred Habeeb Professor and Chairman of
Anesthesiology, Professor of Obstetrics and
Gynecology, University of Alabama at Birmingham,
Birmingham, Alabama
Analgesia During Labor and Delivery

Mercedes A. Concepcion, M.D.
Assistant Professor of Anaesthesia, Harvard Medical
School; Anesthesiologist, Brigham and Women's
Hospital, Boston, Massachusetts
Acute Complications and Side Effects of Regional Anesthesia

Rudolph H. de Jong, M.D.
Professor, University of South Carolina School of
Medicine, Department of Anesthesiology; Director,
Carolina Pain Center, Health South Rehabilitation
Hospital, Columbia, South Carolina
Local Anesthetic Pharmacology

Oscar A. de Leon-Casasola, M.D.
Assistant Professor, Chief, Critical Care Medicine,
Roswell Park Cancer Institute, Buffalo, New York
Outcome After Epidural Anesthesia and Analgesia

John M. De Sio, M.D.
Instructor in Anesthesia, Harvard Medical School;
Department of Anesthesia, Beth Israel Hospital,
Boston, Massachusetts
Benign Pain

Cosmo A. DiFazio, M.D., Ph.D.
Professor, Anesthesiology, University of Virginia
Health Sciences Center, Charlottesville, Virginia
Additives to Local Anesthetic Solutions

M. Joanne Douglas, M.D., F.R.C.P.C.
Clinical Professor, Head, Division of Obstetric
Anaesthesia, University of British Columbia; Head,
Department of Anaesthesia, British Columbia's
Women's Hospital and Health Centre Society,
Vancouver, British Columbia, Canada
Cesarean Section Anesthesia

Kenneth Drasner, M.D.
Associate Professor of Anesthesia, Department of
Anesthesia, University of California, San Francisco,
School of Medicine, San Francisco, California
*Delayed Complications and Side Effects of Regional
Anesthesia*

F. Kayser Enneking, M.D.
Assistant Professor of Anesthesiology, University of
Florida, Gainesville, Florida
Gynecology and Urology

Mary P. Fillinger, M.D.
Assistant Professor of Anesthesiology, Dartmouth
Medical School, Hanover, New Hampshire; Attending
Anesthesiologist, Dartmouth-Hitchcock Medical
Center, Lebanon, New Hampshire
Cardiothoracic and Vascular Surgery

Perry G. Fine, M.D.
Associate Professor, Department of Anesthesiology,
School of Medicine; Associate Medical Director, Pain

Management Center, University of Utah Health Sciences Center, University of Utah, Salt Lake City, Utah
Functional Neuroanatomy

James F. Flynn, M.D., F.R.C.P.C.
Clinical Assistant Professor, Memorial University of Newfoundland; Director of Pain Clinic, General Hospital, Health Sciences Centre, St. John's, Newfoundland, Canada
Head and Neck Regional Blocks

Jeremy M. Geiduschek, M.D.
Assistant Professor, Department of Anesthesiology, University of Washington School of Medicine; Attending Physician, Department of Anesthesia and Critical Care, Children's Hospital and Medical Center, Seattle, Washington
Pediatrics

Patricia Harrison, M.D.
Clinical Assistant Professor, Department of Anesthesiology, State University of New York at Buffalo, School of Medicine and Biomedical Sciences; Clinical Director, Cancer Pain Service, Roswell Park Cancer Institute, Buffalo, New York
Cancer Pain

James E. Heavner, D.V.M., Ph.D.
Professor, Departments of Anesthesiology and Physiology; Director, Anesthesia Research, Texas Tech University Health Sciences Center, Lubbock, Texas
Neurophysiology

Quinn H. Hogan, M.D.
Associate Professor, Director of Pain Management Center, Medical College of Wisconsin, Milwaukee, Wisconsin
Reexamination of Anatomy in Regional Anesthesia

Terese T. Horlocker, M.D.
Assistant Professor of Anesthesiology, Mayo Medical School; Consultant, Department of Anesthesiology, Mayo Clinic and Mayo Foundation, Rochester, Minnesota
Concurrent Medical Problems and Regional Anesthesia

Cynthia Kahn, M.D.
Instructor in Anesthesia, Harvard Medical School; Department of Anesthesia, Beth Israel Hospital, Boston, Massachusetts
Benign Pain

Dan J. Kopacz, M.D.
Staff Anesthesiologist, Virginia Mason Medical Center, Seattle, Washington
Regional Anesthesia of the Trunk

Tim J. Lamer, M.D.
Assistant Professor of Anesthesiology, Mayo Medical School, Rochester, Minnesota; Chair, Division of Pain

Services, Mayo Clinic Jacksonville, Jacksonville, Florida
Sympathetic Nerve Blocks

Craig H. Leicht, M.D., M.P.H.
Associate Professor, School of Medicine, University of Kentucky, Lexington, Kentucky; Chairman, Department of Anesthesiology, Memorial Hospital, Manchester, Kentucky
Postdelivery Analgesia

Mark J. Lema, M.D., Ph.D.
Associate Professor and Vice Chair for Academic Affairs, Department of Anesthesiology, State University of New York at Buffalo, School of Medicine and Biomedical Sciences; Chairman, Department of Anesthesiology, Roswell Park Cancer Institute, Buffalo, New York
Cancer Pain

Timothy R. Lubenow, M.D.
Associate Professor of Anesthesiology, Rush Medical College; Attending Anesthesiologist, Director, Section of Pain Management, Rush-Presbyterian/St. Luke's Medical Center, Chicago, Illinois
Analgesic Techniques

Anne C. P. Lui, M.D.
Assistant Professor, Department of Anaesthesia, University of Ottawa; Active Attending Staff, Ottawa Civic Hospital, Ottawa, Ontario, Canada
Neurosurgery

Johan Lundberg, M.D., Ph.D.
Assistant Professor of Anesthesiology and Critical Care Medicine, Lund University; Attending Anesthesiologist, University Hospital, Lund, Sweden
Cardiothoracic and Vascular Surgery

David C. Mackey, M.D.
Assistant Professor of Anesthesiology, Mayo Medical School, Rochester, Minnesota; Consultant, Division of Anesthesia Services, and Consultant, Division of Pain Medicine, Mayo Clinic Jacksonville, Jacksonville, Florida
Cardiopulmonary Physiology; Physiologic Effects of Regional Block

Dennis J. McMahon, B.S., C.B.E.T.
Chief Anesthesia Technologist, Virginia Mason Hospital, Seattle, Washington
Equipment

Michael F. Mulroy, M.D.
Staff Anesthesiologist, Virginia Mason Medical Center, Seattle, Washington
Outpatients

Joseph M. Neal, M.D.
Clinical Assistant Professor of Anesthesiology,
University of Washington, Staff Anesthesiologist,
Virginia Mason Medical Center; Seattle, Washington
Equipment

Robert S. Neill, M.D.
Consultant Anaesthetist, Glasgow Royal Infirmary,
Glasgow, Scotland
Ophthalmology and Otorhinolaryngology

Kevin J. Nolan, M.D.
Assistant Professor, Department of Anaesthesia,
University of Ottawa; Active Attending Staff, Ottawa
Civic Hospital, Ottawa, Ontario, Canada
Neurosurgery

Robert W. Phelps, M.D., Ph.D.
Associate Professor of Anesthesiology, University of
Colorado Health Sciences Center, Denver, Colorado
Opioid and Nonopioid Analgesics

Somayaji Ramamurthy, M.D.
Professor, Department of Anesthesiology, University of
Texas Health Science Center, San Antonio, Texas
Lower Extremity Blocks

David M. Ransom, M.D.
Fellow in Anesthesiology, Mayo Graduate School of
Medicine, Rochester, Minnesota
Postdelivery Analgesia

Narinder Rawal, M.D., Ph.D.
Visiting Professor, University of Texas Medical School,
Houston, Texas; Senior Consultant, Department of
Anesthesiology and Intensive Care, Örebro Medical
Center Hospital, Örebro, Sweden
*Neuraxial Administration of Opioids and Nonopioids;
Anesthesiology-Based Acute Pain Services: A Contemporary
View*

L. Brian Ready, M.D., F.R.C.P.C.
Professor, Department of Anesthesiology, University of
Washington; Director, University of Washington
Medical Center Pain Service, Seattle, Washington
*Anesthesiology-Based Acute Pain Services: A Contemporary
View*

James N. Rogers, M.D.
Associate Professor, Department of Anesthesiology,
University of Texas Health Science Center, San
Antonio, Texas
Lower Extremity Blocks

Jacob A. Rosenberg, M.D.
Staff Anesthesiologist, Washoe Medical Center, Reno,
Nevada
Functional Neuroanatomy

Per H. Rosenberg, M.D., Ph.D.
Associate Professor of Anesthesiology, Department of
Anesthesiology, Helsinki University Central Hospital,
Helsinki, Finland
Intravenous Regional Anesthesia

John C. Rowlingson, M.D.
Professor of Anesthesiology, University of Virginia
School of Medicine; Director, Pain Management
Center, Department of Anesthesiology, University of
Virginia Health Sciences Center, Charlottesville,
Virginia
Additives to Local Anesthetic Solutions

Robin B. Slover, M.D.
Assistant Professor of Anesthesiology, Director of
Acute Pain Service, University of Colorado Health
Sciences Center; Director of Anesthesia Pain Clinic,
Veterans Administration Medical Center, Denver,
Colorado
Opioid and Nonopioid Analgesics

Ian Smith, B.Sc., M.B.,B.S., F.R.C.A.
Senior Lecturer in Anaesthetics, Keele University,
North Staffordshire Hospital, Stoke-on-Trent, United
Kingdom
Intravenous and Inhaled Adjuncts

Rom A. Stevens, M.D.
Associate Professor of Anesthesiology and Director,
Division of Pain Management, Loyola University,
Stritch School of Medicine, Maywood, Illinois
Neuraxial Blocks

Jeffrey L. Swisher, M.D.
Assistant Professor of Anesthesia, Department of
Anesthesiology, University of California, San
Francisco, School of Medicine, San Francisco,
California
*Delayed Complications and Side Effects of Regional
Anesthesia*

John H. Tucker, M.D., F.R.C.P.C.
Assistant Professor, Department of Anesthesia,
Memorial University of Newfoundland; Staff
Anesthetist, Health Sciences Centre, St. John's
Newfoundland, Canada
Head and Neck Regional Blocks

William F. Urmey, M.D., B.A.
Assistant Professor of Clinical Anesthesiology, Cornell
University Medical College; Medical Director,
Ambulatory Surgery Center, The Hospital for Special
Surgery, New York, New York
Upper Extremity Blocks

Bernadette Th. Veering, M.D., Ph.D.
Senior Lecturer, Medical Faculty, University of Leiden;
Staff Anesthesiologist, Department of Anesthesiology,
University Hospital Leiden, Leiden, The Netherlands
Local Anesthetics

Robert D. Vincent, Jr., M.D.
Associate Professor of Anesthesiology, Director of
Obstetric Anesthesia, University of Mississippi Medical
Center, Jackson, Mississippi
Analgesia During Labor and Delivery

Carol A. Warfield, M.D.
Associate Professor of Anesthesia, Harvard Medical
School; Director, Pain Management Center, Beth
Israel Hospital, Boston, Massachusetts
Benign Pain

Denise J. Wedel, M.D.
Associate Professor of Anesthesiology, Mayo Medical
School; Consultant, Department of Anesthesiology,
Mayo Clinic and Mayo Foundation, Rochester,
Minnesota
Orthopedics

**Paul F. White, Ph.D., M.D., F.F.A.R.A.C.S.,
F.A.N.Z.C.A.**
Professor and Holder of the Margaret Milam
McDermott Distinguished Chair of Anesthesiology;
Department of Anesthesiology and Pain Management,
University of Texas Southwestern Medical School,
Dallas, Texas
Intravenous and Inhaled Adjuncts

Mark P. Yeager, M.D.
Associate Professor of Anesthesiology and Medicine,
Dartmouth Medical School, Hanover, New Hampshire;
Attending Anesthesiologist and Intensivist,
Dartmouth-Hitchcock Medical Center, Lebanon, New
Hampshire
Cardiothoracic and Vascular Surgery

Way Yin, M.D.
Chief, Trauma Anesthesia Services, Director, Regional
Anesthesia Training, Department of Anesthesiology,
PSSA, Wilford Hall Medical Center, Lackland Air
Force Base, Texas
General Surgery and Trauma

Preface

This text is designed to fill the need for a clinically focused textbook of regional anesthesia and analgesia. It will allow physicians-in-training and those physicians whose training is complete to improve their understanding and application of regional techniques in a wide variety of practical clinical situations. Throughout the text, the approach is clinical, with input from physicians around the world who daily practice regional anesthesia and provide analgesia for patients. This text can also be used as a companion to the editor's *Atlas of Regional Anesthesia,* which is an additional source of detailed presentation of practical techniques for performing many of the regional blocks.

The book is divided into five major sections: Development of Regional Anesthesia; Basic Science of Regional Anesthesia; Induction of Regional Anesthesia; Concurrent Medical Problems, Side Effects, and Complications With Regional Anesthesia; and Regional Anesthesia and Analgesia in Practice. The section Regional Anesthesia and Analgesia in Practice includes subsections on regional techniques for surgery, obstetrics, acute pain, and chronic pain. Each of the contributors of clinical chapters has been asked not only to provide a focused clinical summary of the subject but also to detail clinical experience (clinical impressions). The organization of the book minimizes overlap between chapters; however, it was not our intent to completely eliminate overlap. Each chapter can be read without reference to other chapters. For example, chapters covering acute and delayed complications and side effects each contain details about epidural hematoma. This is important because the development of a hematoma can occur acutely or its appearance can be delayed.

The text was edited for uniformity of terminology to minimize confusion among chapters.

The emphasis of this book is on regional anesthesia and analgesia techniques and their clinical application. The scope of pain therapy would necessarily expand this into a much larger text if this topic were included, and it is not my intent to duplicate comprehensive pain texts. Nevertheless, I believe that many of those who use pain texts will benefit from the technical information contained in this work and the insights provided by the contributors, highlighting most major issues in pain care.

This book would not be possible without the creative talents of the contributors and their willingness to participate. The success of the project is theirs. Also important to completion of this work is the administrative support provided by the Mayo Foundation, including the secretarial support provided by Kimberly Krenzke and Mylee Nachtweih and the editorial support of Mary Jane Badker; Carol Kornblith, Ph.D.; Jen Schlotthauer; Roberta Schwartz; Renée Van Vleet; and Sharon Wadleigh. Further, the unequaled abilities of the artist, David Factor, to create the illustrations that helped the more than 40 contributors make their chapters come to life deserve emphasis. He allowed the chapters to be tied together through his talent in conceptually linking the illustrations from chapter to chapter.

Finally, this work would not have been completed without the support and encouragement by the W.B. Saunders team of Bunny Best, Richard Zorab, and Lewis Reines. My thanks to them all.

DAVID L. BROWN

Contents

Note: Color Plates follow pp. 62 and 494.

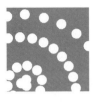

Regional
Anesthesia
and
Analgesia

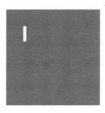

Development of Regional Anesthesia

CHAPTER 1

Observations on Regional Anesthesia

David L. Brown, M.D.

Why Care About Regional
    Anesthesia?
Past Use of Regional Anesthesia

Current Use of Regional Anesthesia
Future of Regional Anesthesia

Why Care About Regional Anesthesia?

Why should anesthesiologists care about the state of regional anesthesia? I believe the major reason is that anesthesiologists are really perioperative risk managers, and regional anesthesia is an important part of individualizing the perioperative risk equation. A second reason anesthesiologists should care about the state of regional anesthesia is the increasing interest by medical professionals and patients in acute and chronic pain control. Pain control relies on effective regional anesthesia and the precision with which the techniques are accomplished.

Every decision we make in our operating room practices involves the estimation of risks and benefits, and this individualization of the risk-benefit equation is what separates a physician with medical judgment from a technician performing a prescription of anesthetic care. A confounding concept is that, even during the safest anesthesia, patients can expect to return to only their preoperative state, not an anesthetically improved one. During the last two decades, our specialty's focus on risk analysis seems to have been to eliminate risks completely during the intraoperative period, such that we often failed to consider how our anesthetic choice impacts patients postoperatively.[1] Although this intraoperative focus has paid dividends, as illustrated by a decrease in liability risk classification for anesthesiologists during the years 1985 to 1990[2] (Fig. 1–1), this intraoperative focus is incomplete and unrealistic for individual patients, and it fails to acknowledge that, for surgical benefits to occur, anesthetic risks and the risks of postoperative recovery (i.e., analgesia) must be incorporated into the patient's risk-benefit equation.

When anesthesiologists are questioned about their preference for anesthetic prescription, they overwhelmingly choose regional anesthesia for themselves.[3-5] Perhaps these anesthesiologists recognize that there is more to anesthetic prescription than the intraoperative period. Accumulating experimental and clinical evidence[6-8] indicates that preventing painful intraoperative neural impulses from reaching the central nervous system minimizes pain transmission in the immediate and distant postoperative periods (Fig. 1–2). Although the clinical application of preemptive analgesia is still maturing, this may be one of the most important reasons to assure our patients that anesthesiol-

ogists are competent to perform a wide variety of regional techniques.

A slightly different conceptual problem in analyzing regional anesthetic risks is that for many the "default mode" of anesthetic practice is general anesthesia. For regional anesthesia to be widely accepted by these physicians, it must clearly be safer than, not simply as safe as, general anesthesia. When the narrow window of the intraoperative period is considered, this focus confounds a clear understanding of anesthetic prescription. Moreover, some anesthetic trainees have not been grounded in regional techniques with the same vigor as general anesthetic techniques,[9, 10] and the training in the techniques during residency does influence the frequency of use in later practice.[5]

Past Use of Regional Anesthesia

Deciding between regional and general anesthesia implies that there is an option for physicians in selecting the safest anesthetic for a patient. It was not until Koller (Fig. 1–3) began placing cocaine into the eye in 1884 that this option existed.[11] For the four decades before 1884, general anesthesia was the only anesthetic technique available. This temporal advantage in developing general anesthetic techniques might have thwarted the development of regional anesthesia, but

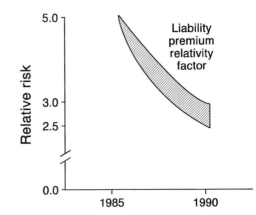

Figure 1–1 Decrease in professional relative liability risks of anesthesiologists as reflected by the insurance industry liability relativity factor range. (Data from Pierce EC Jr: Anesthesia patient safety movement. ASA Newslett 1991; 55: 4–8.)

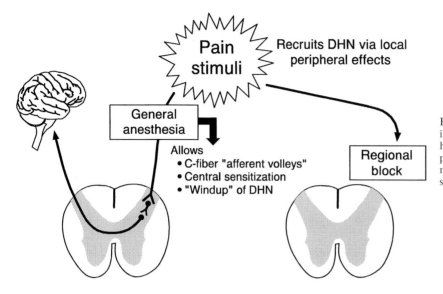

Figure 1–2 Preemptive analgesia concept illustrates that regional blocks can prevent dorsal horn windup and amplification of acute surgical pain by modulating C-fiber afferent volleys and minimizing dorsal horn neuron (DHN) sensitization.

there were zealous surgeons, such as Crile (Fig. 1–4), who understood the advantages of each approach and promoted regional anesthesia.[12] Perhaps these early surgeons were more attuned to the whole of the perioperative period and the advantages regional anesthesia offered. Was this because these surgeons were often the patients' only physician—in concept their primary care physician, internist, anesthesiologist, surgeon, and critical care specialist—from initial contact until the patients returned home? I think this is a likely explanation.

Allen, a colleague of Rudolph Matas, speculated that, "had local analgesia been discovered before general anesthesia, general anesthesia might now be struggling to displace it from its coveted pedestal, and it is not to be doubted but that local anesthesia would have

reached a much higher plane of development, for in all operations suited to its use general anesthesia cannot compare with it in safety and comfort."[13] Allen's belief that regional techniques were unquestionably safer than general anesthetics was not universally shared. Gwathmey[14] suggested, in a retrospective review, that local anesthesia was often unsuitable for major operations, although it appeared safe. He believed that combinations of anesthetics were "safer than any known single anesthetic" and advocated combining regional and general techniques. Crile believed that combining regional and general anesthesia to produce what he termed "anociassociation" was the method of choice (Fig. 1–5). He suggested that the brain must be protected from the psychic strain of operation by use of general anesthesia and that regional analgesia should be used to exclude nociceptive impulses arising from the surgical site.[15]

Lundy's[16] description of balanced anesthesia also incorporated this reasoning, and regional anesthesia was

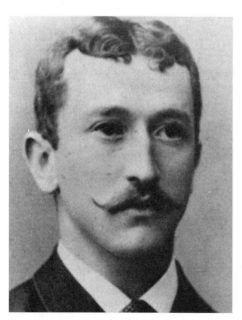

Figure 1–3 Carl Koller (1857–1944), circa 1883. (Photograph courtesy of Wood Library-Museum of Anesthesiology.)

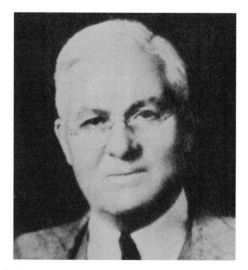

Figure 1–4 George W. Crile (1864–1943). (Photograph courtesy of Wood Library-Museum of Anesthesiology.)

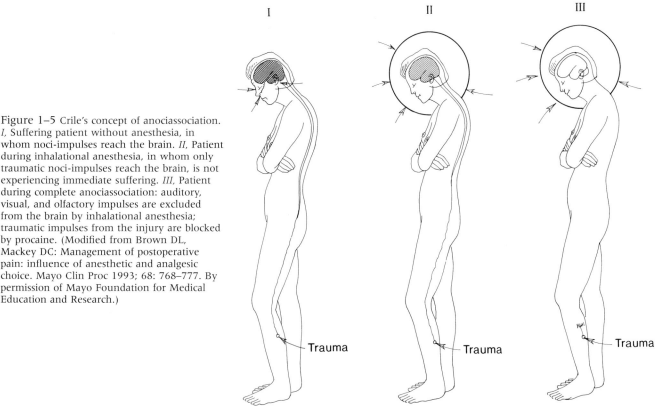

Figure 1–5 Crile's concept of anociassociation. *I*, Suffering patient without anesthesia, in whom noci-impulses reach the brain. *II*, Patient during inhalational anesthesia, in whom only traumatic noci-impulses reach the brain, is not experiencing immediate suffering. *III*, Patient during complete anociassociation: auditory, visual, and olfactory impulses are excluded from the brain by inhalational anesthesia; traumatic impulses from the injury are blocked by procaine. (Modified from Brown DL, Mackey DC: Management of postoperative pain: influence of anesthetic and analgesic choice. Mayo Clin Proc 1993; 68: 768–777. By permission of Mayo Foundation for Medical Education and Research.)

an important component of that anesthetic technique. He advocated intraoperative pain relief by combining premedication, regional analgesia, and light general anesthesia (Fig. 1–6). Sir Robert Macintosh (Fig. 1–7), a European proponent of regional anesthesia, also supported the concept of combining techniques. He stated, "A local analgesic can provide ideal operating conditions when used alone; a fortiori it will afford ideal conditions if a general anesthetic is given at the same time. Local analgesia, alone or combined with general anesthesia, is therefore theoretically justified in every abdominal operation."[17] Moore and Bonica[18] extended the definition of balanced anesthesia when they promoted the concept of combining brachial blocks and spinal anesthetics for upper extremity surgery in which lower extremity harvesting of bone or soft tissue was planned as part of the operation.

Despite these ideas, from the 1950s to the 1970s, pharmaceutical advances led most academic and clini-

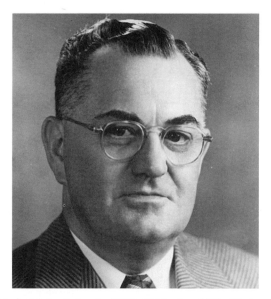

Figure 1–6 John S. Lundy (1894–1973), circa 1960. (Photograph courtesy of Wood Library-Museum of Anesthesiology.)

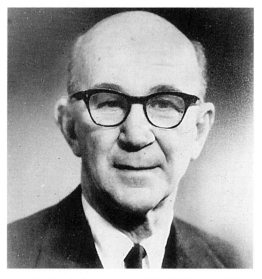

Figure 1–7 Sir Robert Macintosh (1897–1989), circa 1965. (Photograph courtesy of Wood Library-Museum of Anesthesiology.)

Table 1–1 Suggested Reasons Regional Anesthesia Is Used Less Frequently Than Indicated

Patients do not like regional anesthesia
Its performance consumes too much time
There are too many failures
Serious complications can occur
There is a greater medicolegal risk
Most surgeons dislike the method

Adapted from Bonica JJ: Regional anesthesia in private practice. (Editorial.) Anesthesiology 1960; 21: 554–556.

cal anesthesiologists to focus on advancing general anesthesia techniques, and balanced anesthesia came to signify mixtures of inhalational and intravenous medications.[19] It was during this era that mechanical ventilation became commonplace, and deep, opioid-based anesthetics then became possible and were advocated to provide a safer, stress-free anesthetic experience. Anesthesiologists appeared attracted to the intraoperative hemodynamic stability possible with these almost "pure narcotic" anesthetics.[20] It was during this same interval that medicolegal concerns began to significantly impact anesthetic prescription, and the concept that regional anesthesia somehow carried more medicolegal risk was promoted.

In an editorial in *Anesthesiology* in 1960, Bonica[21] suggested that the infrequent use of regional anesthesia in private practice was the result of the factors highlighted in Table 1–1. The medicolegal specter of malpractice remains a concern to many.[22] Some early data indicated that a successful lawsuit might be more likely after regional than general anesthesia, even when community standards were met.[23] However, larger and more recent series do not support this view. The American Society of Anesthesiologists closed claims database suggests that the severity and cost of adverse outcomes with regional and general anesthesia are no different.[24] There are few studies clearly documenting that either regional or general anesthesia is safer for a given surgical patient. Because of the remarkable safety of all intraoperative techniques, it is doubtful that a statistically significant difference between intraoperative anesthetic choices will be shown, except in unusual circumstances.[25–27] This is not the case if decisions about anesthetic prescription include postoperative analgesic plans as part of the original risk-benefit decision.[7, 28, 29]

Current Use of Regional Anesthesia

Anesthesiologists overwhelmingly choose regional anesthesia for their own anesthetic care, but it appears that even physicians completing their training in programs viewed as promoting regional anesthesia (e.g., programs in Seattle at the Virginia Mason Hospital and the University of Washington) use the technique slightly less than 30% of the time.[5] The frequency of use appears to decline compared with the frequency that regional anesthesia was performed during training, as does the range of blocks performed.[5] It has been shown that the regional blocks most frequently per-

formed for surgical anesthesia on entry into private practice, excluding obstetrics, are spinal and axillary block, with epidural block third in frequency.[5] These data are probably slightly different in the mid-1990s, because the introduction of acute pain services has increased the amount of epidural analgesia provided.[10]

In contrast to the data Buffington and colleagues[5] collected on the frequency of regional block use in programs often touted as supporting regional anesthesia training, Kopacz and Bridenbaugh[10] showed that about 29% of anesthesia is performed with regional blocks during anesthetic specialty training nationwide (Fig. 1–8). Even during residency training, the rate of use of regional blocks varied by year of training, with the rate of use of spinal anesthesia decreasing after the first year and many of the peripheral nerve blocks reported during training being performed during pain clinic rotations, not during surgical anesthesia rotations.[10] Although the data from Kopacz and Bridenbaugh[10] (1990 cohort) showed improvements in frequency of regional block use compared with the data from Bridenbaugh[9] (1980 cohort), almost all of the increase was explained by the increase in use of continuous epidural analgesic techniques, primarily for postoperative pain control[10] (Fig. 1–9).

As an example of the disparity in frequency of use between programs, Bridenbaugh[9] identified training programs providing as few as 2.5 spinal anesthetics per resident per year of training in 1980. It is not surprising that some of those trainees feel uncomfortable in providing a comprehensive regional anesthesia practice. Kopacz and Neal[30] showed that more than 40 of each type of block for spinal and epidural anesthesia need to be performed for the physician trainees to sustain improvements in their techniques and become predictably successful with the blocks (Fig. 1–10).

Another aspect of anesthetic practice that confounds a complete understanding of how best to use regional anesthesia is the reluctance by many to combine regional and general anesthetic techniques, despite evi-

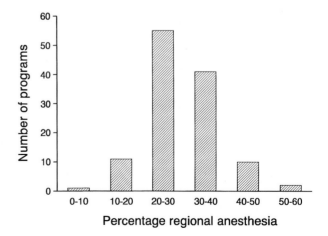

Figure 1–8 Frequency of use of regional block techniques in 1990 by physician trainees in the United States by training programs. (Redrawn from Kopacz DJ, Bridenbaugh LD: Are anesthesia residency programs failing regional anesthesia? The past, present, and future. Reg Anesth 1993; 18: 84–87.)

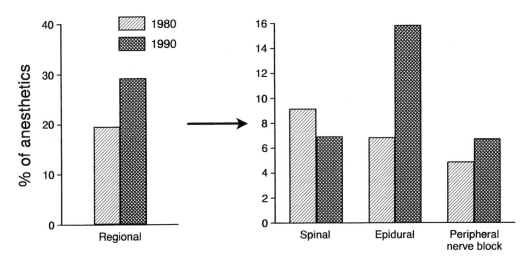

Figure 1–9 Frequency of use of regional block techniques in 1980 and 1990 by physician trainees in United States training programs as a percentage of total anesthetics administered. These data show that most of the increase in regional use was related to the increased use of epidural anesthesia, administered primarily for postoperative analgesia. (From Kopacz DJ, Bridenbaugh LD: Are anesthesia residency programs failing regional anesthesia? The past, present, and future. Reg Anesth 1993; 18: 84–87.)

dence that Crile's early concepts of the benefits of anociassociation have been shown to have neurophysiologic correlates in the dorsal horn of the spinal cord.[8] It is curious that combining regional and general anesthesia or even combining regional anesthesia and something more than minimal sedation in a patient seems to disturb so many contemporary anesthesiologists. This is especially ironic because proponents of general anesthesia often think that combinations of general anesthetic medications are preferable to a single anesthetic drug.[31]

Patients also have ideas about regional anesthesia. Among obstetric patients, the overwhelming reasons parturients refused regional anesthesia compared with general anesthesia were fear of backache, fear of needles, and fear of seeing or hearing intraoperatively.[32] These issues should be addressed directly and compassionately with patients preoperatively, and with knowledge about improved sedatives and advances in anesthetic equipment, most patients' fears should be minimized.

These preoperative discussions may be most effective for patients with higher levels of education. Harders and colleagues[33] showed that patients with advanced education are more willing to accept regional techniques than those with less education after a balanced presentation of the risks and benefits of regional techniques. Perhaps that is why anesthesiologists—the most educated regarding anesthetic risk and benefit—overwhelmingly choose regional anesthesia for themselves. Preoperative psychologic testing of elective surgical patients has shown that advancing age, length of illness leading to surgery, low levels of neuroticism, and high extroversion scores were all positively correlated with acceptance of regional anesthesia.[34]

Future of Regional Anesthesia

The intraoperative anesthetic period has become so safe that comprehensive morbidity or mortality comparisons between regional and general anesthetic regimens are almost impossible to construct or fund.[25–27] Comparisons are more likely to be made among regimens that incorporate regional anesthetic techniques as part of a continuum of perioperative care. It is here that decreases in morbidity, increases in patient satisfaction, and lowered costs of inpatient hospitalization may be realized. These improvements have been demonstrated for high-risk patients undergoing major surgical procedures.[28,29]

It is clear that peripheral regional block techniques should be included in these analgesic comparisons. As an example, Allen and coworkers[35] showed that use of brachial blocks for outpatient hand surgery shortened recovery room stay, decreasing the overall cost of providing outpatient surgery to that group. Another example is the use of femoral nerve block after or as part of

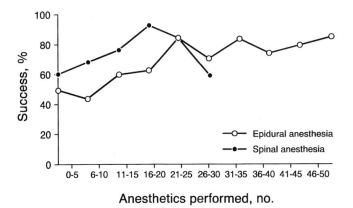

Figure 1–10 Comparison of success with spinal and epidural block by clinical anesthesia year-one resident physicians compared with the number of blocks performed. (From Kopacz DJ, Neal JM: Learning regional anesthesia techniques: how many is enough? [Abstract.] Reg Anesth 1994; 19: S37.)

surgical arthroscopic repair of anterior cruciate ligaments to ease the patient's transfer home on the day of the operation rather than requiring an overnight hospital stay for early pain control.[36]

Patients and physicians need to understand that acceptance of regional anesthesia does not mean that patients will be "awake" during the operation.[32] Well-administered regional anesthesia should provide a balance between the block and supplemental intravenous or inhalational sedation. The introduction of propofol infusions into anesthetic practices allows a combination of rapidly titratable sedation and rapid return of alertness, heretofore not as easily available.[37] The benefits of regional block can be provided in situations in which the laryngeal mask airway is also used, allowing low concentration inhalational anesthesia to be used for sedation without concerns about waste gas scavenging[38] (Fig. 1–11).

Four advances still need to be made in regional anesthesia and analgesia. First, anesthesiologists need to embrace and promote improvements in the "imaging" of regional block anatomy. Our specialty seems to be one of the few areas of medicine in which imaging techniques are not leading to advances in medical practice. This should be changed. Second, work on reversible and longer-acting local anesthetic drug formulations needs to be reenergized. Several investigators are working on reformulating the available local anesthetics to achieve this goal, but further basic work is required before several days' worth of regional block is a reality.[39, 40] Third, improvements in catheters designed for peripheral regional blocks need to continue,

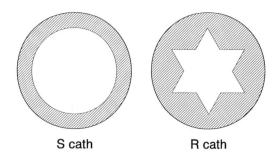

Figure 1–12 Cross section of epidural catheters. S cath is a typical catheter design, and R cath has a lumen that is star shaped, minimizing difficulties with catheter kinking. (Redrawn from Yorozu T, Kondoh M, Morisaki H, et al: An advantage of a new epidural catheter with a unique cross-section. [Abstract.] Anesthesiology 1994; 81: A597.)

allowing anesthesiologists to provide days' worth of effective analgesia[41] (Fig. 1–12). These improved catheters will act as a bridge for clinicians until the longer-acting local anesthetic formulations have been introduced. Fourth, our specialty needs to accept the multimodal approach to perioperative patient care.[42] Far too often, anesthesiologists have focused only on analgesia issues postoperatively and forgotten about the importance of patient satisfaction and adding value to the perioperative period by decreasing the length of stay or medical care costs.

In the remainder of this book, experts in many areas combine their technical expertise with these concepts to offer more comprehensive regional anesthesia to our patients.

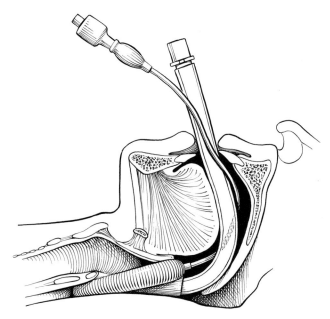

Figure 1–11 Laryngeal mask airway, originally designed by Brain[38] to facilitate airway management in difficult or unusual tracheal intubations, is often used to facilitate combined regional and general anesthesia. This allows "inhalational sedation" during regional anesthesia without worry about contamination of the operating room with inhaled agents. (Adapted from Brain AIJ: The laryngeal mask—a new concept in airway management. Br J Anaesth 1983; 55: 801–804.)

References

1. Keats AS: Anesthesia mortality in perspective. Anesth Analg 1990; 71: 113–119.
2. Pierce EC Jr: Anesthesia patient safety movement—1991. ASA Newslett 1991; 55: 4–8.
3. Katz J: A survey of anesthetic choice among anesthesiologists. Anesth Analg 1973; 52: 373–375.
4. Broadman LM, Mesrobian R, Ruttimann U, et al: Do anesthesiologists prefer a regional or general anesthetic for themselves? (Abstract.) Reg Anesth 1986; 11: A57.
5. Buffington CW, Ready LB, Horton WG: Training and practice factors influence the use of regional anesthesia. Reg Anesth 1985; 10: 2–6.
6. Schulze S, Sommer P, Bigler D, et al: Effect of combined prednisolone, epidural analgesia, and indomethacin on the systemic response after colonic surgery. Arch Surg 1992; 127: 325–331.
7. Tuman KJ, McCarthy RJ, March RJ, et al: Effects of epidural anesthesia and analgesia on coagulation and outcome after major vascular surgery. Anesth Analg 1991; 73: 696–704.
8. Dickenson AH, Sullivan AF: Subcutaneous formalin-induced activity of dorsal horn neurones in the rat: differential response to an intrathecal opiate administered pre or post formalin. Pain 1987; 30: 349–360.
9. Bridenbaugh LD: Are anesthesia programs failing regional anesthesia? Reg Anesth 1982; 7: 26–28.
10. Kopacz DJ, Bridenbaugh LD: Are anesthesia residency programs failing regional anesthesia? The past, present, and future. Reg Anesth 1993; 18: 84–87.
11. Wildsmith JAW: Carl Koller (1857–1944) and the introduction of cocaine into anesthetic practice. Reg Anesth 1984; 9: 161–164.
12. Brown DL, Fink BR: History of neural blockade. In Cousins MJ, Bridenbaugh PO (eds): Neural Blockade in Clinical Anesthesia

and Management of Pain, 3rd ed. Philadelphia, JB Lippincott. (In press.)

13. Allen CW: Local and Regional Anesthesia, 2nd ed, pp 17–25. Philadelphia, WB Saunders Co, 1918.
14. Gwathmey JT: Anesthesia, p 841. New York, D Appleton & Co, 1914.
15. Crile GW: Nitrous oxide anaesthesia and a note on anoci-association, a new principle in operative surgery. Surg Gynecol Obstet 1911; 13: 170–173.
16. Lundy JS: Balanced anesthesia. Minn Med 1926; 9: 399–404.
17. Macintosh RR, Bryce-Smith R: Local Analgesia: Abdominal Surgery. Edinburgh, E & S Livingstone, 1953.
18. Moore DC, Bonica JJ: Combined brachial block and spinal analgesia for bone graft surgery (report of 83 cases). Anesth Analg 1950; 29: 43–50.
19. Little DM, Jr., Stephen CR: Modern balanced anesthesia: a concept. Anesthesiology 1954; 15: 246–261.
20. Lowenstein E, Hallowell P, Levine FH, et al: Cardiovascular response to large doses of intravenous morphine in man. N Engl J Med 1969; 281: 1389–1393.
21. Bonica JJ: Regional anesthesia in private practice. (Editorial.) Anesthesiology 1960; 21: 554–556.
22. Heussner RC Jr: Malpractice plaintiffs' attorneys: the mindset, the methods. Minn Med 1992; 75: 22–27.
23. Solazzi RW, Ward RJ: Analysis of anesthetic mishaps: the spectrum of medical liability cases. Int Anesthesiol Clin 1984; 22: 43–59.
24. Tinker JH, Dull DL, Caplan RA, et al: Role of monitoring devices in prevention of anesthetic mishaps: a closed claims analysis. Anesthesiology 1989; 71: 541–546.
25. Forrest JB, Rehder K, Goldsmith CH, et al: Multicenter study of general anesthesia: I. Design and patient demography. Anesthesiology 1990; 72: 252–261.
26. Forrest JB, Cahalan MK, Rehder K, et al: Multicenter study of general anesthesia: II. Results. Anesthesiology 1990; 72: 262–268.
27. Forrest JB, Rehder K, Cahalan MK, et al: Multicenter study of general anesthesia: III. Predictors of severe perioperative adverse outcomes. Anesthesiology 1992; 76: 3–15.
28. Christopherson R, Beattie C, Frank SM, et al: Perioperative morbidity in patients randomized to epidural or general anesthesia for lower extremity vascular surgery. Anesthesiology 1993; 79: 422–434.
29. Yeager MP, Glass DD, Neff RK, et al: Epidural anesthesia and analgesia in high-risk surgical patients. Anesthesiology 1987; 66: 729–736.
30. Kopacz DJ, Neal JM: Learning regional anesthesia techniques: how many is enough? (Abstract.) Reg Anesth 1994; 19: S37.
31. Kenny GNC, White M: Total intravenous anaesthesia. Recent Adv Anaesth Analg 1993; 10: 1–20.
32. Gajraj NM, Sharma S, Souter AJ, et al: A survey of patients who refuse regional anesthesia. (Abstract.) Anesth Analg 1994; 78: S126.
33. Harders MS, Jorgensen NH, Hullander RM, et al: Patient survey of anesthetic choice: education makes a difference. Anesth Analg 1994; 78: S151.
34. Papanikolaou MN, Voulgart A, Lykouras L, et al: Psychological factors influencing the surgical patients' consent to regional anaesthesia. Acta Anaesth Scand 1994; 38: 607–611.
35. Allen HW, Mulroy MF, Fundis K, et al: Regional versus propofol general anesthesia for outpatient hand surgery. (Abstract.) Anesthesiology 1993; 79: A1.
36. Tierney E, Lewis G, Hurtig JB, et al: Femoral nerve block with bupivacaine 0.25 per cent for postoperative analgesia after open knee surgery. Can J Anaesth 1987; 34: 455–458.
37. Smith I, Monk TG, White PF, et al: Propofol infusion during regional anesthesia: sedative, amnestic, and anxiolytic properties. Anesth Analg 1994; 79: 313–319.
38. Brain AIJ: The laryngeal mask—a new concept in airway management. Br J Anaesth 1983; 55: 801–804.
39. Langerman L, Grant GJ, Zakowski M, et al: Prolongation of epidural anesthesia using a lipid drug carrier with procaine, lidocaine, and tetracaine. Anesth Analg 1992; 75: 900–905.
40. Masters DB, Berde CB, Dutta SK, et al: Prolonged regional nerve blockade by controlled release of local anesthetic from a biodegradable polymer matrix. Anesthesiology 1993; 79: 340–346.
41. Yorozu T, Kondoh M, Morisaki H, et al: An advantage of a new epidural catheter with a unique cross-section. (Abstract.) Anesthesiology 1994; 81: A597.
42. Carpenter RL, Liu SS, Mulroy MF, et al: Multimodal approach to optimize recovery shortens time to discharge after radical retropubic prostatectomy. (Abstract.) Anesthesiology 1994; 81: A1025.

CHAPTER 2

Regional Anesthesia and Chronic Pain Therapy: A History

Douglas R. Bacon, M.D., M.A.

October 16, 1846, the day Morton demonstrated surgical anesthesia induced by the vapors of sulfuric ether, is well known. However, the history of regional anesthesia, the art of anesthetizing a segment of the body to allow an operation to take place or to ameliorate a chronic painful condition, has received considerably less attention. No ceremonies commemorate Koller's first use of cocaine for ophthalmologic surgery, no monument to Koller as the benefactor of all the human race exists as it does for Morton, and Koller's name will not be celebrated as were the names of Crawford Long and Horace Wells. Interestingly, no controversy exists over the discovery of regional anesthesia as it does over the first use of general anesthesia, and many physicians have been content to share the credit for introducing regional anesthesia to the world.

Among the most versatile of techniques, regional anesthesia often permits a patient to remain pain free for long periods after the surgical procedure has been completed. The observation that pain transmission could be interrupted by nerve block forever linked regional anesthesia and pain management. Together, the two fields have helped to deliver on the promise that anesthesiology ". . .knows no limitations; its arms open wide to all those who wish to relieve pain of those who suffer pain."[1]

The modern history of regional anesthesia and pain management began in the late 19th century. Throughout the 20th century, the surgical use of regional anesthesia has expanded, as have the possibilities of cure for those suffering painful conditions. However, the popularity of various techniques has waxed and waned, and the discoveries of new techniques often have been only reintroductions of techniques unknown to younger researchers.

Interest in regional anesthesia has increased and diminished in the 20th century (Fig. 2–1). Spinal anesthesia, as reflected in the citations in the *Quarterly Cumulative Index to the Medical Literature*, enjoyed much investigational interest in the 1930s and again in the 1980s. Major plexus blocks, or conduction anesthesia, increased in popularity in the 1950s, coinciding with concerns about halothane hepatitis. Local and regional techniques have steadily gained in popularity, without the cyclic fluctuations of interest seen for the other citation headings in the literature.

A similar study of pain management citations (Fig. 2–2) revealed a steady, slow increase until the mid-1960s, when an explosion of interest and research took place. The explanation perhaps is linked to the development of the multidisciplinary pain center and the consequent shift in the view of chronic pain as a subdiscipline of many specialties.

As the 20th century has progressed, why has there been an increasing interest in regional anesthesia and pain medicine? What factors have caused physicians to study regional anesthesia and to search for better methods for operative anesthesia and pain control? Moreover, what lessons can be learned that can aid the future development of regional anesthesia?

Early Roots of Regional Anesthesia

Regional anesthesia generally traces its roots to Koller's discovery of the local anesthetic properties of cocaine. However, like general anesthesia, regional techniques have earlier historical roots. In the centuries before Morton's public demonstration, there were many techniques for inducing insensibility, most notably the use of alcohol. William E. Clarke of Rochester, New York, and Crawford Long of Georgia used sulfuric ether to induce anesthesia 4 years before Morton's public work. (For a description of Clarke's work, see Stetson JB: William E. Clarke and his 1842 use of ether. In Fink BR, Morris LE, Stephen CR [eds]: The History of Anesthesia, pp 400–407. Park Ridge, IL, The Wood Library-Museum of Anesthesiology, 1992.)

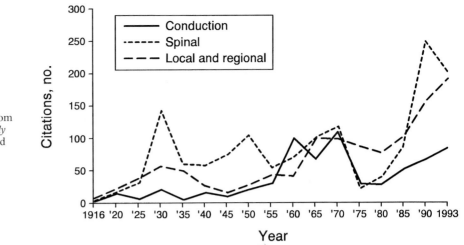

Figure 2–1 Citations in the anesthesia literature specific to regional anesthesia from 1916 to 1993. (Obtained from the *Quarterly Cumulative Index to the Medical Literature* and *Index Medicus.*)

As early as the 11th century, the numbing effects of cold water and ice were known. In England, a Saxon treatment book referred to the practice,[2] but Marco Aurelio Severino of Naples, Italy, in the middle of the 17th century introduced the world to the concept of refrigeration anesthesia. By placing snow in parallel lines across the area to be incised, the area could be made insensible in about 15 min. Never popular, probably because of the difficulty in obtaining snow year round before refrigeration, the technique's greatest use was during the savage Russian-Finnish campaign during the winter of 1939–1940.[3]

Ambroise Paré, the famed 16th century French barber-surgeon, reported that if a firm pressure was applied above the area of operation, less bleeding and pain ensued.[2] James Moore, in 1784, became an advocate of applying pressure to the major nerve trunks to produce anesthesia for amputation (Fig. 2–3). Before the incision, a clamp was tightened on the nerve trunk that supplied the operative area. Pressure on the nerve rendered the area insensible, but the clamp itself produced pain. This tourniquet pain was often significant, and the technique was far from perfect.[3]

Other early discoveries were critical to the development of regional anesthesia and pain management.

Simultaneously, in the two leading medical centers of the 1850s, the syringe and hollow-core needle were developed for subcutaneous injection in humans. In Paris, Charles-Gabriel Pravaz did animal experimentation by using a syringe and a trocar to block peripheral nerves. Alexander Wood, working in Edinburgh, injected a solution of morphine near a nerve trunk to inhibit pain in that nerve's distribution.[4] Before the discovery of a usable local anesthetic, the idea of peripheral nerve block and, indirectly and unrealized, the concept of peripheral opioid receptors had been demonstrated.

The Late 19th Century

In the late 19th century, Vienna had become the mecca for medicine, as Paris and Edinburgh had been earlier in the century. Medical giants were born there, men whose names have been commonplace, such as Theodor Billroth and Sigmund Freud, and in anesthesia, Carl Koller. Koller, a young house officer at the Allgemeines Krankenhaus, observed that cocaine numbed his tongue. As an aspiring ophthalmologist, he and his colleagues were searching for an anesthetic

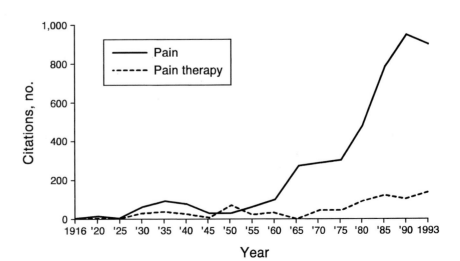

Figure 2–2 Citations in the anesthesia literature specific to pain management from 1916 to 1993. (Obtained from the *Quarterly Cumulative Index to the Medical Literature* and *Index Medicus.*)

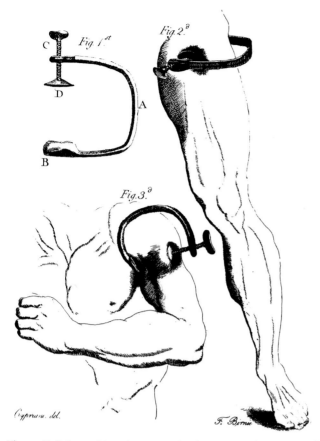

Figure 2–3 James Moore's compression instruments for upper and lower extremities. (Reproduced with permission of the Wellcome Institute Library, London.)

with which to anesthetize only the eye and not the entire patient.

Koller made a conceptual leap: if the tongue was numbed, the cornea should become anesthetized with the topical application of cocaine. He went to the laboratory of Salmon Stricker, a pathologist with whom Koller had been working, and placed the drug on the cornea of a frog and later on that of a guinea pig. After a few moments, Koller found the cornea and conjunctiva insensitive to mechanical, electrical, or chemical stimulation. Koller, enthused by the success of these animal experiments, tried the drug on himself, finding that his cornea was insensitive to instrumentation. He then went to the clinic and began to use his new discovery on patients.[5]

On September 15, 1884, at the Congress of Ophthalmology in Heidelberg, Koller's results were presented to the audience by his colleague Joseph Brettauer. A patient was brought in, and Brettauer anesthetized the eye, probed it, and picked up the conjunctiva and moved the globe in all directions; the patient was pain free![6] The era of local anesthesia had arrived, as dramatically perhaps as Morton's demonstration at the Ether Dome 38 years before.

Koller's work never went beyond topical anesthesia for the eye. However, after the introduction of a definitive local anesthetic, other physicians began to use the drug in new, daring ways that developed regional

anesthesia. Within a year of Koller's report, William Halsted (Fig. 2–4) at the Johns Hopkins Medical School began to block nerves by injecting them with cocaine. During 1884 and 1885, Halsted and his associates reported blocks of the supraorbital, infraorbital, inferior alveolar, and posterior tibial nerves, as well as blocks of the brachial plexus and many other major nerve trunks. He discovered cutaneous anesthesia by injecting cocaine into the intracutaneous tissue.[7] Fascinated by cocaine, Halsted also became addicted to the drug, and because of treatment for this problem, he lost valuable time in the development of regional anesthesia.[8]

In the 16 years between Koller's demonstration of a topical anesthetic and the turn of the 20th century, several major regional blocks were described. In the October 31, 1885, issue of the *New York Medical Journal*, James Leonard Corning (Fig. 2–5) reported a novel application of cocaine to the peridural space. Inferring from the observation that less strychnine, when injected into the subarachnoid space, was needed to produce convulsions than when the drug was injected subcutaneously, Corning thought that the effect of cocaine should be similar. He injected a dog with a 2% solution of cocaine into the "space situated between the spinous processes of two of the inferior dorsal vertebrae." Within 5 min, the hind legs were anesthetized.[9]

Corning proceeded to translate his observations to humans. His first patient suffered from "spinal weakness and seminal incontinence." Corning felt that he could help the patient by abolishing the spinal reflexes. Corning injected a 3% solution "into the space situated between the spinous processes of the eleventh and twelfth dorsal vertebrae." Seeing no effect after 6 to 8 min, he repeated the injection. Within 10 min, the patient felt his lower torso and legs become numb. Using an electric current, Corning found the patient's sensation was abolished; on reexamination the following morning, the patient had returned to normal.[9] Corning never described the aspiration of cerebrospinal

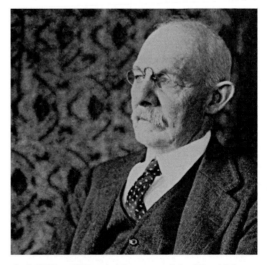

Figure 2–4 William Halsted. (Courtesy of the Wood Library-Museum of Anesthesiology, Park Ridge, IL.)

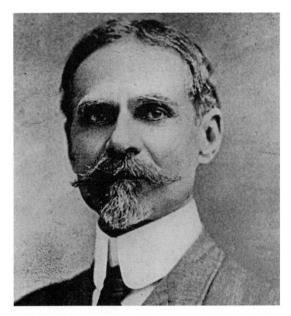

Figure 2–5 James Leonard Corning. (Courtesy of the Wood Library-Museum of Anesthesiology, Park Ridge, IL.)

could be performed and cerebrospinal fluid removed with a hollow-core needle through a paramedian approach without harm to the spinal cord.[10] Schleich described the technique of cocaine infiltration of the skin and soft tissues to the spinal column to anesthetize the tract of the needle before dural puncture.[12]

With the patient in the lateral position, after infiltration, Bier inserted the hollow-core needle. After cerebrospinal fluid had dripped from the needle, a syringe was attached, and 0.01 g of cocaine was injected. Insensibility ensued within 5 min. The first patient so anesthetized was a tuberculous laborer who had had several bad reactions to general anesthesia but needed a palliative procedure. His anesthesia and operation were performed on August 16, 1898. Four more patients would be anesthetized before Bier attempted the anesthetic on himself. Although a technical failure, Bier performed spinal anesthesia on his associate, Dr. Hildebrandt. Both men subsequently developed "spinal headaches" that continued, in Bier's case, for 9 days. In his conclusions, Bier[11] advised bed rest for patients having spinal anesthesia, which may well have been the beginning of this recommendation.

fluid in either injection, leading to the conclusion that he placed the solution in the epidural rather than the subarachnoid space. The onset time of 16 to 20 min tends to support the epidural hypothesis, at least in the human subject.[10]

In 1899, in the German journal *Zeitschrift fur Chirurgie*, Augustus Karl Gustav Bier (Fig. 2–6) reported the use of subarachnoid injection of cocaine to anesthetize patients for operation. His article, entitled (in translation) "Experiments Regarding the Cocainization of the Spinal Cord,"[11] built on the work of two other German physicians, Heinrich Quincke and Carl-Ludwig Schleich. Quincke demonstrated that lumbar puncture

The Early 20th Century

Rudolph Matas (Fig. 2–7), a surgeon in New Orleans, was among the first physicians in the United States to use spinal anesthesia. On November 10, 1899, Matas anesthetized his first patient by using cocaine. Matas found that, with cocaine anesthesia, the level of the block occasionally would increase over what was surgically necessary. In one hemorrhoidectomy, he was able to pinch the skin of the face without the patient feeling it! Fortunately for the patient, the block was incomplete, and the diaphragm and the skin of the abdomen and thorax were not completely anesthetized.[13]

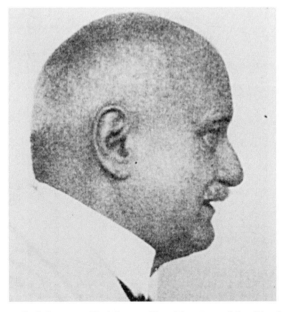

Figure 2–6 Augustus Karl Gustav Bier. (Courtesy of the Wood Library-Museum of Anesthesiology, Park Ridge, IL.)

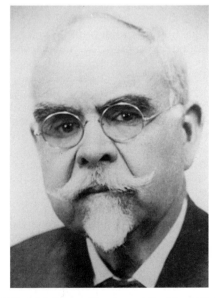

Figure 2–7 Rudolph Matas. (Courtesy of the Wood Library-Museum of Anesthesiology, Park Ridge, IL.)

Matas enthusiastically continued to use cocaine for spinal anesthesia but injected in the low lumbar region. Collecting 50 cases for publication, Matas described severe complications in the last three patients. One had complete respiratory paralysis, which responded to artificial ventilation. High fever developed in another, and the third acquired an intense radiculitis and headache that lasted several months.[13] These incidents convinced Matas to discontinue the use of spinal anesthesia until procaine was introduced in 1905.[14]

As a local anesthetic, cocaine had many drawbacks. At least 13 fatalities were reported[15] in the first 7 years that the drug was in use. The elucidation of the structure of cocaine in 1895 helped fuel the search for a local anesthetic that would not be irritating to the tissues, that was without systemic toxicity, and that did not damage nervous tissue.[16] With cocaine's structure as a base and modifications of the groups attached to it, many new compounds were synthesized. In 1905, Alfred Einhorn[17] created procaine, the first local anesthetic that had few toxic side effects. Although not ideal, procaine was safe, and its synthesis spurred a search that continues today for the ideal local anesthetic.

Procaine was important to regional anesthesia in that many practitioners who had abandoned regional techniques because of the complications now returned to using it. At Matas' Charity Hospital in New Orleans, regional anesthesia resumed. Each surgical admission was evaluated as a possible candidate for a regional anesthetic. Consequently, the surgical staff became expert in the performance of blocks, and the physicians who studied at Charity Hospital took this knowledge with them to other parts of the country. A student of Matas, Carroll W. Allen, published a textbook[18] in 1914 on regional anesthesia that proved popular enough for a second edition in 1918. In this manner, the Charity Hospital and Rudolph Matas played a role in the acceptance of regional anesthesia in America at the turn of the century.[13]

Concurrent with the work at Charity Hospital, a novel application of regional anesthesia was used by the Cleveland Clinic founder and surgeon, George Crile. Combining infiltration and plexus or major regional block with light general anesthesia, Crile was able to blunt the patient's stress response. Crile and Lower's description[19] of anociassociation sounded like classic anesthetic teaching in that Crile believed that the procedure began long before the patient entered the operating room and that premedication with morphine and scopolamine was desirable. He further stated that care must be taken during the procedure to ensure that tissues were not roughly handled and that surgical technique was as swift and gentle as possible. Postoperative care was equally important, and Crile believed that no detail was too small for the surgeon's attention.

Gaston Labat Popularizes Regional Anesthesia

One of the seminal events in the history of regional anesthesia and pain management in America began in

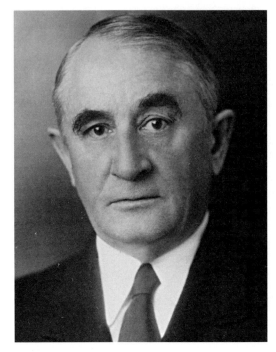

Figure 2–8 Charles Mayo. (Courtesy of the Wood Library-Museum of Anesthesiology, Park Ridge, IL.)

Paris. Charles Mayo (Fig. 2–8) was in Paris to visit the famed French surgeon Victor Pauchet. Impressed by the skill of the anesthesiologist taking care of the patient, Mayo asked Pauchet if he could invite the young man to the United States to teach regional anesthesia techniques to the Mayo Clinic surgeons. Gaston Labat (Fig. 2–9) agreed and arrived at the Mayo Clinic on September 29, 1920. In the course of his year in Roch-

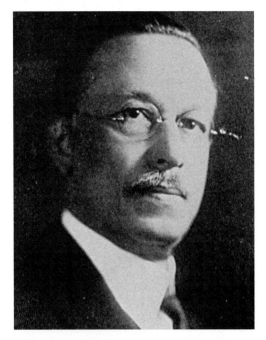

Figure 2–9 Gaston Labat. (Courtesy of the Wood Library-Museum of Anesthesiology, Park Ridge, IL.)

ester, Minnesota, Labat[20] gave lectures, built a strong foundation for regional anesthesia at the Clinic, and began work on his classic text, *Regional Anesthesia: Its Technic and Clinical Application*.[21]

Labat's book was an outgrowth of *L'Anesthésie Régionale*,[22] for which Labat was a contributing author to its 1921 edition, although it was published with Pauchet as the first author. (There are three editions of Pauchet's book. The third edition lists Labat as third author.) There is a striking similarity between the illustrations of *L'Anesthésie Régionale* and *Regional Anesthesia*. Many of the illustrations are transpositions; a right foot in Pauchet's book becomes a left foot in Labat's. In revising the illustrations, Labat[20] also made changes, such as needle placement, to illustrate more clearly how the block should be performed.

What was most important about Labat's book was its popularity. The first printing of 2500 in 1922 was quickly followed by another press run of 3000. A second printing larger than the first is highly unusual for any book, especially a medical text. Another 2000 copies of the first edition were published in 1924, for a total 7500.[23] In this book, regional anesthetic techniques were illustrated and accessible to a large number of physicians for the first time.

Labat left the Mayo Clinic on October 1, 1921, and took up residence in New York City. He soon obtained privileges at several New York hospitals (Fig. 2–10) and began to teach a 3-week course on regional anesthesia. Courses were offered four times each year—October, December, February, and April[24]—and gave physicians an opportunity to learn regional anesthetic techniques by demonstration and practical application.

Within 2 years of his arrival in New York, the American Society of Regional Anesthesia (ASRA) was organized, ostensibly to honor Labat. Serving as the first president of this multispecialty organization, Labat strove to make the society a forum for new discoveries in regional anesthesia despite the fact that the membership consisted of surgeons, neurosurgeons, neurologists, and anesthesiologists.[25] During the first 3 years of its existence, papers from eight meetings appeared in *Current Researches in Anesthesia and Analgesia*, the only journal devoted to the practice of anesthesia at the time. Francis Hoeffer McMechan, as editor, published many of these articles under the heading of the "Official Proceedings of the American Society of Regional Anesthesia."[26]

The ASRA jointly sponsored meetings with other anesthesia societies, which gave the society a national scope. Although most meetings were held in the New York Academy of Medicine, the October 27, 1925, meeting was held in Philadelphia, and the Eastern and Midwestern societies jointly sponsored the meeting with the ASRA. A year later, the Canadian and Eastern societies along with the ASRA jointly sponsored a meeting. Even when meeting in New York, physicians from such distant places as Rochester, Minnesota (John Lundy); Lamar, Colorado (Lanning E. Likes); and Madison, Wisconsin (Arnold Jackson), appeared before the society to present their work. Because these were only the papers published in *Current Researches in Anesthesia and Analgesia*, there may have been a more diverse group of physicians presenting their work.[26]

After 1929, the Proceedings ceased to be published in the journal. In 1933, when Paul Wood (Fig. 2–11) was elected secretary of the society, he began the practice of mimeographing the minutes and sending them to members across the country. This brought the society closer to its well-dispersed members and continued to allow the society to function as a sounding board for regional anesthesia. (The 1937 ASRA Directory lists members from all across the country, including California, Wisconsin, Minnesota, Massachusetts, and Pennsylvania in addition to New York State. ASRA Directory 1937. *The Collected Papers of Paul Wood, M.D.*, The Wood Library-Museum of Anesthesiology Collection, Park Ridge, IL.)

Labat's Legacy

In 1935, Emery Rovenstine (Fig. 2–12) was appointed Chairman of the Anesthesia Department at

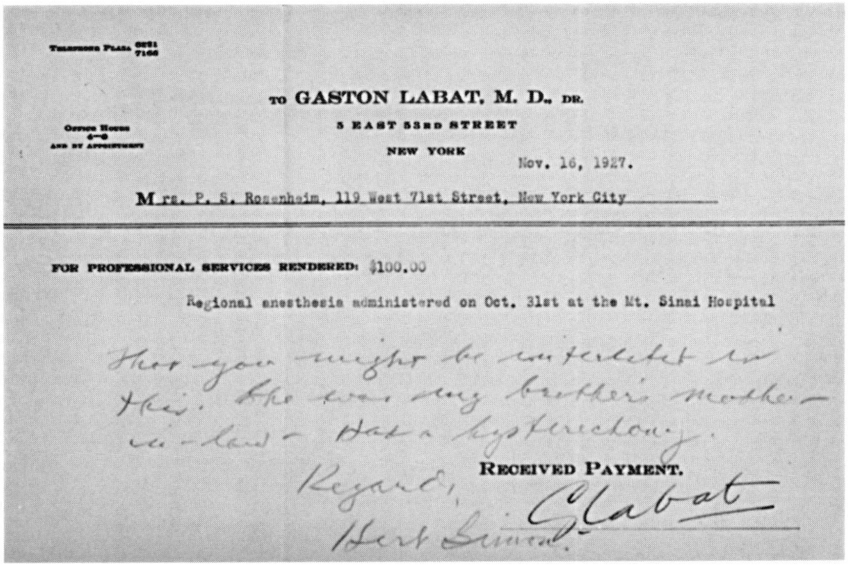
TO GASTON LABAT, M. D., DR.
5 EAST 53RD STREET
NEW YORK
Nov. 16, 1927.
Mrs. P. S. Rosenheim, 119 West 71st Street, New York City
FOR PROFESSIONAL SERVICES RENDERED: $100.00
Regional anesthesia administered on Oct. 31st at the Mt. Sinai Hospital
RECEIVED PAYMENT.

Figure 2–10 Bill from Gaston Labat to Mrs. P. S. Rosenheim for services rendered. (Courtesy of the Wood Library-Museum of Anesthesiology, Park Ridge, IL.)

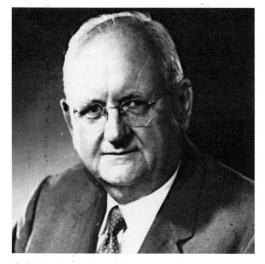

Figure 2–11 Paul Wood. (Courtesy of the Wood Library-Museum of Anesthesiology, Park Ridge, IL.)

Bellevue Hospital. Although Labat had died the previous October, Rovenstine quickly and enthusiastically embraced Labat's teaching and traditions. Along with Hippolyte Wertheim, a Bellevue surgeon and practitioner of Labat's methods of regional anesthesia, Rovenstine undertook the study of the application of regional anesthesia to painful conditions. Rovenstine and Wertheim continued the Bellevue courses in regional anesthesia. Rovenstine eventually became noted for his expertise in block anesthesia and his private block clinic.[27]

As the 1930s progressed, a subtle change occurred in the papers presented before the society. In the early years, original papers were mostly concerned with which regional technique was appropriate for which operation. There were also the important reports concerning the thousands of regional anesthetic procedures that proved the safety and the efficacy of regional anesthesia. Perhaps this interest reflected the multidisciplinary nature of the organization and the desire of the surgeons to secure the best anesthesia for their patients.

The 1937 ASRA Membership Directory does not list one member who was not also a member of the American Society of Anesthesiologists. By the late 1930s, the ASRA membership was almost entirely anesthesiologists (Fig. 2–13), and there was a new importance placed on the use of regional anesthesia for the relief of chronic painful conditions. By 1937, ASRA president Rovenstine[28] declared that the society was more or less concerned with advancing chronic pain management. ASRA was also considered an important enough organization to cosponsor with other anesthesia organizations the Silver Jubilee meeting of the Associated Anesthetists of the United States and Canada.[29]

In addition to the Rovenstine and Bellevue tradition of Labat, there is another. In his 12-month tenure at the Mayo Clinic, Labat also set up courses for the surgeons in regional anesthesia. One of them, W. L. Meeker, trained John Lundy when he arrived at the Clinic to head the Section of Anesthesia in 1924. Lundy

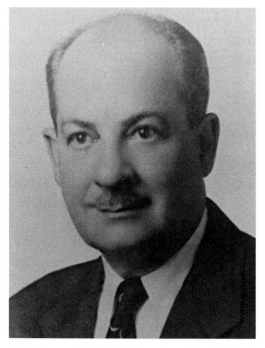

Figure 2–12 Emery Rovenstine. (Courtesy of the Wood Library-Museum of Anesthesiology, Park Ridge, IL.)

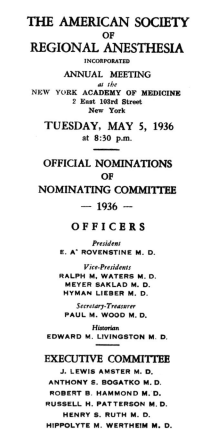

THE AMERICAN SOCIETY
OF
REGIONAL ANESTHESIA
INCORPORATED

ANNUAL MEETING
at the
NEW YORK ACADEMY OF MEDICINE
2 East 103rd Street
New York

TUESDAY, MAY 5, 1936
at 8:30 p.m.

———

OFFICIAL NOMINATIONS
OF
NOMINATING COMMITTEE

— 1936 —

OFFICERS

President
E. A. ROVENSTINE M. D.

Vice-Presidents
RALPH M. WATERS M. D.
MEYER SAKLAD M. D.
HYMAN LIEBER M. D.

Secretary-Treasurer
PAUL M. WOOD M. D.

Historian
EDWARD M. LIVINGSTON M. D.

———

EXECUTIVE COMMITTEE

J. LEWIS AMSTER M. D.
ANTHONY S. BOGATKO M. D.
ROBERT B. HAMMOND M. D.
RUSSELL H. PATTERSON M. D.
HENRY S. RUTH M. D.
HIPPOLYTE M. WERTHEIM M. D.

Figure 2–13 American Society of Regional Anesthesia Program, May 5, 1936. (Courtesy of the Wood Library-Museum of Anesthesiology, Park Ridge, IL.)

was soon offering postgraduate courses for physicians in regional anesthesia. When his residency training program was established, Lundy trained those physicians in regional anesthesia, establishing the Mayo Clinic tradition.[30]

The American Society of Regional Anesthesia and the American Board of Anesthesiology

The involvement of anesthesiologists such as Paul Wood, John Lundy, Ralph Waters, and Emery Rovenstine in the ASRA was important because of the emphasis it placed on regional anesthesia and pain management in the American Board of Anesthesiology (ABA). By 1936, McMechan and the American Society of Anesthetists (ASA) had become antagonists. Working within the American Medical Association (AMA) and with the American Board of Surgery (ABS), the ASA had developed all the necessary criteria to define a specialist in anesthesiology. The AMA, however, required two national anesthesia organizations to sponsor the board.[31]

At the time, the Associated Anesthetists of the United States and Canada was a national anesthesia organization under the control of McMechan. Approached by the ASA, he rebuffed the offer of joining in sponsorship of the ABA because of his long-standing feud with the AMA. The ASA then approached the ASRA to become the second national sponsor of the ABA. Because Rovenstine, a principal in the ASA, was also president of ASRA at the time, the society agreed. The seal of the ABA bears testimony to that fact, because the initials of the four groups (i.e., ASA, ASRA, AMA, ABS) form the cross in the familiar seal of the ABA.[31]

The first examination of the ABA had a preponderance of questions based on regional anesthesia (Tables 2–1 and 2–2). For developing criteria for acceptable residency training in anesthesiology, a clinic where patients with pain problems were diagnosed and treated was essential. The ASRA had a tremendous influence in the formative years of the infrastructure of modern anesthesiology.[31]

Table 2–1 Regional Anesthesia Sample Questions From the First Written Examination of the American Board of Anesthesiology

PATHOLOGY SECTION
1. Discuss how Raynaud's disease may be differentiated from thromboangiitis obliterans by anesthetic methods.

PHARMACOLOGY SECTION
1. Discuss the advisability of using spinal anesthesia in the presence of pernicious anemia.
2. List the toxic effects of procaine hydrochloride.

Reprinted by permission of the publisher from Bacon DR, Lema MJ: To define a specialty: a brief history of the American Board of Anesthesiology's first written examination. J Clin Anesth 1992; 4: 489–497. Copyright 1992 by Elsevier Science Inc.

Table 2–2 Regional Anesthesia Sample Questions From the First Written Examination of the American Board of Anesthesiology

ANATOMY SECTION
1. What landmarks are used and how is the plexus approached in performing a brachial plexus block by the supraclavicular route?
2. Describe a method for producing block anesthesia for a surgical procedure involving a bunion.
3. What is Horner's syndrome and how may it be produced?
4. Following a successful caudal and transsacral block, what structures are anesthetized?

Reprinted by permission of the publisher from Bacon DR, Lema MJ: To define a specialty: a brief history of the American Board of Anesthesiology's first written examination. J Clin Anesth 1992; 4: 489–497. Copyright 1992 by Elsevier Science Inc.

The Death of the American Society of Regional Anesthesia and the World's Fair of 1939

The late 1930s were unkind to the ASRA. By 1939, only eight members had paid their dues for the year. The society was dying. Emery Rovenstine called an emergency meeting of the officers of the organization, and it was decided that the ASRA would amalgamate with the ASA. The treasury was donated (Fig. 2–14) to the ASA as a trust to set up an annual Labat award to the physician who had done the most to promote regional anesthesia. However, this never came to pass.[32]

For the field of pain management, the late 1930s and early 1940s were good. The World's Fair was held in New York City, attracting more than a million visitors. In the Hall of Man, for all the world to see and alongside all the other medical specialties, was an exhibition on anesthesia. One of the central points of this display was the Lundy model of regional anesthesia. A schematic model displaying the human nervous system turned the region of the body anesthetized by a block a different color. In this exhibit, the public could learn about regional anesthesia firsthand.[33]

In another part of the exhibition, there was a continuous slide show. The descriptions of the education and training of an anesthesiologist and the field were displayed. Within the definition of anesthesiology, regional anesthesia played a large role. The dichotomy between surgical anesthesia and therapeutic block techniques is evident, and for 1939, it is surprising to see thoracic epidural procedures so prominently mentioned.[33]

The significance of regional anesthesia at the World's Fair lies not with which blocks or techniques were described to the public. It is the central role that regional anesthesia played in the exhibit that is important. By that time, regional anesthesia was an important therapeutic modality in the hands of the anesthesiologist. By publicly displaying the various regional anesthetic techniques, the public was educated and, it was hoped, more receptive when and if a regional technique was recommended.

David Kaliski, then health commissioner for the city of New York, began corresponding with Paul Wood

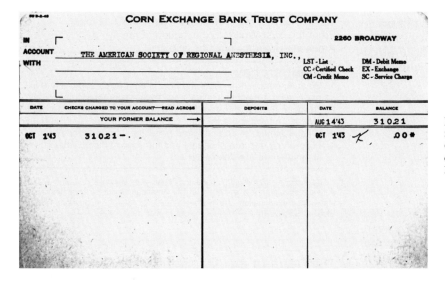

Figure 2–14 Final withdrawal of the American Society of Regional Anesthesia funds from the Corn Exchange Bank, October 1, 1943. (Courtesy of the Wood Library-Museum of Anesthesiology, Park Ridge, IL.)

about compensation for treating painful conditions. Wood and Kaliski agreed on fees for blocks, including the necessity for repeated blocks to treat certain conditions. Kaliski and Wood also developed a list of physicians who were considered capable of performing these procedures.[34] On the eve of World War II, the treatment of painful conditions by regional anesthetic techniques was recognized by the Workmen's Compensation Board of the city of New York.

World War II

On the home front, Robert Hingson, working in a United States Public Health Service Hospital, was charged with caring for the pregnant wives of Coast Guard seamen. Concerned about the effects of morphine-scopolamine, Hingson looked to find a safe and painless method to deliver the infants of these women. His answer came with a malleable needle placed sacrally deep to the peridural ligament: continuous caudal anesthesia. It proved safe and effective and may well have started epidural analgesia for labor and delivery.[30]

America's entry into World War II generated a personnel crisis in anesthesiology. There were insufficient physicians to staff field hospitals and other places where anesthesiologists were needed. Ninety-day courses were established to train physicians to administer anesthetics—a rushed introduction to anesthesiology, but one that included the basics of regional anesthesia. Manuals were developed to guide the novice specialists in the care of the wounded. The "dos and don'ts" included anesthesia. Helpful suggestions were included, such as the amount of local anesthetic necessary to produce adequate anesthesia for a particular operation, and another section described the strength and amount of local anesthetic that could safely be administered.[35]

Regional anesthesia was not relegated to the European theater of operations. Samuel L. Lieberman, then a young captain in the United States Army Medical

Corps, cared for battle casualties during the New Georgia and Bougainville campaigns. As the commanding officer of B Company, 118th Medical Battalion from January 1, 1945, to June 1, 1945, Lieberman worked in a clearing station. Of the soldiers brought in with abdominal wounds, only 12.5% died after he switched from the more conventional inhalation anesthetic (mortality rate of 46%) to continuous spinal anesthesia with Lemmon's malleable spinal needle. For his work, Lieberman was awarded the Legion of Merit, the highest decoration bestowed on a medical officer.[36]

The Rise of the Pain Center

War unfortunately produces many injuries and, with them, chronic, painful conditions. John J. Bonica (Fig. 2–15) began his study of pain at the Madigan Army Hospital in Tacoma, Washington. He confronted patients with reflex sympathetic dystrophy, causalgia, phantom limb pain, and many other complex and puzzling conditions. Blocks were successful in only some cases; others required consultation with colleagues in other disciplines.[37]

It soon became apparent that communication between all parties was somewhat inefficient. Bonica realized that, by bringing all the specialists together, a meaningful dialogue could begin and hopefully new and effective therapeutic options for the patient would result. The anesthesiologist's desire to help war casualties resulted in the beginnings of the multidisciplinary pain center.[37]

Bonica's role was far greater than establishing a multidisciplinary pain center. Bonica's pen was equally important. His book, *The Management of Pain*,[38] remains a comprehensive text in pain management. It emphasizes the use of regional anesthesia for the management of painful conditions. Bonica's willing participation in the refresher courses offered at the ASA annual meeting helped educate anesthesiologists about the importance of pain management.[39] As his career progressed, he would become President of the American Society

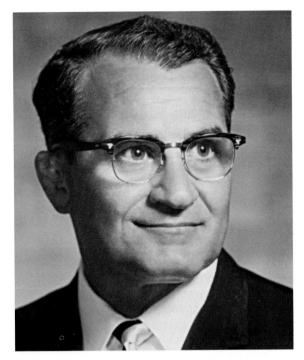

Figure 2–15 John Bonica. (Courtesy of the Wood Library-Museum of Anesthesiology, Park Ridge, IL.)

of Anesthesiologists and later President of the World Federation of Societies of Anesthesiology. These roles helped regional anesthesia to gain visibility in the national and world communities and to bring attention to the benefits of regional anesthesia and pain management.

Bonica's West Coast associate, Daniel C. Moore (Fig. 2–16), also played an enormous role in popularizing regional anesthesia. Through his work at the Virginia Mason Clinic, he established a premier surgical regional anesthesia center. His book, *Regional Block: A Handbook for Use in the Clinical Practice of Medicine and Surgery*,[40] was designed as a how-to manual for physicians. Like Bonica, Moore was an active participant in the ASA annual meeting, and as a scientific exhibitor, he related his experience with regional anesthesia and complications with the techniques to the anesthesiology community. As President of the American Society of Anesthesiologists, he argued for the purchase of land on which the ASA headquarters now resides.

The story of regional anesthesia in the postwar period is greater than both Bonica and Moore. Many physicians began to study regional anesthetic techniques in an attempt to understand the myriad complications and address them. Leroy Vandam and Robert Dripps[41] published their classic article on spinal anesthesia in 1956 in the *Journal of the American Medical Association*. They studied the complications associated with subarachnoid block and for the first time delineated the incidence of postdural puncture headache and related it to needle size.

During this period, Nicholas Greene also studied spinal anesthetics. He determined the baricity of local anesthetic solutions relative to the cerebrospinal fluid.

In his classic book, *Physiology of Spinal Anesthesia*,[42] Greene described the now common hypobaric, isobaric, and hyperbaric anesthetic solutions and how they affect the height and spread of the block.

The New American Society of Regional Anesthesia

In 1975, Alon Winnie (Fig. 2–17) and colleagues began to see the need for a society to promote regional anesthetic techniques and pain management. Interest in regional anesthesia was growing, and to sustain that interest and to benefit patients, the American Society of Regional Anesthesia was formed, without prior knowledge of the New York City group formed around Labat. The purpose was similar: to educate physicians and patients about the benefits of regional anesthesia.[43]

Like its predecessor, the new ASRA began to hold meetings as a forum for the presentation of research results and to demonstrate techniques to other physicians. The Labat group was a multidisciplinary group, but the new ASRA was anesthesiology based. The teachings of Labat, filtered through Lundy's program at the Mayo Clinic and Rovenstine at Bellevue Hospital, and the emphasis placed by the American Board of Anesthesiology ensured that anesthesiologists were the practitioners of regional anesthesia in America.

The ASRA meetings began in 1976 in Phoenix, Arizona, 6 months after the society was organized.[43] Linked at first with the International Anesthesia Research Society, meeting the day before, the ASRA

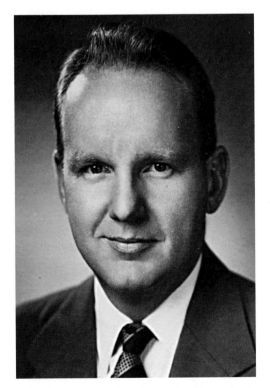

Figure 2–16 Daniel Moore. (Courtesy of the Wood Library-Museum of Anesthesiology, Park Ridge, IL.)

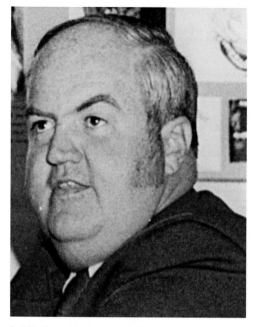

Figure 2–17 Alon Winnie. (Courtesy of the Wood Library-Museum of Anesthesiology, Park Ridge, IL.)

membership gradually increased (Fig. 2–18) and became independent from the International Anesthesia Research Society. Today, the ASRA Annual Meeting is a well-attended (Fig. 2–19), 3-day affair with lectures, workshops, and paper presentations. In 1977, the Labat Lectureship was established to honor those who had contributed to the field of regional anesthesia. The list included Daniel Moore, John Bonica, Sir Robert Macintosh, Torsten Gordh, John Adriani, Alon Winnie, Nicholas Greene, P. Prithvi Raj, B. Raymond Fink, and Sol Schnider.

In 1987, the society established a distinguished service award. Winners of this prestigious honor include L. Donald Bridenbaugh, Gertie Marx, Jess Weiss, and Jordan Katz. A year later, the society established another named lectureship to honor John Bonica. Distinguished scientists who have delivered that lecture in-

clude Michael Cousins, Tony Yaksh, Stephen Abram, and Henrik Kehlet.

One of ASRA's most innovative programs has been the regional workshops. In addition to lectures about advances in regional anesthetic technique, there is often a chance to practice on mannequins under the supervision of renowned experts. Numerous events each year held in different geographic parts of the country ensure that the message about regional anesthesia is heard in the anesthetic community.

Regional Anesthesia, the ASRA's peer-reviewed journal, began publication in 1977, only a year after the founding of the society. It has served as a forum for issues related to regional anesthesia. Results of scientific inquiry into problems of interest in regional anesthesia are published there, permitting the readership access to the latest data on new drugs and techniques. Meeting announcements are part of the advertisement section, giving anesthesiologists information on where to present the results of their work and where to go to increase the fund of knowledge concerning regional anesthesia and pain management.

Conclusion

The history of regional anesthesia and pain management has developed in ways that could never have been envisioned by Carl Koller as he probed the frog's anesthetized eye in Vienna. Unlike general anesthesia, for which the therapeutic relevancy is relegated to the operating room, regional anesthesia has helped anesthesiologists branch out beyond the surgical suite. With techniques established throughout its history, regional anesthesia has had significant impact in labor and delivery rooms and in pain clinics. The efficacy of blocks for pain management, when combined with other treatment modalities and assistance from colleagues in different specialties, has exceeded many expectations.

Pioneers in regional anesthesia throughout its history have struggled to popularize techniques that might improve the patient's surgical or labor experience. Teach-

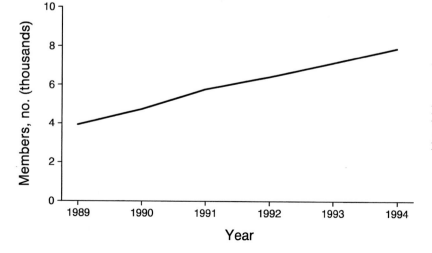

Figure 2–18 Membership (American members) in the American Society of Regional Anesthesia (1989–1994). (Courtesy of John A. Hinckley, Executive Secretary, ASRA.)

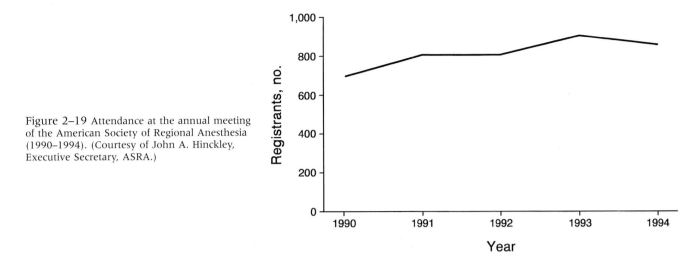

Figure 2–19 Attendance at the annual meeting of the American Society of Regional Anesthesia (1990–1994). (Courtesy of John A. Hinckley, Executive Secretary, ASRA.)

ers like Labat, although perhaps not credited with an important "first," need to be remembered as educators of large numbers of physicians. Labat's teaching endured beyond the confines of the Mayo Clinic or Bellevue Hospital; his textbook remains a classic and is still sought out by serious regional anesthesiologists.

The work of Moore and Bonica should also be emphasized. Innovators in bringing together many different specialists to treat pain patients and popularizing regional anesthetics in the operating rooms, these men helped boost the popularity of regional anesthesia and created a systematic, effective form of pain management. Their prominent role in the medical politics of anesthesia nationally and internationally helped bring much needed recognition to the field.

The resurgence of the ASRA has provided American anesthesiology, and perhaps the world, with an organization dedicated to the advancement of the field. Through meetings, workshops, and *Regional Anesthesia*, the society works to further physicians' knowledge. The impact of these meetings can be seen in the delivery room, the operating suite, and the pain clinic, where the results benefit the most important member of the anesthesia team, the patient.

References

1. McMechan FH: Morton bust presentation address. Anesth Analg 1929; 8: 4–10.
2. Madigan SR, Raj PP: History and current status of pain management. In Raj PP (ed): Practical Management of Pain, 2nd ed, pp 3–15. St. Louis, Mosby-Year Book, 1992.
3. Robinson V: Victory Over Pain: A History of Anesthesia, pp 40–44. Oxford, Schuman, 1946.
4. Fink BR: History of neural blockade. In Cousins MJ, Bridenbaugh PO (eds): Neural Blockade in Clinical Anesthesia and Management of Pain, 2nd ed, pp 3–21. Philadelphia, JB Lippincott, 1988.
5. Koller C: Personal reminiscences of the first use of cocain as local anesthetic in eye surgery. Anesth Analg 1928; 7: 9–11.
6. Robinson V: Victory Over Pain: A History of Anesthesia, pp 248–250. Oxford, Schuman, 1946.
7. Halsted WS: Practical comments on the use and abuse of cocaine; suggested by its invariably successful employment in more than a thousand minor surgical operations. N Y Med J 1885; 42: 294.
8. Olch PD: William S. Halsted and local anesthesia: Contributions and complications. Anesthesiology 1975; 42: 479–486.
9. Corning JL: Spinal anaesthesia and local medication of the cord. N Y Med J 1885; 42: 483–485.
10. Vandam LD: On the origins of intrathecal anesthesia. Int Anesthesiol Clin 1989; 27: 2–7.
11. Bier A: Experiments regarding the cocainization of the spinal cord. Zeitschr Chir 1899; 51: 361–369. In Little DM, Jr: Classical file. Surv Anesthesiol 1981; 25: 340–353.
12. Goerig M, Schulte am Esch J: Carl-Ludwig Schleich and the scandal during the annual meeting of the German surgical society in Berlin in 1892. In Fink BR, Morris LE, Stephen CR (eds): The History of Anesthesia, pp 216–222. Park Ridge, IL, The Wood Library-Museum of Anesthesiology, 1992.
13. Adriani J: Labat's Regional Anesthesia: Techniques and Clinical Applications, pp 691–709. St. Louis, Warren H Green, 1985.
14. Cohn I, Deutsch HB: Rudolph Matas: A Biography of One of the Great Pioneers in Surgery, p 279. Toronto, Doubleday, 1960.
15. De Jong RH: Local Anesthetics, pp 1–8. St. Louis, Mosby-Year Book, 1994.
16. Ritchie JM, Greene NM: Local anesthetics. In Gilman AG, Rall TW, Nies AS, et al (eds): Goodman and Gilman's The Pharmacological Basis of Therapeutics, 8th ed, pp 311–331. New York, Pergamon Press, 1990.
17. Lund PC: Reflections upon the historical aspects of spinal anesthesia. Reg Anesth 1983; 8: 89–98.
18. Allen CW: Local and Regional Anesthesia. Philadelphia, WB Saunders, 1914.
19. Crile GW, Lower WE: Surgical Shock and the Shockless Operation Through Anoci-Association, 2nd ed, pp 125–138. Philadelphia, WB Saunders, 1920.
20. Brown DL, Winnie AP: Biography of Louis Gaston Labat, M.D. Reg Anesth 1992; 17: 249–262.
21. Labat G: Regional Anesthesia; Its Technic and Clinical Application. Philadelphia, WB Saunders, 1922.
22. Pauchet V, Sourdat P, Labat G: L'Anesthésie Régionale, 3rd ed. Paris, Octave Doin, 1921.
23. Lee JA: Some foundations on which we have built. Reg Anesth 1985; 10: 99–109.
24. Advertisement. Anesth Analg 1925; 4: XIII.
25. Betcher AM, Ciliberti BJ, Wood PM, et al: The jubilee year of organized anesthesia. Anesthesiology 1956; 17: 226–264.
26. Articles appearing in Current Researches in Anesthesia and Analgesia, 1924–1928.
27. Papper EM: Regional anesthesia: a critical assessment of its place in therapeutics. E. A. Rovenstine Memorial Lecture. Anesthesiology 1967; 28: 1074–1084.
28. Minutes of Meeting of the ASRA, February 27, 1937. In The Collected Papers of Paul Wood, M.D. Park Ridge, IL, The Wood Library-Museum of Anesthesiology.
29. Program of the Silver Jubilee Meeting of the Associated Anesthetists of the United States and Canada, June 7–11, 1937, Atlantic

City, New Jersey. Park Ridge, IL, The Wood Library-Museum of Anesthesiology.

30. Hingson RA: The pathway across half a century of development of safe control of obstetric pain in childbirth. Reg Anesth 1981; 6: 62–66.

31. Bacon DR, Lema MJ: To define a specialty: a brief history of the American Board of Anesthesiology's first written examination. J Clin Anesth 1992; 4: 489–497.

32. Minutes of Meeting of the American Society of Regional Anesthesia, 1939, 1940, and 1943. In The Collected Papers of Paul Wood, M.D. Park Ridge, IL, The Wood Library-Museum of Anesthesiology.

33. Bacon DR, Lema MJ, Yearley CK: For all the world to see: anesthesia at the 1939 New York World's Fair. J Clin Anesth 1993; 5: 252–258.

34. Correspondence between David J. Kaliski, M.D. and Paul M. Wood, M.D., 1939–1940. In The Collected Papers of Paul Wood, M.D. Park Ridge, IL, The Wood Library-Museum of Anesthesiology.

35. Manual of Therapy: European Theater of Operations. In The Collected Papers of Henry Ruth. Park Ridge, IL, The Wood Library-Museum of Anesthesiology.

36. Bacon DR, Lema MJ: Standing on the promises: the career of Samuel L. Lieberman, M.D. Sphere 1989; 42: 20–24.

37. Thompson D: Pain relief's founding father. *Time,* June 11, 1984.

38. Bonica JJ: The Management of Pain. Philadelphia, Lea & Febiger, 1953.

39. American Society of Anesthesiologists Annual Meeting Programs, 1950–1994. Park Ridge, IL, The Wood Library-Museum of Anesthesiology.

40. Moore DC: Regional Block: A Handbook for Use in the Clinical Practice of Medicine and Surgery. Springfield, Illinois, Charles C Thomas, 1953.

41. Vandam LD, Dripps RD: Long-term follow-up of patients who received 10,098 spinal anesthetics. JAMA 1956; 161: 586–591.

42. Greene NM: Physiology of Spinal Anesthesia. Baltimore, Williams & Wilkins, 1959.

43. Winnie A: Nothing new under the sun. Reg Anesth 1982; 7: 95–102.

II

Basic Science of Regional Anesthesia

PART A
Anatomy

CHAPTER 3
Functional Neuroanatomy

Perry G. Fine, M.D., Jacob Rosenberg, M.D.

This chapter on neuroanatomy is intended to provide a concise and functionally oriented review of the extremely complex human nervous system as a practical resource for anesthesiologists. The emphasis is on sensory inputs to the central nervous system, with clinically significant implications for pain management or regional anesthesia noted in each subsection. The architecture of the somatic sensory system is described from the periphery to the cortex, and descending pathways of pain control are outlined. Visceral innervation, which includes the autonomic system and its function with regard to pain, is also described.

Overview

The peripheral nerves are composed of axons from the somatic and visceral (i.e., autonomic) systems, with afferent (i.e., sensory) and efferent (i.e., motor) components in each system.[1-3] Somatic motor nerves have cell bodies in the anterior horn of the spinal cord or in the motor nuclei of cranial nerves. These axons exit the cord in the ventral root, fuse with the dorsal root, and contribute to spinal and peripheral nerves supplying striated muscle. Autonomic motor fibers have cell bodies in the motor nuclei of the brain stem or in the intermediolateral column of the spinal cord. The autonomic system is divided into two parts: the sympathetic (i.e., thoracolumbar) and the parasympathetic (i.e., craniosacral) systems. Sympathetic cell bodies are located from T-1 to L-2 or L-3. Parasympathetic cell bodies reside in the S-2, S-3, and S-4 segments of spinal cord and in the autonomic motor nuclei of the brain stem[4-6] (Table 3–1).

The efferent autonomic axons are located near ventral roots (or cranial nerves) and the spinal nerves, synapsing in the peripheral ganglia. Sympathetic nerves leave the spinal nerves by means of white rami communicantes to join the paravertebral sympathetic chain. They may synapse at that level or course up or down the chain before synapsing and rejoining spinal nerves through the gray rami communicantes. Some axons do not synapse in the paravertebral chain or return to spinal nerves. They synapse in prevertebral ganglia (e.g., celiac, mesenteric, hypogastric ganglia). Axons are then distributed to effector sites by distributing with arterial vasculature. Unlike the unipolar somatic motor cells, the preganglionic and postganglionic fibers of the autonomic nervous system are multipolar. The autonomic efferent system consists of a two-neuron chain instead of the one-neuron pattern of the somatic efferent system (Figs. 3–1 and 3–2).

Table 3–1 Classification of Nerve Fibers by Function

Somatic efferent: motor to striated muscle of myotomes (cell bodies in the ventral horn cells in the cord and motor nuclei of cranial nerves III, IV, VI, XII)

Somatic afferent: sensory from skin, limbs, and body wall (cell bodies in the dorsal horn of cord and nuclei of V, VII, IX, X)

Special somatic afferent: vestibular and cochlear (cell bodies in the VIII nucleus)

Special visceral efferent: motor to striated muscle of branchial arch mesoderm (cell bodies in the motor nuclei of V, VII, and the nucleus ambiguus of X)

General visceral efferent: motor to smooth muscle and glands (cell bodies in the intermediolateral cell column of T-1 to L-2 [sympathetic] and S-2 to S-4 [parasympathetic] and in the Edinger-Westphal nucleus of III, superior salivatory nucleus of VII, inferior salivatory nucleus of IX, and dorsal motor nucleus of X)

General visceral afferent: sensory from internal organs (cell bodies in the dorsal horn of cord and the tractus solitarius for afferents from VII, IX, X)

Special visceral afferent: taste, olfaction

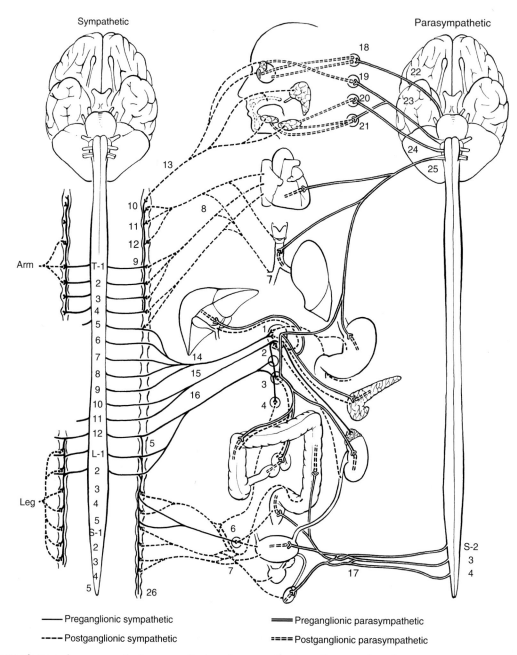

Sympathetic

Parasympathetic

Arm

Leg

——— Preganglionic sympathetic
----- Postganglionic sympathetic

══ Preganglionic parasympathetic
==== Postganglionic parasympathetic

Figure 3–1 Sympathetic and parasympathetic preganglionic and postganglionic outflow. 1, celiac plexus; 2, aorticorenal plexus; 3, superior mesenteric plexus; 4, inferior mesenteric plexus; 5, lumbar paravertebral sympathetic chain; 6, superior hypogastric plexus; 7, inferior hypogastric plexus; 8, cardiac nerves; 9, stellate ganglion; 10, superior cervical ganglion; 11, middle cervical ganglion; 12, intermediate cervical ganglion; 13, carotid nerve; 14, greater splanchnic nerve; 15, lesser splanchnic nerve; 16, least splanchnic nerve; 17, nervi erigentes and pelvic nerves; 18, ciliary ganglia; 19, pterygopalatine ganglia; 20, otic ganglia; 21, submandibular ganglia; 22, cranial nerve (CN) III; 23, CN VII; 24, CN IX; 25, CN X; and 26, ganglion of impar. (Modified from Woodburne RT: Essentials of Human Anatomy, 7th ed, p 32. New York, Oxford University Press, 1983.)

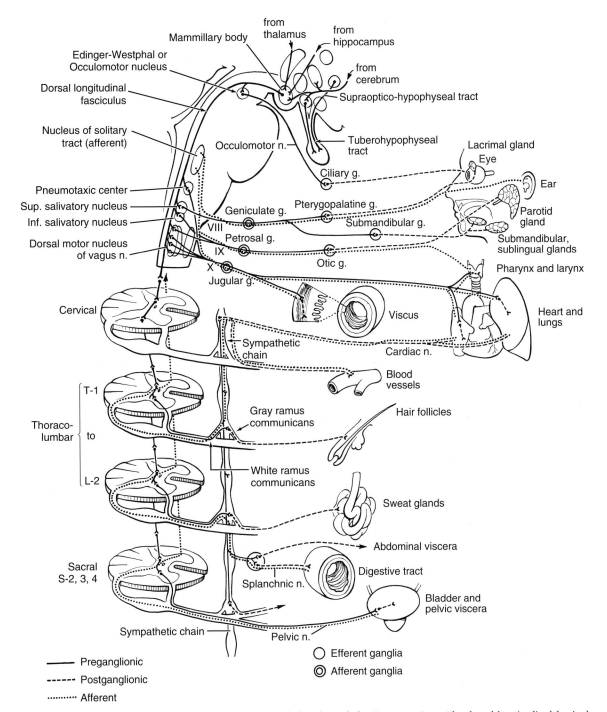

Figure 3–2 Schematic representation of autonomic pathways, including hypothalamic connections. The dorsal longitudinal fasciculus provides descending inhibitory modulation. g., ganglion; inf., inferior; n., nerve; sup., superior. (Redrawn from Bonica JJ: The Management of Pain, 2nd ed, vol I, p 148. Philadelphia, Lea & Febiger, 1990.)

Transmission of afferent (i.e., sensory) input is initiated by activation of peripheral receptors and subsequent depolarization of their axons. These axons relay information to their cell bodies located in the dorsal root ganglion, which is proximal to the intervertebral foramen but just lateral to the spinal cord.[2, 6] Central dendritic processes of these first-order neurons synapse in the dorsal horn, where sensory input is modulated. Sensory information moves cephalad by means of ascending columns such as the anterolateral funiculi (i.e.,

spinothalamic tracts) and the posterior columns to synapse in the reticular system and the thalamus, finally projecting to the cerebral cortex (Fig. 3–3).[7-9]

Clinical Note: *Somatic sensory fibers from several spinal nerves often fuse to form peripheral nerves. Nevertheless, each spinal nerve still conveys cutaneous input from a conceptually discrete area of skin. These areas, or dermatomes,*

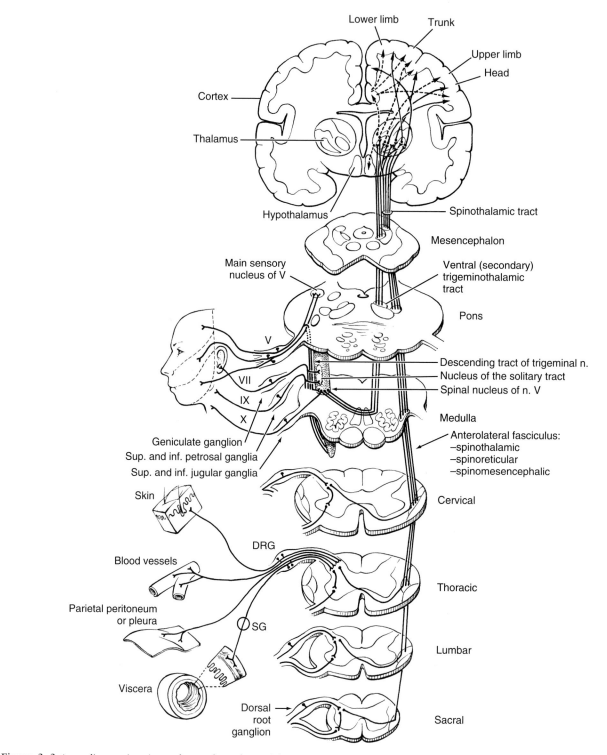

Figure 3–3 Ascending nociceptive pathways from the periphery via autonomic and somatic primary afferents. DRG, dorsal root ganglion; inf., inferior; n., nerve; SG, sympathetic ganglion; sup., superior. (Redrawn from Bonica JJ: The Management of Pain, 2nd ed, vol I, p 29. Philadelphia, Lea & Febiger, 1990.)

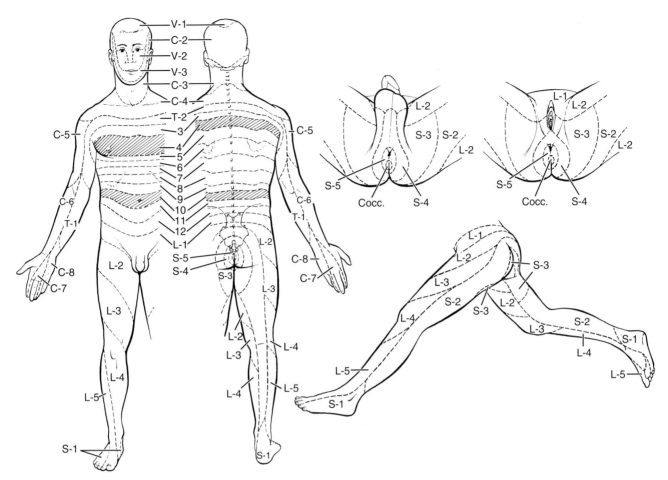

Figure 3–4 Mapping of the dermatomes.

provide a clinically useful sensory map of the body surface. The cutaneous somatic input retains a radicular organization, as do the bone (i.e., sclerotomes) and muscle (i.e., myotomes) afferents (Figs. 3–4 through 3–7 and Table 3–2).

Visceral afferents traverse the prevertebral ganglia without synapsing and course through the sympathetic chain and then gray rami communicantes and the dorsal root to their cell bodies in the dorsal root ganglia. From there, they project to the cerebral cortex in a manner similar to the somatic sensory fibers.[4, 6]

Periphery

Sensory axons are generally classified by size, which correlates with conduction velocity and function (Table 3–3). Fiber diameter is a function of the degree of myelination of the axons.[10] A-delta and C fibers are responsible for the transmission of nociceptive impulses. A-delta fibers primarily transmit sharp initial pain, and C fibers transmit so-called second pain, which is qualitatively dull, aching, or burning and persists longer than the noxious stimulus.[11, 12] In cutaneous tissue, there are subtypes of receptors, including

mechanoreceptors, polymodal nociceptors, and several types of thermoreceptors.[13] The A-delta mechanoreceptors respond to intense mechanical stimulation. Their receptive fields consist of multiple discrete spots that are less than 1 mm². As many as 20 spots may be grouped over an area from 1 mm² to 8 cm² to create a receptive field for a single neuron.[13] However, most of the nociceptive input (95% of fibers) from cutaneous tissue is from polymodal nociceptor C fibers. They respond to intense mechanical, thermal, and chemical stimuli. Polymodal nociceptors respond differently to different stimuli. For example, although repeated mechanical stimuli produce fatigue, repeated thermal stimuli produce sensitization (i.e., lowered threshold to a subsequent stimulus).[13, 14] Temporal summation also may be necessary to produce pain. Thresholds for stimulation of polymodal nociceptors by temperature stimuli are below conscious pain thresholds. However, multiple or prolonged temperature stimuli eventually produce a response above the conscious pain threshold.[15]

Deep tissues also have nociceptive afferents that are A-delta and C fibers. Muscle C fibers produce deep, aching, poorly localized pain. Pain fibers are responsive to various degrees of pressure, violent contraction or stretch, ischemia, and inflammation.[15–20]

In joints, in addition to the A-alpha and A-gamma

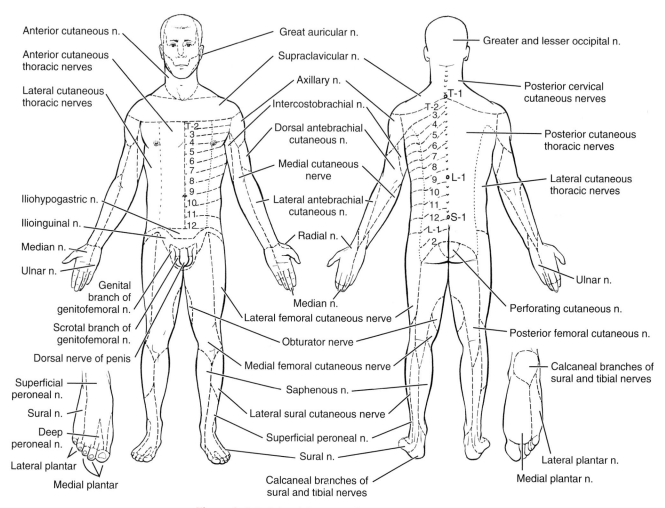

Figure 3–5 Peripheral dermatomal innervation. n., nerve.

fibers responsive to tendon stretch, afferents respond to noxious movements of the joint and chemical inflammation. Inflammation promotes sensitization and accounts for the pain that occurs with minimal motion in chronic arthritis.[21, 22]

Periosteum has the lowest pain threshold of all deep tissue and is supplied by a dense plexus of A-delta and C fibers. Cancellous bone is well supplied, but cortex and marrow have little nociceptive supply.[23]

Somatic Sensory System

Most visceral and somatic sensory afferents reach the spinal cord through the dorsal root. Their cell bodies are in the dorsal root ganglia, and the central dorsal root contains the neuron's dendritic processes.[9] Between 60% and 70% of dorsal root ganglion cells have axons that are small-diameter myelinated or unmyelinated fibers (i.e., A-delta or C fibers).[9]

As the dorsal root approaches the spinal cord, it divides into many rootlets. At the dorsal root entry zone, the small nociceptive fibers migrate to the lateral side.[24, 25]

Lissauer's tract is a dense system of predominantly propriospinal fibers that extend longitudinally from the periphery of the dorsal horn to the cord's surface. Its fibers project to laminae I, II, and III of the dorsal horn.[7]

Clinical Note: *Sindou and colleagues[24] developed a selective posterior rhizotomy based on the fact that pain fibers seem to move laterally before entering the spinal cord. When considering dorsal rhizotomy as a definitive means of pain control, it is important to recognize the accumulating evidence of the presence of pain fibers in the ventral root. Stimulation of the ventral root produces pain that can be blocked by local anesthetic applied to the dorsal root ganglion.[26] Presumably, cell bodies in the dorsal root ganglion send axonal or central processes through the ventral root. This may account for the failure of selective rhizotomy or dorsal root entry zone lesions for treatment of chronic pain.*

Dorsal Horn

The dorsal horn is a processing center for incoming information. The dorsal horn consists of six distinctive

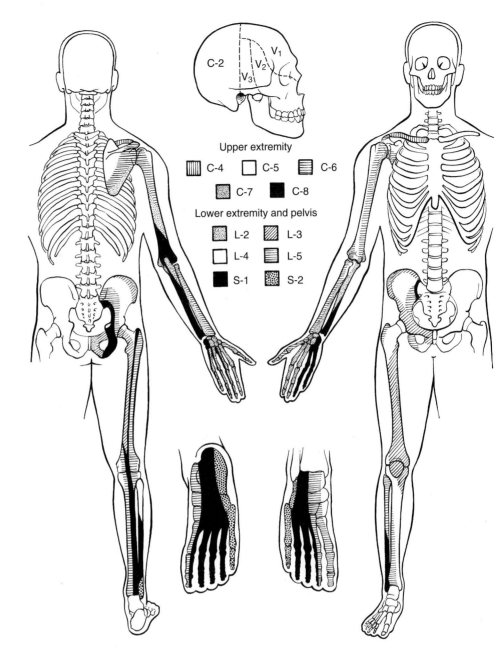

Figure 3–6 Mapping of the sclerotomes.

layers of neurons differentiated morphologically and functionally, as originally described by Rexed.[27] Lamina I is referred to as the marginal layer; lamina II, the substantia gelatinosa; and laminae III through V, the nucleus proprius. This structure is maintained throughout the spinal cord.[28]

Lamina I is a thin layer at the lateral cap of the dorsal horn. It receives a high concentration of nociceptive input, and many of its cell bodies are nociceptive specific (i.e., sensitive only to noxious input). Other sources of input to lamina I include Lissauer's tract and, by relay, interneuronal connections from deeper layers of the dorsal horn. Muscle afferents and cutaneous afferents converge on lamina I nociceptive-specific cell bodies. Presumably, this convergence accounts for cutaneous tenderness associated with painful muscular stimuli. Other cells receive input from thermal receptors, and still others receive input from wide dynamic range neurons, which are cells responding to noxious and innocuous stimuli. Differentiation of input occurs by a higher frequency of discharge by wide dynamic range neurons to noxious stimuli. Projections from lamina I ascend through long tracts, and they also form shorter interconnections with other spinal segments.[28, 29]

Lamina II is subdivided into inner (IIi) and outer (IIo) layers. The IIo cells respond to noxious stimuli, and the IIi cells respond to innocuous tactile stimuli.[28–30] Input to IIo cells comes from nociceptive afferents and descending inhibitory axons. Islet cells in laminae IIi and IIo seem to function as inhibitory neurons.[30, 31] These neurons interface with lamina I cells, other lamina II neurons, and lamina III. Projections to lamina I plus various patterns of tonic dis-

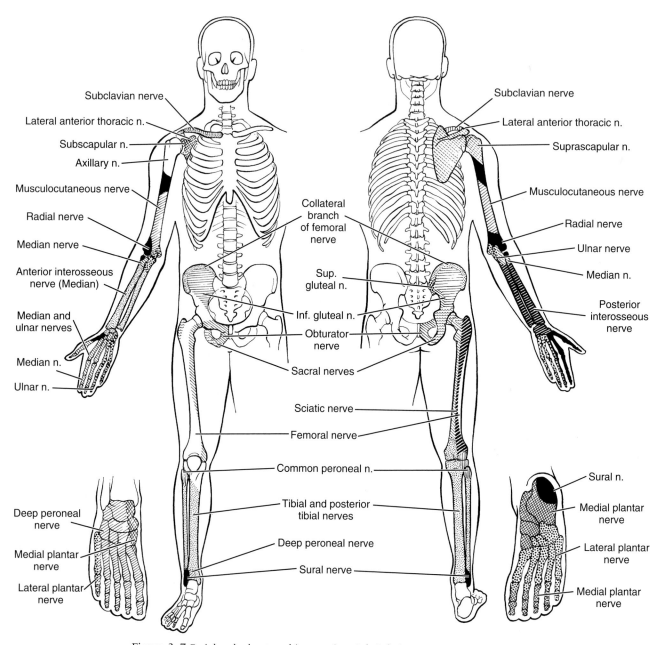

Figure 3–7 Peripheral sclerotomal innervation. Inf., inferior; n., nerve; Sup., superior.

charge implicate lamina II as a modulating influence on afferent impulses.[3] Some lamina II cells are inhibited by innocuous input, and some are inhibited by nociceptive stimuli. Others are stimulated by noxious stimuli, and still others are stimulated by innocuous input. These cells act to raise or lower stimulus thresholds in other cells.[28]

Laminae III and IV project to ascending tracts and to the dorsal columns. Input appears to be primarily from low threshold mechanical cutaneous receptors (which are not nociceptive), although some input is from the wide dynamic range neurons.[28, 29]

Lamina V receives input from A-delta and C-nociceptive fibers and projects to the spinothalamic and spinomesencephalic tracts.[28] Wide dynamic range neurons receive input from various mechanical, thermal,

and chemical receptors. Wide dynamic range neurons from laminae V and I appear to contribute 30% to 50% of the ascending system fibers.[29] Typically, a wide dynamic range neuron has a large receptive field with a central area responsive to noxious and tactile stimuli, but the periphery is responsive only to noxious stimuli. An inhibitory receptive field may surround the excitatory area, and there is overlap of receptive fields with other wide range dynamic neurons.[29] Inputs to lamina V also arise from descending tracts and interneuronal connections from other laminae. Nociceptive input may be from visceral, muscle, or cutaneous afferents.[31, 32]

Lamina VI is most prevalent at lumbosacral and cervical cord segments.[27] These cells receive convergent input from limb musculature and cutaneous afferents.[28]

Table 3–2 Somatic Motor Innervation

REGION, ACTION, AND PRIMARY MUSCLE(S)	SPINAL OR CRANIAL ROOT*	PERIPHERAL NERVE SUPPLY
Head		
Muscles of mastication (masseter, temporalis, and pterygoids)	CN 5	Mandibular nerve
Neck and Head		
Flexion		
Longus colli	C-2 to C-6	APDSN
Longus capitis	C-1 to C-3	APDSN
Rectus capitis	C-1,2	APDSN
Thoracolumbar Region		
Flexion and rotation		
Rectus abdominus	T-6 to T-12	APDSN
External oblique	T-6 to T-12	APDSN
Internal oblique	T-7 to T-12	APDSN
Transverse abd.	T-7 to T-12	APDSN
Extension		
Iliocostocervicalis (cerv, thorac, lumb)	C-2 to L-5	PPDSN
Longissimus (capit, cerv, thorac)	C-2 to L-5	PPDSN
Spinales (capit, cerv, thorac)	C-2 to T-12	PPDSN
Semispinales	C-2 to T-12	PPDSN
Multifidus	C-2 to T-12	PPDSN
Respiration		
Intercostals	T-1 to T-12	Intercostals
Diaphragm	C-2 to C-4	Phrenic
Shoulder Rotator Cuff		
Supraspinatus	C-5,6	Suprascapular
Infraspinatus	C-5,6	Suprascapular
Subscapularis	C-5,6	N. to subscapularis
Teres minor	C-5,6	Axillary
Scapular Motion		
Elevation		
Levator scapulae	C-4,5	Dorsal scapular
Rhomboideus	C-4,5	Dorsal scapular
Trapezius (sup. fibers)	CN XI	Spinal accessory
Depression		
Trapezius (inf. fibers)	CN XI	Spinal accessory
Pectoralis major	C-5 to T-1	Med and lat pectorals
Subclavius	C-5,6	N. to subclavius
Upward rotation		
Serratus anterior	C-5 to C-7	Long thoracic
Trapezius (upper, lower fibers)	CN XI	Spinal accessory
Downward rotation		
Levator scapulae	C-4,5	Dorsal scapular
Rhomboideus	C-4,5	Dorsal scapular
Pectoralis major, minor	C-5 to T-1	Lat and med pectorals
Latissimus dorsi	C-6 to C-8	Thoracodorsal
Abduction (protraction)		
Serratus anterior	C-5 to C-7	Long thoracic
Pectoralis major	C-5 to T-1	Lat and med pectorals
Adduction (retraction)		
Trapezius (middle fibers)	CN XI	Spinal accessory
Rhomboideus	C-4,5	Dorsal scapular
Latissimus dorsi	C-6 to C-8	Thoracodorsal
Arm Motion		
Flexion		
Pectoralis major (clavic. head)	C-5 to T-1	Med and lat pectorals
Deltoid (ant. fibers)	C-5,6	Axillary
Coracobrachialis	C-6,7	Musculocutaneous
Biceps brachii	C-5,6	Musculocutaneous
Extension		
Latissimus dorsi	C-6 to C-8	Thoracodorsal
Teres major	C-6	Subscapular
Deltoid (post. fiber)	C-5,6	Axillary
Triceps brachii	C-7,8	Radical
Abduction		
Deltoid (middle fibers)	C-5,6	Axillary
Supraspinatus	C-5,6	Suprascapular
Infraspinatus	C-5,6	Suprascapular
Teres minor	C-5,6	Axillary
Adduction		
Pectoralis major, minor	C-5 to T-1	Med and lat pectorals
Latissimus dorsi	C-6 to C-8	Thoracodorsal
Teres major	C-5,6	Subscapular

Table continued on following page

Table 3–2 Somatic Motor Innervation *Continued*

REGION, ACTION, AND PRIMARY MUSCLE(S)	SPINAL OR CRANIAL ROOT*	PERIPHERAL NERVE SUPPLY
Arm Motion *Continued*		
Medial rotation		
Subscapularis	C-5,6	N. to subscapularis
Latissimus dorsi	C-6 to C-8	Thoracodorsal
Pectoralis major, minor	C-5 to T-1	Med and lat pectorals
Lateral rotation		
Infraspinatus	C-5,6	Suprascapular
Teres minor	C-5,6	Axillary
Elbow and Forearm Motion		
Extension		
Triceps brachii	C-6 to C-8	Radial
Anconeus	C-7,8	Radial
Flexion		
Biceps brachii	C-5,6	Musculocutaneous
Brachialis	C-5,6	Musculocutaneous
Brachioradialis	C-5,6	Radial
Wrist Motion		
Flexion		
Flexor carpi radialis	C-6,7	Median
Flexor carpi ulnaris	C-7,8	Ulnar
Palmaris longus	C-7,8	Median
Extension		
Extensor carpi radialis, longus and brevis	C-6,7	Radial
Extensor carpi ulnaris	C-7,8	Radial (post. inteross.)
Radial deviation		
Flexor carpi radialis	C-6,7	Median
Extensor carpi radialis, longus and brevis	C-6,7	Radial
Ulnar deviation		
Flexor carpi ulnaris	C-7,8	Ulnar
Extensor carpi ulnaris	C-7,8	Radial (post. inteross.)
Digits (2-5)		
Flexion		
Flexor digit superficialis	C-7 to T-1	Median
Flexor digit profundus	C-7 to T-1	Median (ant. inteross.)
Extension		
Extensor digit communis	C-7,8	Radial (post. inteross.)
Extensor digit minimi	C-7,8	Radial (post. inteross.)
Extensor indicis	C-7,8	Radial (post. inteross.)
Abduction		
Dorsal interossei	C-8, T-1	Ulnar
Adduction		
Palmar interossei	C-8, T-1	Ulnar
Motion of Thumb		
Flexion		
Flexor pollicis longus	C-7,8	Median (ant. inteross.)
Extension		
Extensor pollicis longus	C-7,8	Radial (post. inteross.)
Extensor pollicis brevis	C-7,8	Radial (post. inteross.)
Abductor pollicis longus	C-7,8	Radial (post. inteross.)
Adduction		
Adductor pollicis	C-8, T-1	Ulnar
Abduction		
Abductor pollicis brevis	C-8, T-1	Median
Opponens pollicis	C-8, T-1	Median
Opposition		
Opponens pollicis	C-8, T-1	Median
Hypothenar Group (motion of 5th finger)		
Abductor digiti minimi	C-8, T-1	Ulnar
Flexor digiti brevis	C-8, T-1	Ulnar
Opponens digiti minimi	C-8, T-1	Ulnar
Hip and Thigh		
Extension		
Gluteus maximus	L-5 to S-2	Inferior gluteal
Semitendinosus	L-5, S-1	Tibial
Semimembranosus	L-5, S-1	Tibial
Biceps femoris	L-5, S-1	Tibial
Biceps femoris (shorthead)	L-5, S-1	Peroneal
Flexion		
Iliopsoas	L-2 to L-4	Branches fr. lumb. plexus and femoral
Rectus femoris	L-2 to L-4	Femoral
Adductor brevis	L-2 to L-4	Obturator
Sartorius	L-2 to L-4	Femoral
Abductor longus	L-2 to L-4	Obturator
Tensor fasciae latae	L-4 to S-1	Superior gluteal

Table continued on opposite page

Table 3–2 Somatic Motor Innervation *Continued*

REGION, ACTION, AND PRIMARY MUSCLE(S)	SPINAL OR CRANIAL ROOT*	PERIPHERAL NERVE SUPPLY
Hip and Thigh *Continued*		
Abduction		
Gluteus medius	L-4 to S-1	Superior gluteal
Gluteus minimus	L-4 to S-1	Superior gluteal
Tensor fasciae latae	L-4 to S-1	Superior gluteal
Gluteus maximus	L-5, S-1	Superior gluteal
Adduction		
Adductor longus	L-2 to L-4	Obturator
Adductor brevis	L-2 to L-4	Obturator
Adductor magnus	L-3 to L-5	Obturator and tibial
Gluteus maximus	L-5 to S-2	Inferior gluteal
Pectineus	L-2 to L-4	Femoral
Medial rotation		
Tensor fasciae latae	L-4 to S-1	Superior gluteal
Gluteus minimus	L-4 to S-1	Superior gluteal
Gluteus medius (ant. fibers)	L-4 to S-1	Superior gluteal
Semitendinosus	L-5, S-1	Tibial
Semimembranosus	L-5, S-1	Tibial
Lateral rotation		
Gluteus maximus	L-5 to S-2	Inferior gluteal
Knee and Leg		
Extension		
Rectus femoris	L-2 to L-4	Femoral
Vastus medialis, intermed, and lateralis	L-2 to L-4	Femoral
Sartorius	L-2 to L-4	Femoral
Leg flexion		
Semitendinosus	L-5 to S-2	Tibial
Semimembranosus	L-5, S-1	Tibial
Biceps femoris (longhead)	L-5 to S-2	Tibial
Gracilis	L-2,3	Obturator
Biceps femoris (shorthead)	S-1 to S-3	Peroneal
Gastrocnemius	S-1,2	Tibial
Ankle and Foot		
Dorsiflexion		
Tibialis anterior	L-4 to S-1	Deep peroneal
Peroneus longus, brevis	L-4 to S-1	Superficial peroneal
Plantar flexion		
Gastrocnemius	S-1,2	Tibial
Soleus	S-1,2	Tibial
Eversion		
Peroneus longus, brevis	L-4 to S-1	Superficial peroneal
Inversion		
Tibialis anterior	L-4 to S-1	Deep peroneal
Tibialis posterior	L-5, S-1	Tibial
Toes		
Flexion		
Flexor digiti longus, brevis	L-5, S-1	Tibial
Flexor hallucis longus, brevis	L-5, S-1	Tibial
Flexor digiti minimi brevis	L-5, S-1	Medial plantar
Quadratus plantae	L-5, S-1	Lateral plantar
Extension		
Extensor digiti longus brevis	L-5, S-1	Deep peroneal
Extensor hallucis longus	L-5, S-1	Lateral plantar
Lumbricales	L-5, S-1	Medial plantar
Dorsal inteross.	S-1, S-2	Lateral plantar
Abduction		
Abductor hallucis	L-5, S-1	Lateral plantar
Abductor digiti minimi	S-1, S-2	Lateral plantar
Dorsal inteross.	S-1, S-2	Lateral plantar
Adduction		
Adductor hallucis	S-1, S-2	Lateral plantar
Plantar inteross.	S-1, S-2	Lateral plantar
Pelvis and Perineum		
Levator ani	S-2 to S-4	Pudendal nerve
Anal and urethral sphincters	S-2 to S-4	Pudendal nerve

*Notice the extensive overlap of muscular innervation by spinal nerves. The progressively distal migration of musculature during embryogenesis carries the nerve supply along with it.

Abd., abdominis; ant., anterior; APDSN, anterior primary division of spinal nerve; capit, capitis; cerv, cervicis; clavic., clavicular; CN, cranial nerve; digit, digitorum; fr. lumb., from lumbar; inf., inferior; intermed, intermedius; inteross., interossei; lat, lateral; lumb, lumborum; med, medial; N., nerve; post., posterior; PPDSN, posterior primary division of spinal nerve; sup., superior; thorac, thoracis.

Modified from Bonica JJ: The Management of Pain, 2nd ed, vol I, pp 142–143. Philadelphia, Lea & Febiger, 1990.

Table 3–3 Classification of Peripheral Nerve Fibers

NERVE FIBER TYPE	INNERVATION	DIAMETER RANGE (μm)	CONDUCTION VELOCITY RANGE (m/s)
Aα	Primary muscle spindle motor to skeletal muscles	12–20	70–120
Aβ	Cutaneous touch and pressure afferents	5–15	30–70
Aγ	Motor to muscle spindle	6–8	15–30
Aδ	Mechanoreceptors, nociceptors, thermoreceptors	1–4	12–30
B	Sympathetic preganglionic	1–3	3–15
C	Mechanoreceptors, nociceptors, thermoreceptors, sympathetic postganglionic	0.5–1.5	0.5–2

Some data from Hursh JB: Conduction velocity and diameter of nerve fibers. Am J Physiol 1939; 127:131–139.

Laminae VII, VIII, and IX are in the ventral horn and project to spinothalamic and spinoreticular tracts. Input is from interneuronal connections from other laminae.[28]

Lamina X consists of a group of cells surrounding the spinal canal. Input is received bilaterally and is nociceptive and high-intensity specific. Projections are to other laminae throughout the length of the spinal cord.[33]

Clinical Note: *Nocifensive reflexes can be described as suprasegmental and cortical or spinal segmental (Table 3–4). Spinal reflexes are generated by nociceptive impulses being transmitted through the laminae of the dorsal horn to somatomotor or autonomic neurons at various spinal levels. These provoke responses such as paralytic ileus, vasoconstriction, tachycardia (through propriospinal impulses up the cord to cardiac accelerator fibers), or muscle spasm.[34, 35] Suprasegmental reflexes are transmitted through the ascending tracts to the brain stem, hypothalamus, and cortex, where withdrawal reflexes, autonomic responses, and conscious responses are generated. Blocking afferent input decreases these potentially harmful somatic responses and possibly decreases morbidity.[36, 37] This is one of the theoretical constructs behind preemptive analgesia clinical interventions and research studies.[38]*

The dense interneuronal connections in the dorsal horn provided a framework for the gate control theory by Melzack and Wall.[28] Descending systems of endorphinergic and serotonergic transmitters provide inhibition of dorsal horn cells receiving nociceptive input.[39] Other descending systems may enhance nociceptive

transmission. Interconnections among cells, particularly the wide dynamic range neurons, provide modulating control over which inputs are perceived as painful. Inhibitory fields surrounding central excitatory fields of wide dynamic range neurons block general stimuli from being perceived as noxious. The lamina IIi cells, which are activated by innocuous stimuli, may inhibit responsiveness of other neurons to noxious input if the inhibitory outflow from lamina IIi is not itself inhibited by the noxious input.[28, 29]

The dorsal horn of the spinal cord serves as a complex neuronal switching station. It acts as an integration system where sensory input is filtered, attenuated, or amplified before being relayed to other spinal segments or to the cortex.

Ascending Pathways

Ascending pathways from the dorsal horn to the brain consist of the lateral spinothalamic tract, the spinoreticular tract, spinomesencephalic tract, the dorsal column postsynaptic spinomedullary system, and the propriospinal multisynaptic ascending system (see Fig. 3–3).[3, 40]

The spinothalamic tract is the most important pathway for nociceptive transmission. Lesions that interrupt the spinothalamic tract (i.e., anterolateral quadrant of spinal cord) cause loss of pain sensation in the contralateral side below the level of the lesion.[41] These lesions also interrupt spinomesencephalic and spinoreticular tracts. Cell bodies are in laminae I and V through VIII of the dorsal horn.[40, 42] Axons cross the midline in the ventral commissure within two spinal segments of their origin and ascend as the lateral spinothalamic tract.[7, 40] Laminae I and V axons synapse in the ventroposterolateral nucleus of the thalamus and the posteromedial thalamus, where they then project to somatosensory cortex.[43–45] Laminae VI through VIII project through the lateral spinothalamic tract to the reticular formation of the medulla, pons, midbrain, periaqueductal gray, hypothalamus, and medial and intralaminar thalamic nuclei. These ultimately project to the limbic forebrain with diffuse cortical connections.[43–45]

As the spinothalamic tract ascends cephalad, it adds fibers to its anteromedial border, producing a somatotopic organization. Sacral segments are dorsolateral; cervical segments are anteromedial.[7, 30] Spinothalamic tract fibers terminating in the ventroposterolateral nucleus of the thalamus remain somatotopically oriented, but other terminations (e.g., reticular formation, medial thalamus) lose their orientation.[40, 43] The spinothalamic tract transmits nociceptive-specific impulses, proprioceptive input, light touch, and innocuous thermal stimuli.[29]

Clinical Note: *An important distinction is that input from wide dynamic range neurons is not somatotopically organized, but nociceptive-specific impulses generally are. The input from wide dynamic range neurons may be perceived as vague*

Table 3–4 Reflex Responses to Nociceptive Input*

I. Segmental and suprasegmental reflex responses and potential pathophysiologic consequences
  A. Increased general sympathetic tone due to increases in hypothalamic activity, segmental sympathetic reflexes (i.e., norepinephrine), and adrenal medullary secretion (i.e., epinephrine and norepinephrine), which results in:
    1. Vasoconstriction in skin, splanchnic region, and nonpriority organs produces an increase in peripheral resistance and decreased venous capacitance
    2. Increased stroke volume and heart rate lead to increased cardiac output
    3. Increased blood pressure and consequent increased myocardial work
    4. Increased metabolic rate and oxygen consumption
    5. Decreased gastrointestinal tone leads to decreased gastric emptying which may progress to ileus
    6. Decrease in urinary tract tone leads to urinary retention
  B. Increased skeletal muscle tone which may progress to spasm
    1. Increased tone of skeletal muscles of the trunk leads to a decrease in chest wall compliance and increased intraabdominal pressure, leading to alveolar and arterial mismatch, producing hypoxemia and possible pneumonitis
II. Endocrine responses
  A. Catabolic: increases in corticotropin, cortisol, antidiuretic hormone, growth hormone, cyclic adenosine monophosphate, catecholamines, renin, angiotensin II, aldosterone, glucagon, and interleukin-1
  B. Anabolic: decreases in insulin and testosterone

III. Metabolic responses
  A. Carbohydrate: epinephrine and glucagon release lead to hyperglycemia and glucose intolerance; insulin resistance due to increases in hepatic glycogenolysis leads to growth hormone, cortisol, free fatty acids, epinephrine, and glucagon release, producing gluconeogenesis; decreases in insulin secretion or action
  B. Protein: increased muscle protein metabolism provides alanine for gluconeogenesis due to increases in cortisol, glucagon, epinephrine, and interleukin-1
  C. Fat: increased lipolysis and oxidation of tissue fat provide increases in free fatty acids, leading to gluconeogenesis due to increases in catecholamines, glucagon, cortisol, and growth hormone
IV. Water and electrolyte responses
  A. Retention of water and sodium and increased excretion of potassium due to increases in aldosterone, antidiuretic hormone, and cortisol
  B. Decreased functional extracellular fluid as it shifts to vascular and cellular compartments due to increases in catecholamines, antidiuretic hormone, angiotensin II, and prostaglandin
V. Respiratory responses
  A. Suprasegmental stimulation of respiratory center with consequent hyperventilation counteracted by hypoventilation caused by splinting and skeletal muscle spasm
VI. Diencephalic and cortical responses
  A. Anxiety and fear increase hypothalamic response, causing a further increase in general sympathetic tone, catecholamines, and other systems
  B. Increased blood viscosity, clotting time, fibrinolysis, and platelet aggregation increase the risk of thromboembolism and other dysfunction
  C. Pain stimulates psychologic mechanisms with deleterious emotional effects

*Continued or intense nociceptive input increases the likelihood of recruiting additional spinal levels of input and suprasegmental reflexes. Anxiety and fear also increase suprasegmental responses. The rationale for preemptive analgesia and attentiveness to postoperative pain control is to decrease or eliminate complications such as atelectasis, hypoxemia, pneumonia, ileus, and thrombosis by decreasing detrimental segmental and suprasegmental reflexes.
Modified from Bonica JJ: The Management of Pain, 2nd ed, vol I, p 177. Philadelphia, Lea & Febiger, 1990.

diffuse pain, unlike the more specific nociceptive input from the lateral spinothalamic tract. Intense stimulation of just the central area of wide dynamic range neurons may refer pain to a wider area.[43, 46] This is a plausible mechanism for the referred pain of myofascial trigger points.

The spinoreticular tract is an important component of nocifensive reflexes, because it is a direct link between reticular arousal centers and the dorsal horn.[47, 48] Most spinoreticular neurons in the dorsal horn have input from wide dynamic range neurons. This implicates the spinoreticular tract in suprasegmental pain reflexes such as autonomic reflexes and aversive drive.[47, 48]

Spinomesencephalic tract fibers run parallel and lateral to the spinoreticular tract. Cell bodies are predominantly located in lamina I or V and seem to be nociceptive specific.[28] Terminations are in the periaqueductal gray and other midbrain nuclei.[48–50] It is possible that the spinomesencephalic tract activates a system of descending pain inhibition beginning at the periaqueductal gray.[49, 50]

Mehler[45, 49, 50] considered the spinomesencephalic, spinoreticular, and medial projecting spinothalamic tracts to be the paleospinothalamic tract and the lateral thalamic projecting spinothalamic tract to be the neospinothalamic tract. The neospinothalamic tract conveys more rapid, discrete, and localized nociceptive impulses than the paleospinothalamic tract. The paleospinothalamic tract and its projections to the periaqueductal gray, hypothalamus, medial and intralaminar thalamic nuclei, and reticular system provoke more affective responses to pain, such as vague unpleasantness, emotive drive, autonomic reflexes, and endocrine responses.[43, 45, 49–51]

Clinical Note: *Surgical lesioning of the spinothalamic tract, which is clinically referred to as cordotomy, may be useful as a definitive pain-relieving procedure in patients with terminal disease, but these interventions often fail to provide long-term benefit. After a year, pain redevelops in about 50% of patients. On average, analgesia recedes caudad at a rate of one spinal level per*

month. This observation has led to the suggestion that there are alternative pathways involved over time in the transmission of nociceptive input. The pathways implicated in alternative pain transmission include the dorsal columns and the propriospinal multisynaptic ascending system.[52] Propriospinal multisynaptic ascending system pathways consist of multisynaptic interneuronal connections that ascend around the center of the spinal cord. Basbaum[52] demonstrated that isolated polysynaptic pathways are able to transmit pain up to the cortex.

The dorsal columns course cephalad to terminate in the nucleus gracilis (for lumbar fibers) and nucleus cuneatus (for cervical fibers) of the medulla.[7, 8] Axons then cross the midline to form the medial lemniscus, which terminates in the ventroposterolateral thalamus. The dorsal horn cells of origin are in laminae III and IV.[51, 53] They appear to transmit mostly proprioceptive and innocuous touch information.[53] However, the dorsal columns may play a role in modulating nociceptive information in the spinothalamic tract and in providing discriminatory information to localize pain.[54] Melzack and Wall[54] proposed that dorsal column input acts as a trigger to prepare the cerebral cortex for incoming nociceptive data. The cortex then turns on appropriate descending systems that help modulate the dorsal horn response to nociceptive data. The lateral neospinothalamic tract then provides rapid precise localization of nociceptive data that activates suprasegmental and cortical reflexes. Concurrently, paleospinothalamic tract input acts to arouse the whole organism to ongoing tissue damage, activating the neuroendocrine, emotional, and autonomic reflexes associated with pain.[39, 51, 54]

Clinical Note: *Wall and Melzack's gate control theory[54] for the dorsal columns provides a partial explanation for the efficacy of dorsal column stimulation in relieving certain neuropathic pains. Presumably, pain-producing discharges propagate cephalad through the anterolateral spinothalamic pathways of the neospinothalamic, paleospinothalamic, spinomesencephalic, and spinoreticular tracts. Dorsal column stimulation could block or scramble signals going to thalamic nuclei and decrease sensitization to nociceptive input by increasing transmission through the dorsal columns. Alternatively, in chronic neuropathic pain, the dorsal columns may be more directly involved in nociceptive transmission, blocking transmission in the spinothalamic tract. Dorsal column stimulation has also been implicated in antidromic stimulation of the dorsal horn, because cutting the dorsal column caudal to stimulation prevents analgesia. Naloxone does not reverse dorsal column stimulation analgesia as it does with periaqueductal gray stimulation, suggesting that nonopioid systems act as neurochemical mediators of this stimulus-response modality.[55-57]*

Trigeminal Sensory System

The central portion of the trigeminal system is composed of the trigeminal mesencephalic nucleus, the main sensory nucleus, and the spinal trigeminal nucleus.[58, 59] The trigeminal mesencephalic nucleus consists of cell bodies that relay proprioceptive impulses from the temporomandibular joint, the masticatory and ocular muscles, and the oropharynx. Central branches project to the motor nucleus of cranial nerve V, a pattern that is analogous to the anterior horn. Other primary afferents have cell bodies in the gasserian ganglion, like dorsal root ganglia, with projections through the sensory trigeminal root to the brain stem terminating in the main sensory nucleus and spinal trigeminal nucleus. The trigeminal tract runs longitudinally along the brain stem from the pons to caudal medulla in the same fashion as Lissauer's tract in the spinal cord. The axons of the gasserian ganglion cells form the peripheral trigeminal nerve. The main sensory nucleus is at the level of the pons, but the spinal trigeminal nucleus extends as far caudad as C-2. The entire trigeminal sensory system is somatotopically organized.[58, 59]

The upper cervical dorsal root fibers and sensory (i.e., somatic) roots of cranial nerves VII, IX, and X (i.e., innervating posterior tongue, tonsils, pharynx, tympanic membranes, external auditory canals) primarily synapse in the spinal trigeminal nucleus. The caudal spinal trigeminal nucleus is similar to the dorsal horn and contains laminae I through IV. Lamina V is represented by part of the lateral reticular formation.[59, 60]

Ascending sensory projections include proprioceptive information transmitted from the main sensory nucleus and rostral spinal trigeminal nucleus. These fibers are analogous to the medial lemniscus. They cross the midline at the level of the pons and form the ventral trigeminal lemniscus, which terminates in the ventroposteromedial nucleus of thalamus.[58, 61] From there, projections reach the sensory cortex, having maintained somatotopic organization. Pain pathways follow the trigeminothalamic tract projecting to the ventroposteromedial thalamic nucleus and then to the somatosensory cortex. This is analogous to the neospinothalamic tract, which is also somatotopically organized.[58, 61] Other neurons from caudal spinal trigeminal nucleus (forming an analogue of paleospinothalamic tract) project ipsilaterally and contralaterally to the hypothalamus, periaqueductal gray, and medial and intralaminar thalamic nuclei. This system is not somatotopically organized.[58, 61]

Supraspinal Pain Pathways

Supraspinal systems play a significant role in transmitting pain information.[3, 6, 62] The reticular system has myriad projections, including those to the cortex, hypothalamus, and intralaminar thalamus. The connections to multiple autonomic centers, including cardiac, respiratory, neuroendocrine, and somatomotor centers, in addition to the periaqueductal gray region, implicate the reticular formation in pain modulation.[48, 51] The medial thalamus and hypothalamus also have input to the limbic system, contributing to the emotional and affective responses in pain.[51] Limbic lesions have been shown to attenuate the unpleasantness of pain without changing discriminative ability.[63]

The hypothalamus itself is often considered part of the limbic system. The medial hypothalamus controls autonomic nervous functions by means of connections to the dorsal motor nucleus of the vagus and the dorsolateral funiculus, which provides input to the spinal cord.[64] The ventromedial hypothalamus regulates pituitary function, and the lateral hypothalamus is intimately connected with the limbic system.[64, 65] The limbic system is concerned with the emotive content of a stimulus and therefore with incentives to action.[51] The interconnections among multiple nuclei of the limbic system and their interconnections with the periaqueductal gray, hypothalamus, thalamic nuclei, reticular system, and cortex are complex and important but beyond the scope of this chapter to explore.[51, 65, 66]

Thalamus

The thalamus can be divided into paleothalamus and neothalamus. The paleothalamus includes the medial and intralaminar nuclei. It is not somatotopically organized and receives input from paleospinothalamic tract and spinoreticular formation. These nuclei project to wide areas of the cortex, particularly the limbic system. Lesions in these nuclei seem to alter the affective component of pain.[51, 63, 66, 67] The neothalamus consists of the ventral basal complex, which is subdivided into the ventroposterolateral and ventroposteromedial nuclei. The ventroposterolateral nucleus is somatotopically organized with input primarily from the medial lemniscus (i.e., contralateral dorsal columns), the neospinothalamic tract, the periaqueductal gray, and the descending fibers from somatosensory cortex. Projections are to somatosensory cortex (i.e., areas SI and SII). The ventroposteromedial nucleus receives input from the somatotopically organized trigeminal pathways. Projections are similar to those of the ventroposterolateral nucleus.[66–68]

Cerebral Cortex

The cerebral cortex receives sensory input in the primary (SI) and secondary (SII) somatosensory areas. SI is located in the postcentral gyrus and receives projections from the ventroposterolateral and ventroposteromedial nuclei. SII is in the parietal lobe on the superior aspect of the suprasylvian fissure.[69] SI is the larger and more important of the areas. It is somatotopically organized. It appears that there are at least two (and probably three) complete representations of the body within SI, each receiving different types of input (i.e., deep pressure, cutaneous stimulation, and joint motion).[69] SII does not seem to be somatotopically

organized. This area receives projections from the paleothalamic tracts. Other cortical connections are diffuse and extensive, including descending fibers to the thalamus and interconnections with the limbic system and periaqueductal gray.[68, 69]

Clinical Note: *Cerebrovascular disease or injury (e.g., strokes) in the thalamus or the cortex can produce a central neuropathic pain syndrome. Tasker[70] demonstrated that the thalamus could be involved in generating chronic pain, particularly deafferentation pain. Tasker also demonstrated that thalamic stimulation can relieve deafferentation pain but not nociceptive pain.[71, 72] Thalamic stimulation may provide pain relief when spinal cord stimulation does not—when a destructive peripheral or spinal nervous system lesion (e.g., herpes zoster infection) decreases the number of fibers available for stimulation in the spinal cord—but these anatomic changes do not extend to the thalamus.[73]*

Deep brain stimulation can also be used to facilitate descending inhibition of nociceptive impulses by placing electrodes in the periaqueductal gray or periventricular gray. Basbaum and Fields[74–76] concluded that the nucleus raphe magnus and other medullary nuclei receive input from the periaqueductal gray, which transmits descending nociceptive inhibitory signals to the dorsal horn. This central endorphinergic output is linked to serotonergic fibers that are located in the dorsolateral funiculus and project to laminae I and V in the dorsal horn.[29, 74–76]

Descending Pathways of Pain Modulation

As early as 1902, Sherrington[77] emphasized the importance of the interaction between inhibitory and excitatory systems, but it was not until 1965 that Melzack and Wall[54] proposed their gate control theory of pain modulation. They presented a basic model for sensory modulation within the dorsal horn region by extrinsic stimuli (i.e., peripheral afferent impulses) and internal regulation (i.e., supraspinal descending inhibitory systems). Subsequent work on stimulation-produced analgesia and the discovery of enkephalins originally supported this theory, which was later deemed overly simplistic.[78, 79] Experiments demonstrated that stimulation-produced analgesia was enkephalin-mediated from the periaqueductal gray through midline raphe nuclei of the medulla (particularly the nucleus raphe magnus) to the dorsal horn by inhibitory serotonergic fibers in the dorsolateral funiculus.[75] Lesions within the nucleus raphe magnus blocked stimulation-produced analgesia, but stimulation of the nucleus raphe magnus produced analgesia.[75] Fields and colleagues[80] further elaborated this regulatory model through the demonstration of pain-modulating descending systems emanating from the brain stem.

Descending control systems that begin in the somatosensory cortex with corticospinal fibers course along the dorsal lateral funiculus and terminate in dorsal horn laminae I and II. These fibers exert direct control on dorsal horn neurons.[81] These fibers probably enhance the inhibitory functions of other descending systems.

Although stimulation of the periventricular gray and ventroposterolateral plus ventroposteromedial nuclei of the thalamus can produce analgesia, the most important descending system appears to begin in the periaqueductal gray.[75, 76] Input is from frontal and insular cortex, limbic system, and hypothalamus, in addition to the reticular system, locus coeruleus, and spinal cord.[82] Descending connections are to rostral medulla, especially the nucleus raphe magnus and reticular nuclei, and directly to the medullary and spinal dorsal horn by means of the dorsal lateral funiculus.[82] Multiple reticular nuclei (including the nucleus raphe magnus) then project directly to the dorsal horn by means of the dorsal lateral funiculus. Multiple neurotransmitters are involved. Each neuron may receive input from several transmitters, and each neuron may release multiple neurotransmitters.[81]

The descending fibers that modulate nociception occur at various sites throughout the central nervous system. The most important pathways appear to be serotonergic or noradrenergic and originate in the periaqueductal gray, with relays through medullary reticular nuclei to the dorsal horn through the dorsal lateral funiculus. The neurochemistry at each level appears to be extraordinarily complex, allowing for subtle adjustments in the system.

Visceral Pain Phenomena

Stimuli required to produce pain vary among visceral structures, but an adequately intense and specific stimulus must be applied to generate a response.[83–85] For example, the myocardium is sensitive to ischemia but not to mechanical stimulation. Intestine can be cut, crushed, or burned without pain, but traction, distension, and contractions against obstruction produce severe pain.[84] Generally, serosa is sensitive to traction, distension, and chemical irritation, and mucosa is sensitive to inflammatory processes. The type of stimulus required to incite pain reflects a major neurophysiologic difference between ectodermal (e.g., skin, mucous membranes) and mesodermal (e.g., serosa, muscle, bone) structures.[83, 85, 86]

The quality of visceral pain is often different from that of somatic pain. Ectodermal pain is initially sharp and followed by localized burning or throbbing. Visceral and deep muscle pain tend to be poorly localized and are experienced as dull, aching sensations. Perhaps this is because the ratio of A to C fibers is 1:10 in visceral afferents but 1:2 in cutaneous afferents. Visceral nociceptive fibers innervate a much larger area than somatic afferents and have extensive overlap between receptive fields.[86]

Like visceral pain, deep muscle and ligament nociception can give rise to pain in segmental patterns analogous to dermatomes and referred to as sclerotomes and myotomes.[87] Deep somatic pain generates secondary hyperalgesia, reflex muscle spasm, referred pain, and sympathetic hyperactivity (Fig. 3–8).[87, 88] For example, Lewis and Kellgren[88] demonstrated that pain caused by injection of L-1 interspinous ligament produced a pattern similar to the pain of ureteral colic, and just as with renal colic, testicular retraction occurred (i.e., autonomic reflex involving L-1 sympathetic fibers).

A hallmark of visceral pain is intense autonomic activity such as sweating, nausea, emesis, hypotension, and bradycardia. The phenomena of secondary hyperalgesia, referred pain, reflex skeletal muscle spasm, and autonomic reflexes are all associated with visceral pain.[35, 85, 88]

True visceral pain is vague in character and location, and it produces referred pain. For example, the early pain of appendicitis is periumbilical.[4, 6] This referral occurs because the visceral afferents supplying small bowel serosa pass through the celiac ganglia and splanchnic nerves to the sympathetic chain and gray rami to enter the spinal cord at about T-10. Pain is perceived as emanating from the T-10 dermatome.[4, 6] As appendicitis progresses, pain localizes to the right lower quadrant because of inflammation spreading to the parietal peritoneum. Because parietal peritoneum has the same nerve supply as the overlying somatic structures, pain is felt in the dermatome and myotome supplied by that nerve. Referred pain is accompanied by secondary hyperalgesia, tenderness, and reflex skeletal muscle spasm.[4, 6, 85] Secondary hyperalgesia (i.e., increased sensitivity in convergent cutaneous derma-

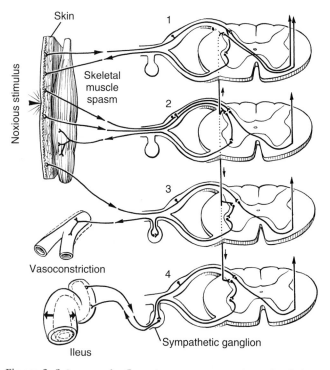

Figure 3–8 Segmental reflexes in response to noxious stimulation. (Modified from Bonica JJ: The Management of Pain, 2nd ed, vol I, p 52. Philadelphia, Lea & Febiger, 1990.)

tomes) probably results from changes in dorsal horn neurochemistry leading to sensitization of dorsal horn nociceptive neurons, particularly wide dynamic range neurons.[85]

Clinical Note: *With visceral pain, the extent and intensity of reflex muscle spasm are related to the intensity and duration of the painful stimulus. Particularly persistent and intense nociceptive impulses produce prolonged excitability in the dorsal horn, along with expanding receptive fields and lowered depolarization thresholds.[89, 90] Increased duration and intensity of nociceptive stimuli cause the reflex spasm to spread beyond the spinal roots supplying the initial source of pain.[89, 90] For instance, pancreatitis may cause an initial spasm in the T-8 to T-10 musculature, but unabated, this visceral stimulus may eventually spread to involve the entire chest wall. Similarly, a herniated disk at L-5 may initially produce radicular symptoms, and it eventually may produce muscular spasm and tenderness in adjacent myotomes and dermatomes. Autonomic reflexes account for vasovagal responses or tachycardia, local piloerection and vasoconstriction, sweating, and a plethora of central neuroendocrine responses.[91] It is postulated that these physiologic responses create secondary pain "generators" that may outlast the original nociceptive impulse and reinforce the secondary response (see Fig. 3–8).[90]*

Several mechanisms have been postulated for how referred pain occurs. Experimental data support a model of visceral and cutaneous afferent fibers converging onto neurons in laminae V through VIII of the dorsal horn. In this model, only small myelinated and unmyelinated fibers converge (i.e., only nociceptive input from cutaneous and visceral afferents converges).[92] Visceral and somatic fibers converge in the dorsal horn, the thalamus, and the sensory cortex.[93]

A second explanation implicates cells in the dorsal root ganglion that have bifurcated axons. One branch goes to skin and the other to muscle or viscera.[93–95] Several researchers have demonstrated that a single dorsal root ganglion cell can be stimulated from two different peripheral nerves or sometimes from the sympathetic chain (i.e., visceral afferent) and a cutaneous nerve. These findings hold even after dorsal rhizotomy, which indicates that convergence is not mediated through central interneuronal connections.[93–95]

Visceral-cutaneous convergence, bifurcation of dorsal root ganglion axons, and segmental responses to nociception seem to account for phenomena of referred pain.[93–95] Noxious stimulus-induced changes in dorsal horn neurochemistry, segmental reflexes, and suprasegmental reflexes promote the prolongation and spread of pain. The suprasegmental-cortical reflexes support increased general sympathetic tone, increased secretion of cortisol, corticotropin, glucagon, growth hormone, antidiuretic hormone, increased blood vis-

cosity, increased clotting time, fibrinolysis, platelet aggregation, ileus, and decreased renal blood flow, which teleologically appear to be acute survival adaptations (see Table 3–4).[35–37, 89, 91]

Autonomic Nervous System

The autonomic nervous system is composed of efferent (i.e., motor) and afferent (i.e., sensory) fibers. The sensory fibers are similar to those in the somatic afferent system.[65, 96]

The efferent pathway is composed of a two-neuron chain, unlike the somatic efferents, which have a single neuron in the anterior horn of the spinal cord (see Figs. 3–1 and 3–2). The central neuron is located in the intermediolateral cell column, from T-1 to L-2 for the sympathetic efferents.[4, 5, 97] The parasympathetic system has central neurons in the visceral efferent nuclei of the brain (i.e., dorsal motor nucleus of the vagus, salivatory nuclei, and oculomotor or Edinger-Westphal nucleus) and the sacral segments S-2, S-3, and S-4 of the intermediolateral column.[4, 5, 97]

The sacral parasympathetics leave the spinal cord with the anterior spinal roots and then branch off as the pelvic splanchnic nerves (i.e., nervi erigentes). They pass through the hypogastric plexus and synapse in terminal ganglia in end organs, such as the bladder, uterus, descending colon, genitalia (Fig. 3–9). Afferent fibers from pelvic viscera course with the nervi erigentes but terminate in dorsal root ganglia at S-2, S-3, and S-4.[4, 5, 97] The cranial portion of the parasympathetic system consists of central cell bodies in the oculomotor, facial, and vagal nuclei. The physiologic effects of the autonomic system are listed in Table 3–5.

The oculomotor nerve (i.e., Edinger-Westphal nucleus) sends axons to synapse in the ciliary ganglion, which then supplies the ciliary muscle (e.g., accommodation) and the iris sphincter (e.g., constricts iris). The salivatory nucleus supplies the presynaptic fibers to the facial nerve by way of the pterygopalatine and submandibular ganglia and to the glossopharyngeal nerve through the otic ganglion. Postganglionic fibers control secretions of the mucous membranes; pharynx; and lacrimal, parotid, sublingual, and submandibular glands.[4, 5, 97] The dorsal motor nucleus of the vagus supplies preganglionic fibers to thoracic and abdominal viscera by means of the vagus nerve. Parasympathetic ganglia are usually located in the visceral structures and have short postganglionic fibers. The vagus and glossopharyngeal nerves also provide somatic efferent fibers to the larynx, pharynx, and soft palate musculature.[3, 4, 65, 97]

Afferent parasympathetics transmit somatosensory input from the ear, pharynx, and larynx through cranial nerves VII, IX, and X. Vagal afferents, comprising 80% of the vagal fibers, transmit sensory information from thoracic and abdominal organs. Cell bodies are in the inferior and superior jugular ganglia (i.e., vagus), geniculate ganglia (i.e., facial), and petrosal ganglia (i.e., glossopharyngeal). All of these ganglia can be likened to the dorsal root ganglia inasmuch as they

Table 3–5 Physiologic Responses to Autonomic Stimulation

STRUCTURE	SYMPATHETIC RESPONSE	PARASYMPATHETIC RESPONSE	PARASYMPATHETIC PATH
Eye			
Ciliary muscle	Relaxes	Contracts	Oculomotor nucleus to ciliary ganglion via oculomotor nerve
Pupillary muscle	Dilates (mydriasis)	Contracts (miosis)	
Lacrimal glands		↑ Secretions	Nucleus of cranial nerve VII to pterygopalatine ganglion to lacrimal nerve
Levator palpebrae	Ptosis		
Salivary glands			
Parotid	↓ Secretions secondary to ↓ blood flow	Profuse serous secretions	Inferior salivatory nucleus Cranial nerve IX to otic ganglion
Sublingual	Same as above	Same as above	Superior salivatory nucleus
Submaxillary			Cranial nerve VII, chorda tympani
Thyroid	Stimulates		
Bronchial tree			
Musculature	Relaxes	Constricts	Dorsal motor nucleus of vagus
Glands		↑ Secretions	
Heart			
Rate	↑	↓	As above
Contractility	↑	↓	
Esophagus sphincter	Contracts	Relaxes	As above
Motility	↓	↑	
Secretions	Inhibits	↑	
Liver	Glycogenolysis Gluconeogenesis		
Gallbladder	Relaxes	Contracts	Dorsal motor nucleus of vagus
Pancreas			
Insulin secretion	↓	↑	As above
Intestine			
Motility	↓	↑	As above
Secretions	↓	↑	
	Relaxes	Contracts	
Colon			
Internal sphincter	Contracts		
Adrenal gland	80% Epinephrine 20% Norepinephrine		
Genitalia			
Seminal vesicle	Contraction Ejaculation		
Vas deferens	Contraction		
Penile erectile tissue		Relaxes—causes erection	Pelvic splanchnic nervi erigentes
Uterus	Relaxation		
Arteries			
Coronary	Constricts		
Skeletal muscle	Relaxes		
Skin	Constricts		
Viscera	Constricts		
Veins	Constricts		

↑, increased; ↓, decreased.
Data from Bonica JJ: The Management of Pain, 2nd ed, vol I, pp 133–158. Philadelphia, Lea & Febiger, 1990 and Guyton AC: Textbook of Medical Physiology, 5th ed, pp 768–783. Philadelphia, WB Saunders, 1976.

house primary sensory cell bodies only.[4, 5, 65, 98] These ganglionic neurons project to the nucleus solitarius tract and then to the thalamus.[4, 98] Sacral parasympathetics provide sensations of nociception and distension (e.g., triggering reflex arcs) from pelvic viscera. They project to the dorsal horn and then to the thalamus.[65]

The sympathetic nervous system consists of cell bodies in the T-1 to L-2 intermediolateral cell column whose axons exit the cord with the anterior spinal roots. The axons leave the spinal nerve by means of the white rami communicantes from T-1 to L-2 or L-3 to synapse outside the central neuraxis in paravertebral ganglia, prevertebral ganglia, and adrenal glands.[65, 99, 100]

After leaving the spinal nerves, preganglionic axons form the paravertebral sympathetic chain. These bilateral structures fuse distally in the ganglion of impar (i.e., midline and anterior to the sacrococcygeal juncture) and terminate cephalad at the C-2 level in the bilateral superior cervical ganglia.

The cervical ganglia lie ventral to the medial base of the transverse processes. The thoracic ganglia lie anterior to the heads of ribs, and the lumbar ganglia lie along the anterolateral surfaces of the vertebral bodies. The sacral ganglia lie on the anterior surface of the sacrum medial to anterior sacral foramina. There are usually four somewhat distinct cervical ganglia: superior, middle, intermediate, and stellate (often a fusion

Figure 3–9 Autonomic innervation of pelvic viscera (male). Inf., inferior; n., nerve. (Modified from Bonica JJ: The Management of Pain, 2nd ed, vol II, p 1290. Philadelphia, Lea & Febiger, 1990.)

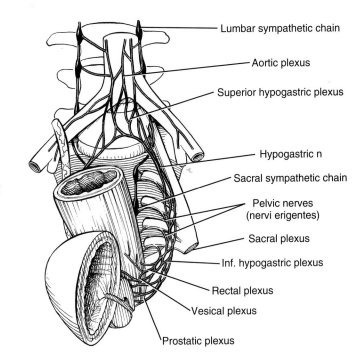

- Lumbar sympathetic chain
- Aortic plexus
- Superior hypogastric plexus
- Hypogastric n
- Sacral sympathetic chain
- Pelvic nerves (nervi erigentes)
- Sacral plexus
- Inf. hypogastric plexus
- Rectal plexus
- Vesical plexus
- Prostatic plexus

of inferior cervical and T-1 ganglia). Below these are segmental ganglia, with considerable interindividual variability, consisting of 10 to 12 thoracic, 3 to 5 lumbar, and 4 sacral ganglia and the terminal ganglion of impar.

Postganglionic fibers from paravertebral ganglia can rejoin spinal nerves at any level through the gray rami for distribution to skin and muscle. Unlike white rami, gray rami are present for each spinal nerve.[4, 5, 99] In addition to gray rami, postganglionic sympathetic fibers are distributed by the three cardiac nerves to thoracic viscera, including the heart. Postganglionic sympathetic fibers (e.g., carotid nerve) are distributed to the head along with the carotid artery and its branches. A few preganglionic fibers synapse in the carotid plexus and then continue cephalad with the artery.

Distally, preganglionic fibers from the T-5 to T-10 segments traverse the sympathetic chain, exiting to form the greater splanchnic nerve, which synapses in the celiac ganglion and superior mesenteric ganglion. Postganglionic fibers course with blood vessels to supply abdominal organs. Fibers from T-10 to T-12 form the lesser splanchnic nerve, and fibers from T-10 to L-2 form the (variably present) least splanchnic nerve. These nerves synapse in the inferior mesenteric, aortic-renal, and renal ganglia. Postganglionic fibers supply small and large intestine, kidneys, ureters, and genitalia by distributing with the vascular supply. Some fibers do not synapse in the prevertebral (e.g., celiac, mesenteric, corticorenal) ganglia but synapse directly with chromaffin cells in the adrenal gland.[57, 65]

Still more distally, preganglionic fibers from L-1 to L-3 run caudally down the sympathetic chain and may exit, without synapsing, to form the superior, middle, and inferior hypogastric plexus. After synapsing in the hypogastric plexus, postganglionic fibers supply descending colon and pelvic viscera. The pelvic viscera

are also supplied by postganglionic fibers, which leave the sympathetic chain after synapsing in paravertebral lumbosacral ganglia and then traverse the hypogastric plexus.[65, 99]

Clinical Note: *There are gray rami at every spinal level connecting the sympathetic chain back to spinal (i.e., somatic) nerves for distribution. The upper extremity is supplied by middle, intermediate, stellate, T-2, and T-3 ganglia, although fibers may come from sites as distal as T-2 to T-8. Gray rami connect with the roots of the brachial plexus at C-5 to T-2. Consequently, to block the sympathetic nerve supply to the upper extremity, local anesthetic must reach T-1 or T-2 ganglia.[99, 100]*

Similarly, the lower extremity is supplied by L-1 to S-3 paravertebral ganglia, reconnecting with spinal roots L-1 to S-3 by gray rami. However, paravertebral ganglia caudal to L-3 have preganglionic fibers from T-10 to L-3 cell bodies only. A lower extremity lumbar sympathetic block can be achieved by blocking L-1, L-2, and L-3 ganglia. Any paravertebral ganglia caudal to L-3 is blocked because its preganglionic fibers must pass through the paravertebral chain from L-1, L-2, and L-3. For the upper extremity, a similar effect can be achieved by blocking T-1 and T-2, because cervical preganglionic fibers enter the sympathetic chain at T-1 or caudad. However, because a thoracic paravertebral block is technically more difficult, a cervical block (i.e., stellate ganglion block) is performed, and hopefully local anesthetic spreads caudally through fascial planes to T-2 ganglia.[100]

In addition to this already complicated distribution system, there are anomalous and accessory ganglia. Some synapses take place in spinal nerves, white rami, and ventral roots, bypassing the sympathetic trunk.[14] These pathways are most common in lower cervical and upper thoracic segments and in the lower thoracic and upper lumbar regions. Presumably, this could account for the incomplete results after surgical sympathectomy compared with those after chemical sympathetic block because of extensive diffusion of local anesthetic solutions.[100]

Sympathectomy also affects autonomic afferents. For example, a celiac plexus block produces deafferentation of the abdominal viscera, and theoretically, such a patient would not be aware of pain emanating from, for example, gastric ulceration or appendicitis until parietal peritoneum and somatic innervation became involved. This is one of the

theoretic reasons for limiting this useful technique to selected cases involving terminal illness in which benefits clearly outweigh risks.

Central projections of autonomic afferents from the dorsal root ganglia are to the dorsal horn, anterior horn (i.e., skeletal motor cells), and intermediolateral cell column (i.e., sympathetic efferents). These pathways complete reflex arcs, producing muscle spasm and enhancement of sympathetic tone.[6, 7] Table 3–6 provides a list of visceral autonomic innervation, including nociceptive fibers.

The hypothalamus coordinates autonomic nervous activity with input from the cortex, limbic system, thalamus, and reticular activating system. The major de-

Table 3–6 Autonomic and Visceral Afferent Innervation*

REGION AND STRUCTURE	SYMPATHETIC NERVE SUPPLY			NOCICEPTIVE PATHWAYS	
	Location of Cell Body in Spinal Cord and Course of Preganglionic Neurons	Site of Synapse of Preganglionic with Postganglionic Neurons	Course of Postganglionic Axons	Location of Primary Afferent Pathway	Entrance into Central Nervous System
Head and Neck					
Meninges and arteries of brain	T-1,2 (3)† To and through cervical sympathetic chain	All cervical sympathetic ganglia	Plexuses around internal carotid and vertebral arteries	CN V, IX, X C-1 to C-3	Trigeminal subnucleus caudalis C-1 to C-3 spinal segments
Eye	T-1 to T-3 (4) To and through cervical sympathetic chain	Superior cervical ganglion and ganglia in internal carotid plexus	Internal carotid and cavernosus plexuses → ciliary ganglion or nasociliary nerve → ciliary nerves or along ophthalmic artery	Ophthalmic branch of CN V	Trigeminal subnucleus caudalis
Lacrimal gland‡	T-1,2 To and through cervical sympathetic ganglia	Superior cervical sympathetic ganglion	Internal carotid plexus → vidian nerve → sphenopalatine ganglion → maxillary nerve → zygomatic and lacrimal nerves	Lacrimal nerve → ophthalmic branch of CN V	As above
Parotid gland‡	As above	All cervical sympathetic ganglia	External carotid plexus → internal maxillary and middle meningeal plexus → auriculotemporal nerve and plexus and the parotid arterial plexuses	Parotid nerve → auriculotemporal nerve of mandibular division of CN V	As above
Submandibular and sublingual glands‡	As above	As above	External carotid plexus → facial plexus → submandibular ganglion → direct glandular filaments or via lingual nerves or directly to glands along vessels	Submandibular branch of lingual nerve → mandibular division of CN V	As above
Thyroid gland	As above	Middle and inferior cervical sympathetic ganglia	Perivascular sympathetic plexuses accompanying superior and inferior thyroid arteries	Afferents accompanying sympathetic pathways	T-1 and T-2 spinal cord segments
Blood vessels of skin and somatic structures (e.g., sweat glands, hair follicles)	T-1 to T-4 To and through cervical sympathetic chain	All cervical sympathetic ganglia	In perivascular plexuses accompanying various branches of external and internal carotid arteries	Afferents accompanying sympathetic nerves CN V, IX, X; C-2 to C-4	T-1 to T-4 spinal cord Subnucleus caudalis C-2 to C-4 spinal cord segments

Table continued on opposite page

Table 3–6 Autonomic and Visceral Afferent Innervation* *Continued*

	SYMPATHETIC NERVE SUPPLY			NOCICEPTIVE PATHWAYS	
REGION AND STRUCTURE	**Location of Cell Body in Spinal Cord and Course of Preganglionic Neurons**	**Site of Synapse of Preganglionic with Postganglionic Neurons**	**Course of Postganglionic Axons**	**Location of Primary Afferent Pathway**	**Entrance into Central Nervous System**
Thoracic Viscera					
Heart	T-1 to T-4 (5) To upper thoracic and cervical sympathetic chain	All cervical and upper four (five) thoracic ganglia	Superior, middle, and inferior cervical cardiac nerves and the four (five) thoracic cardiac nerves → cardiac plexuses	Afferents in middle and inferior cervical cardiac and thoracic cardiac nerves	T-1 to T-4 (5)
Larynx	T-1,2 To and through cervical sympathetic chain	Superior cervical ganglion	Laryngeal branch of superior cervical ganglion → superior laryngeal nerve	Superior laryngeal nerve	Trigeminal subnucleus caudalis
Trachea, bronchi, and lungs	T-2 to T-6 (7) To upper thoracic sympathetic chain	T-2 to T-6 (7) Sympathetic ganglia	Pulmonary branches from sympathetic trunk → pulmonary plexuses	Afferents with sympathetics Afferents with vagus	T-2 to T-6 (7) N. tractus solitarius (medulla)
Esophagus					
Cervical	T-2 to T-4 To and through upper thoracic sympathetic chain	All cervical sympathetic ganglia and pharyngeal plexus	From cervical ganglia to recurrent laryngeal nerve	Afferents in vagus Afferents with sympathetics	N. tractus solitarius T-2 to T-4 (?)
Thoracic	T-3 to T-6 To and through upper thoracic sympathetic chain	Stellate and upper thoracic ganglia	Direct esophageal branches and through cardiac sympathetic nerves	Afferents with vagus Afferents with sympathetics	N. tractus solitarius T-3 to T-6 (?)
Abdominal	T-5 to T-8 To thoracic sympathetic chain → superior thoracic splanchnic nerve	Celiac ganglia	Via plexuses around left gastric and inferior phrenic arteries	Afferents with sympathetics Afferents with vagus	T-5 to T-8 N. tractus solitarius
Thoracic aorta	T-1 to T-5 (6) To thoracic sympathetic chain	Synapse upper 5 (6) thoracic sympathetic ganglia	Branches from cardiac sympathetic nerves and direct fibers from thoracic sympathetic chain	Afferents with sympathetic pathways	T-1 to T-5 (6)
Abdominal Viscera					
Abdominal aorta	T-5 to L-2 Some through splanchnic nerves and direct branches	Celiac ganglia and paravertebral sympathetic chain	Fibers that contribute to the aortic plexus	Afferents associated with sympathetics	T-5 to L-2
Stomach and duodenum	T-(5) 6 to T-9 (10) (11) Superior (greater) and middle (lesser) thoracic splanchnic nerves and celiac plexus	Celiac ganglia	Right and left gastric and gastroepiploic plexuses	Afferents with sympathetics	T-(5) 6 to T-9 (10) (11)
Gallblader and bile ducts	T-(5) 6 to T-9 (10) Superior thoracic (greater) splanchnic nerves and celiac plexus	Celiac ganglia	Hepatic and gastroduodenal plexuses	Afferents associated with sympathetics	T-(5) 6 to T-9 (10)
Liver	T-(5) 6 to T-9 (10) Superior thoracic (greater) splanchnic nerves and celiac plexus	Celiac ganglia	Hepatic plexus	Afferents associated with sympathetics	T-(5) 6 to T-9 (10)
Pancreas	T-(5) 6 to T-10 (11) Superior thoracic (greater) splanchnic nerves and celiac plexus	Celiac ganglia	Direct branches from celiac plexus and offshoots from splenic, gastroduodenal, and pancreaticoduodenal plexuses	Afferents associated with sympathetics	T-5 to T-10 (11)
Small intestines	T-8 to T-12 right T-8 to T-11 left To superior (greater) and middle (lesser) thoracic splanchnic nerves to celiac plexus	Celiac and superior mesenteric ganglia	Superior mesenteric plexus → nerves alongside jejunal and ileal arteries	Follow sympathetic pathways through celiac and inferior mesenteric plexuses	T-(8) 9, 10 T-10,11
Cecum and appendix‡	T-10 to T-12 Superior (greater) and middle (lesser) thoracic splanchnic nerves → celiac and superior mesenteric plexuses	Celiac and superior mesenteric ganglia	Nerves alongside ileocolic artery	Accompanying sympathetic pathways	T-10 to T-12

Table continued on following page

Table 3–6 Autonomic and Visceral Afferent Innervation* *Continued*

REGION AND STRUCTURE	SYMPATHETIC NERVE SUPPLY			NOCICEPTIVE PATHWAYS	
	Location of Cell Body in Spinal Cord and Course of Preganglionic Neurons	Site of Synapse of Preganglionic with Postganglionic Neurons	Course of Postganglionic Axons	Location of Primary Afferent Pathway	Entrance into Central Nervous System
Abdominal Viscera Continued					
Colon to splenic flexure‡	T-10 to L-1 Middle (lesser) and inferior (least) thoracic and first lumbar splanchnic nerves	Superior and inferior mesenteric ganglia	Mesenteric plexus → nerves alongside right, middle, and superior left colic arteries	Associated with sympathetic, pass through superior and inferior mesenteric plexuses and splanchnic nerves and to spinal cord	T-10 to L-1
Splenic flexure to rectum‡	L-1,2 (left side) S-2 to S-4 Lumbar and sacral splanchnic nerves → inferior mesenteric and inferior hypogastric pelvic plexuses	Inferior mesenteric ganglion and ganglia in superior and inferior hypogastric plexuses	Nerves alongside inferior left colic and rectal arteries	Afferents with parasympathetic nerves and pudendal nerves	S-2,3,5
Suprarenal (adrenal) glands‡	T-(7) 8 to L-1 (2) Superior (greater), middle (lesser), and inferior (least) thoracic splanchnic nerves and first (2nd) lumbar splanchnic nerves	Chromaffin cells of adrenal medulla	Within the gland	Afferents with sympathetics	L-1,2 (left)
Kidneys‡	T-10 to T-12, L-1 (2) Middle (lesser) and inferior (least) thoracic splanchnic nerves and first (2nd) lumbar splanchnic nerves → celiac and renal plexuses	Celiac and aorticorenal ganglia	Along renal plexus	Accompanies sympathetic pathways	T-10 to T-12 (L-1,2)
Ureters‡					
Upper two thirds	T-(10) 11 to L-2 Middle and inferior thoracic splanchnic and upper two lumbar splanchnic nerves	Celiac and aorticorenal ganglia	Superior mesenteric and renal plexuses → superior and middle ureteric nerves	Associated with sympathetics	T-10 to T-12 (L-2)
Lower one third	T-11 to L-1, S-2 to S-4	Aorticorenal ganglion and sacral sympathetic ganglia	Aortic, superior hypogastric, and inferior hypogastric (pelvic) plexuses and sacral splanchnic nerves	Accompany sympathetic and parasympathetic nerves	T-10 to T-12
Pelvic Viscera					
Bladder	T-(11) 12 to L-2 Middle and inferior thoracic splanchnic nerves	Inferior mesenteric ganglion and sacral paravertebral ganglia	Superior and inferior hypogastric plexuses and sacral splanchnic nerves to vesical plexus	Predominantly afferents of parasympathetic nerves; also some sympathetic afferents	S-2 to S-4
Uterus	T-(6-9) 10 to L-1 (2) Splanchnic nerves to aortic and ovarian plexuses and superior and inferior hypogastric plexuses	Celiac ganglion and various paravertebral ganglia	Lumbar and sacral splanchnic nerves, superior, middle, and inferior hypogastric plexuses → uterine plexus	Accompanying sympathetic pathways	T-11 to L-2
Testes, ductus deferens, epididymis, seminal vesicles, prostate	T-10 to L-1 inclusive Splanchnic nerves → aortic and superior hypogastric plexus	Paravertebral ganglia and inferior mesenteric ganglion	Follow various vascular plexuses in sacral splanchnic nerves	Testes (ovaries); prostate; parasympathetic afferents	T-10 S-2 to S-4
Trunks and Limbs (vessels, sweat glands, and hair follicles)					
Trunk	T-1 to T-12	T-1 to T-12 paravertebral sympathetic ganglia	Gray rami communicantes → thoracic spinal nerves	Primary afferents in spinal nerves	T-2 to L-1

Table continued on opposite page

Table 3–6 Autonomic and Visceral Afferent Innervation* *Continued*

REGION AND STRUCTURE	SYMPATHETIC NERVE SUPPLY			NOCICEPTIVE PATHWAYS	
	Location of Cell Body in Spinal Cord and Course of Preganglionic Neurons	Site of Synapse of Preganglionic with Postganglionic Neurons	Course of Postganglionic Axons	Location of Primary Afferent Pathway	Entrance into Central Nervous System
Trunks and Limbs Continued					
Upper extremities	T-2 to T-8 (9) To and through upper thoracic and lower cervical sympathetic chain	Middle and stellate ganglia; T-2 and T-3 ganglia	Gray rami communicantes to roots of brachial plexus → brachial plexus and its major nerves; some directly to plexuses around subclavian, axillary, and upper brachial arteries	Brachial plexus and its branches	C-5 to T-1
Lower extremities	T-10 to L-2 To and through lumbar and upper sacral sympathetic chain	L-1 to S-3 paravertebral ganglia	Gray rami communicantes → lumbosacral plexus and its major nerves; direct branches to perivascular plexuses as far as upper femoral artery	Lumbosacral plexus	L-1 to S-3

*Because referred pain is most likely the result of visceral-somatic convergence, one way to diagnose visceral injury is to correlate dermatomal pain patterns with visceral innervation. Dermatomal hypersensitivity and sensations of cutaneous pain can be caused by nociceptive processes involving viscera or deep somatic structures.

†Segments in parentheses are inconstant.

‡Unilateral innervation.

CN, cranial nerve; N., nerve.

Modified from Bonica JJ: The Management of Pain, 2nd ed, vol I, pp 154–156. Philadelphia, Lea & Febiger, 1990.

scending control pathway is the dorsal longitudinal fasciculus, which supplies cranial nuclei, intermediolateral cell columns (i.e., parasympathetic and sympathetic), and reticular formation.[64]

References

1. Snell R: Clinical Neuroanatomy for Medical Students, 3rd ed, pp 91–121. Boston, Little, Brown, 1992.
2. Barr ML, Kiernan JA: The Human Nervous System: An Anatomical Viewpoint, 6th ed, pp 67–85. Philadelphia, JB Lippincott, 1993.
3. Bonica JJ: The Management of Pain, 2nd ed, vol I, p 28. Philadelphia, Lea & Febiger, 1990.
4. Snell R: Clinical Neuroanatomy for Medical Students, 3rd ed, pp 485–518. Boston, Little, Brown, 1992.
5. Barr ML, Kiernan JA: The Human Nervous System: An Anatomical Viewpoint, 6th ed, pp 364–376. Philadelphia, JB Lippincott, 1993.
6. Gilman S, Newman SW: Manter and Gatz's Essentials of Clinical Neuroanatomy and Neurophysiology, 7th ed, pp 38–47. Philadelphia, FA Davis, 1987.
7. Snell R: Clinical Neuroanatomy for Medical Students, 3rd ed, pp 363–380. Boston, Little, Brown, 1992.
8. Barr ML, Kiernan JA: The Human Nervous System: An Anatomical Viewpoint, 6th ed, pp 293–312. Philadelphia, JB Lippincott, 1993.
9. Fitzgerald M: The course and termination of primary afferent fibers. In Wall PD, Melzack R (eds): Textbook of Pain, pp 34–48. Edinburgh, Churchill Livingstone, 1984.
10. Hursh JB: Conduction velocity and diameter of nerve fibers. Am J Physiol 1939; 127: 131–139.
11. LaMotte RH, Campbell JN: Comparison of responses of warm and nociceptive C-fiber afferents in monkey with human judgments of thermal pain. J Neurophysiol 1978; 41: 509–528.
12. Dubner R, Price DD, Beitel RE, et al: Peripheral neural correlates of behavior in monkey and human related to sensory-discriminative aspects of pain. In Anderson DJ, Matthews B (eds): Pain in the Trigeminal Region, pp 57–66. Amsterdam, Elsevier/North-Holland, 1977.
13. Burgess PR, Perl ER: Cutaneous mechanoreceptors and nociceptors. In Iggo A (ed): Handbook of Sensory Physiology, vol 2: Somatosensory System, pp 29–78. Berlin, Springer-Verlag, 1973.
14. White JC: Sensory innervation of the viscera: studies on visceral afferent neurones in man based on neurosurgical procedures for relief of intractable pain. Res Nerv Ment Dis 1942; 23: 373–390.
15. Lynn B: The detection of injury and tissue damage. In Wall PD, Melzack R (eds): Textbook of Pain, pp 19–33. Edinburgh, Churchill Livingstone, 1984.
16. Paintal AS: Functional analysis of group III afferent fibres of mammalian muscles. J Physiol (Lond) 1960; 152: 250–270.
17. Mense S: Nervous outflow from skeletal muscle following chemical noxious stimulation. J Physiol (Lond) 1977; 267: 75–88.
18. Mense S, Stahnke M: Responses in muscle afferent fibres of slow conduction velocity to contractions and ischaemia in the cat. J Physiol (Lond) 1983; 342: 383–397.
19. Mense S: Sensitization of group IV muscle receptors to bradykinin by 5-hydroxytryptamine and prostaglandin E2. Brain Res 1981; 225: 95–105.
20. Kniffki KD, Mense S, Schmidt RF: Responses of group IV afferent units from skeletal muscle to stretch, contraction and chemical stimulation. Exp Brain Res 1978; 31: 511–522.
21. Schaible HG, Schmidt RF: Activation of groups III and IV sensory units in medial articular nerve by local mechanical stimulation of knee joint. J Neurophysiol 1983; 49: 35–44.
22. Coggeshall RE, Hong KA, Langford LA, et al: Discharge characteristics of fine medial articular afferents at rest and during passive movements of inflamed knee joints. Brain Res 1983; 272: 185–188.
23. Hurrell DJ: The nerve supply of bone. J Anat 1937; 72: 54–61.
24. Sindou M, Quoex C, Baleydier C: Fiber organization at the posterior spinal cord-rootlet junction in man. J Comp Neurol 1974; 153: 15–26.
25. Ransom SW: An experimental study of Lissauer's tract and the dorsal roots. J Comp Neurol 1914; 24: 531–545.
26. Frykholm R, Hyde J, Norlén G, et al: On pain sensations pro-

duced by stimulation of ventral roots in man. Acta Physiol Scand Suppl 1953; 106: 455–469.

27. Rexed B: A cytoarchitectonic atlas of the spinal cord in the cat. J Comp Neurol 1954; 100: 297–379.

28. Wall PD: The dorsal horn. In Wall PD, Melzack R (eds): Textbook of Pain, pp 80–87. Edinburgh, Churchill Livingstone, 1984.

29. Dubner R, Bennett GJ: Spinal and trigeminal mechanisms of nociception. Annu Rev Neurosci 1983; 6: 381–418.

30. Gobel S: Golgi studies of the neurons in layer I of the dorsal horn of the medulla (trigeminal nucleus caudalis). J Comp Neurol 1978; 180: 375–393.

31. Adriaensen H, Gybels J, Handwerker HO, et al: Response properties of thin myelinated (A-delta) fibers in human skin nerves. J Neurophysiol 1983; 49: 111–122.

32. Pomeranz B, Wall PD, Weber WV: Cord cells responding to fine myelinated afferents from viscera, muscle and skin. J Physiol (Lond) 1968; 199: 511–532.

33. Basbaum AI: Anatomical substrates of pain and pain modulation and their relationship to analgesic drug action. In Kuhar MJ, Pasternak GW (eds): Analgesics: Neurochemical, Behavioral, and Clinical Perspectives, pp 97–123. New York, Raven Press, 1984.

34. Zimmerman M: Peripheral and central nervous mechanisms of nociception, pain, and pain therapy: facts and hypotheses. Adv Pain Res Ther 1979; 3: 3–32.

35. Melzack R, Wall PD, Ty TC: Acute pain in an emergency clinic: latency of onset and descriptor patterns related to different injuries. Pain 1982; 14: 33–43.

36. Kehlet H: Influence of epidural analgesia on the endocrine-metabolic response to surgery. Acta Anaesthesiol Scand Suppl 1978; 70: 39–42.

37. Kehlet H: Pain relief and modification of the stress response. In Cousins MJ, Phillips GD (eds): Acute Pain Management, pp 49–75. New York, Churchill Livingstone, 1986.

38. Kehlet H, Dahl JB: Preemptive analgesia. In Stanley TH, Ashburn MA (eds): Anesthesiology and Pain Management, pp 189–195. Dordrecht, The Netherlands, Kluwer Academic Publishers, 1994.

39. Dennis SG, Melzack R: Pain-signalling systems in the dorsal and ventral spinal cord. Pain 1977; 4: 97–132.

40. Willis WD: The origin and destination of pathways involved in pain transmission. In Wall PD, Melzack R (eds): Textbook of Pain, pp 88–99. Edinburgh, Churchill Livingstone, 1984.

41. Kerr FWL, Lippman HH: The primate spinothalamic tract as demonstrated by anterolateral cordotomy and commissural myelotomy. Adv Neurol 1974; 4: 147–156.

42. Willis WD, Kenshalo DR Jr, Leonard RB: The cells of origin of the primate spinothalamic tract. J Comp Neurol 1979; 188: 543–573.

43. Ralston HJ III: Synaptic organization of the spinothalamic tract projections to the thalamus, with special reference to pain. Adv Pain Res Ther 1984; 6: 183–195.

44. Kerr FW: The ventral spinothalamic tract and other ascending systems of the ventral funiculus of the spinal cord. J Comp Neurol 1975; 159: 335–356.

45. Mehler WR: The anatomy of the so-called "pain tract" in man: an analysis of the course and distribution of the ascending fibers of the fasciculus anterolateralis. In French JD, Porter RW (eds): Basic Research in Paraplegia, pp 26–55. Springfield, IL, Charles C Thomas, 1962.

46. Giesler GJ Jr, Yezierski RP, Gerhart KD, et al: Spinothalamic tract neurons that project to medial and/or lateral thalamic nuclei: evidence for a physiologically novel population of spinal cord neurons. J Neurophysiol 1981; 46: 1285–1308.

47. Bowsher D: Role of the reticular formation in responses to noxious stimulation. Pain 1976; 2: 361–378.

48. Casey KL: Supraspinal mechanisms in pain: the reticular formation. In Kosterlitz HW, Terenius LY (eds): Pain and Society, pp 183–200. Weinheim, Chemie, 1980.

49. Mehler WR: Some observations on secondary ascending afferent systems in the central nervous system. In Knighton RS, Dumke PR (eds): Pain, pp 11–32. Boston, Little, Brown, 1966.

50. Mehler WR: Some neurological species differences—a posteriori. Ann N Y Acad Sci 1969; 167: 424–468.

51. Melzack R, Casey KL: Sensory, motivational and central control determinants of pain: a new conceptual model. In Kenshalo DR Jr (ed): The Skin Senses, pp 423–443. Springfield, IL, Charles C Thomas, 1968.

52. Basbaum AI: Conduction of the effects of noxious stimulation by short-fiber multisynaptic systems of the spinal cord in the rat. Exp Neurol 1973; 40: 699–716.

53. Rustioni A, Hayes NL, O'Neill S: Dorsal column nuclei and ascending spinal afferents in macaques. Brain 1979; 102: 95–125.

54. Melzack R, Wall PD: Pain mechanisms: a new theory. Science 1965; 150: 971–979.

55. Foreman RD, Beall JE, Coulter JD, et al: Effects of dorsal column stimulation on primate spinothalamic tract neurons. J Neurophysiol 1976; 39: 534–546.

56. Richardson DE, Dempsey CW: Monoamine turnover in CSF of patients during dorsal column stimulation for pain control. (Abstract) Pain Suppl 1984; 2: S224.

57. Meyerson BA: Electrostimulation procedures: effects, presumed rationale, and possible mechanisms. Adv Pain Res Ther 1983; 5: 495–534.

58. Darian-Smith I: The trigeminal system. In Iggo A (ed): Handbook of Sensory Physiology, vol 2: Somatosensory System, pp 271–314. Berlin, Springer-Verlag, 1973.

59. Olszewski J: On the anatomical and functional organization of the trigeminal nucleus. J Comp Neurol 1950; 92: 401–409.

60. Price DD, Dubner R, Hu JW: Trigeminothalamic neurons in nucleus caudalis responsive to tactile, thermal, and nociceptive stimulation of monkey's face. J Neurophysiol 1976; 39: 936–953.

61. Smith RL: Axonal projections and connections of the principal sensory trigeminal nucleus in the monkey. J Comp Neurol 1975; 163: 347–375.

62. Foltz EL, White LE Jr: Pain "relief" by frontal cingulumotomy. J Neurosurg 1962; 19: 89–100.

63. Melzack R, Stotler WA, Livingston WK: Effects of discrete brainstem lesions in cats on perception of noxious stimulation. J Neurophysiol 1958; 21: 353–367.

64. Snell R: Clinical Neuroanatomy for Medical Students, 3rd ed, pp 471–483. Boston, Little, Brown, 1992.

65. Jänig W: The autonomic nervous system. In Schmidt RF, Thews G (eds): Human Physiology, pp 111–144. New York, Springer-Verlag, 1983.

66. Albe-Fessard D, Berkley KJ, Kruger L, et al: Diencephalic mechanisms of pain sensation. Brain Res 1985; 356: 217–296.

67. Willis WD: Thalamocortical mechanisms of pain. Adv Pain Res Ther 1985; 9: 245–267.

68. Jones EG, Friedman DP: Projection pattern of functional components of thalamic ventrobasal complex on monkey somatosensory cortex. J Neurophysiol 1982; 48: 521–544.

69. Kaas JH, Nelson RJ, Sur M, et al: Multiple representations of the body within the primary somatosensory cortex of primates. Science 1979; 204: 521–523.

70. Tasker RR, Tsuda T, Hawrylyshyn P: Clinical neurophysiological investigation of deafferentation pain. Adv Pain Res Ther 1983; 5: 713–738.

71. Tasker RR: Thalamic procedures. In Schaltenbrand G, Walker AE (eds): Stereotaxy of the Human Brain: Anatomical Physiological and Clinical Applications, pp 484–497. New York, Thieme-Stratton, 1982.

72. Tasker RR: Identification of pain processing systems by electrical stimulation of the brain. Hum Neurobiol 1982; 1: 261–272.

73. Loeser JD, Ward AA Jr, White LE Jr: Chronic deafferentation of human spinal cord neurons. J Neurosurg 1968; 29: 48–50.

74. Basbaum AI: Functional analysis of the cytochemistry of the spinal dorsal horn. Adv Pain Res Ther 1985; 9: 149–175.

75. Basbaum AI, Fields HL: Endogenous pain control systems: brainstem spinal pathways and endorphin circuitry. Annu Rev Neurosci 1984; 7: 309–338.

76. Basbaum AI, Fields HL: Endogenous pain control mechanisms: review and hypothesis. Ann Neurol 1978; 4: 451–462.

77. Sherrington CS: The Integrative Action of the Nervous System. New York, Charles Scribner, 1906.

78. Mayer DJ, Wolfle TL, Akil H, et al: Analgesia from electrical stimulation in the brainstem of the rat. Science 1971; 174: 1351–1354.

79. Hughes J, Smith TW, Kosterlitz HW, et al: Identification of two related pentapeptides from the brain with potent opiate agonist activity. Nature 1975; 258: 577–580.

80. Fields HL, Bry J, Hentall I, et al: The activity of neurons in the rostral medulla of the rat during withdrawal from noxious heat. J Neurosci 1983; 3: 2545–2552.

81. Ruda MA, Bennett GJ, Dubner R: Neurochemistry and neural circuitry in the dorsal horn. Prog Brain Res 1986; 66: 219–268.

82. Hammond DL: Control systems for nociceptive afferent processing: the descending inhibitory pathways. In Yaksh TL (ed): Spinal Afferent Processing, pp 363–390. New York, Plenum Press, 1986.

83. Cervero F: Persistent Pain: Modern Methods of Treatment, vol IV, pp 1–20. New York, Grune & Stratton, 1983.

84. Hertz AF: The Goulstonian lectures on the sensibility of the alimentary canal in health and disease. Lancet 1911; 1: 1051, 1118, 1187.

85. Cervero F: Deep and visceral pain. In Kosterlitz HW, Terenius LY (eds): Pain and Society, pp 263–282. Weinheim, Chemie, 1980.

86. Jänig W, Morrison JFB: Functional properties of spinal visceral afferents supplying abdominal and pelvic organs, with special emphasis on visceral nociception. Prog Brain Res 1986; 67: 87–114.

87. Kellgren JH: On the distribution of pain arising from deep somatic structures with charts of segmental pain areas. Clin Sci 1939; 4: 35–46.

88. Lewis T, Kellgren JH: Observations relating to referred pain, viscero-motor reflexes and other associated phenomena. Clin Sci 1939; 4: 47–71.

89. Cook AJ, Woolf CJ, Wall PD, et al: Dynamic receptive field plasticity in rat spinal cord dorsal horn following C-primary afferent input. Nature 1987; 325: 151–153.

90. Woolf CJ, Wall PD: Relative effectiveness of C primary afferent fibers of different origins in evoking a prolonged facilitation of the flexor reflex in the rat. J Neurosci 1986; 6: 1433–1442.

91. Wilmore DW, Long JM, Mason AD, et al: Stress in surgical patients as a neurophysiologic reflex response. Surg Gynecol Obstet 1976; 142: 257–269.

92. Cervero F: Somatic and visceral inputs to the thoracic spinal cord of the cat: effects of noxious stimulation of the biliary system. J Physiol (Lond) 1983; 337: 51–67.

93. Bahr R, Blumberg H, Jänig W: Do dichotomizing afferent fibers exist which supply visceral organs as well as somatic structures? A contribution to the problem of referred pain. Neurosci Lett 1981; 24: 25–28.

94. Pierau FK, Taylor DC, Abel W, et al: Dichotomizing peripheral fibres revealed by intracellular recording from rat sensory neurones. Neurosci Lett 1982; 31: 123–128.

95. Kruger L, Mantyh PW: Changing concepts in the anatomy of pain. Semin Anesth 1985; 4: 209–217.

96. Bonica JJ: Autonomic innervation of the viscera in relation to nerve block. Anesthesiology 1968; 29: 793–813.

97. Gilman S, Newman SW: Manter and Gatz's Essentials of Clinical Neuroanatomy and Neurophysiology, 7th ed, pp 182–190. Philadelphia, FA Davis, 1987.

98. Gilman S, Newman SW: Manter and Gatz's Essentials of Clinical Neuroanatomy and Neurophysiology, 7th ed, pp 87–95. Philadelphia, FA Davis, 1987.

99. Bonica JJ: The Management of Pain, 2nd ed, vol I, p 147. Philadelphia, Lea & Febiger, 1990.

100. Bonica JJ, Buckley FP: Regional analgesia with local anesthetics. In Bonica JJ (ed): The Management of Pain, 2nd ed, vol II, pp 1883–1966. Philadelphia, Lea & Febiger, 1990.

CHAPTER 4

Reexamination of Anatomy in Regional Anesthesia

Quinn Hogan, M.D.

Anatomy is to physiology as geography is to history—it describes the theater of events.

Jean Frennel (1497–1558)

Introduction

Successful management of regional anesthesia requires attention to physiology and principles of safe medical practice, but at its core it is an exercise in applied anatomy. Analgesia occurs only if the anesthetic solution is delivered in suitable proximity to the desired neural structures, and complications follow passage of solution into unintended zones. Ability to visualize internal anatomy characterizes anesthesiologists who are skillful at regional anesthesia.

How Anatomic Data Are Acquired

The most obvious method of anatomic investigation is dissection, but this has problems. Preservation of specimens produces artifactual changes in delicate tissues such as nerves and their adjacent soft tissues. Some misleading concepts of connective tissue anatomy are perpetuated in current texts from original work in the 19th century on desiccated cadavers, which produced illusory fibrous barriers from condensed fat, such as in the intervertebral foramen. Dissection of fresh or even living material, as during operation, is also not an ideal source of anatomic information. In order to observe the structures of interest, dissection must destroy neighboring layers, which produces distorted relationships. This is especially so in the spinal canal where insubstantial and semifluid structures are surrounded by a massive wall or in regions where subatmospheric pressures act on soft tissues, as

in the chest and the spinal canal. The limited resolution of dissection is a further problem and is particularly apparent in the examination of nerves. Modern techniques of retrograde labeling of neurons and histochemical staining of whole-mount specimens[1] have exposed a rich complexity of small fibers and alternative axonal pathways unsuspected by earlier authorities. (Although dissection has probably been exhausted as a research tool, time spent in the autopsy or cadaver laboratory rewards clinicians seeking to improve their regional anesthesia skills with an improved appreciation of internal three-dimensional relationships.)

Anatomy revealed through the injection of solutions should likewise be interpreted cautiously. Endoscopy[2, 3] requires the creation of an air- or fluid-filled cavity where one may not naturally exist, such as in the epidural space. Injecting contrast material for radiographic imaging[4–7] or a substance that solidifies to make a cast[8, 9] also distorts the native anatomy. Cryomicrotome sectioning[10] of cadavers frozen in toto avoids distortion artifacts, but changes may occur with death. Magnetic resonance imaging and computed tomography lack comparable detail, but they approach the ideal of an artifact-free depiction of actual anatomy.

Importance of Imaging

When regional anesthesia is used for surgical and obstetric analgesia, accurate needle placement is readily evident by the successful production of a block. Injection for the diagnosis and treatment of pain is more problematic, because smaller doses of solution are used and documentation of successful injection is less clear. Studies consistently demonstrate that erroneous needle placement is a common feature of lumbar sympathetic blocks,[11, 12] paravertebral nerve blocks,[11, 12] and caudal canal injections.[13, 14] Even if the needle tip or catheter arrives at the desired location, the passage of solution through the body is controlled by subtle and unpredictable pressures and connections between tissues. Imaging reveals an unexpected variety of pathways by which solution may travel within the body (Fig. 4–1; see Color Plate 1), even after injections with concrete end points that are usually performed without imaging, such as subarachnoid and stellate ganglion blocks.[15, 16]

In addition to the uncertainty of using surface observation or palpation of structures with the needle tip to direct needle placement, further uncertainty arises from the natural variability of anatomy.[17, 18] Like any biologic variable, the location, size, shape, and even number of anatomic structures are predictable only within a certain range. Although certain features may vary by sex or race,[19, 20] most of the variability cannot be anticipated, and anatomic patterns (e.g., location of vessels, neural routes, and connections) commonly differ on opposite sides of an individual. For these reasons, the author believes radiologic imaging is imperative when the accuracy of a block must be ensured.

Those who have dissected or inspected much have at least learn'd to doubt when others, who are ignorant of anatomy, and do not take the trouble to attend it, are in no doubt at all.
Giovanni Battista Morgagni (1682–1771)

Future Developments in Anatomy

One could expect that most anatomic details have been elucidated. Anatomy is the oldest of medical sciences, and departments at medical schools are rapidly turning from anatomy per se toward cell biology. However, clinical issues pose new anatomic questions. An example is the development of cauda equina syndrome after spinal anesthesia. Maldistribution of anesthetic is proposed as the basis for this neuropathic injury, but the shape of the spine, the volume of cerebrospinal fluid (CSF) and its longitudinal distribution, and the degree of interindividual variability of these measures are not adequately known. Clinical investigators should take the lead in this type of anatomic study.

Meanwhile, new methods of anatomic research are revealing unanticipated complexity in structural organization. Histochemical and immunologic labeling techniques improve anatomic resolution to the extent that connections of individual neurons can be followed and their chemical fingerprints recognized. With the incorporation of dynamic considerations into anatomy, such as the direction of flow in segments of the anterior spinal artery or the stimuli necessary to activate cells in various parts of the spinal dorsal horn, anatomy has begun to merge with other basic sciences in explaining biologic function.

Structural details of anatomy germane to particular blocks are covered in the relevant chapters. This chapter focuses on organizational anatomic concepts, neglected but important details, and new or changing ideas.

Vertebral Column

Vertebral Bones

The vertebral column is the bony reference for various blocks used in surgery, obstetrics, and pain management, including spinal and epidural anesthetics, blocks of paravertebral and prevertebral sympathetic structures, blocks of segmental nerves emerging from the vertebral column, and injections into the joints of the vertebral column. It is the most clearly metameric portion of human anatomy, with 7 cervical vertebrae, 12 thoracic, 5 lumbar, 5 sacral, and 4 coccygeal. Clinical ability to estimate segmental level from palpable landmarks is often overestimated. The most prominent spinous process is usually the 7th cervical; the 7th thoracic spine is usually opposite the inferior angle of the scapula; and the line connecting the iliac crests (Tuffier's line) crosses the vertebral column most often at the L4-5 disk, but these indices are not reliable owing to natural variability in anatomic parameters (Fig. 4–2).[17] For instance, the first thoracic vertebral spine may be more prominent than the 7th cervical, and Tuffier's line may cross the vertebral column as high as the L3-4 disk or as low as the L5-S1 disk.[21 – 23] For this reason, the accuracy of predicting the vertebral level of needle insertion is about 50% at best when unaided by radiologic imaging.[24 – 26]

An archetypal vertebral bone consists of posterior elements forming a vertebral arch and the body anteriorly (Fig. 4–3). The lumbar vertebral bodies are hourglass shaped with a diameter 15% less at the middle than at the end plates.[27] Stout pedicles arise on the posterolateral aspects of the body and fuse with the plate-like laminae to enclose the vertebral foramen, and in sequence they form the vertebral canal. In the cervical and lumbar regions, the canal approaches a triangular shape; in the thoracic vertebrae, it is circular

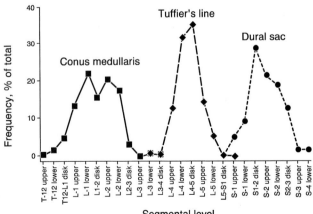

Figure 4–2 The expected values for anatomic parameters, such as the termination of the spinal cord and dural sac and the location of Tuffier's line, are approximately normally distributed, demonstrating the variability of anatomic parameters. (Modified from Hogan QH: Tuffier's line: the normal distribution of anatomic parameters. [Letter to the editor.] Anesth Analg 1993; 78: 194–195.)

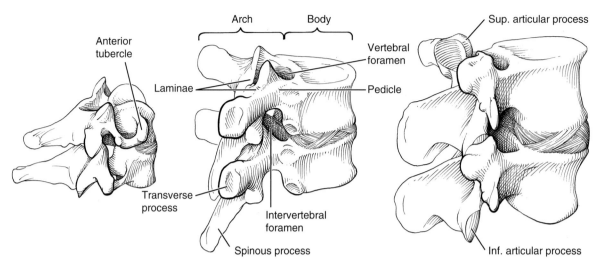

Figure 4–3 Principal elements of the vertebral bones, comparing cervical (left), thoracic (middle), and lumbar (right) types. The cervical vertebrae show C-6 with an anterior tubercle and C-7 without an anterior tubercle. Inf., inferior; Sup., superior.

and smaller. Canal width between the pedicles is about 22 mm at L-1 and enlarges progressively to about 27 mm at L-5. It is fairly constant at about 17 mm in the thoracic region and expands to 25 mm throughout the cervical canal.[20, 28–32] Anteroposterior diameters of the vertebral foramina are uniform at 15 to 16 mm throughout the vertebral column.[33] The pedicles form the lateral wall of the vertebral canal but leave a gap called the intervertebral foramen or, more suitably, the nerve root canal because it contains the segmental nerves as well as other neural and vascular structures. The transverse process is based at the junction of the pedicle and lamina and passes laterally. The spinous process projects posteriorly from the midline junction of the laminae, is often bifid in the cervical column, and may not be in the midline at other levels.

Childhood sacral vertebrae are connected by cartilage but progress to bony fusion after puberty. In the adult, only a narrow residue of the sacral disks persists. An abrupt increase in the lumbar lordotic curve occurs at the L-5 to S-1 junction, accentuating the prominence of the anterior S-1 vertebral body. Anomalous patterns of vertebral segmentation are restricted to the lumbosacral spine.[34] This parallels the interspecies stability of mammalian cervical and thoracic segmentation and the marked variability in the number of lumbar vertebrae, even among primates.[35] The last lumbar or first sacral vertebra is often indeterminate in configuration, with fusion of L-5 to S-1 in 6.2% of subjects (sacralization of L-5, bilateral in 1.5%) or incomplete fusion of S-1 to S-2 in 5.3% (lumbarization of S-1, bilateral in 4.1%).[34] Developmental defects in a lumbar vertebral arch occur in 3.9% of subjects.

The sacrum is the least predictable portion of vertebral anatomy (Fig. 4–4). Adult sacral canal volume may vary from 12 to 65 mL.[36] Fusion of the posterior roof of the sacral vertebral canal is typically complete down to the S-5 level, where the sacral hiatus remains open. However, no posterior bony roof or virtually complete closure of the sacral vertebral canal is found in about 8% of subjects.[19] In 5% of adult sacral bones,

the anteroposterior diameter of the canal at the hiatus is 2 mm or less.[36] Fortunately, access through the sacral hiatus is consistent in children. The coccyx represents the last four vertebrae joined into a single structure.

Joints and Ligaments

Movement of the vertebral column is made possible by articulations of several types and is constrained by various ligaments (Fig. 4–5). The vertebral bodies are joined at their end plates by fibrocartilaginous disks that have an avascular gelatinous core, the nucleus pulposus, surrounded by collagenous lamellae of the annular ligament. The broad anterior longitudinal ligament reinforces the ventral aspect of the disk and binds the vertebral bodies together. The posterior longitudinal ligament does the same in the vertebral canal posterior to the vertebral bodies, but it is formed into a narrow band, spreading only as it merges with outer layers of the disk. This ligament may ossify and produce spinal stenosis, particularly at cervical and thoracic levels.[37] With aging, the disk loses hydration and resiliency. Because the posterior longitudinal ligament reinforces the midline portion of the disk, rents usually form in the paramedian posterior disk, from which extruded nuclear material may egress to produce compression of the spinal cord or nerves in the vertebral canal. The lateral upper edge of cervical vertebral bodies extends as the uncinate process to articulate with the body of the next cephalad vertebra at the uncovertebral joint (of Luschka). Arthritic changes of this joint or process may encroach on the cervical nerve root canals.

Adjacent posterior elements articulate by true diarthrodial joints, the zygapophyseal (facet) joints. The inferior articular process projecting caudally overlaps the superior articular process from the next most caudal vertebra. In the cervical and lumbar column, the facet joints are posterior to the transverse processes, whereas the thoracic facets are anterior to the trans-

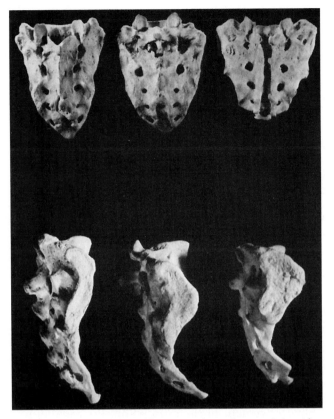

Figure 4–4 The highly variable nature of sacral anatomy is evident in the different degrees of closure of the posterior bony covering of the spinal canal and the sacral cornua as well as different curvatures of the sacral canal. (From Bergman RA, Thompson SA, Afifi AK, et al: Catalogue of Human Anatomic Variation, 2nd ed, p 553. © Williams & Wilkins, Baltimore, 1988.)

anterior portion in an almost coronal plane. The transition from the characteristic thoracic- to lumbar-type articulation is gradual in 54% of subjects with intermediate articular orientation at T11-12.[39] Otherwise, the change is abrupt, with a coronal superior facet and a curved, sagittal inferior facet on a single vertebra at T-12 (29%), T-11 (16%), or L-1 (0.5%) with frequent asymmetry. The thoracolumbar transition is also marked by an amplification in the size of the mammillary process, a bony protuberance extending rostrally and posteriorly from the upper posterior aspect of the superior articular process. By overhanging the facet surface of the superior articular process, the mammillary processes at the thoracolumbar transition encircle the inferior articular processes from the vertebra above, locking it in a mortice-like joint.[40, 41] This probably stiffens the articulation and decreases motion, especially during extension.

The orientation of the facets dictates the movements possible between two vertebrae. Minimal rotation is allowed at lumbar levels because of the sagittally opposing portions. Thoracic facets limit flexion but permit rotation. In the cervical column, movement in all planes is less restricted and includes translation (anteroposterior or sliding) between adjacent vertebrae controlled by the uncinate processes as lateral guide rails.[38] Movement in the sagittal plane (flexion and extension) is maximal in the cervical region and at L5-S1. As well as restricting motion, the facets are weight bearing in the cervical region[42] and lumbosacral joint.[43] Lumbar posterior joints may transmit load, in part, by the tip of the inferior articular process contacting the lamina of the vertebra below.[44]

The capsule of the facets is loose and redundant at the inferior and superior ends of the joint, and injection of the joints is often accompanied by leakage of the solution into the epidural space from medial disruption of the capsule.[45–47] Rudimentary fibroadipose menisci and synovial folds cushion the superior and inferior poles of the lumbar zygapophyseal joints,[48] but with

verse processes. Joint surfaces are midway between axial and coronal planes in the cervical region and much more vertical and almost coronal at thoracic levels.[38] Lumbar facet joints are distinctly curved, the posterior portion parallel to the sagittal plane and the

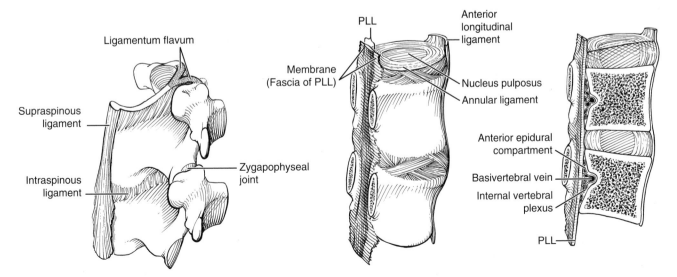

Figure 4–5 Basic fibrous components of the vertebral column. PLL, posterior longitudinal ligament.

age these typically disappear and the cartilage on the joint surfaces thins.[49] Although facet menisci are innervated by small myelinated nerves[50] and an entrapment syndrome has been proposed,[48] there is no clear evidence to implicate them in the production of back pain.

A heavy band, the supraspinous ligament, joins the tips of the spinous processes but thins and vanishes in the lower lumbar region,[51] perhaps to allow greater flexion there. The interspinous ligament is a narrow web between the spinous processes, with fibers running in a posterocranial direction. It may have a slit-like midline cavity filled with fat.[51] Because these two fibrous structures are composed largely of collagen, a needle passing through them generates a characteristic snapping sensation as the fibers are parted. The ligamentum flavum, in contrast, is 80% elastin, and its dense homogeneous texture is readily appreciated as a needle passes through it. Tension in the ligamentum flavum is evident as it retracts to half its length when cut. It spans from the anterior surface of the cephalad lamina of an adjacent pair of vertebrae to the posterior aspect of the lower lamina. The right and left halves meet at an angle of less than 90°, and a gap may be present in the midline.[10] Its lateral edges wrap anteriorly around the medial margin of the facet joints, reinforcing the joint capsule. Bone may grow into the margins of the ligamentum flavum even in young individuals (Fig. 4–6; see Color Plate 2).[37, 52, 53] This is a normal feature at mid and lower thoracic levels and less common in lumbar segments. Because the peak incidence of flaval ossification is at the most inferior thoracic-type (coronally oriented) facet articulation,[40, 54] ossifications probably represent a response to the increased rotatory strains at these levels. Fine bone spurs in the ligamentum flavum may impede the progress of a spinal or epidural needle and may be mistaken for fracture fragments on radiographic images.

Mechanical failure of the intervertebral disk usually precedes facet disease,[55] leading to loss of disk height and pathologically increased overlap of the facets. This decreases the longitudinal dimensions of the intervertebral foramen and foreshortens the ligamentum flavum, causing it to buckle into the foramen, contributing to foraminal narrowing (Fig. 4–7; see Color Plate 2). Facet arthritis with periarticular exostoses is another source of cord and nerve compression,[56] and medial expansion of pathologic facets may interfere with epidural or spinal needle placement as well.

Epidural Space

The epidural space is the area outside the dural sac but inside the vertebral canal. Walls of the vertebral canal are vertebral bodies and disks anteriorly, pedicles laterally, and laminae and ligamenta flava posteriorly. Contents of the epidural space include nerves and vessels, but the majority is fat. Whereas the brain is protected by a rigid case, the spinal cord must exist in the flexible vertebral column. A biomechanical accommodation is provided by a padding of epidural fat that is nearly fluid in texture and has nonadherent surfaces

to permit gliding movement of the neural structures. The distance from the skin to the lumbar epidural space in the midline is on average about 5 cm, but it may be as small as 3 cm and rarely greater than 8 cm. The distance loosely correlates with weight and is somewhat greater at L3-4 than at other lumbar levels.[57–62]

Depictions of epidural anatomy in anesthesia texts typically show a space of uniform width completely encircling the dura. However, in its undisturbed state as revealed by cryomicrotome sections[10] (Figs. 4–8 and 4–9; see Color Plates 3 to 5) and in vivo imaging, the lumbar vertebral canal is filled mostly by the dural sac and the epidural space is empty (a "potential space") in large areas where dura contacts bone and ligament. Epidural contents are contained in a series of metamerically and circumferentially discontinuous compartments separated by zones where the dura contacts the canal wall (Fig. 4–10). Inferior to the L4-5 disk and in the sacral canal, the dural sac tapers to a smaller diameter and does not fill the canal as completely, so there is a proportionate increase in the abundance of epidural fat.

The posterior compartment of the epidural space is filled by a fat pad that is triangular in axial section. It lies between the dura and ligamenta flava, but it extends slightly under the caudalmost portion of the lamina above. It is not adherent to these structures, which allows movement of the dura within the canal during spinal flexion.[63–67] Additionally, catheters or fluid may pass between the surfaces of the fat, canal wall, and dura. The extent of inflammation and fibrosis surrounding a chronic epidural catheter varies according to whether it is adjacent to fat or between dura and canal wall.[68] The fat pad is attached to the posterior midline by a vascular pedicle that enters through the gap between the right and left ligamenta flava (Fig. 4–11; see Color Plate 6). This mesentery-like attachment and the accompanying fat pad may be seen as a midline filling defect in radiologic studies with contrast medium[4, 5, 7] and as an incomplete "membrane" during epiduroscopy.[2, 3] Claims of midline fibrous septa differ from cryomicrotome[10] and histologic[69] examinations that show no fibrous elements in the epidural space. In fact, the epidural fat is unique in the body in having virtually no fibrous content.[70, 71] Asymmetric development of cutaneous anesthesia after epidural local anesthetic injection is often attributed to a hypothetic median septum, but a technical error of needle or catheter insertion is the proper explanation because reinsertion in these cases results in complete block.[72]

Posterior epidural fat may enter the facet joint space through gaps in the ligamentum flavum.[73] Lipomatous expansion of the epidural fat during systemic steroid therapy or endogenous Cushing's syndrome is well recognized (Fig. 4–12; see Color Plate 6) and may produce neurologic compromise.[74, 75] Whether direct application of glucocorticoid to the epidural fat after epidural steroid treatment of radiculopathy produces a similar response has not been examined. Symptomatic epidural lipomatosis may also occur in morbid obesity[76] or in a normal individual.[77] The normal posterior epi-

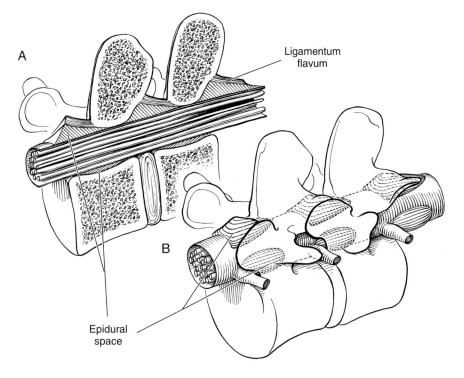

Figure 4–10 Extensive portions of the epidural space are empty. These regions where the dura is in contact with the spinal canal wall separate the epidural contents into discontinuous compartments (crosshatched areas).

Ligamentum flavum

Epidural space

dural fat displaced by facet arthropathy contributes to central vertebral canal stenosis.[78]

Isolation of epidural contents into compartments may have subtle influences on pharmacokinetics of lipid-soluble agents and on tissue mechanics. The epidural space behaves like a Starling resistor,[79] with pressures decreasing to a nonzero plateau after injection,[80] independent of the volume injected.[81] This may be due to the apposition of dura and bone, which injected fluid must pass to escape the posterior epidural space. As in the joint spaces and pleural cavity, the rigid enclosure of the posterior epidural space allows the tissues to generate a subatmospheric tissue fluid pressure,[82] owing to the usual action of lymphatics and the balance of osmotic and hydrostatic forces across the capillary endothelium (Starling forces). Alteration of epidural space during needle insertion may further lower epidural pressure. These actions produce the force that aspirates a hanging drop into the needle hub as the tip enters the compartment.

Segmental nerves, vessels, and fat fill the lateral epidural compartment that forms just medial to each intervertebral foramen. Except in advanced degenerative disease, the intervertebral foramina are widely open and allow the free egress of solution injected within the vertebral canal. Because of the extent to which the lateral epidural wall is incomplete and the lack of a rigid barrier in the intervertebral foramina, the pressure in the epidural space closely reflects abdominal pressure, and increased abdominal pressure, such as during a cough or pregnancy, is readily transmitted to the epidural space.[83] There is no reason to believe that veins passing through the intervertebral foramina in some way play a special role in conducting pressure changes from the abdomen to the vertebral canal.

Stretching laterally from the posterior longitudinal

ligament is a fine membrane that completely separates the anterior epidural compartment from the rest of the vertebral canal (see Fig. 4–5). This anterior space is almost entirely occupied by a nearly confluent internal vertebral plexus, from which the basivertebral vein originates as it penetrates into the vertebral body. Above the L4-5 disk, the anterior epidural compartment is obliterated at the level of each disk by attachment of the posterior longitudinal ligament to the disk. Caudal to this level, and especially in the caudal canal, the anterior epidural space widens to a capacious fat-filled cavity as the dural sac diminishes in size. This may contribute to difficulty in delivering local anesthetic to the L-5 and sacral nerve roots during epidural anesthesia because solution is not confined in close proximity with neural structures at these levels, unlike elsewhere in the vertebral column.

The behavior of solutions and catheters within the epidural space can be explained by anatomic findings. As a needle tip passes anterior to the ligamentum flavum, injected air or saline enters into the plane between the nonadherent dorsal fat pad and canal wall. This is the loss of resistance noted when the syringe plunger suddenly yields to pressure exerted during needle advancement. Solution or air injected into the epidural space readily distributes between the surfaces of the various structures and encircles the dura, with only an occasional impediment in the dorsal midline where the dura may adhere to the lamina or fat. Less often, the needle might pass into the substance of the dorsal fat pad, making catheter passage difficult.

The distance that a needle must travel after entering the epidural space within the ligamentum flavum before contacting the dura is a maximum of about 8 mm at the cephalad extent of the interlaminar space and in the midline.[84] If the needle enters the spinal canal away

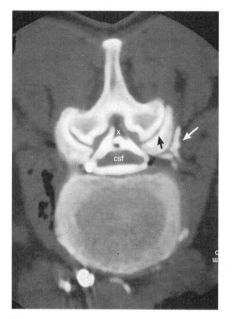

Figure 4–13 Computed tomographic scan of lumbar epidural catheter at typical location at internal aspect of an intervertebral foramen (straight white arrow). Injection of 10 mL of contrast medium shows uniform spread surrounding and compressing the cerebrospinal fluid (csf) and out the contralateral foramen (curved arrow). ×, posterior epidural fat; black arrow, facet joint space. An air bubble is evident in the posterior epidural space between the dura and fat.

from the midline, it may encounter the dura with no further advancement because the dorsal epidural fat pad thins toward its lateral attenuations. As a catheter is passed through the needle, there may be a brief resistance to advancement as the tip impinges on the dura. Computed tomography (Fig. 4–13) shows that a catheter tip inserted 3 cm into the vertebral canal most frequently travels laterally to the internal aspect of an intervertebral foramen, but injected solution still surrounds the dura circumferentially (see Fig. 4–1D and E; see Color Plate 1). Even when the catheter tip lies exterior to the intervertebral foramen in the paravertebral space, distribution of the injectant is preferentially back into the vertebral canal. This is because the muscular confines of the perivertebral space cause high pressures to develop with injection, whereas the adjacent spinal canal has a maximum pressure set by the CSF pressure (about 15 cm H_2O) and accepts flow by displacing CSF. Fluid injected during any block around the vertebral column can enter the epidural space. This has been demonstrated for brachial plexus blocks,[85–87] stellate ganglion and lumbar sympathetic chain blocks,[88, 89] and especially intercostal[90] and paravertebral spinal nerve blocks.[91]

Catheters that transgress anteriorly through the membrane that isolates the anterior epidural space are likely to enter a vein, often with a perceptible sudden yield ("pop"). If a more cephalad needle angle is used, as is done with thoracic epidural catheterization or during a paramedian approach, the catheter is less apt to advance anteriorly where the majority of large epidural veins are located.

Meninges and Cerebrospinal Fluid

Spinal dura mater is a connective tissue sac that extends from the skull, where its fusion with the foramen magnum terminates the epidural space, to its caudal terminus at about the S-2 level. Other attachments are weak except fibrous slips to the posterior longitudinal ligament, particularly in the lumbar region,[92] and anchors from the dural nerve root sleeves to the epineural tissue in the intervertebral foramen. A dorsal fold, termed a "plica dorsalis medianalis," has been observed when epidural injectant (air or solution) compresses the dural sac because scattered attachments tether the dura to the dorsal epidural fat and lamina. The undisturbed dura, however, is circular or oval in axial section.[10] Cheng[93] observed that the dura is thickest in the dorsal midline and thinner in the lumbar area than more rostrally, but few data are offered. Lumbar dura is nonetheless tough enough to prevent puncture by epidural catheters in most instances.[94]

Dura is composed of lamellae made up predominantly of collagen and some elastin elements, separated by clefts filled with ground substance,[95] which accounts for dural permeability.[96] Fibrous strands are oriented in both circumferential and longitudinal fashion,[95] with more running lengthwise.[97] Dura is somewhat elastic, especially in the circumferential dimension,[97] and is freely compressible. Dynamic changes in shape and volume accommodate shifts in CSF from the intracranial space or between different sections of the vertebral dural sac. The Valsalva maneuver dramatically and immediately collapses the lumbar and thoracic dural sac, displacing CSF rostrally (Fig. 4–14).[98–101] The displaced CSF does not enter the calvaria, which is a confined space and is pressurized comparable with the thoracoabdominal cavity, but distends the cervical dural sac, which is not surrounded by a pressurized chamber. Tensing of the dura with flexion of the vertebral column, especially at cervical levels, causes an increased CSF pressure[102] and a rostral shift of the dural sac within the vertebral canal of close to 2 cm.[63–67]

Arachnoid mater is a thin membrane within the dura that encloses the subarachnoid space and the CSF. Arachnoid cells, tight intracellular junctions, and basal lamina together with those of the pia contribute to a physiologically active barrier.[103] The arachnoid layer is only loosely attached to the inner aspect of the dura. Whereas the substantial dura can be cleanly punctured, the arachnoid is velamentous and filmy in texture and withdraws from an advancing needle. Injections of radiographic contrast medium intended for the subarachnoid space commonly flow in part into the subdural space. This is probably a misnomer, because the cleft that most easily forms when arachnoid is pulled away from dura is not between the dura and arachnoid membranes, but more properly between layers of arachnoid.[104] Planar radiographic images showing a thin layer of contrast medium surrounding the dura without lateral spread along the nerve roots have been used to support claims in anesthetic case reports of the subdural passage of injected solution. There is, however, no evidence to support the contention that epi-

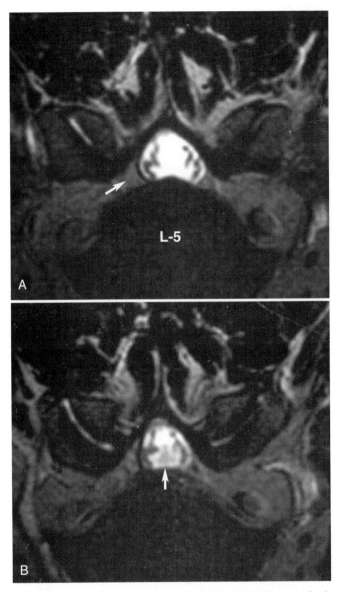

A

L-5

B

Figure 4–14 Axial magnetic resonance images of lumbar vertebral canal, using fast spin-echo sequence to highlight the cerebrospinal fluid (CSF). *A*, During control conditions, the cross sectional area of CSF is greater than during abdominal compression *(B)*, principally because of inward displacement of foraminal contents and lateral epidural space (arrow in *A*). Also evident are triangular darkened areas in the CSF (arrow in *B*), indicating amplified flow artifact, owing to the extended longitudinal oscillation of CSF with increased abdominal pressure. Both of these phenomena may contribute to increased local anesthetic spread when abdominal contents are compressed, such as with obesity and pregnancy.

cisterns at the base of the brain. Most CSF then flows along the convexities of the brain toward the arachnoid granulations (also called pacchionian bodies) along the sagittal sinus. These are macroscopic defects in the dura through which arachnoid membrane herniates and probably account for much of the CSF absorption back into the venous circulation, although other mechanisms participate.[109] Particulate matter as large as 7 μ may pass through the granulations from CSF into venous blood,[110] and electron microscopy has confirmed widened intracellular spaces[111] and transcellular fenestrations[112] in arachnoid granulations. These passages open only when exposed to a CSF pressure in excess of the venous pressure, which ensures that flow will be only from CSF to veins. The pressure-sensing feature of arachnoid granulations regulates CSF pressure to about 10 to 20 cm H_2O in the lateral position.[113]

A small amount of CSF produced leaves the cranial cavity and enters the spinal subarachnoid space to pass downward posterior to the cord and return upward anterior to the cord. Superimposed on this bulk flow is a longitudinal oscillation of the CSF column (see Fig. 4–14) in synchrony with the pulsations of the arteries in the skull.[114] The amplitude of this movement is about 9 mm per cycle in the cervical CSF and about 4 mm at the thoracolumbar junction, with minimal movement in the distal lumbar sac. Oscillatory CSF pulsation is a possible but unexplored mechanism for local anesthetic distribution after subarachnoid injection. Material injected into the lumbar CSF ascends to the basal cisterns within an hour.[115]

Little is known about the volume of CSF or about correlations of this variable with height, weight, body mass index, or age, despite its key role as the diluting volume for subarachnoid anesthetic solutions. Of the entire 140 mL of CSF, estimates for the share in the spinal subarachnoid space range from 30 to 80 mL,[116, 117] with a large variation among individuals. The composition of CSF[118] is similar to that of serum but with a lower pH (7.32), potassium value (2.9 mEq/L), and glucose value (about two thirds of concurrent serum concentration) and a higher P_{CO_2} (47 mm Hg) and concentrations of magnesium (2.2 mEq/L), sodium (145 mEq/L), and chloride (125 mEq/L). Protein concentrations are much less than in serum, with greater concentrations in lumbar CSF (300 mg/L) than in ventricular CSF (170 mg/L). The specific gravity of lumbar CSF is about 1.006.

In contrast to the anterior subarachnoid space, which is empty of structures, the posterior subarachnoid space is crowded with membranous elements (Fig. 4–17).[119–121] These are the residue of the embryologic connective tissue that develops into the subarachnoid space by gradually decreasing cellularity and increasing intercellular space, progressing from anterior to posterior around the cord.[122] Remnants of the tissue form a mesh of trabeculae, especially in the young, that spans the space from arachnoid to join the pia mater (the meningeal layer that envelops the surface of the cord and nerve roots). (Because of the intimate relationship, common embryologic origin, and similar microscopic

dural injectant cannot travel in such a way (Fig. 4–15), and a study of intentional subdural injection showed that solution preferentially passes out along the nerve roots.[105] A dural-based loculation on computed tomography does, however, prove a subdural injection (Fig. 4–16).

About 500 mL of CSF is formed each day,[106, 107] principally by the choroid plexuses of the cerebral ventricles, with an uncertain contribution from ependyma, pia, and brain parenchyma.[108, 109] Bulk flow distributes the fluid from the cerebral ventricular system to the

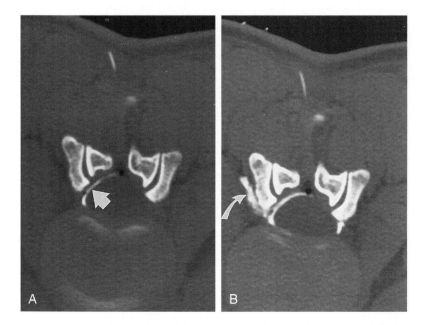

Figure 4–15 Subdural injection is a difficult diagnosis to make, even with computed tomography. *A*, This lumbar image appears to qualify for a subdural pattern of spread, because the layer of injectant exclusively follows the dural contour (arrow). *B*, However, further injection shows contrast material passing out the intervertebral foramen (curved arrow) and even through the contralateral foramen.

structure of the inner two meninges, they are often designated jointly as pia-arachnoid or leptomeninges.)

Denticulate ligaments, more substantial than trabeculae, extend laterally from the sides of the cord to suspend it within the dural sac. A variably fenestrated partition, the subarachnoid septum or septum posticum, extends from the posterior midline of the cord to the inner aspect of the arachnoid. Dissection reveals a distinct and continuous membrane at lumbar levels in 28% of cadavers and virtually always at thoracic and cervical levels.[120] The degree to which these membranes affect distribution of anesthetic solutions is unknown. Although large-volume injections of myelogram dye are rarely confined by these structures, drainage of CSF during pneumoencephalography may be impeded by other membranes that extend from each posterior nerve root to the septum posticum and dorsolateral arachnoid, forming a lateral oblique cul-de-sac.[119]

More problematic for the anesthesiologist is the occurrence of cysts within the subarachnoid space (Fig. 4–18). These saccular dilatations of the septum posticum are actually diverticula because their rostral ends communicate with the subarachnoid space. They attract little attention from radiologists and surgeons because they opacify promptly with modern contrast

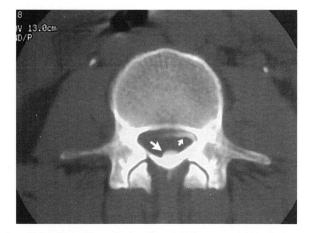

Figure 4–16 This computed tomographic image provides clear evidence of partial subdural injectant distribution, creating a bleb within the dural sac (straight arrow). At least part of the solution has spread around the dural sac in the epidural space (curved arrow). Unexpected rupture of such a subdural bleb containing local anesthetic could happen after many uneventful injections, creating the impression of catheter "migration" into the subarachnoid space.

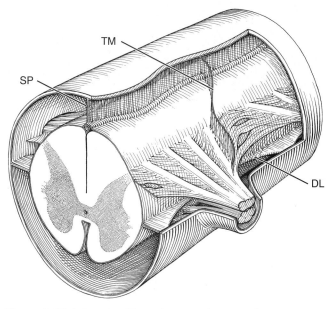

Figure 4–17 Subarachnoid membranous elements. The subarachnoid septum appears like a variably fenestrated curtain following the posterior vein. Dentate ligaments (DL) span to the lateral dural sac, whereas variable transverse membranes (TM) may connect the septum posticum (SP) to the membrane spanning the posterior nerve roots, creating a cul-de-sac. (Reprinted by permission of the publisher from Nauta HJW, Dolan E, Yasargil MG: Microsurgical anatomy of spinal subarachnoid space. Surg Neurol 19: 431–437. © 1983 by Elsevier Science Inc.)

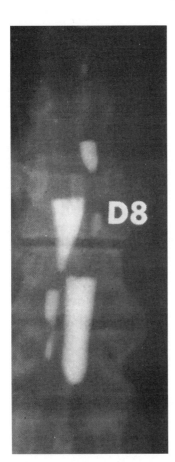

Figure 4–18 Multiple subarachnoid cysts within the thoracic dural sac at the T-8 to T-10 levels, highlighted by radiographic contrast material. The horizontal interface in this sitting subject is due to settling of the dense oily contrast material. (From Teng P, Papatheodorou C: Spinal arachnoid diverticula. Br J Radiol 1966; 39: 249–254.)

agents and are unlikely to produce symptoms. However, use of large amounts of oily radiographic contrast medium delineates loculated CSF in 45% [123] to 84% [124] of films of upright healthy subjects. Because the mixing of the cystic fluid with the rest of the CSF is often slow and influenced by posture, injection into cysts is a potential cause of inadequate spinal anesthesia.

As nerve roots exit the dural sac, they carry with them a tubular extension of the arachnoid membrane, subarachnoid space, and CSF as far as the proximal pole of the posterior root ganglion (Fig. 4–19). [125] At the lateral end of this nerve root sheath, which averages about 6 mm long at L-1 to about 15 mm long at S-1 and S-2, [126] the subarachnoid space is obliterated as a cul-de-sac by the reflection of the arachnoid back along the nerve root. In this area, the dural sleeve is invaded by villi of arachnoid, which are typically not apparent to the unaided eye. Progressively with age, arachnoid villi may distend with CSF and herniate outside the dura to form macroscopic arachnoid granulations similar to those in the intracranial dural sinuses. [127–129] Particulate ink injected into the CSF collects as a cuff at the furthest lateral extent of the CSF space along the posterior root ganglion and nerve roots, and it even stains the epidural fat and lymphatics,

indicating egress of CSF and trapping of particulate matter at these sites. [130]

Spinal arachnoid granulations are not plentiful even in adulthood and lack the surrounding connective tissue cleft and accompanying venous confluence evident with cerebral granulations, so other imperfections in the meninges at the nerve root sleeve must account for the passage of material out of the CSF at the ink cuff. [131] Specifically, the lateral recess of the subarachnoid space terminates as a maze of lacunae filled with cellular debris and macrophages, [132] and it probably provides an important drainage and cleansing site. Root sleeves may also be a portal for the entry of local anesthetic from the epidural space into the CSF because the nerve roots are close at hand and the surface area of the dural root sleeve is large compared with the minimal CSF available at this site to dilute the anesthetic. This explains the segmental onset of epidural anesthesia despite a CSF site of action: other nerve roots lying in the central pool of CSF and passing to more caudal intervertebral foramina would not be as directly affected.

Distension of root sheath arachnoid granulations can lead to saccular subarachnoid diverticula outside the dural sac proper (Fig. 4–20A). [133] These occasionally expand into the vertebral canal (usually lower thoracic [134]) where they are termed "extradural cysts." However, they usually occupy the intervertebral foramina and are referred to as nerve root sheath or perineural cysts. Their cause is probably congenital. Rexed and Wennström [135] found proliferation of arachnoid tissue with invasion of the adjacent dura and cystic degeneration in 37% of lumbar spines obtained at autopsy from subjects with no clinically evident back disease, whereas other studies [136–138] have documented saccular diverticula of thoracic, lumbar, and sacral nerve root sheaths in from 9% to 18% of asymptomatic subjects. Diverticula are usually multiple and symmetric in a given subject, and they often erode adjacent bone. Perineural cysts at the sacral level, termed "Tarlov's cysts," are the largest and most common, reaching several centimeters in diameter and destroying sacral bone. These occasionally expand into the pelvic cavity, presenting as anterior sacral meningoceles [139] that may be familial. [140] Cystic sheath lesions are also observed at cervical vertebral levels in 30% of older healthy subjects, especially at C-6 to C-8, but these do not exceed 7 mm in diameter. [141]

At other than sacral levels, it is exceptional for either the normal nerve root sheath [142] or sheath diverticula [137] to extend lateral to the dorsal root ganglion and intervertebral foramen. Therefore, injection into such a sheath or cyst after a paravertebral needle insertion is likely only if the needle is mistakenly advanced into the intervertebral foramen. An unintended subarachnoid injection could also follow needle placement into a diverticulum in the vertebral canal during epidural anesthesia. Although unproved, both events could produce extensive spinal anesthesia, possibly with a delayed onset because of the slow exchange of CSF with the main subarachnoid compartment.

A similar but much less common form of fluid-filled

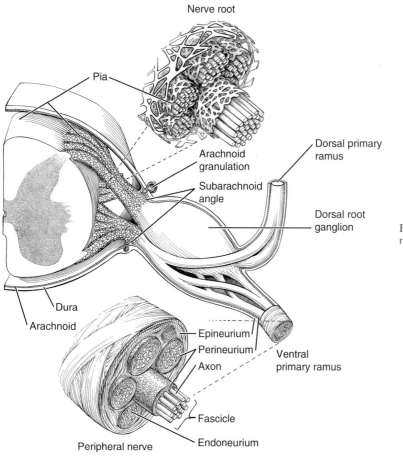

Figure 4–19 Structure of nerve roots and peripheral nerve, and the continuity of various layers.

vertebral canal mass originates as a dilatation of the capsule of a degenerating facet joint on its anterior and medial aspect (Fig. 4–20B). These are termed "synovial or ganglion cysts," depending on whether a synovium is evident on histologic examination. They are characteristically found in axial images and at dissection to be broadly based on a degenerating facet joint at a lower lumbar (usually L-4 or L-5) level, where they compress the dural sac from its posterolateral aspect,[143, 144] possibly producing radiculopathy. They may be gas filled, and the thickened cyst rim often enhances with gadolinium during magnetic resonance imaging. Facet joint arthrography might demonstrate a connection to the joint space. Even less commonly, ganglion cysts have been noted to arise from the posterior or anterior longitudinal ligaments, dura mater, or ligamentum flavum. Because the cavities of ganglion cysts do not communicate with the subarachnoid space, they could be the rare cause of inadequate spinal or epidural anesthesia.

Cord and Nerve Roots

The adult spinal cord measures 41 to 48 cm long from C-1 to its end and weighs between 24 and 36 g.[145] It is about 10 mm in diameter, with expansion in the lateral dimension at the cervical (14 mm) and lumbosacral (12 mm) levels to accommodate the greater gray matter for the limbs. Flexion of the verte-

bral column stretches parts of the spinal cord by as much as 18% to 24%.[64, 65] The tapered end, called the conus medullaris, usually lies at about the level of the L1-2 intervertebral disk, although this is variable and it may be as low as L-3.[146–148] Rootlets along the cord fuse into anterior and posterior spinal roots.

The law of Bell and Magendie dictates that afferent (sensory) fibers are in the posterior root and efferent (motor) fibers in the anterior root. Electron microscopy, however, has revealed plentiful unmyelinated afferent fibers in the anterior root,[149] comprising between 15% and 30% of all fibers.[150] Initial theories proposed that these are axonal loops of afferents that ultimately pass to the cord in the posterior root,[151] but more recent study has revealed no such fibers.[152] Rather, most of the nonmyelinated afferents in the anterior root project exclusively in the anterior root. Although many seem to end blindly in its midportion before reaching the cord,[153] sufficient fibers enter the cord by this anterior path to explain the failure of posterior rhizotomy to reliably eliminate pain. A minority of anterior root afferent fibers convey pial sensitivity of the anterior root itself[151] and project to the cord via the posterior root. After peripheral nerve injury, the number of anterior root afferents increases, which may represent recurrent nerve sprouts from peripheral sources.[154]

As rootlets emerge from the cord and join together as a root, each takes along a thin layer of pia that

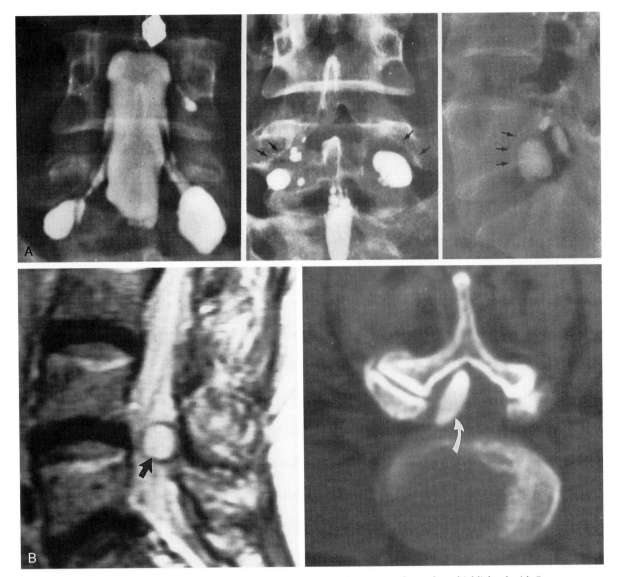

Figure 4–20 Cysts in the epidural space. *A,* Root sheath cysts, also called Tarlov's cysts, shown here highlighted with Pantopaque myelography. As in this case, they are usually sacral and often multiple, and they may erode the pedicle (arrows in center) or vertebral body (arrows in right). (*A* from Taveras JM, Wood EH: Diagnostic Neuroradiology, 2nd ed, p 1144. Baltimore, Williams & Wilkins, 1976.) *B,* Sagittal T2-weighted magnetic resonance image without gadolinium enhancement (left) and axial computed tomographic images (right) of a ganglion cyst (arrows) of the L4-5 facet joint, encroaching on the vertebral canal of a 78-year-old woman. The image on right followed the injection of contrast material into the facet joint at its posterolateral margin. (*B,* Images courtesy of Forrest T. Bates, M.D., Appleton, WI.)

continues the entire length of the root, separating the root into fascicles. Rather than the unitary structure often portrayed in texts, the roots are an association of up to five such fascicles held together loosely by an even more frail outer layer of pia.[155–157] These meningeal coverings of the roots (sometimes, confusingly, also referred to as the nerve root sheath) and their basement membrane are notably mesh-like and porous (see Fig. 4–19). Unlike the peripheral nerves, which protect their contents with sturdy and selectively permeable barriers, the axons in the nerve roots are freely bathed by the surrounding CSF, which gives ready access to drugs and particulate matter from the subarachnoid space.

Segments that contribute to a plexus innervating the upper or lower extremity have roots considerably larger in diameter than at other levels. Galindo and colleagues[158] examined the correlation of epidural anesthesia onset with nerve size by measuring the diameter of the proximal mixed spinal nerve and its sheath but did not study the roots, which are more relevant as a site of anesthetic action. Several old studies[159] used preserved specimens and unreliable measures of cross sectional area, but they confirmed the greater size of cervical and lumbosacral roots. The present author's observations concur that L-5 through S-2 roots are largest, with a fair degree of interindividual variation. Large roots may be the most resistant to local anesthetic, contributing to delayed or absent block at L-5 through S-2 and variable results among individuals.

Because the cord is much shorter than the entire vertebral canal, lumbar and sacral roots acquire a long oblique course within the dural sac and together compose the cauda equina. These nerve roots, which are about 7 cm in length at L-1, 17 cm at S-1, and 27 cm at S-5,[160] tend to gravitate toward the most dependent part of the dural sac, regardless of posture,[161] with the anterior root medial as well as anterior to the posterior root.[162] Marked lengthening and redundancy of the sacral roots often accompany lumbar spinal canal stenosis.[163]

Within the dural sac, multiple connections between adjacent roots are found in all specimens, with between three and nine such intersegmental anastomoses at the upper cervical region and a similar number at the lumbosacral level.[164, 165] Nerve roots pivot tightly around the inner and caudal aspect of the pedicle as they exit the vertebral canal. Flexion of the vertebral column, especially of the neck, lengthens the vertebral canal by several millimeters, so that the lumbosacral roots are tensed compared with their relaxed and redundant condition during spinal extension.[65] Anterior and posterior roots perforate the dural sac through a common aperture at each intervertebral foramen. Anomalous patterns of distribution at the foramina are discovered in dissections of 14% of normal subjects[166] and include two root pairs exiting at one level with an adjacent empty foramen.[167–169] These variations occur because the dorsal root ganglia develop from a continuous sheet of neural crest tissue, and separation into segments is imprecise. Myelography has revealed a much lower incidence because resolution is limited and only the subarachnoid contents are seen.[166] The clinical consequence of occasionally aberrant arrangements is the development of anesthesia in an unexpected distribution after foraminal injection for intended nerve root block.[168] The posterior root dissociates into its component fascicles just before arriving at the posterior root ganglion, which contains sensory neuron somata. The ganglion occurs in the foramen directly inferior to the pedicle in the lumbar region,[126] further into or beyond the foramen in the cervical region, and in the vertebral canal in the sacrum.

There are eight cervical neural segments; the 8th spinal nerve emerges between the 7th cervical and 1st thoracic vertebrae, whereas the other cervical nerves emerge above their same numbered vertebral bones, and the thoracic, lumbar, and sacral nerves exit the vertebral column below their same numbered bony segment. Because the disks lie opposite the caudal end of the intervertebral foramen, disk disease usually affects the nerve that exits at the next foramen. As an example, the L-4 nerve would exit the L4-5 foramen safely cephalad to nuclear material extruded from the L4-5 disk, but the L-5 nerve, drawn laterally by its imminent exit through the L5-S1 foramen, is liable to be irritated.

Neural Supply of the Vertebral Column

Sensory innervation of the vertebral column[170–174] remains an active area of research because the origin of back pain is uncertain. The medial branch of the dorsal primary ramus of the spinal nerve supplies the dorsal vertebral structures, including the supraspinous

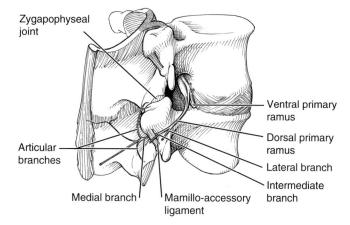

Figure 4–21 Innervation of facet joints and the route of the medial branch of the posterior primary ramus of the peripheral nerve.

and intraspinous ligaments, periosteum, and fibrous capsule of the facet joint (Fig. 4–21). Of these, only the facet joint is consistently well innervated, including nociceptive fibers penetrating the capsule as well and into the synovial folds.[175] Because a single segmental nerve sends branches to the facet joint above and below it, somatotopic localization of stimulation is vague. The ligamentum flavum has few nerve endings that are found only on its surface. It is possible that, like the costovertebral joints, all fibers innervating these posterior skeletal structures pass through the sympathetic chain on their afferent course to the cord.[174]

The innervation of the anterior longitudinal ligament, vertebral bodies, disks, and structures within the spinal canal is derived from cells with their somas in neighboring dorsal root ganglia,[176] the axons of which are delivered to these sites entirely by sympathetic pathways,[174] including perivascular nerve plexuses, the sympathetic chain, and its ramifications. Up to five sinuvertebral nerves, also called the recurrent nerves, meningeal rami, or the nerves of Luschka, course through each intervertebral foramen anterior to the dorsal root ganglion on their passage into the vertebral canal (Fig. 4–22).[174, 177] They originate from plexiform branches of the rami communicantes near where the rami join the anterior primary ramus of the spinal nerve. Distribution is limited to the anterior vertebral canal, especially to an extensive plexus that follows the posterior longitudinal ligament, which in turn passes fibers (coiled to allow relative movement) to the anterior dura. Other filaments supply the posterior aspect of the disk, penetrating perhaps one third the thickness of the anulus fibrosus.[173, 174, 178, 179] The inner anulus, center of the disk, and vertebral end plates have no nerves, although the interior of a degenerating disk may develop free nerve endings.[180, 181] Ascending and descending branches from the sinuvertebral nerve span as many as eight vertebral segments and cross the midline.[173, 174, 176, 177, 182] This polysegmental and bilateral innervation of vertebral elements may explain the wide distribution of pain from stimulation of nerve endings in the disk, posterior longitudinal ligament, or dura by disk protrusion at a single level.

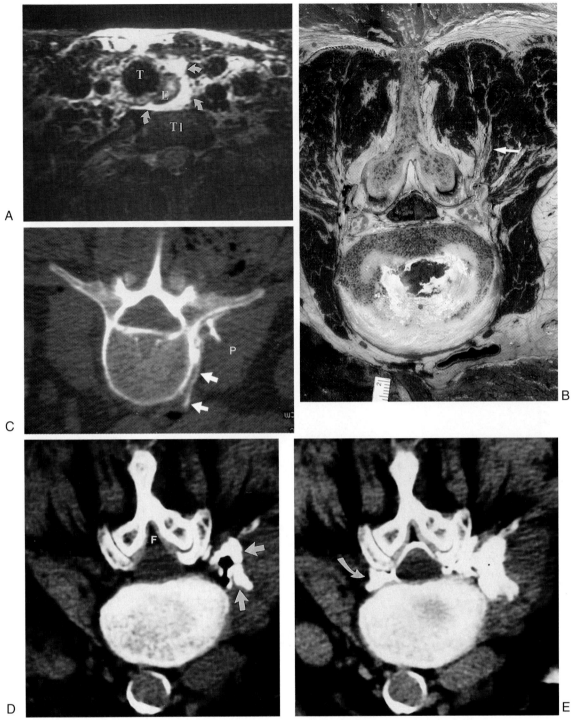

Figure 4–1 Unexpected patterns of injectant distribution are a common observation. *A,* Injection at the right C-6 anterior tubercle passed entirely to the contralateral side, shown here in magnetic resonance image at the T-1 level (anatomic left on right of image; arrows delineate solution). E, esophagus; T, trachea. *B,* Green ink injected into the lumbar epidural space of a cadaver demonstrates posterior distribution into the paraspinous muscles (arrow), which may contribute to back pain when EDTA (ethylenediaminetetraacetic acid) is included in the anesthetic solution. *C,* Injection through a normally functioning epidural catheter shows passage of solution through the intervertebral foramen into the psoas muscle (P) and anterior around the vertebral body (arrows) to the region of the sympathetic chain. This could variably contribute to intense sympathetic block. *D,* An epidural catheter that produced a normal block, after 0.5-mL injection of radiographic contrast medium, shows the tip of the catheter in the psoas muscle (arrows) after exiting through the intervertebral foramen. F, epidural fat. *E,* Injection of 10 mL of contrast medium through the catheter shown in *D* produces spread into the spinal canal, around the dura in the epidural space, and even out the contralateral intervertebral foramen (arrow).

PLATE 1

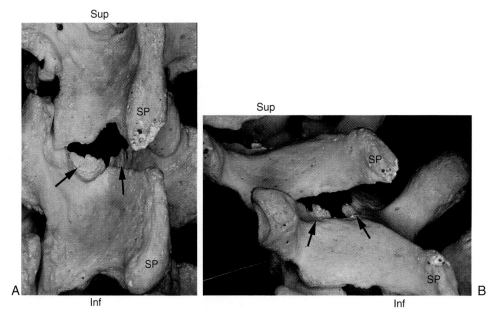

Figure 4–6 Ossification of the ligamenta flava (arrows) at L1-2 *(A)* and T2-3 *(B)* forms substantial shelves of bone in the path of spinal and epidural needles. Inf., inferior; SP, spinous process; Sup., superior.

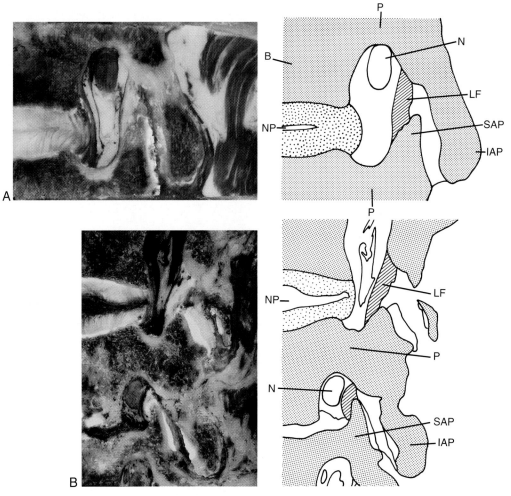

Figure 4–7 *A*, Sagittal cryomicrotome sections and key drawings of normal intervertebral foramen. *B*, Foramen after disk collapse. Overlap of superior and inferior articular processes (SAP and IAP) and bunching of ligamentum flavum (LF) result in crowding and possibly irritation of the peripheral nerve (N) at its origin in the foramen. B, body; NP, nucleus pulposus; P, pedicle. (Cryomicrotome images courtesy of Bruce H. Nowicki, B.S.)

PLATE 2

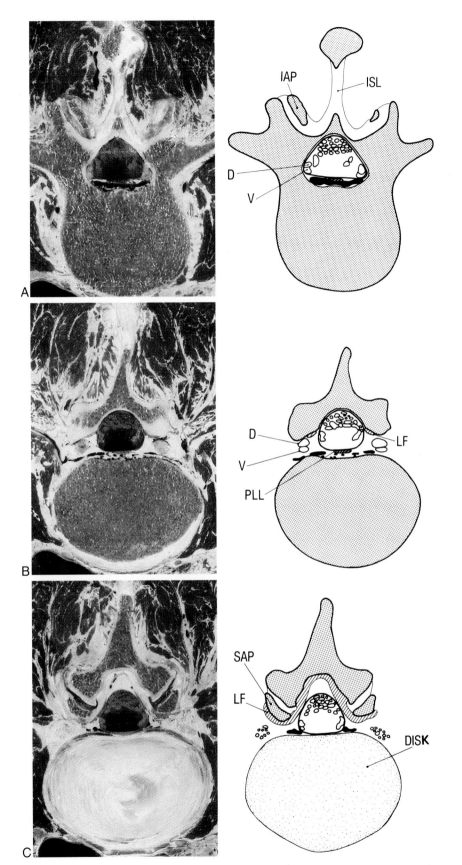

Figure 4–8 *A*, Axial cryomicrotome sections and key drawings through the pedicles of L-3. *B*, Caudal portion of L-3. *C*, L3-4 disk.

Illustration continued on following page

PLATE 3

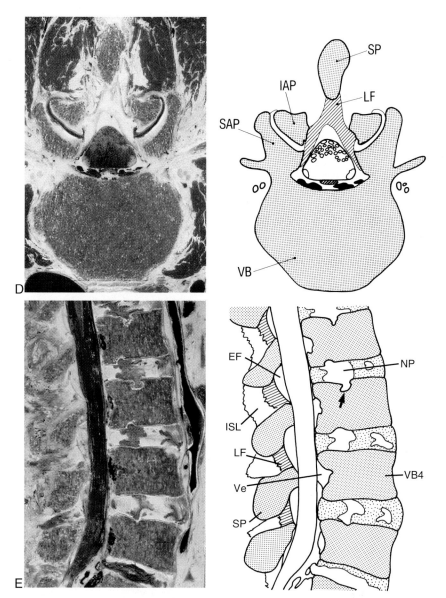

Figure 4–8 *Continued D,* Rostral edge of the L-4 pedicles. The image varies greatly through the metameric cycle, because the epidural contents are not uniform in distribution. The dura is in contact with the spinal canal wall over much of its extent. *E,* Midline sagittal view demonstrates the structures through which a needle must pass to enter the epidural space: interspinous ligament (ISL), ligamentum flavum (LF), and posterior epidural fat (EF). The posterior epidural space has its greatest anteroposterior dimension at its rostral end. D, dorsal root; IAP, inferior articular process; NP, nucleus pulposus; PLL, posterior longitudinal ligament; SAP, superior articular process; SP, spinous process; V, ventral root; VB4, vertebral body of L-4; Ve, veins; arrow, Schmorl's node.

PLATE 4

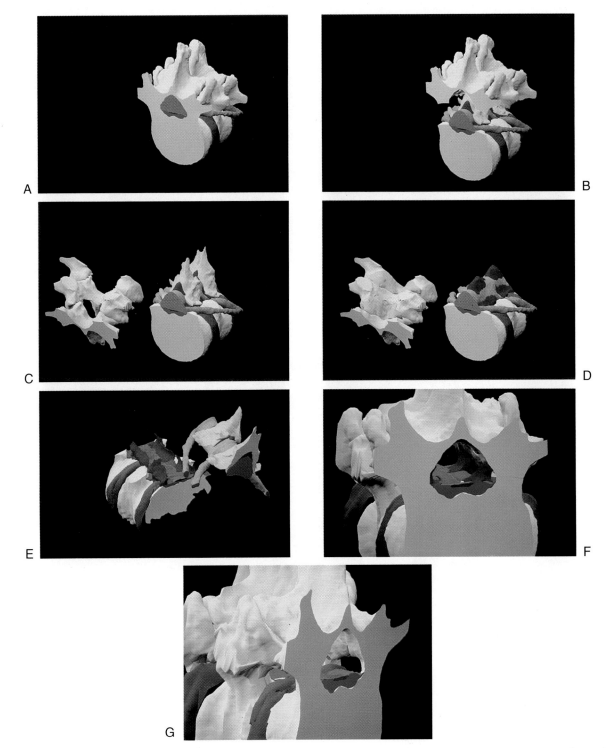

Figure 4–9 For improved examination and manipulation, the exact planar anatomy can be encoded and digitally reconstructed into three dimensions, maintaining perfect original relationships. (Software developed by University of Washington Department of Biological Structures.) *A,* All of L-4 and parts of L-3 and L-5 from a rostral, posterior, lateral oblique perspective (light blue, bone; brown, disk and ligaments; blue, veins; yellow, ligamentum flavum; red, fat; orange, neural structures). The posterior elements are separated through the pedicles *(B)* and inverted *(C)* to reveal the ligamenta flava straddling the posterior epidural fat. *D,* Placing the ligamenta flava with the posterior elements shows the circumferentially and longitudinally discontinuous distribution of epidural contents. *E,* From a caudal oblique perspective, removal of the dural sac and ligamenta flava reveals the anterior and lateral epidural space in contact with the dura, including the posterior longitudinal ligament (separating the dura from the venous bed) and the lateral fat compartments. *F,* A longitudinal view from above down the spinal canal shows the smoothed surfaces provided by epidural fat. *G,* With the fat removed, structures in the intervertebral foramen that could impinge on the passing nerves include pedicle superiorly, ligamentum flavum and facet joint posteriorly, and disk inferiorly and anteriorly as well as veins.

PLATE 5

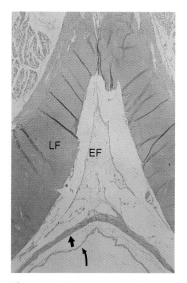

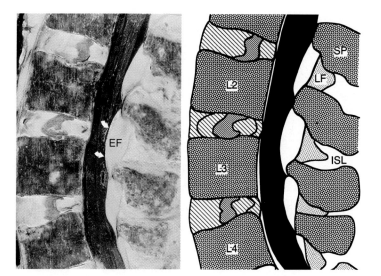

Figure 4–11 Human dorsal epidural space axial section shows the epidural fat (EF) with no fibrous content, mostly nonadherent to the internal aspect of the ligamentum flavum (LF) and the external aspect of the dura (straight arrow). Striations in the LF are artifactual folds during preparation. Curved arrow, arachnoid mater. (Hematoxylin and eosin.)

Figure 4–12 Midline sagittal cryomicrotome section and key drawing of lumbar vertebrae of a man who received systemic steroid therapy. Expansion of the posterior epidural fat (EF) (arrows) causes encroachment into the vertebral canal. ISL, interspinous ligament; LF, ligamentum flavum; SP, spinous process.

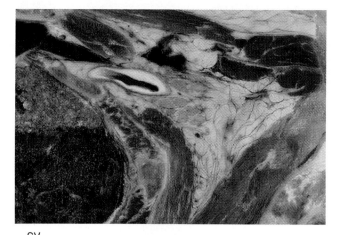

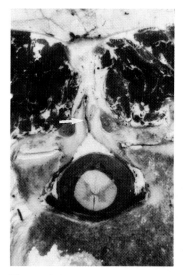

Figure 4–25 Low thoracic axial cryomicrotome section shows a midline posterior vein (arrow) entering the posterior epidural space between the two ligamenta flava.

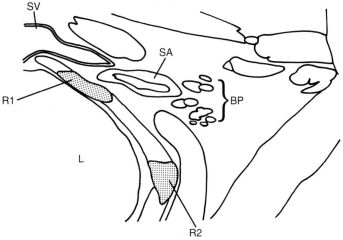

Figure 4–26 Axial cryomicrotome section and key drawing of the brachial plexus (BP) as it enters the axilla, having passed over the first rib (R1). No sheath is evident, and fat septation freely enters among the components of the plexus. L, lung; R2, second rib; SA, subclavian artery; SV, subclavian vein.

PLATE 6

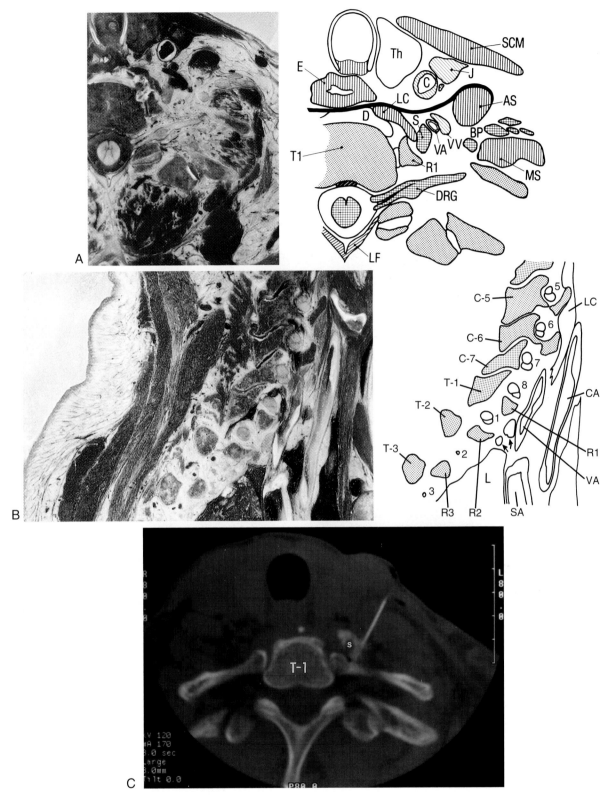

Figure 4–31 *A,* Axial cryomicrotome section through the first thoracic vertebral body and index drawing. *B,* Paramedian sagittal cryomicrotome section of the neck and index drawing delineates the anatomy surrounding the stellate ganglion (S in *A* and arrows in *B*). C-5 through T-3 = vertebral bones; R1 through R3 = ribs 1 through 3; numerals 5 through 8 and 1 through 3 = segmental nerves of cervical 5 through 8 and thoracic 1 through 3. AS, anterior scalene muscle; BP, brachial plexus; CA, carotid artery; D, disk; DRG, dorsal root ganglion; E, esophagus; J, jugular vein; L, lung; LC, longus colli muscle; LF, ligamentum flavum; MS, middle scalene muscle; SA, subclavian artery; SCM, sternocleidomastoid muscle; Th, thyroid; VA, vertebral artery; VV, vertebral vein. *C,* An in vivo demonstration of the location of the stellate ganglion(s) surrounded by contrast material injected during computerized tomography–guided stellate block. (From Hogan QH, Erickson SJ, Abram SE: Computerized tomography–guided stellate ganglion blockade. Anesthesiology 1992; 77: 596–599.)

PLATE 7

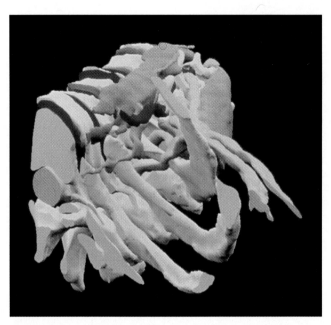

Figure 4–33 Computer reconstruction of axial cryomicrotome data demonstrates proximity of the sympathetic chain and stellate ganglion to the brachial plexus. Light blue, bone; brown, disk and ligaments; blue, veins; red, vertebral artery; yellow, brachial plexus and dural sac; lavender, muscles; green, sympathetic chain. The perspective is from within the left chest, looking cephalad and mesial.

PLATE 8

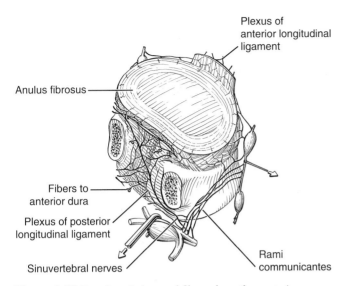

Plexus of
anterior longitudinal
ligament

Anulus fibrosus

Fibers to
anterior dura

Plexus of posterior
longitudinal ligament

Sinuvertebral nerves

Rami
communicantes

Figure 4–22 Drawing of plexus of fibers along the posterior longitudinal ligament and anterior dura within the vertebral canal, the sinuvertebral nerves feeding this system, and the rami communicantes. The complexity exhibited in these details is derived from studies using acetylcholinesterase histochemical staining. (Modified from Groen GJ, Baljet B, Drukker J: Nerves and nerve plexuses of the human vertebral column. Am J Anat 1990; 188: 282–296. Copyright © 1990. Reprinted by permission of Wiley-Liss, Inc, a subsidiary of John Wiley & Sons.)

The investing pial membrane of the anterior and posterior roots has sensory innervation,[183] as does the pia of the cord.[184] From nerve endings in the pia of the anterior root, impulses reach the spinal cord by traveling laterally in the anterior root to the posterior root ganglion and then medially via the posterior root.[152, 154, 185] Injury to the root leads to increased small fiber innervation of the pia.[186] The costovertebral joints are exclusively innervated by a plexus of minute fibers derived from branches of the adjacent sympathetic trunk.[187]

Few fibers are seen in the posterior spinal canal or dura,[182, 188] accounting for the lack of sensations from these tissues during anesthetic procedures. Fine branches from the rami communicantes and sympathetic trunk contribute to a plexus along the anterior longitudinal ligament and the anterior and lateral aspects of the disks. Only perivascular nerves enter the vertebral body.

Several lines of evidence indicate a sensory function for fibers innervating the vertebral column:

1. Only a few of the neurons terminate on motor structures such as vessels.

2. Excision of the dorsal root ganglia eliminates fibers in the nerve plexuses of the posterior and anterior longitudinal ligaments.[176]

3. Characteristic sensory endings are evident. Some complex unencapsulated (pressure-sensing) and encapsulated (proprioceptive) nerve terminations are found,[171, 189–191] but most are bare nociceptors. Even on facet joints, however, the fiber density is low and receptive fields are large.[192]

4. Substance P, a polypeptide neurotransmitter characteristic of small nociceptive fibers, is found in nerves of the posterior longitudinal ligament,[193, 194] dura,[195] pia on the anterior aspect of the cord and on the ventral roots,[196] supraspinous ligament,[197] annular ligament of the disk,[194] and facet joint capsule[197, 198] and is present[199] but rare[200] in facet menisci and absent in the central disk and ligamentum flavum.[193, 194, 198]

5. Various methods have been used to test sensitivity of vertebral structures in humans, such as mechanical stimulation with needles and hypertonic saline[190, 201–206] in surgery during local anesthesia[171, 207–212] or afterward by using threads that had been attached to various tissues during the operation.[213] These reports indicate that the posterior longitudinal ligament and anterior dura are especially sensitive and produce deep pain at or adjacent to the midline of the back and into the buttock. Manipulation of these structures at cervical levels can induce chest pain. Irritation of the surface of the disk or the inner portion of a degenerated disk produces typical deep back pain with radiation to the pelvis and abdomen and only rarely radiation into the lower extremity. Mechanical stimulation of the posterior root produces an electric sensation, whereas manipulation of the anterior root evokes a deep ache; inflamed roots consistently produce pain when manipulated. Facet joint stimulation creates low back pain that radiates into the thigh, with extensive overlap of referral areas from the various joints even when L1-2 and L4-5 joints are compared. Interspinous and supraspinous ligaments produce only minimal local and sometimes referred pain, and the ligamentum flavum, posterior dura, lamina, vertebral body, and spinous process are essentially insensitive.

6. Physiologic recordings in laboratory animals have documented mechanoreceptive sensory fields in facet joints,[214, 215] disk, dura, ligaments, periosteum, paraspinous muscles,[214, 216, 217] and the pial surface of the ventral roots,[152] for which stretching is the most potent stimulus.[185] The receptive field of a single cell or axon with vertebral innervation is typically large and always includes multiple tissues.

Afferent pathways for deep somatic sensation of midline structures are predominantly in sympathetic rami and trunks. This is evident from the pattern of nerve connections, from retrograde neural labeling studies,[218] and from detection of evoked activity in the sympathetic rami and trunks during stimulation of vertebral structures.[216, 219] Electrical stimulation of the sympathetic chain or rami in awake human subjects provokes localized back pain[220, 221] or extremity pain.[222] These observations indicate that blocks or ablation of the chain might have therapeutic potential in back pain, but only preliminary observations are available.[206, 221, 223]

Vascular Supply of the Vertebral Column

The vertebral column and the enclosed neural structures derive their arterial supply from segmental spinal arteries, which are branches of the thyrocervical and costocervical trunks and the vertebral artery in the neck and branches of the aorta more inferiorly, includ-

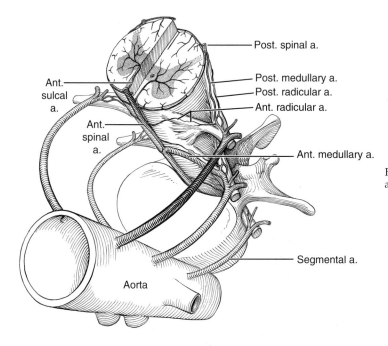

Figure 4–23 Arterial supply of the cord. a., artery; Ant., anterior; Post., posterior.

ing the intercostal and lumbar arteries (Fig. 4–23). Small branches of these vessels are distributed to the vertebral bones[224] and musculature. The nucleus pulposus of the intervertebral disk is avascular and receives its nutrition by flow of tissue fluid generated through a pumping mechanism of alternating compression and expansion with movement.[225] Fluid is expelled from axial loading in the upright posture, with a typical loss of about 2 cm in height through the day.[226]

At every intervertebral foramen, the segmental artery gives off radicular arteries that enter the spinal canal with each posterior and anterior root and provide nutrient flow to them. In addition, a major medullary feeder artery delivering flow to the intrinsic system of the cord travels along about 8 of the anterior and 12 of the posterior roots.[227] Previous descriptions stated that every radicular vessel makes at least a minor anastomotic contribution to the longitudinal vessels of the cord[228] or that the medullary feeders were simply enlarged radicular vessels, but more recent kinetic study of flow patterns has dispelled these views.[229] The anterior feeders split at the anterior median fissure of the cord into ascending and descending divisions that link to make an anastomotic chain, the anterior median longitudinal arterial trunk of the spinal cord (or anterior spinal artery). Similar linking of posterior medullary feeders produces right and left posterolateral longitudinal arterial trunks (or posterior spinal arteries) just posterior to the origin of the posterior nerve roots. The two systems join only at the conus medullaris. Penetrating midline branches (sulcal arteries) from the anterior spinal artery ramify in the anterior two thirds of the spinal cord whereas the posterior arteries supply the posterior one third, with negligible overlap or capillary anastomosis between the fields. A circumferential pial network probably contributes minimal nutrient flow to the cord.[230]

The longitudinal arteries of the cord, which are the sole source of medullary perfusion, should not be pictured as substantial and continuous throughout the length of the cord (Fig. 4–24).[231, 232] Along the length of these arteries, which are the longest in the body, the direction of blood flow is not uniform but depends on the proximity of the nearest contributing feeder,[233] and flow direction at any point may change in response to physiologic and pathologic influences.[234] Therefore, although the anterior arterial system of the cord is usually anatomically continuous, it is functionally a longitudinal series of independent vascular beds centered on the regional medullary feeder.[235] For this reason, the term anastomotic "trunk" may be preferable to "artery" for the longitudinal channels. The details of segmental contributions to the trunks are critical to delineating areas of the cord particularly sensitive to ischemia. Numerous descriptions of the pattern of medullary feeders have identified dominant vessels at certain levels in a highly variable pattern. Typically, a major contribution is made by a single anterior medullary feeder, known as the artery of Adamkiewicz, that enters at a level between T-7 and L-4, usually on the left. Often, however, a uniquely conspicuous artery is not apparent; the site and size of a dominant feeder to the lumbosacral cord are so unpredictable[236] that the concept is clinically unreliable. Without specific anatomic detail about an individual,[237] any segment of the cord must be considered at risk and any segmental artery must be considered critical.[238]

In general, the anterior and deep portions of the cord supplied by the anterior spinal artery are most prone to damage during ischemia, even during systemic hypotension or hypoxia without vascular damage.[239–241] This may be due partly to an inherent sensitivity of the anterior horn motor neurons,[240, 242, 243] and flaccid paralysis is commonly found at the level of the

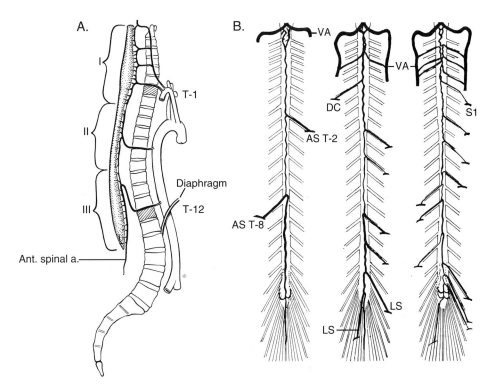

Figure 4–24 Contributions to the anterior (Ant.) spinal artery (a.). *A,* The anterior spinal artery, depicted schematically, receives inflow at various levels, typically divided into I, cervicothoracic; II, midthoracic; and III, thoracolumbar areas, with flow in the anterior spinal artery away from the feeders. However, as demonstrated in human neonatal specimens (*B*), there is a wide variability of anterior medullary feeder locations and sizes. AS, aortic segmental artery; DC, deep cervical artery; LS, lateral sacral artery; SI, superior intercostal artery; VA, vertebral artery. (*A* redrawn from Lazorthes G, Gouaze A, Zadeh JO, et al: Arterial vascularization of the spinal cord: recent studies of the anastomotic substitution pathways. J Neurosurg 1971; 35: 253–262. *B* redrawn from Dommisse GF: The Arteries and Veins of the Human Spinal Cord From Birth, p 23. Edinburgh, Churchill Livingstone, 1975.)

ischemic injury. Infarction of the anterior cord additionally produces loss of pain sensation and motor changes (spastic paralysis) distal to the injury as a result of dysfunction of the spinothalamic and pyramidal tracts.[244] Vascular anatomy contributes to making the anterior cord prone to ischemic injury. Anterior medullary feeders are larger but fewer than their posterior counterparts,[238] producing stretches of anterior spinal cord with precarious blood supply far downstream from feeders along the anterior trunk. Clinical and experimental ischemic injuries, however, are rarely limited to the anterior two thirds of the cord, which is considered the classic zone of anterior spinal cord infarction.[245] Rather, injury is greatest in the deep gray matter, with more extensive lesions expanding in a concentric fashion, including the dorsal horns. Distal nonpainful sensation is usually intact to some degree after any subtotal vascular injury to the cord because at least some of the superficial dorsal columns survive. It is this conspicuous clinical feature that gives rise to the common, although inexact, diagnosis of anterior spinal artery syndrome, despite the infrequent confirmation of the anatomic lesion of anterior spinal cord infarction by autopsy.[246]

Vulnerable watershed areas of the anterior arterial supply of the cord occur especially in the midthoracic zone[247] where feeders are most rare. Furthermore, this zone has the lowest density of penetrating branches from the anterior trunk,[231, 232] and the intercostal arteries providing feeder vessels in the thorax lack the extensive interconnections that provide alternative supply to the extraspinal arteries in the neck and lumbosacral region.[246] As a result, the most common levels for nonsurgical spinal stroke are T-3 to T-9.[241] Ischemic injury of the anterior cord, however, can occur at any level.[244] Cord infarction after thoracolumbar aortic operation is typically at a thoracic segmental level,[248] whereas conus and lumbosacral ischemic injuries may follow disruption of spinal arteries during abdominal aortic operation. Experiments indicate that injury is predictable only after anterior spinal artery ligation just caudal to the entrance of a major thoracolumbar feeder, and not after ligating the dominant feeder itself, indicating inadequate alternative supply caudally.[249] However, predicting responses to vascular interruption in clinical situations is impossible because the sites and adequacy of feeders vary.

The arterial supply to the nerve roots has been intensively studied to understand the pathophysiology of lumbar radiculopathy and neural claudication from spinal stenosis.[250, 251] Like the anterior spinal trunk, the radicular arteries appear as a single continuous vessel from the intervertebral foramen to the cord but are in fact functionally two vessels with flow originating both at the cord end and in the intervertebral foramen, converging toward a watershed in the middle.[229, 251] This is fortuitous, because an obstruction from a pathologic compression will not block flow to either side but only in the compressed area. The radicular arteries branch within the root to supply the separate fascicles of the root, and they are markedly coiled at the origin of each branch to allow relative movement of the loosely bound fascicles.[156] The capillary network in the roots is much less developed than in peripheral nerves,[156] and there is no collateral arterial inflow along the course of the roots, which may be 20 cm long. It is fortunate, then, that transport of nutrients can take place from the ambient CSF through the gauze-like membranes surrounding the roots,[252] and that the P_{O_2} of the CSF, at about 67 mm Hg, exceeds that of the nerve root.[251] This alternative path for the exchange of nutrients is probably of greater importance than the vascular route.

Venous occlusion may also play a role in the genesis of radicular pain.[253] The arteries of roots are tolerant to chronic compression and maintain patency,[254] but venous obliteration and nerve root edema follow even a brief interval of root compression.[255] Roots have much less fibrous content than peripheral nerves.[256] This and the absence of a perineurium make them prone to damage by stretching,[257] which then results in venous stasis.[250] Crowding of the intervertebral foramen by disk or facet disease produces venous obstruction before impinging on the nerve and leads to fibrosis of the roots[258] and therefore diminished nutrient exchange with the CSF. Because posterior root ganglia are enclosed in a capsule, edema after ganglion compression causes a compartment syndrome with increased tissue pressure.[259]

Large and tortuous venous trunks are found on the anterior and posterior midline of the cord surface and drain to medullary veins that exit through the intervertebral foramina. Veins of the epidural space form a primitive, valveless plexus[260] composed of high-capacitance and thin-walled vessels that are exceedingly frail.[261, 262] This archaic system interconnects the deep veins of the pelvis, abdomen, chest, and head and conducts flow in any direction dictated by the relative pressures in these cavities.[263] Batson[261] and others[264] have highlighted the possibility of the distribution of venous metastasis via this route during caval occlusion. It is often claimed that conditions that cause generalized increased intra-abdominal pressure such as pregnancy and obesity will divert systemic venous flow into the vertebral canal. This is unlikely because epidural pressure increases in tandem with intra-abdominal pressure. Selective occlusion of the vena cava, however, does encourage venous flow into the alternative pathway of the epidural system by increasing venous pressures distal to the block,[265, 266] and flow reversal during caval occlusion by external abdominal compression has been observed.[267–269] There is no direct evidence of epidural venous distension during pregnancy or other clinical conditions.

The internal vertebral veins of the anterior epidural space are usually depicted as a double system with a medial and a lateral component, but dissection,[270] venography,[271] and cryomicrotome section[10] show a virtually confluent pool except at disk levels where the vessels are displaced laterally by the apposition of the dura and posterior longitudinal ligament with the disk (see Fig. 4–8A; Color Plate 3). Other than a tiny vascular pedicle entering the posterior fat in the midline between the ligamenta flava (Fig. 4–25; see Color Plate 6), there are essentially no veins in the posterior epidural space,[269] except caudal to the L5-S1 disk where the veins are widely distributed.[271]

There has been little study of the lymphatic system of the vertebral column. Epidural ink injection in rabbits shows that lymphatics begin draining particulate matter from the epidural space within 5 min.[272] Lymphatics play a minor role in the uptake of epidural drugs,[273]

but the dissipation of extruded disk material[274, 275] and blood injected for the treatment of post–lumbar puncture headache[276] indicates an active lymphatic system.

Peripheral Nervous System

Spinal Nerves

Lateral to the posterior root ganglion, the anterior and posterior spinal nerve roots break into small fascicles that then reassemble as the anterior and posterior primary rami of the segmental spinal nerve (see Fig. 4–19). This rearrangement via a miniature plexus distributes sensory and motor elements to both primary rami. The spinal nerve, defined as the united posterior and anterior spinal roots, exists only as this network of fascicles between the roots and primary rami.[277]

Because they supply only the skin and muscles along the vertebral column, the posterior primary rami are typically smaller than the anterior rami at the same level. The C-2 posterior rami are an exception; they innervate much of the scalp via the greater occipital nerve. Not all posterior primary rami have branches to the skin, including C-6 through C-8 (sometimes C-5) and L-4 and L-5. Skin branches from the other posterior rami descend steeply to their dermatomal field, so that the T-12 distal branches reach the iliac crest, T-10 supplies the skin over the L-2 and L-3 spinous processes, and L-1 supplies skin over the upper sacrum.[278] This is an important consideration in evaluating back pain or in planning regional anesthesia for back operation.

Ventral rami supply the rest of the trunk and limbs as well as the viscera via rami communicantes. The simple segmental arrangement of the trunk is distorted by the complicated morphogenesis of the neck and limbs, leading to union and division of the anterior primary rami at those levels. Exact connections within the plexuses and the distribution of segmental contributions are widely variable among subjects. For example, 28% of lumbosacral plexuses have central connections shifted proximally ("prefixed") or distally ("postfixed") along the vertebral column compared with the usual pattern.[279] Examination of 63 bodies showed seven major configurations of the brachial plexus, with none having more than 57% representation and 61% of bodies differing in type between right and left.[280] By means of plexuses, fibers from various cord segments are distributed to the necessary peripheral nerves. The anterior primary rami of the spinal nerves that give rise to a plexus are often referred to as the "roots" of that plexus. It is inaccurate and confusing, however, to use the term "spinal nerve root" for the neural structures external to the intervertebral foramen, as in "nerve root injection" (properly a paravertebral, foraminal, or segmental spinal nerve injection).

The various plexuses have been described as occupying fascial envelopes that contain the spread of anesthetic solution, although there is little evidence to support this. The brachial plexus originates between the anterior and middle scalene muscles, whose fascia overlies the origins of the plexus. More laterally, rather than lying freely within a dense fibrous container, the nerves[281] are enmeshed in loosely organized areolar tissue. Dissection is a technique prone to creating connective tissue planes where they are expected; areolar connective tissue can be dissected away until the nerves are evident, whereupon the remaining connective tissue is proclaimed a sheath. No sheath is evident on cryomicrotome sections (Fig. 4–26; see Color Plate 6).[282, 283] The illusion of a surrounding tubular sheath is, in part, due to the pattern of injectant spread. Direction is given to injected solution boluses and catheters, however, by adjacent structures and the grain of the connective tissue. The lumbar plexus is contained within the substance of the psoas muscle[284] rather than being in a fascial compartment, as is often claimed. No discernible sheath encloses the femoral nerve, so solution injected at the femoral nerve simply spreads out beneath the iliac muscle without reaching the lumbar plexus.[285]

Dermatomes

There is no segmentation evident on the surface of the spinal cord or by histologic examination of its substance. It is only by the grouping of rootlets into rootlet bundles bound for a common dorsal root ganglion and intervertebral foramen that a pattern of segments is superimposed on connections of the peripheral system with the central nervous system (CNS).

Because of interconnections of rootlets and roots, applying the concept of segmentation to the cord results in overlapping and oblique (nonaxial) separations between successive segments.[164, 165] With the exception of C-1, each vertebral segment is associated with a dermatome, defined as the cutaneous area supplied by that one spinal nerve. No sensory area has been identified for the first cervical segment, but fine C-1 posterior root fibers are found and produce orbital and forehead pain when mechanically or electrically stimulated during operation with local anesthesia.[286]

There is clearly extensive overlap between consecutive peripheral dermatomes, because the division of an individual root rarely produces an appreciable loss of sensibility.[287] Rootlets that contribute to a root innervate serially overlapping portions of the greater root dermatome; rootlets are ordered in sequence from the cephalad to caudal end of the dermatome according to their order along the cord.[288] The segmental distribution of fibers to the skin has been studied by mapping zoster eruptions, residual sensation after sectioning the roots on either side of an intact segment, absent sensation after root section or anesthesia, vasodilatation during stimulation of roots, and pain with nerve root compression and visceral disease.[278] The resulting diagrams, however, show considerable disagreement (Fig. 4–27).[289] Also, variability among subjects has been noted, perhaps owing to interconnections between roots. As a consequence, the sensory innervation of a particular site cannot be assigned with certainty to any segmental level. The dermatome for pain and temperature sensibility usually exceeds the dimensions of the

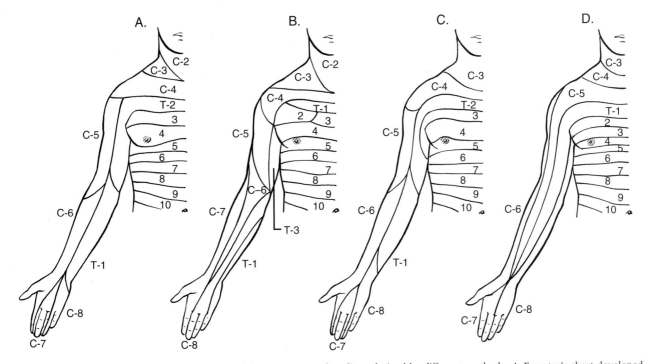

Figure 4–27 Examples of dermatome charts show different segmental outlines derived by different methods. *A*, Foerster's chart developed by root sections and observation of vasodilatation from stimulation of nerve stumps. *B*, Dermatomes according to Head, using distribution of herpes zoster lesions. *C*, Bonica's composite chart derived from nerve blocks and radiation of mechanical paresthesias. *D*, Pattern of hypalgesia observed by Keegan from clinical radiculopathy and after rhizotomy and local anesthetic injection. (Redrawn from Bonica JJ: The Management of Pain, 2nd ed, pp 133–140. Philadelphia, Lea & Febiger, 1990.)

dermatome for touch for the same root.[287] Furthermore, plasticity is evident in the connections of skin primary afferents to the CNS. The extent of cutaneous innervation of an isolated segmental spinal nerve is fully apparent only on section of longitudinal fibers of Lissauer's tract in the spinal cord above and below the test nerve, after which responses can be elicited from skin two segments away. Each sensory point is innervated by fibers from as many as five different roots.[290] After peripheral nerve section[291] or even epidural anesthesia,[292] CNS neurons develop novel proximal receptive fields at cutaneous sites where stimulation before nerve interruption produced no response. Receptive fields also expand to incorporate nearby regions of cutaneous injury at sites previously outside the innervated area.[293] Evidently, individual second-order sensory neurons in the cord have extensive suppressed, latent synapses with cutaneous nerves that are unmasked only after the loss of a dominant source of peripheral input. Facilitatory influences from adjacent segments have also been described.[294] This may explain the elusive nature of reliably defining peripheral or CNS connections (or both) and the inconsistency of dermatomal mapping.

Tests of peripheral motor manifestations of spinal segmentation may also result in confusion, because there is inconsistency in the segmental innervation of extremity muscles. Marked departure from the usual distribution of L-5 and S-1 motor fibers is found in 16% of subjects,[295] in whom stimulation of L-5 produces movement typical of S-1 and vice versa.

As limb buds elongate in utero, the nerves of the midportion of the plexus maintain their cutaneous representation in the hands and feet but become buried in the proximal limb (see Fig. 4–2). This produces an axial line on both surfaces of the limb where nonsequential dermatomes abut. For instance, C-4 and T-2 dermatomes adjoin on the chest and anterior shoulder, and C-6 contacts T-1 on the palmar forearm; the intervening nerves have grown out into the limbs and have no residual dermal representation proximally. A similar arrangement is evident in the lower limb. (A detailed discussion is available in *Gray's Anatomy*.[296]) Determination of the level of anesthesia achieved during spinal or epidural anesthesia requires careful attention to these discontinuities.

Peripheral Nerves

The outermost layer of a peripheral nerve, the epineurium, is made of loose connective tissue in continuity at the intervertebral foramen with the dura of the nerve root sleeve (see Fig. 4–19). Within this inert supporting tissue, the individual axons are organized into fascicles by a surrounding sheath, the perineurium. The endoneurium within the fascicles provides the connective tissue between the axons. As well as being a substantial structural element, the perineurium includes multiple layers of metabolically active epithelium.[297] Cells of the perineurium share common histologic and enzyme histochemical features with the pia-

arachnoid membranes, so it is highly probable that the perineurium controls the endoneural milieu in the same fashion as the pia-arachnoid does for the CNS.[298] By providing a diffusion barrier, the endothelium of the endoneurial vessels[299] and the perineurium[297] act as a "blood-nerve barrier" for the fascicles. Peripheral nerves are much more tolerant to vascular compromise than nerve roots[156] because of frequent collateral contributions and redundant routes of flow in the epineural and perineural layers.[298]

It has been recognized for many years that nerve fascicles may serve as a passive conduit for distribution of infectious agents or injected solution from the periphery to the CNS.[300] Injection outside the perineurium makes a local bleb on the nerve. However, after chance placement of the needle into a fascicle, solution enters with an ease similar to intravascular injection[301] and can travel great distances inside the perineural tube (Fig. 4–28).[302] Perineurium of the peripheral nerve is in proximal continuity with the porous inner layer of the nerve root meninges[303] and ends as an open-ended tube at the proximal end of the root.[304] Topologically, therefore, the interior of a peripheral nerve fascicle is separated from the CSF by only the attenuated

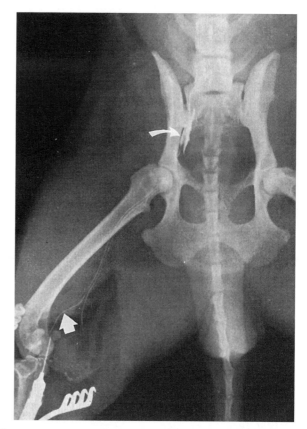

Figure 4–28 Injectant introduced into the distal perineural tube readily travels proximally. In this experimental example, solution injected into the peripheral nerve of the lower extremity of a dog (straight arrow) extended to the lumbosacral plexus (curved arrow) and even crossed into other fascicles to travel distally again. Some contrast material has also entered the subarachnoid space. (From French JD, Strain WH, Jones GE: Mode of extension of contrast substances injected into peripheral nerves. J Neuropathol Exp Neurol 1948; 7: 47–58.)

layers of overlying nerve root pia. By this route, intrafascicular peripheral injections travel in minutes to hours into the subpial space of the roots and then into the CSF or spinal cord.[305, 306] Damage to the cord or delayed spill into the CSF has been demonstrated.[301, 302] Although Moore and associates[301] recognized the clinical potential of intraneural injections to produce cord injury and spinal anesthesia, this pathway is infrequently considered as a mechanism of unexpected spinal anesthesia during perivertebral or more peripheral blocks. Injection into CSF in a nerve root sleeve is more often credited for such events but is a less likely cause of central spread.

Autonomic Nervous System

General Concepts

Autonomic mechanisms play a central role in maintaining stability during anesthesia, and in other cases they produce adverse phenomena. Because of this, a clear understanding of autonomic function is essential to the management of every anesthetic. The distribution of autonomic activity and the location of autonomic structures are especially pertinent in the use of regional anesthesia for surgical procedures and pain management. The broad outlines have been recognized for many years. However, there is a growing appreciation of complexity in the autonomic system that has outgrown the schematized presentation customary in general texts.

Originally, the autonomic nervous system was defined as neural elements that had no obvious connection to the central nervous system, particularly the large sympathetic trunks and deep neural plexuses. This distinction became less clear with the discovery of the rami communicantes, which connect the sympathetic trunks to the CNS, and of the influence of the brain on autonomic function. The autonomic system is viewed conventionally as controlling involuntary visceral activity, but exact boundaries of the autonomic nervous system are ambiguous and hard to delineate. Two features consistently distinguish the autonomic nervous system:

1. Efferent autonomic pathways from the CNS to the effector organs always include two neurons in series, the preganglionic and postganglionic fibers, that synapse in ganglia. (The adrenal gland is an exception.) Somatic motor signals follow a single cell pathway from cord to motor end plate.

2. Preganglionic autonomic neurons are organized in the CNS in compact nuclei, with cell bodies that are histologically distinct from somatic motor neurons.

Some neural pathways are not easily classified as either autonomic or somatic. Even though swallowing and phonation are mediated by the vagus nerve, which is commonly considered part of the parasympathetic system, these are largely voluntary functions. Also, the innervation of the larynx and pharynx is somatic in pattern, with a single cell path from the CNS to striated muscle, and therefore it should not be considered an autonomic component despite its route. (The vagus is similarly mixed with regard to afferent fibers, including both visceral afferents from internal organs and somatic afferents from the skin of the ear.) The internal plexus of nerves in the gut functions independently and also receives autonomic input; it is often considered separately as the enteric nervous system. Afferent fibers should not be included in the autonomic system.

Distinction between the two types of autonomic efferents, the sympathetic and parasympathetic systems, was originally based on the distribution of nerves to the effector organs (Langley, in Jänig and McLachlan[307]). Global functional patterns were attributed to the two systems in the early part of this century, with opposing roles described for each organ. In this formulation, stimulation and heightened activity characterize the sympathetic system (subserving fight or flight), whereas vegetative homeostasis is maintained by the parasympathetic system (rest and digest). Closer inspection, however, does not support a simple antagonism of the two systems. Some organs, such as the sweat glands, liver, and spleen, have only sympathetic innervation, whereas in the eye and bladder the sympathetic system plays a minor role and parasympathetic activity almost entirely determines activity.

Although simple functional antagonism is not a consistent feature distinguishing parasympathetic from sympathetic systems, some reliable distinctions can be made between the two autonomic divisions:

1. Site of preganglionic neuron cell body. Parasympathetic cell bodies are in the cranial nerve nuclei and in the intermediolateral cell column of the 2nd through 4th sacral spinal cord segments. The parasympathetic system can also be referred to as the craniosacral system. The sympathetic preganglionic cell bodies are in spinal cord segments T-1 through L-2, making this the thoracolumbar system.

2. Site of the preganglionic-postganglionic synapse. In the parasympathetic system, this is close to the innervated organ or actually in it, whereas the synapse and postganglionic cell bodies of the sympathetic system are in ganglia at a distance from the final destination (except the adrenal gland).

3. Neurotransmitter. Although preganglionic to postganglionic transmission is mediated principally by acetylcholine in both systems, the postganglionic neurotransmitter at the effector organ differs. Acetylcholine is the principal transmitter at all parasympathetic sites and at eccrine sweat glands (the neurotransmitter at apocrine glands is uncertain) and skeletal muscle vasodilator sites in the sympathetic system. The principal neurotransmitter at other sympathetic effector sites is norepinephrine.

Parasympathetic System

Preganglionic fibers of the parasympathetic system pass directly to the organ of destination. The vagus nerve is involved in 75% of all parasympathetic trans-

Table 4–1 Actions of the Parasympathetic System

Eye: pupillary constriction and accommodation
Lacrimal and salivary glands: secretion
Heart: bradycardia and decreased inotropy
Lungs: bronchoconstriction and secretion
Stomach and large and small intestine: secretion and peristalsis
Ureter and bladder: contraction
Genitalia: vasodilatation and erection

mission and distributes fibers as far distal in the digestive tract as the transverse colon. These axons terminate on ganglion cells embedded in plexuses in the walls of the target organs and produce actions summarized in Table 4–1.

Parasympathetic motor fibers in the oculomotor nerve synapse in the ciliary ganglion behind the eye, giving rise to short ciliary nerves to the iris. Salivary and lacrimal glands are innervated by parasympathetic fibers of the facial and glossopharyngeal nerves. Sacral parasympathetic fibers form the pelvic nerves and pass to the bladder, genitals, descending and sigmoid colon, and rectum where they synapse with postganglionic cells. There are no parasympathetic fibers in peripheral nerves to the extremities.

Sympathetic Nervous System

The golden age for the study of sympathetic nervous system anatomy was the 1930s through the 1950s. Enthusiasm for surgical neuroablative procedures for painful conditions and vascular insufficiency fueled research on histologic and anatomic features. Virtual abandonment of sympathetic surgery also led to a diminished appreciation of this anatomy. Advances in microscopy, neural labeling, and histochemical approaches have revealed new details of sympathetic structure and function.

Sympathetic Neural Pathways

The hypothalamus coordinates sympathetic activity, with various identifiable centers controlling temperature and circulatory regulation, metabolism, and fluid balance. Other important integrative sites are in the ventrolateral medulla, which in turn gives rise to poorly localized uncrossed descending tracts to the spinal cord. The preganglionic sympathetic cell bodies are clustered in the intermediolateral cell column and to a lesser extent more medially (the intermediomedial nucleus); they are much smaller than the motor neurons of the ventral horn. About 8% of the preganglionic cell population is lost per decade, perhaps contributing to the dysautonomia of the elderly.[308]

To some extent, preganglionic somata are distributed according to their target organs, so that at any segmental level, cells innervating viscera are grouped medially to those sending fibers to somatic destinations.[218] These cells are distributed in a somatotopic pattern longitudinally in the cord. However, because of the contracted span of segments containing preganglionic neurons

compared with the length of the entire cord, the destination of sympathetic activity initiated at a given spinal level does not superimpose on the sensory dermatome or myotome of that spinal level. Intermediolateral cells that produce sympathetic activity in the eye, lacrimal glands, and salivary glands are found at spinal levels corresponding to dermatomal segments T-1 to T-2; skin and muscles of the head and neck, T-1 to T-4; upper extremity, T-2 to T-8; and lower extremity, T-10 to L-2. (There is no exact agreement among authorities about these levels.[309]) Even though the preganglionic fibers in a single spinal nerve originate from only a limited ipsilateral region of the cord,[310] there is so much overlap of peripheral projections of the fibers that no clearly discernible sympathetic dermatomes can be identified.

Sympathetic efferent centers in the spinal cord for internal organs generally match the segmental destination of general visceral afferents from these sites (heart, T-1 to T-4 and perhaps T-5; lungs and bronchi, T-2 to T-6; stomach, pancreas, and small intestine, T-6 to T-10; colon up to the splenic flexure, T-10 to L-1; uterus and kidney, T-10 to T-11; distal colon, ureter, and bladder, L-1 and L-2).[311]

Rami Communicantes

Traditional teaching offers a standardized sympathetic wiring diagram (Fig. 4–29). Myelinated preganglionic fibers leave the spinal cord in the anterior roots of segments T-1 through L-2 and course from the spinal nerve to the paravertebral chain in the white rami communicantes. The fibers synapse in the paravertebral ganglia on the lateral aspects of the vertebral column, ascend or descend in the paravertebral chain to synapse at sites remote from their entry into the chain, or course medially in splanchnic nerves to synapse in prevertebral ganglia. The customary formulation further states that unmyelinated postganglionic axons rejoin the spinal nerves via the gray rami to innervate somatic structures. Some debate has centered on whether there are sympathetic efferents from the 8th cervical spinal segment or segments caudal to L-2, but the evidence is uncertain. Sympathetic innervation is not limited to segmental levels with spinal cord visceral efferents and white rami (T-1 to L-2) because the paravertebral chain and gray rami distribute postganglionic sympathetic fibers to spinal nerves at cervical, low lumbar, and sacral segments as well.

Despite their names, the gray and white rami communicantes are indistinguishable on gross examination.[187, 312, 313] The general schema described above dates to work that was performed before the use of electron microscopy, when identification of unmyelinated fibers was difficult. Modern findings diverge from the idealized view in important ways. Rather than all being myelinated B fibers, half[314] or more[315] of preganglionic axons are unmyelinated,[316–318] and some of the postganglionic fibers in the gray rami are myelinated.[314] Furthermore, the white rami carry not only preganglionic fibers but also an approximately equal number of postganglionic fibers,[314] and the gray rami also convey

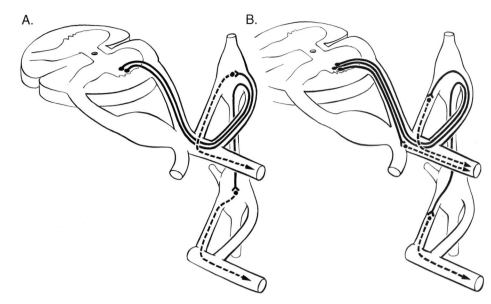

Figure 4–29 *A,* Conventional schematic diagram for sympathetic cell bodies and fiber routes. *B,* Ganglion cells, however, are also found at intermediate ganglia along the rami and peripheral nerve.

preganglionic axons.[308] Sensory axons from visceral sites are now known to reach the spinal cord via gray rami as well as white rami.[319] At the margins of the thoracolumbar sympathetic outflow, mixed rami contain both gray and white components.[320] Somatic motor fascicles may be found in cervical gray rami, in which they course to the strap muscles of the neck.

Conventional illustrations from dissections depict a single white and gray ramus at each thoracic level, but modern techniques show unexpected complexity and variability.[187, 321] The rami can have an ascending, descending, or transverse course from spinal nerve to sympathetic chain, where they join either at the ganglia or connecting segments. There are up to five rami per vertebral segment, and because they may cross en route to the sympathetic chain, segments within the chain overlap.

In addition to distributing fibers to limbs and body wall, gray rami contribute sympathetic efferent fibers to the posterior root ganglion and the anterior roots.[322, 323] Their function is unknown, but they markedly proliferate after peripheral nerve injury in that segment.[324]

Ganglia

The sympathetic ganglia (Greek for "knot") are fusiform expansions of the paravertebral chains and condensations in the prevertebral plexuses where the cell bodies of most postganglionic nerves reside. Most ganglion cells receive synaptic input from several preganglionic axons. These inputs have a variable ability to depolarize the ganglion cell, which may respond to a single strong input or multiple weak inputs by summation. Alternative sites, termed "intermediate ganglia," also contain ganglion cells and can be found throughout the cervical trunk, vertebral nerve, gray and white rami, and peripheral nerves.[325–329]

Somatotopic organization is evident in the ganglia, with cells of different morphology and peripheral destinations clustered in different parts of the ganglion.[330, 331] Another level of organization has been revealed by

histochemical typing of preganglionic and postganglionic cells. Although acetylcholine is the principal neurotransmitter in the ganglia, there is a large variety of substances released by preganglionic cells that influence synaptic function. These have been identified by immunoreactivity and include leu-enkephalin, neurotensin, substance P, somatostatin, vasoactive intestinal peptide, calcitonin gene–related peptide, and corticotropin-releasing factor.[332–335] Typically, acetylcholine is released at low stimulation frequencies and peptides are released at high stimulation frequencies.[336] A primary function of these regulatory peptides may be to alter neuronal excitability and thereby modulate the effectiveness of synaptic transmission for an hour or more.[335]

The neurotransmitters released by postganglionic cells at their effector sites are also diverse and specific to the innervated tissue and function.[337] About 15% of paravertebral ganglion cells have cholinergic sudomotor or vasodilator fibers (and may simultaneously release vasoactive intestinal peptide), but only 1% of prevertebral ganglion cells release acetylcholine at their terminus. At high firing rates, many of the adrenergic neurons corelease neuropeptide Y (vasoconstrictor fibers) or somatostatin (gut secretomotor fibers) and less often substance P, calcitonin gene–related peptide, or neurotensin. Inhibitory motor innervation of the gut and pilomotor fibers typically releases norepinephrine alone. These various cells in turn associate with preganglionic fibers that also have distinctive neuropeptide immunoreactivity.[338] This histochemical complexity may provide therapeutic opportunities.[339] Morphologic coding is similarly evident, because postganglionic fibers with different roles also group by size.[340]

As in other parts of the nervous system, ganglion function is subject to plasticity,[341–343] part of which may be due to changes in dendritic anatomy. Individual ganglion cells have been observed to sprout or retract dendritic branches over periods as short as 2 weeks.[344]

Ganglion cells, especially those in the prevertebral

ganglia, receive synapses from sensory fibers. The stellate ganglion also can integrate sensory information and function independently of the CNS.[345] Specifically, in a decentralized ganglion produced by sectioning the sympathetic chain on either side of the ganglion and all rami from the cord, mechanical and chemical stimulation of the heart still produces reflex stimulation of postganglionic efferents to the heart by way of synaptic contact in the ganglion. Integrative neural processing such as this is not accounted for by the traditional notion of sympathetic ganglia as sites for hard-wired monosynaptic relays. These investigations also indicate that there are visceral afferent neurons that have cell bodies not in the dorsal root ganglion but in the periphery, probably in the stellate ganglion.[346, 347]

Paravertebral Chains

Not all fibers leave the ganglia at the level at which they enter. In order to convey sympathetic fibers to the pelvis and legs, the ganglia on each side of the spinal column are joined into a chain by segments containing axons diverging longitudinally. To provide sympathetic innervation to the pelvis and lower extremities, lumbar and sacral chains continue caudally beyond the most inferior white ramus at L-2. Similarly, although central connections cease at T-1, the chain continues cephalad into the neck as the cervical trunk to deliver sympathetic fibers to the arms and head. There is usually less than one ganglion per body segment at thoracic levels,[187] and segmentation of the paravertebral chain is even less predictable at other levels.

The lumbar chain provides a site for therapeutic intervention, because chemical or surgical interruption at or below L-2 may completely deprive the lower extremities of sympathetic innervation. Even though fibers have been discovered crossing the midline anterior to the vertebral bodies from one chain to the other,[348, 349] these are rare. Unlike the thoracic chain, which passes along the head of the ribs in the posterior part of the chest, the lumbar chain lies against the vertebral column on its anterolateral aspect, along the insertion of the psoas muscle on the vertebral bodies. Because the psoas is more substantial at L-4 than at more cephalad levels, the sympathetic chain lies more anterior in the lower lumbar spine than at L-1 where it enters the abdomen under the medial arcuate ligament. At the L-5 level, the psoas diverges laterally away from the vertebral column, and the sympathetic chain plunges posteriorly to join the sacrum on its anterior surface.

Dense fibrous tissue ensheaths the vertebral column and also tightly encases the lumbar chain. The hourglass shape of the lumbar vertebral bodies[27] produces a tunnel where the connective tissue and chain span the pinched-in waist of the vertebral body (Figs. 4–1C; see Color Plate 1; and 4–30). This passage conducts the segmental vessels and rami communicantes to the intervertebral foramina, but it also allows solution injected against the vertebra at the midvertebral level to pass posteriorly to the foramina. Thus, the ideal needle position for lumbar sympathetic block is close

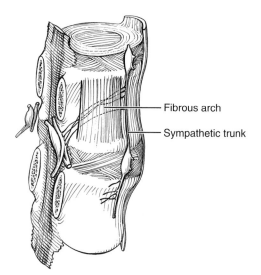

Figure 4–30 The rami communicantes pass from the intervertebral foramen anteriorly to the sympathetic chain beneath the fascia of the psoas muscle, which spans from the vertebral body end plates over the more narrow waist, making a fibrous tunnel. The segmental vessels (not shown) have the same route. Solution injected in the middle of the anterolateral vertebral body can pass through this tunnel to the intervertebral foramen and epidural space.

to or within the perivertebral fascia, just anterior to the psoas muscle, and adjacent to one of the vertebral end plates.

Distribution of ganglia in the rostral paravertebral chain is highly variable and may differ from side to side within one subject. Most often, there is one inferior cervical ganglion fused with the first thoracic ganglion to form the stellate, or thoracocervical, ganglion. The inferior cervical and first thoracic ganglia rarely fail to fuse,[325, 350] although a constriction in the middle of the stellate ganglion may represent vestigial segmentation. The chain continues cephalad as the cervical trunk assembled from strands emerging from the stellate ganglion that pass around the vertebral artery, often forming a vertebral ganglion. A middle cervical ganglion usually occurs at about the C-6 vertebral level, and a large superior cervical ganglion is found on the anterior surface of the C-1 and C-2 lateral masses.

The most frequent site for injection during cervicothoracic sympathetic block is the anterior tubercle of the vertebral transverse process of C-6 or C-7. These levels are chosen for safety and the clarity of the landmarks, not because this is the location of the ganglion. In vivo imaging with magnetic resonance shows the ganglion anterior to the inferior margin of the head of the first rib (Fig. 4–31; see Color Plate 7).[282] From dissections, a position is described at the seventh transverse process or between the seventh transverse process and the first rib. This higher location may be due to artifact from the loss of the downward traction of the lung when dissection opens the tissue planes.

Just medial to the stellate ganglion is the longus colli muscle, which inserts into the anterolateral aspect of the first three thoracic vertebral bodies. As it ascends into the neck, the muscle assumes a position anterior to the cervical transverse processes. The sympathetic chain likewise swings anterior as it passes cephalad, resting on the anterior surface of the longus colli muscle in the neck, enmeshed in the prevertebral fascia. The vertebral artery lies anterior to the stellate ganglion in the chest, but it must pass posteriorly into the foramen transversarium on ascending into the neck. Because of the crossing paths of the vessel and the sympathetic chain, the vertebral artery often actually penetrates between the strands that join the stellate ganglion to the cervical sympathetic chain. At and above the C-6 level, the vertebral artery is protected within the transverse process, whereas the artery passes anterior to the transverse process of C-7 (Fig. 4–32). Consequently, injection at C-7 may result in a greater risk of a systemic toxic response to local anesthetic. Occasionally (about 8% of necks[351]), the vertebral artery is exposed anterior to the transverse process of C-6 and C-5 as well. Because solution injected into the vertebral artery passes directly to the brain stem without dilution in the systemic blood, less than 1 mL of local anesthetic may produce a seizure.

The stellate ganglion is immediately adjacent to the C-8 and T-1 roots of the brachial plexus (Fig. 4–33; see Color Plate 8) with no fibrous barrier between them.[282] For this reason and because paratracheally injected solution passes readily into the epidural space,[88] it is impossible to eliminate the possibility of a subtle component of somatic block during a stellate block.

Local anesthetic injected just superficially to the prevertebral fascia at the sixth cervical vertebral anterior tubercle produces a block of the cervical sympathetic trunk that traverses this site, predictably resulting in Horner's syndrome. Inferiorly, the solution tracks down

into the mediastinum,[16, 352] in the same way that a retropharyngeal abscess dissects into the mediastinum via the same tissue planes. This carries the solution anterior to the stellate ganglion. Although sympathetic fibers heading to the upper roots of the plexus are well blocked where they originate from the middle cervical ganglion, most of the sympathetic input to the brachial plexus is carried to the inferior trunk by gray rami from the stellate ganglion inferiorly,[312] so sympathetic block of the arm is not a consistent result of anterior paratracheal injections.[353–355]

Other routes deliver sympathetic fibers to the head and upper extremity. The vertebral nerve originates from the stellate ganglion and ascends with the vertebral artery into the neck where it provides gray rami to the cervical nerve roots up to the C-3 level[313, 326, 327, 356] and intracranial innervation following the basilar artery.[357] This pathway includes preganglionic fibers that may actually outnumber the fibers ascending in the cervical sympathetic trunk[327] as well as ganglion cells. For these reasons, the vertebral nerve may be considered a deep system in parallel with the cervical sympathetic trunk. The plexus accompanying the carotid artery may similarly deliver sympathetic fibers to the third through fifth cervical levels.[327, 358] Linked branches of the sinuvertebral nerves in the vertebral canal also provide ascending sympathetic innervation in parallel with the sympathetic chain.[359] Sympathetic fibers can reach the brachial plexus without passing through the stellate ganglion or sympathetic chain via branches of the second and third intercostal nerves.[360] These nerves of Kuntz are identified only occasionally by gross inspection, but with modern staining techniques, numerous large nerves and small connecting fibers, many with ganglion cells, have been discovered in most[187] or all specimens.[321] Other sympathetic traffic bypasses the paravertebral chain when preganglionic neurons synapse in intermediate ganglia in the spinal nerve with ganglion cells that send postganglionic fibers directly to the peripheral nerves.[328] The importance of these alternative paths is that sympathetic nerve blocks or surgical ablative procedures may in fact produce incomplete sympathetic interruption.[361]

The accumulating bulk of evidence points strongly to the existence of a sympathetic supply to the upper limb so extensive that no practical operation . . . can be relied on to effect an absolutely complete denervation.

B.S. Ray (1953)

Prevertebral Plexuses

The gray rami are lateral branches from the paravertebral sympathetic chain that deliver sympathetic fibers to the body wall and extremities. As many as 11 medial branches per segment[187] also leave the chain to provide sympathetic innervation to intrathoracic and intra-abdominal viscera. Postganglionic fibers, some myelinated, are found in these medial branches.[331] Most, however, are preganglionic fibers (usually unmyelinated[331]) that synapse with ganglion cells among the neural mesh that forms a nearly continuous plexus along the great arteries of the chest and abdomen. Portions of

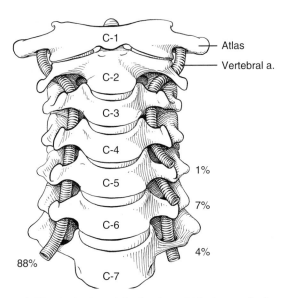

Figure 4–32 Distribution of the level at which the vertebral artery (a.) enters the transverse process. Most common is at C-6, shown on the anatomic right side of this compound image. However, other entry sites are not rare (12% of total). (From Bergman Thompson SA, Afifi AK, et al: Catalog of Human Anatomic Variation, 2nd ed, p 368. © Williams & Wilkins, Baltimore, 1988.)

this network and adjacent groups of ganglion cells (prevertebral ganglia) are named for the vessel they surround, but clear boundaries are not evident. Important medial sympathetic branches from the paravertebral chains include the cardiac nerves from the superior, stellate, and especially the middle cervical ganglion, leading to the cardiac plexus; the greater splanchnic nerve (T-5 to T-9) to the celiac ganglion; the lesser splanchnic nerve (T-9 to T-10) to the aorticorenal ganglion; the least splanchnic nerve (T-11 to T-12; often absent) to the renal plexus; the lumbar splanchnic nerves to the celiac and mesenteric plexuses and superior hypogastric plexus; and median branches from the sacral chain to the inferior hypogastric plexus. The two paravertebral chains terminate by joining in the single midline ganglion impar.

As in the stellate ganglion, prevertebral ganglia integrate sensory information. Visceral afferents from the gut alter postganglionic efferent activity in the prevertebral mesenteric ganglia, producing a viscerosympathetic reflex independent of the spinal cord[362] and mediated by synapses from branches of visceral afferents on their way to the cord. Parasympathetic preganglionic fibers also contribute to the formation of the prevertebral plexuses. Vagal elements intermix in the cardiac and celiac plexuses and may even synapse within the prevertebral ganglia to gate efferent sympathetic activity.[363] Sacral parasympathetic fibers are brought to the inferior hypogastric plexuses by the pelvic splanchnic nerves (twigs from S-2 to S-4) and further ascend to the superior hypogastric and inferior mesenteric plexuses.

Adrenal Gland

The adrenal gland is composed of large chromaffin cells, homologous with ganglion cells elsewhere in the sympathetic system. Preganglionic fibers, many of them nonmyelinated, innervate the gland, distributing from their origin in spinal segments T-8 to L-1 through the greater splanchnic nerve and celiac plexus and to some degree the lesser splanchnic nerve. Unlike other sympathetic circuits, the postganglionic cells of the adrenal gland release epinephrine as well as norepinephrine.

Peripheral Distribution of Sympathetic Fibers

Virtually all arteries and arterioles are surrounded by sympathetic nerve axons. Veins in the extremities have negligible innervation, but visceral veins are extensively supplied with sympathetic terminals and participate in control of vascular capacitance.[364] Innervation of most vessels in the limbs is by postganglionic axons branching off from peripheral nerves, as is the sympathetic supply to piloerector muscles and sweat glands of the skin, rather than by extension of sympathetic axons that accompany the large arteries of the trunk. In the peripheral nerve, sympathetic postganglionic axons are bundled together by Schwann cells and make up about 23% of the total fiber count.[365] Efferent sympathetic fibers supplying a cutaneous region do not necessarily arrive by the same pathway as the sensory

afferents supplying that area. For instance,[366] the radial aspect of the dorsum of the hand receives sensory and sudomotor innervation via the radial nerve but vasomotor innervation from the median nerve. Similarly, the lateral aspect of the foot may receive its sympathetic input from peroneal branches but transmit sensory information in the sural nerve.[367]

Each sympathetic fiber ends in a series of several hundred varicosities that, in the past, were thought to form only distant and poorly organized contact with effector cell membranes that were generally responsive to norepinephrine. Careful microscopic imaging has revealed, however, that almost all varicosities form close, specialized synaptic contact resembling the neuromuscular junction.[368] Electrophysiologic studies have also confirmed quantal transmission at sympathetic synapses.[307, 369]

Sympathetic Function

Sympathetic effects (Table 4–2) underlie homeostatic integration of thermal and fluid balance, respiration, metabolism, and circulation. Much of this is achieved through vascular mechanisms that are complex and include widely distributed vasoconstrictor and vasodilator[370] fibers influenced by numerous reflexes.

Early authors described the pattern of sympathetic activation as a simultaneous all-or-none response of the entire system in a widely distributed manner, unlike the detailed and localized discharge of parasympathetic elements. This was supported by the discovery of extensive divergence of sympathetic impulses in the ganglia, where between 28 and 176 postganglionic cells are found for every arriving preganglionic axon, compared with a ratio of about 1:5 for parasympathetic ganglia. More recent study, however, has revealed graded and differential patterns of activity in sympathetic fibers bound for different effectors or different organs. For instance, muscle vasoconstrictor fibers, unlike cutaneous vasoconstrictor fibers, are under baroreceptor and respiratory control.[307] Distinct patterns of spontaneous and reflex activity characterize vasodilator, pilomotor, sudomotor, and various motility neurons, and sympathetic activity to different vascular beds may respond in opposite ways to reflex stimuli.[371] Reflex patterns are organized by connections in the spinal cord and persist in spinal animals.[372] It is evidently not appropriate to speculate about an overall sympathetic

Table 4–2 Sympathetic Actions at Specific Organs

Skin: piloerector and sudomotor
Eye: pupillary dilatation
Salivary glands: viscid secretion and vasoconstriction
Heart: increased inotropy and chronotropy
Lungs: bronchodilatation
Stomach and small and large intestine: inhibition of secretion and peristalsis, increased sphincter tone
Ureter and bladder: inhibited contraction except increased trigone and sphincter tone
Genitalia: ejaculation
Metabolism: hepatic gluconeogenesis and glycogenolysis and decreased pancreatic insulin production

tone that might characterize all aspects of sympathetic activity.[307] Anatomic and physiologic evidence instead depicts a system of distinct functional pathways with focal, graded effects.

Visceral Afferents

Regulatory and nociceptive information from the internal organs of the thorax and abdomen and from peripheral blood vessels is transmitted by visceral afferent fibers. Their axons are A-δ and C fibers that end with simple free terminals and respond to increased wall or capsule tension, inflammation, or ischemia. In addition to signaling information through propagated membrane depolarizations, axonal transport in these sensory fibers may deliver important trophic substances. Visceral afferent fibers in the vagus have cell bodies in the nodose ganglion and transmit nonconscious regulatory stimuli as well as sensations of fullness and nausea but not pain. (An exception is conscious sensations, including irritation, conveyed from the hypopharynx and upper airway by the superior and recurrent laryngeal branches of the vagus.) Stimulation of vagal afferents may, however, cause generalized inhibitory[373] or stimulatory[374] effects on spinal neurons that transmit nociceptive information. The balance of this discussion centers on noncranial visceral afferents.

Except for certain peripheral sensory cells forming closed reflex loops in the sympathetic ganglia, the cell bodies of noncranial visceral afferents, like somatic afferents, reside in the spinal dorsal root ganglia. Visceral sensory axons characteristically are located in sympathetic pathways. Fibers converge on the prevertebral ganglia, continue without synapses to the paravertebral chain via the splanchnic nerves and other medial branches of the chain, and join the segmental nerves of levels T-1 to L-2 through the white rami communicantes and sometimes the gray rami.[319] They then pass into the spinal cord through the dorsal root. Some visceral afferent traffic alternatively reaches the cord through the ventral root; 30% of axons in feline S-1 anterior root are unmyelinated afferents.[149] There are no afferents entering the thoracolumbar cord from the head.[372] An unresolved question is the extent and importance of afferents from the extremities and body wall that pass through the sympathetic chain. Sensory pathways from the vessels of the extremities through the white rami might transmit vascular sensibility.[375] Most of these fibers join peripheral nerves, but some may follow arteries to the sympathetic chain. It has been argued[376] that painful conditions commonly referred to as causalgia or reflex sympathetic dystrophy are not related to aberrant sympathetic efferent activity but are simply nociception mediated by visceral afferents from the extremities. Solid evidence supports a sympathetic pathway for deep somatic afferents from the chest wall[377, 378] and vertebral column.

Because visceral sensory neurons pass through the sympathetic chain, and in many cases play a role in modulating sympathetic efferent activity, these neu-

rons are often included as part of the sympathetic nervous system. Various features make this an awkward grouping. First of all, not all visceral sensation passes centrally through sympathetic structures.[379] From the sigmoid colon, rectum, neck of the bladder, prostate, and cervix of the uterus, most visceral afferent fibers retrace the route of parasympathetic efferent neurons, entering the cord in the posterior roots of S-2 to S-4. A few fibers from these organs ascend in the prevertebral plexuses to enter at L-1 or L-2 and have an uncertain role. Afferents from thoracic organs, pancreas, and biliary tree ascend in the phrenic nerve as well as passing to the thoracic cord via medial branches of the sympathetic chain.

Second, the boundary between somatic and visceral afferent systems is not simple. There is a growing recognition that most primary visceral afferent fibers synapse in the spinal dorsal horn with second-order cells that also receive input from somatic structures.[379, 380] The response of a single cell to stimulation at both somatic (usually skin) and visceral receptive fields, known as viscerosomatic convergence, is likewise common at more cephalad sites in the brain stem. Visceral afferent fibers are few in number and have large and overlapping receptive fields, which results in a poor ability to characterize and localize visceral stimuli. Although visceral afferents comprise less than 10% of all fibers entering the thoracolumbar spinal cord, 75% of thoracic dorsal horn cells receive visceral sensory input,[381] and the stimulation of a single visceral nerve, unlike stimulation of a somatic nerve, is followed by neuronal excitation in widespread segments of the cord.[379] In a teleologic sense, viscerosomatic convergence and extensive central divergence of visceral information provide an efficient means for the small number of fibers to produce an ascending signal, using structures usually conducting somatic information until an intense internal stimulus intervenes. Referred pain is probably explained by this anatomic arrangement, because ascending signals from cells most often activated by skin primary afferents create a perception of skin sensation on the less frequent occasions when they are activated by visceral input.

Finally, categorizing visceral afferents as part of the sympathetic system ignores similarities between visceral and deep somatic sensory organization:[380]

1. Deep somatic fibers, like visceral afferents, converge on secondary neurons that are multireceptive with skin input. This is particularly true of the innervation of the vertebral column[217]; dorsal horn cells that respond to vertebral stimulation not only receive input from multiple deep midline and truncal sites but also always have convergent input from the skin, sometimes bilaterally. This hyperconvergence contributes to the clinical challenge of diagnosing back and extremity pain.

2. Visceral afferents and deep somatic afferents end in dorsal horn laminae I and V, unlike skin fibers, which distribute more widely in the cord gray matter.

3. Whereas dorsal horn neurons that receive input only from skin afferents may respond exclusively to

nociceptive stimuli or exclusively to low-threshold stimuli, visceral and deep somatic circuits always respond to a broad range of stimuli in a graded fashion (wide dynamic range); because no purely nociceptive visceral or deep somatic afferents are found, pain is probably encoded by stimulus intensity and cell firing rate.

4. Visceral and deep somatic stimuli produce a similar quality of poorly localized discomfort, referred pain, and a generalized increase in CNS excitability with motor and autonomic reflexes. Visceral afferents are not a natural part of the sympathetic system and are not distinct in a simple way from the somatic system.

Conclusions

Anatomic themes of particular importance in regional anesthesia include the following:

1. Variability. Few structures are strictly consistent in size, location, or design among individuals or even between the opposite sides of an individual (e.g., plexus layout, vertebral segmentation).

2. Complexity. The closer anatomy is examined, the more elaborate it appears (e.g., paravertebral chain connections, arachnoid membranes in the posterior subarachnoid space).

3. Plasticity. Anatomy, especially of neural elements, changes with time and conditions (e.g., afferent terminations of myelinated sensory axons,[382] synapses within sympathetic ganglia, cutaneous receptive fields of CNS neurons).

References

1. Baljet B, Drukker J: An acetylcholinesterase method for in toto staining of peripheral nerves. Stain Technol 1975; 50: 31–36.
2. Blomberg R: The dorsomedian connective tissue band in the lumbar epidural space of humans: an anatomical study using epiduroscopy in autopsy cases. Anesth Analg 1986; 65: 747–752.
3. Blomberg RG, Olsson SS: The lumbar epidural space in patients examined with epiduroscopy. Anesth Analg 1989; 68: 157–160.
4. Luyendijk W, van Voorthuisen AE: Contrast examination of the spinal epidural space. Acta Radiol Diagn (Stockh) 1966; 5: 1051–1066.
5. Hatten HP Jr: Lumbar epidurography with metrizamide. Radiology 1980; 137: 129–136.
6. Reynolds AF Jr, Roberts PA, Pollay M, et al: Quantitative anatomy of the thoracolumbar epidural space. Neurosurgery 1985; 17: 905–907.
7. Savolaine ER, Pandya JB, Greenblatt SH, et al: Anatomy of the human lumbar epidural space: new insights using CT-epidurography. Anesthesiology 1988; 68: 217–220.
8. Husemeyer RP, White DC: Topography of the lumbar epidural space. A study in cadavers using injected polyester resin. Anaesthesia 1980; 35: 7–11.
9. Harrison GR, Parkin IG, Shah JL: Resin injection studies of the lumbar extradural space. Br J Anaesth 1985; 57: 333–336.
10. Hogan QH: Lumbar epidural anatomy. A new look by cryomicrotome section. Anesthesiology 1991; 75: 767–775.
11. Ferrer-Brechner T, Brechner VL: Accuracy of needle placement during diagnostic and therapeutic nerve blocks. Adv Pain Res Ther 1975; 1: 679–683.
12. Jain S, Shah N, Bedford R: Needle position for paravertebral and sympathetic nerve blocks: radiologic confirmation is needed. (Abstract.) Anesth Analg 1991; 72: S125.
13. White AH, Derby R, Wynne G: Epidural injections for the diagnosis and treatment of low-back pain. Spine 1980; 5: 78–86.
14. Renfrew DL, Moore TE, Kathol MH, et al: Correct placement of epidural steroid injections: fluoroscopic guidance and contrast administration. Am J Neuroradiol 1991; 12: 1003–1007.
15. Ross BK, Coda B, Heath CH: Local anesthetic distribution in a spinal model: a possible mechanism of neurologic injury after continuous spinal anesthesia. Reg Anesth 1992; 17: 69–77.
16. Hogan QH, Erickson SJ, Haddox JD, et al: The spread of solutions during stellate ganglion block. Reg Anesth 1992; 17: 78–83.
17. Hogan QH: Tuffier's line: the normal distribution of anatomic parameters. (Letter to the editor.) Anesth Analg 1994; 78: 194–195.
18. Bergman RA, Thompson SA, Afifi AK, et al: Compendium of Human Anatomic Variation: Text, Atlas, and World Literature, 2nd ed. Baltimore, Urban & Schwarzenberg, 1988.
19. Norenberg A, Johanson DC, Gravenstein JS: Racial differences in sacral structure important in caudal anesthesia. Anesthesiology 1979; 50: 549–551.
20. Amonoo-Kuofi HS: Maximum and minimum lumbar interpedicular distances in normal adult Nigerians. J Anat 1982; 135: 225–233.
21. Edwards EA: Operative anatomy of the lumbar sympathetic chain. Angiology 1951; 2: 184–198.
22. MacGibbon B, Farfan HF: A radiologic survey of various configurations of the lumbar spine. Spine 1979; 4: 258–266.
23. Quinnell RC, Stockdale HR: The use of in vivo lumbar discography to assess the clinical significance of the position of the intercrestal line. Spine 1983; 8: 305–307.
24. Sjögren P, Gefke K, Banning AM, et al: Lumbar epidurography and epidural analgesia in cancer patients. Pain 1989; 36: 305–309.
25. Gielen MJ, Slappendel R, Merx JL: Asymmetric onset of sympathetic blockade in epidural anaesthesia shows no relation to epidural catheter position. Acta Anaesthesiol Scand 1991; 35: 81–84.
26. Van Gessel EF, Forster A, Gamulin Z: Continuous spinal anesthesia: where do spinal catheters go? Anesth Analg 1993; 76: 1004–1007.
27. Ericksen MF: Some aspects of aging in the lumbar spine. Am J Phys Anthropol 1976; 45: 575–580.
28. Berry JL, Moran JM, Berg WS, et al: A morphometric study of human lumbar and selected thoracic vertebrae. Spine 1987; 12: 362–367.
29. Scoles PV, Linton AE, Latimer B, et al: Vertebral body and posterior element morphology: the normal spine in middle life. Spine 1988; 13: 1082–1086.
30. Hurme M, Alaranta H, Aalto T, et al: Lumbar spinal canal size of sciatica patients. Acta Radiol 1989; 30: 353–357.
31. Panjabi MM, Takata K, Goel V, et al: Thoracic human vertebrae. Quantitative three-dimensional anatomy. Spine 1991; 16: 888–901.
32. Panjabi MM, Duranceau J, Goel V, et al: Cervical human vertebrae. Quantitative three-dimensional anatomy of the middle and lower regions. Spine 1991; 16: 861–869.
33. Amonoo-Kuofi HS: The sagittal diameter of the lumbar vertebral canal in normal adult Nigerians. J Anat 1985; 140: 69–78.
34. Willis TA: An analysis of vertebral anomalies. Am J Surg 1929; 6: 163–168.
35. Todd TW: Numerical significance in the thoraco-lumbar vertebrae of the mammalia. Anat Rec 1922; 24: 261–286.
36. Trotter M: Variations of the sacral canal: their significance in the administration of caudal analgesia. Anesth Analg 1947; 26: 192–202.
37. Miyasaka K, Kaneda K, Ito T, et al: Ossification of spinal ligaments causing thoracic radiculomyelopathy. Radiology 1982; 143: 463–468.
38. Milne N: The role of zygapophysial joint orientation and uncinate processes in controlling motion in the cervical spine. J Anat 1991; 178: 189–201.
39. Singer KP, Breidahl PD, Day RE: Variations in zygapophyseal

joint orientation and level of transition at the thoracolumbar junction. Preliminary survey using computed tomography. Surg Radiol Anat 1988; 10: 291–295.

40. Davis PR: The thoraco-lumbar mortice joint. J Anat 1955; 89: 370–377.

41. Singer KP: Thoracolumbar mortice joint: radiological and histological observations. Clin Biomech 1989; 4: 137–143.

42. Pal GP, Routal RV: A study of weight transmission through the cervical and upper thoracic regions of the vertebral column in man. J Anat 1986; 148: 245–261.

43. Davis PR: Human lower lumbar vertebrae: some mechanical and osteological considerations. J Anat 1961; 95: 337–344.

44. Yang KH, King AI: Mechanism of facet load transmission as a hypothesis for low-back pain. Spine 1984; 9: 557–565.

45. Dory MA: Arthrography of the lumbar facet joints. Radiology 1981; 140: 23–27.

46. Raymond J, Dumas J-M: Intraarticular facet block: diagnostic test or therapeutic procedure? Radiology 1984; 151: 333–336.

47. Moran R, O'Connell D, Walsh MG: The diagnostic value of facet joint injections. Spine 1988; 13: 1407–1410.

48. Bogduk N, Engel R: The menisci of the lumbar zygapophyseal joints. A review of their anatomy and clinical significance. Spine 1984; 9: 454–460.

49. Wang ZL, Yu S, Haughton VM: Age-related changes in the lumbar facet joints. Clin Anat 1989; 2: 55–62.

50. Giles LG, Taylor JR: Human zygapophyseal joint capsule and synovial fold innervation. Br J Rheumatol 1987; 26: 93–98.

51. Heylings DJ: Supraspinous and interspinous ligaments of the human lumbar spine. J Anat 1978; 125: 127–131.

52. Williams DM, Gabrielsen TO, Latack JT: Ossification in the caudal attachments of the ligamentum flavum. An anatomic and computed tomographic study. Radiology 1982; 145: 693–697.

53. Williams DM, Gabrielsen TO, Latack JT, et al: Ossification in the cephalic attachment of the ligamentum flavum. An anatomical and CT study. Radiology 1984; 150: 423–426.

54. Maigne JY, Ayral X, Guerin-Surville H: Frequency and size of ossifications in the caudal attachments of the ligamentum flavum of the thoracic spine. Role of rotatory strains in their development. An anatomic study of 121 spines. Surg Radiol Anat 1992; 14: 119–124.

55. Butler D, Trafimow JH, Andersson GB, et al: Discs degenerate before facets. Spine 1990; 15: 111–113.

56. Epstein JA, Epstein BS, Lavine LS, et al: Lumbar nerve root compression at the intervertebral foramina caused by arthritis of the posterior facets. J Neurosurg 1973; 39: 362–369.

57. Cork RC, Kryc JJ, Vaughan RW: Ultrasonic localization of the lumbar epidural space. Anesthesiology 1980; 52: 513–516.

58. Palmer SK, Abram SE, Maitra AM, et al: Distance from the skin to the lumbar epidural space in an obstetric population. Anesth Analg 1983; 62: 944–946.

59. Rosenberg H, Keykhak MM: Distance to the epidural space in nonobstetric patients. (Letter to the editor.) Anesth Analg 1984; 63: 539–540.

60. Currie JM: Measurement of the depth to the extradural space using ultrasound. Br J Anaesth 1984; 56: 345–347.

61. Harrison GR, Clowes NW: The depth of the lumbar epidural space from the skin. Anaesthesia 1985; 40: 685–687.

62. Sutton DN, Linter SP: Depth of extradural space and dural puncture. Anaesthesia 1991; 46: 97–98.

63. Greene HM: Lumbar puncture and the prevention of postpuncture headache. JAMA 1926; 86: 391–392.

64. Smith CG: Changes in length and position of the segments of the spinal cord with changes in posture in the monkey. Radiology 1956; 66: 259–265.

65. Reid JD: Effects of flexion-extension movements of the head and spine upon the spinal cord and nerve roots. J Neurol Neurosurg Psychiatr 1960; 23: 214–221.

66. Breig A, Marions O: Biomechanics of the lumbosacral nerve roots. Acta Radiol (Diagn) 1963; 1: 1141–1160.

67. Kubik S, Muntener M: Zur Topographie der spinalen Nervenwurzeln. II. Der Einfluss des Wachstums des Duralsackes, sowie der Krummungen und der Bewegungen der Wirgelsaule auf die Verlaufsrichtung der spinalen Nervenwurzeln. Acta Anat (Basel) 1969; 74: 149–168.

68. Williams CR, Grafe MR, Mathews S: The long-term epidural tissue reaction to three different catheter materials. (Abstract.) Reg Anesth 1994; 19(Suppl): 18.

69. Hogan Q, Lynch K, Lacitis I: Histologic features of epidural soft tissue and its relation to the dura and canal wall. (Abstract.) Reg Anesth 1993; 18(Suppl): 54.

70. Ramsey HJ: Fat in the epidural space of young and adult cats. Am J Anat 1959; 104: 345–380.

71. Ramsey HJ: Comparative morphology of fat in the epidural space. Am J Anat 1959; 105: 219–232.

72. Asato F, Hirakawa N, Oda M, et al: A median epidural septum is not a common cause of unilateral epidural blockade. Anesth Analg 1990; 71: 427–429.

73. Singer KP, Giles LG, Day RE: Intra-articular synovial folds of thoracolumbar junction zygapophyseal joints. Anat Rec 1990; 226: 147–152.

74. George WE Jr, Wilmot M, Greenhouse A, et al: Medical management of steroid-induced epidural lipomatosis. N Engl J Med 1983; 308: 316–319.

75. Quint DJ, Boulos RS, Sanders WP, et al: Epidural lipomatosis. Radiology 1988; 169: 485–490.

76. Badami JP, Hinck VC: Symptomatic deposition of epidural fat in a morbidly obese woman. AJNR 1982; 3: 664–665.

77. Bednar DA, Esses SI, Kucharczyk W: Symptomatic lumbar epidural lipomatosis in a normal male. A unique case report. Spine 1990; 15: 52–53.

78. Herzog RJ, Kaiser JA, Saal JA, et al: The importance of posterior epidural fat pad in lumbar central canal stenosis. Spine 1991; 16 (6 Suppl): S227–S233.

79. Rocco AG, Scott DA, Boas RA, et al: The epidural space behaves as a Starling resistor and inflow resistance is elevated in a diseased epidural space. (Abstract.) Reg Anesth 1990; 15(Suppl): 39.

80. Usubiaga JE, Wikinski JA, Usubiaga LE: Epidural pressure and its relation to spread of anesthetic solutions in epidural space. Anesth Analg 1967; 46: 440–446.

81. Paul DL, Wildsmith JA: Extradural pressure following the injection of two volumes of bupivacaine. Br J Anaesth 1989; 62: 368–372.

82. Guyton AC, Granger HJ, Taylor AE: Interstitial fluid pressure. Physiol Rev 1971; 51: 527–563.

83. Shah JL: Influence of cerebrospinal fluid on epidural pressure. Anaesthesia 1981; 36: 627–631.

84. Nickalls RW, Kokri MS: The width of the posterior epidural space in obstetric patients. (Letter to the editor.) Anaesthesia 1986; 41: 432–433.

85. Kumar A, Battit GE, Froese AB, et al: Bilateral cervical and thoracic epidural blockade complicating interscalene brachial plexus block: report of two cases. Anesthesiology 1971; 35: 650–652.

86. Scammell SJ: Case report: inadvertent epidural anaesthesia as a complication of interscalene brachial plexus block. Anaesth Intensive Care 1979; 7: 56–57.

87. Lombard TP, Couper JL: Bilateral spread of analgesia following interscalene brachial plexus block. Anesthesiology 1983; 58: 472–473.

88. Evans JA, Dobben GD, Gay GR: Peridural effusion of drugs following sympathetic blockade. JAMA 1967; 200: 573–578.

89. Moore DC: Complications of Regional Anesthesia: Etiology—Signs and Symptoms—Treatment, pp 53–54. Springfield, IL, Charles C Thomas, 1955.

90. Middaugh RE, Menk EJ, Reynolds WJ, et al: Epidural block using large volumes of local anesthetic solution for intercostal nerve block. Anesthesiology 1985; 63: 214–216.

91. Krempen JF, Smith BS, DeFreest LJ: Selective nerve root infiltration for the evaluation of sciatica. Orthop Clin North Am 1975; 6: 311–315.

92. Blikra G: Intradural herniated lumbar disc. J Neurosurg 1969; 31: 676–679.

93. Cheng PA: The anatomical and clinical aspects of epidural anesthesia. Anesth Analg 1963; 42: 398–415.

94. Hardy PA: Can epidural catheters penetrate dura mater? An anatomical study. Anaesthesia 1986; 41: 1146–1147.

95. Fink BR, Walker S: Orientation of fibers in human dorsal lumbar dura mater in relation to lumbar puncture. Anesth Analg 1989; 69: 768–772.

96. Bernards CM, Hill HF: Morphine and alfentanil permeability through the spinal dura, arachnoid, and pia mater of dogs and monkeys. Anesthesiology 1990; 73: 1214–1219.

97. Patin DJ, Eckstein EC, Harum K, et al: Anatomic and biomechanical properties of human lumbar dura mater. Anesth Analg 1993; 76: 535–540.

98. Reitan H: On movements of fluid inside the cerebro-spinal space. Acta Radiol 1941; 22: 762–779.

99. Scott WG, Furlow LT: Myelography with pantopaque and a new technic for its removal. Radiology 1944; 43: 241–249.

100. Epstein BS: The effect of increased interspinal pressure on the movement of iodized oil within the spinal canal. Am J Roentgenol 1944; 52: 196–199.

101. Martins AN, Wiley JK, Myers PW: Dynamics of the cerebrospinal fluid and the spinal dura mater. J Neurol Neurosurg Psychiatr 1972; 35: 468–473.

102. Watanabe S, Yamaguchi H, Ishizawa Y: Level of spinal anesthesia can be predicted by the cerebrospinal fluid pressure difference between full-flexed and non–full-flexed lateral position. Anesth Analg 1991; 73: 391–393.

103. Shanthaveerappa TR, Bourne GH: The "perineural epithelium," a metabolically active, continuous, protoplasmic cell barrier surrounding peripheral nerve fasciculi. J Anat 1962; 96: 527–537.

104. Shantha TR: Subdural space: What is it? Does it exist? (Abstract.) Reg Anesth 1992; 17(Suppl): 85.

105. Mehta M, Maher R: Injection into the extra-arachnoid subdural space. Experience in the treatment of intractable cervical pain and in the conduct of extradural (epidural) analgesia. Anaesthesia 1977; 32: 760–766.

106. Rubin RC, Henderson ES, Ommaya AK, et al: The production of cerebrospinal fluid in man and its modification by acetazolamide. J Neurosurg 1966; 25: 430–436.

107. Cutler RW, Page L, Galicich J, et al: Formation and absorption of cerebrospinal fluid in man. Brain 1968; 91: 707–720.

108. Milhorat TH: The third circulation revisited. J Neurosurg 1975; 42: 628–645.

109. Oreskovic D, Whitton PS, Lupret V: Effect of intracranial pressure on cerebrospinal fluid formation in isolated brain ventricles. Neuroscience 1991; 41: 773–777.

110. Welch K, Pollay M: Perfusion of particles through arachnoid villi of the monkey. Am J Physiol 1961; 201: 651–654.

111. Gomez DG, Potts DG: The surface characteristics of arachnoid granulations. Arch Neurol 1974; 31: 88–93.

112. Levine JE, Povlishock JT, Becker DP: The morphological correlates of primate cerebrospinal fluid absorption. Brain Res 1982; 241: 31–41.

113. Gilland O: Normal cerebrospinal-fluid pressure. N Engl J Med 1969; 280: 904–905.

114. Enzmann DR, Pelc NJ: Normal flow patterns of intracranial and spinal cerebrospinal fluid defined with phase-contrast cine MR imaging. Radiology 1991; 178: 467–474.

115. Di Chiro G: Observations on the circulation of the cerebrospinal fluid. Acta Radiol Diagn (Stockh) 1966; 5: 988–1002.

116. Millen JW, Woollam DHM: The Anatomy of the Cerebrospinal Fluid, p 26. London, Oxford Press, 1962.

117. Fink BR, Gerlach R, Richards T, et al: Improved magnetic resonance (MR) imaging method for measurement of spinal fluid volume in normal subjects: use of fast spin echo pulse sequence. (Abstract.) Anesthesiology 1992; 77: A875.

118. Lentner C: Geigy Scientific Tables, 8th ed, vol 1, pp 165–177. Basel, Ciba-Geigy, 1981.

119. Jirout J: Pneumomyelography, 2nd ed, pp 27–41. Springfield, IL, Charles C Thomas, 1969.

120. Di Chiro G, Timins EL: Supine myelography and the septum posticum. Radiology 1974; 111: 319–327.

121. Nauta HJ, Dolan E, Yasargil MG: Microsurgical anatomy of spinal subarachnoid space. Surg Neurol 1983; 19: 431–437.

122. Osaka K, Handa H, Matsumoto S, et al: Development of the cerebrospinal fluid pathway in the normal and abnormal human embryos. Childs Brain 1980; 6: 26–38.

123. Teng P, Papatheodorou C: Spinal arachnoid diverticula. Br J Radiol 1966; 39: 249–254.

124. Teng P, Rudner N: Multiple arachnoid diverticula. Arch Neurol 1960; 2: 348–356.

125. Brierley JB: The penetration of particulate matter from the cerebrospinal fluid into the spinal ganglia, peripheral nerves, and perivascular spaces of the central nervous system. J Neurol Neurosurg Psychiatr 1950; 13: 203–215.

126. Cohen MS, Wall EJ, Brown RA, et al: 1990 AcroMed Award in basic science. Cauda equina anatomy. II: extrathecal nerve roots and dorsal root ganglia. Spine 1990; 15: 1248–1251.

127. Basmajian JV: The depressions for the arachnoid granulations as a criterion of age. Anat Rec 1952; 112: 843–846.

128. Grossman CB, Potts DG: Arachnoid granulations: radiology and anatomy. Radiology 1974; 113: 95–100.

129. Shantha TR, Evans JA: The relationship of epidural anesthesia to neural membranes and arachnoid villi. Anesthesiology 1972; 37: 543–557.

130. Brierley JB, Field EJ: The connexions of the spinal sub-arachnoid space with the lymphatic system. J Anat 1948; 82: 153–166.

131. Hassin GB: Villi (pacchionian bodies) of the spinal arachnoid. Arch Neurol Psychiatr 1930; 23: 65–78.

132. Himango WA, Low FN: The fine structure of a lateral recess of the subarachnoid space in the rat. Anat Rec 1971; 171: 1–19.

133. Nabors MW, Pait TG, Byrd EB, et al: Updated assessment and current classification of spinal meningeal cysts. J Neurosurg 1988; 68: 366–377.

134. Gortvai P: Extradural cysts of the spinal canal. J Neurol Neurosurg Psychiatr 1963; 26: 223–230.

135. Rexed BA, Wennström KG: Arachnoidal proliferation and cystic formation in the spinal nerve-root pouches of man. J Neurosurg 1959; 16: 73–84.

136. Tarlov IM: Sacral Nerve-Root Cysts, Another Cause of the Sciatic or Cauda Equina Syndrome. Springfield, IL, Charles C Thomas, 1953.

137. Smith DT: Cystic formations associated with human spinal nerve roots. J Neurosurg 1961; 18: 654–660.

138. Larsen JL, Smith D, Fossan G: Arachnoidal diverticula and cystlike dilatations of the nerve-root sheaths in lumbar myelography. Acta Radiol Diagn (Stockh) 1980; 21: 141–145.

139. North RB, Kidd DH, Wang H: Occult, bilateral anterior sacral and intrasacral meningeal and perineurial cysts: case report and review of the literature. Neurosurgery 1990; 27: 981–986.

140. Thomas M, Halaby FA, Hirschauer JS: Hereditary occurrence of anterior sacral meningocele: report of ten cases. Spine 1987; 12: 351–354.

141. Holt S, Yates PO: Cervical nerve root "cysts." Brain 1964; 87: 481–490.

142. Lindblom K: The subarachnoid spaces of the root sheaths in the lumbar region. Acta Radiol 1948; 30: 419–426.

143. Hemminghytt S, Daniels DL, Williams AL, et al: Intraspinal synovial cysts: natural history and diagnosis by CT. Radiology 1982; 145: 375–376.

144. Knox AM, Fon GT: The appearances of lumbar intraspinal synovial cysts. Clin Radiol 1991; 44: 397–401.

145. Barson AJ, Sands J: Regional and segmental characteristics of the human adult spinal cord. J Anat 1977; 123: 797–803.

146. McCotter RE: Regarding the length and extent of the human medula spinalis. Anat Rec 1916; 10: 559–564.

147. Needles JH: The caudal level of termination of the spinal cord in American whites and American Negroes. Anat Rec 1935; 63: 417–424.

148. Reimann AF, Anson BJ: Vertebral level of termination of the spinal cord with report of a case of sacral cord. Anat Rec 1944; 88: 127–138.

149. Coggeshall RE, Coulter JD, Willis WD Jr: Unmyelinated axons in the ventral roots of the cat lumbosacral enlargement. J Comp Neurol 1974; 153: 39–58.

150. Coggeshall RE: Law of separation of function of the spinal roots. Physiol Rev 1980; 60: 716–755.

151. Risling M, Dalsgaard CJ, Cukierman A, et al: Electron microscopic and immunohistochemical evidence that unmyelinated ventral root axons make U-turns or enter the spinal pia mater. J Comp Neurol 1984; 225: 53–63.

152. Habler HJ, Jänig W, Koltzenburg M, et al: A quantitative study of the central projection patterns of unmyelinated ventral root afferents in the cat. J Physiol (Lond) 1990; 422: 265–287.

153. Risling M, Hildebrand C: Occurrence of unmyelinated axon

profiles at distal, middle and proximal levels in the ventral root L7 of cats and kittens. J Neurol Sci 1982; 56: 219–231.

154. Risling M, Hildebrand C, Cullheim S: Invasion of the L7 ventral root and spinal pia mater by new axons after sciatic nerve division in kittens. Exp Neurol 1984; 83: 84–97.

155. Haller FR, Low FN: The fine structure of the peripheral nerve root sheath in the subarachnoid space in the rat and other laboratory animals. Am J Anat 1971; 131: 1–19.

156. Parke WW, Watanabe R: The intrinsic vasculature of the lumbosacral spinal nerve roots. Spine 1985; 10: 508–515.

157. Kaar GF, Fraher JP: The sheaths surrounding the attachments of rat lumbar ventral roots to the spinal cord: a light and electron microscopical study. J Anat 1986; 148: 137–146.

158. Galindo A, Hernandez J, Benavides O, et al: Quality of spinal extradural anaesthesia: the influence of spinal nerve root diameter. Br J Anaesth 1975; 47: 41–47.

159. Ingbert C: An enumeration of the medullated nerve fibers in the dorsal roots of the spinal nerves of man. J Comp Neurol 1903; 13: 53–120.

160. Sunderland S: Avulsion of nerve roots. In Vinken PJ, Bruyn GW (eds): Handbook of Clinical Neurology, vol 25, pp 393–435. Amsterdam, North-Holland Publishing, 1976.

161. Fink BR, Gerlach R, Maravilla KR, et al: Postdural mobility of cauda equina: evidence from fast sequence magnetic resonance imaging (MRI). (Abstract.) Anesthesiology 1993; 79: A828.

162. Wall EJ, Cohen MS, Massie JB, et al: Cauda equina anatomy. I: Intrathecal nerve root organization. Spine 1990; 15: 1244–1247.

163. Suzuki K, Takatsu T, Inoue H, et al: Redundant nerve roots of the cauda equina caused by lumbar spinal canal stenosis. Spine 1992; 17: 1337–1342.

164. Pallie W: The intersegmental anastomoses of posterior spinal rootlets and their significance. J Neurosurg 1959; 16: 188–196.

165. Pallie W, Manuel JK: Intersegmental anastomoses between dorsal spinal rootlets in some vertebrates. Acta Anat (Basel) 1968; 70: 341–351.

166. Kadish LJ, Simmons EH: Anomalies of the lumbosacral nerve roots. An anatomical investigation and myelographic study. J Bone Joint Surg Br 1984; 66: 411–416.

167. Kikuchi S, Hasue M, Nishiyama K, et al: Anatomic and clinical studies of radicular symptoms. Spine 1984; 9: 23–30.

168. Nitta H, Tajima T, Sugiyama H, et al: Study on dermatomes by means of selective lumbar spinal nerve block. Spine 1993; 18: 1782–1786.

169. Neidre A, MacNab I: Anomalies of the lumbosacral nerve roots. Review of 16 cases and classification. Spine 1983; 8: 294–299.

170. Stilwell DL: The nerve supply of the vertebral column and its associated structures in the monkey. Anat Rec 1956; 125: 139–162.

171. Edgar MA, Ghadially JA: Innervation of the lumbar spine. Clin Orthop 1976; 115: 35–41.

172. Bogduk N: The innervation of the lumbar spine. Spine 1983; 8: 286–293.

173. Forsythe WB, Ghoshal NG: Innervation of the canine thoracolumbar vertebral column. Anat Rec 1984; 208: 57–63.

174. Groen GJ, Baljet B, Drukker J: Nerves and nerve plexuses of the human vertebral column. Am J Anat 1990; 188: 282–296.

175. Giles LG, Taylor JR, Cockson A: Human zygapophyseal joint synovial folds. Acta Anat (Basel) 1986; 126: 110–114.

176. Kojima Y, Maeda T, Arai R, et al: Nerve supply to the posterior longitudinal ligament and the intervertebral disc of the rat vertebral column as studied by acetylcholinesterase histochemistry. I. Distribution in the lumbar region. J Anat 1990; 169: 237–246.

177. Kimmel DL: Innervation of spinal dura mater and dura mater of the posterior cranial fossa. Neurology 1961; 11: 800–809.

178. Bogduk N, Tynan W, Wilson AS: The nerve supply to the human lumbar intervertebral discs. J Anat 1981; 132: 39–56.

179. Kojima Y, Maeda T, Arai R, et al: Nerve supply to the posterior longitudinal ligament and the intervertebral disc of the rat vertebral column as studied by acetylcholinesterase histochemistry. II. Regional differences in the distribution of the nerve fibres and their origins. J Anat 1990; 169: 247–255.

180. Shinohara H: Lumbar disc lesion, with special reference to the histological significance of nerve endings of the lumbar discs.

(Japanese.) Nippon Seikeigeka Gakkai Zasshi 1970; 44: 553–570.

181. Coppes MH, Marani E, Thomeer RT, et al: Innervation of annulus fibrosis in low back pain. (Letter to the editor.) (Published erratum appears in Lancet 1990; 4: 324.) Lancet 1990; 336: 189–190.

182. Groen GJ, Baljet B, Drukker J: The innervation of the spinal dura mater: anatomy and clinical implications. Acta Neurochir (Wien) 1988; 92: 39–46.

183. Hromada J: On the nerve supply of the connective tissue of some peripheral nervous system components. Acta Anat 1963; 55: 343–351.

184. Clark SL: Innervation of the pia mater of the spinal cord and medulla. J Comp Neurol 1931; 53: 129–145.

185. Jänig W, Koltzenburg M: Receptive properties of pial afferents. Pain 1991; 45: 77–85.

186. Raine CS, Brown AM, McFarlin DE: Heterotopic regeneration of peripheral nerve fibres into the subarachnoid space. J Neurocytol 1982; 11: 109–118.

187. Groen GJ, Baljet B, Boekelaar AB, et al: Branches of the thoracic sympathetic trunk in the human fetus. Anat Embryol (Berl) 1987; 176: 401–411.

188. Edgar MA, Nundy S: Innervation of the spinal dura mater. J Neurol Neurosurg Psychiatr 1966; 29: 530–534.

189. Malinský J: The ontogenetic development of nerve terminations in the intervertebral discs of man. Acta Anat 1959; 38: 96–113.

190. Hirsch C, Ingelmark B-E, Miller M: The anatomical basis for low back pain. Acta Orthop Scand 1963; 33: 1–17.

191. Jackson HC II, Winkelmann RK, Bickel WH: Nerve endings in the human lumbar spinal column and related structures. J Bone Joint Surg Am 1966; 48: 1272–1281.

192. McLain RF: Mechanoreceptor endings in human cervical facet joints. Spine 1994; 19: 495–501.

193. Korkala O, Gronblad M, Liesi P, et al: Immunohistochemical demonstration of nociceptors in the ligamentous structures of the lumbar spine. Spine 1985; 10: 156–157.

194. Konttinen YT, Gronblad M, Antti-Poika I, et al: Neuroimmunohistochemical analysis of peridiscal nociceptive neural elements. Spine 1990; 15: 383–386.

195. Edvinsson L, Rosendal-Helgesen S, Uddman R: Substance P: localization, concentration and release in cerebral arteries, choroid plexus and dura mater. Cell Tissue Res 1983; 234: 1–7.

196. Dalsgaard CJ, Risling M, Cuello C: Immunohistochemical localization of substance P in the lumbosacral spinal pia mater and ventral roots of the cat. Brain Res 1982; 246: 168–171.

197. el-Bohy A, Cavanaugh JM, Getchell ML, et al: Localization of substance P and neurofilament immunoreactive fibers in the lumbar facet joint capsule and supraspinous ligament of the rabbit. Brain Res 1988; 460: 379–382.

198. Ashton IK, Ashton BA, Gibson SJ, et al: Morphological basis for back pain: the demonstration of nerve fibers and neuropeptides in the lumbar facet joint capsule but not in ligamentum flavum. J Orthop Res 1992; 10: 72–78.

199. Giles LG, Harvey AR: Immunohistochemical demonstration of nociceptors in the capsule and synovial folds of human zygapophyseal joints. Br J Rheumatol 1987; 26: 362–364.

200. Gronblad M, Korkala O, Konttinen YT, et al: Silver impregnation and immunohistochemical study of nerves in lumbar facet joint plical tissue. Spine 1991; 16: 34–38.

201. Kellgren JH: On the distribution of pain arising from deep somatic structures with charts of segmental pain areas. Clin Sci 1939; 4: 35–46.

202. Sinclair DC, Feindel WH, Weddell G, et al: The intervertebral ligaments as a source of segmental pain. J Bone Joint Surg Br 1948; 30: 515–521.

203. Hockaday JM, Whitty CW: Patterns of referred pain in the normal subject. Brain 1967; 90: 481–496.

204. Mooney V, Robertson J: The facet syndrome. Clin Orthop 1976; 115: 149–156.

205. McCall IW, Park WM, O'Brien JP: Induced pain referral from posterior lumbar elements in normal subjects. Spine 1979; 4: 441–446.

206. El-Mahdi MA, Abdel Latif FY, Janko M: The spinal nerve root "innervation," and a new concept of the clinicopathological

interrelations in back pain and sciatica. Neurochirurgia (Stuttg) 1981; 24: 137–141.

207. Falconer MA, McGeorge M, Begg AC: Observations on the cause and mechanism of symptom-production in sciatica and low-back pain. J Neurol Neurosurg Psychiatr 1948; 11: 13–26.

208. Wiberg G: Back pain in relation to the nerve supply of the intervertebral disc. Acta Orthop Scand 1949; 19: 211–221.

209. Frykholm R, Hyde J, Norlén G, et al: On pain sensations produced by stimulation of ventral roots in man. Acta Physiol Scand Suppl 1953; 106: 455–469.

210. Fernström U: A discographical study of ruptured lumbar intervertebral discs. Acta Chirurg Scand Suppl 1960; 258: 1–60.

211. Murphey F: Sources and patterns of pain in disc disease. Clin Neurosurg 1968; 15: 343–351.

212. Kuslich SD, Ulstrom CL, Michael CJ: The tissue origin of low back pain and sciatica: a report of pain response to tissue stimulation during operations on the lumbar spine using local anesthesia. Orthop Clin North Am 1991; 22: 181–187.

213. Smyth MJ, Wright V: Sciatica and the intervertebral disc: an experimental study. J Bone Joint Surg Am 1958; 40: 1401–1418.

214. Cavanaugh JM, el-Bohy A, Hardy WN, et al: Sensory innervation of soft tissues of the lumbar spine in the rat. J Orthop Res 1989; 7: 378–388.

215. Yamashita T, Cavanaugh JM, el-Bohy AA, et al: Mechanosensitive afferent units in the lumbar facet joint. J Bone Joint Surg Am 1990; 72: 865–870.

216. Bahns E, Ernsberger U, Jänig W, et al: Discharge properties of mechanosensitive afferents supplying the retroperitoneal space. Pflugers Arch 1986; 407: 519–525.

217. Gillette RG, Kramis RC, Roberts WJ: Characterization of spinal somatosensory neurons having receptive fields in lumbar tissues of cats. Pain 1993; 54: 85–98.

218. Jänig W, McLachlan EM: Identification of distinct topographical distributions of lumbar sympathetic and sensory neurons projecting to end organs with different functions in the cat. J Comp Neurol 1986; 246: 104–112.

219. Gillette RG, Kramis RC, Roberts WJ: Sympathetic activation of cat spinal neurons responsive to noxious stimulation of deep tissues in the low back. Pain 1994; 56: 31–42.

220. Walker AE, Nulson F: Electrical stimulation of the upper thoracic portion of the sympathetic chain in man. (Abstract.) Arch Neurol Psychiatr 1948; 59: 559–560.

221. Sluijter ME: The use of radiofrequency lesions for pain relief in failed back patients. Int Disabil Stud 1988; 10: 37–43.

222. Echlin F: Pain responses on stimulation of the lumbar sympathetic chain under local anesthesia: a case report. J Neurosurg 1949; 6: 530–533.

223. Brena SF, Wolf SL, Chapman SL, et al: Chronic back pain: electromyographic, motion and behavioral assessments following sympathetic nerve blocks and placebos. Pain 1980; 8: 1–10.

224. Ratcliffe JF: The arterial anatomy of the adult human lumbar vertebral body: a microarteriographic study. J Anat 1980; 131: 57–79.

225. Holm S, Nachemson A: Variations in the nutrition of the canine intervertebral disc induced by motion. Spine 1983; 8: 866–874.

226. Tyrrell AR, Reilly T, Troup JD: Circadian variation in stature and the effects of spinal loading. Spine 1985; 10: 161–164.

227. Dommisse GF: The arteries, arterioles, and capillaries of the spinal cord. Surgical guidelines in the prevention of postoperative paraplegia. Ann R Coll Surg Engl 1980; 62: 369–376.

228. Crock HV, Yoshizawa H: The Blood Supply of the Vertebral Column and Spinal Cord in Man, p 26. New York, Springer-Verlag, 1977.

229. Parke WW, Gammell K, Rothman RH: Arterial vascularization of the cauda equina. J Bone Joint Surg Am 1981; 63: 53–62.

230. Koyanagi I, Tator CH, Lea PJ: Three-dimensional analysis of the vascular system in the rat spinal cord with scanning electron microscopy of vascular corrosion casts. Part 1: normal spinal cord. Neurosurgery 1993; 33: 277–284.

231. Woollam DHM, Millen JW: The arterial supply of the spinal cord and its significance. J Neurol Neurosurg Psychiatr 1955; 18: 97–102.

232. Lazorthes G, Gouaze A, Zadeh JO, et al: Arterial vascularization of the spinal cord: recent studies of the anastomotic substitution pathways. J Neurosurg 1971; 35: 253–262.

233. Fried LC, Doppman JL, Di Chiro G: Direction of blood flow in the primate cervical spinal cord. J Neurosurg 1970; 33: 325–330.

234. Di Chiro G, Fried LC: Blood flow currents in spinal cord arteries. Neurology 1971; 21: 1088–1096.

235. Suh TH, Alexander L: Vascular system of the human spinal cord. Arch Neurol Psychiatr 1939; 41: 659–677.

236. Dommisse GF: The Arteries and Veins of the Human Spinal Cord From Birth. Edinburgh, Churchill Livingstone, 1975.

237. Savader SJ, Williams GM, Trerotola SO, et al: Preoperative spinal artery localization and its relationship to postoperative neurologic complications. Radiology 1993; 189: 165–171.

238. Ross RT: Spinal cord infarction in disease and surgery of the aorta. Can J Neurol Sci 1985; 12: 289–295.

239. Krogh E: The effect of acute hypoxia on the motor cells of the spinal cord. Acta Physiol Scand 1950; 20: 263–292.

240. Gilles FH, Nag D: Vulnerability of human spinal cord in transient cardiac arrest. Neurology 1971; 21: 833–839.

241. Silver JR, Buxton PH: Spinal stroke. Brain 1974; 97: 539–550.

242. Gelfan S, Tarlov IM: Differential vulnerability of spinal cord structures to anoxia. J Neurophysiol 1955; 18: 170–188.

243. van Harreveld A, Schadé JP: Nerve cell destruction by asphyxiation of the spinal cord. J Neuropathol Exp Neurol 1962; 21: 410–423.

244. Foo D, Rossier AB: Anterior spinal artery syndrome and its natural history. Paraplegia 1983; 21: 1–10.

245. Fried LC, Aparicio O: Experimental ischemia of the spinal cord. Histologic studies after anterior spinal artery occlusion. Neurology 1973; 23: 289–293.

246. Turnbull IM: Blood supply of the spinal cord: normal and pathological considerations. Clin Neurosurg 1973; 20: 56–84.

247. Dommisse GF: The Arteries and Veins of the Human Spinal Cord From Birth, p 19. Edinburgh, Churchill Livingstone, 1975.

248. Mawad ME, Rivera V, Crawford S, et al: Spinal cord ischemia after resection of thoracoabdominal aortic aneurysms: MR findings in 24 patients. AJR 1990; 155: 1303–1307.

249. Fried LC, Di Chiro G, Doppman JL: Ligation of major thoracolumbar spinal cord arteries in monkeys. J Neurosurg 1969; 31: 608–614.

250. Rydevik B, Brown MD, Lundborg G: Pathoanatomy and pathophysiology of nerve root compression. Spine 1984; 9: 7–15.

251. Yoshizawa H, Kobayashi S, Hachiya Y: Blood supply of nerve roots and dorsal root ganglia. Orthop Clin North Am 1991; 22: 195–211.

252. Rydevik B, Holm S, Brown MD, et al: Diffusion from the cerebrospinal fluid as a nutritional pathway for spinal nerve roots. Acta Physiol Scand 1990; 138: 247–248.

253. Parke WW: The significance of venous return impairment in ischemic radiculopathy and myelopathy. Orthop Clin North Am 1991; 22: 213–221.

254. Watanabe R, Parke WW: Vascular and neural pathology of lumbosacral spinal stenosis. J Neurosurg 1986; 64: 64–70.

255. Olmarker K, Rydevik B, Holm S: Edema formation in spinal nerve roots induced by experimental, graded compression. An experimental study on the pig cauda equina with special reference to differences in effects between rapid and slow onset of compression. Spine 1989; 14: 569–573.

256. Gamble HJ: Comparative electron-microscopic observations on the connective tissues of a peripheral nerve and a spinal nerve root in the rat. J Anat 1964; 98: 17–25.

257. Sunderland S, Bradley KC: Stress-strain phenomena in human spinal nerve roots. Brain 1961; 84: 120–124.

258. Hoyland JA, Freemont AJ, Jayson MI: Intervertebral foramen venous obstruction. A cause of periradicular fibrosis? Spine 1989; 14: 558–568.

259. Rydevik BL, Myers RR, Powell HC: Pressure increase in the dorsal root ganglion following mechanical compression. Closed compartment syndrome in nerve roots. Spine 1989; 14: 574–576.

260. Abrams HL: The vertebral and azygos venous systems, and some variations in systemic venous return. Radiology 1957; 69: 508–526.

261. Batson OV: The function of the vertebral veins and their role in the spread of metastases. Ann Surg 1940; 112: 138–149.

262. Dommisse GF: The Arteries and Veins of the Human Spinal

Cord From Birth, pp 90–92. Edinburgh, Churchill Livingstone, 1975.

263. Herlihy WF: Revision of the venous system: the role of the vertebral veins. Med J Aust 1947; 1: 661–672.

264. Coman DR, deLong RP: The role of the vertebral venous system in the metastasis of cancer to the spinal column: experiments with tumor-cell suspensions in rats and rabbits. Cancer 1951; 4: 610–618.

265. Anderson R: Diodrast studies of the vertebral and cranial venous systems: to show their probable role in cerebral metastases. J Neurosurg 1951; 8: 411–422.

266. Nordenström B: A method of angiography of the azygos vein and the anterior internal venous plexus of the spine. Acta Radiol 1955; 44: 201–208.

267. Helander CG, Lindbom A: Sacrolumbar venography. Acta Radiol 1955; 44: 410–416.

268. Schobinger RA, Krueger EG, Sobel GL: Comparison of intraosseous vertebral venography and pantopaque myelography in the diagnosis of surgical conditions of the lumbar spine and nerve roots. Radiology 1961; 77: 376–397.

269. Gershater R, St. Louis EL: Lumbar epidural venography. Review of 1,200 cases. Radiology 1979; 131: 409–421.

270. Crock HV, Yoshizawa H: The Blood Supply of the Vertebral Column and Spinal Cord in Man, p 51. New York, Springer-Verlag, 1977.

271. Meijenhorst GC: Computed tomography of the lumbar epidural veins. Radiology 1982; 145: 687–691.

272. Nohara Y, Brown MD, Eurell JC: Lymphatic drainage of epidural space in rabbits. Orthop Clin North Am 1991; 22: 189–194.

273. Durant PA, Yaksh TL: Distribution in cerebrospinal fluid, blood, and lymph of epidurally injected morphine and inulin in dogs. Anesth Analg 1986; 65: 583–592.

274. Saal JA, Saal JS, Herzog RJ: The natural history of lumbar intervertebral disc extrusions treated nonoperatively. Spine 1990; 15: 683–686.

275. Bush K, Cowan N, Katz DE, et al: The natural history of sciatica associated with disc pathology. A prospective study with clinical and independent radiologic follow-up. Spine 1992; 17: 1205–1212.

276. DiGiovanni AJ, Galbert MW, Wahle WM: Epidural injection of autologous blood for postlumbar-puncture headache. II. Additional clinical experiences and laboratory investigation. Anesth Analg 1972; 51: 226–232.

277. Kostelic JK, Haughton VM, Sether LA: Anatomy of the lumbar spinal nerves in the intervertebral foramen. Clin Anat 1991; 4: 366–372.

278. Bonica JJ: The Management of Pain, 2nd ed, vol 1, pp 133–146. Philadelphia, Lea & Febiger, 1990.

279. Horwitz MT: The anatomy of the lumbosacral nerve plexus—its relation to variations of vertebral segmentation and the posterior sacral nerve plexus. Anat Rec 1939; 74: 91–107.

280. Kerr AT: The brachial plexus of nerves in man, the variations in its formation and branches. Am J Anat 1918; 23: 285–395.

281. Thompson GE, Rorie DK: Functional anatomy of the brachial plexus sheaths. Anesthesiology 1983; 59: 117–122.

282. Hogan QH, Erickson SJ: MR imaging of the stellate ganglion: normal appearance. (Published erratum appears in AJR 1992; 158: 1320.) AJR 1992; 158: 655–659.

283. Kellman GM, Kneeland JB, Middleton WD, et al: MR imaging of the supraclavicular region: normal anatomy. AJR 1987; 148: 77–82.

284. Farny J, Drolet P, Girard M: Anatomy of the posterior approach to the lumbar plexus block. Can J Anaesth 1994; 41: 480–485.

285. Ritter J, Zimpfer M: Inguinal paravascular "3-in-1" block technique does not block the lumbar plexus. (Abstract.) Reg Anesth 1994; 19(Suppl): 7.

286. Kerr FWL: A mechanism to account for frontal headache in cases of posterior-fossa tumors. J Neurosurg 1961; 18: 605–609.

287. Foerster O: The dermatomes in man. Brain 1933; 56: 1–39.

288. Kuhn RA: Organization of tactile dermatomes in cat and monkey. J Neurophysiol 1953; 16: 169–182.

289. Keegan JJ, Garrett FD: The segmental distribution of the cutaneous nerves in the limbs of man. Anat Rec 1948; 102: 409–437.

290. Denny-Brown D, Kirk EJ, Yanagisawa N: The tract of Lissauer in relation to sensory transmission in the dorsal horn of spinal cord in the macaque monkey. J Comp Neurol 1973; 151: 175–200.

291. Devor M, Wall PD: Effect of peripheral nerve injury on receptive fields of cells in the cat spinal cord. J Comp Neurol 1981; 199: 277–291.

292. Metzler J, Marks PS: Functional changes in cat somatic sensory-motor cortex during short-term reversible epidural blocks. Brain Res 1979; 177: 379–383.

293. McMahon SB, Wall PD: Receptive fields of rat lamina 1 projection cells move to incorporate a nearby region of injury. Pain 1984; 19: 235–247.

294. Kirk EJ, Denny-Brown D: Functional variation in dermatomes in the macaque monkey following dorsal root lesions. J Comp Neurol 1970; 139: 307–320.

295. Young A, Gety J, Jackson A, et al: Variations in the pattern of muscle innervation by the L5 and S1 nerve roots. Spine 1983; 8: 616–624.

296. Williams PL, Warwick R, Dyson M, et al: Gray's Anatomy, 37th ed, pp 1150–1153. Edinburgh, Churchill Livingstone, 1989.

297. Shanthaveerappa TR, Bourne GH: Perineural epithelium: a new concept of its role in the integrity of the peripheral nervous system. Science 1966; 154: 1464–1467.

298. Lundborg G: Structure and function of the intraneural microvessels as related to trauma, edema formation, and nerve function. J Bone Joint Surg Am 1975; 57: 938–948.

299. Olsson Y: Studies on vascular permeability in peripheral nerves. IV. Distribution of intravenously injected protein tracers in the peripheral nervous system of various species. Acta Neuropathol (Berl) 1971; 17: 114–126.

300. Brierley JB, Field EJ: The fate of intraneural injection as demonstrated by the use of radio-active phosphorus. J Neurol Neurosurg Psychiatr 1949; 12: 86–99.

301. Moore DC, Hain RF, Ward A, et al: Importance of the perineural spaces in nerve blocking. JAMA 1954; 156: 1050–1053.

302. Sullivan WE, Mortensen OA: Visualization of the movement of a brominized oil along peripheral nerves. Anat Rec 1934; 59: 493–501.

303. McCabe JS, Low FN: The subarachnoid angle: an area of transition in peripheral nerve. Anat Rec 1969; 164: 15–33.

304. Haller FR, Haller C, Low FN: The fine structure of cellular layers and connective tissue space at spinal nerve root attachments in the rat. Am J Anat 1972; 133: 109–123.

305. French JD, Strain WH, Jones GE: Mode of extension of contrast substances injected into peripheral nerves. J Neuropathol Exp Neurol 1948; 7: 47–58.

306. Selander D, Sjostrand J: Longitudinal spread of intraneurally injected local anesthetics. An experimental study of the initial neural distribution following intraneural injections. Acta Anaesthesiol Scand 1978; 22: 622–634.

307. Jänig W, McLachlan EM: Specialized functional pathways are the building blocks of the autonomic nervous system. J Auton Nerv Syst 1992; 41: 3–13.

308. Low PA, Dyck PJ: Splanchnic preganglionic neurons in man. III. Morphometry of myelinated fibers of rami communicantes. J Neuropathol Exp Neurol 1978; 37: 734–740.

309. Renck H: Management of Abdominoviscberal Pain by Nerve Block Techniques, pp 28–32. Fribourg, Switzerland, Mediglobe, 1992.

310. Rubin E, Purves D: Segmental organization of sympathetic preganglionic neurons in the mammalian spinal cord. J Comp Neurol 1980; 192: 163–174.

311. Bonica JJ: Autonomic innervation of the viscera in relation to nerve block. Anesthesiology 1968; 29: 793–813.

312. Sunderland S: The distribution of sympathetic fibers in the brachial plexus in man. Brain 1948; 71: 88–102.

313. Sheehan D: On the innervation of the blood-vessels of the upper extremity: some anatomical considerations. Br J Surg 1933; 20: 412–424.

314. Coggeshall RE, Hancock MB, Applebaum ML: Categories of axons in mammalian rami communicantes. J Comp Neurol 1976; 167: 105–123.

315. Kuo DC, Yang GC, Yamasaki DS, et al: A wide field electron microscopic analysis of the fiber constituents of the major splanchnic nerve in cat. J Comp Neurol 1982; 210: 49–58.

316. Foley J: Composition of the cervical sympathetic trunk. Proc Soc Exp Biol Med 1943; 52: 212–214.

317. Jänig W, Schmidt RF: Single unit responses in the cervical sympathetic trunk upon somatic nerve stimulation. Pflugers Arch 1970; 314: 199–216.

318. Kamosinska B, Nowicki D, Szulczyk A, et al: Spinal segmental sympathetic outflow to cervical sympathetic trunk, vertebral nerve, inferior cardiac nerve and sympathetic fibres in the thoracic vagus. J Auton Nerv Syst 1991; 32: 199–204.

319. Coggeshall RE, Galbraith SL: Categories of axons in mammalian rami communicantes. Part II. J Comp Neurol 1978; 181: 349–359.

320. Pick J, Sheehan D: Sympathetic rami in man. J Anat 1946; 80: 12–20.

321. van Rhede van der Kloot E, Drukker J, Lemmens HA, et al: The high thoracic sympathetic nerve system—its anatomic variability. J Surg Res 1986; 40: 112–119.

322. Stevens RT, Hodge CJ Jr, Apkarian AV: Catecholamine varicosities in cat dorsal root ganglion and spinal ventral roots. Brain Res 1983; 261: 151–154.

323. Kummer W, Gibbins IL, Stefan P, et al: Catecholamines and catecholamine-synthesizing enzymes in guinea-pig sensory ganglia. Cell Tissue Res 1990; 261: 595–606.

324. McLachlan EM, Jang W, Devor M, et al: Peripheral nerve injury triggers noradrenergic sprouting within dorsal root ganglia. Nature 1993; 363: 543–546.

325. Wrete M: The anatomy of the sympathetic trunks in man. J Anat 1959; 93: 448–459.

326. Skoog T: Ganglia in the communicating rami of the cervical sympathetic trunk. Lancet 1947; 2: 457–460.

327. Hoffman HH: An analysis of the sympathetic trunk and rami in the cervical and upper thoracic regions in man. Ann Surg 1957; 145: 94–103.

328. Alexander WF, Kuntz A, Henderson WP, et al: Sympathetic ganglion cells in ventral nerve roots: their relation to sympathectomy. Science 1949; 109: 484.

329. Pick J: The identification of sympathetic segments. Ann Surg 1957; 145: 355–364.

330. Bosnjak ZJ, Kampine JP: Electrophysiological and morphological characterization of neurons in stellate ganglion of cats. Am J Physiol 1985; 248: R288–R292.

331. Kuo DC, Oravitz JJ, DeGroat WC: Tracing of afferent and efferent pathways in the left inferior cardiac nerve of the cat using retrograde and transganglionic transport of horseradish peroxidase. Brain Res 1984; 321: 111–118.

332. Dun NJ, Karczmar AG: Actions of substance P on sympathetic neurons. Neuropharmacology 1979; 18: 215–218.

333. Konishi S, Tsunoo A, Otsuka M: Enkephalins presynaptically inhibit cholinergic transmission in sympathetic ganglia. Nature 1979; 282: 515–516.

334. Bosnjak ZJ, Seagard JL, Roerig DL, et al: The effects of morphine on sympathetic transmission in the stellate ganglion of the cat. Can J Physiol Pharmacol 1986; 64: 940–946.

335. Campbell G: Cotransmission. Annu Rev Pharmacol Toxicol 1987; 27: 51–70.

336. Furness JB, Morris JL, Gibbins IL, et al: Chemical coding of neurons and plurichemical transmission. Annu Rev Pharmacol Toxicol 1989; 29: 289–306.

337. Benarroch EE: Neuropeptides in the sympathetic system: presence, plasticity, modulation, and implications. Ann Neurol 1994; 36: 6–13.

338. Gibbins IL: Vasoconstrictor, vasodilator and pilomotor pathways in sympathetic ganglia of guinea-pigs. Neuroscience 1992; 47: 657–672.

339. Fine PG, Ashburn MA: Effect of stellate ganglion block with fentanyl on postherpetic neuralgia with a sympathetic component. Anesth Analg 1988; 67: 897–899.

340. Gibbins IL: Vasomotor, pilomotor and secretomotor neurons distinguished by size and neuropeptide content in superior cervical ganglia of mice. J Auton Nerv Syst 1991; 34: 171–183.

341. Bachoo M, Ciriello J, Polosa C: Effect of preganglionic stimulation on neuropeptide-like immunoreactivity in the stellate ganglion of the cat. Brain Res 1987; 400: 377–382.

342. Gallego R, Geijo E: Chronic block of the cervical trunk increases synaptic efficacy in the superior and stellate ganglia of the guinea-pig. J Physiol (Lond) 1987; 382: 449–462.

343. Bachoo M, Polosa C: Long-term potentiation of nicotinic transmission by a heterosynaptic mechanism in the stellate ganglion of the cat. J Neurophysiol 1991; 65: 639–647.

344. Purves D, Hadley RD: Changes in the dendritic branching of adult mammalian neurones revealed by repeated imaging in situ. Nature 1985; 315: 404–406.

345. Bosnjak ZJ, Seagard JL, Kampine JP: Peripheral neural input to neurons of the stellate ganglion in dog. Am J Physiol 1982; 242: R237–R243.

346. Bosnjak ZJ, Kampine JP: Cardiac sympathetic afferent cell bodies are located in the peripheral nervous system of the cat. Circ Res 1989; 64: 554–562.

347. Kummer W, Oberst P: Neuronal projections to the guinea pig stellate ganglion investigated by retrograde tracing. J Auton Nerv Syst 1993; 42: 71–80.

348. Kleiman A: Causalgia: evidence of the existence of crossed sensory sympathetic fibers. Am J Surg 1954; 87: 839–841.

349. Webber RH: An analysis of the cross communications between the sympathetic trunks in the lumbar region in man. Ann Surg 1957; 145: 365–370.

350. Kuntz A: Distribution of the sympathetic rami to the brachial plexus: its relation to sympathectomy affecting the upper extremity. Arch Surg 1927; 15: 871–877.

351. Bergman RA, Thompson SA, Afifi AK, et al: Compendium of Human Anatomic Variation: Text, Atlas, and World Literature, 2nd ed, p 378. Baltimore, Urban & Schwarzenberg, 1988.

352. Guntamukkala M, Hardy PA: Spread of injectate after stellate ganglion block in man: an anatomical study. Br J Anaesth 1991; 66: 643–644.

353. Hardy PA, Wells JC: Extent of sympathetic blockade after stellate ganglion block with bupivacaine. Pain 1989; 36: 193–196.

354. Malmqvist EL, Bengtsson M, Sorensen J: Efficacy of stellate ganglion block: a clinical study with bupivacaine. Reg Anesth 1992; 17: 340–347.

355. Hogan Q, Taylor ML, Goldstein M, et al: Success rates in producing sympathetic blockade by paratracheal injection. Clin J Pain 1994; 10: 139–145.

356. Chen XQ, Bo S, Zhong SZ: Nerves accompanying the vertebral artery and their clinical relevance. Spine 1988; 13: 1360–1364.

357. Arbab MA, Wiklund L, Delgado T, et al: Stellate ganglion innervation of the vertebro-basilar arterial system demonstrated in the rat with anterograde and retrograde WGA-HRP tracing. Brain Res 1988; 445: 175–180.

358. Kimmel DL: Rami communicantes of cervical nerves and the vertebral plexus in the human embryo. (Abstract.) Anat Rec 1955; 121: 321–322.

359. van Buskirk C: Nerves in the vertebral canal: their relation to the sympathetic innervation of the upper extremities. Arch Surg 1941; 43: 427–432.

360. Kirgis HD, Kuntz A: Inconstant sympathetic neural pathways: their relation to sympathetic denervation of the upper extremity. Arch Surg 1942; 44: 95–102.

361. Lemmens HA, Drukker J: Thoracodorsal sympathectomy en bloc: anatomical variations versus results. Acta Neurochir 1985; 74: 152–153.

362. Szurszewski JH: Physiology of mammalian prevertebral ganglia. Ann Rev Physiol 1981; 43: 53–68.

363. Berthoud H-R, Powley TL: Characterization of vagal innervation to the rat celiac, suprarenal and mesenteric ganglia. J Auton Nerv Syst 1993; 42: 153–169.

364. Hainsworth R: Vascular capacitance: its control and importance. Rev Physiol Biochem Pharmacol 1986; 105: 101–173.

365. Schmalbruch H: Fiber composition of the rat sciatic nerve. Anat Rec 1986; 215: 71–81.

366. Campero M, Verdugo RJ, Ochoa JL: Vasomotor innervation of the skin of the hand: a contribution to the study of human anatomy. J Anat 1993; 182: 361–368.

367. Hoffert MJ, Greenberg RP, Wolskee PJ, et al: Abnormal and collateral innervations of sympathetic and peripheral sensory fields associated with a case of causalgia. Pain 1984; 20: 1–12.

368. Luff SE, McLachlan EM, Hirst GD: An ultrastructural analysis of the sympathetic neuromuscular junctions on arterioles of the submucosa of the guinea pig ileum. J Comp Neurol 1987; 257: 578–594.

369. Hirst GD, Edwards FR: Sympathetic neuroeffector transmission in arteries and arterioles. Physiol Rev 1989; 69: 546–604.

370. Kawarai M, Koss MC: Neurogenic cutaneous vasodilation in the cat forepaw. J Auton Nerv Syst 1992; 37: 39–46.

371. Dean C, Seagard JL, Hopp FA, et al: Differential control of sympathetic activity to kidney and skeletal muscle by ventral medullary neurons. J Auton Nerv Syst 1992; 37: 1–10.

372. Jänig W: The sympathetic nervous system in pain: physiology and pathophysiology. In Stanton-Hicks M (ed): Pain and the Sympathetic Nervous System, pp 17–89. Dordrecht, Kluwer Academic Publishers, 1990.

373. Chandler MJ, Hobbs SF, Bolser DC, et al: Effects of vagal afferent stimulation on cervical spinothalamic tract neurons in monkeys. Pain 1991; 44: 81–87.

374. Ren K, Randich A, Gebhart GF: Spinal serotonergic and kappa opioid receptors mediate facilitation of the tail flick reflex produced by vagal afferent stimulation. Pain 1991; 45: 321–329.

375. Kuntz A: Afferent innervation of peripheral blood vessels through sympathetic trunks: its clinical implications. South Med J 1951; 44: 674–678.

376. Schott GD: Visceral afferents: their contribution to "sympathetic dependent" pain. Brain 1994; 117: 397–413.

377. Holmes R, Torrance RW: Afferent fibres of the stellate ganglion. Q J Exp Physiol 1959; 44: 271–281.

378. Downman CBB, Hazarika NH: Somatic nerve pathways through some thoracic rami communicantes. J Physiol 1962; 163: 340–346.

379. Ness TJ, Gebhart GF: Visceral pain: a review of experimental studies. Pain 1990; 41: 167–234.

380. Jänig W: Neuronal mechanisms of pain with special emphasis on visceral and deep somatic pain. Acta Neurochir Suppl (Wien) 1987; 38: 16–32.

381. Cervero F: Visceral pain. In Dubner R, Gebhart GF, Bond MR (eds): Proceedings of the Vth World Congress on Pain, pp 216–226. Amsterdam, Elsevier Science Publishers, 1988.

382. Woolf CJ, Shortland P, Coggeshall RE: Peripheral nerve injury triggers central sprouting of myelinated afferents. Nature 1992; 355: 75–78.

CHAPTER 5

Neurophysiology

James E. Heavner, D.V.M., Ph.D.

Introduction

Overview

Interruption of communication among neurons in sensory (afferent) pathways is the general effect of drugs used to produce regional anesthesia or analgesia. More specifically, these drugs either stop the communication process within primary afferent axons or alter the communication between primary afferent axons and second-order (spinal cord) neurons in afferent pathways.

The neuronal communication process begins in primary afferent neurons (Fig. 5–1) with a stimulus (chemical, mechanical, or thermal) to the distal nerve terminal (sensory nerve ending, sensory receptor) that elicits graded depolarization of the terminal membrane. The depolarization spreads passively to the axon proper, where an all-or-none action potential is generated if the transmembrane potential reaches the required threshold voltage. The action potential then propagates along the axon membrane (propagated action potential) to the neuron's proximal end in the spinal cord. The action potential invades the proximal terminal and produces a graded depolarization that is responsible for initiating neurotransmitter release. The released neurotransmitter crosses the synaptic cleft and initiates a graded depolarization in the second-order neuron (Fig. 5–1).

The proximal primary afferent nerve terminal and the second-order neuron generally are subjected to several other neural inputs (presynaptic, postsynaptic) that either (1) add to the depolarization (excitation) induced by the action potential that invades the proximal terminal or the action of the neurotransmitter on the second-order neuron or (2) antagonize the excitation, i.e., have inhibitory influences.

In this chapter, important concepts are discussed related to excitable membranes and synaptic transmission that contribute to the understanding of how local anesthetics and analgesics act when used to produce regional anesthesia or analgesia.

Historical Perspectives

The ancient Egyptians discarded the brain during the mummification process because they considered it and peripheral nerves to be of so little importance. Galen (AD 200) considered the nervous system to be a system of pneumatic tubes conducting animal spirits to various parts of the body from the cerebral ventricles. The source of animal spirits was natural spirits derived from food digested by the liver and subsequently converted to vital spirits in the heart. Vital spirits were pumped to the ventricle of the brain where animal spirits were formed. This was accepted as fact for 1500 years.[1]

Luigi Galvani then suggested that "nerve power" was electricity after finding that electrical shocks cause a muscle to twitch. This remained a speculation until 1840, when Du Bois-Reymond measured injury current in nerves by using a galvanometer. He subsequently measured a small transient change in electric current when an undamaged nerve was stimulated.

This led to formulation of the membrane theory by Julius Bernstein[2] in 1902 to explain basic mechanisms of electrical activity seen in both nerve and muscle. According to the theory, a resting excitable cell has a measurable voltage difference across its membrane—the resting potential. The potential is due to unequal distribution of Na^+ and K^+ between the inside and

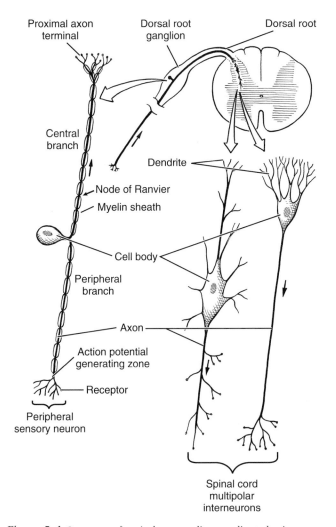

Figure 5–1 Structure of typical mammalian myelinated primary afferent axon and second-order (multipolar) interneurons. *Arrows* indicate the normal (orthodromic) direction of impulse conduction in axons. The relationship between the interneuron and the primary afferent neuron is shown within the context of general anatomy of the spinal cord and some related structures. (From MOLECULAR CELL BIOLOGY 2/E by Darnell, Lodish and Baltimore. Copyright © 1990 by Scientific American Books. Used with permission of W.H. Freeman and Company.)

outside of the cell and a high membrane permeability to K[+] but not Na[+]. "Membrane breakdown" was a term he assigned to the transient loss of the selective membrane permeability that generated an action potential. Equipment and techniques that would permit measurement of these potentials to test Bernstein's theory had not been developed at this time.

Rediscovery of the giant squid axon by J. Z. Young[3] in 1936 set the stage for experiments by Hodgkin, Huxley, and Katz and by Curtis and Cole. Results of these experiments are the basis for contemporary ideas and research regarding the electrical properties of excitable cells. The diameter of a giant squid axon is approximately 0.5 to 1 mm (~100 times larger than other nerves). It is relatively easy to insert an electrode into the squid axon and record transmembrane electrical events.

Bernstein applied the Nernst equation to explain

transmembrane potentials of excitable cells.[4] The Nernst equation is derived from equations that describe the chemical forces and the electrical forces present when charged molecules are separated by a selectively permeable membrane. The Nernst equation is used to calculate the equilibrium potential for an ion.

Hodgkin[5] and Katz[4] and also Curtis and Cole[6] tested Bernstein's theory by measuring the value of the resting potential of the giant squid axon as a function of the extracellular K[+] concentration. The transmembrane potential measured followed the theoretic equilibrium potential for K[+] except at low external K[+] concentration. The results were interpreted to indicate that the axon membrane is primarily K[+] selective at rest but is also slightly permeable to other ions. An expanded equation, the Goldman-Hodgkin-Katz equation, was formulated to describe the transmembrane potential of membranes permeable to several ionic species (e.g., nerve axon).

This equation illustrated that the actual value of the transmembrane potential is set by the concentrations of each ion and its respective permeability coefficient. If several ions are distributed across a membrane that is permeable to only one of the ion species, the transmembrane potential equals the equilibrium potential of the permeant ion.

Bernstein's hypothesis predicted that the action potential is generated by a transient total breakdown in the ionic selectivity of the membrane, causing the membrane potential to go to 0 mV. However, Hodgkin and Katz and also Curtis and Cole found that during the action potential the membrane potential went to +30 to +50 mV. Hodgkin and Katz changed the extracellular Na[+] concentration and discovered that the resting potential is relatively insensitive to [Na[+]]out but the amplitude of the action potential and the speed of depolarization decreased when [Na[+]]out was decreased. From the experimental outcomes, Hodgkin and Katz rejected Bernstein's proposal that the membrane goes from being K[+] selective to nonselective during the action potential. Instead, it goes from K[+] selective to Na[+] selective to generate the action potential (sodium hypothesis). The amount of Na[+] that must cross the membrane to cause a large (>100 mV) change in membrane potential was calculated to be approximately 10^{-12} mol Na[+]/cm^2 of membrane, changing the intracellular Na[+] concentration by less than 10^{-7} M in the squid axon.

Studies of action potentials provide substantial information about excitable membranes, but they do not allow easy study of the mechanisms that underlie permeability changes. Another technique, called the voltage clamp, was used by Hodgkin and Huxley[7] in a series of experiments to study the permeability changes in the giant squid axon during excitation. In essence, the voltage clamp involves using a control circuit to adjust transmembrane potential to a desired level and hold it there while measuring the electric current that flows. This is analogous to injecting heat into a room to maintain the room at a constant temperature set on a thermostat. The current measured in a voltage clamp experiment is a measure of the permeability of the membrane to ions. Information about the permeability changes can be obtained by detailed analysis of the properties of the currents.

When Hodgkin and Huxley changed the squid axon membrane potential from -65 mV to 0, a large transient inward current followed by a maintained outward current was seen. Using a series of different voltages, they observed that the early transient current could be detected in response to depolarizations more positive than -40 mV. Peak amplitude of the current was reached at approximately -10 mV, and then it decreased until the current polarity reversed at approximately the sodium equilibrium potential ($+50$ mV). The late maintained outward current became evident at membrane potentials more positive than -20 mV and became larger as the voltage became more positive. Subsequently, it was proved that the early current was carried by Na^+ moving into the axon and the later maintained current was carried by K^+ moving out of the axon. The term "activation" was used for the process that led to the opening of the Na^+ pathway, and "inactivation" was applied to the slower process that led to closing of the Na^+ pathway. It was subsequently shown that the K^+ process also involved voltage-dependent activation, but there was no inactivation process.

Hodgkin and Huxley formulated a mathematical model to describe the properties of the voltage-clamp currents and to predict action potentials. A starting assumption for the model was the existence of separate channels for Na^+, K^+, and other ions. The model included an activation variable *(m)* and an inactivation variable *(h)*, both of which were time and voltage dependent and varied from 0 to 1. The *m* and *h* were the forerunners of the concepts of gates regulating the flow of ions through channels and of gating currents measured during channel activation and inactivation.

Composition of Neuronal Membranes

It is important to emphasize that neuronal membranes are complex structures. They have a basic framework (lipids) with specialized components (proteins) somewhat randomly located within or closely associated with the basic organization. Specialized components particularly relevant to the subject of this chapter include ion channels, ion pumps, enzymes (e.g., adenosine triphosphatase), and neurotransmitter receptors. The membranes give form to neurons and prevent cellular contents from floating into the surrounding medium. They have the features essential for creation and maintenance of a transmembrane potential and those essential for graded depolarization, generation of an action potential, and membrane repolarization.[8]

The basic structure of the neuronal membrane is a lipid bilayer. The major lipids are phospholipids, cholesterol, and glycolipids. One part of the lipid molecule, the head group, seeks water (hydrophilic), while the other, the tail group, seeks a nonpolar environment (hydrophobic). In schematic drawings, the head group

of the phospholipid, phosphatidylcholine, is often drawn as a ball with two wiggly chains hanging from it (Fig. 5–2). The head groups of the common phospholipids have either a net negative charge or a negative and positive charge together.

Proteins that are part of the membrane are immersed in the lipid bilayer in definite and fixed orientation (Fig. 5–2). They serve transport, signaling, catalytic, and structural roles. The primary, secondary, and tertiary structures of neuronal proteins are known with some precision. Some membrane proteins are glycosylated (sugar residues are added). As much as 30% of the dry weight of the Na^+ channel molecule is carbohydrate.

Transmembrane Potential and Excitability

One fundamental feature of neurons that is essential for communication in the nervous system is that the neuronal membrane is polarized. Indeed, a transmembrane potential difference of about -60 mV is recorded from neurons with a microelectrode inserted inside the cell and a reference electrode placed in the extracellular fluid (Fig. 5–3).

Transmembrane Potential

The charge separation (transmembrane electrical potential) results because the neuronal membrane is selectively permeable to certain ions.[9] This point is illustrated by what happens when two different concentrations of KCl are placed in two compartments separated by a membrane permeable to K^+ but not to Cl^-. The concentration in compartment 1 is higher than in compartment 2. K^+ will move down its concentration gradient. This movement causes a potential difference to develop between the two compartments. The higher the potential gets, the harder it is for the K^+ ions to move against the electrical gradient. Finally, when the electrical gradient just balances the chemical or concentration gradient, there is no net movement of ions and the equilibrium potential for potassium is established. The Nernst equation includes factors for the concentration and electrical gradients and can be used to calculate the equilibration potential for an ion species.

The equation for the chemical potential is:

$$\Delta Gchem = RTln\frac{C2}{C1}$$

and the equation for the electrical potential is:

$$\Delta Gelect = zF(V2 - V1)$$

At equilibrium, $\Delta Gelect + \Delta Gchem = \phi$.

A series of mathematical manipulations (substitution, rearrangement, conversion from ln to log, and reduction of constants to simplest form) produces the Nernst equation, e.g., for potassium:

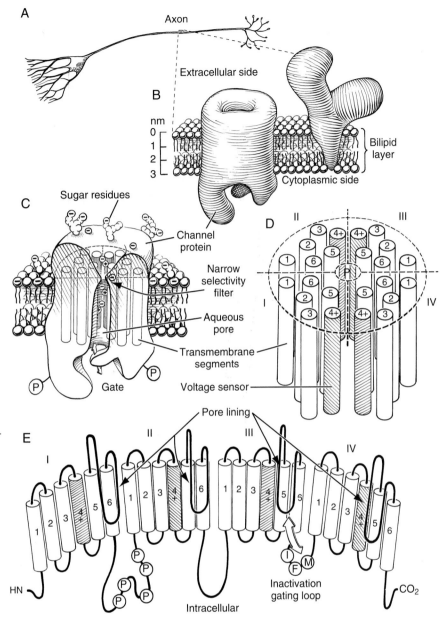

Figure 5–2 A, Interneuron drawing is included for orientation. B, Schematic drawings of lipid bilayer. C, Working hypothesis for a channel. The channel is drawn as a transmembrane macromolecule with a hole through the center. The external surface of the molecule is glycosylated. The functional regions, selectivity filter, gate, and voltage sensor are deduced from voltage clamp experiments and are beginning to be charted by structural studies. P, phosphate. (C modified from Hille B: Ionic Channels of Excitable Membranes, 2nd ed, p 66. Sunderland, MA, Sinauer Associates, 1992.) D, Highly schematic presentation of channel as viewed looking across a membrane. The Roman numerals indicate the four repeating α subunits of the channel protein. S_{1-6} represent the six α-helical transmembrane segments in each of the four repeating amino acid chains that form a pore. P indicates the pore formed by the four subunits. E, Linear presentation of the four repeating α subunits of an Na^+ channel. Note that segment 4 contains + symbols. This segment corresponds to the voltage sensor shown in A. P shows phosphorylation sites. The loop between 5 and 6 forms the pore lining. (D and E modified from Wann KT: Neuronal sodium and potassium channels: structure and function. Br J Anaesth 1993; 71: 2–14.)

$$E_K = -59\log\left(\frac{[K]in}{[K]ext}\right)$$

If the intracellular concentration of K^+ is 10 times that of the extracellular, $E_K = -59$ mV. C = concentration; V = voltage; E_K = the potential difference in mV across the membrane; R = gas constant, 8.314 joules/degree per mole; T = absolute temperature (°K + 273 + ambient temperature, °C); z = charge on the ion; and F = Faraday's constant, 96,500 coulombs/mole.

Table 5–1 shows the equilibrium potential for some ions present in excitable cells calculated by using the Nernst equation and the ion concentrations in the external and internal milieu.

The axon membrane is primarily K^+ selective at rest, but it is also slightly permeable to other ions. The Goldman-Hodgkin-Katz equation mathematically de-

scribed (e.g., axonal) membranes that are permeable to different degrees to several ion species.

The Goldman-Hodgkin-Katz equation is as follows:

$$V_m = \left(\frac{RT}{F}\right) \times ln\frac{P_K[K]ext + P_{Na}[Na]ext + P_{Cl}[Cl]in}{P_K[K]in + P_{Na}[Na]in + P_{Cl}[Cl]ext}$$

P = permeability coefficient for ion species.

In actual conditions, maintenance of the membrane potential requires, in addition to the passive concentration and electromotive forces, an active process. This active process, often called the sodium pump, is necessary to maintain the concentration gradient for Na^+, the principal cation in the extracellular fluid. The axon membrane is somewhat permeable to Na^+ during resting conditions, allowing some passive movement of Na^+ into the axon. If the sodium pump does not re-

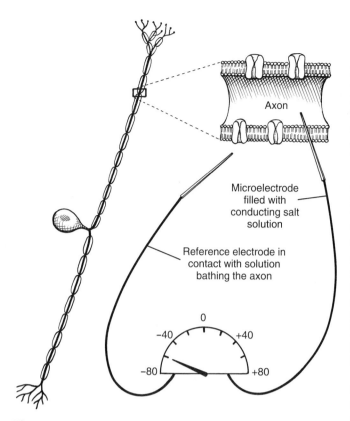

Figure 5–3 Measurement of the electric potential across an axonal membrane. A microelectrode, constructed by filling a glass tube of extremely small diameter with a conducting fluid such as KCl, is inserted into an axon. A reference electrode is placed in the bathing medium. A potentiometer connecting the two electrodes registers the potential: in this case, a resting potential of −60 mV.

move Na^+ at the same rate as Na^+ enters the axon, the transmembrane potential slowly disappears.

In summary, the primary factors responsible for the transmembrane potential of neurons are (1) a membrane that is somewhat selectively permeable to ion species, (2) a concentration gradient across the membrane, (3) charged ions that distribute unevenly across the membrane, and (4) an active process that removes Na^+ from inside the neuron at the same rate as the Na^+ passively enters it.

Depolarization and Repolarization

The electrical messages of excitable cells are changes of the electrical potential difference across the cell sur-

Table 5–1 Ionic Concentrations and Equilibrium Potentials for the Squid Giant Axon

ION	[X]in, mM	[X]ext, mM	E_x, mV
Na^+	72	455	+48
K^+	345	10	−90
Cl^-	61	540	−55
Ca^{2+}	$<10^{-7}$	10	$>+64$

ext, extracellular; in, intracellular; x, ion species.

face membrane. In analyzing the electrical signals of the nervous system, neurophysiologists distinguish between action potentials and slow potentials. Action potentials are used to send messages rapidly and usually over long distances (e.g., along nerve axons in a nerve trunk). They are transmitted as brief, depolarizing changes of membrane potential at a constant speed and with no loss of amplitude. The only stimulus for an action potential is a membrane depolarization larger than the threshold level.

Slow potentials, on the other hand, do not propagate at constant amplitude or over long distances. They are responses of highly localized transducing mechanisms, with amplitude and duration determined by the amplitude and duration of the stimulus. Unlike action potentials, slow potentials have no threshold. They originate at chemical synapses, in response to the chemical transmitter, or presynaptically, in response to action potentials invading the presynaptic terminus, and at sensory or other receptors in response to appropriate stimuli. Some slow potentials are depolarizing, and some are hyperpolarizing. Whenever an action potential is initiated in normal situations, it is triggered by a depolarizing slow potential of sufficient amplitude.

Slow potentials result from structural rearrangement of membrane protein that culminates in a change in the ionic permeability of the cell membrane. For instance, interaction of a neurotransmitter with its receptor initiates the structural rearrangement that leads to ion permeability change.

Action potentials normally are initiated by depolarizing slow potentials. At threshold, a process termed "activation" leads to the opening of the Na^+ permeability pathway, and an inward (Na^+) current is generated. At the same time, a slower process termed "inactivation" is initiated, and this leads to closing of the Na^+ permeability pathway. The net result is a transient inward current. Once activated, the Na^+ permeability pathway cannot be reactivated until the membrane potential has returned to its resting value for a brief period.[10]

The Na^+ conductance changes are accompanied by outward flow of K^+ related to voltage-dependent activation of a K^+ permeability pathway. The K^+ process is slower than the Na^+ process and has no inactivation process.

Because both activation and inactivation of the Na^+ pathway are faster than the activation process for K^+ permeability, there is an initial inward flow of Na^+ producing the action potential. As the Na^+ current starts to decay as a result of the Na^+ inactivation process, the more slowly developing outward K^+ current that produces repolarization of the membrane appears. As the membrane voltage returns to its resting value, the voltage-dependent K^+ permeability pathway is inactivated.

Although action potentials are normally initiated by slow depolarization, the rapid propagation of action potentials along an axon is self-generating owing to the voltage dependence of processes that produce the action potential. Said another way, an action potential in one area of an axon depolarizes the adjacent membrane to threshold. More precisely, this is how action potentials are propagated in C fibers. The mechanism of impulse propagation is slightly different for myelinated fibers.

Recall that myelinated axons are surrounded by myelin formed by Schwann cells wrapped tightly around the axon. This provides an insulating layer that is broken every 0.2 to 1 mm for a length of about 5 μm in regions called "nodes of Ranvier." Na^+ channels are concentrated in this nodal region, and this is where action potentials are generated. The change in membrane potential caused by the action potential in one node extends to the next node and elicits an action potential in that node. This process is termed "saltatory conduction."

Ion Channels

The concept of ionic channels as discrete, ion selective, molecular pores is universally accepted. Channels such as the Na^+ pore that can change from being primarily nonconductive to being conductive are called "gated channels." If the conductance state change is induced by electrical forces, the channel is said to be "voltage gated." If the conductance change is initiated by the binding of a ligand to a receptor, the channel is said to be "ligand gated."[11] Voltage-gated sodium and potassium channels are the ones of greatest importance in terms of depolarization and repolarization of axonal membranes.[12] The voltage-gated Na^+ channel is generally accepted as the target of local anesthetics.

Structure

Voltage-gated channels have been subjected to intense investigation by scientists. As a result, there is much known about these channels, including their genetic code and hence molecular structure. Structure-function drawings of voltage-gated ion channels are readily available (see Fig. 5–2C). The basic form of these drawings has not changed much during the last 10 or more years. What *has* changed is the detail added to the drawing. For instance, the drawing in Figure 5–2C contains some detail about a voltage sensor. There are strong functional analogies among the different ion channels. The striking differences are thought to arise as variations on a common structural and functional theme.[13] Understanding the molecular basis for voltage-dependent activation, rapid inactivation, and selective and efficient ion conductance is a major goal of current research on ion channel proteins.

Na^+ channels have four repeating α subunits and a β_1 and a β_2 subunit. Focus here is on α subunits because they are able to perform channel function. The β subunits apparently have a modulatory influence on the α subunits. Each of the four α subunits is composed of six α-helical transmembrane segments that are repeating amino acid chains (see Fig. 5–2D and 5–2E). The locations of the voltage sensor, inactivation gating loop, and pore lining are shown in Figure 5–2. The

primary feature that determines ion specificity apparently is the amino acid sequence in the amino acid chains.

Channel States

Voltage-gated ion channels exist in different states depending on the transmembrane potential and recent functional history. For instance, at negative membrane potentials, most Na^+ channels are in closed, resting states. In response to membrane depolarization, the channels convert to the open state, resulting in Na^+ influx through the channel, and then they convert to a nonconducting, inactive state.[14] The local anesthetic receptor in the Na^+ channel apparently has a higher affinity when channels are open or inactivated than when the channels are resting; hence the terms "state-dependent block" and "modulated receptor."

Electrophysiologic Measurements of Gating Currents

If ionic currents are blocked by substitution of permeant ions or by using open-channel blockers, currents can still be measured when the membrane potential is changed (Fig. 5–4E). These currents are gating currents and are caused by the movement of protein-bound charges. Charge movement in the voltage sensor of the Na^+ channel is thought to produce the gating current. Local anesthetics decrease the fraction of "on" charge movements associated with Na^+ channel activation.[15]

Classification of Mammalian Axons

There are two major classes of mammalian axons: myelinated and unmyelinated (Fig. 5–5). The myelinated axons are divided into two groups, A and B, and the unmyelinated form a single C group (Table 5–2). There are four subclasses of A fibers: α, β, γ, δ. The classification is based on structure, size, conduction velocity, and function of the axons. Differences in how action potentials are propagated in the two major classes of axons have already been mentioned (saltatory and nonsaltatory).

Physiologic Perspectives on Other Potential Local Anesthetic Targets

Given the structural similarities between Na^+, K^+, and Ca^{2+} channels, it is reasonable to expect that the effects of local anesthetics may not be exerted selectively on Na^+ channels. One example of an effect of local anesthetics on Ca^{2+} channels that might contribute to spinal anesthesia was reported by Sugiyama and Muteki.[16] Using cultured cells from rat dorsal root ganglion, they demonstrated that tetracaine depressed two types of Ca^{2+} channels: the high-voltage activated

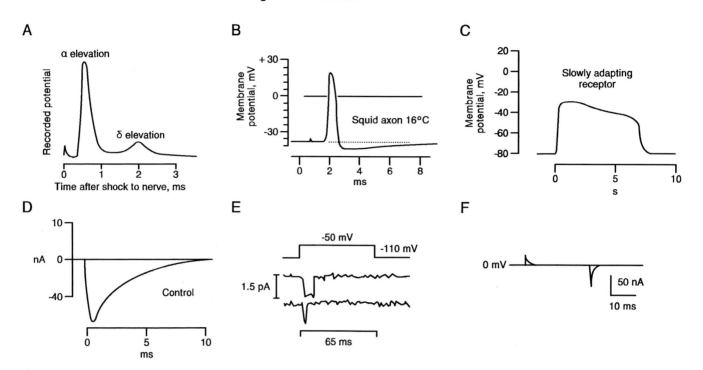

Figure 5–4 Sequence of recordings representing different levels of electrical activity recorded from axons or primary sensory receptors. *A,* Compound action potential recorded from a nerve trunk. *B,* Single action potential recorded with intra-axonal electrode. A compound action potential is the summation of many single action potentials. *C,* Slow depolarization recorded with electrode in a slowly adapting sensory receptor. The slow depolarization generates one or more action potentials in an individual axon. *D,* Ionic currents (Na+ down, K+ up) recorded from an axon that are generated during depolarization and repolarization. *E,* Single-channel currents, many of which form the current trace shown in *D. F,* Gating currents recorded when ionic currents are prevented during membrane depolarization. Note different units and scales on axes.

and the low-voltage activated. They suggested that inhibition by local anesthetics of Ca^{2+} influx through voltage-gated Ca^{2+} channels might interfere with neurotransmitter release because the release depends on Ca^{2+} flux. Such release would block synaptic transmission. Tabatabai and Booth[17] demonstrated that nerve cell soma isolated from the rat superior cervical ganglia was more sensitive than presynaptic nerve fibers to lidocaine. They concluded that when local anesthetics are injected into areas where cell bodies and processes (axons and dendrites) are present together, such as

during stellate ganglion block, lumbar sympathetic block, celiac plexus block, and intrathecal administration for spinal anesthesia, the cell bodies and the processes are all affected.

Sotgiu et al[18] reported that intravenous administration of lidocaine has a selective effect on the transmitter-receptor systems involved in the processing of nociceptive information in the spinal cord dorsal horn. Their findings and those by Woolf and Wiesenfeld-Hallin[19] showed that intravenous administration of lidocaine suppresses the responses of wide dynamic

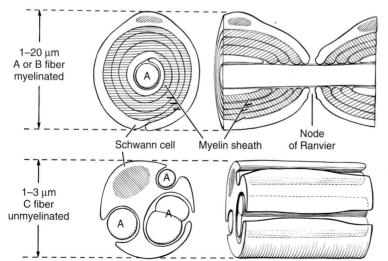

Figure 5–5 Schematic drawing of unmyelinated and myelinated axons (A) enveloped in Schwann cells. The vertebrate C fiber usually has several axons surrounded by one Schwann cell. The myelinated fiber has one axon wrapped in a myelin sheath formed by a spiral wrapping of Schwann cell membranes. At periodic intervals, the myelin sheath is interrupted, forming the node of Ranvier.

Table 5–2 Classification of Fibers in Peripheral Nerves

FIBER TYPE	DIAMETER, μm	MYELIN	CONDUCTION VELOCITY (MEAN), m/s	FUNCTION
A				
α	12–20	Yes	100	Proprioception, motor or skeletal muscle
β	5–12	Yes	50	Cutaneous touch, motor
γ	3–6	Yes	20	Muscle tone (motor to muscle spindles)
δ	2–5	Yes	15	Pain, temperature, touch
B	1–4	Yes	7	Preganglionic autonomic
C	0.3–1.2	No	1	Pain and postganglionic autonomic

range neurons in the dorsal horn of rats to noxious but not to non-noxious stimulation. The *Veratrum* alkaloid veratridine apparently inhibits impulse propagation in C fibers of the rabbit, with some selectivity and in a use-dependent manner.[20] Veratridine binds to and selectively stabilizes an open configuration of the Na^+ channel. This produces a persistent increase in Na^+ permeability and subsequently in membrane depolarization. The investigators suggested that the *Veratrum* alkaloids may be a useful means of providing peripheral analgesia.

Concluding Comments

This chapter focuses almost exclusively on those events leading to sensory perception that depend on voltage-gated ion channels, with emphasis on voltage-gated Na^+ channels in peripheral axons because these generally are accepted as being the target of local anesthetics. Receptors on or near ligand-dependent ion channels are generally accepted as being the targets of other drugs (e.g., α_2-adrenergic agonists, opioids) used to produce regional analgesia.

References

1. White MM: Excitability and conduction. In Frazer A, Molinoff PB, Winokur A (eds): Biological Bases of Brain Function and Disease, pp 19–32. New York, Raven Press, 1994.
2. Hille B: Introduction to physiology of excitable cells. In Patton HD, Fuchs AF, Hille B, et al (eds): Textbook of Physiology: Excitable Cells and Neurophysiology, 21st ed, pp 1–20. Philadelphia, WB Saunders Co, 1989.
3. Young JZ: Structure of nerve fibres and synapses in some invertebrates. Cold Spring Harbor Symp Quant Biol 1936; 4: 1–12.
4. Katz B: Nerve, Muscle, and Synapse. New York, McGraw-Hill, 1966.
5. Hodgkin AL: The Conduction of the Nervous Impulse. Springfield, IL, Charles C Thomas, 1964.
6. Curtis HJ, Cole KS: Transverse impedance of the giant squid axon. J Gen Physiol 1938; 21: 757–765.
7. Hodgkin AL, Huxley AF: A quantitative description of membrane current and its application to conduction and excitation in nerve. J Physiol (Lond) 1952; 117: 500–544.
8. Gardner D (ed): Forty years of membrane current in nerve. Physiol Rev 1992; 72(suppl): S1–S186.
9. Hille B: Membrane excitability: action potential propagation in axons. In Patton HD, Fuchs AF, Hille B, et al (eds): Textbook of Physiology: Excitable Cells and Neurophysiology, 21st ed, pp 49–79. Philadelphia, WB Saunders Co, 1989.
10. Stühmer W: Structure and function of sodium channels. Cell Physiol Biochem 1993; 3: 277–282.
11. North RA (ed): Ligand- and Voltage-Gated Ion Channels. Boca Raton, FL, CRC Press, 1995.
12. Hille B: Voltage-gated channels and electrical excitability. In Patton HD, Fuchs AF, Hille B, et al (eds): Textbook of Physiology: Excitable Cells and Neurophysiology, 21st ed, pp 80–97. Philadelphia, WB Saunders Co, 1989.
13. Catterall WA: Structure and function of voltage-gated ion channels. Trends Neurosci 1993; 16: 500–506.
14. Ragsdale DS, McPhee JC, Scheuer T, et al: Molecular determinants of state-dependent block of Na^+ channels by local anesthetics. Science 1994; 265: 1724–1728.
15. Bekkers JM, Greeff NG, Keynes RD, et al: The effect of local anaesthetics on the components of the asymmetry current in the squid giant axon. J Physiol (Lond) 1984; 352: 653–668.
16. Sugiyama K, Muteki T: Local anesthetics depress the calcium current of rat sensory neurons in culture. Anesthesiology 1994; 80: 1369–1378.
17. Tabatabai M, Booth AM: Effects of lidocaine on the excitability and membrane properties of the nerve cell soma. Clin Physiol Biochem 1990; 8: 289–296.
18. Sotgiu ML, Lacerenza M, Marchettini P: Selective inhibition by systemic lidocaine of noxious evoked activity in rat dorsal horn neurons. Neuroreport 1991; 2: 425–428.
19. Woolf CJ, Wiesenfeld-Hallin Z: The systemic administration of local anaesthetics produces a selective depression of C-afferent fibre evoked activity in the spinal cord. Pain 1985; 23: 361–374.
20. Schneider M, Datta S, Strichartz G: A preferential inhibition of impulses in C-fibers of the rabbit vagus nerve by veratridine, an activator of sodium channels. Anesthesiology 1991; 74: 270–280.

CHAPTER 6
Cardiopulmonary Physiology

David C. Mackey, M.D.

The Pulmonary System

The principal purpose of the pulmonary system is to maintain the oxygen and carbon dioxide content of the arterial blood within a narrow physiologic range, despite a constantly varying rate of metabolism. This is achieved by pulmonary gas exchange, which is under tight neurochemical control and is composed of three processes: ventilation, or the movement of alveolar gas to and from the external environment; diffusion, or the transfer of alveolar gas between the alveolus and the capillary blood; and perfusion, or the distribution of pulmonary blood flow to the alveoli for optimal gas exchange. A basic understanding of pulmonary physiology and the more common disturbances in its component homeostatic functions is essential for the anesthesiologist to maximize the therapeutic efficacy and minimize the risk of regional anesthetic and analgesic procedures.

The Larynx

The adult larynx lies anterior to the third through sixth cervical vertebrae and connects the pharynx superiorly to the trachea inferiorly. This hollow organ lined by mucous membrane is composed of cartilage, ligaments, muscles, and membranes. Successful execution of various topical and regional anesthetic procedures involving this structure requires familiarity with its function and innervation (Fig. 6–1). Although phonation is the most prominent purpose of the larynx, the anesthesiologist is primarily concerned with its role in airway protection and obstruction. The narrowest portion of the larynx is at the level of the vocal cords in adults and at the level of the cricoid cartilage in young children. It is here that the presence of foreign objects and of mucosal edema secondary to instrumentation or anaphylaxis is most likely to cause upper airway obstruction. Bilateral recurrent laryngeal nerve paralysis, resulting in flaccid, approximated vocal cords, and laryngospasm may also cause upper airway obstruction.

Laryngeal airway protection is achieved by means of the swallow, gag, and cough reflexes.[1, 2] These reflexes are elicited by tactile and noxious chemical laryngeal stimulation, which initiates vagal afferent impulses that are transmitted to the medulla for processing and which produce the stereotypic efferent protective swallow, gag, and cough responses. Stimulation of the trachea and lower airway structures also produces the vagal-mediated cough reflex. Airway stimulation may provoke a substantial neuroendocrine stress response,[3, 4] and the protective airway reflexes may be deliberately blunted or abolished for diagnostic and therapeutic purposes by topical application of local anesthetics to the mucosa of the upper airway or by specific nerve blocks. However, even in the absence of topical or regional anesthesia, the anesthesiologist must remain vigilant to the possibility of depressed airway reflexes, with the attendant risk of pulmonary aspiration, in the settings of abnormal levels of consciousness, advanced age, general debility, and administration of volatile anesthetics, opioids, and other systemic anesthetic and analgesic agents.

Sensory innervation of the posterior portion of the tongue, pharynx, and tonsils is furnished by the glossopharyngeal nerve, and mucosal sensory innervation

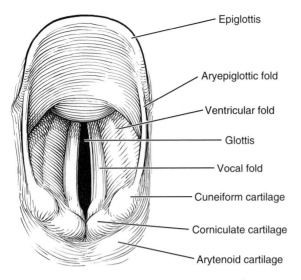

Figure 6–1 Laryngeal structures visible during direct laryngoscopy in the adult patient.

Epiglottis

Aryepiglottic fold

Ventricular fold

Glottis

Vocal fold

Cuneiform cartilage

Corniculate cartilage

Arytenoid cartilage

from the epiglottis to the vocal cords is provided by the superior laryngeal nerve branch of the vagus nerve. Sensory innervation from the vocal cords to the upper region of the trachea is furnished by the recurrent laryngeal branch of the vagus nerve. With the exception of the cricothyroid muscle and a portion of the transverse arytenoid muscle, which are supplied by the external branch of the superior laryngeal nerve and which tense and approximate the vocal cord, respectively, all motor innervation of the larynx is provided by the recurrent laryngeal nerve. Injury or local anesthetic block of a recurrent laryngeal nerve results in hoarseness, with the ipsilateral vocal cord positioned midline as a result of unopposed action of the cricothyroid and transverse arytenoid muscles. Bilateral recurrent laryngeal nerve injury or block results in midline approximation of both vocal cords and possible ventilatory obstruction.

Anatomy of the Lung

The respiratory tract is divided into conducting and respiratory portions. The conducting system conveys the inspired and expired gases to and from the respiratory portion of the lung, where gaseous exchange with the blood occurs. The conducting system begins with the trachea, a flexible tube approximately 11 cm long and 2 cm in diameter in adults, which extends from the cricoid cartilage, corresponding to the level of the sixth cervical vertebra, to its bifurcation at the carina at the level of the fifth thoracic vertebra into the two main stem bronchi. The trachea is lined with ciliated epithelium and mucus-secreting goblet cells. Its patency is maintained by a series of C-shaped cartilage rings closed posteriorly by smooth muscle. Distal to the trachea, the conducting portion of the respiratory tract continues as an arborescent system of tubular structures beginning as the two main stem bronchi and

ending approximately 16 generations of branching later as the terminal bronchioles.

The respiratory portion of the respiratory tract is the site of gaseous exchange between inspired air and pulmonary capillary blood.[5, 6] It begins with the branching of the terminal bronchioles into the respiratory bronchioles and continues for approximately another seven generations of arborization to end with the alveoli. There are approximately 300 million alveoli in the lungs, with each alveolus having an average diameter of approximately 0.2 mm. Alveolar type II pneumonocytes secrete surfactant, a phospholipid substance that lowers the surface tension of fluid lining the alveoli and prevents their collapse.[7-9] The alveolar walls are immediately adjacent to the surrounding pulmonary capillaries, and it is here that most of the gaseous exchange between inspired air and pulmonary blood takes place (Fig. 6–2). The large total surface area of the alveolar septa forms a respiratory membrane of approximately 70 m^2.

The Pleura

Each hemithorax is lined by parietal pleura, a serous membrane rich in blood and lymphatic vessels, which is reflected over each lung as the visceral pleura.[10] A thin layer of fluid lines the interpleural space and lubricates the movement of the lungs. The elastic recoil of the lung created by the surface tension of the fluid lining the alveoli and by the elastin and collagen fibers of the lung parenchyma itself opposes the outward expansion of the chest wall and creates a negative pressure in the interpleural space of approximately 5 cm H_2O during breathing at rest. Lung collapse (i.e., pneumothorax) of variable degree secondary to its property of elastic recoil occurs if air is introduced into

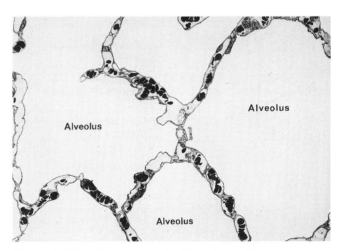

Figure 6–2 The photomicrograph of lung tissue with erythrocyte-filled pulmonary capillaries immediately adjacent to alveoli illustrates the large surface area of the respiratory membrane and the extremely thin diffusion barrier between inspired air and pulmonary capillary blood. (Original investigator, Peter Gehr.) (From Fawcett DW: A Textbook of Histology, 11th ed, p 747. Courtesy of Gehr P: By permission of Chapman & Hall, New York.)

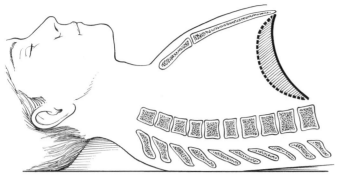

Figure 6–3 Normal diaphragmatic displacement (shaded area) and end-expiratory position (broken line) in an awake, supine, spontaneously breathing person at rest.

the interpleural space through a hole in the chest wall or, more commonly, during administration of regional anesthetics by needle penetration of the extremely delicate lung tissue.

The Muscles of Ventilation

During normal inspiration, the lungs are expanded by downward excursion of the diaphragm and by elevation of the ribs, which lengthens chest cavity and increases its anteroposterior diameter, respectively (Figs. 6–3 and 6–4).[11, 12] During resting inspiration, the contribution of intercostal muscle contraction is small, with more than 75% of the effort supplied by contraction of the diaphragm. The diaphragm is anatomically divided into a crural part, composed of fibers arising from paravertebral ligaments; a costal part, composed of fibers arising from the lower ribs; and a fibrous central tendon.

Resting expiration is a passive phenomenon, with compression of the lung tissue by the elastic recoil of the thoracic wall, the abdomen, and the lungs themselves and by diaphragmatic relaxation. Most of the work of breathing at rest is normally expended during inspiration, overcoming the elastic recoil of the lungs and chest, but at increased ventilatory rates or in conditions of narrowed airways, the increase in gas flow resistance demands a much larger percentage of ventilatory effort. In these situations, diaphragmatic inspiratory effort is augmented by the external intercostal muscles, which elevate the rib cage and increase the anteroposterior diameter of the thoracic cavity approximately 20% at maximal exertion. The sternocleidomastoid, anterior serratus, and scalene muscles assist the external intercostals by also providing tension force to elevate the ribs.[13]

During active expiration, the elastic recoil forces of the thoracic and abdominal structures acting to compress the lungs are augmented by contraction of the internal intercostal muscles and by the muscles of the abdominal wall (i.e., rectus abdominis, transversus abdominis, and internal and external obliques), which pull the rib cage downward to decrease the anteroposterior dimension of the thoracic cavity and which put upward pressure on the diaphragm by increasing intraabdominal pressure.[14]

Innervation of the Muscles of Ventilation

Motor innervation of the diaphragm is provided by the phrenic nerves (i.e., C-3 to C-5). The diaphragm is

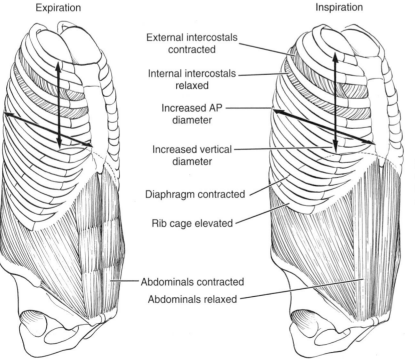

Expiration

Inspiration

External intercostals contracted

Internal intercostals relaxed

Increased AP diameter

Increased vertical diameter

Diaphragm contracted

Rib cage elevated

Abdominals contracted
Abdominals relaxed

Figure 6–4 Effect of intercostal muscles on expansion and contraction of the thoracic cavity during inspiration and expiration, respectively. AP, anteroposterior.

differentially innervated, allowing the costal and crural sections to contract independently. Sensory innervation of the diaphragm is provided by the phrenic and the lower intercostal nerves.

The intercostal nerves supply the chest wall and much of the abdominal wall, providing motor innervation to the internal and external intercostal muscles and most of the abdominal musculature. Accurate knowledge of the anatomic distribution and origin of the intercostal nerves is essential for efficacious regional blocks and for appreciation of possible complications of the blocks.[15] Shortly after the dorsal and ventral roots combine to form the segmental nerve at each spinal cord level, the segmental nerve divides into a dorsal ramus, which supplies vertebral and paravertebral structures, and a ventral ramus, or intercostal nerve (Fig. 6–5). Each intercostal nerve is closely accompanied by an intercostal artery and vein and lies in the costal groove as it courses laterally until it reaches the rib angle. At approximately that point, it leaves the groove to lie initially deep to and then within the substance of the internal intercostal muscle as it courses through the thoracic wall from the vertebral column to the sternum (Fig. 6–6).

Only the third through the sixth intercostal nerves follow this stereotypic distribution. The first thoracic nerve contributes to the brachial plexus and provides only a small intercostal nerve, which frequently possesses no lateral or anterior cutaneous branches. The 7th through 11th intercostal nerves leave their respective intercostal spaces to supply the abdominal wall musculature, and the 12th thoracic segmental nerve is the subcostal nerve, which also supplies abdominal wall musculature.

Motor innervation of the accessory muscles of ventilation is provided by several nerves. The sternocleidomastoid muscles are supplied by the spinal accessory nerve (i.e., cranial nerve XI) and by the second cervical nerve of the cervical plexus. Motor innervation of the scalene muscles is provided directly by ventral rami of the cervical nerves. The anterior serratus muscles are innervated by the long thoracic nerve (i.e., C-5 to C-7), which originates from the brachial plexus.

Autonomic Innervation of the Thorax and Lungs

Each intercostal nerve connects to the sympathetic chain through white and gray rami communicantes. The preganglionic sympathetic neuron cell bodies reside in the intermediolateral horn of the spinal cord. Preganglionic sympathetic fibers exit the spinal cord through the anterior spinal nerve root to enter the corresponding spinal nerve. Each preganglionic sympathetic fiber then enters a paravertebral sympathetic chain ganglion through a white ramus communicans. Most preganglionic sympathetic fibers synapse with a postganglionic neuron in the ganglion they have entered. However, some extend up or down the sympathetic chain to synapse in one of the other chain ganglia, and others pass through the paravertebral gan-

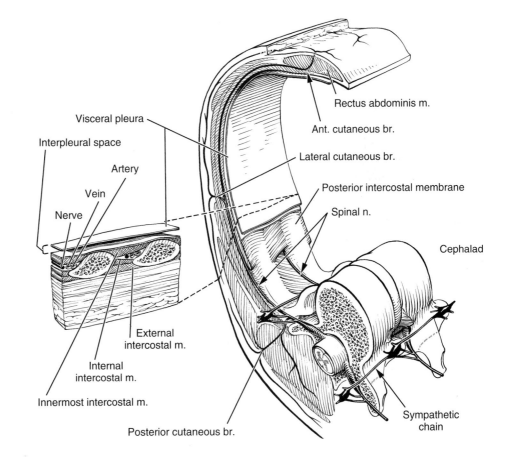

Figure 6–5 Typical course of an intercostal nerve (i.e., ventral ramus of a thoracic segmental nerve). Ant., anterior; br., branch; m., muscle; n., nerve.

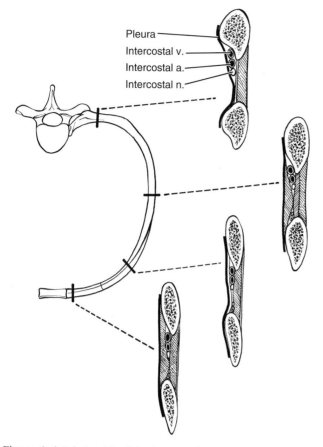

Pleura
Intercostal v.
Intercostal a.
Intercostal n.

Figure 6–6 Relationship of the intercostal neurovascular bundle to an adjacent rib and intercostal muscles as it courses through the thoracic wall from the vertebral column to the sternum. a., artery; n., nerve; v., vein.

glion chain to synapse on postganglionic neurons located in collateral ganglia near the visceral structures they innervate. Postganglionic fibers exit the sympathetic chain ganglia to reenter the spinal nerves through the gray rami communicantes and then continue to their effector organ by means of the spinal nerve, or the fibers pass through the sympathetic chain or collateral ganglia to the structure they innervate through sympathetic nerves.

The trachea and lungs are innervated by afferent and efferent sympathetic and parasympathetic fibers, and autonomic regulation is an important factor for modulation of pulmonary ventilation and pulmonary perfusion.[16–20] Sympathetic innervation originates at the spinal cord level of T-1 through T-4, and parasympathetic innervation is contributed by the vagus nerves. Pulmonary autonomic fibers have been found as far distally as the alveolar ducts and alveolar walls.

Parasympathetic autonomic innervation of the upper and lower airways and of the respiratory portion of the lungs is accomplished through preganglionic fibers whose cell bodies are located in the medulla. These fibers course through the vagus nerves to synapse with postganglionic neurons located within the thoracic structures they innervate.

The autonomic nervous system is an important factor

in bronchospastic disease.[21–23] The walls of the bronchi and bronchioles contain more smooth muscle than any other portion of the respiratory tract, and they receive sympathetic and parasympathetic innervation.[24] β_2-Adrenergic stimulation causes bronchodilation and decreased bronchial secretion; cholinergic stimulation causes bronchoconstriction. Nonadrenergic, noncholinergic innervation of the respiratory tract promotes bronchodilation, possibly mediated by vasoactive intestinal peptide.[25, 26] Inflammatory mediators such as the leukotrienes produce bronchoconstriction. Some pulmonary nerve fibers contain substance P and other neuropeptides, the significance of which is unknown.

Autonomic nervous system activity is also a key factor in neurogenic pulmonary edema, which is a relatively common, although only partially understood, phenomenon occurring with central nervous system injury such as intracranial hemorrhage, seizure, or trauma. This process is mediated by massive centrally mediated sympathetic discharge and perhaps other autonomic activity, and it involves increased pulmonary vascular pressure and pulmonary capillary leak.[27–30]

Metabolic and Pharmacokinetic Functions of the Lungs

Although the primary purpose of the lungs is gas exchange between the atmosphere and blood, the organs also serve several nonrespiratory functions. These processes include the ability to synthesize, activate, inactivate, or sequester many substances, including local anesthetics (Table 6–1).[31, 32]

Regulation of Ventilation

Precise autonomic neural control of ventilation in response to the variations in metabolic rate is main-

Table 6–1 Metabolic and Pharmacokinetic Functions of the Lungs

Synthesized and released into the blood
Prostaglandins
Histamine
Kallikrein
von Willebrand factor
Tissue plasminogen activator
Partially removed from the blood
Prostaglandins
Bradykinin
Serotonin
Norepinephrine
Acetylcholine
Fentanyl
Propranolol
Lidocaine
Atrial natriuretic factor
Adenosine
Imipramine
Activated in the lung
Angiotensin I
Arachidonic acid

Modified from Stoelting RK: Pharmacology and Physiology in Anesthetic Practice, 2nd ed, p 730. Philadelphia, JB Lippincott, 1991.

tained by the respiratory center located in the pons and medulla (Fig. 6–7).[33] Two groups of medullary neurons, a dorsal group composed primarily of inspiratory neurons and a ventral group composed of inspiratory and expiratory neurons, provide the basic, underlying reciprocal inspiratory and expiratory drive. Normally, at rest inspiration is an active process driven by phrenic motor innervation of the diaphragm, and expiration is a passive process initiated by cessation of phrenic efferent motor traffic and thus diaphragmatic relaxation. The pneumotaxic center in the dorsal pons regulates inspiration by its inhibitory influence on the inspiratory neuron group of the dorsal medulla. Ventilatory signals from the respiratory center are influenced by neural input from stretch receptors located in the walls of the bronchi and bronchioles and from chemoreceptors located in the medulla and in the carotid and aortic bodies. Cortical modulation by corticospinal tracts also affects the activity of the respiratory center.

Contribution of Thoracic Anatomy to Risk in Regional Anesthetic Procedures

The proximity of the intercostal nerves to the adjacent interpleural space and underlying lung tissue presents the risk of pneumothorax in intercostal and paravertebral nerve block procedures. For the same reason, pneumothorax is also a principal risk of brachial plexus blocks performed near the first rib and directed to the level of the nerve trunks and divisions because of the proximity of the lung apex. Brown and colleagues[34] described a technique of supraclavicular block derived from cadaveric and magnetic resonance imaging study of regional anatomic structures and designed to minimize this risk (Fig. 6–8).

At the intervertebral foramen, the dura, arachnoid, and pia membranes fuse and become continuous with the epineurium of the peripheral segmental nerves. Local anesthetic and neurolytic solutions injected intra-

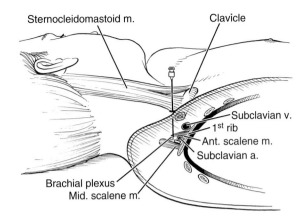

Figure 6–8 The supraclavicular block technique of Brown and colleagues was designed to minimize risk of pneumothorax by avoidance of the lung apex. The needle insertion point is immediately adjacent to the superior margin of the clavicle, at the lateral border of the insertion of the clavicular head of the sternocleidomastoid muscle (m.) onto the clavicle. Paresthesias are sought by needle movement confined to a parasagittal plane situated at the needle insertion site, first through a 30° arc cephalad and then through a 30° arc caudad. a., artery; Ant., anterior; Mid., middle; v., vein. (Modified from Brown DL, Cahill DR, Bridenbaugh LD: Supraclavicular nerve block: anatomic analysis of a method to prevent pneumothorax. Anesth Analg 1993; 76: 530–534.)

neurally during intercostal nerve block may spread centrally by means of this potential conduit into the cerebrospinal fluid if the block procedure is performed near the vertebral column or if the volume of injectant is greater than 2 to 3 mL.[35–38] In addition to spreading within the intercostal space, the loose structure of the innermost intercostal muscle provides a pathway for intercostal injections to spread to adjacent intercostal spaces, with the extent of spread dependent on the volume injected.[39] The proximity of vascular structures to each intercostal nerve and its branches enhances systemic local anesthetic absorption, increasing the relative risk of local anesthetic systemic toxicity with intercostal nerve block.[40, 41] The rich vascularity of the upper airway mucosa also facilitates local anesthetic uptake and increases the risk of local anesthetic systemic toxicity with topical anesthesia of the larynx and trachea.

Regional block procedures that affect the intercostal or phrenic nerve (or both) and, to a lesser extent, the accessory muscles of ventilation have an effect on ventilatory mechanics that depends on the extent of the block. The appreciable plasma levels of local anesthetics which accompany certain regional anesthetic procedures and the sedation used as an adjunct to regional blocks also may have an effect on ventilation.[42, 43] The significance of these risks depends on the degree of patient debility.[44–49] Cough is a protective mechanism for removal of bronchopulmonary secretions, particularly in the setting of abnormal mucociliary function or excessive secretions.[50–52] The effectiveness of this protective reflex may be diminished or abolished by block of its afferent sensory limb or its efferent motor limb.

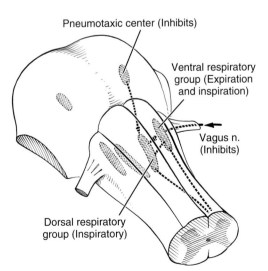

Figure 6–7 Ventral depiction of the respiratory center, which is located bilaterally in the pons and medulla. n., nerve.

The Cardiovascular System

The function of the heart and circulatory system is to transport blood, which carries oxygen and nutrients to the peripheral tissues and removes metabolic by-products. The anesthesiologist should possess a basic understanding of the physiology of this system, because regional anesthetic procedures may influence normal cardiovascular function directly or indirectly through effects on its neural control mechanisms. Underlying pathologic changes in the cardiovascular system may profoundly affect the physiologic results of regional anesthetic techniques. Regional anesthesia may be tailored to a specific disease state and surgical procedure in an attempt to improve perioperative outcome.

The Heart as a Circulatory Pump

The heart is a four-chamber muscular organ that can be considered as two functionally separated pumps: the right side of the heart and the left side of the heart. Each side of the heart consists of a ventricle, which contracts forcefully to propel blood through the pulmonary and systemic circulations, and an atrium, which is a conduit and reservoir that receives venous blood and contracts to prime the ventricle. The right side of the heart receives deoxygenated venous blood from the systemic circulation and pumps it through the pulmonary circulation; the left side of the heart receives oxygenated blood from the pulmonary veins and pumps it through the systemic circulation. Four valves, two in each side of the heart, maintain forward blood flow.

The coronary arteries originate from the aortic root and supply almost all of the nutritive blood supply to the myocardium, with the right coronary artery supplying most of the right ventricle and the posterior portion of the left ventricle and the left coronary artery supplying the anterior and lateral portions of the left ventricle. Unlike other vascular beds of the body, capillary blood flow to the left ventricular myocardium decreases to a relatively low value during systole instead of diastole because of compression of the left ventricular intramyocardial blood vessels by the forceful contraction of the left ventricular myocardium in systole. Tachycardia, in which the myocardium spends relatively more of the cardiac cycle in systole, may be accompanied by lower coronary blood flow at a time when myocardial metabolic demands are increased. Most of the venous blood from the left ventricle returns to the central circulation through the coronary sinus, and most of the venous blood from the right ventricle empties directly into the right atrium through the anterior cardiac veins. The thebesian veins return a small portion of the venous coronary blood flow directly into all four chambers of the heart.

Coronary blood flow is controlled principally by local tissue autoregulation by means of vasodilator metabolites such as adenosine. However, the autonomic nervous system affects coronary blood flow by regulation of systemic arterial blood pressure and by regulation of heart rate. The coronary vasculature also receives rich autonomic innervation. Although the coronary vasculature contains α- and β-adrenergic receptors, the direct effect of sympathetic stimulation is probably limited to vasoconstriction. Parasympathetic stimulation may provide a weak, direct vasodilator effect.[53]

Cardiac Electrophysiology

The heart is a muscular organ with a fibrous connective tissue skeleton. The cardiac muscle fibers form a tightly knit syncytium that allows electrical impulses to propagate easily throughout the mass of the organ (Fig. 6–9). Coordinated muscular contraction is initiated and propagated by specialized pacemaker and conduction muscle tissue. Rhythmic discharge of the sinus, or sinoatrial, node, located near the superior vena cava in the superior lateral wall of the right atrium, initiates the cardiac cycle. Electrical impulses from the sinus node are transmitted across the atria and to the atrioventricular node by the interconnected atrial myocytes and by internodal pathways composed of specialized conducting atrial muscle fibers.

The atrioventricular node, which is located in the septal wall of the right atrium posteriorly near the ostium of the coronary sinus, delays the electrical impulse slightly before conducting it to the atrioventricular bundle of His. The cardiac impulse then is transmitted by means of the atrioventricular bundle across the fibrous cardiac skeleton, which electrically isolates the atria from the ventricles, to the ventricular muscle. The atrioventricular bundle subsequently divides into the right and left bundles of Purkinje and then arborizes throughout the ventricular muscle mass, allowing the cardiac impulse to depolarize the ventricular muscle fibers in a rapid coordinated manner.

The action potential of cardiac fibers is typical of that of other excitable membranes in that it can be characterized by electrochemical phases that are represented by changes in membrane potential

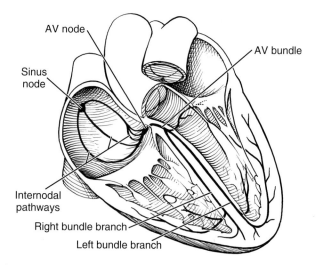

Figure 6–9 The sinus node, atrioventricular (AV) node, and cardiac conduction system.

(Fig. 6–10).[54–56] Phase 4 represents the resting potential of the myocyte membrane. Phase 0 represents opening, or activation, of fast Na^+ channels and decreased K^+ permeability, with rapid movement of Na^+ into the cell. Phase 1, or early rapid repolarization, represents inactivation of the Na^+ channels and a brief increase in K^+ permeability, with movement of K^+ out of the cell. Activation of slow Ca^{2+} channels, allowing movement of Ca^{2+} into the cell, occurs during phase 2. Phase 3, characterized by inactivation of Ca^{2+} channels, increased permeability to K^+, and movement of K^+ out of the cell, marks the completion of repolarization and the return to the baseline resting potential. Although the basic electrochemical action potential physiology is similar for all excitable cardiac cells, the mechanisms vary sufficiently to result in characteristic action potential morphologies for each of the different types of cardiac muscle fibers (see Fig. 6–10).

The cardiac impulse ordinarily is initiated by the sinoatrial node, which is the pacemaker of the heart. Constant leakage of Na^+ into the sinus node fibers gradually raises the resting potential (i.e., phase 4) of the fiber to a threshold voltage of approximately -40 mV, at which point activation of calcium-sodium channels allows rapid entry of Ca^{2+} and Na^+ into the cell interior (i.e., phase 0), initiating an action potential (Fig. 6–11). Although the atrioventricular node and Purkinje fibers possess the same properties of self-excitation (i.e., automaticity) and repetitive discharge (i.e., rhythmicity) as the sinus node, the sinus node fibers normally discharge more rapidly, depolarizing the other potential pacemaker cells before their spontaneous depolarization can occur. Conditions that slow or interrupt the discharge rate of the sinoatrial node, which ordinarily depolarizes at a rate of 70 to 80 beats/min and suppresses other potential pacemaker tissue that discharges at a slower rate, may allow the atrioventricular node, which discharges at a rate of 40 to 60 beats/min, or Purkinje fibers, which discharge at a rate of 15 to 40 beats/min, to emerge as the cardiac pacemaker.

Effect of Local Anesthetic Agents on the Cardiovascular System

Like cells of the peripheral and central nervous system, the property of excitability possessed by myocardial fibers renders them susceptible to the effects of local anesthetics.[57–60] This pharmacologic susceptibility may result in therapeutic or toxic effects as a consequence of the direct action of the local anesthetic agent on the myocardial cells, with dose-related decreases in cardiac contractility and conduction, or the effect of the local anesthetic agent on neural cardiac control mechanisms.[61–70] Local anesthetics may cause contraction or dilation of vascular smooth muscle.[71–73] Cocaine may produce myocardial ischemia and infarction through induction of coronary vasoconstriction.[74–76] Systemic epinephrine from epinephrine-containing local anesthetic solutions used in regional anesthesia may have therapeutic or adverse cardiovascular effects.[77–82]

Cardiac Output

Cardiac output is defined as the volume of blood pumped per minute; it is further defined as the product of the heart rate and the stroke volume.

$$\text{Cardiac output} = \text{heart rate} \times \text{stroke volume}$$

Cardiac output is frequently expressed relative to body surface area as the cardiac index.

$$\text{Cardiac index} = \text{cardiac output} \div \text{body surface area}$$

The normal value for the cardiac index is 2.5 to 4.2 L/min per m². Just as cardiac output is determined by the heart rate and stroke volume, stroke volume is determined by the variables of preload, afterload, and inotropic state of the myocardium. Ventricular preload depends on venous return, and at a constant heart rate, the cardiac output is normally directly proportional to the venous return (i.e., Frank-Starling law of the heart). Venous tone is usually the most influential factor affecting venous return, but patient positioning, pericardial fibrosis or effusion, and alterations in intrathoracic pressure may also be clinically important. An excessively high heart rate, loss of the ventricular priming effect of the atrial contraction, or abnormally low ventricular compliance can adversely affect ventricular preload and cardiac output. Ventricular afterload is determined mainly by systemic vascular resistance, which

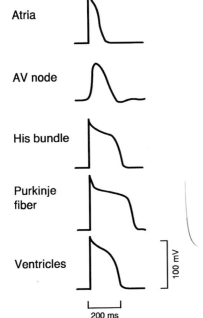

Figure 6–10 Characteristic action potential morphology from different cardiac cells. The action potential lengthens until reaching a maximum duration in the Purkinje fibers, and then it shortens. AV, atrioventricular. (From Marriott HJL, Boudreau Conover MH: Advanced Concepts in Arrhythmias, 2nd ed. St Louis, CV Mosby, 1989.)

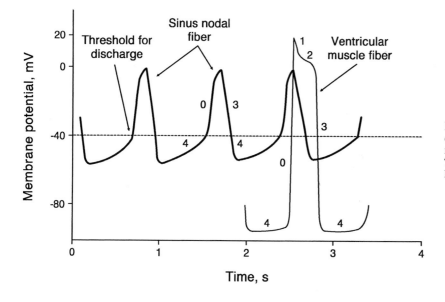

Figure 6–11 Comparison of the action potentials of sinus node fibers with those of ventricular muscle fibers. (Modified from Guyton AC: Textbook of Medical Physiology, 8th ed, p 112. Philadelphia, WB Saunders Co, 1991.)

is influenced principally by arteriolar tone. Variations in contractility are determined by humoral, neural, and myocardial disease processes.

Neural Control of the Heart

The autonomic nervous system maintains tight control of the heart and circulation through sympathetic and vagal efferent pathways that are modulated by arterial baroreflexes, cardiac reflexes, and arterial chemoreflexes (Fig. 6–12).[83–90] A basic understanding of cardiovascular control mechanisms is important to appreciate the potential for regional anesthesia to induce perturbations in hemodynamic and electrophysiologic homeostasis.

Cardiac output is heavily influenced by the balanced effect of sympathetic and parasympathetic outflow on heart rate, preload, afterload, and myocardial contractility (Fig. 6–13). Heart rate is normally set by the spontaneous depolarization rate of the sinus node, which is subject to neural and humoral influence. Neural control of the sinus node discharge rate is determined by the tonic balance of its sympathetic noradrenergic and parasympathetic cholinergic innervation, with the latter normally predominating. Resting sympathetic tone normally maintains the heart rate at approximately 30% greater than the heart rate in the setting of total sympathetic withdrawal, and strong sympathetic stimulation can increase the heart rate of young persons to as high as 200 to 250 beats/min. Administration of parasympatholytic drugs such as atropine increases the normal resting heart rate from 70 to between 150 and 180 beats/min because of unopposed resting sympathetic tone, and strong vagal stimulation can induce cardiac standstill. The heart rate increases to approximately 100 beats/min in normal resting persons under conditions of complete noradrenergic and cholinergic block.

Although reflex control of the sinus rate typically depends on afferent traffic from extracardiac receptors,

mechanisms influencing the sinus rate may also be initiated locally. Stretch of the right atrial wall initiates a neural reflex, the Bainbridge reflex, which increases the rate of sinus node depolarization, and stretch of the sinus node itself also increases its rate of discharge.[91, 92]

In addition to the influence of tonic sympathetic-parasympathetic balance on heart rate, these opposing autonomic influences also affect cardiac conductivity

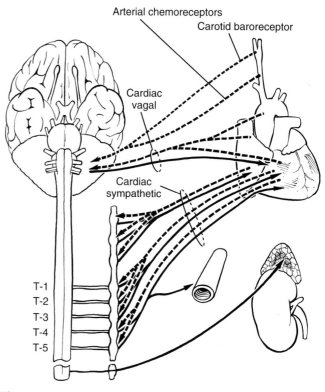

Figure 6–12 Afferent (dashed lines) and efferent (solid lines) pathways of cardiovascular mechanoreflexes and chemoreflexes involved in blood pressure control. (Modified from Smith ML, Carlson MD, Thames MD: Reflex control of the heart and circulation: implications for cardiovascular electrophysiology. J Cardiovasc Electrophysiol 1991; 2: 441–449.)

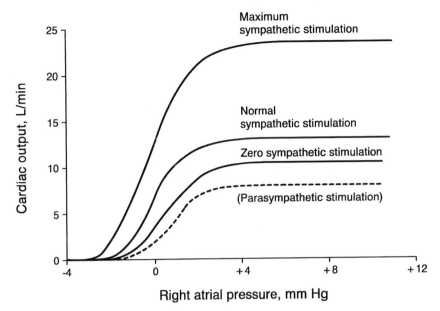

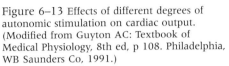

Figure 6–13 Effects of different degrees of autonomic stimulation on cardiac output. (Modified from Guyton AC: Textbook of Medical Physiology, 8th ed, p 108. Philadelphia, WB Saunders Co, 1991.)

and contractility: sympathetic discharge increases atrioventricular nodal and His-Purkinje ventricular conduction and increases atrial and ventricular contractility, and parasympathetic discharge has the opposite effect.

Control of Vasomotion

Factors influencing arteriolar and venous tone include the autoregulatory effects of the intrinsic smooth muscle contractile response to distension of the vessel wall and the vasodilator or vasoconstrictor effects of products of local tissue metabolism. Other determinants of vascular tone include systemically secreted hormones, humoral substances secreted by the endothelium, and neural control mechanisms (Table 6–2).

Table 6–2 Factors Affecting Vasomotion

CONSTRICTION	DILATION
Increased noradrenergic discharge	Decreased noradrenergic discharge
Circulating catecholamines (except epinephrine in skeletal muscle and liver)	Circulating epinephrine in skeletal muscle and liver
Angiotensin II	Atrial natriuretic peptide
Vasopressin	Histamine
Locally released serotonin	Kinins
Endothelin-1	Substance P
Neuropeptide Y	CGRPα
Decreased local temperature	Vasoactive intestinal peptide
Circulating Na$^+$-K$^+$ ATPase inhibitor	Lactate, K$^+$, adenosine
	Increased CO$_2$ tension
	Decreased pH
	Decreased O$_2$ tension
	Increased local temperature
	Nitric oxide (endothelium-derived relaxing factor)
	Activation of cholinergic dilators in skeletal muscle

ATPase, adenosine triphosphatase; CGRPα, calcitonin gene-related peptide α. Modified from Ganong WF: Review of Medical Physiology, 17th ed, p 547. Norwalk, CT, Appleton & Lange, 1995.

In general, the arterial resistance vessels regulate arterial blood pressure and tissue blood flow, and the venous capacitance vessels store blood. Approximately two-thirds of the body's entire blood volume is in the systemic veins, with approximately 15% in the systemic arteries and an additional 7% in the systemic arterioles and capillaries. The remainder of the body's blood volume is normally contained in the heart and pulmonary vessels. The sympathetic nervous system plays a major role in vasomotor control.[93–96] All blood vessels except capillaries and venules contain smooth muscle supplied by noradrenergic sympathetic motor fibers, which course from the spinal cord to visceral blood vessels through specific sympathetic nerves and to the somatic tissues through the spinal nerves. The small arteries and arterioles are the most densely innervated, but with the exception of the splanchnic veins, venous innervation is relatively sparse. A generalized increase in sympathetic vascular tone increases cardiac venous return by decreasing venous capacitance and increases systemic vascular resistance by stimulating arteriolar constriction, thereby increasing both cardiac output and blood pressure. Other than its effect on the heart, the parasympathetic nervous system plays relatively little role in circulatory regulation.

The resistance vessels of skeletal muscle tissue are also innervated by cholinergic sympathetic fibers which cause vasodilatation. In contrast to the noradrenergic sympathetic vasoconstrictor fibers, these cholinergic vasodilator fibers do not exhibit resting tonic activity. These vasodilator fibers probably play little role in normal circulatory control. However, their activation, along with activation of cholinergic cardioinhibitory fibers and withdrawal of noradrenergic sympathetic outflow, is the mechanism of vasovagal syncope.[97–100]

Control of Vasomotor Activity

Although spinal cord reflex activity provides some modulation of cardiovascular homeostasis, the principal site of cardiovascular autonomic control is the vasomotor center, which is located in the reticular substance of the medulla and lower pons. Descending tracts from the cerebral cortex and other higher centers project to the vasomotor center and are responsible for the increase in heart rate and blood pressure that accompanies emotions. Afferent traffic projecting to the vasomotor center also arises from several cardiopulmonary receptor sites. Arterial baroreceptors located in most large arteries of the thorax and neck, but particularly abundant in the carotid sinus and aortic arch, increase or decrease their firing activity in direct proportion to the arterial blood pressure.[101] An increase in baroreceptor activity in response to an increase in blood pressure reflexively decreases heart rate and contractility and leads to peripheral vasodilatation. A decrease in baroreceptor activity accompanying a decrease in blood pressure has the opposite effect. Arterial chemoreceptors located in the aortic arch and in the carotid bodies are stimulated by hypoxia and acidosis, and their afferent barrage leads to activation of the vasomotor center.[102-104] Additional sensory receptors, which are located diffusely in cardiopulmonary vessels and supply afferent fibers that course with the sympathetic nerves, may provide nociception. Their activation generally results in an increase in sympathetic activity and a decrease in parasympathetic outflow.[105]

Vagal Cardiopulmonary Receptors

Receptors with myelinated and nonmyelinated vagal afferent fibers are located throughout the cardiopulmonary circulation, especially within the heart, and they are associated with various incompletely understood phenomena.[106-108] Activation of nonmyelinated vagal afferents located primarily in the inferoposterior left ventricle increases vagal activity and inhibits sympathetic outflow, leading to vasodilatation, bradycardia, and hypotension. This depressor reflex, the Bezold-Jarisch reflex, is associated with various clinical scenarios involving hypotension and bradycardia or asystole, including syncope, sudden death, myocardial infarction, coronary arteriography and reperfusion, hypoxemia, hypovolemia, and spinal anesthesia.[109-122]

Sympathetic-Parasympathetic Autonomic Balance and Heart Rate Variability

The sinus rhythm exhibits continuous fluctuations around the mean heart rate, a phenomenon resulting from periodic inhibition of vagal tone by afferent barrages from the medullary respiratory center and from baroreceptors and thoracic stretch receptors (Fig. 6–14).[123-126] Quantification of heart rate variability, the degree of heart rate deviation from the mean heart rate, is a valuable tool to assess the degree of sympathetic-parasympathetic autonomic balance, which may be detrimentally altered in disorders such as coronary artery disease, hypertension, diabetes, brain damage, Guillain-Barré syndrome, uremic neuropathy, sudden infant death syndrome, and antepartum fetal distress.[126,127]

Cardiac sympathetic-parasympathetic autonomic balance is clinically important because it is a primary determinant of cardiac electrical stability. Increased sympathetic tone promotes arrhythmias by decreasing ventricular refractoriness and fibrillation thresholds and by generating late potentials. Because increased vagal tone counters the proarrhythmic manifestations of increased sympathetic stimulation, it is protective.[128,129] Clinical assessment of the sympathetic-parasympathetic balance provides important prognostic informa-

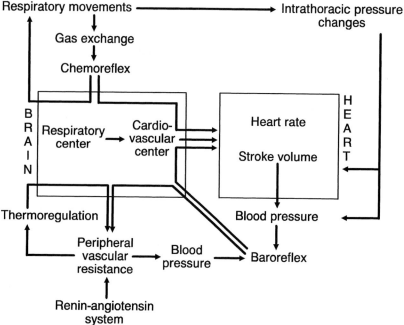

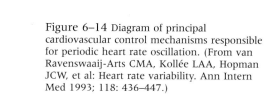

Figure 6–14 Diagram of principal cardiovascular control mechanisms responsible for periodic heart rate oscillation. (From van Ravenswaaij-Arts CMA, Kollée LAA, Hopman JCW, et al: Heart rate variability. Ann Intern Med 1993; 118: 436–447.)

tion regarding the risk of sudden cardiac death in postinfarction patients and may prove to be equally valuable in assessing other disease processes associated with autonomic dysfunction and increased morbidity and mortality.[130-144] General and regional anesthesia are associated with altered autonomic balance.[145-148] Autonomic dysfunction related to cardiovascular disease and diabetes, as assessed by heart rate variability studies, has been shown to correlate with perioperative morbidity.[149-151]

Sympathetic Imbalance and Cardiac Electrophysiologic Stability

Just as sympathetic-parasympathetic autonomic balance has an effect on the cardiac impulse, the relationship between right and left cardiac sympathetic tone affects the cardiac electrophysiology: left cardiac sympathetic dominance causes prolongation of the QT interval, which is closely associated with reentrant arrhythmias and sudden death.[152-154] Clinical processes associated with sudden death in which left-sided cardiac sympathetic dominance has been implicated as an etiologic factor include the congenital long QT syndromes (i.e., Jervell and Lange-Nielsen and Romano-Ward syndromes), sudden infant death syndrome, and psychologic stress.[143, 155-160] Because of the propensity for arrhythmias, the anesthesiologist must be aware of the anesthetic implications of prolonged QT syndromes.[161, 162]

β-Blockade is the principal therapy for congenital long QT syndrome, and left-sided cardiac sympathetic denervation is the treatment of choice for those patients who do not improve on medical therapy.[163, 164] Although the anesthesiologist may be asked to perform a prognostic or therapeutic left stellate ganglion block in these patients, there is no evidence that a right stellate ganglion block in a patient without a history of cardiac disease can create a situation of left stellate dominance and pose a risk of arrhythmia induction.[165-167]

The Heart as an Endocrine Organ

Various hormonal mechanisms are involved in the regulation of myocardial function in health and disease. Atrial natriuretic factor is the best known substance involved in these processes, but others include vasopressin, the renin-angiotensin system, and perhaps substance P.[168-171] Atrial natriuretic factor is a peptide secreted principally by the atrial myocytes in response to atrial distension, but it has also been found in the brain and peripheral nervous system. This hormone acts on the kidney by stimulating urine flow and sodium excretion, but it also has actions at other sites, promoting vasodilatation directly and by decreasing overall sympathetic tone, inhibiting release of aldosterone and vasopressin, and opposing the effect of angiotensin II.[172-177]

The Athletic Heart Syndrome

Highly trained athletes often have several cardiovascular adaptations to vigorous physical exercise, including increased ventricular wall thickness, increased chamber size, and increased resting vagal tone.[178-180] Resting sinus bradycardia, sinus pauses exceeding 2 s, first and second degree atrioventricular blocks (i.e., Mobitz type I and type II), ST-segment and T-wave repolarization changes, and electrocardiographic criteria diagnostic of right and left ventricular hypertrophy are relatively common.[181, 182] Although the electrocardiographic patterns of this population may be considered normal variants rather than abnormal, it has been suggested that these patients may be at increased risk for life-threatening, anesthesia-related cardiac events.[183, 184]

Regional Anesthesia in the Setting of Coexisting Cardiopulmonary Disease

Although regional anesthesia often involves less physiologic trespass than general anesthesia, it is incumbent on the anesthesiologist to understand the pathophysiology of coexisting thoracic and cardiovascular disease and to comprehend their anesthetic implications. Potential interactions may involve the procedure for needle insertion, the resultant neuromuscular or autonomic block, or the accompanying sedation.

Summary

A thorough understanding of basic cardiopulmonary anatomy, physiology, and disease states is important for planning the optimal anesthetic for the patient. This knowledge allows the practitioner to tailor the block procedure, minimize the anesthetic risk in relation to a given operation, and use regional anesthetic modalities as actual therapy, as in the case of acute and chronic pain management.

References

1. Sant'Ambrogio G, Mathew OP: Control of upper airway muscles. News Physiol Sci 1988; 3: 167–172.
2. Bartlett D Jr: Respiratory functions of the larynx. Physiol Rev 1989; 69: 33–57.
3. Bedford RF, Feinstein B: Hospital admission blood pressure: a predictor for hypertension following endotracheal intubation. Anesth Analg 1980; 59: 367–370.
4. Shribman AJ, Smith G, Achola KJ: Cardiovascular and catecholamine responses to laryngoscopy with and without tracheal intubation. Br J Anaesth 1987; 59: 295–299.
5. Gil J: Organization of microcirculation in the lung. Annu Rev Physiol 1980; 42: 177–186.
6. Wagner PD: Ventilation-perfusion relationships. Annu Rev Physiol 1980; 42: 235–247.
7. Bourbon J, Rieutort M: Pulmonary surfactant: biochemistry, physiology and pathology. News Physiol Sci 1987; 2: 129–132.
8. Van Golde LM, Batenburg JJ, Robertson B: The pulmonary surfactant system: biochemical aspects and functional significance. Physiol Rev 1988; 68: 374–455.

9. Notter RH, Finkelstein JN: Pulmonary surfactant: an interdisciplinary approach. J Appl Physiol 1984; 57: 1613–1624.

10. Hills BA: The pleural interface. Thorax 1985; 40: 1–8.

11. De Troyer A: The mechanism of the inspiratory expansion of the rib cage. J Lab Clin Med 1989; 114: 97–104.

12. De Troyer A, Estenne M: Functional anatomy of the respiratory muscles. Clin Chest Med 1988; 9: 175–193.

13. De Troyer A, Estenne M: Coordination between rib cage muscles and diaphragm during quiet breathing in humans. J Appl Physiol 1984; 57: 899–906.

14. De Troyer A, Sampson M, Sigrist S, et al: How the abdominal muscles act on the rib cage. J Appl Physiol 1983; 54: 465–469.

15. Moore DC: Anatomy of the intercostal nerve: its importance during thoracic surgery. Am J Surg 1982; 144: 371–373.

16. Barnes PJ: Neural control of human airways in health and disease. Am Rev Respir Dis 1986; 134: 1289–1314.

17. Nadel JA, Barnes PJ: Autonomic regulation of the airways. Annu Rev Med 1984; 35: 451–467.

18. Downing SE, Lee JC: Nervous control of the pulmonary circulation. Annu Rev Physiol 1980; 42: 199–210.

19. Dawson CA: Role of pulmonary vasomotion in physiology of the lung. Physiol Rev 1984; 64: 544–616.

20. Bergofsky EH: Humoral control of the pulmonary circulation. Annu Rev Physiol 1980; 42: 221–233.

21. Undem BJ: Neural-immunologic interactions in asthma. Hosp Pract (Off Ed) 1994; 29: 59–65, 69-70.

22. Dueck R: Anesthesia for the asthmatic patient. Semin Anesth 1987; 6: 2–9.

23. Barnes PJ: Autonomic control of airway function in asthma. Chest 1987; 91(Suppl 5): 45S–48S.

24. Gabella G: Innervation of airway smooth muscle: fine structure. Ann Rev Physiol 1987; 49: 583–594.

25. Barnes PJ: The third nervous system in the lung: physiology and clinical perspectives. (Editorial.) Thorax 1984; 39: 561–567.

26. Barnes PJ: Non-adrenergic non-cholinergic neural control of human airways. Arch Int Pharmacodyn Ther 1986; 280(Suppl 2): 108-228.

27. Pender ES, Pollack CV Jr: Neurogenic pulmonary edema: case reports and review. J Emerg Med 1992; 10: 45–51.

28. Simon RP: Neurogenic pulmonary edema. Neurol Clin 1993; 11: 309–323.

29. Ell SR: Neurogenic pulmonary edema: a review of the literature and a perspective. Invest Radiol 1991; 26: 499–506.

30. Bekemeyer WB, Pinstein ML: Neurogenic pulmonary edema: new concepts of an old disorder. South Med J 1989; 82: 380–383.

31. Bakhle YS: Pharmacokinetic and metabolic properties of lung. Br J Anaesth 1990; 65: 79–93.

32. Jorfeldt L, Lewis DH, Löfström JB, et al: Lung uptake of lidocaine in man. Reg Anesth 1980; 5: 6–7.

33. Duffin J, Hung S: Respiratory rhythm generation. Can Anaesth Soc J 1985; 32: 124–137.

34. Brown DL, Cahill DR, Bridenbaugh LD: Supraclavicular nerve block: anatomic analysis of a method to prevent pneumothorax. Anesth Analg 1993; 76: 530–534.

35. Moore DC, Hain RF, Ward A, et al: Importance of the perineural spaces in nerve blocking. JAMA 1954; 156: 1050–1053.

36. Moore DC: Intercostal nerve block: spread of India ink injected to the rib's costal groove. Br J Anaesth 1981; 53: 325–329.

37. Benumof JL, Semenza J: Total spinal anesthesia following intrathoracic intercostal nerve blocks. Anesthesiology 1975; 43: 124–125.

38. Sury MR, Bingham RM: Accidental spinal anaesthesia following intrathoracic intercostal nerve blockade. A case report. Anaesthesia 1986; 41: 401–403.

39. Crossley AW, Hosie HE: Radiographic study of intercostal nerve blockade in healthy volunteers. Br J Anaesth 1987; 59: 149–154.

40. Tucker GT, Mather LE: Clinical pharmacokinetics of local anaesthetics. Clin Pharmacokinet 1979; 4: 241–278.

41. Moore DC, Bush WH, Scurlock JE: Intercostal nerve block: a roentgenographic anatomic study of technique and absorption in humans. Anesth Analg 1980; 59: 815–825.

42. Gross JB, Caldwell CB, Shaw LM, et al: The effect of lidocaine on the ventilatory response to carbon dioxide. Anesthesiology 1983; 59: 521–525.

43. Gross JB, Caldwell CB, Shaw LM, et al: The effect of lidocaine infusion on the ventilatory response to hypoxia. Anesthesiology 1984; 61: 662–665.

44. Freund FG, Bonica JJ, Ward RJ, et al: Ventilatory reserve and level of motor block during high spinal and epidural anesthesia. Anesthesiology 1967; 28: 834–837.

45. Hecker BR, Bjurstrom R, Schoene RB: Effect of intercostal nerve blockade on respiratory mechanics and CO_2 chemosensitivity at rest and exercise. Anesthesiology 1989; 70: 13–18.

46. Wahba WM, Craig DB, Don HF, et al: The cardio-respiratory effects of thoracic epidural anaesthesia. Can Anaesth Soc J 1972; 19: 8–19.

47. McCarthy GS: The effect of thoracic extradural analgesia on pulmonary gas distribution, functional residual capacity and airway closure. Br J Anaesth 1976; 48: 243–248.

48. Cory PC, Mulroy MF: Postoperative respiratory failure following intercostal block. Anesthesiology 1981; 54: 418–419.

49. Riley RH: Respiratory arrest following interpleural block in a narcotized patient. (Letter to the editor.) Can J Anaesth 1990; 37: 487–488.

50. Irwin RS, Rosen MJ, Braman SS: Cough. A comprehensive review. Arch Intern Med 1977; 137: 1186–1191.

51. Banner AS: Cough: physiology, evaluation, and treatment. Lung 1986; 164: 79–92.

52. McCool FD, Leith DE: Pathophysiology of cough. Clin Chest Med 1987; 8: 189–195.

53. Thomas JX Jr, Jones CE, Randall WC: Neural modulation of coronary blood flow. In Randall WC (ed): Nervous Control of Cardiovascular Function, pp 178–198. New York, Oxford University Press, 1984.

54. Tsien RW: Calcium channels in excitable cell membranes. Annu Rev Physiol 1983; 45: 341–358.

55. Armstrong CM: Sodium channels and gating currents. Physiol Rev 1981; 61: 644–683.

56. Hille B: Ionic channels: molecular pores of excitable membranes. Harvey Lect 1986–1987; 82: 47–69.

57. Bean BP, Cohen CJ, Tsien RW: Lidocaine block of cardiac sodium channels. J Gen Physiol 1983; 81: 613–642.

58. Wheeler DM, Bradley EL, Woods WT Jr: The electrophysiologic actions of lidocaine and bupivacaine in the isolated, perfused canine heart. Anesthesiology 1988; 68: 201–212.

59. Moller RA, Covino BG: Cardiac electrophysiologic effects of lidocaine and bupivacaine. Anesth Analg 1988; 67: 107–114.

60. Butterworth JF IV, Strichartz GR: Molecular mechanisms of local anesthesia: a review. Anesthesiology 1990; 72: 711–734.

61. Hondeghem LM, Katzung BG: Antiarrhythmic agents: The modulated receptor mechanism of action of sodium and calcium channel-blocking drugs. Annu Rev Pharmacol Toxicol 1984; 24: 387–423.

62. Hondeghem LM: Antiarrhythmic agents: modulated receptor applications. Circulation 1987; 75: 514–520.

63. Clarkson CW, Hondeghem LM: Mechanism for bupivacaine depression of cardiac conduction: fast block of sodium channels during the action potential with slow recovery from block during diastole. Anesthesiology 1985; 62: 396–405.

64. Nancarrow C, Rutten AJ, Runciman WB, et al: Myocardial and cerebral drug concentrations and the mechanisms of death after fatal intravenous doses of lidocaine, bupivacaine, and ropivacaine in the sheep. Anesth Analg 1989; 69: 276–283.

65. Rutten AJ, Nancarrow C, Mather LE, et al: Hemodynamic and central nervous system effects of intravenous bolus doses of lidocaine, bupivacaine, and ropivacaine in sheep. Anesth Analg 1989; 69: 291–299.

66. Butterworth JF IV, Brownlow RC, Leith JP, et al: Bupivacaine inhibits cyclic-3',5'-adenosine monophosphate production. A possible contributing factor to cardiovascular toxicity. Anesthesiology 1993; 79: 88–95.

67. Heavner JE: Cardiac dysrhythmias induced by infusion of local anesthetics into the lateral cerebral ventricle of cats. Anesth Analg 1986; 65: 133–138.

68. Thomas RD, Behbehani MM, Coyle DE, et al: Cardiovascular toxicity of local anesthetics: an alternative hypothesis. Anesth Analg 1986; 65: 444–450.

69. Bernards CM, Artru AA: Effect of intracerebroventricular picrotoxin and muscimol on intravenous bupivacaine toxicity: evi-

dence supporting central nervous system involvement in bupi-vacaine cardiovascular toxicity. Anesthesiology 1993; 78: 902–910.

70. Chang KS, Yang M, Andresen MC: Clinically relevant concentrations of bupivacaine inhibit rat aortic baroreceptors. Anesth Analg 1994; 78: 501–506.

71. Fleisch JH, Titus E: Effect of local anesthetics on pharmacologic receptor systems of smooth muscle. J Pharmacol Exp Ther 1973; 186: 44–51.

72. Johns RA, DiFazio CA, Longnecker DE: Lidocaine constricts or dilates rat arterioles in a dose-dependent manner. Anesthesiology 1985; 62: 141–144.

73. Johns RA, Seyde WC, DiFazio CA, et al: Dose-dependent effects of bupivacaine on rat muscle arterioles. Anesthesiology 1986; 65: 186–191.

74. Lange RA, Cigarroa RG, Yancy CW Jr, et al: Cocaine-induced coronary-artery vasoconstriction. N Engl J Med 1989; 321: 1557–1562.

75. Kalsner S: Cocaine sensitization of coronary artery contractions: mechanism of drug-induced spasm. J Pharmacol Exp Ther 1993; 264: 1132–1140.

76. Welder AA, Grammas P, Melchert RB: Cellular mechanisms of cocaine cardiotoxicity. Toxicol Lett 1993; 69: 227–238.

77. Kennedy WF Jr, Bonica JJ, Ward RJ, et al: Cardiorespiratory effects of epinephrine when used in regional anesthesia. Acta Anaesthesiol Scand Suppl 1966; 23: 320–333.

78. Freyschuss U, Hjemdahl P, Juhlin-Dannfelt A, et al: Cardiovascular and metabolic responses to low dose adrenaline infusion: an invasive study in humans. Clin Sci (Colch) 1986; 70: 199–206.

79. Tarnow J, Muller RK: Cardiovascular effect of low-dose epinephrine infusions in relation to the extent of preoperative beta-adrenoceptor blockade. Anesthesiology 1991; 74: 1035–1043.

80. Moore DC, Scurlock JE: Possible role of epinephrine in prevention or correction of myocardial depression associated with bupivacaine. Anesth Analg 1983; 62: 450–453.

81. Toyoda Y, Kubota Y, Kubota H, et al: Prevention of hypokalemia during axillary nerve block with 1% lidocaine and epinephrine 1:100,000. Anesthesiology 1988; 69: 109–112.

82. Lunn JJ, Narr BJ: Prevention of hypokalemia during axillary nerve block. (Letter to the editor) Anesthesiology 1989; 70: 365–366.

83. Armour JA, Hopkins DA: Anatomy of the extrinsic efferent autonomic nerves and ganglia innervating the mammalian heart. In Randall WC (ed): Nervous Control of Cardiovascular Function, pp 20–45. New York, Oxford University Press, 1984.

84. Wurster RD: Central nervous system regulation of the heart: an overview. In Randall WC (ed): Nervous Control of Cardiovascular Function, pp 307–320. New York, Oxford University Press, 1984.

85. James TN: Clinical significance of neural control of the heart. In Randall WC (ed): Nervous Control of Cardiovascular Function, pp 435–463. New York, Oxford University Press, 1984.

86. Smith ML, Carlson MD, Thames MD: Reflex control of the heart and circulation: implications for cardiovascular electrophysiology. J Cardiovasc Electrophysiol 1991; 2: 441–449.

87. Feldman JL, Ellenberger HH: Central coordination of respiratory and cardiovascular control in mammals. Annu Rev Physiol 1988; 50: 593–606.

88. Talman WT, Kelkar P: Neural control of the heart. Central and peripheral. Neurol Clin 1993; 11: 239–256.

89. Benarroch EE: The central autonomic network: functional organization, dysfunction, and perspective. Mayo Clin Proc 1993; 68: 988–1001.

90. Kent KM, Cooper T: The denervated heart: a model for studying autonomic control of the heart. N Engl J Med 1974; 291: 1017–1021.

91. Bainbridge FA: The influence of venous filling upon the rate of the heart. J Physiol (Lond) 1915; 1: 65–84.

92. Pathak CL: Autoregulation of chronotropic response of the heart through pacemaker stretch. Cardiology 1973; 58: 45–64.

93. Henriksen O: Local sympathetic reflex mechanism in regulation of blood flow in human subcutaneous adipose tissue. Acta Physiol Scand Suppl 1977; 450: 1–48.

94. Wallin BG, Fagius J: Peripheral sympathetic neural activity in conscious humans. Annu Rev Physiol 1988; 50: 565–576.

95. Calaresu FR, Yardley CP: Medullary basal sympathetic tone. Annu Rev Physiol 1988; 50: 511–524.

96. Rosell S: Neuronal control of microvessels. Annu Rev Physiol 1980; 42: 359–371.

97. Epstein SE, Stampfer M, Beiser GD: Role of the capacitance and resistance vessels in vasovagal syncope. Circulation 1968; 37: 524–533.

98. Ziegler MG, Echon C, Wilner KD, et al: Sympathetic nervous withdrawal in the vasodepressor (vasovagal) reaction. J Auton Nerv Syst 1986; 17: 273–278.

99. Wallin BG, Sundlof G: Sympathetic outflow to muscles during vasovagal syncope. J Auton Nerv Syst 1982; 6: 287–291.

100. Goldstein DS, Spanarkel M, Pitterman A, et al: Circulatory control mechanisms in vasodepressor syncope. Am Heart J 1982; 104: 1071–1075.

101. Mancia G, Grassi G, Bertinieri G, et al: Arterial baroreceptor control of blood pressure in man. J Auton Nerv Syst 1984; 11: 115–124.

102. Somers VK, Mark AL, Zavala DC, et al: Contrasting effects of hypoxia and hypercapnia on ventilation and sympathetic activity in humans. J Appl Physiol 1989; 67: 2101–2106.

103. Somers VK, Mark AL, Zavala DC, et al: Influence of ventilation and hypocapnia on sympathetic nerve responses to hypoxia in normal humans. J Appl Physiol 1989; 67: 2095–2100.

104. Somers VK, Mark AL, Abboud FM: Interaction of baroreceptor and chemoreceptor reflex control of sympathetic nerve activity in normal humans. J Clin Invest 1991; 87: 1953–1957.

105. Malliani A: Cardiovascular sympathetic afferent fibers. Rev Physiol Biochem Pharmacol 1982; 94: 11–74.

106. Donald DE, Shepherd JT: Reflexes from the heart and lungs: physiological curiosities or important regulatory mechanisms. Cardiovasc Res 1978; 12: 446–469.

107. Zucker IH: Left ventricular receptors: physiological controllers or pathological curiosities? Basic Res Cardiol 1986; 81: 539–557.

108. Thoren P: Role of cardiac vagal C-fibers in cardiovascular control. Rev Physiol Biochem Pharmacol 1979; 86: 1–94.

109. Lee TM, Kuo JS, Chai CY: Central integrating mechanism of the Bezold-Jarisch and baroceptor reflexes. Am J Physiol 1972; 222: 713–720.

110. Mark AL: The Bezold-Jarisch reflex revisited: clinical implications of inhibitory reflexes originating in the heart. J Am Coll Cardiol 1983; 1: 90–102.

111. Abboud FM: Ventricular syncope: is the heart a sensory organ? (Editorial.) N Engl J Med 1989; 320: 390–392.

112. Milstein S, Buetikofer J, Lesser J, et al: Cardiac asystole: a manifestation of neurally mediated hypotension-bradycardia. J Am Coll Cardiol 1989; 14: 1626–1632.

113. Robertson D, Hollister AS, Forman MB, et al: Reflexes unique to myocardial ischemia and infarction. J Am Coll Cardiol 1985; 5(Suppl 6): 99B–104B.

114. Perez-Gomez F, Garcia-Aguado A: Origin of ventricular reflexes caused by coronary arteriography. Br Heart J 1977; 39: 967–973.

115. Koren G, Weiss AT, Ben-David Y, et al: Bradycardia and hypotension following reperfusion with streptokinase (Bezold-Jarisch reflex): a sign of coronary thrombolysis and myocardial salvage. Am Heart J 1986; 112: 468–471.

116. Sanders JS, Ferguson DW: Profound sympathoinhibition complicating hypovolemia in humans. Ann Intern Med 1989; 111: 439–441.

117. Nemerovski M, Shah PK: Syndrome of severe bradycardia and hypotension following sublingual nitroglycerin administration. Cardiology 1981; 67: 180–189.

118. Johnson AM: Aortic stenosis, sudden death, and the left ventricular baroceptors. Br Heart J 1971; 33: 1–5.

119. Berk JL, Levy MN: Profound reflex bradycardia produced by transient hypoxia or hypercapnia in man. Eur Surg Res 1977; 9: 75–84.

120. Simpson RJ Jr, Podolak R, Mangano CA Jr, et al: Vagal syncope during recurrent pulmonary embolism. JAMA 1983; 249: 390–393.

121. Fullerton DA, St. Cyr JA, Clarke DR, et al: Bezold-Jarisch reflex

in postoperative pediatric cardiac surgical patients. Ann Thorac Surg 1991; 52: 534–536.

122. Mackey DC, Carpenter RL, Thompson GE, et al: Bradycardia and asystole during spinal anesthesia: a report of three cases without morbidity. Anesthesiology 1989; 70: 866–868.

123. Eckberg DL: Human sinus arrhythmia as an index of vagal cardiac outflow. J Appl Physiol 1983; 54: 961–966.

124. Hirsch JA, Bishop B: Respiratory sinus arrhythmia in humans: How breathing pattern modulates heart rate. Am J Physiol 1981; 241: H620–H629.

125. Levy MN, Martin P: Parasympathetic control of the heart. In Randall WC (ed): Nervous Control of Cardiovascular Function, pp 68–94. New York, Oxford University Press, 1984.

126. Van Ravenswaaij-Arts CM, Kollée LA, Hopman JC, et al: Heart rate variability. Ann Intern Med 1993; 118: 436–447.

127. Kamath MV, Fallen EL: Power spectral analysis of heart rate variability: a noninvasive signature of cardiac autonomic function. Crit Rev Biomed Eng 1993; 21: 245–311.

128. Lown B, Verrier RL: Neural activity and ventricular fibrillation. N Engl J Med 1976; 294: 1165–1170.

129. Esler M: The autonomic nervous system and cardiac arrhythmias. Clin Auton Res 1992; 2: 133–135.

130. Vanoli E, Schwartz PJ: Sympathetic-parasympathetic interaction and sudden death. Basic Res Cardiol 1990; 85(Suppl 1): 305–321.

131. Ewing DJ: Heart rate variability: an important new risk factor in patients following myocardial infarction. Clin Cardiol 1991; 14: 683–685.

132. Seale WL, Gang ES, Peter CT: The use of signal-averaged electrocardiography in predicting patients at high risk for sudden death. PACE Pacing Clin Electrophysiol 1990; 13: 796–807.

133. Simson MB: The role of signal averaged electrocardiography in identifying patients at high risk for lethal ventricular tachyarrhythmias. PACE Pacing Clin Electrophysiol 1991; 14: 944–952.

134. Odemuyiwa O, Malik M, Farrell T, et al: Comparison of the predictive characteristics of heart rate variability index and left ventricular ejection fraction for all-cause mortality, arrhythmic events and sudden death after acute myocardial infarction. Am J Cardiol 1991; 68: 434–439.

135. Farrell TG, Bashir Y, Cripps T, et al: Risk stratification for arrhythmic events in postinfarction patients based on heart rate variability, ambulatory electrocardiographic variables and the signal-averaged electrocardiogram. J Am Coll Cardiol 1991; 18: 687–697.

136. Casolo GC, Stroder P, Signorini C, et al: Heart rate variability during the acute phase of myocardial infarction. Circulation 1992; 85: 2073–2079.

137. Schwartz PJ, La Rovere MT, Vanoli E: Autonomic nervous system and sudden cardiac death: experimental basis and clinical observations for post-myocardial infarction risk stratification. Circulation 1992; 85(Suppl 1): I77–I91.

138. Anema JR, Heijenbrok MW, Faes TJ, et al: Cardiovascular autonomic function in multiple sclerosis. J Neurol Sci 1991; 104: 129–134.

139. Malpas SC, Whiteside EA, Maling TJ: Heart rate variability and cardiac autonomic function in men with chronic alcohol dependence. Br Heart J 1991; 65: 84–88.

140. Broadstone VL, Roy T, Self M, et al: Cardiovascular autonomic dysfunction: Diagnosis and prognosis. Diabet Med 1991; 8(Spec No): S88–S93.

141. Leipzig TJ, Lowensohn RI: Heart rate variability in neurosurgical patients. Neurosurgery 1986; 19: 356–362.

142. Kuroiwa Y, Shimada Y, Toyokura Y: Postural hypotension and low R-R interval variability in parkinsonism, spino-cerebellar degeneration, and Shy-Drager syndrome. Neurology 1983; 33: 463–467.

143. Perticone F, Ceravolo R, Maio R, et al: Heart rate variability and sudden infant death syndrome. PACE Pacing Clin Electrophysiol 1990; 13: 2096–2099.

144. Pincus SM, Viscarello RR: Approximate entropy: a regularity measure for fetal heart rate analysis. Obstet Gynecol 1992; 79: 249–255.

145. Kato M, Komatsu T, Kimura T, et al: Spectral analysis of heart rate variability during isoflurane anesthesia. Anesthesiology 1992; 77: 669–674.

146. Latson TW, McCarroll SM, Mirhej MA, et al: Effects of three anesthetic induction techniques on heart rate variability. J Clin Anesth 1992; 4: 265–276.

147. Kimura T, Komatsu T, Hirabayashi A, et al: Autonomic imbalance of the heart during total spinal anesthesia evaluated by spectral analysis of heart rate variability. Anesthesiology 1994; 80: 694–698.

148. Fleisher LA, Frank SM, Shir Y, et al: Cardiac sympathovagal balance and peripheral sympathetic vasoconstriction: epidural versus general anesthesia. Anesth Analg 1994; 79: 165–171.

149. Burgos LG, Ebert TJ, Asiddao C, et al: Increased intraoperative cardiovascular morbidity in diabetics with autonomic neuropathy. Anesthesiology 1989; 70: 591–597.

150. Fleisher LA, Pincus SM, Rosenbaum SH: Approximate entropy of heart rate as a correlate of postoperative ventricular dysfunction. Anesthesiology 1993; 78: 683–692.

151. Latson TW, Ashmore TH, Reinhart DJ, et al: Autonomic reflex dysfunction in patients presenting for elective surgery is associated with hypotension after anesthesia induction. Anesthesiology 1994; 80: 326–337.

152. Schwartz PJ: Sympathetic imbalance and cardiac arrhythmias. In Randall WC (ed): Nervous Control of Cardiovascular Function, pp 225–252. New York, Oxford University Press, 1984.

153. Malliani A, Schwartz PJ, Zanchetti A: Neural mechanisms in life-threatening arrhythmias. Am Heart J 1980; 100: 705–715.

154. Schwartz PJ, Moss AJ: Prolonged Q-T interval: what does it mean? J Cardiovasc Med 1982; 7: 1317–1330.

155. Crampton R: Preeminence of the left stellate ganglion in the long Q-T syndrome. Circulation 1979; 59: 769–778.

156. Schwartz PJ: Idiopathic long QT syndrome: progress and questions. Am Heart J 1985; 109: 399–411.

157. Stramba-Badiale M, Lazzarotti M, Schwartz PJ: Development of cardiac innervation, ventricular fibrillation, and sudden infant death syndrome. Am J Physiol 1992; 263(Pt 2): H1514–H1522.

158. Verrier RL, Lown B: Autonomic nervous system and malignant cardiac arrhythmias. In Weiner H, Hofer MA, Stunkard AJ (eds): Brain, Behavior, and Bodily Disease, pp 273–291. New York, Raven Press, 1981.

159. Talman WT: Cardiovascular regulation and lesions of the central nervous system. Ann Neurol 1985; 18: 1–13.

160. Lane RD, Schwartz GE: Induction of lateralized sympathetic input to the heart by the CNS during emotional arousal: a possible neurophysiologic trigger of sudden cardiac death. Psychosom Med 1987; 49: 274–284.

161. Strickland RA, Stanton MS, Olsen KD: Prolonged QT syndrome: Perioperative management. Mayo Clin Proc 1993; 68: 1016–1020.

162. Galloway PA, Glass PS: Anesthetic implications of prolonged QT interval syndromes. Anesth Analg 1985; 64: 612–620.

163. Schwartz PJ, Stone HL: Unilateral stellectomy and sudden death. In Schwartz PJ, Brown AM, Malliani A, et al (eds): Neural Mechanisms in Cardiac Arrhythmias, pp 107–122. New York, Raven Press, 1978.

164. Schwartz PJ, Locati EH, Moss AJ, et al: Left cardiac sympathetic denervation in the therapy of congenital long QT syndrome. A worldwide report. Circulation 1991; 84: 503–511.

165. Yanagida H, Kemi C, Suwa K: The effects of stellate ganglion block on the idiopathic prolongation of the Q-T interval with cardiac arrhythmia (the Romano-Ward syndrome). Anesth Analg 1976; 55: 782–787.

166. Kashima T, Tanaka H, Minagoe S, et al: Electrocardiographic changes induced by the stellate ganglion block in normal subjects. J Electrocardiol 1981; 14: 169–174.

167. Gardner MJ, Kimber S, Johnstone DE, et al: The effects of unilateral stellate ganglion blockade on human cardiac function during rest and exercise. J Cardiovasc Electrophysiol 1993; 4: 2–8.

168. Frohlich ED: The heart. An endocrine organ (revisited). Arch Intern Med 1985; 145: 809–811.

169. De Hert SG, Gillebert TC, Andries LJ, et al: Role of the endocardial endothelium in the regulation of myocardial function. Physiologic and pathophysiologic implications. Anesthesiology 1993; 79: 1354–1366.

170. Urata H, Healy B, Stewart RW, et al: Angiotensin II receptors in normal and failing human hearts. J Clin Endocrinol Metab 1989; 69: 54–66.

171. Fuller RW, Maxwell DL, Dixon CM, et al: Effect of substance P on cardiovascular and respiratory function in subjects. J Appl Physiol 1987; 62: 1473–1479.

172. Genest J, Cantin M: The atrial natriuretic factor: Its physiology and biochemistry. Rev Physiol Biochem Pharmacol 1988; 110: 1–145.

173. Athanassopoulos G, Cokkinos DV: Atrial natriuretic factor. Prog Cardiovasc Dis 1991; 33: 313–328.

174. Adams SP: Structure and biologic properties of the atrial natriuretic peptides. Endocrinol Metab Clin North Am 1987; 16: 1–17.

175. Samson WK: Atrial natriuretic factor and the central nervous system. Endocrinol Metab Clin North Am 1987; 16: 145–161.

176. Debinski W, Kuchel O, Buu NT: Atrial natriuretic factor is a new neuromodulatory peptide. Neuroscience 1990; 36: 15–20.

177. Harris PJ, Skinner SL: Intra-renal interactions between angiotensin II and atrial natriuretic factor. Kidney Int Suppl 1990; 30: S87–S91.

178. George KP, Wolfe LA, Burggraf GW: The "athletic heart syndrome." A critical review. Sports Med 1991; 11: 300–330.

179. Bryan G, Ward A, Rippe JM: Athletic heart syndrome. Clin Sports Med 1992; 11: 259–272.

180. Dixon EM, Kamath MV, McCartney N, et al: Neural regulation of heart rate variability in endurance athletes and sedentary controls. Cardiovasc Res 1992; 26: 713–719.

181. Hanne-Paparo N, Drory Y, Schoenfeld Y, et al: Common ECG changes in athletes. Cardiology 1976; 61: 267–278.

182. Viitasalo MT, Kala R, Eisalo A: Ambulatory electrocardiographic recording in endurance athletes. Br Heart J 1982; 47: 213–220.

183. Frerichs RL, Campbell J, Bassell GM: Psychogenic cardiac arrest during extensive sympathetic blockade. Anesthesiology 1988; 68: 943–944.

184. Kreutz JM, Mazuzan JE: Sudden asystole in a marathon runner: The athletic heart syndrome and its anesthetic implications. Anesthesiology 1990; 73: 1266–1268.

CHAPTER 7

The Stress Response and Regional Anesthesia

M. Soledad Cepeda, M.D., Daniel B. Carr, M.D.

Definition

The integrated, adaptive living web of neuroendocrine, immunologic, and intercellular biochemical signals evoked in higher organisms by tissue injury is termed the "stress response." The concept of stress as a shared feature common to many dissimilar external and internal challenges that evoke a uniform syndrome of general adaptation originated with Selye.[1] In his comprehensive monograph, Selye summarized work of the preceding century, detailing numerous stress responses evident in many organs, particularly the endocrine system, after various stressors including tissue injury and environmental challenges such as exercise, infection, water deprivation, and starvation.

Through the introduction and refinement of sensitive, quantitative hormone assays during the past three decades, the stress response has become identified operationally with neuroendocrine phenomena. These phenomena include pituitary-adrenal stimulation, catecholamine release from the adrenal medulla, and other blood-borne hormonal responses that regulate carbohydrate, protein, and lipid metabolism. Much evidence implicates these benchmark indices of stress as effectors of the body's response to operation or trauma. The classic narrow focus on these markers and mediators of disturbed homeostasis has enlarged to include immune and cardiovascular changes during pain or trauma.[2] Moreover, oxidative stress—intracellular metabolic dysfunction and injury as a result of excessive free radical levels—during pain or trauma is now understood to be harmful globally and particularly within neural pain pathways.[3] Within such pathways, pain-induced generation of oxygen radicals is associated with excessive, persistent neuronal activation, followed if unchecked by cell degeneration and death.

This chapter surveys neural and classic hormonal aspects of the stress response, along with emerging data on immunologic and intracellular metabolic sequelae of pain and trauma. Although this highly conserved system of responses must be important in the natural setting, in the hospitalized patient it is associated with catabolism, increased cardiac work, arrhythmogenesis, hypercoagulability, and immunosuppression. Hence, a stress-free perioperative course has been advanced as a clinical goal.[4] A pain-free perioperative course, achievable preemptively through regional anesthesia and attractive per se to patients, deprives stress responses of an important (but not exclusive) trigger.

Because this survey is presented in relation to the potential impact of regional anesthesia on clinical outcome, we will consider evidence that avoidance of the normal physiologic response to operation, trauma, or pain improves clinical outcomes. However, until an investigator infuses exogenous stress hormones to simulate typically high (conventional) blood levels in a postoperative patient group otherwise kept stress- and pain-free by regional anesthesia, the precise contribution of these stress responses to clinical outcomes will remain uncertain.

Stress Response: Neural Afferent Limb

Afferent neural pathways convey signals of pain and tissue injury to central sites of sensory, autonomic, and neuroendocrine integration, resulting in the classic neuroendocrine stress response.[3] Nociceptive stimuli are transmitted from the surgical incision or site of trauma to the spinal cord through A-δ (myelinated, fast) and C (unmyelinated, slow) fibers. Some evidence indicates that the fast-conducting fibers may also, via a recently described spinohypothalamic tract, participate in the hypothalamic activation characteristic of the initial endocrine response to operation.[5]

Most C fiber nociceptors respond to noxious mechanical, thermal, and chemical stimuli and so are termed "C polymodal nociceptors." The receptive field for the spinal cord dorsal horn neuron activated by a C polymodal nociceptor may be quite large, in contrast to spinal cord neurons supplied by A-δ nociceptors, whose receptive fields tend to be small clusters of spots.[5] After local injury, peripheral nociceptors become hypersensitive to noxious stimuli as a result of accumulation of algesiogenic substances in the periphery. This peripheral sensitization is augmented by important biologic processes that result in central sensitization of the spinal cord and rostral sites.[6-8]

Even during experimental conditions that preclude sensitization of C polymodal nociceptors in the periphery, spinal cord nociceptive neurons become sensitized by repeated brief stimulation that leads to prolonged spontaneous discharge or "windup."[6-9] Windup and concurrent hyperalgesia depend on intracellular metabolic changes caused by excitatory amino acids acting on the N-methyl-D-aspartate and related receptors,[10] followed by the intraneural generation of oxygen-derived free radicals such as nitric oxide.[3, 11, 12] These intraneural stress responses are a microcosm of previously recognized systemic sequelae of macroscopic tissue injury due to free radical generation during trauma or ischemia.[13] Later in this overview, we present emerging evidence that regional anesthesia inhibits not only classic, systemic neuroendocrine stress responses but also these increasingly studied intracellular stress responses within the spinal cord.

Nociceptive afferent fibers enter the spinal cord dorsal horn primarily through the dorsal roots, then ascend or descend one or two segments in Lissauer's tract and synapse within the six anatomically distinct layers of the dorsal horn. Cutaneous nociceptive afferents project to laminae I, II, and V, whereas visceral and muscle nociceptive fibers end mainly in laminae I and V.[14, 15] After decussation, pain fibers ascend in the anterolateral quadrant of the spinal cord, mainly in the spinothalamic and spinoreticulothalamic tracts (Fig. 7–1). As the spinothalamic tract approaches the thalamus, it separates into medial and lateral divisions. The lateral spinothalamic tract is not present in lower animals and so is termed the "neospinothalamic tract." It appears to provide sensory and discriminative features of painful stimuli.[5] The medial spinothalamic tract is found in lower animals and is termed "paleospinothalamic." The medial spinothalamic tract projects to the brain stem reticular formation, medial thalamus, periaqueductal gray matter, and hypothalamus, and it is believed to mediate arousal, autonomic responses, and emotional and affective aspects of pain.[14] The spinothalamic tracts project in a somatotopically organized manner to the primary somatosensory cortex of the parietal lobe, which mediates sensory and discriminative aspects of pain.[5] The frontal lobes, which receive diffuse projections from the medial thalamic nuclei, are concerned with affective and motivational aspects of pain perception.

The spinoreticulothalamic tract has been implicated in the neuroendocrine response to pain and the genesis of the surgical stress response.[5, 16] Axons of the spinoreticular tract ascend intermixed with the spinothalamic tract, terminate bilaterally in the brain stem reticular formation, and enter the hypothalamus, where they join the medial forebrain bundle and reach the hypothalamic paraventricular nucleus. The paraventricular nucleus is the major integrating center for nociceptive afferent signals and global hormonal, behavioral, and autonomic responses.[3, 17] Neurons containing vasopressin and corticotropin-releasing hormone are located within the paraventricular nucleus.[17, 18] Vasopressin is transported from the paraventricular nucleus and stored in the posterior pituitary until it is secreted into blood. Corticotropin-releasing hormone is released into the portal circulation of the pituitary stalk, where it is carried to corticotroph cells that secrete adrenocorticotropic hormone (ACTH), β-endorphin, and related peptides that are the hallmarks of the hypothalamic-pituitary-adrenal response to stress.

Stress Response: Hormonal Efferent Limb

Two linked efferent hormonal axes dominate the systemic neuroendocrine response to surgical stress: hypothalamic-pituitary-adrenocortical and sympathoadrenomedullary (Fig. 7–2). Activation of these two major axes, through both direct and indirect effects on target organs, causes blood levels of catabolic hormones such as catecholamines, cortisol, and glucagon to increase and levels of anabolic hormones such as insulin to decline.

With respect to the first axis, trophic hormones released from the hypothalamus during stress stimulate the pituitary to release ACTH, growth hormone, and prolactin.[19] Circulating ACTH stimulates adrenal synthesis and secretion of cortisol and aldosterone. ACTH and β-endorphin[20-22] are derived from the same precursor, pro-opiomelanocortin.[23] Pro-opiomelanocortin undergoes a series of regulated, ordered proteolytic cleavages and modifications in the corticotrophs of the anterior pituitary to yield not only ACTH but also β-lipoprotein—the precursor of β-endorphin[24]—and other daughter molecules.[25] Interestingly, although not itself derived from pro-opiomelanocortin, delta-sleep-inducing peptide is colocalized and cosecreted with ACTH from pituitary corticotrophs in response to administration of corticotropin-releasing hormone and appears to have a role in hypothalamic-pituitary-adrenocortical regulation during stress.[26] In light of the widespread disruption of sleep after surgical and other forms of stress and the adverse consequences of such deprivation, measures such as afferent block that preserve hypothalamic-pituitary-adrenocortical function may positively impact sleep patterns.[27]

Hypothalamic regulation of anterior pituitary secretion of pro-opiomelanocortin–derived peptides is multihormonal, principally by corticotropin-releasing hor-

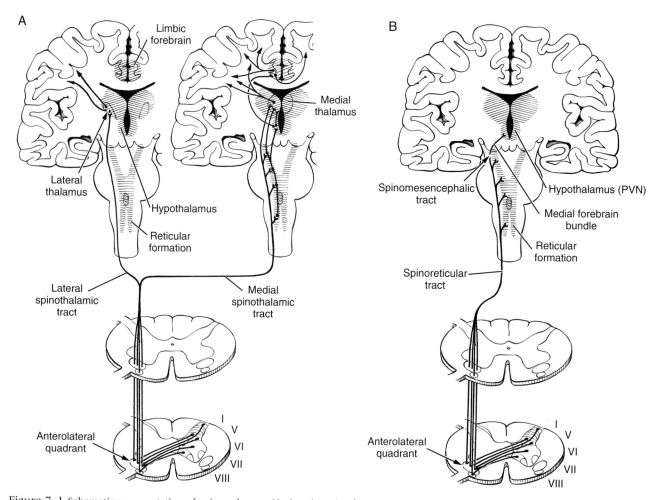

Figure 7–1 Schematic representation of pain pathways. Nociceptive stimuli are transmitted through A-δ and C fibers, enter the spinal cord via the dorsal root, ascend or descend one or two segments, and synapse within the six layers of the dorsal horn. Axons from second-order neurons decussate and ascend in the anterolateral quadrant of the spinal cord in the spinothalamic and spinoreticulothalamic tracts. *A,* The spinothalamic tract separates into lateral and medial divisions. These project, respectively, to the lateral thalamus or to the reticular formation, periaqueductal gray matter, hypothalamus, medial thalamus, and somatosensory cortex. *B,* Axons of the spinoreticular tract ascend intermixed with the spinothalamic tract, terminate bilaterally in the brain stem reticular formation, and enter the hypothalamus, where they join the medial forebrain bundle and reach the hypothalamic paraventricular nucleus (PVN).

mone and vasopressin.[28–30] These two neurally derived hormones exert synergistic actions. Corticotropin-releasing hormone is produced in many brain regions, including the paraventricular nucleus of the hypothalamus, the brain stem, the limbic system, and the cortex.[16, 31, 32] The major influence that corticotropin-releasing hormone has on the global stress response extends into neuroendocrine, autonomic, and behavioral components. Central administration of corticotropin-releasing hormone generates a coordinated series of responses that include pituitary-adrenal and sympathetic nervous system activation, anorexia, decreased libido, hypothalamic hypogonadism, and changes in motor activity.[31, 32]

Vasopressin amplifies the pro-opiomelanocortin–related cascade evoked by corticotropin-releasing hormone from pituitary corticotrophs and potentiates the associated adrenocortical response.[33, 34] Increases in central vasopressin secretion (unrelated to plasma osmolarity) may mediate incremental pituitary-adrenal activation when new stressors are encountered during chronic physiologic stress,[29] thereby enabling the hypothalamic-pituitary-adrenocortical axis to maintain adequate responsiveness to increased functional demands. Angiotensin II, prostaglandins, catecholamines, histamine, and oxytocin also figure prominently in the central regulation of ACTH and β-endorphin secretion.[35, 36] Oxytocin stimulates ACTH secretion when given alone,[33, 37] has a synergistic effect with corticotropin-releasing hormone on ACTH release, and has an additive effect with vasopressin on ACTH release.[37]

Circulating ACTH acts on cell membrane receptors in the zona fasciculata and zona reticularis of the adrenal cortex to activate adenylate cyclase, which in turn elicits the synthesis and secretion of cortisol and aldosterone.[38] Increasing levels of cortisol exert negative feedback on the synthesis and release of both corticotropin-releasing hormone and ACTH.[38–40] On the other hand, cortisol exerts a longer-term facilitatory action on catecholamine synthetic enzymes of the adrenal medulla.[41] In vivo, the net balance of positive and negative feedback effects within the hypothalamic-pituitary-

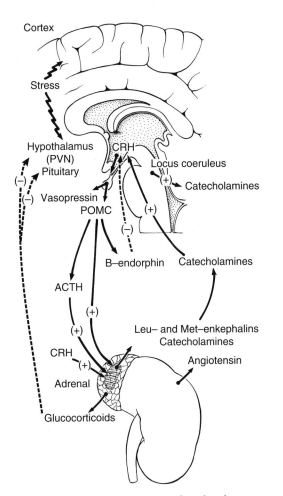

Figure 7–2 The hypothalamic-pituitary-adrenal and sympathoadrenomedullary axes. These two linked efferent hormonal axes dominate the systemic neuroendocrine response to surgical stress. The paraventricular nucleus (PVN) of the hypothalamus is the key integrative site of these responses. Secretion of corticotropin-releasing hormone (CRH) from the PVN is multihormonally regulated. Adrenocorticotropic hormone (ACTH) elicits the synthesis and secretion of cortisol, which exerts negative feedback on the synthesis of CRH and ACTH. CRH also directly stimulates steroidogenesis in the adrenal medulla. Activation of the locus coeruleus causes release of catecholamines in the adrenal medulla and within the central nervous system, augmenting the hypothalamic-pituitary-adrenal response. + indicates positive feedback. − indicates inhibition. POMC, proopiomelanocortin.

existence of an entirely intra-adrenal corticotropin-releasing hormone and ACTH mechanism that responds to stress and hence locally replicates the hypothalamic-pituitary-adrenal response.[43]

The second major stress hormone axis is typified by circulating catecholamines that are released from a wide variety of sources during stress. There is heterogeneity for both the origins of and regulatory mechanisms governing distinct plasma catecholamines. Plasma epinephrine levels chiefly (but not exclusively) reflect adrenomedullary activity, which also results in the release of leu- and met-enkephalins into the circulation.[44, 45] Plasma levels of norepinephrine are less clearly indicative of adrenomedullary activity, because they reflect aggregate "spillover" from regional peripheral sympathetic nerves, e.g., in vasculature of skeletal muscle, kidney, and other viscera.

Central norepinephrine levels principally derive from the terminal efferent projections of the locus coeruleus, the principal cluster of noradrenergic cell bodies in the central nervous system.[46] Efferent pathways emanating from these neurons send a dense network of terminal fields to many disparate regions in the brain, including hypothalamus, limbic system, hippocampus, and cerebral cortex.[46] The paraventricular nucleus, a key central site of neuroendocrine and autonomic integration, is densely innervated by noradrenergic terminals originating mainly from clusters of cells in the medulla oblongata and to a smaller extent in the locus coeruleus.[47] Central corticotropin-releasing hormone and norepinephrine systems constitute a positive feedback loop in which each system reinforces the function of the other. Identification of noradrenergic synapses on corticotropin-releasing hormone–containing cells in the paraventricular nucleus suggests a substrate according to which central noradrenergic activity modulates hypothalamic-pituitary-adrenocortical function, consistent with the known contribution of paraventricular nucleus catecholamines to hypothalamic-pituitary-adrenocortical activation during stress.[47] Conversely, in the rat, local application of corticotropin-releasing hormone onto locus coeruleus neurons markedly increases their firing rate, and norepinephrine is a potent stimulus to the in vitro release of corticotropin-releasing hormone from pituitary corticotrophs. Inhibitory feedback controls on these positively reverberating corticotropin-releasing hormone–norepinephrine systems include glucocorticoids, gamma-aminobutyric acid, ACTH, and the endogenous opioids.[46]

Increases in circulating levels of growth hormone and prolactin have also been described during and after operation.[48, 49] Growth hormone secretion is influenced by numerous hormones, including ACTH, vasopressin, cortisol, and catecholamines.[48] Mediators such as prostaglandin E_2 stimulate growth hormone release by activating the receptor for growth hormone–releasing hormone. Opioids exert negative feedback on the stress-related synthesis and release not only of corticotropin-releasing hormone and ACTH but also of growth hormone and prolactin.[44] On the other hand, when opioids are administered to subjects during basal (un-

adrenocortical system during chronic reexposure to acute stress clearly favors the former. Hypothalamic-pituitary-adrenocortical responsiveness is maintained indefinitely during chronic reexposure to acute stressors, leading to the concept that prior stress induces a "facilitatory trace" in the neural components of the hypothalamic-pituitary-adrenocortical system.[42]

Corticotropin-releasing hormone is also able to stimulate adrenal steroidogenesis independent of pituitary ACTH release through mechanisms that involve intra-adrenal production of ACTH. Some adrenal medullary chromaffin cells possess high-affinity binding sites for corticotropin-releasing hormone and contain and corelease pro-opiomelanocortin–derived peptides along with catecholamines. Limited data further support the stressed) conditions, levels of growth hormone and prolactin increase acutely.[20]

Pituitary secretion of gonadotropins and thyrotropin typically declines during stress. The pattern of synthesis of triiodothyronine (T_3) shifts during acute illness such that an inactive isomer (reverse T_3) predominates, but patients remain clinically euthyroid.[22, 48]

The Immuno-Hypothalamic-Pituitary-Adrenocortical Axis During Stress

Abundant clinical and experimental evidence points to the prime importance of afferent neurogenic stimuli in eliciting classic stress responses after operation or trauma.[50, 51] In his original description of the generalized adaptation syndrome, however, Selye[1] himself raised the possibility that tissue factors per se might be capable of evoking this syndrome. Selye and many others pursued this speculation as to the existence of a "tissue corticotropin-releasing factor" having a chemical structure distinct from hypothalamic peptides and manifest even in deafferented sites of injury. Observations that tissue injury elicits a pituitary-adrenal response in animals after autotransplantation of the pituitary into the renal capsule (and hence without any brain-pituitary connection) confirm the importance of extraneural factors in this response.[52]

Circulating corticotropin-releasing hormone–like activity evoked by tissue trauma is now identified with a cascade of inflammatory cytokines, chiefly tumor necrosis factor–alpha, interleukin-1, and interleukin-6.[53, 54] Each of these three inflammatory cytokines is recognized as a potent stimulator of the hypothalamic-pituitary-adrenocortical axis at each of its three levels. High doses of interleukin-6 also appear to stimulate vasopressin,[55] possibly explaining the occasional postinfectious or postoperative development of the syndrome of inappropriate antidiuretic hormone secretion. Other products of an activated immune system such as interleukin-2 and interferon-alfa or interferon-gamma also stimulate the hypothalamic-pituitary-adrenocortical axis, presumably by inducing the secretion of tumor necrosis factor–alpha, interleukin-1, and interleukin-6.[56–59] The now-abandoned endotoxin stimulation test of hypothalamic-pituitary-adrenocortical responsiveness and the well-recognized hypothalamic-pituitary-adrenocortical activation during bacterial infection[60] are now viewed as consequences of the "immunoneuroendocrine" interaction.[61]

The central nervous system and pituitary contain receptors for cytokines such as interleukin-1[46] and interleukin-6.[62] It is not yet clear whether peripheral and central sources of interleukin-1α or interleukin-1β interact with each other or whether circulating interleukin-1 and interleukin-6 cross the blood-brain barrier to exert their effect.[63] Cytokine stimulation of the hypothalamic-pituitary-adrenocortical axis is mediated, at least in part, through prostaglandins such as prostaglandin E_2 and related compounds such as platelet-activating factor. Interleukin-1 stimulation of endothelial cell prostaglandin E_2 secretion within circum-

ventricular organs, for example, could cause the release of corticotropin-releasing hormone from the nerve terminals of the median eminence, which lies outside the blood-brain barrier.[63] It has also been shown that the action of interleukin-1 on its receptors in the area postrema, which also lies outside the blood-brain barrier, leads to noradrenergic-mediated corticotropin-releasing hormone release from hypothalamic neurons. In addition, peripherally derived cytokines may gain access to the brain during disease states such as infection or inflammation, because blood-brain barrier integrity is impaired in these conditions.[46]

In patients, operation evokes a systemic cytokine response, the magnitude of which correlates with the magnitude of surgical trauma.[64] Interleukin-1β and interleukin-6 responses increase with the severity of the surgical insult, interleukin-6 levels being maximal in patients in whom major complications develop.[64] This form of correlation does not prove causation. Several laboratories have reported that human peripheral blood mononuclear cells secrete pro-opiomelanocortin peptides, including ACTH, that can stimulate adrenocortical function directly via a "lymphoid adrenal axis" independent of the hypothalamic-pituitary-adrenocortical axis.[65–67] However, evidence against this concept has emerged from findings that human peripheral blood mononuclear cells do not express pro-opiomelanocortin transcripts that are translated into pro-opiomelanocortin peptides,[68] although this study could not exclude pro-opiomelanocortin expression from other immune cells or compartments.[69]

Apart from ACTH, other peptide neurotransmitters present within central nervous system pathways responsive to pain and stress also appear to act at peripheral sites of inflammation. For example, neuropeptides such as substance P, corticotropin-releasing hormone, and the endorphins have immunomodulatory roles.[70–73] Substance P, present in peripheral terminals of sensory afferents, augments inflammatory processes by binding and stimulating immune cells, induces histamine release from mast cells, and enhances expression of the mRNA for interleukin-1β, interleukin-6, and tumor necrosis factor–alpha.[70, 74] Substance P is released within the joint space and stimulates synovial cells to secrete prostaglandins and collagenase.[75]

Corticotropin-releasing factor has been identified in cells of the immune system, in sensory afferent neurons, and in inflamed tissue.[71, 72] Its presence within the joint space of patients with rheumatoid arthritis may reflect local synthesis or delivery to the joint through sensory and sympathetic terminals.[71] Sympathetic nerves innervate immune organs such as thymus and spleen.[76] Within the joint space, corticotropin-releasing hormone appears to have a proinflammatory effect because local passive immunoneutralization of corticotropin-releasing hormone decreases both the volume and cellularity of the inflammatory exudate.[72] Many immune cell types, including lymphoid cells, express specific receptors for various neuropeptides in addition to substance P and corticotropin-releasing hormone, and they respond to neuropeptide exposure by proliferation and cytokine release.[58, 67, 77]

Ample preclinical and clinical evidence points to frankly impaired humoral and cellular immune mechanisms after operation, trauma, or pain. Such impairment has been observed, for example, in responsiveness to mitogens or antigens, lymphocyte-mediated cytotoxicity, delayed hypersensitivity, skin graft rejection, antibody response, and natural killer cell activity.[58, 78, 79]

Glucocorticoids have the clearest role as mediators of hypothalamic-pituitary-adrenocortical–induced immunosuppression. They inhibit the immune cascade at virtually every level: macrophage antigen presentation to lymphocytes, lymphocyte proliferation, lymphocyte differentiation to effector cell subtypes, migration of leukocytes, and production of phospholipid-derived mediators[39] and cytokines.[46, 56] Two distinct intracellular receptors for adrenal steroids have been cloned.[80] The type I receptor is also known as the mineralocorticoid receptor because of its high affinity for aldosterone, although it has an equally high affinity for corticosterone. The type II receptor, also known as the glucocorticoid receptor, has a 6-fold to 10-fold lower affinity for corticosterone than does the type I but hardly binds to mineralocorticoids. The varied responsiveness of different cells to acute exposure to different corticosteroids reflects not only systemic glucocorticoid levels that are subject to diurnal or stress regulation but also each cell's differential expression of type I and type II receptors and the bioavailability of hormone to surrounding tissue.[81]

Other stress hormones also contribute to the immunosuppression seen with stress. Macrophage cell membranes express α_1- and α_2-adrenoreceptors. Catecholamines decrease chemotactic and phagocytic activity, block the activation of macrophages to a tumoricidal and antiviral state, and inhibit the production of reactive oxygen intermediates.[76, 82] Growth hormone and prolactin act as endogenous restorative agents that counteract stress-induced immunosuppression. Lymphocytes have growth hormone and prolactin receptors whose occupation stimulates cytokine production. Prolactin is an essential growth factor in one line of lymphoid cells.[83]

Endogenous opioids play many roles in stress-induced alterations of the immune system.[84] For example, the decreased natural killer cell activity observed during stress-induced analgesia[85, 86] appears to result from central endogenous opioid release and is blocked by opioid antagonists. However, analgesic doses of morphine block the surgery-induced increase in metastases, apparently by increasing natural killer cell activity.[79]

Stress-related signaling between the nervous and immune systems is reciprocal, is highly regulated,[24] and uses common signals in both directions[83] (Fig. 7–3). Broadly speaking, the immuno-hypothalamic-pituitary-adrenocortical response is governed by "long-loop" negative feedback.[83] Inflammatory mediators[87] stimulate each of the three levels of the hypothalamic-pituitary-adrenocortical response, thereby increasing plasma ACTH, β-endorphin, and glucocorticoid levels, dampening the immune response.[46, 83] "Peripheral cor-

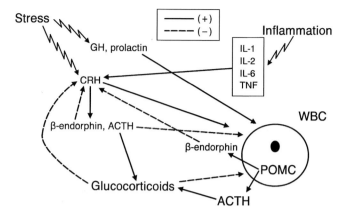

Figure 7–3 Bidirectional communication between the endocrine and immune systems. Trauma such as major operation evokes both neuroendocrine and cytokine responses. Trophic hormones released by the hypothalamus stimulate the pituitary to release adrenocorticotropic hormone (ACTH), prolactin, and growth hormone (GH), among other hormones. Tumor necrosis factor (TNF) and interleukins (IL) stimulate the hypothalamic-pituitary-adrenocortical axis. Peripheral white blood cells (WBC) (see text for details) may directly stimulate the adrenal cortex by secreting ACTH and other pro-opiomelanocortin (POMC) peptides. WBC also express receptors for other pituitary hormones besides ACTH, such as GH and prolactin, that modulate the immune response. CRH, corticotropin-releasing hormone.

ticotropin-releasing hormone" may possibly provide a local, proinflammatory counterbalance within this long loop.[50, 71, 72, 88–90] The importance of the hypothalamic-pituitary-adrenocortical axis in holding stress-induced immune responses under control has given rise to the concept that prevention of overexuberant immune reactions is an important function of the hypothalamic-pituitary-adrenocortical response.[83] Genetic, surgical, or pharmacologic disruptions of these signals are, in both animal models and clinical studies, associated with enhanced susceptibility to or severity of immune-related systemic disease.[46, 91, 92] However, adverse metabolic sequelae and clinical outcomes in the postoperative setting appear to be averted through the use of regional anesthesia to deprive the stress response of its neural afferent trigger.

Metabolic Responses to Stress

More than 50 years ago, Cuthbertson described a disturbance of metabolism produced by bony and nonbony injury and divided this disturbance into "ebb" and "flow" phases.[93, 94] This description is still recognized as valid today. The ebb phase is a hypometabolic state in which neither metabolic rate nor oxygen consumption increases to the extent permitted by substrate availability. Depending on many factors such as the severity of the injury and the treatment applied, the ebb phase typically lasts no more than a day.[93, 95] Plasma concentrations of catecholamines, cortisol, glucagon, and growth hormone are generally high during this phase, whereas plasma insulin concentrations are depressed in relation to plasma glucose.[93]

The ebb phase evolves into a more prolonged flow phase in which catabolism predominates. Metabolic rate, core temperature, pulse rate, oxygen consumption, urinary excretion of nitrogen, and other indices of protein breakdown, such as 3-methylhistidine, zinc, and creatinine,[96] all increase during the flow phase. The duration and intensity of these catabolic changes vary according to the severity and nature of the injury.

Although there is no question that both hypothalamic-pituitary-adrenocortical and sympathomedullary responses produce major metabolic shifts during stress, cytokines are increasingly recognized as modulators of carbohydrate, protein, and lipid metabolism.[97] Interleukin-1 and tumor necrosis factor inhibit lipoprotein lipase, thereby causing increases in triglyceride concentration.[97, 98] Both tumor necrosis factor and interleukin-1 stimulate thermogenesis and acute phase protein synthesis.[59, 99, 100] Interleukin-1 inhibits the secretion of insulin and glucagon and thus appears to contribute to an increase in glucose production.[101] Tumor necrosis factor causes mobilization of amino acids from peripheral tissues and acts in concert with interleukin-1 to decrease peripheral glucose uptake.[98]

Glucose Metabolism

After injury, several mechanisms disrupt normal regulation of release and uptake of glucose. Hyperglycemia after operation results from impairment of dual regulatory processes through which, in unstressed subjects, increased plasma glucose levels inhibit hepatic gluconeogenesis and increase peripheral glucose use.[94, 102] Hepatic gluconeogenesis after injury is stimulated by an increase in substrate supply, particularly amino acids such as alanine from skeletal muscle,[102] glycerol released from adipose tissue lipolysis, and lactate derived from ischemic tissues and areas of inflammation.[96, 103]

In uninjured individuals, increased plasma glucose concentration stimulates pancreatic insulin secretion, with various end-organ actions, particularly on liver, adipose, and muscle. Insulin enhances the activity of enzymes involved in glycolysis, glucose oxidation, and glucose synthesis and also increases blood flow to muscle by selective vasodilation.[104] Yet immediately after injury, high circulating catecholamine levels decrease pancreatic insulin secretion. Later, plasma insulin increases to levels that are inappropriately high for the plasma glucose concentration.[105] The delayed increase in insulin levels reflects both the decreased adrenergic restraint on secretion and the stimulation of insulin release by amino acids, particularly arginine, a potent insulin secretagogue.[93, 106] Despite the increased insulin concentration at this point after injury, insulin fails to exert its expected anabolic effect ("insulin resistance"). Thus, postoperative glucose production is enhanced, glucose storage is decreased, fat mobilization and oxidation are increased, and protein turnover is also resistant to the normal anabolic effect of insulin.

Studies[93] to evaluate the role of epinephrine, cortisol, and glucagon in altering glucose metabolism, by means of concurrent infusions of unstressed subjects, indicate that these three hormones act synergistically to promote and sustain hepatic glucose production, increase metabolic rate, and lower glucose clearance. During the initial phase of such infusions, as shortly after trauma, the increase in insulin is blunted in relation to the level of hyperglycemia.[93, 94, 106] At present, there is growing concern over possibly deleterious effects of hyperglycemia on the brain and heart after operation, and clinical studies[107] are being performed to determine whether tight control of perioperative glucose levels can improve outcome of cardiac operation.

Lipid Metabolism

An increase in free fatty acids and glycerol concentration as a result of lipolysis in adipose tissue can be demonstrated intraoperatively, e.g., during open cholecystectomy, provided that sensitive collection methods such as catheter microdialysis are used.[108] Increased fat oxidation continues into the flow phase, when fat provides the major part of the energy requirement. The number of adipose-derived calories correlates positively with the severity of the injury.[94, 109] Adipose tissue lipolysis is acutely stimulated by epinephrine and potentiated by cortisol, glucagon, and growth hormone.[110] Increased circulating levels of these catabolic hormones impair the ability of insulin to inhibit lipolysis effectively, leading to increased fatty acid turnover.[109] Indeed, fat continues to be mobilized after trauma or operation, even when sufficient glucose is given to meet energy requirements. Cortisol appears to play a major, if not the major, role in this mobilization because of its marked stimulatory effect on lipoprotein lipase activity within adipose tissue.[111]

Protein Metabolism

Protein synthesis and degradation both increase after injury.[103, 112] Breakdown of protein stores predominates, particularly in skeletal muscle, but also in loose connective tissue and intestinal viscera.[113] A partial exception is the liver, in which stress increases the synthesis of acute phase proteins and decreases synthesis of other proteins such as albumin and transferrin.[96, 103, 112] In parallel with findings for inflammatory mediator release or other hormone effects on metabolism, the magnitude of protein catabolism varies with the severity of the trauma.[114] Also, as is true for glucose and fat metabolism, cortisol and other glucocorticoids antagonize insulin's antiproteolytic effect on skeletal muscle.[115] After trauma or operation, there is a marked increase in the peripheral oxidation of branched chain amino acids to provide substrates for gluconeogenesis. These amino acids are rendered unavailable for reincorporation into body protein.[95] Hence, nitrogen is excreted as urinary urea, and body protein stores are progressively depleted.[102, 112] 3-Methylhistidine, derived from myofibrillar protein, has proved useful as a marker of global protein breakdown in studies of post-surgical stress responses.[103]

Regional Anesthesia and Analgesia and Clinical Stress Responses

Operation during general anesthesia elicits a neuro-endocrine response that encompasses virtually all the features described above: increased plasma concentrations of catecholamines, prolactin, growth hormone, vasopressin, ACTH, β-endorphin, cortisol, vasopressin, and cytokines, with resultant catabolism, immunosuppression, hyperglycemia, water retention, and other undesirable sequelae.[49, 116–119] The magnitude of these global responses depends on the surgical site, the extent and duration of anesthesia, and the postoperative analgesic technique.[49, 114, 117, 120] Because neural stimuli and inflammatory mediators together trigger the stress response, modifying these inputs should, in theory, lead to the stress response's partial or total suppression. Although specific interleukin antagonists are now available, their use has not yet progressed into the clinical postoperative period. Accordingly, this discussion is limited to those techniques currently available to the anesthesiologist (Fig. 7–4) and the impact of these techniques on clinical outcome.[121]

Epidural Local Anesthesia and Analgesia

Extensive data support the efficacy of local anesthetic epidural block to T-4 in suppressing completely the hypothalamic-pituitary-adrenocortical response to lower extremity orthopedic and lower abdominal surgery[117, 122] as well as blocking the increased concentration of cytokines seen after lower extremity orthopedic surgery.[117] Suppression of hypothalamic-pituitary-adrenocortical responses in this context also preserves nitrogen balance postoperatively, when otherwise it would be grossly negative. Higher dermatomal levels and longer duration of sensory block lead to more complete attenuation of the stress response.[123, 124] Epidural local anesthetic block for less than 4 h has only a transient inhibitory effect on the adrenocortical and hyperglycemic response to operation,[125] which can still emerge after block lasting less than 24 h.[126] On the other hand, the inhibitory effects of afferent block for a full 24 h after operation remain evident for 4 days.[126]

When the operative site is the upper abdomen or thorax, epidural block with local anesthetics is at best only partially effective in blocking hypothalamic-pituitary-adrenocortical or cytokine responses.[117, 120, 127–129] Even during laparoscopic cholecystectomy, local anesthetic epidural block fails to eliminate the stress response, despite an adequate anesthetic level and excellent analgesia.[116] The failure of local anesthetic epidural block (even at seemingly appropriate dermatomal levels) to inhibit the stress response to thoracic or upper abdominal operation is still not explained. It has been proposed that afferent nociceptive activity may persist below the threshold for conscious perception of pain, yet be sufficient to evoke neuroendocrine responses. The observation that somatosensory potentials evoked by thoracic sensory stimulation persist despite thoracic epidural anesthesia supports this hypothesis.[130] Other neural afferent pathways that may remain active to evoke hormonal responses despite clinically adequate somatic anesthesia during local anesthetic epidural block include sympathetic, vagal, and phrenic afferents.[51, 128]

Epidural local anesthesia and analgesia are associated with systemic beneficial effects that may result, at least in part, from inhibition of hypothalamic-pituitary-adrenocortical or sympathomedullary responses. One such effect is to decrease postoperative hypercoagulability.[131] The effects of epidural anesthesia and analgesia on coagulation are complex and not fully elucidated. Local anesthetics by themselves decrease platelet reactivity. Epidural infusion of local anesthetic (plus fentanyl) prevents the typical postoperative decline in fibrinolysis[132] by blunting the normal increase in plasminogen activator levels. Infusion of a stress hormone "cocktail" (epinephrine, cortisol, and glucagon) in normal volunteers increases platelet reactivity and fibrinogen levels, but it does not reproduce the typical postoperative decrease in fibrinolytic activity.[133] Hence, a reduction in humoral markers of stress may explain some, although not all, of the postoperative benefits of epidural local analgesia on hypercoagulability.

Other effects of local anesthetic epidural block implicated in these benefits include blunting of the usual postoperative increases of factor VIII and von Willebrand factor, decrease in fibrinogen values,[131, 134] and improvement of blood flow in the calves and femoral

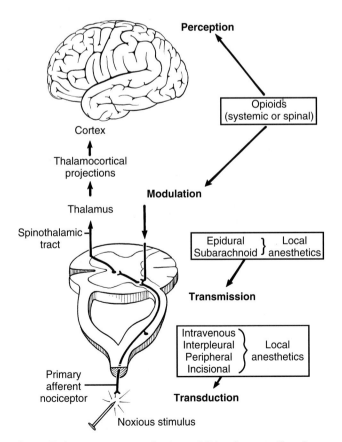

Figure 7–4 Perioperative analgesic modalities that can affect the neuroendocrine response to pain and surgery.

veins. These mechanisms are distinct from the decrease in intraoperative bleeding attributed to lower venous pressures during epidural compared with general anesthesia.[135, 136]

Differences in the effects of regional and general anesthesia on immune function (other than complement activation) are not yet well studied. Neutrophils extracted from peripheral blood during spinal anesthesia for hip surgery migrate more rapidly toward a complement-derived attractant than neutrophils during the same operation performed during general anesthesia, correlating with lower intraoperative levels of epinephrine.[137] The clinical implications of these effects on in vitro neutrophil activity are unknown, but one may speculate that if regional anesthetic techniques prove to impair immune function less than general anesthesia, this effect may help to explain seemingly unrelated clinical benefits of regional anesthesia on clinical outcome, such as a decrease in postoperative pulmonary infections.[138, 139]

Effects of epidural local anesthesia and analgesia in infants appear to be similar to those in adults. Lumbar epidural local anesthetics, in concentrations lower than those needed for adults, blunt the hormonal stress response during surgical procedures in the lower part of the body.[124] Also as in adults, intraoperative epidural local anesthesia with continued infusion to provide acceptable postoperative analgesia in children undergoing upper abdominal operations does not inhibit increases in epinephrine, glucose, ACTH, and cortisol, although norepinephrine levels are lower during epidural analgesia.[118]

Neuraxial Administration of Opioids

The effects of neuraxial administration of opioids on the surgical stress response, despite yielding good pain relief, are less both in magnitude and duration than the inhibition of this response produced by neuraxial local anesthetics. Trends toward decreased levels of catecholamines, cortisol, antidiuretic hormone, and glucose have been reported during analgesia with opioids given neuraxially.[120, 127, 129, 140, 141] Addition of morphine given epidurally to epidural administration of bupivacaine does not appear to augment the effectiveness of epidural administration of bupivacaine in suppressing postoperative increases in the concentration of glucose and cortisol,[120] and morphine does not improve catabolism even when administered for 72 h postoperatively.[142]

If we compare neuraxial with intravenous administration of opioids for analgesia, opioids given neuraxially seem to have greater potency in decreasing the stress response to operation. Equianalgesic doses of fentanyl given epidurally or intravenously produced disparate effects on peak β-endorphin levels and duration of plasma cortisol increase after operation, with the epidural group showing reductions in both measurements despite lower dose requirements.[49]

Because epidural administration of opioids achieves substantial plasma levels,[143] the enhanced potency of

neuraxial compared with systemic administration of opioids in stress hormone inhibition may simply reflect concurrent increases in plasma and cerebrospinal fluid opioid levels achieved during spinal administration. Many reports[144, 145] indicate that high doses of systemically administered opioids inhibit intraoperative and early postoperative endocrine and metabolic responses to abdominal and cardiac surgery. However, such single-dose effects do not extend beyond about 8 h,[104, 125] and reductions in hypothalamic-pituitary-adrenocortical responses during high-dose systemic administration of opioids do not prove that analgesia has been satisfactory.

The hypothalamic-pituitary-adrenocortical axis is subject to negative feedback control by endogenous opioids or their exogenous surrogates (see Fig. 7–2), and many pains are recognized as resistant or refractory to opioids.[24] Conversely, patient-controlled analgesia with systemic administration of opioid provides effective postoperative analgesia[138] but has little influence on the hypothalamic-pituitary-adrenocortical response to operation.[119, 146] It is possible though that certain elements of the global stress response, such as immune impairment, may be blocked by analgesic doses of opioids that are subthreshold to influence hypothalamic-pituitary-adrenocortical reactivity.[79]

Peripheral Regional Block

Because of the importance of neural afferent activity in initiating the perioperative stress response, it is logical to suppose that peripheral nerve blocks might prevent this response. However, clinical trials of various perioperative nerve blocks have shown a general lack of effect despite achieving good pain control in many cases. For example, intraoperative paravertebral blocks during abdominal surgery attenuate the early stress response minimally despite providing pain relief for 1 to 6 h.[147]

Intercostal nerve blocks have a modest inhibitory effect on postoperative hyperglycemia but little other effect.[50] Interpleural analgesia, achieved by administration of local anesthetic between visceral and parietal pleurae,[148] provides good pain relief after cholecystectomy, renal surgery, and multiple unilateral rib fractures (although less so after thoracotomy), but it too is insufficient to decrease postoperative stress responses.[124] The dissociation between good analgesia after peripheral nerve blocks for upper abdominal or thoracic surgery and a lack of stress response inhibition parallels findings for epidural local anesthesia, and it suggests once again that unperceived afferent stimuli and input through unblocked pathways sustain stress responses to operations at these sites.

The potential of peripheral regional blocks at more caudal locations to inhibit stress responses is not as well studied, but again, as for epidural local anesthesia, it may be greater than for operations more proximally. Dorsal penile nerve block for neonatal circumcision is effective in decreasing not only behavioral distress but also the adrenocortical stress response.[149] On the other hand, innovative techniques such as continuous intra-peritoneal infusion of bupivacaine fail to influence systemic stress responses.[150]

The Spinal Cord Stress Response: Neuronal Sensitization and Reorganization

Until quite recently, the significance of the spinal cord as a stress-responsive organ was overlooked. As investigators' attention focused exclusively on the hypothalamic-pituitary-adrenocortical and adrenomedullary responses, the spinal cord was viewed as a mere relay for afferent nociceptive signals on their way from the periphery to the hypothalamus. Ongoing research has now shown that pain is a dynamic process, the biochemical and molecular aspects of which share many features with memory, and that the spinal cord is a key site of this adaptive process.[8, 151] Just as brief traumatic experiences can forever change one's perceptions, brief nociceptive stimulation can cause dorsal horn neuronal sensitization (decrease in pain threshold and widening of cutaneous receptive fields) and long-lasting, even permanent synaptic reorganization.[9, 152–154] The sensory consequence of this central sensitization is not only "primary" hyperalgesia in the area of tissue injury but also "secondary" hyperalgesia[155] in the surrounding area (Fig. 7–5).

Although the physiology of nociception is covered elsewhere in this text, it is appropriate to note here these new advances in its understanding for three reasons. First, these adaptive responses within individual neurons of the dorsal horn (Fig. 7–6) are literally "stress responses" in Selye's initial meaning, and so their description is a direct extension of prior work on physiologic responses to "diverse nocuous agents."[1] Second, the processes by which spinal cord neurons

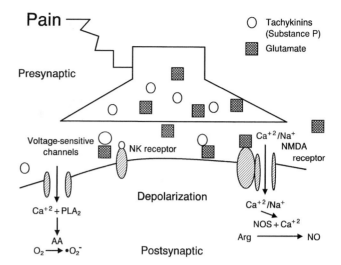

Figure 7–6 Schematic representation of intracellular stress responses within single nociceptive neurons of the spinal cord dorsal horn. C fibers release glutamate (an excitatory amino acid) along with substance P and related tachykinins (excitatory peptides). Glutamate acts through *N*-methyl-D-aspartate (NMDA) receptors to produce an influx of calcium and sodium, causing depolarization followed by activation of voltage-dependent calcium channels, in turn permitting the influx of more calcium. Elevated levels of intracellular calcium stimulate nitric oxide synthase (NOS) and also catalyze arachidonic acid (AA) formation. Oxidative phosphorylation, triggered both by binding of tachykinins to neurokinin (NK) receptors and glutamate to "metabotropic" glutamate receptors, generates intracellular free radicals such as peroxide. Arg, arginine. (Modified from Woolf CJ, Chong MS: Preemptive analgesia—treating postoperative pain by preventing the establishment of central sensitization. Anesth Analg 1993; 77: 362–379.)

become sensitized or even reorganize their synaptic connections depend on intracellular "oxidative stress"[13]: the generation of free radicals, particularly nitric oxide.[156–158] Nitric oxide not only subserves hyperalgesia[159–162] but also in high concentrations can lead to neuronal injury or death.[11, 163] Another form of intracellular stress response in dorsal horn neurons, expression of the *c-fos* proto-oncogene, has been observed immediately after peripheral nerve injury[164] and also may regulate synaptic reorganization and death.[165, 166] Third, because excitatory neurotransmitters such as glutamate[167, 168] evoke long-term hyperexcitability in the spinal cord by stimulating the synthesis of nitric oxide,[160, 169–171] and free radicals in turn regulate the function of the *N*-methyl-D-aspartate receptor,[12] research in this area has provided a strong theoretic underpinning for preemptive analgesia. Clinical trials of preemptive analgesia commonly use regional anesthetic techniques to prevent afferent impulses from reaching the spinal cord, with the goals of controlling both acute postoperative pain and long-term chronic pain[8, 151, 172] (Fig. 7–7).

The enthusiasm for preemptive analgesia based on preclinical grounds[173, 174] appeared to be supported in early studies that often involved small numbers of patients, insufficient controls, or other design flaws such as failure to sustain analgesia intraoperatively or postoperatively.[175, 176] Other studies have shown less striking results,[177] but as Kehlet[178] has pointed out, they

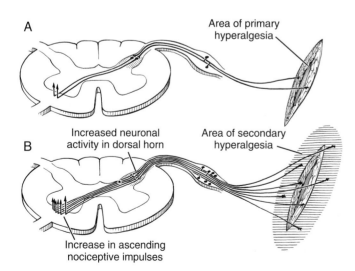

Figure 7–5 Neural mechanisms of primary and secondary hyperalgesia. *A,* Primary hyperalgesia may include sensitization of peripheral nociceptors and central neurons. *B,* Secondary hyperalgesia is based on an altered central processing, with reduction in pain threshold, expansion of receptive fields, and even long-lasting permanent synaptic reorganization.

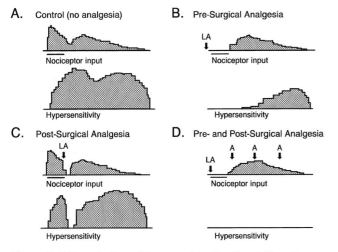

A. Control (no analgesia)

Nociceptor input

Hypersensitivity

B. Pre-Surgical Analgesia

LA

Nociceptor input

Hypersensitivity

C. Post-Surgical Analgesia

LA

Nociceptor input

Hypersensitivity

D. Pre- and Post-Surgical Analgesia

LA   A   A   A

Nociceptor input

Hypersensitivity

Figure 7–7 Hypothetic model prepared by Woolf and Chong[8] to present the rationale for aggressive pain control. *A,* Central hypersensitivity evoked by nociceptive afferent input during (horizontal line) and after operation. *B,* Preoperative local anesthesia (LA) eliminates intraoperative afferent input only until the anesthetic wears off, after which time sensitization can still take place. *C,* Postoperative LA briefly shuts off nociceptor input, but hypersensitivity has already become established and soon reappears. *D,* The combination of preemptive LA plus repeated doses of postoperative systemic analgesia (A) (e.g., opioid or nonsteroidal anti-inflammatory drug) is most effective in averting central sensitization. (Redrawn from Woolf CJ, Chong MS: Preemptive analgesia—treating postoperative pain by preventing the establishment of central sensitization. Anesth Analg 1993; 77: 362–379.)

have tended to place an inordinate amount of emphasis on single dimensions such as stress hormone suppression or pain control, rather than evaluating an integrated, multimodal approach to improving clinical outcomes.

Regional Anesthesia, Stress Suppression, and Outcome

Paralleling the greater effectiveness of regional anesthesia at suppressing stress responses during lower abdominal versus upper abdominal or thoracic surgery, regional anesthesia tends to have a more clearly favorable impact on operative morbidity when applied to procedures below the umbilicus versus upper abdominal, thoracic, or abdominal aortic operations.[135, 179–181] Epidural anesthesia and analgesia offer striking benefits over general anesthesia for peripheral vascular surgery.[134] Patients undergoing peripheral vascular surgery are at increased risk of postoperative cardiovascular complications and early arterial graft failure[131] owing to a perioperative hypercoagulable state. Epidural local anesthesia and analgesia are associated with a lower incidence of reoperation for inadequate tissue perfusion,[182] fewer thrombotic events, and, in some studies, lower rates of cardiovascular, infectious, and total postoperative complications as well as shorter intensive care unit stays.[131]

Clinical outcomes in high-risk groups, such as the

grossly obese[183] or American Society of Anesthesiologists class III patients having aortic surgery,[184] likewise appear to favor patients given epidural local anesthesia and postoperative analgesia. In a provocative pilot study,[184] patients who received regional anesthesia had earlier mobilization; were more alert; and had more rapid recovery of bowel function, less cardiovascular and infectious morbidity, a decreased duration of tracheal intubation, and earlier dismissal from the intensive care unit and the hospital. These findings suggest that in the high-risk population, epidural local anesthesia and analgesia may offer clinical advantages over general anesthesia and conventional analgesia, even for operation in the upper abdomen.

Whether epidural anesthesia and postoperative analgesia have particular value for patients with ischemic heart disease is controversial. The cardiac sympathetic block achieved by thoracic epidural anesthesia appears to increase the diameter of stenotic epicardial coronary artery segments in patients with coronary artery disease, which may improve regional perfusion of ischemic areas without causing dilatation of coronary resistance vessels. This avoids maldistribution of coronary blood flow (coronary steal) and may be beneficial to patients with coronary artery disease.[185] Improved left ventricular wall motion and ejection fraction have been observed with epidural block but disappear after volume loading.[186] Other investigators have demonstrated that intraoperative epidural anesthesia (with light general anesthesia) plus postoperative epidural administration of morphine decreases the risk of postoperative myocardial ischemia in patients with coronary artery disease compared with general anesthesia and conventional analgesia, but they do not lower the overall risk of postoperative cardiac morbidity.[187] Still others, however, find more frequent, longer, and more severe silent ischemic events in the 24 h after spinal analgesia for minor surgery compared with a reference day of normal daily activities.[188]

The difficulties in interpreting studies that compare analgesia or stress response suppression when opioids are given via systemic versus epidural routes extend to studies of the cardiac effects of opioids given epidurally versus systemically. Opioids are known to act centrally to shift the baroreceptor reflex response and raise the ventricular fibrillation threshold and peripherally on innervated myocardium to attenuate catecholamine-induced inotropy and chronotropy.[2] Not surprisingly, postoperative "intensive analgesia" achieved with high doses of systemically administered sufentanil after coronary artery bypass grafting is associated with diminished severity of ischemic episodes.[189] Further prospective controlled trials are needed to define the incidence of perioperative ischemia and other cardiac morbidity in patients with coronary artery disease receiving either regional anesthesia or general anesthesia with or without high doses of opioids.[190]

Conclusion

The complex, linked group of physiologic responses to pain or trauma has been studied since the 19th century, but investigation in this area is, if anything, increasing in pace as the present century draws to a close. Concurrently, as biologic research fields and subfields have proliferated, the meaning of the term "stress response" has broadened to the point of referring to environmentally evoked reactions at every level of organization from subcellular to the whole body. This observation is not meant pejoratively, because a defining feature of all life, from unicellular to individual levels, is continuous adaptation to environmental challenges!

Historically and hormonally, the dominant neuroendocrine responses to pain and trauma are hypothalamic-pituitary-adrenocortical and sympathoadrenal. Activation of these axes, particularly the hypothalamic-pituitary-adrenocortical, is accomplished through nociceptive afferents and circulating cytokines, and continued bidirectional signaling between neural and immune systems governs the evolution of the hypothalamic-pituitary-adrenocortical response from onset to remission. Together, the hypothalamic-pituitary-adrenocortical and sympathoadrenal efferent limbs modulate nearly all physiologic systems, particularly those involved in analgesia, cardiopulmonary, metabolic, and immune function. Because of the integrated nature of pain and stress responses,[3] the clinical technique of dense afferent nociceptive block to achieve preemptive analgesia (particularly for operations below the umbilicus) often blunts hormonal stress responses as well.

It is not yet clear whether an aggressive approach to suppression of stress responses by inhibiting cytokine generation as well as the central nervous system's learned facilitation of hormonal secretion is clinically possible, but emerging data suggest that such an approach is both feasible and useful. Reasoning that it is an oversimplification to expect that all dimensions of the bodily response to operation or trauma will remain dormant if pain alone is suppressed, Kehlet[178] and Møiniche et al[191] have separately suppressed postoperative pain and inflammation along with other detrimental aspects of "normal" convalescence such as prolonged immobilization or fasting through an integrated, multimodal protocol. Their remarkable initial successes in preventing postoperative fatigue and pulmonary impairment as well as achieving early dismissal of their patients are sure to influence the next several years of clinical studies of regional anesthesia in this era of cost-effective, outcome-driven medical care.[121]

In addition to clinical outcomes research to evaluate improved management protocols constructed on the basis of physiologic knowledge, controlled trials will yield new knowledge on optimal sites, techniques, drugs, and delivery methods to use for different operations, and the timing to best do so. The goal of these trials will be to uncouple surgical procedures, which we as anesthesiologists can rarely dictate, from their normal nociceptive, catabolic, and immunologic sequelae that increasingly are under our control.

References

1. Selye H: A syndrome produced by diverse nocuous agents. Nature 1936; 138: 32.

2. Carr DB, Verrier RL: Opioids in pain and cardiovascular responses: overview of common features. J Cardiovasc Electrophysiol 1991; 2 Suppl: s34.

3. Agnati LF, Tiengo M, Ferraguti F, et al: Pain, analgesia, and stress: an integrated view. Clin J Pain 1991; 7 Suppl 1: S23–S37.

4. Kehlet H: The surgical stress response: should it be prevented? Can J Surg 1991; 34: 565–567.

5. Katz N, Ferrante FM: Nociception. In Ferrante FM, VadeBoncouer TR (eds): Postoperative Pain Management, pp 17–67. New York, Churchill Livingstone, 1993.

6. Dubner R, Ren K: Central mechanisms of thermal and mechanical hyperalgesia following tissue inflammation. In Boivie J, Hansson P, Lindblom U (eds): Touch, Temperature, and Pain in Health and Disease: Mechanisms and Assessments, pp 267–277. Seattle, IASP Press, 1994.

7. Woolf CJ: The dorsal horn: state-dependent sensory processing and the generation of pain. In Wall PD, Melzack R (eds): Textbook of Pain, 3rd ed, pp 101–112. Edinburgh, Churchill Livingstone, 1994.

8. Woolf CJ, Chong MS: Preemptive analgesia—treating postoperative pain by preventing the establishment of central sensitization. Anesth Analg 1993; 77: 362–379.

9. Cook AJ, Woolf CJ, Wall PD, et al: Dynamic receptive field plasticity in rat spinal cord dorsal horn following C-primary afferent input. Nature 1987; 325: 151–153.

10. Meller ST: Thermal and mechanical hyperalgesia: a distinct role for different excitatory amino acid receptors and signal transduction pathways. Am Pain Soc J 1994; 3: 215–231.

11. Marzatico F, Cafe C: Oxygen radicals and other toxic oxygen metabolites as key mediators of the central nervous system tissue injury. Funct Neurol 1993; 8: 51–66.

12. Aizenman E, Hartnett KA, Reynolds IJ: Oxygen free radicals regulate NMDA receptor function via a redox modulatory site. Neuron 1990; 5: 841–846.

13. McCord JM: Oxygen-derived free radicals in postischemic tissue injury. N Engl J Med 1985; 312: 159–163.

14. Bonica JJ: Anatomic and physiologic basis of nociception and pain. In Bonica JJ (ed): The Management of Pain, 2nd ed, Vol 1, pp 28–94. Philadelphia, Lea & Febiger, 1990.

15. Fields HL (ed): Pain Syndromes in Neurology, pp 1–18. Stoneham, MA, Butterworth-Heinemann, 1990.

16. Palkovits M, Mezey E, Csiffary A, et al: Chemical neuroanatomy of brain structures involved in the stress-response with special reference to corticotropin-releasing factor. In Kvetňanský R, McCarty R, Axelrod J (eds): Stress: Neuroendocrine and Molecular Approaches, Vol 1, pp 3–14. New York, Gordon and Breach Science Publishers, 1992.

17. Swanson LW, Sawchenko PE, Lind RW, et al: The CRH motoneuron: differential peptide regulation in neurons with possible synaptic, paracrine, and endocrine outputs. Ann N Y Acad Sci 1987; 512: 12–23.

18. Antoni FA: Receptors mediating the CRH effects of vasopressin and oxytocin. Ann N Y Acad Sci 1987; 512: 195–204.

19. Jurcovicova J, Kvetňanský R, Dobrakovova M, et al: Prolactin response to immobilization stress and hemorrhage: the effect of hypothalamic deafferentations and posterior pituitary denervation. Endocrinology 1990; 126: 2527–2533.

20. Carr DB: Opioids. Int Anesthesiol Clin 1988; 26: 273–287.

21. Morley JE: The endocrinology of the opiates and opioid peptides. Metabolism 1981; 30: 195–209.

22. Oyama T, Wakayama S: The endocrine responses to general anesthesia. Int Anesthesiol Clin 1988; 26: 176–181.

23. Eipper BA, Mains RE: Structure and biosynthesis of pro-adrenocorticotropin/endorphin and related peptides. Endocr Rev 1980; 1: 1–27.

24. Cepeda MS, Carr DB: The neuroendocrine response to postoperative pain. In Ferrante FM, VadeBoncouer TR (eds): Postoperative Pain Management, pp 79–106. New York, Churchill Livingstone, 1993.

25. Carr DB, Lipkowski AW, Silbert BS: Biochemistry of the opioid peptides. In Estafanous FG (ed): Opioids in Anesthesia, pp 3–19. Stoneham, MA, Butterworth-Heinemann, 1991.

26. Friedman TC, Garcia-Borreguero D, Hardwick D, et al: Diurnal rhythm of plasma delta-sleep-inducing peptide in humans: evidence for positive correlation with body temperature and nega-

tive correlation with rapid eye movement and slow wave sleep. J Clin Endocrinol Metab 1994; 78: 1085–1089.

27. Gottschlich MM, Jenkins ME, Mayes T, et al: A prospective clinical study of the polysomnographic stages of sleep after burn injury. J Burn Care Rehabil 1994; 15: 486–492.

28. Plotsky PM: Regulation of hypophysiotropic factors mediating ACTH secretion. Ann N Y Acad Sci 1987; 512: 205–217.

29. Bartanusz V, Jezova D, Bertini LT, et al: Stress-induced increase in vasopressin and corticotropin-releasing factor expression in hypophysiotrophic paraventricular neurons. Endocrinology 1993; 132: 895–902.

30. Aguilera G, Kiss A, Hauger R, et al: Regulation of the hypothalamic-pituitary-adrenal axis during stress: role of neuropeptides and neurotransmitters. In Kvetňanský R, McCarty R, Axelrod J (eds): Stress: Neuroendocrine and Molecular Approaches, Vol 1, pp 365–382. New York, Gordon and Breach Science Publishers, 1992.

31. Fisher LA: Corticotropin-releasing factor: endocrine and autonomic integration of responses to stress. Trends Pharmacol Sci 1989; 10: 189–193.

32. Dunn AJ, Berridge CW: Is corticotropin-releasing factor a mediator of stress responses? Ann N Y Acad Sci 1990; 579: 183–191.

33. Kjaer A, Knigge U, Bach FW, et al: Permissive, mediating and potentiating effects of vasopressin in the ACTH and beta-endorphin response to histamine and restraint stress. Neuroendocrinology 1993; 58: 588–596.

34. Scaccianoce S, Muscolo LA, Cigliana G, et al: Evidence for a specific role of vasopressin in sustaining pituitary-adrenocortical stress response in the rat. Endocrinology 1991; 128: 3138–3143.

35. Axelrod J: The relationship between the stress hormones, catecholamines, ACTH and glucocorticoids. In Usdin E, Kvetňanský R, Axelrod J (eds): Stress: The Role of Catecholamines and Other Neurotransmitters, Vol. 1, pp 3–13. New York, Gordon and Breach Science Publishers, 1983.

36. Mezey E, Reisine T, Brownstein MJ, et al: Peripheral catecholamines regulate in vivo ACTH release through adrenergic receptors in the rat anterior pituitary. In Usdin E, Kvetňanský R, Axelrod J (eds): Stress: The Role of Catecholamines and Other Neurotransmitters, Vol. 1, pp 225–231. New York, Gordon and Breach Science Publishers, 1983.

37. Link H, Dayanithi G, Fohr KJ, et al: Oxytocin at physiological concentrations evokes adrenocorticotropin (ACTH) release from corticotrophs by increasing intracellular free calcium mobilized mainly from intracellular stores: oxytocin displays synergistic or additive effects on ACTH-releasing factor or arginine vasopressin-induced ACTH secretion, respectively. Endocrinology 1992; 130: 2183–2191.

38. Negro-Vilar A, Johnston C, Spinedi E, et al: Physiological role of peptides and amines on the regulation of ACTH secretion. Ann N Y Acad Sci 1987; 512: 218–236.

39. Munck A, Guyre PM, Holbrook NJ: Physiological functions of glucocorticoids in stress and their relation to pharmacological actions. Endocr Rev 1984; 5: 25–44.

40. Keller-Wood ME, Dallman MF: Corticosteroid inhibition of ACTH secretion. Endocr Rev 1984; 5: 1–24.

41. Smelik PG: Factors determining the pattern of stress responses. In Usdin E, Kvetňanský R, Axelrod J (eds): Stress: The Role of Catecholamines and Other Neurotransmitters, Vol 1, pp 17–24. New York, Gordon and Breach Science Publishers, 1983.

42. Akana SF, Dallman MF, Bradbury MJ, et al: Feedback and facilitation in the adrenocortical system: unmasking facilitation by partial inhibition of the glucocorticoid response to prior stress. Endocrinology 1992; 131: 57–68.

43. Andreis PG, Neri G, Mazzocchi G, et al: Direct secretagogue effect of corticotropin-releasing factor on the rat adrenal cortex: the involvement of the zona medullaris. Endocrinology 1992; 131: 69–72.

44. Grossman A: Opioids and stress in man. J Endocrinol 1988; 119: 377–381.

45. Zaloga GP: Catecholamines in anesthetic and surgical stress. Int Anesthesiol Clin 1988; 26: 187–198.

46. Sternberg EM, Chrousos GP, Wilder RL, et al: The stress response and the regulation of inflammatory disease. Ann Intern Med 1992; 117: 854–866.

47. Pacak K, Palkovits M, Kvetňanský R, et al: Stress-induced norepinephrine release in the paraventricular nucleus of rats with brainstem hemisections: a microdialysis study. Neuroendocrinology 1993; 58: 196–201.

48. Frohman LA, Krieger DT: Neuroendocrine physiology and disease. In Felig P, Baxter JD, Broadus AE, et al (eds): Endocrinology and Metabolism, 2nd ed, pp 185–247. New York, McGraw-Hill, 1986.

49. Salomaki TE, Leppaluoto J, Laitinen JO, et al: Epidural versus intravenous fentanyl for reducing hormonal, metabolic, and physiologic responses after thoracotomy. Anesthesiology 1993; 79: 672–679.

50. Wei ET, Kiang JG, Buchan P, et al: Corticotropin-releasing factor inhibits neurogenic plasma extravasation in the rat paw. J Pharmacol Exp Ther 1986; 238: 783–787.

51. Kehlet H: Modification of responses to surgery by neural blockade: clinical implications. In Cousins MJ, Bridenbaugh PO (eds): Neural Blockade in Clinical Anesthesia and Management of Pain, 2nd ed, pp 145–188. Philadelphia, JB Lippincott, 1988.

52. Carr DB, Ballantyne JC, Osgood PF, et al: Pituitary-adrenal stress response in the absence of brain-pituitary connections. Anesth Analg 1989; 69: 197–201.

53. Moses AM: Comments on some clinical implications of the release of adrenocorticotropin and vasopressin by interleukin-6 and other cytokines. (Editorial.) J Clin Endocrinol Metab 1994; 79: 932–933.

54. Späth-Schwalbe E, Born J, Schrezenmeier H, et al: Interleukin-6 stimulates the hypothalamus-pituitary-adrenocortical axis in man. J Clin Endocrinol Metab 1994; 79: 1212–1214.

55. Mastorakos G, Weber JS, Magiakou M-A, et al: Hypothalamic-pituitary-adrenal axis activation and stimulation of systemic vasopressin secretion by recombinant interleukin-6 in humans: potential implications for the syndrome of inappropriate vasopressin secretion. J Clin Endocrinol Metab 1994; 79: 934–939.

56. Cambronero JC, Rivas FJ, Borrell J, et al: Interleukin-2 induces corticotropin-releasing hormone release from superfused rat hypothalami: influence of glucocorticoids. Endocrinology 1992; 131: 677–683.

57. Dantzer R, Kelley KW: Stress and immunity: An integrated view of relationships between the brain and the immune system. (Abstract.) Life Sci 1989; 44: 1995.

58. Matta S, Singh J, Newton R, et al: The adrenocorticotropin response to interleukin-1 beta instilled into the rat median eminence depends on the local release of catecholamines. Endocrinology 1990; 127: 2175–2182.

59. Billingham ME: Cytokines as inflammatory mediators. Br Med Bull 1987; 43: 350–370.

60. Carr DB, Bergland R, Hamilton A, et al: Endotoxin-stimulated opioid peptide secretion: two secretory pools and feedback control in vivo. Science 1982; 217: 845–848.

61. Kakucska I, Qi Y, Clark BD, et al: Endotoxin-induced corticotropin-releasing hormone gene expression in the hypothalamic paraventricular nucleus is mediated centrally by interleukin-1. Endocrinology 1993; 133: 815–821.

62. Ohmichi M, Hirota K, Koike K, et al: Binding sites for interleukin-6 in the anterior pituitary gland. Neuroendocrinology 1992; 55: 199–203.

63. Saper CB, Breder CD: The neurologic basis of fever. N Engl J Med 1994; 330: 1880–1886.

64. Baigrie RJ, Lamont PM, Kwiatkowski D, et al: Systemic cytokine response after major surgery. Br J Surg 1992; 79: 757–760.

65. Harbour-McMenamin D, Smith EM, Blalock JE: Bacterial lipopolysaccharide induction of leukocyte-derived corticotropin and endorphins. Infect Immun 1985; 48: 813–817.

66. Smith EM, Meyer WJ, Blalock JE: Virus-induced corticosterone in hypophysectomized mice: a possible lymphoid adrenal axis. Science 1982; 218: 1311–1312.

67. Cavagnaro J, Waterhouse GA, Lewis RM: Neuroendocrine-immune interactions: immunoregulatory signals mediated by neurohumoral agents. Year Immunol 1988; 3: 228–246.

68. van Woudenberg AD, Metzelaar MJ, van der Kleij AA, et al: Analysis of proopiomelanocortin (POMC) messenger ribonucleic acid and POMC-derived peptides in human peripheral blood mononuclear cells: no evidence for a lymphocyte-derived POMC system. Endocrinology 1993; 133: 1922–1933.

69. Sharp B, Linner K: What do we know about the expression of proopiomelanocortin transcripts and related peptides in lymphoid tissue? (Editorial.) Endocrinology 1993; 133: 1921a–1921b.

70. Ansel JC, Brown JR, Payan DG, et al: Substance P selectively activates TNF-alpha gene expression in murine mast cells. J Immunol 1993; 150: 4478–4485.

71. Crofford LJ, Sano H, Karalis K, et al: Corticotropin-releasing hormone in synovial fluids and tissues of patients with rheumatoid arthritis and osteoarthritis. J Immunol 1993; 151: 1587–1596.

72. Karalis K, Sano H, Redwine J, et al: Autocrine or paracrine inflammatory actions of corticotropin-releasing hormone in vivo. Science 1991; 254: 421–423.

73. Payan D: Neuropeptides and inflammation: the role of substance P. Annu Rev Med 1989; 40: 341–352.

74. Okamoto Y, Shirotori K, Kudo K, et al: Cytokine expression after the topical administration of substance P to human nasal mucosa: the role of substance P in nasal allergy. J Immunol 1993; 151: 4391–4398.

75. Joyce TJ, Yood RA, Carraway RE: Quantitation of substance-P and its metabolites in plasma and synovial fluid from patients with arthritis. J Clin Endocrinol Metab 1993; 77: 632–637.

76. Felten DL, Felten SY, Bellinger DL, et al: Noradrenergic sympathetic neural interactions with the immune system: structure and function. Immunol Rev 1987; 100: 225–260.

77. Weigent DA, Carr DJ, Blalock JE: Bidirectional communication between the neuroendocrine and immune systems: common hormones and hormone receptors. Ann N Y Acad Sci 1990; 579: 17–27.

78. Saba TM, Scovill WA: Effect of surgical trauma on host defense. Surg Annu 1975; 7: 71–102.

79. Page GG, Ben-Eliyahu S, Yirmiya R, et al: Morphine attenuates surgery-induced enhancement of metastatic colonization in rats. Pain 1993; 54: 21–28.

80. Reul JM, de Kloet ER: Two receptor systems for corticosterone in rat brain: microdistribution and differential occupation. Endocrinology 1985; 117: 2505–2511.

81. Spencer RL, Miller AH, Moday H, et al: Diurnal differences in basal and acute stress levels of type I and type II adrenal steroid receptor activation in neural and immune tissues. Endocrinology 1993; 133: 1941–1950.

82. Tecoma ES, Huey LY: Psychic distress and the immune response. Life Sci 1985; 36: 1799–1812.

83. Reichlin S: Neuroendocrine-immune interactions. N Engl J Med 1993; 329: 1246–1253.

84. Morley JE, Benton D, Solomon GF: The role of stress and opioids as regulators of the immune response. In McCubbin JA, Kaufmann PG, Nemeroff CB (eds): Stress, Neuropeptides, and Systemic Disease, pp 221–231. San Diego, Academic Press, 1991.

85. Morley JE, Kay NE, Solomon GF, et al: Neuropeptides: conductors of the immune orchestra. Life Sci 1987; 41: 527–544.

86. Shavit Y, Lewis JW, Terman GW, et al: Opioid peptides mediate the suppressive effect of stress on natural killer cell cytotoxicity. Science 1984; 223: 188–190.

87. Cepeda MS, Lipkowski AW, Langlade A, et al: Local increases of subcutaneous beta-endorphin immunoactivity at the site of thermal injury. Immunopharmacology 1993; 25: 205–213.

88. Wei ET, Kiang JG: Inhibition of protein exudation from the trachea by corticotropin-releasing factor. Eur J Pharmacol 1987; 140: 63–67.

89. Hargreaves KM, Dubner R, Costello AH: Corticotropin releasing factor (CRF) has a peripheral site of action for antinociception. Eur J Pharmacol 1989; 170: 275–279.

90. Hargreaves KM, Costello AH, Joris JL: Release from inflamed tissue of a substance with properties similar to corticotropin-releasing factor. Neuroendocrinology 1989; 49: 476–482.

91. Yirmiya R, Shavit Y, Ben-Eliyahu S, et al: Modulation of immunity and neoplasia by neuropeptides released by stressors. In McCubbin JA, Kaufmann PG, Nemeroff CB (eds): Stress, Neuropeptides, and Systemic Disease, pp 261–286. San Diego, Academic Press, 1991.

92. Sternberg EM, Wilder RL, Chrousos GP, et al: Stress responses and the pathogenesis of arthritis. In McCubbin JA, Kaufmann PG, Nemeroff CB (eds): Stress, Neuropeptides, and Systemic Disease, pp 287–300. San Diego, Academic Press, 1991.

93. Frayn KN: Hormonal control of metabolism in trauma and sepsis. Clin Endocrinol (Oxf) 1986; 24: 577–599.

94. Hensle TW, Askanazi J: Metabolism and nutrition in the perioperative period. J Urol 1988; 139: 229–239.

95. Brown JM, Grosso MA, Harken AH: Cytokines, sepsis and the surgeon. Surg Gynecol Obstet 1989; 169: 568–575.

96. Cerra FB: Hypermetabolism-organ failure syndrome: a metabolic response to injury. Crit Care Clin 1989; 5: 289–302.

97. Zamir O, Hasselgren PO, Kunkel SL, et al: Evidence that tumor necrosis factor participates in the regulation of muscle proteolysis during sepsis. Arch Surg 1992; 127: 170–174.

98. Bone RC: The pathogenesis of sepsis. Ann Intern Med 1991; 115: 457–469.

99. Beutler B: Cachectin in tissue injury, shock, and related states. Crit Care Clin 1989; 5: 353–367.

100. Simpson SQ, Casey LC: Role of tumor necrosis factor in sepsis and acute lung injury. Crit Care Clin 1989; 5: 27–47.

101. Bendtzen K, Mandrup-Poulsen T, Nerup J, et al: Cytotoxicity of human pI 7 interleukin-1 for pancreatic islets of Langerhans. Science 1986; 232: 1545–1547.

102. Wolfe RR: Carbohydrate metabolism in the critically ill patient. Implications for nutritional support. Crit Care Clin 1987; 3: 11–24.

103. Cerra FB: Metabolic manifestations of multiple systems organ failure. Crit Care Clin 1989; 5: 119–131.

104. Tappy L, Randin D, Vollenweider P, et al: Mechanisms of dexamethasone-induced insulin resistance in healthy humans. J Clin Endocrinol Metab 1994; 79: 1063–1069.

105. Douglas RG, Shaw JH: Metabolic response to sepsis and trauma. Br J Surg 1989; 76: 115–122.

106. Lange MP, Dahn MS, Jacobs LA: The significance of hyperglycemia after injury. Heart Lung 1985; 14: 470–472.

107. Kennedy DJ, Butterworth JF IV: Endocrine function during and after cardiopulmonary bypass: recent observations. J Clin Endocrinol Metab 1994; 78: 997–1002.

108. Fellander G, Nordenstrom J, Tjader I, et al: Lipolysis during abdominal surgery. J Clin Endocrinol Metab 1994; 78: 150–155.

109. Wiener M, Rothkopf MM, Rothkopf G, et al: Fat metabolism in injury and stress. Crit Care Clin 1987; 3: 25–56.

110. Copeland KC, Nair KS: Acute growth hormone effects on amino acid and lipid metabolism. J Clin Endocrinol Metab 1994; 78: 1040–1047.

111. Ottosson M, Vikman-Adolfsson K, Enerback S, et al: The effects of cortisol on the regulation of lipoprotein lipase activity in human adipose tissue. J Clin Endocrinol Metab 1994; 79: 820–825.

112. Elwyn DH: Protein metabolism and requirements in the critically ill patient. Crit Care Clin 1987; 3: 57–69.

113. Wilmore DW: Catabolic illness: strategies for enhancing recovery. N Engl J Med 1991; 325: 695–702.

114. Chernow B, Alexander HR, Smallridge RC, et al: Hormonal responses to graded surgical stress. Arch Intern Med 1987; 147: 1273–1278.

115. Louard RJ, Bhushan R, Gelfand RA, et al: Glucocorticoids antagonize insulin's antiproteolytic action on skeletal muscle in humans. J Clin Endocrinol Metab 1994; 79: 278–284.

116. Rademaker BM, Ringers J, Odoom JA, et al: Pulmonary function and stress response after laparoscopic cholecystectomy: comparison with subcostal incision and influence of thoracic epidural analgesia. Anesth Analg 1992; 75: 381–385.

117. Naito Y, Tami S, Shingu K, et al: Responses of plasma adrenocorticotropic hormone, cortisol, and cytokines during and after upper abdominal surgery. Anesthesiology 1992; 77: 426–431.

118. Wolf AR, Eyres RL, Laussen PC, et al: Effect of extradural analgesia on stress responses to abdominal surgery in infants. Br J Anaesth 1993; 70: 654–660.

119. Moller IW, Dinesen K, Sondergard S, et al: Effect of patient-controlled analgesia on plasma catecholamine, cortisol and glucose concentrations after cholecystectomy. Br J Anaesth 1988; 61: 160–164.

120. Scott NB, Mogensen T, Bigler D, et al: Continuous thoracic extradural 0.5% bupivacaine with or without morphine: effect on quality of blockade, lung function and the surgical stress response. Br J Anaesth 1989; 62: 253–257.

121. Carr DB: The evolving practice of regional anesthesia. Curr Opin Anesthesiol 1994; 7: 427–429.

122. Ramanathan J, Coleman P, Sibai B: Anesthetic modification of hemodynamic and neuroendocrine stress responses to cesarean delivery in women with severe preeclampsia. Anesth Analg 1991; 73: 772–779.

123. Moller IW, Hjortso E, Krantz T, et al: The modifying effect of spinal anaesthesia on intra- and postoperative adrenocortical and hyperglycaemic response to surgery. Acta Anaesthesiol Scand 1984; 28: 266–269.

124. Scott NB, Mogensen T, Bigler D, et al: Comparison of the effects of continuous intrapleural vs epidural administration of 0.5% bupivacaine on pain, metabolic response and pulmonary function following cholecystectomy. Acta Anaesthesiol Scand 1989; 33: 535–539.

125. Blunnie WP, McIlroy PD, Merrett JD, et al: Cardiovascular and biochemical evidence of stress during major surgery associated with different techniques of anaesthesia. Br J Anaesth 1983; 55: 611–618.

126. Brandt MR, Fernades A, Mordhorst R, et al: Epidural analgesia improves postoperative nitrogen balance. Br Med J 1978; 1: 1106–1108.

127. Scheinin B, Scheinin M, Asantila R, et al: Sympatho-adrenal and pituitary hormone responses during and immediately after thoracic surgery—modulation by four different pain treatments. Acta Anaesthesiol Scand 1987; 31: 762–767.

128. Traynor C, Paterson JL, Ward ID, et al: Effects of extradural analgesia and vagal blockade on the metabolic and endocrine response to upper abdominal surgery. Br J Anaesth 1982; 54: 319–323.

129. Rutberg H, Hakanson E, Anderberg B, et al: Effects of the extradural administration of morphine, or bupivacaine, on the endocrine response to upper abdominal surgery. Br J Anaesth 1984; 56: 233–238.

130. Lund C, Hansen OB, Mogensen T, et al: Effect of thoracic epidural bupivacaine on somatosensory evoked potentials after dermatomal stimulation. Anesth Analg 1987; 66: 731–734.

131. Tuman KJ, McCarthy RJ, March RJ, et al: Effects of epidural anesthesia and analgesia on coagulation and outcome after major vascular surgery. Anesth Analg 1991; 73: 696–704.

132. Rosenfeld BA, Beattie C, Christopherson R, et al: The effects of different anesthetic regimens on fibrinolysis and the development of postoperative arterial thrombosis. Anesthesiology 1993; 79: 435–443.

133. Rosenfeld BA, Faraday N, Campbell D, et al: Hemostatic effects of stress hormone infusion. Anesthesiology 1994; 81: 1116–1126.

134. Steele SM, Slaughter TF, Greenberg CS, et al: Epidural anesthesia and analgesia: implications for perioperative coagulability. (Editorial.) Anesth Analg 1991; 73: 683–685.

135. Scott NB, Kehlet H: Regional anaesthesia and surgical morbidity. Br J Surg 1988; 75: 299–304.

136. Gunter JB, Forestner JE, Manley CB: Caudal epidural anesthesia reduces blood loss during hypospadias repair. J Urol 1990; 144: 517–519.

137. Erskine R, Janicki PK, Ellis P, et al: Neutrophils from patients undergoing hip surgery exhibit enhanced movement under spinal anaesthesia compared with general anaesthesia. Can J Anaesth 1992; 39: 905–910.

138. Acute Pain Management Guideline Panel: Acute pain management: operative or medical procedures and trauma. Clinical practice guideline. AHCPR Pub. No. 92-0032. Rockville, MD, Agency for Health Care Policy and Research, Public Health Service, United States Department of Health and Human Services, February 1992.

139. Hendolin H, Lahtinen J, Lansimies E, et al: The effect of thoracic epidural analgesia on respiratory function after cholecystectomy. Acta Anaesthesiol Scand 1987; 31: 645–651.

140. Bormann B, Weidler B, Dennhardt R, et al: Influence of epidural fentanyl on stress-induced elevation of plasma vasopressin (ADH) after surgery. Anesth Analg 1983; 62: 727–732.

141. Kehlet H: Surgical stress: the role of pain and analgesia. Br J Anaesth 1989; 63: 189–195.

142. Tsuji H, Shirasaka C, Asoh T, et al: Effects of epidural administration of local anesthetics or morphine on postoperative nitrogen loss and catabolic hormones. Br J Surg 1987; 74: 421–425.

143. Loper KA, Ready LB, Downey M, et al: Epidural and intravenous fentanyl infusions are clinically equivalent after knee surgery. Anesth Analg 1990; 70: 72–75.

144. Mangano DT, Siliciano D, Hollenberg M, et al: Postoperative myocardial ischemia: therapeutic trials using intensive analgesia following surgery. Anesthesiology 1992; 76: 342–353.

145. Anand KJS, Hickey PR: Halothane-morphine compared with high-dose sufentanil for anesthesia and postoperative analgesia in neonatal cardiac surgery. N Engl J Med 1992; 326: 1–9.

146. Wasylak TJ, Abbott FV, English MJ, et al: Reduction of postoperative morbidity following patient-controlled morphine. Can J Anaesth 1990; 37: 726–731.

147. Giesecke K, Hamberger B, Jarnberg PO, et al: Paravertebral block during cholecystectomy: effects on circulatory and hormonal responses. Br J Anaesth 1988; 61: 652–656.

148. Murphy DF: Interpleural analgesia. Br J Anaesth 1993; 71: 426–434.

149. Stang HJ, Gunnar MR, Snellman L, et al: Local anesthesia for neonatal circumcision. Effects on distress and cortisol response. JAMA 1988; 259: 1507–1511.

150. Scott NB, Mogensen T, Greulich A, et al: No effect of continuous i.p. infusion of bupivacaine on postoperative analgesia, pulmonary function and the stress response to surgery. Br J Anaesth 1988; 61: 165–168.

151. Dahl JB: Neuronal plasticity and pre-emptive analgesia: implications for the management of postoperative pain. Dan Med Bull 1994; 41: 434–442.

152. Dubner R: Hyperalgesia and expanded receptive fields. (Editorial.) Pain 1992; 48: 3–4.

153. Hu JW, Sessle BJ, Raboisson P, et al: Stimulation of craniofacial muscle afferents induces prolonged facilitatory effects in trigeminal nociceptive brain-stem neurones. Pain 1992; 48: 53–60.

154. Dubner R, Ruda MA: Activity-dependent neuronal plasticity following tissue injury and inflammation. Trends Neurosci 1992; 15: 96–103.

155. LaMotte RH, Shain CN, Simone DA, et al: Neurogenic hyperalgesia: psychophysical studies of underlying mechanisms. J Neurophysiol 1991; 66: 190–211.

156. Moncada S, Palmer RM, Higgs EA: Nitric oxide: physiology, pathophysiology, and pharmacology. Pharmacol Rev 1991; 43: 109–142.

157. Snyder SH: Nitric oxide: first in a new class of neurotransmitters. Science 1992; 257: 494–496.

158. Moncada S, Higgs A: The L-arginine–nitric oxide pathway. N Engl J Med 1993; 329: 2002–2012.

159. Meller ST, Gebhart GF: Nitric oxide (NO) and nociceptive processing in the spinal cord. Pain 1993; 52: 127–136.

160. Coderre TJ, Katz J, Vaccarino AL, et al: Contribution of central neuroplasticity to pathological pain: review of clinical and experimental evidence. Pain 1993; 52: 259–285.

161. Ren K: Wind-up and the NMDA receptor: from animal studies to humans. (Editorial.) Pain 1994; 59: 157–158.

162. Montague PR, Gancayco CD, Winn MJ, et al: Role of NO production in NMDA receptor-mediated neurotransmitter release in cerebral cortex. Science 1994; 263: 973–977.

163. Coyle JT, Puttfarcken P: Oxidative stress, glutamate, and neurodegenerative disorders. Science 1993; 262: 689–695.

164. Draisci G, Iadarola MJ: Temporal analysis of increases in c-fos, preprodynorphin and preproenkephalin mRNAs in rat spinal cord. Brain Res Mol Brain Res 1989; 6: 31–37.

165. Smeyne RJ, Vendrell M, Hayward M, et al: Continuous c-fos expression precedes programmed cell death in vivo. Nature 1993; 363: 166–169.

166. Bokesch PM, Marchand JE, Connelly CS, et al: Dextromethorphan inhibits ischemia-induced c-fos expression and delayed neuronal death in hippocampal neurons. Anesthesiology 1994; 81: 470–477.

167. Woolf CJ, Thompson SW: The induction and maintenance of central sensitization is dependent on N-methyl-D-aspartic acid receptor activation; implications for the treatment of post-injury pain hypersensitivity states. Pain 1991; 44: 293–299.

168. Chapman V, Haley JE, Dickenson AH: Electrophysiologic analysis of preemptive effects of spinal opioids on N-methyl-D-aspartate receptor-mediated events. Anesthesiology 1994; 81: 1429–1435.

169. Dawson VL, Dawson TM, London ED, et al: Nitric oxide mediates glutamate neurotoxicity in primary cortical cultures. Proc Natl Acad Sci U S A 1991; 88: 6368–6371.

170. Garthwaite J: Glutamate, nitric oxide and cell-cell signalling in the nervous system. Trends Neurosci 1991; 14: 60–67.

171. Kitto KF, Haley JE, Wilcox GL: Involvement of nitric oxide in spinally mediated hyperalgesia in the mouse. Neurosci Lett 1992; 148: 1–5.

172. Wall PD: The prevention of postoperative pain. (Editorial.) Pain 1988; 33: 289–290.

173. Jebeles JA, Reilly JS, Gutierrez JF, et al: The effect of pre-incisional infiltration of tonsils with bupivacaine on the pain following tonsillectomy under general anesthesia. Pain 1991; 47: 305–308.

174. Tverskoy M, Cozacov C, Ayache M, et al: Postoperative pain after inguinal herniorrhaphy with different types of anesthesia. Anesth Analg 1990; 70: 29–35.

175. Niv D, Devor M: Does the blockade of surgical pain preempt postoperative pain and prevent its transition to chronicity? IASP Newsletter 1993, November-December: 1–6.

176. McQuay HJ, Carroll D, Moore RA: Postoperative orthopaedic pain—the effect of opiate premedication and local anaesthetic blocks. Pain 1988; 33: 291–295.

177. Dierking GW, Dahl JB, Kanstrup J, et al: Effect of pre- vs postoperative inguinal field block on postoperative pain after herniorrhaphy. Br J Anaesth 1992; 68: 344–348.

178. Kehlet H: Postoperative pain relief—a look from the other side. Reg Anesth 1994; 19: 369–377.

179. Baron JF, Bertrand M, Barre E, et al: Combined epidural and general anesthesia versus general anesthesia for abdominal aortic surgery. Anesthesiology 1991; 75: 611–618.

180. Bredtmann RD, Herden HN, Teichmann W, et al: Epidural analgesia in colonic surgery: results of a randomized prospective study. Br J Surg 1990; 77: 638–642.

181. Jayr C, Thomas H, Rey A, et al: Postoperative pulmonary complications: epidural analgesia using bupivacaine and opioids versus parenteral opioids. Anesthesiology 1993; 78: 666–676.

182. Christopherson R, Beattie C, Frank SM, et al: Perioperative morbidity in patients randomized to epidural or general anesthesia for lower extremity vascular surgery. Anesthesiology 1993; 79: 422–434.

183. Rawal N, Sjostrand U, Christoffersson E, et al: Comparison of intramuscular and epidural morphine for postoperative analgesia in the grossly obese: influence on postoperative ambulation and pulmonary function. Anesth Analg 1984; 63: 583–592.

184. Yeager MP, Glass DD, Neff RK, et al: Epidural anesthesia and analgesia in high-risk surgical patients. Anesthesiology 1987; 66: 729–736.

185. Blomberg S, Emanuelsson H, Kvist H, et al: Effects of thoracic epidural anesthesia on coronary arteries and arterioles in patients with coronary artery disease. Anesthesiology 1990; 73: 840–847.

186. Baron JF, Coriat P, Mundler O, et al: Left ventricular global and regional function during lumbar epidural anesthesia in patients with and without angina pectoris: influence of volume loading. Anesthesiology 1987; 66: 621–627.

187. Beattie WS, Buckley DN, Forrest JB: Epidural morphine reduces the risk of postoperative myocardial ischaemia in patients with cardiac risk factors. Can J Anaesth 1993; 40: 532–541.

188. Christensen EF, Sogaard P, Egebo K, et al: Myocardial ischaemia and spinal analgesia in patients with angina pectoris. Br J Anaesth 1993; 71: 472–475.

189. Mangano DT, Siliciano D, Hollenberg M, et al: Postoperative myocardial ischemia: therapeutic trials using intensive analgesia following surgery. The Study of Perioperative Ischemia (SPI) Research Group. Anesthesiology 1992; 76: 342–353.

190. Reilly CS: Regional analgesia and myocardial ischaemia. (Editorial.) Br J Anaesth 1993; 71: 467–468.

191. Møiniche S, Dahl JB, Rosenberg J, et al: Colonic resection with early discharge after combined subarachnoid-epidural analgesia, preoperative glucocorticoids, and early postoperative mobilization and feeding in a pulmonary high-risk patient. Reg Anesth 1994; 19: 352–356.

CHAPTER 8

Local Anesthetic Pharmacology*

Rudolph H. de Jong, M.D.

PART ONE Fundamentals

Local anesthetics are sodium channel–blocking drugs that halt impulse conduction in excitable tissues such as peripheral nerves and spinal roots. The conduction block is reversible, dissipating with time as drug is released from channel receptors. Applied to an accessible neural structure, local anesthetics dull sensation in the innervated part distal to the block without altering sensation in other body parts or depressing consciousness. Local anesthetics are conceptually and technically different from general anesthetics, depressant drugs that dull sensation and allow invasive therapy anywhere.

History

The mouth-numbing properties of cocaine, an extract from the leaves of the coca shrub grown in the Andean foothills, have been known for centuries. In 1855, Gaedicke extracted the alkaloid erythroxyline from coca leaves. Albert Niemann isolated cocaine from the erythroxyline extract in 1860 and sagely observed that the bitter crystals numbed his tongue.

Sigmund Freud, the founder of psychoanalysis, became intrigued by the new drug's medicinal properties and shared his insights with Carl Koller, a fellow intern. Koller realized that anesthesia of the eye might become a reality. The first report of such anesthesia was in 1884. News of the discovery spread like wildfire through the medical world, and cocaine soon was tested on the upper airway for ear, nose, and throat surgery. Although his contribution to ophthalmology is uncontested, Koller failed to receive the coveted Assistantship to the Vienna Eye Clinic. He died in 1944, a bitter man.[1]

Erdtman from Sweden, testing the alkaloid gramine in the 1940s, noticed that the substance numbed the tongue. The potential for local anesthesia was apparent from the similarities to the history of cocaine. Löfgren, his assistant, synthesized lidocaine from a series of aniline derivatives in 1943. Lidocaine, a potent and stable local anesthetic, combines high tissue penetrance with acceptably low toxicity. To this day, Sweden remains the birthplace of many new local anesthetics (e.g., long-acting bupivacaine and ropivacaine).

---

*Reprinted in part from de Jong RH: Local Anesthetics. St. Louis, Mosby–Year Book, 1994.

Pharmacodynamics

As detailed in Chapter 5 (see also reviews[2] or texts[3]), the key to local anesthetic action is locked in the lipo-protein membrane that separates a nerve's internal stable axoplasm from the more turbulent extraneural environment; the membrane functions like the casing of a sausage. Traversing the nerve membrane are sparsely distributed, protein-lined, ion-conducting channels. A nerve's resting potential is generated by the potassium ion concentration gradient, and the action potential is generated by the sodium ion concentration gradient. The metabolically fueled sodium-potassium pump restores and maintains these cross-membrane ionic gradients by continuously pumping sodium out and potassium in.

Local Anesthetic Action

Deactivation of the sodium channel is the heart of local anesthetic blockade. Local anesthetics stop impulse generation and halt signal propagation by preventing initiation of an action potential. This is brought about by rendering transmembrane sodium channels, which normally provide conducting pathways, impermeable to the inward surge of sodium ions during depolarization. The resting potential is unaffected, and the blocked nerve remains polarized. Local anesthetic blockade is a nondepolarizing (i.e., stabilizing) type of block, somewhat comparable to neuromuscular block by curare.

The sodium channel has a polar local anesthetic binding site that becomes accessible during voltage-induced conformational changes of the channel protein configuration. Electrostatic binding, probably to charged fatty acid tails, locks the movement of helical protein subunits that normally open and close (i.e., gate) the channel to transmembrane sodium ion traffic. The channel binding site is accessible to the local anesthetic cation only through the inner (i.e., axoplasmic) pore, requiring initial passage by the lipophilic local anesthetic base through the lipid nerve membrane (Fig. 8–1).

The uncharged local anesthetic base also contributes to the sodium channel block. The local anesthetic base is lipid soluble and serves as the carrier vehicle that traverses the nerve membrane. On emergence at the inner surface of the membrane, the base dissociates, and the cation locks the sodium channel. The local anesthetic base also diffuses laterally through the membrane to reach the sodium channel binding site by means of the membrane-channel interface. This route does not require pore transit and functions independently of the channel state.

Minimum Blocking Concentration

Bupivacaine is severalfold more potent than lidocaine, which is severalfold more potent than procaine. To offer a measure of relative potency, the minimum

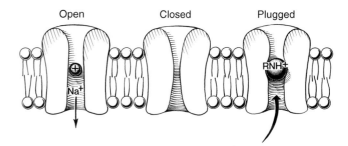

Figure 8–1 Channel entry. On the left is an open channel, inward permeant to sodium ions. The center channel is in the resting closed configuration; although impermeant to sodium ions here, the channel remains voltage responsive. The channel on the right, although in open configuration, is impermeant to sodium ions because it has a local anesthetic cation (RNH^+) bound to the gating receptor site. Notice that the local anesthetic enters the sodium channel from the axoplasmic (lower) side; the channel filter precludes direct entry through the external mouth. Because the local anesthetic renders the membrane impermeant to sodium ions and therefore inexcitable to local action currents, the nerve is blocked. (Modified from de Jong RH: Local Anesthetics, p 49. St. Louis, Mosby–Year Book, 1994.)

blocking concentration (C_m) of local anesthetic is defined as the drug concentration that just halts impulse traffic; this is the concentration that blocks the nerve and provides regional anesthesia.

However, in myelinated axons, the electrical impulse can skip over one, two, or even three solidly blocked nodes of Ranvier. At the C_m of a local anesthetic, propagation of a single impulse is halted by bathing three successive nodes of a myelinated axon or the same length (5 to 6 mm) of a nonmyelinated fiber. For the sake of standardization and convenience, the C_m commonly is expressed for a 10-mm length of nerve.

In contrast with previously held beliefs, the experimental C_m appears to be independent of fiber diameter at steady-state conditions and at slow rates of nerve stimulation. The C_m represents a dynamic equilibrium between channel-bound and channel-released drug, such that the net sodium current is decreased below the firing threshold level. Clinically, variables such as nerve length, rate of impulse traffic, speed of drug diffusion, and concentration and volume of local anesthetic solution considerably complicate idealized laboratory situations.

Frequency-Dependent Nerve Block

Local anesthetic preferentially binds to sodium channels in the open state, but it is released faster than it is bound by channels in the resting state. The receptor accessibility status of the channel state (i.e., open, inactivated, closed, or resting) itself affects the quality or depth of the block. This membrane polarity-dependent variability in the quality of the block is called a state-dependent block.

When the frequency of stimulation is increased, membrane ion channels are open and exposed to local anesthetic more frequently. Accordingly, opportunities are enhanced for sodium channel drug binding and reduced for drug release, and a frequency-dependent (i.e., use-dependent or phasic) nerve block ensues. The faster the nerve is made to fire, the more profound is the block that develops. State and frequency dependence are useful concepts for understanding the cardiotoxicities of local anesthetics such as lidocaine and bupivacaine.

Critical Blocking Length

Nerve impulses can skip over one, two, or even three blocked nodes. Anatomically, the thicker a nerve fiber, the longer is the distance between one node and the next; the internodal interval is much greater in large-diameter motor fibers than in small, thin pain-conducting fibers. Each nerve fiber has a critical blocking length (CBL), which is proportional to the diameter, spanning three nodes that must be coated by local anesthetic to ensure a complete impulse block.

Differential Nerve Block

As explained in Chapters 3 and 5, the CBL of a large-diameter nerve fiber is several times that of a small-diameter nerve fiber. A large A-alpha motor fiber may remain functional, but pain-related barrages in thin A-delta and C fibers are halted. During such a differential nerve block, the patient, although pain free, can still perceive touch and pressure and contract muscles (Fig. 8–2).

The CBL of spinal B fibers (i.e., preganglionic autonomic axons) approximates that of the smallest sensory (i.e., cold) fibers. The sympathetic block that inevitably accompanies spinal or epidural anesthesia extends several segments higher and lingers longer than analgesia; it can be approximated by testing for cold sensation. Similar considerations of low C_m and small CBL apply to postganglionic fibers in the sympathetic chains.

Because an impulse can skip over two blocked inexcitable nodes, at least 5 mm (preferably 8 mm or more) of nerve length must be bathed in local anesthetic solution to ensure a dense block of even the thickest nerve fibers. Because the internodal distance increases with the diameter of the axon, uneven longitudinal diffusion further contributes to erratic drug distribution, leading to a differential block of small and large myelinated fibers. Obstructed radial penetration toward, and erratic axial spread through, the core of a major nerve trunk are additional causes for incomplete anesthesia, a differential block of sensory and motor fibers, or both.

Physicochemical Considerations

Local anesthetics are organic amines, with an intermediary ester or amide linkage separating the lipophilic ring-linked head from the hydrophilic hydrocarbon tail. The weakly basic local anesthetic amine is lipid soluble but water insoluble and unstable. Crystalline salts of the local anesthetic base, conversely, are water soluble and stable but lipid insoluble.

When dissolved in water, the salt crystals ionize to yield local anesthetic cations and chloride or other acid anions. The local anesthetic cation (i.e., positively charged quaternary amine) is in dissociation equilibrium with the local anesthetic base (i.e., uncharged amine). The proportions of cation and base are governed by the drug's fixed pK_a and the variable ambient pH. The more acid the solution, the greater is the proportion of cation and the lesser that of local anesthetic base, according to the equation

$$\log\left(\frac{[\text{cation}]}{[\text{base}]}\right) = pK_a - pH$$

in which [cation] and [base] denote the concentration of local anesthetic cation and base, respectively.

Drug Dissociation

The lipid-soluble uncharged local anesthetic base species diffuses from the extraneural injection site through the nerve sheath toward individual nerve fibers, and it eventually penetrates the neural membrane. Once through the axonal membrane, the local anesthetic base reverts to a cation that interacts with sodium channel binding sites to barricade sodium ion traffic and block impulse conduction. The cation to base ratio, as determined from the previous equation, is critical to a successful nerve conduction block. If too little base and too few local anesthetic molecules reach the neural target, too few cations are available for binding and too few sodium channels close to ion

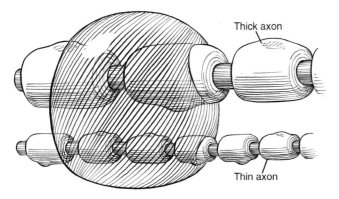

Thick axon

Thin axon

Figure 8–2 Nodal interval longitudinal (length-dependent) blockade. Two side-by-side axons—one thin, one thick—are bathed in a puddle of local anesthetic at the minimum blocking concentration (C_m); the internode (i.e., internodal interval) of the thick fiber is twice that of the thin one. The local anesthetic solution covers three successive nodes of the thin axon *(bottom)* but only one node of the thick axon *(top)*. Impulses can skip easily over one and even two inexcitable nodes, enabling conduction along the thick axon to continue uninterrupted. In the thin axon, with its three nodes covered by local anesthetic, impulse conduction is halted. Sufficient volume should be injected to coat at least three successive nodes (~1 cm) of even the thickest axon. A longitudinal block is the main operand in a threshold differential block of thin nerve bundles (e.g., spinal roots). (Modified from de Jong RH: Local Anesthetics, p 68. St. Louis, Mosby–Year Book, 1994.)

Table 8–1 Dissociation Constants

LOCAL ANESTHETIC	pK$_a$*
Benzocaine	3.5
Mepivacaine	7.7
Lidocaine	7.8
Etidocaine	7.9
Prilocaine	7.9
Ropivacaine	8.1
Bupivacaine	8.1
MEGX (monoethylglycine xylidide)	8.1
Tetracaine	8.4
Pipecolyl xylidide	8.6
Cocaine	8.6
Dibucaine	8.8
Procaine	8.9
Chloroprocaine	9.1
Hexylcaine	9.3
Procainamide	9.3
Piperocaine	9.8

*The dissociation constants are rounded.
From de Jong RH: Local Anesthetics, p 109. St. Louis, Mosby–Year Book, 1994.

traffic. The dissociation constants of local anesthetics are shown in Table 8–1.

The tissue acidosis accompanying infection or the limited buffering capacity of mucous membrane hampers base dissociation, yielding incomplete anesthesia. A local anesthetic with low pK$_a$ (e.g., benzocaine), conversely, is virtually undissociated at physiologic pH and provides excellent mucosal penetrance. However, because of an ultra-low pK$_a$, few cations dissociate to consummate the block, and a high concentration of benzocaine (10% to 20%) is needed to numb the submucosal nerve endings.

Pharmacokinetics

Absorption diverts local anesthetic into the bloodstream, which distributes it throughout the organism. A portion of the blood-borne local anesthetic is bound to plasma albumin and globulin fractions (mainly α_1-acid glycoprotein) that limit the amount of freely diffusible unbound drug. Most organs have greater affinity and larger storage volume for local anesthetic than plasma compartments and represent a vast static reservoir that buffers the blood level. During continuous local anesthetic infusion, these buffers eventually become saturated (about 2 days in the case of bupivacaine), sharply raising the drug's blood level and the risk of drug toxicity.

The plasma concentration–time profile provides a snapshot of the shifting balance among local anesthetic absorption from the injection site, interim uptake by tissue reservoirs, drug biotransformation, and ultimate excretion. Pharmacokinetic equations are derived from sequential plasma drug concentrations, permitting construction of drug disposition models. The terminology is a bit arcane, but what follows are explanations applicable to clinical practice.

The combined volume of organ reservoirs represents the apparent volume of drug distribution. Clearance expresses the rate at which local anesthetic is removed from this reservoir. Half-time is a convenient composite measure describing how quickly or slowly the local anesthetic plasma concentration is halved. After four or five half-times, the drug is cleared from storage sites for all practical purposes.

Absorption

The rate of local anesthetic absorption depends on the vascularity of the injection site. The more vascular the tissue, the faster the absorption, the higher the blood level, and the sooner the blood level peaks. For any given site, absorption depends on drug dose delivered and on tissue perfusion; absorption is essentially concentration independent. Local vasoconstriction, as with epinephrine, slows absorption, and more local anesthetic is retained for a longer time at the target site, generating a more profound and prolonged impulse block.

Disposition

Local anesthetic disposition in humans is approximated by a two-compartment model: one phase of rapid dilution into blood and well-perfused organs (e.g., brain), followed by a slower steady phase of distribution into the capacious buffer of less-perfused organs (e.g., muscle). Two half-times are defined: one (alpha) for the rapid initial dilution phase and a second (beta) for the slow but steady distribution phase. The second (or beta) phase parameters have greater clinical application because they represent steady-state conditions. Rapid lowering of blood level (i.e., short half-time) is a desirable trait, because it shortens the duration of a toxic reaction.

Amino amide local anesthetics rely on hepatic blood flow for clearance. Incompletely protein-bound drugs such as lidocaine or mepivacaine have a major free plasma fraction; their disposition is hepatic and flow dependent. Drugs that are bound strongly to plasma protein such as bupivacaine or ropivacaine have little free (unbound) drug to donate to hepatic clearance; their elimination rate depends on the concentration of the free fraction. Urinary and fecal elimination are minor routes for intact local anesthetic; the drug metabolites and conjugates are largely excreted renally.

Diffusion

To reach the neural target site, local anesthetic must diffuse through tissue barriers. In a peripheral nerve, the main diffusion barrier is the perineurium. In transmeningeal diffusion, the arachnoid mater is the principal barrier.[4] Intravenous regional anesthesia results from reverse diffusion of local anesthetic across the blood-nerve barrier. The blocking agent reaches nerve trunks and terminal nerve branches. The threshold local anesthetic block so attained is bolstered by an ischemic conduction block.[5]

Tachyphylaxis to local anesthetics turns out to be a mechanical rather than a pharmacodynamic phenomenon: it is seen only with staggered injections. In contrast, continuous infusion enhances local anesthetic potency by raising the nerve to a supra-C_m steady state level. Over time, the quantity of local anesthetic required for a continuous infusion block decreases as drug absorption matches drug disposition. A gradual decrease of the concentration of infused local anesthetic to the near-C_m range can maintain adequate analgesia for days with little or no motor block and without risking spillover from saturated tissue buffers.

Molecular Configuration

Local anesthetics form a remarkably homogeneous class of drugs with respect to their biologic properties and molecular structure. Other than chemical variations on a common structural theme, three distinguishing features individualize local anesthetics. One is the drug's linkage (i.e., ester or amide), which separates the aromatic lipophilic head from the hydrophilic tail. Second is the drug's binding to lipids and proteins, which controls spread, penetration, duration, and toxicity. Third is the drug's pK_a (see Table 8–1), which governs the proportions of local anesthetic base and cation at any given pH.

Most injectable local anesthetics in common use are weakly basic tertiary amines; prilocaine (a partner, with lidocaine, in a eutectic mixture of local anesthetics [EMLA] cream) and articaine are secondary amines. Conceptually, a tertiary amine is derived from ammonia (NH_3), with each of the three hydrogen atoms replaced by organic substitutes. The general configuration of local anesthetic amines (Fig. 8–3) comprises two key structural components: a lipophilic aromatic head and a hydrophilic aminoalkyl tail. The two are joined by an intermediate carboxy linkage, which is an ester or an amide configuration.

The bulky aromatic head commonly is derived from benzoic acid (i.e., ester family) or aniline (i.e., aminoacyl family). The hydrophilic hydrocarbon tail, containing dissociable nitrogen, is less easily characterized; amino derivatives of ethyl alcohol, acetic acid, or ringed piperidine are common. Compounds lacking the hydrophilic tail are almost insoluble in water (e.g., 1 part benzocaine dissolves in 2500 parts water) and are unsuitable for injection, although quite satisfactory for topical application to mucosal surfaces.

Ester and Amide Linkages

The 0.6- to 0.9-nm separation of the lipophilic and hydrophilic fractions by an intermediate chain of four or five atoms has proved to be critical in providing proper planar orientation for the molecule's characteristic binding to sodium channel receptors. Other compounds, such as antihistaminic and anticholinergic drugs, share this general structure (except for linkage composition) but exhibit weak local anesthetic effects at best. The linkage also determines the course of biotransformation, an important feature underscored by the classification of local anesthetics as ester-linked or amide-linked compounds.

Ester-linked local anesthetics, as characterized by procaine, are readily hydrolyzed by appropriate plasma esterases. Amide-linked local anesthetics, as characterized by lidocaine, generally require prior enzymatic dismantling to ready them for eventual hepatic hydrolysis. Consequently, amino amides more often are excreted partially or almost intact.

The linkage's reactive carbonyl group (C=O), common to ester and amide local anesthetics, is essentially planar, because it is stabilized by considerable resonance energy. The linkage also keeps the head and tail of the molecule stretched apart while retaining the spatially flexible orientation that allows molding to the ion channel receptors.

Structural Characteristics

Of the hundreds of local anesthetics synthesized, few have survived outside the pharmaceutical laboratory and even fewer have survived clinical trials. Some initially promising drugs proved to be highly toxic systemically or irritating to tissues; others were too insoluble in water or too unstable in solution. The proper balance among high potency, low toxicity, and adequate solubility in water and lipids seems to be attained with intermediate linkages of one to three carbon atoms.

Lengthening the para-amino chain of the aromatic ring makes the compound more resistant to hydrolysis, offering a longer duration of action but greater toxicity, as for tetracaine. Substitution elsewhere along the aromatic ring alters the three-dimensional configuration of the molecule and imparts new features. The methyl groups occupying the two ortho positions of the xylidine ring convey great stability to the molecule (e.g., lidocaine, bupivacaine). Their bulk also shields the amide linkage, rendering it resistant to enzymatic hydrolysis.

When the four valences of a carbon atom each are linked to a different atom or group, the carbon atom is said to be asymmetric or chiral, because the molecule can be configured around the chiral carbon in two three-dimensional mirror images. The resultant stereoisomers have different physicochemical and often different biologic properties, including rotation of the axis of polarization of a light beam in a counterclockwise (left) or clockwise (right) direction.

The two structural variants are designated as S (sinis-

Linkage

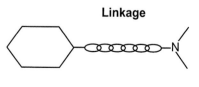

Lipophilic Part   **Hydrophilic Part**

Figure 8–3 Basic assembly of a local anesthetic molecule, with aromatic and amino fractions joined by an amino ester or amino amide "linkage." (From de Jong RH: Local Anesthetics, p 99. St. Louis, Mosby–Year Book, 1994.)

ter or left) and *R* (rectus or right) enantiomers, with the axis of light rotation shown as (−) for counterclockwise and (+) for clockwise deflection. Notice that the optical axis does not necessarily follow the steric configuration; *S*(+)-mepivacaine compares with *S*(−)-ropivacaine.

Many local anesthetics (e.g., bupivacaine, prilocaine) contain a chiral carbon and both have *S* and *R* configurations. During synthesis, equal proportions of the two enantiomers are generated, and the mixture is said to be racemic because the effects of opposite light-polarizing axes cancel each other. Cocaine, the naturally derived original local anesthetic, is a pure levorotatory enantiomer, designated as β-cocaine; a dextrorotatory cocaine, named α-cocaine or pseudococaine, was said in the 1920s to be twice as potent, more thermostable, and less toxic than naturally occurring cocaine.

The stereospecificity of local anesthetics was not seriously explored until bupivacaine cardiotoxicity was investigated. *R*(+)-bupivacaine has a much longer dwell time in cardiac sodium channels than the *S*(−) form, accounting for the considerably greater cardiotoxicity of *R*(+)-bupivacaine.[6] Of additional significance is the more potent depressant effect on brain-stem cardiorespiratory neurons of *R*(+)-bupivacaine compared with its *S*(−) enantiomer.[7]

Metabolism

The intramolecular linkage determines a drug's cardinal properties, which include direction and rapidity of the first stage of metabolism. Ester-linked local anesthetics (e.g., procaine, tetracaine) are readily hydrolyzed in plasma to the parent aromatic acid and amino alcohol, but amide-linked tertiary amines (e.g., lidocaine) resist direct plasma hydrolysis and require one or more preliminary degradation steps before eventual hepatic hydrolysis. Other amino amides with a nonlinear cyclic amino tail (e.g., mepivacaine, bupivacaine) are eliminated as intermediaries with the amide linkage still intact, defying any attempt at hydrolytic cleavage.

The resistance of the amide bond to nonenzymatic hydrolysis is shown by the ability of amino amide local anesthetics to withstand considerable physicochemical abuse; they can be autoclaved with supersaturated steam without a significant loss of potency. Procaine, conversely, tolerates autoclaving only briefly, and poorly at that, before becoming biologically inert; its shelf life too is less than that of lidocaine. Tetracaine, probably because it is hydrolyzed much more slowly than procaine, can be autoclaved repeatedly with little loss of potency.

The cardiotherapeutic use of lidocaine given systemically permitted biochemical mapping of its fate in humans, which was not feasible in studies using volunteers. Study of bupivacaine disposition in humans has been spurred by long-term infusion in the control of postoperative and chronic pain. As a result, differences between biotransformation in laboratory animals and in humans have become apparent.

PART TWO Clinical Pharmacology

Amino Ester Local Anesthetics

One major class of local anesthetics (Fig. 8–4) has an ester linkage to benzoic acid or its derivatives in common. Because cocaine, the first local anesthetic, is a benzoic acid ester, subsequent synthetic local anesthetics (e.g., procaine) all were developed from that mold. Not until about 60 years later was a whole new class of local anesthetics—the amide-linked (amino amide) group—introduced.

Ester-linked local anesthetics are cleaved by hydrolysis at the ester linkage, but the rates of the reaction vary considerably among amino esters. Tetracaine, for example, is hydrolyzed four or five times more slowly than procaine in human plasma, and other amino esters are affected more by hepatic than by plasma enzymes. As a rule, esters of para-aminobenzoic acid or its derivatives (e.g., procaine, tetracaine) are more readily hydrolyzed by plasma enzymes than by liver enzymes compared with local anesthetic esters of other aromatic acids (e.g., piperocaine), which are hydrolyzed more readily in the liver than in plasma. Cocaine, a double ester, straddles the divide and requires both plasma and liver cholinesterases for disposition.

Procaine

Procaine, the first in the synthetic para-aminobenzoic acid ester family, was synonymous with local anesthesia for a long time. Its relatively low toxicity permitted extensive regional block procedures, with up to 1000 mg being considered an acceptable dose. It has long since been replaced by more potent, longer-acting, and more readily diffusible ester- and amide-linked local anesthetics.

The primary step in human procaine metabolism is hydrolysis by plasma enzymes to form para-aminobenzoic acid and diethylaminoethanol. Procainesterase is indistinguishable from serum pseudocholinesterase, which also hydrolyzes succinylcholine; patients with low plasma pseudocholinesterase levels could suffer protracted procaine toxicity. If this deficiency is a possibility, a nonhydrolyzable local anesthetic such as lidocaine may be the better choice.

Chloroprocaine

Rather trivial alterations of the procaine molecule can introduce major changes in biologic activity. To illustrate, chloroprocaine (2-chloroprocaine; see Fig. 8–4) is hydrolyzed some four times faster than procaine in human plasma; it is less toxic after intravenous injection than procaine. In obstetric analgesia, in particular, fetal metabolism of chloroprocaine (although half as fast as in maternal plasma) still ensures fast clearance with minimal residual effect. However, nag-

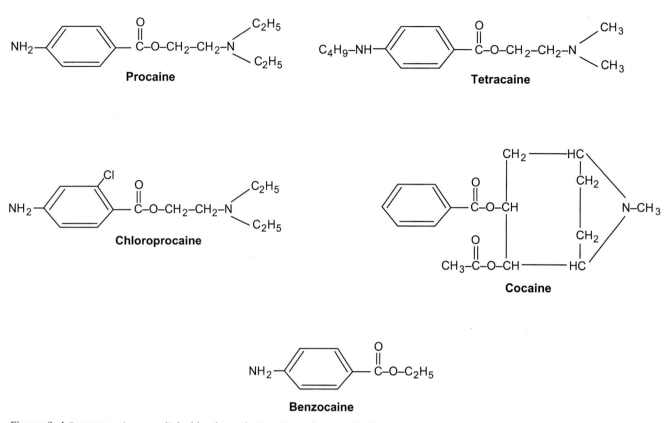

Figure 8–4 Representative ester-linked local anesthetics. (From de Jong RH: Local Anesthetics, p 178. St. Louis, Mosby–Year Book, 1994.)

ging issues about potential myelotoxicity and neurotoxicity caused chloroprocaine to yield ground again to bupivacaine.

The Chloroprocaine Riddle

When word spread in the 1970s that intrathecally delivered chloroprocaine solution might be neurotoxic, attention focused on what was previously considered an innocuous drug of low toxicity. The formulation of Nesacaine was unusual in that it contained an acid stabilizer (i.e., sodium metabisulfite) that prevented oxidation and ensured a stable shelf life. In vivo experiments soon showed that the chloroprocaine formulation caused neural damage, whereas lidocaine, bupiva-

caine, and saline proved innocuous.[8] The prevailing opinion was that the local anesthetic was benign but the stabilizer was not.[9, 10]

Because strong demand continued for a local anesthetic that rapidly hydrolyzed in the fetal circulation, the product was reformulated by substituting ethylenediaminetetraacetic acid (EDTA) as a stabilizer antioxidant. Soon after the switch from bisulfite to EDTA stabilizer, reports appeared in the 1980s of severe lumbar muscle spasm after uneventful epidural analgesia with chloroprocaine, probably secondary to the calcium-chelating action of EDTA.[11] Table 8–2 shows that large (>40 mL) volumes of EDTA-containing solution greatly increase the incidence of lumbar back pain but that chloroprocaine alone contributes to a lesser extent.

Table 8–2 Lumbar Back Pain After Epidural Chloroprocaine Injection

LOCAL ANESTHETIC	VOLUME, mL	EDTA	pH	NO PAIN (INCIDENCE)	NEEDLE TRACK PAIN (INCIDENCE)*	LUMBAR PAIN (INCIDENCE)*
2% Lidocaine	≥40	No	6.3	14/20	6/20	0/20
3% Chloroprocaine	≥20	Yes	3.3	13/20	6/20	1/20
3% Chloroprocaine	≥40	Yes	3.3	6/20	2/20	12/20
3% Chloroprocaine	≥40	No	2.9	10/20	7/20	3/20
3% Chloroprocaine	≥40	Yes	7.3	8/20	6/20	6/20

*Localized needle track pain versus general lumbar ache, 1 day after epidural injection.
EDTA, ethylenediaminetetraacetic acid.
Adapted from Stevens RA, Urmey WF, Urquhart BL, et al: Back pain after epidural anesthesia with chloroprocaine. Anesthesiology 1993; 78: 492–497; in de Jong RH: Local Anesthetics, p 362. St. Louis, Mosby–Year Book, 1994.

Lidocaine, even in a large volume (>40 mL), caused, at most, needle track discomfort but no lumbar muscle spasm pain.

Premature Obituary?

If the dual obstacles of an innocuous stabilizer and high acidity could be resolved, chloroprocaine might well emerge again as a clinically relevant local anesthetic. Potential advantages are its favorable blocking potency, high diffusibility, fast onset, and extremely rapid metabolism that limits toxicity. Further setting it apart from currently favored amino amide local anesthetics is its rapid disposition by fetus and newborn, offering all the makings of a potentially ideal obstetric analgesic.

Tetracaine

Substituting a butylamino radical for the para-amino group on procaine's aromatic ring and shortening the alkylamino tail yields tetracaine. This rather simple modification (see Fig. 8–4) spawns a totally different local anesthetic that is 10 times more potent and hydrolyzed three to four times more slowly than procaine. However, it also is about 10 times more toxic systemically. Nevertheless, the therapeutic advantages of tetracaine over procaine are considerably longer duration of action and more intense neural blockade; it remains a staple for subarachnoid anesthesia because of a proven track record of safety, predictable duration of action, and rapid onset.

As a spinal anesthetic, 10 to 15 mg of tetracaine offers a solid block to midthoracic dermatomes, lasting 2 to 3 hours. The duration of action can be prolonged by about 50% with the addition of epinephrine. Doses for vaginal or abdominal delivery should be decreased by one third or more to avoid excessively high spread. Bupivacaine is a solid contender for drug of choice in spinal anesthesia, with approximately equal duration of action. Its unique advantage is a long duration of nerve block without resorting to a vasoconstrictor, a potentially important consideration in selected patients.

Tetracaine is hydrolyzed completely by cleavage at the ester linkage; hydrolysis products appear first in the bile and then, after reabsorption from the intestinal tract, in the urine. Although the speed of tetracaine hydrolysis is four times slower than that of procaine, it still is fast compared with amino amide local anesthetics. The hydrolysis products are para-butylaminobenzoic acid and dimethylaminoethanol, neither of which is thought to be toxic. Whether these metabolites are excreted as such, conjugated, or further modified is unknown.

Benzocaine

The ethyl ester of para-aminobenzoic acid (see Fig. 8–4) differs from injectable amino esters in that it lacks the characteristic hydrophilic amine tail. Even so, it possesses the essential anesthesiophoric configuration. As a weak base ($pK_a = 3.5$), benzocaine exists almost entirely as the uncharged (i.e., neutral) free base species at physiologic pH. Accordingly, it is barely soluble in water (1 part in 2500) and causes tissue irritation when injected. Benzocaine is used extensively as a wound-dusting powder or as a topical anesthetic in products like burn nostrums, hemorrhoid salves, or throat lozenges. The probable metabolic pathway is hydrolysis to para-aminobenzoic acid and ethanol, but whether this takes place and to what extent remain uncertain.

Benzocaine is used in upper airway manipulation to anesthetize the trachea with products such as Hurricaine or Cetacaine. It was noticed serendipitously that spraying the tracheal stoma of goats with benzocaine caused pronounced methemoglobinemia (up to 32%).[12] Further analysis of clinical reports suggested a direct toxic drug (or metabolite) action, rather than an idiosyncratic reaction, as ruled earlier by an expert panel from the Food and Drug Administration. Neonates may be particularly susceptible because fetal hemoglobin is more readily oxidized than the adult form.

Amino Amide Local Anesthetics

The amide-linked local anesthetics (Fig. 8–5) are much more resistant to hydrolysis at the linkage joint than their ester-linked cousins; their longer duration of action is an immediate benefit. In most instances, a tertiary amino amide must be converted first to a simpler, secondary amine form before the linkage can be cleaved. A common first step is dealkylation of the amino nitrogen, transforming a tertiary to a secondary amine: for example, lidocaine to monoethyl-glycine xylidide (MEGX). A secondary amine such as prilocaine is more readily hydrolyzed by amidases than are tertiary amines.

Subclassification

The two different ways by which an amide linkage is pieced together influence the resultant amino amide's metabolism and its duration of action. The amide linkage is formed by fusing an aromatic amine with an alkyl-amino acid or, the other way around, by joining an aromatic acid to an alkyl-amino alcohol compound (Fig. 8–6). The former approach yields an aminoacyl amide, typified by lidocaine and mepivacaine; the latter yields an aminoalkyl amide, represented by dibucaine and procainamide. Differences in rate and route of biotransformation between the aminoacyl and aminoalkyl amides are that the aminoacyl local anesthetics are metabolized faster and more completely than the aminoalkyl local anesthetics.

Within the dominant aminoacyl class there is a further distinction based on whether the hydrophilic amino tail is a straight carbon chain (e.g., lidocaine) or the amino nitrogen is captured within a ringed struc-

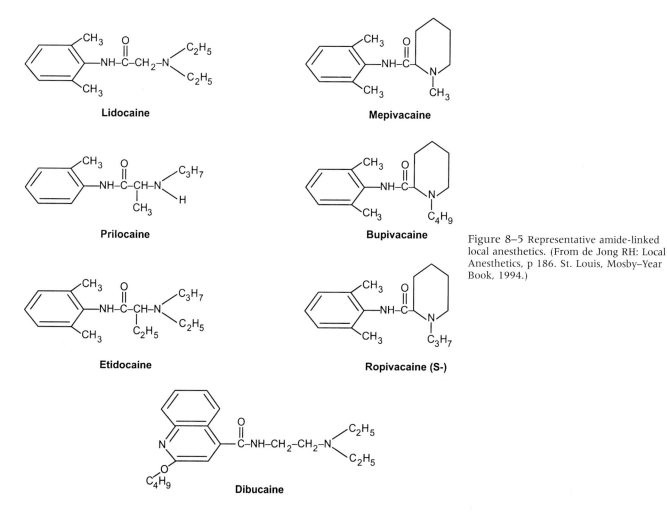

Figure 8–5 Representative amide-linked local anesthetics. (From de Jong RH: Local Anesthetics, p 186. St. Louis, Mosby–Year Book, 1994.)

ture (e.g., mepivacaine). The lipophilic aromatic head is a ringed carbon product.

The pipecolyl xylidide ringed local anesthetics (e.g., mepivacaine) differ from the aminoalkyl xylidide class (e.g., lidocaine) by being even more strongly resistant to hydrolytic cleavage of the amide linkage. The massive piperidine ring evidently shields them from enzymatic access.[13] The resistance to amide linkage cleavage of pipecolyl xylidides presents a particular problem for local anesthetic disposition in neonates.

Aminoacyl Amides

Because the bulk of the local anesthetic molecule remains essentially intact during initial metabolic steps, questions remain about the biologic activity and toxicity of complex intermediary products. Lidocaine and bupivacaine metabolism are singled out, because these local anesthetics commonly are given as a continuous infusion spanning days or longer periods. Efficient disposition of the infused drug is desirable because, if it is not cleared, the parent drug or metabolites may accumulate, causing unwanted and perhaps unexpected toxic side effects.

Aminoalkyl Xylidides: The Lidocaine Family

Lidocaine. In the half century since its discovery, lidocaine has supplanted procaine as the standard local anesthetic. Although its activity to toxicity ratio is not much different from that of procaine, lidocaine diffuses farther and faster, yields a more solid and longer-lasting block, and seldom raises concern about allergy.

Widespread use and varied applications (e.g., antiarrhythmic, anticonvulsant) of lidocaine led to a detailed study, and more is known about its fate in humans than that of any other local anesthetic. Its duration of action is several hours, which is a desirable attribute for rapid recovery (e.g., ambulatory surgery) but less desirable when prolonged anesthesia or pain relief is needed. One approach is to slow drug absorption with a vasoconstrictor; another is repeated injection or continuous catheter infusion.

Vasoconstrictor. The addition of a vasoconstrictor to the local anesthetic solution theoretically decreases blood flow in the target region, slowing drug absorption. If the drug stays longer on target, this prolongs the duration of the nerve block by as much as 50% (in the case of lidocaine). There are other advantages as well. Because more drug molecules are available, with less dilution by tissue fluid, the nerve block is more intense. It is possible to obtain the same depth of block

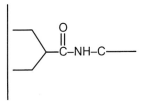

Aminoalkyl Amide

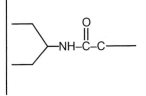

Aminoacyl Amide

Figure 8–6 The amide linkage of local anesthetics is expressed in two varieties. Dibucaine and procainamide are aminoalkyl amides, and lidocaine and bupivacaine are aminoacyl amides. (From de Jong RH: Local Anesthetics, p 187. St. Louis, Mosby–Year Book, 1994.)

with a lower drug concentration, decreasing the total drug dose; alternatively, a larger volume of more dilute drug can be used to achieve a wider spread of analgesia, as in epidural anesthesia.

By analogous reasoning, systemic toxicity is decreased because less drug is absorbed per unit time, and the total absorptive process is slowed. The net result is a lower peak blood level (compared with the same dose of plain lidocaine) that occurs later. The enhanced margin of safety is shown by manufacturer-suggested recommended maximum drug doses: for plain lidocaine, 5 mg/kg body weight, compared with 7 mg/kg for lidocaine with epinephrine (Table 8–3).

Although numerous vasoconstrictors and adrenergic agents have been tested (e.g., phenylephrine, octapressin, clonidine), epinephrine has remained the first choice. The usual amount of epinephrine is 5 μg/mL (also expressed as 1:200,000). More epinephrine (i.e., 10 μg/mL) provides little or no extended duration of action and raises the possibility of side effects from epinephrine injection.

Therapeutic Uses. Lidocaine has found other therapeutic uses, especially the suppression of ventricular arrhythmias. Lidocaine is a fast-acting, sodium channel–blocking class Ib agent, widely used to treat post-myocardial infarction ventricular dysrhythmias. Rapid unbinding from the cardiac sodium channel during diastole places lidocaine in the fast-in, fast-out category, quite unlike the persistent conduction-blocking effect of bupivacaine. An intriguing laboratory finding is paradoxic agonism, in which lidocaine displaces bupivacaine from cardiac sodium channel binding sites.[14] If confirmed, this may help explain the unexpected observation that lidocaine reverses bupivacaine-induced cardiac arrhythmias.[15, 16]

There appears to be solid, albeit old evidence that a

moderate systemic dose of lidocaine decreases intensity and duration of experimentally induced and clinically manifested seizures. Anticonvulsant therapy with lidocaine remains an option in Scandinavia; it has proved effective, even for conventional, therapy-resistant newborn convulsions.[17]

Intravenous Regional Anesthesia. Intravenous regional anesthesia, filling the venous tree of a vascularly isolated limb with dilute local anesthetic solution, differs from conventional nerve block in that it generates a core-to-mantle diffusion gradient in nerve trunks. Superimposed on that action is direct local anesthetic access to nerve terminals and small cutaneous nerve filaments,[18] combined with ischemic conduction block of large-diameter motor nerves that, with time, supplements local anesthetic block.[5]

Lidocaine has resumed its drug-of-choice status for intravenous regional anesthesia in North America because other contenders have not fared as well. Prilocaine would be an ideal choice, because of near-equal potency yet lower systemic toxicity, were it not for hemotoxic metabolites that cause delayed onset methemoglobinemia. Bupivacaine, because it is more strongly tissue bound, also looked promising initially. Analgesia remained after tourniquet deflation, but systemic cardiotoxicity removed bupivacaine from consideration. Perhaps ropivacaine will fare better.

Systemic Analgesia. A fascinating application, with growth potential in management of central pain, is lidocaine-induced systemic analgesia. Lidocaine is an effective, albeit short-duration suppressant of the cough reflex during tracheal intubation,[19] suggesting an effect on peripheral nociceptors and on central impulse conduction. Infusion of lidocaine (5 mg/kg body weight) over a 30-minute span relieved the burning foot pain of diabetic neuropathy for 3 to 21 days in 11 of 15 patients.[20]

Lidocaine given orally has poor bioavailability because of pronounced hepatic first-pass extraction. More resistant derivatives were developed for antiarrhythmic therapy, and these are finding niche application in pain management. Diabetic neuropathy, for instance, responds to mexiletine given orally. A commonly used dose of mexiletine is 750 mg/d, with considerable comfort produced at an average blood level of 3.4 μmol/L.[21] A similar mexiletine dose of 10 mg/kg/d relieved various neuropathic pain syndromes, including amputation stump pain and chemotherapeutic and postirradiation neuralgias.[22] Holding out hope for therapy-resistant central pain syndromes is a report[23] of relief from thalamic pain syndrome in eight of nine patients treated with mexiletine at a dose of 10 mg/kg/d.

Metabolism. Lidocaine is metabolized in the liver by microsomal mixed-function oxidases and amidases. The oxidative pathway requires cytochrome P-450, which is present even in neonatal liver.[24] The liver is the chief (probably the sole) organ for lidocaine biotransformation; lidocaine metabolism is limited by hepatic blood flow. With lidocaine's high extraction ratio, only advanced hepatic disease hampers its metabolism, causing the blood level to increase.[25]

Species- and route-dependent pathways of lidocaine

biotransformation have been postulated (Fig. 8–7). In humans, direct hydrolysis of the amide linkage can be considered minor at best.[26] However, oxidative metabolism of the various intermediary products of lidocaine is brisk. Almost 80% of a single dose of lidocaine can be accounted for as hydroxylated products in human urine.

Biotransformation of lidocaine starts with oxidative de-ethylation of the amino nitrogen to an intermediary secondary amine. De-ethylation of diethylglycine xylidide (i.e., lidocaine) yields MEGX and acetaldehyde (see Fig. 8–7). MEGX, which is much more readily hydrolyzed than lidocaine, yields ethylglycine and ortho-xylidine. MEGX is then further dismantled by shearing the remaining ethyl radical from the amino nitrogen. Two-step de-ethylation of lidocaine eventually yields glycine xylidide, a primary amine, that makes a late appearance in human plasma and urine. The plasma half-life of glycine xylidide is quite long (i.e., traces can still be detected 2 days after a lidocaine bolus), and once formed, glycine xylidide continues to

be excreted long after lidocaine and MEGX have faded away. The potential for glycine xylidide accumulation during continuous lidocaine infusion is quite real.[27]

MEGX is excreted renally, and the kidney seems amply capable of keeping up with the metabolite load during infusion; decreased renal function raises neither lidocaine nor MEGX blood levels.[25] Only frank renal failure could present the hazard of drug and primary metabolite accumulation. Surprisingly, given its simpler chemical structure, renal capacity for glycine xylidide elimination is much more marginal than for MEGX. Glycine xylidide accumulates slowly during continuous lidocaine infusion, because it is much closer to renal transport saturation; reduction in renal function that is well short of frank renal failure leads to further glycine xylidide accumulation.[25] Glycine xylidide accumulation is of some clinical concern because it, like lidocaine, blocks cardiac sodium channels and competes with the parent drug for channel occupancy.[24]

MEGX retains much of lidocaine's cardiovascular activity and is comparable to lidocaine in its potential to

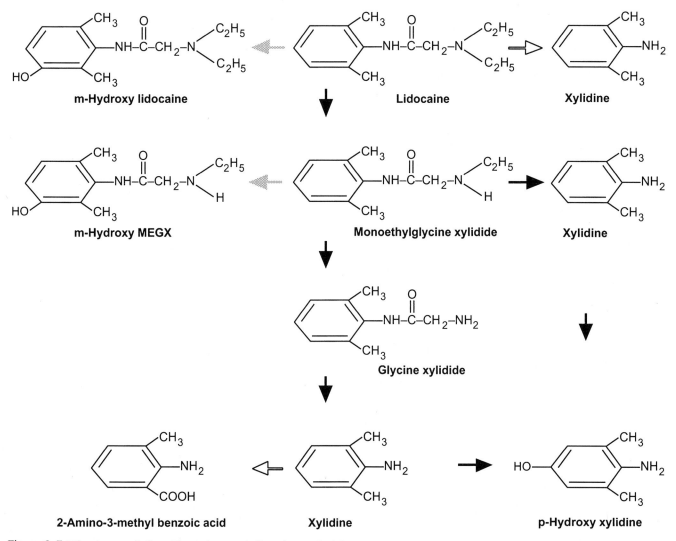

Figure 8–7 Lidocaine metabolism. The major metabolic pathways for lidocaine in humans are shown with solid arrows; the minor routes are indicated with stippled arrows. Unfilled arrows point to products in nonhuman species. MEGX, monoethyl-glycine xylidide. (From de Jong RH: Local Anesthetics, p 189. St. Louis, Mosby–Year Book, 1994.)

induce convulsions at increased blood levels. Although glycine xylidide alone does not induce convulsions, it does retain the latent convulsant potential of its lidocaine precursor. When glycine xylidide coexists with lidocaine or MEGX, it potentiates the convulsant property of the other two. Signs of central nervous system toxicity could occur—even if the lidocaine blood level is subconvulsant—when substantial quantities of MEGX or glycine xylidide, or both, accumulate.[27]

Because lidocaine readily crosses the placenta, consideration of drug disposition in the newborn is germane to selecting an obstetric anesthetic. Because of near-adult cytochrome P-450 levels, oxidative dealkylation and hydroxylation of lidocaine proceed together, with MEGX as the first step, although proportions could vary.[26] The newborn can dispose adequately of lidocaine. Mepivacaine, however, fares less well; it is cleared three times slower than lidocaine from the fetal circulation. Unlike lidocaine, mepivacaine is metabolized very little by the immature liver; its disposition instead relies mainly on renal excretion of intact drug.

Prilocaine. Prilocaine, a lidocaine homologue (see Fig. 8–5), is a secondary amine local anesthetic. When first introduced, prilocaine received considerable notice because it is approximately as potent as lidocaine yet has remarkably lower intravenous toxicity. Because the fetus tolerates prilocaine better than lidocaine, prilocaine was viewed as the replacement for lidocaine in obstetric anesthesia. Aromatic hydroxylation is accomplished by microsomal oxidation, a pathway that involves cytochrome P-450 and is present in neonates, suggesting rapid prilocaine disposition after birth.[26]

Biotransformation proved to be problematic for prilocaine, because its aminophenol metabolites oxidize hemoglobin to methemoglobin. Although minor degrees of methemoglobinemia occasionally follow the use of lidocaine or benzocaine, prilocaine consistently decreases the blood's oxygen-carrying capacity, sometimes sufficiently to cause visible cyanosis. Despite its undeniable advantages, prilocaine is infrequently used for regional anesthesia because of its metabolites.

Prilocaine has made a comeback because of another physicochemical attribute: miscibility. When mixed in equal proportions, lidocaine and prilocaine crystals form an oily substance with a melting point lower than either of its parents. This EMLA is picked up by the transdermal transport system to anesthetize terminal afferent nerve fibers. The resultant dermal analgesia allows painless venipuncture in children and other superficial dermal procedures. The main drawback is slow absorption; dermal analgesia requires 1 hour's application under an occluded skin dressing.

Because of its impulse-generation blocking action on subdermal nerve endings, application to spontaneously discharging neurons seems a logical therapeutic extension. In early informal clinical trials, we and others have used EMLA cream with encouraging results in the treatment of postherpetic allodynia, superficial scar neuromas, and atypical facial pain. Although encouraging, the uncertainties of prolonged aminophenol metabolite exposure must first be dispelled before long-term treatment can be recommended.

Articaine. Articaine was introduced in the 1970s as a low-toxicity replacement for lidocaine. It has found favor as a regional anesthetic in dentistry, but dependence on epinephrine addition (without it, an articaine block can be unpredictable) negated evanescent advantages in regional anesthesia of other body parts. The efficacy, safety, kinetic properties, and physicochemical attributes are close to those of lidocaine in a peripheral or epidural nerve block.[28] Overall, articaine with epinephrine has little to distinguish it from lidocaine or mepivacaine, whose proven track records give them the advantage.

Articaine is an aminoacyl amide-linked local anesthetic that is unique in two ways. First, it is a secondary amine, like prilocaine. Second, unlike the prevalent 6-member xylidine aromatic ring in other aminoacyls, it has a 5-member sulfur-containing thiophene ring. Also different is its metabolism, which oxidizes the thiophene ring rather than the secondary amino nitrogen tail. Articaine's cardiotoxicity is on the order of that of lidocaine but with less frequency dependence.[29] The drug seems to have found a comfortable niche in dentistry, where the addition of epinephrine is an advantage.

Etidocaine. Etidocaine, derived from lidocaine (see Fig. 8–5), initially seemed promising because of its long duration of action (i.e., on the order of bupivacaine), short latency (i.e., similar to lidocaine), and intense motor blockade. However, like bupivacaine, etidocaine was cursed with early cardiotoxicity.[30] Worse yet, etidocaine selectively blocked motor fibers more intensely than sensory fibers, giving rise to the anomalous situation of a weak patient with unsatisfactory analgesia, especially undesirable in patients in labor.

Etidocaine's great lipid solubility and near-total plasma protein binding theoretically give it strong advantages of long duration, low toxicity, and minor placental transfer. However, the clinical impression negated any potential advantages, and the drug is little used in North America. A niche market remains in regional anesthesia for surgery of the eye, in which profound cycloplegia is a distinct asset.[31] Metabolic information, because of etidocaine's rare use, is sketchy.

Pipecolyl Xylidides: the Mepivacaine Family

The pipecolyl xylidide family, like the aminoalkyl xylidide family, traces its roots to Sweden in the 1950s. Although structurally different in tail assembly, the common amide linkage conveys clinical qualities comparable to mepivacaine and lidocaine for surgical anesthesia. Differences arise from the more complex and bulky nitrogen-containing piperidine ring compared with the simpler straight-chained aminoalkyl portion.

The metabolism is more circuitous and less complete because of extensive shielding of the amide linkage by a ringed structure at either end (see Fig. 8–5). This becomes evident in neonates, whose immature hepatic enzyme system may be overwhelmed by mepivacaine, clearing it much more slowly than lidocaine. The second difference is that the carbon atom connecting the piperidine ring to the amide linkage is chiral, and pipecolyl xylidides exist in two structural configurations: *R* and *S*. Experimentally, the *S* enantiomer is less cardiotoxic than the *R* antipode.

Mepivacaine. Although it has a cyclic piperidine rather than a linear alkyl-amino hydrophilic tail (see Fig. 8–5), mepivacaine resembles lidocaine in many clinical respects, such as impulse blocking potency and toxicity. Mepivacaine's duration of action may be slightly longer than that of lidocaine, although the difference is not sufficiently pronounced to often warrant selection of one agent over the other. The 1.5% solution of mepivacaine has become a popular choice for major nerve blocks (e.g., brachial plexus) because of rapid onset of analgesia, predictable diffusion, adequate motor block, and duration of action sufficient for ambulatory surgery, yet not so long as to require prolonged recovery room stay.

Although marketing claims for intrinsic vasoconstriction have been made, in practice, epinephrine (5 μg/mL) commonly is added to decrease absorption and to prolong duration. Mepivacaine also lends itself well to mixture with a long-acting agent such as bupivacaine. The resultant "supercaine" theoretically combines the best features of both drugs to provide rapid onset with long duration of block for postsurgical pain relief. The toxicity of "supercaine" is approximately the sum of its local anesthetic constituents.

Mepivacaine has not fared as well as lidocaine in obstetric anesthesia because of poor hepatic handling of the complex double-ringed structure. Otherwise, few significant differences between mepivacaine and lidocaine appear in clinical studies, and the selection of one over the other for regional anesthesia is more a matter of personal experience and price negotiation than of major pharmacologic distinction. The commercial product is the racemic, optically neutral, balanced mixture of *R* and *S* enantiomers.

R-mepivacaine has threefold greater affinity for, and fourfold slower diastolic release from, the cardiac sodium channel than *S*-mepivacaine.[32] The former is the more cardiotoxic fast-in, slow-out component of racemic (*R-S*) mepivacaine; in humans, mepivacaine cardiotoxicity has not been as troublesome as with bupivacaine. Metabolism also may be stereoselective.

Mepivacaine's bicyclic structure, like that of bupivacaine and ropivacaine, guides it down a metabolic trail that differs from lidocaine. The chief or sole metabolic activity resides in the liver, with metabolites appearing as such and as conjugates with glucuronic acid in the bile. The greater portion of metabolites excreted in the bile subsequently is reabsorbed from the intestinal tract to be renally eliminated. Only a tiny fraction of the original mepivacaine input ultimately is recoverable from feces.

A major product of mepivacaine metabolism (Fig. 8–8) in adult humans is obtained by *N*-demethylation of the piperidine nucleus to pipecolyl xylidide (i.e., desmethyl mepivacaine), which has proved remarkably

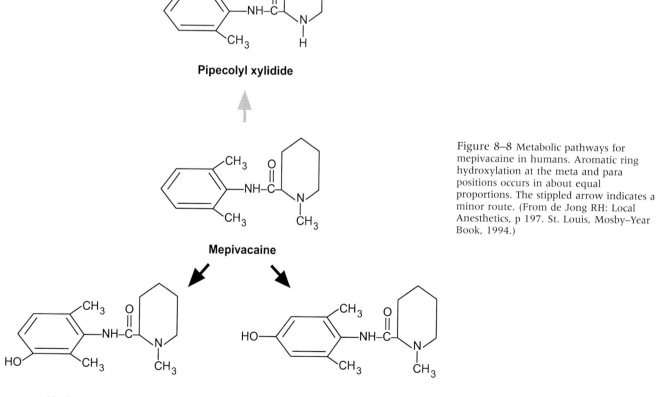

Pipecolyl xylidide

Mepivacaine

m-Hydroxy mepivacaine

p-Hydroxy mepivacaine

Figure 8–8 Metabolic pathways for mepivacaine in humans. Aromatic ring hydroxylation at the meta and para positions occurs in about equal proportions. The stippled arrow indicates a minor route. (From de Jong RH: Local Anesthetics, p 197. St. Louis, Mosby–Year Book, 1994.)

resistant to further degradation.[3] An alternative route, more productive with mepivacaine than with bupivacaine, is ring hydroxylation to meta- and para-hydroxy mepivacaine. Because *R*-mepivacaine and *S*-mepivacaine clear at different rates, hepatic meta- and para-hydroxylation may be site specific, the racemic commercial product yielding equal amounts of each.[32]

Mepivacaine illustrates the metabolic attempts at lowering local anesthetic toxicity. Although desmethyl mepivacaine is about two thirds as toxic as mepivacaine, para-hydroxy mepivacaine is only one third as toxic. And subsequent breakdown or conjugation, or both, further lower the toxicity of mepivacaine fragments. Because mepivacaine resists attempts at degradation beyond *N*-dealkylation, conjugation to water-soluble renally excreted nontoxic glucuronides clearly is the detoxification avenue of choice.

Bupivacaine. Bupivacaine is representative of a second-generation of longer-acting local anesthetics. It is closely related to mepivacaine (see Fig. 8–5), as is ropivacaine. Lengthening the methyl tail of mepivacaine's piperidine ring to a four-carbon butyl chain imparts longer duration of action and enhances potency, albeit with greater toxicity as the trade-off. Bupivacaine analgesia lasts two to three times longer than that provided by lidocaine or mepivacaine. Repeated administration or continuous infusion may cause drug and by-product accumulation as a result of saturation of storage reservoirs; blood levels increase. The local anesthetic is quite lipid soluble, is extensively bound to plasma proteins, and has a favorable maternal-to-fetal gradient.

By all appearances, bupivacaine was well on the way to even wider use, until an editorial linked hitherto scattered clinical and anecdotal reports of sudden cardiac arrest after regional anesthesia with long-lasting agents; worse yet, most of the adverse outcomes occurred in term-pregnant women.[33] Eventually, 0.75% bupivacaine was withdrawn from obstetric use. The potent 0.75% solution remains available for nonobstetric use; it is a preferred local anesthetic for ophthalmic blocks, because it combines solid analgesia with profound relaxation of orbital and periorbital muscles.[31]

The 0.25% and 0.5% solutions of bupivacaine are used most often in regional anesthesia. The latter is used when muscle relaxation and analgesia are required (e.g., brachial plexus block for shoulder operation or fracture repair); 0.25% solution is used for routine analgesia techniques or in the elderly. Regardless of concentration, it is the total mass of bupivacaine used that sets the limit on dosing: the manufacturer recommends 1 to 2 mg/kg body weight or 150 to 200 mg for a fit adult. As highlighted later in the chapter, these dosing recommendations may need to be tailored to individual circumstances. For example, the upper limit of bupivacaine dose used during epidural anesthesia should be less than that used during combined femoral and sciatic nerve block. A cautious approach is simple to implement; the injection is fractionated while the patient's voice is monitored for early warning signs of slurred speech.

Although bupivacaine is well absorbed from the injection site, strong tissue binding ensures buffering from too-rapid peaks and long duration of action. Used for perineural analgesia, a bupivacaine block may last from 4 to 6 or more hours. The duration of action in the epidural space is about 2 to 3 hours; a longer duration of analgesia requires catheter placement for infusion. Epinephrine has not significantly reduced blood levels of absorbed bupivacaine or notably prolonged analgesia. Mostly, epinephrine side effects are produced without benefit of longer duration of action. Experimentally, epinephrine could aggravate bupivacaine cardiotoxicity.[34] However, epinephrine may be beneficial as a marker of intravascular injection and has been added to bupivacaine used during regional block, despite minimal prolongation of the block or reduction in bupivacaine blood levels after regional block.

Bupivacaine has become widely used—perhaps as drug of choice in North America—for extended labor or postoperative analgesia by continuous catheter infusion. After a period of "soaking" with concentrated solution, the infusate can be diluted gradually to 0.1% or less. For extended relief of pain, the synergistic analgesic action of opioid with local anesthetic is particularly useful because it permits pain relief without significant muscle weakness. Tachyphylaxis in response to local anesthetics (i.e., the drug becomes increasingly less effective, mandating more frequent injection of ever larger volumes) has become a curiosity of the past, because intermittent injection was replaced by continuous infusion. With continuous infusion, the opposite of tachyphylaxis is seen, and clinical local anesthetic concentrations eventually approach the experimental C_m.

Bupivacaine's amide linkage, well sheltered by piperidine at one end and by xylidine at the other end, is virtually hydrolysis resistant in humans.[13] The initial metabolic process instead turns to dealkylation of the piperidine nitrogen to yield pipecolyl xylidide (i.e., desmethyl mepivacaine), which is also the dealkylation product of mepivacaine and ropivacaine metabolism; similarities between the fate of the three local anesthetics may be noticed. Debutylation (Fig. 8–9) is a genuine detoxification process: pipecolyl xylidide is only one eighth as lethal as the bupivacaine parent.

Because bupivacaine is widely used for prolonged epidural or peripheral infusion, metabolites not previously encountered with administration of a single dose have been uncovered. Of these, para-hydroxy (4-OH) bupivacaine is best characterized. Pipecolyl xylidide and para-hydroxy bupivacaine accumulate slowly when bupivacaine is infused at a rate sufficient to provide pain relief. As with the parent drug, buffer reservoir saturation may take 1 to 2 days, after which blood levels are a function of clearance rates.[35] Although bupivacaine levels during infusion can rise quite high (>5 μg/mL), signs of overt toxicity are rare.[36] Because in the central nervous system of humans the acute toxic level of bupivacaine is on the order of 2 μg/mL, it appears that it is not so much the absolute bupivacaine blood level as it is the rate of change in plasma concentration that provokes signs of toxicity.[3]

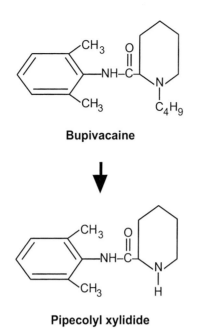

Bupivacaine

Pipecolyl xylidide

Figure 8–9 Bupivacaine biotransformation. (From de Jong RH: Local Anesthetics, p 199. St. Louis, Mosby–Year Book, 1994.)

Like mepivacaine and ropivacaine, bupivacaine has an asymmetric chiral carbon atom. The concepts of chirality and stereospecificity are clarified by an everyday example. The right hand (Fig. 8–10)—one member of a left-right pair—slides into only a right glove to conform to a specific fit. The right foot, conversely, nonselectively fits either one of a pair of socks.

Stereospecificity of the cardiac sodium channel has been especially well studied, demonstrating a threefold tighter affinity for $R(+)$- than for $S(-)$-bupivacaine.[37] The $R(+)$-bupivacaine enantiomer appears to be the fast-in, slow-out partner of the racemic bupivacaine isomer pair, and the $S(-)$ enantiomer is the less cardio-

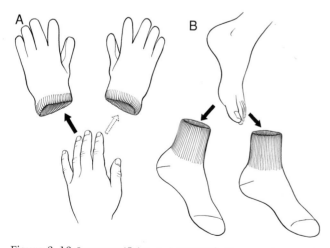

Figure 8–10 Stereospecificity. *A,* A stereoselective receptor accepts only the matching *R-* or *S-*configuration enantiomer, much like a left-hand glove fits only the left hand. The right-hand glove does not match at all with ("rejects") the left hand. *B,* A nonselective receptor accepts either of the two steric antipodes, much like the left foot fits either one of a pair of socks.

toxic of the two. The issue is more complex, because in comparing the effects of bupivacaine enantiomers on medullary control neurons, R-bupivacaine had severalfold greater cardiorespiratory depressant effects than the S enantiomer.[7] Bupivacaine cardiotoxicity is precipitated by a direct myocardial and an indirect central component. The net result of these two actions remains a lively issue that may help resolve the puzzling cardiac sensitivity to bupivacaine at term pregnancy.

These stereoselective findings culminated in the introduction of ropivacaine, the $S(-)$ enantiomer of the propyl homologue of mepivacaine and bupivacaine. Ropivacaine's channel association and dissociation constants may not be quite those of lidocaine, but they are a considerable step forward compared with those of racemic bupivacaine.[38] Theory and in vitro analysis aside, ropivacaine is a remarkable advance in decreasing in vivo cardiotoxicity.

Ropivacaine. The newest member of the pipecolyl xylidide amino amide family is ropivacaine, the propyl (C_3H_7) derivative of pipecolyl xylidide (see Fig. 8–5). Its pharmacologic properties lie between those of bupivacaine and mepivacaine, leaning closer to the former than the latter. Like its cousins, ropivacaine has an asymmetric chiral carbon atom where the carboxyamide linkage joins the piperidine ring. The chiral carbon allows for two mirror-imaged steric twins of the molecule: one is the left-rotating $S(-)$ enantiomer, and the other is the right-rotating $R(+)$ enantiomer (Fig. 8–11). Although mepivacaine and bupivacaine are dispensed as the optically inactive (i.e., left-rotation nullifies right-rotation) racemic R-S mixture, ropivacaine is the optically active (left-rotating) pure $S(-)$ isomer.

Far from being a me-too drug, ropivacaine takes unique advantage of the high-potency, low-toxicity profile of the left-rotary form compared with the right-rotary enantiomer. In vitro studies comparing $S(-)$- with $R(+)$-ropivacaine show the former to be severalfold less arrhythmogenic than the latter. The lethality of $S(-)$ is also less than that of $R(+)$-ropivacaine but nerve impulse blocking potency and duration of action compare favorably with racemic bupivacaine. Some unknowns, such as myotoxicity relative to bupivacaine, remain to be determined. Even so, obstetric regional anesthesia practice should reap immediate benefits in labor and delivery applications.

Clinically meaningful vasoconstriction appears to accompany ropivacaine injection, unlike mepivacaine. Blanching and decreased cutaneous blood flow are observed with ropivacaine infiltration, making it a good candidate for surgical field blocks.[39] Epidural blood flow and drug uptake are decreased by ropivacaine.[40] By the same token, vasoconstriction begs the question of uterine blood flow and placental circulation. Reassuringly, ropivacaine blood levels as high as 2.5 μg/mL did not affect ovine placental blood flow, fetal outcome, or maternal or fetal toxic responses.[41]

Pipecolyl xylidide appears to be the primary metabolic product of hepatic dealkylation, with toxicity about one-eighth that of the parent compound (see Fig. 8–9). Renal excretion of unchanged ropivacaine is

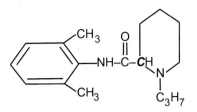

S-Ropivacaine

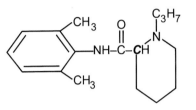

R-Ropivacaine

Figure 8–11 Ropivacaine is the propylpipecolyl xylidide homologue of mepivacaine (methylpipecolyl xylidide) and bupivacaine (butylpipecolyl xylidide). All three have a chiral asymmetric carbon atom (dense C in figure) where the aminoacyl linkage joins the piperidine ring. Two mirror-image optical isomers coexist: *S*-ropivacaine (sinister; *top*) and *R*-ropivacaine (rectus; *bottom*). Unlike its cousin homologues, formulated as the racemic [*RS*(±); optically neutral] mixture, only the *S*(−) enantiomer of ropivacaine is used clinically; the *R*(+) enantiomer proved more cardiotoxic than the *S*(−) form. (From de Jong RH: Local Anesthetics, p 385. St. Louis, Mosby–Year Book, 1994.)

a small percentage of parent drug, but that of pipecolyl xylidide, although about 50%, appears to be rate limited; metabolite accumulation is possible during extended ropivacaine infusion.[13] From the metabolism of mepivacaine and bupivacaine, hydroxylated ropivacaine, pipecolyl xylidide, or both may be expected, as well as conjugation products. Limited studies in human subjects confirm the rapid disposition and low systemic toxicity of ropivacaine.[42]

Aminoalkyl Amides

Of the two better-known aminoalkyl amides, only procainamide has been studied in detail. Dibucaine, the first aminoalkyl amide local anesthetic to be synthesized, has found only limited use, mostly as a spinal or topical anesthetic.

Procainamide

Procainamide is a weak local anesthetic and irritating on injection; it has found no application in regional anesthesia. Conversely, it is widely used by cardiologists in the oral prophylaxis and therapy of cardiac arrhythmias. More than one half of the procainamide administered orally is excreted unchanged in human urine; concern over metabolic accumulation has not been as intense as in the case of lidocaine. Procainamide is hydrolyzed spontaneously in human plasma;

the blood level slowly declines by 10% to 15% per hour.

Dibucaine

The biodegradation of dibucaine is sluggish compared with that of other amide-linked local anesthetics. Limited use, high toxicity, and a complex heterocyclic molecule have stifled investment in the sensitive analytic methodology needed to trace its fate in humans. Whatever the by-products, dibucaine metabolism is slow and incomplete, and the dominant excretory product is unchanged local anesthetic in the urine.[3]

Adverse Effects

Untoward responses to local anesthetics are systemic or localized. Systemic reactions occur when organ systems distant to the injection site respond to blood-borne drug. Localized reactions occur when the drug injures the structures it contacts directly. Because local anesthetic is injected perineurally in concentrations severalfold greater than the theoretical minimum to offset gross inefficiency of the delivery system, cells or tissues in direct contact with this strong solution can be harmed.

Systemic Toxicity

Systemic reactions, except allergy, are dose dependent: the higher the local anesthetic concentration in the blood, the more pronounced the response. Measures aimed at lowering the local anesthetic blood level, such as using the lowest dose in the weakest solution plus minimizing absorption with a vasoconstrictor, go a long way toward decreasing the incidence of systemic reactions in the patient population. A special concern is that local anesthetic absorbed into the maternal bloodstream may harm the fetus or depress the newborn infant.

Between localized and systemic responses are global reactions that can be precipitated by minute quantities of drug in previously sensitized or genetically atopic individuals. Although local anesthetics enjoy an enviable record of safety, familiarity with the various manifestations of toxicity provides early warning that something may be amiss, thereby minimizing the more unpleasant complications.

Overdosage

The higher the plasma level and the faster it increases, the more likely that an adverse systemic response is about to happen. Most toxic reactions are straightforward time- and dose-dependent phenomena. The more molecules attached to a receptor configuration, the more pronounced is the response.

Some field-proven guidelines are provided in Table 8–3, but physicians should heed the term "suggested"

Table 8–3 Manufacturers' Suggested Perineural Local Anesthetic Doses*

LOCAL ANESTHETIC	DOSE BY BODY WEIGHT, mg/kg	AVERAGE ADULT DOSE, mg
Procaine (Novocain)	14	1000
Prilocaine (Citanest)	10	600
Lidocaine (Xylocaine)	7†	500†
Mepivacaine (Carbocaine)	7†	500†
Tetracaine (Pontocaine)	1.5	100
Ropivacaine (tentative)	1–2	150–200
Bupivacaine (Marcaine, Sensorcaine)	1–2	150

*Manufacturer-suggested dose limits for perineural (extravascular and extrathecal) use. This table in no way implies that these dosages are safe or absolute maxima. Systemic reactions can be encountered with much smaller doses, but much larger doses, used judiciously, have been administered without ill effects.
†With 5 μg/mL of 1:200,000 epinephrine.
Adapted from Moore DC, Bridenbaugh LD, Thompson GE, et al: Factors determining dosages of amide-type local anesthetic drugs. Anesthesiology 1977; 47: 263–268; in de Jong RH: Local Anesthetics, p 353. St. Louis, Mosby–Year Book, 1994.

in the table. The values are estimates for reasonably fit patients; they may be too high for the elderly or infirm or too low for the healthy. The data reflect the implicit assumption of perineural placement; unintended intravascular or intrathecal injection of so large a dose has the potential for grave adverse effects on heart, brain, and circulation.

Most so-called drug-related reactions are not related to the drug. In this category are the needle-shy patients who respond with hyperventilation, sweating, or vasovagal reaction. Common too are reactions related to the additive rather than the local anesthetic. Sodium bisulfite is a frequent culprit, as are preservatives of the paraben (para-aminobenzoic acid) family, such as methylparaben or propylparaben.

Allergy

Allergy to a given drug is an exception to the rule relating toxicity with drug mass. Allergy is defined as an adverse reaction to a substance after previous sensitization to that same compound or to a closely related one. After the individual is sensitized, minute quantities of the offending drug (i.e., antigen) can trigger a massive allergic response when the person encounters the immunoglobulin antibody. The mating of antigen and antibody initiates a cascading sequence of reactions. An immediate (i.e., systemic, anaphylactic) reaction occurs when humoral antibodies have been synthesized. If the antibody is formed by tissue-resident lymphoid cells, a delayed (i.e., localized) reaction develops, with skin a prominent target.

The causative mechanism of an allergic reaction affects the speed of onset and severity of reaction. The type I immunoglobulin E–mediated antibody response is swiftly progressive and severe; it is true anaphylaxis. Circulating bioamines, released by mast cell degranulation, trigger a massive systemic defense reaction: airway edema, bronchospasm, and hypotension are particularly pernicious. The slower-onset type IV allergic reaction follows non–immunoglobin E–mediated release of histamine and other reactive products from sensitized lymphocytes. Depending on the amount of mediator released, severity of reaction can vary from

rapid anaphylactoid shock to slowly progressive contact dermatitis.

Although true allergy to amino amides (e.g., lidocaine, bupivacaine) is exceedingly rare, the anesthesiologist cannot ignore the warning, and testing is needed. There is little doubt that cross sensitivity between amino esters (e.g., procaine, benzocaine, tetracaine) exists and extends to other para-aminobenzoic acid esters, such as sunscreen lotions or preservatives of the paraben (e.g., methylparaben, propylparaben) family. Whether amino amide local anesthetics cross-react within the group is far less certain. Most so-called allergies to local anesthetic represent adverse reactions to preservatives and additives.

Convulsions

Convulsions occur when focal excitation of a subcortical limbic site (possibly amygdala) propagates beyond its bounds to spread globally. As local anesthetic blood levels increase, limbic discharges fan out through the brain, precipitating synchronous epileptiform bursts characteristic of a grand mal seizure. Paradoxically, local anesthetics are used as anticonvulsants at lower blood levels.

A short-acting neuromuscular blocking agent such as succinylcholine has been advocated to stop the convulsive muscle spasms of a seizure.[43] The paralyzing agent does not stop the brain's electrical seizure discharges; it merely stops their external muscular manifestations. The primary indication for a paralyzing agent is an inability to adequately ventilate a convulsing patient; its use meets the increased oxygen demand of the convulsing brain and contracting muscles, and it lowers the arterial carbon dioxide tension, raising the brain's seizure threshold to local anesthetics.

Benzodiazepines have proved to be specific and effective in subcortical seizure management. They play a prime role in preventing and in treating local anesthetic-induced convulsions in humans. Benzodiazepines, by decreasing limbic excitability, preclude activation of the focal seizure generator and may be useful in preventing central local anesthetic toxicity.[3] When contemplating the use of high doses of local anesthetic close to presumed toxic limits, as in a brachial plexus block, benzodiazepine premedication may be advisable.

Neurotoxicity

In the laboratory, local anesthetics are effective sodium current blockers and destructive neurotoxins, at concentrations severalfold lower than those used clinically. This may seem worrisome, but there is a comfortable 50-fold margin between the median blocking and toxic concentrations.[44] This is a considerably more generous therapeutic window than that available for most other drugs. It appears that the optimal conditions of the laboratory environment are miniature models of more rugged clinical conditions. A more concentrated local anesthetic solution is needed for regional block in humans, but the neurotoxic concentration is commensurately higher.

Perhaps the one clinical situation equivalent to an isolated nerve stretched in a test chamber is spinal anesthesia. Bare spinal rootlets float in an enclosed sac of fluid and may be more readily blocked and more readily injured. Chloroprocaine or its stabilizers, or both, were implicated in the past. Attention in the 1990s has focused on spinal anesthesia with concentrated (5%) lidocaine made hyperbaric with syrup (7.5% dextrose). Although neural injury was initially thought to result from mechanical stasis from fine-bore spinal catheters, the drug combination now is coming under scrutiny, and the device has been recast in the lesser role of accessory.[45]

Cardiotoxicity

As in nerve, local anesthetics decrease the cardiac action potential by limiting the inward flow of sodium current. Cardiac tissue is rendered less excitable and more frequency dependent, such that impulse propagation can be slowed; lidocaine and congeners such as mexiletine are widely used antiarrhythmics. Lidocaine is a fast-in, fast-out sodium channel blocker that reaches steady-state blockade in one or two beats. Bupivacaine is a fast-in but slow-out local anesthetic whose blocking action increases with successive beats and with faster rates; this sets the stage for malignant reentrant cardiac arrhythmias. For reasons yet unclear, the heart is further sensitized to bupivacaine at term pregnancy.

Local anesthetics with an asymmetric chiral carbon atom (e.g., mepivacaine, bupivacaine) show stereoselectivity for the cardiac sodium channel binding site. The R enantiomer has greater receptor affinity than the S isopode. Ropivacaine, a pure $S(-)$ enantiomer, is considerably less cardiotoxic than racemic bupivacaine.

Cardiovascular effects of local anesthetics arise, in part, with a magnitude yet unknown, from central action on medullary autonomic control sites. Arrhythmias and blood pressure changes are produced by intracerebral injection of minute amounts of bupivacaine; medullary cardiorespiratory control sites also show stereoselectivity. That arrhythmias in unanesthetized humans or animals often precede convulsions further points to a centrally mediated component. Prior medication with a known central nervous system suppressant, such as a benzodiazepine, is suggested; a dilemma is the risk-benefit balance between maternal and fetal welfare.

Because experimental work with induction, prevention, modification, or treatment of bupivacaine-induced arrhythmias has been done mostly in isolated hearts or in surgically anesthetized animals, the clinical impact is far from clear. First, experiments on isolated hearts may point the way but need to be refined in the intact organism. Second, because regional anesthesia is practiced on awake patients, experiments need to be conducted on previously instrumented awake animals. Until these standards are met, no specific drug therapy for bupivacaine cardiotoxicity can be recommended.

Expectations are high that ropivacaine will circumvent the curse of racemic bupivacaine cardiotoxicity; whether ropivacaine will prove as hardy a local anesthetic still is unanswered. The $S(-)$-bupivacaine enantiomer bears watching. Its longer butyl side chain, compared with ropivacaine's propyl tail, may make for greater potency and longer staying power. Whether these attributes are outweighed by greater toxicity determines which of the two cousins will be the front-runner, whether each will fill a practical niche, or whether one will fade from use.

References

1. Wildsmith JAW: Carl Koller (1857–1944) and the introduction of cocaine into anesthetic practice. Reg Anesth 1984; 9: 161–164.
2. Butterworth JF IV, Strichartz GR: Molecular mechanisms of local anesthesia: a review. Anesthesiology 1990; 72: 711–734.
3. de Jong RH: Local Anesthetics. St. Louis, Mosby–Year Book, 1994.
4. Bernards CM, Hill HF: The spinal nerve root sleeve is not a preferred route for redistribution of drugs from the epidural space to the spinal cord. Anesthesiology 1991; 75: 827–832.
5. Rosenberg PH: 1992 ASRA lecture. Intravenous regional anesthesia: nerve block by multiple mechanisms. Reg Anesth 1993; 18: 1–5.
6. Boban M, Stowe DF, Gross GJ, et al: Potassium channel openers attenuate atrioventricular block by bupivacaine in isolated hearts. Anesth Analg 1993; 76: 1259–1265.
7. Denson DD, Behbehani MM, Gregg RV: Enantiomer-specific effects of an intravenously administered arrhythmogenic dose of bupivacaine on neurons of the nucleus tractus solitarius and the cardiovascular system in the anesthetized rat. Reg Anesth 1992; 17: 311–316.
8. Raymond SA, Strichartz GR: Further comments on the failure of impulse propagation in nerves marginally blocked by local anesthetic. (Letter to the editor.) Anesth Analg 1990; 70: 121–122.
9. de Jong RH: The chloroprocaine controversy. Am J Obstet Gynecol 1981; 140: 237–239.
10. Ready LB, Plumer MH, Haschke RH, et al: Neurotoxicity of intrathecal local anesthetics in rabbits. Anesthesiology 1985; 63: 364–370.
11. Stevens RA, Urmey WF, Urquhart BL, et al: Back pain after epidural anesthesia with chloroprocaine. Anesthesiology 1993; 78: 492–497.
12. Severinghaus JW, Xu FD, Spellman MJ Jr: Benzocaine and methemoglobin: recommended actions. (Letter to the editor.) Anesthesiology 1991; 74: 385–387.

13. Rosenberg PH, Heavner JE: Acute cardiovascular and central nervous system toxicity of bupivacaine and desbutylbupivacaine in the rat. Acta Anaesthesiol Scand 1992; 36: 138–141.

14. Starmer CF: Theoretical characterization of ion channel blockade: competitive binding to periodically accessible receptors. Biophys J 1987; 52: 405–412.

15. de Jong RH, Davis NL: Treating bupivacaine arrhythmias: preliminary report. Reg Anesth 1981; 6: 99–103.

16. Kytta J, Heavner JE, Badgwell JM, et al: Cardiovascular and central nervous system effects of co-administered lidocaine and bupivacaine in piglets. Reg Anesth 1991; 16: 89–94.

17. Hellström-Westas L, Westgren U, Rosen I, et al: Lidocaine for treatment of severe seizures in newborn infants: I. Clinical effects and cerebral electrical activity monitoring. Acta Paediatr Scand 1988; 77: 79–84.

18. Heavner JE, Leinonen L, Haasio J, et al: Interaction of lidocaine and hypothermia in Bier blocks in volunteers. Anesth Analg 1989; 69: 53–59.

19. Yukioka H, Hayashi M, Terai T, et al: Intravenous lidocaine as a suppressant of coughing during tracheal intubation in elderly patients. Anesth Analg 1993; 77: 309–312.

20. Kastrup J, Angelo H, Petersen P, et al: Treatment of chronic painful diabetic neuropathy with intravenous lidocaine infusion. Br Med J 1986; 292: 173.

21. Dejgard A, Petersen P, Kastrup J: Mexiletine for treatment of chronic painful diabetic neuropathy. Lancet 1988; 1: 9–11.

22. Tanelian DL, Brose WG: Neuropathic pain can be relieved by drugs that are use-dependent sodium channel blockers: lidocaine, carbamazepine, and mexiletine. Anesthesiology 1991; 74: 949–951.

23. Awerbuch GI, Sandyk R: Mexiletine for thalamic pain syndrome. Int J Neurosci 1990; 55: 129–133.

24. Bennett PB, Woosley RL, Hondeghem LM: Competition between lidocaine and one of its metabolites, glycylxylidide, for cardiac sodium channels. Circulation 1988; 78: 692–700.

25. Arthur GR: Pharmacokinetics of local anesthetics. In Strichartz GR (ed): Local Anesthetics, pp 165–186. Berlin, Springer-Verlag, 1987.

26. Denson DD, Mazoit JX: Physiology, pharmacology, and toxicity of local anesthetics: adult and pediatric considerations. In Raj PP (ed): Clinical Practice of Regional Anesthesia, pp 73–105. New York, Churchill Livingstone, 1991.

27. Hellström-Westas L, Svenningsen NW, Westgren U, et al: Lidocaine for treatment of severe seizures in newborn infants: II. Blood concentrations of lidocaine and metabolites during intravenous infusion. Acta Paediatr 1992; 81: 35–39.

28. van Oss GECJM, Vree TB, Baars AM, et al: Pharmacokinetics, metabolism, and renal excretion of articaine and its metabolite articainic acid in patients after epidural administration. Eur J Anaesthesiol 1989; 6: 49–56.

29. Moller RA, Covino BG: Cardiac electrophysiologic effects of articaine compared with bupivacaine and lidocaine. Anesth Analg 1993; 76: 1266–1273.

30. de Jong RH, Ronfeld RA, DeRosa RA: Cardiovascular effects of convulsant and supraconvulsant doses of amide local anesthetics. Anesth Analg 1982; 61: 3–9.

31. Sarvela PJ: Comparison of regional ophthalmic anesthesia produced by pH-adjusted 0.75% and 0.5% bupivacaine and 1% and 1.5% etidocaine, all with hyaluronidase. Anesth Analg 1993; 77: 131–134.

32. Vree TB, Beumer EM, Lagerwerf AJ, et al: Clinical pharmacokinetics of R(+)- and S(-)-mepivacaine after high doses of racemic mepivacaine with epinephrine in the combined psoas compartment/sciatic nerve block. Anesth Analg 1992; 75: 75–80.

33. Albright GA: Cardiac arrest following regional anesthesia with etidocaine or bupivacaine. (Editorial.) Anesthesiology 1979; 51: 285–287.

34. Kinney WW, Kambam JR, Wright W: Propranolol pretreatment reduces cardiorespiratory toxicity due to plain, but not epinephrine-containing, intravenous bupivacaine in rats. Can J Anaesth 1991; 38(4 Pt 1): 533-536.

35. Pere P, Tuominen M, Rosenberg PH: Cumulation of bupivacaine, desbutylbupivacaine and 4-hydroxybupivacaine during and after continuous interscalene brachial plexus block. Acta Anaesthesiol Scand 1991; 35: 647–650.

36. Richter O, Klein K, Abel J, et al: The kinetics of bupivacaine (Carbostesin) plasma concentrations during epidural anesthesia following intraoperative bolus injection and subsequent continuous infusion. Int J Clin Pharmacol Ther Toxicol 1984; 22: 611–617.

37. Tucker GT, Lennard MS: Enantiomer specific pharmacokinetics. Pharmacol Ther 1990; 45: 309–329.

38. Arlock P: Actions of three local anaesthetics: lidocaine, bupivacaine and ropivacaine on guinea pig papillary muscle sodium channels (V_{max}). Pharmacol Toxicol 1988; 63: 96–104.

39. Guinard JP, Carpenter RL, Morell RC: Effect of local anesthetic concentration on capillary blood flow in human skin. Reg Anesth 1992; 17: 317–321.

40. Dahl JB, Simonsen L, Mogensen T, et al: The effect of 0.5% ropivacaine on epidural blood flow. Acta Anaesthesiol Scand 1990; 34: 308–310.

41. Santos AC, Arthur GR, Roberts DJ, et al: Effect of ropivacaine and bupivacaine on uterine blood flow in pregnant ewes. Anesth Analg 1992; 74: 62–67.

42. Scott DB, Lee A, Fagan D, et al: Acute toxicity of ropivacaine compared with that of bupivacaine. Anesth Analg 1989; 69: 563–569.

43. Moore DC, Bridenbaugh LD: Oxygen: The antidote for systemic toxic reactions from local anesthetic drugs. JAMA 1960; 174: 842–847.

44. Bainton C, Wingrove D, Strichartz G: Irreversible conduction block in isolated peripheral nerve by high concentrations of lidocaine. Anesthesiology 1993; 79(Suppl): A872.

45. de Jong RH: Last round for a "heavyweight"? (Editorial; comment). Anesth Analg 1994; 78: 3–4.

CHAPTER 9

Opioid and Nonopioid Analgesics

Robin B. Slover, M.D., Robert W. Phelps, M.D., Ph.D.

Background

The word opium is derived from the Greek word for juice, referring to the juice of the poppy, *Papaver somniferum*, which has been used for thousands of years. Opium contains more than 20 distinct alkaloids, the best known being morphine, named for Morpheus, the Greek god of dreams. Opioid use as an adjuvant to anesthesia has continued to develop since 1665, when Johan Sigismund Elsholtz produced anesthesia and analgesia by injecting crude opium into a dog's veins.[1] The recognition of opiate binding sites in 1973[2] led to the use of intrathecally and epidurally administered opiates in 1979[3, 4] for analgesia. Spinal administration of opioids is now widely used for the management of postoperative pain and to manage severe cancer and chronic pain.

Traditionally, the naturally occurring alkaloids of opium have been called opiates or morphine-like drugs. Opioids are compounds with morphine-like properties. This generic term can refer to natural or synthetic substances and to endogenous peptides. The term "narcotic" is derived from the Greek word for stupor and, strictly speaking, refers to any substance that can induce sleep. In the legal context, the word "narcotic" refers to any substance that can cause dependence.[1] However, the term is often used to refer to opiates and opioids. This usage, although technically incorrect, is widespread, and most opioids are interchangeably referred to as narcotics.

Not all of the opiates derived from opium have analgesic properties. The opiate alkaloids can be divided into two distinct chemical classes: phenanthrenes and benzylisoquinolines. Phenanthrene alkaloids include morphine and codeine. Benzylisoquinoline alkaloids include papaverine (a vasodilator) and noscapine, which lack morphine-like properties.

Exogenous Opioids

Historically, opioids have been classified as naturally occurring, synthetic, and semisynthetic. This classification is now artificial because all opioids can be synthesized. However, for many of the naturally occurring compounds, it is cheaper to isolate these from a plant extract than to synthesize them. The endogenous peptides—enkephalins, endorphins, and dynorphins–are also opioids.

Morphine is the prototypic opioid (Fig. 9–1). The heavy lines in Figure 9–1 represent the part of the structure that is common among opiates.[5] Morphine has five interlocking rings that make up its molecular skeleton. By modifying various functional groups on this skeleton, semisynthetic narcotics such as hydro-

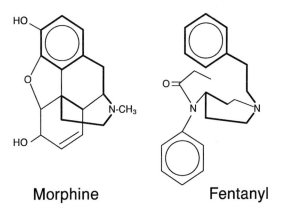

Morphine   **Fentanyl**

Figure 9–1 The chemical structure of morphine and fentanyl. The essential portion of the structure of morphine related to receptor activation is indicated by solid lines. Fentanyl has been drawn to emphasize its similarity to morphine. (From Phelps R: Factors influencing perioperative parenteral narcotic analgesics. Probl Anesth 1988; 2: 362–375.)

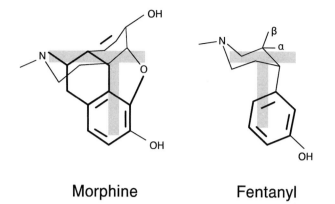

Morphine   Fentanyl

Figure 9–2 The T-shaped core of opioids.

morphone and oxycodone are formed; the structural modifications create different pharmacologic properties. Synthetic opioids such as meperidine and fentanyl are formed by a progressive reduction of the number of fused rings. The structure of fentanyl is also shown in Figure 9–1, configured to show its similarities to morphine. Although chemically different, the three-dimensional configurations of these compounds are similar enough that opioid receptors respond to the compounds in nearly identical fashion.

All opioids are envisaged to show a common core: a T-shaped structure with a piperidine ring, thought to confer "opioid-like" properties, as the crossbar and a hydroxylated phenyl group as the vertical axis[6] (Fig. 9–2). Potent opioids also share other structural characteristics: a quaternary carbon, a tertiary amine nitrogen, and a phenolic hydroxyl (e.g., morphine derivatives) or ketone group (e.g., methadone, meperidine).[7]

Endogenous Opioids

The body makes endogenous opioids that function as neurotransmitters, neuromodulators, and hormones. These compounds are involved in the perception of pain, modulation of behavior, and regulation of autonomic and neuroendocrine function.[8]

Different endogenous opioids are generated from three prohormones or major precursor molecules: prepro-opiomelanocortin, preproenkephalin, and prepro-dynorphin (Table 9–1). Prepro-opiomelanocortin is a polyfunctional prohormone, containing the β-endorphin structure and the sequences for corticotropin and melanocyte-stimulating hormone. β-Endorphin is the most potent of the endogenous opioids and is distributed in the pituitary, hypothalamus, thalamus (anterior and intermediate lobes),[9] periaqueductal gray matter, amygdala, ventromedial hypothalamic nuclei, reticular formation, stria terminalis, and locus coeruleus.[10]

The peptide structures generated from preproenkephalin are leu- and met-enkephalin. These structures are distributed more widely than β-endorphin. Enkephalins are found throughout the gastrointestinal tract, sympathetic nervous system, adrenal medulla, and in most areas in the brain important for antinociception, such as the periaqueductal gray, rostral ventral medulla, caudate nucleus, amygdala, hypothalamus, and posterior pituitary lobe. In the spinal cord, enkephalins are found in Rexed's layers I, II, III, and VII[11] (Fig. 9–3).

Each preproenkephalin molecule contains four met-enkephalin and one leu-enkephalin sequence. However, the ratio between met-enkephalin and leu-enkephalin varies from one brain region to another. The processing of a preproenkephalin molecule may differ between the periphery and the brain and among different neuronal populations.[12]

Cleavage of preprodynorphin produces dynorphin A, dynorphin B, neuroendorphin, and leu-morphine. Leu-enkephalin has been shown to be a product of preprodynorphin and of preproenkephalin.[13,14] Dynorphins are found in the hypothalamus, area postrema, superior olive in the pons, nucleus tractus solitarius in the medulla oblongata, and dorsal horn of the spinal cord.[15] In the dorsal horn, dynorphin-containing cells are found in layers I and V.

Endogenous opioids control nociception primarily at the level of the periaqueductal gray, medulla, and spinal cord. All three endogenous opioid peptides are found in the periaqueductal gray. Activation of the periaqueductal gray activates multiple medullary controls involving serotonin, norepinephrine, and other bulbospinal descending systems. Proenkephalin and prodynorphin cells are found in several layers of the

Table 9–1 Endogenous Opioid Specificity

PRECURSOR	PEPTIDE	RECEPTOR SPECIFICITY
Prepro-opiomelanocortin	β-Endorphin	$\mu = \delta > \epsilon >> \kappa$
Preproenkephalin	Leu-enkephalin	$\delta >> \mu$
	Met-enkephalin	$\delta >> \mu$
Preprodynorphin	Dynorphin A and B	$\kappa >> \mu$

Modified from Hedner T, Nordberg G. In Rawal N, Coombs DW (eds): Spinal Narcotics, pp 1–31. Reprinted by permission of Kluwer Academic Publishers, 1990.

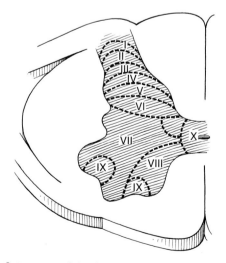

Figure 9–3 Structure of the dorsal horn shows the various lamina.

dorsal horn (i.e., I, V, VII), where they have actions on nociceptive afferents and second-order neurons.[16–18]

Opioid Receptors

Endogenous and exogenous opioids appear to act at several types of specific receptors within the central nervous system. The recognition site is a highly specific proteolipid structure. Only levorotatory isomers can attach to the binding site.[2] Each opioid receptor is coupled to a G protein, which modulates the changes in ion flux and membrane polarity leading to an antinociceptive effect.

Opioid receptors have been labeled with Greek letters. On the basis of neurophysiologic and behavioral evidence from animal studies, μ, δ, κ, σ, ϵ, and λ receptors have been postulated[19–22] (Table 9–2). Approximately 50% of the amino acid sequences making up the receptor structures are identical for μ, δ, and κ receptors.[23]

Mu Receptors

Morphine is the prototype μ agonist, and β-endorphin is the endogenous opioid that predominantly binds with μ receptors. Aside from the agonists-antagonists, all clinically useful spinal opioids are μ agonists. Activation of μ receptors effectively blunts somatic and visceral pain.[22, 24] Mu receptors are coupled to G proteins, and activation of μ receptors leads to neuronal hyperpolarization from an increase in potassium conductance. The G protein–mediated effect directly counters the decrease in potassium permeability caused by substance P.[24] The μ receptors may also be functionally coupled to adenylate cyclase.[25] The μ receptors are associated with the descending inhibitory norepinephrine tract and can inhibit norepinephrine release.[26]

The μ receptor has been subdivided into μ_1 and μ_2 subtypes. The μ_1 receptor is a high-affinity site responsible for analgesia but not respiratory depression. The μ_1 subtype constitutes 40% of spinal opioid receptors.[22] The μ_2 receptors are low-affinity receptors responsible for respiratory depression, ileus, and bradycardia. Unfortunately, there is no therapeutic agent that binds to μ_1 receptors only.

Delta Receptors

The δ agonists are more potent spinal analgesics than morphine and also cause respiratory depression.[27] Like μ receptors, activation of δ receptors also blunts somatic pain, but they are unable to blunt visceral pain. [D-Ala^2, D-Leu^5]-enkephalin has demonstrated considerable antinociceptor activity in animals and humans[28, 29]; however, enkephalins are rapidly degraded by peptidases on administration, which limits their clinical usefulness. A clinically effective δ selective agonist is not available.

The δ receptors are also coupled to G proteins. Activation of δ receptors changes potassium conductance, similar to μ receptors, but δ receptors have not been linked to adenylate cyclase. Thirteen types of G-coupled potassium ion channels have been identified.

The binding of δ receptors has been postulated to potentiate μ receptor analgesia by facilitating G protein coupling with μ receptors.[30] Synergism has been shown between δ and μ agents.[31] The δ receptors inhibit acetylcholine release.[24] Analgesic cross-tolerance between μ and δ ligands does not occur.

The δ receptors have two subtypes: δ_1 and δ_2.[32] These receptors are distributed throughout the brain (espe-

Table 9–2 Opioid Receptor Classification

RECEPTOR SUBTYPE	ANALGESIC ACTIVITY	AGONIST	ANTAGONIST	OTHER ACTIONS
μ		Morphine DAMGO	Naloxone	
μ_1	Supraspinal	Morphine = β-endorphin	Naloxonazine	Prolactin release Acetylcholine Tumor
μ_2	Spinal	Morphine > β-endorphin	β-Funaltrexamine	Respiratory depression Inhibition of gastrointestinal transit
δ		Enkephalins	Naloxone	
δ_1	Spinal	Leu-enkephalin DADL DPDPE	DALCE	Tumor
	Supraspinal	Met-enkephalin Deltorphins	Naltrindole	
κ		Dynorphin A Ethylketocyclazocine	Naloxone	
κ_1	Spinal	Dynorphin B α-Neoendorphin		Diuresis Sedation
κ_2	Supraspinal			
κ_3	Supraspinal	Nalorphine		

DADL, [D-Ala^2, D-Leu^5] enkephalin; DALCE, [D-Ala^2, Leu^5, Cys^6] enkephalin; DAMGO, [D-Ala^2, Me Phe^4, Gly (ol)] enkephalin; DPDPE, [D-Pen^2, D-Pen^5] enkephalin.
Modified from Hedner T, Nordberg G. In Rawal N, Coombs DW (eds): Spinal Narcotics, pp 1–31. Reprinted by permission of Kluwer Academic Publishers, 1990; and from Pleuvry BJ: Opioid receptors and their relevance to anaesthesia. Br J Anaesth 1993; 71: 119–126.

cially in limbic structures) and spinal cord. The δ_1 receptors are predominantly found in the spinal cord,[33] accounting for 10% of spinal opioid receptors.[22] The δ_2 receptors are supraspinal. Both enkephalins are the prototypic ligands for δ receptors: leu-enkephalin for δ_1 and met-enkephalin for δ_2. Glyburide, believed to block adenosine triphosphate–sensitive potassium channels in the central nervous system, antagonizes δ_1-induced analgesia and morphine-induced analgesia. Tetraethylammonium blocks δ_2-induced analgesia but has no effect on δ_1- or morphine-induced analgesia.[34]

Kappa Receptors

The κ receptors are effective in blunting viscerochemical input but ineffectual in blunting somatic pain.[35] Dynorphins are the prototypical endogenous opioids binding to κ receptors in the spinal cord. Morphine can activate κ receptors, but it has a 200 times greater affinity for μ receptors than for κ receptors.[36] Activation of κ receptors causes a voltage-dependent reduction in Ca^{2+} conductance, leading to decreased Ca^{2+} entry into the cell.[37] The κ receptors have been shown to inhibit dopamine release.[24] The spinal analgesic activity of opioid agonists-antagonists results from κ receptor activation, but clinical use of these drugs is hampered by their μ antagonistic properties.

Three subtypes of κ receptors have been postulated: κ_1, κ_2, and κ_3. The κ_1 receptors are located in the spinal cord; activation causes analgesia and sedation,[28] although there is less concomitant respiratory depression. The κ_2 receptors are not well characterized. No specific agonist has been found; instead, κ_2 receptors are defined by antagonist-binding studies. The κ_3 receptors are located supraspinally. Their density in the brain is twice as high as μ or δ receptors.[28] Their regional distribution is similar to that of μ receptors; however, there is a much lower density of κ_3 receptors than μ receptors in the periaqueductal gray.[28] Nalorphine primarily acts through κ_3 receptors to produce analgesia.[28]

Other Receptor Types

A separate epsilon (ϵ) receptor has been proposed on the basis of in vitro binding experiments with [³H]ethylketocyclazocine in the rat vas deferens.[38] β-Endorphin has a high affinity for this receptor, which does not appear to respond to μ-, δ-, or κ-receptor agonists. This receptor has also been found in the brains of rat, guinea pig, cow, pig, and chicken. In the animal species examined, it is more abundant than μ, δ, or κ_1 receptors. It is hypothesized to mediate the supraspinal analgesic effects of β-endorphin, and further studies to characterize its importance in humans are needed. There is some speculation that κ_2 receptors may be the same as ϵ receptors on the basis of binding studies.[32]

Sigma receptors (σ) were originally proposed by Martin and colleagues[19] as being responsible for the mental changes (e.g., dysphoria, mania, hallucina-

tions), mydriasis, tachypnea, and tachycardia seen with opioids. N-allyl-norcyclazocine (SKF10.047) is the typical experimental agonist used to identify this receptor. However, SKF10.047 is not specific to σ receptors; it binds to μ receptors as well.[23]

Psychotropic drugs such as phencyclidine, haloperidol, and droperidol can also bind to σ receptors, as can such diverse agents as cocaine, progesterone, dextromethorphan, and pentazocine.[39] Naloxone is inactive at σ receptors.[40] Many newer antipsychotic drugs used to treat mental illness (e.g., schizophrenia) bind to the σ receptor. The σ receptors have been identified in the central nervous system and as part of the immune and endocrine systems. The evidence[41] suggests that the σ receptor may play a major role in the regulation of the glutaminergic system by means of the N-methyl-D-aspartate receptors (NMDA).

The σ receptor exists in several forms: a high-affinity form, a low-affinity form, and a phencyclidine subtype. The phencyclidine receptor subtype is located in the ion channel gated by NMDA.[32]

The lambda receptor (λ) is postulated on the basis of binding studies in the rat brain.[42] This receptor is not well characterized, and further studies need to be done before its place in human opioid regulation will be fully understood.

Interactions of Opioids at Receptors

Opioid interactions at specific receptor subtypes are important in producing analgesia (Fig. 9–4). Opioids appear to have both presynaptic and postsynaptic activity in the dorsal horn. Presynaptic inhibition of substance P release occurs with μ and δ agonists.[43] Postsynaptic inhibition of second-order neurons also has been shown. Systemic administration of opioids has been shown to depress activation of wide dynamic range neurons in a dose-dependent, naloxone-reversible fashion. Wide dynamic range neurons are found

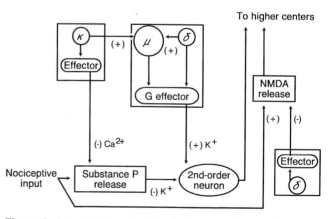

Figure 9–4 Modulation of nociceptive impulses by opioid receptor activation. NMDA, N-methyl-D-aspartate. (From Sinatra RS: Pharmacokinetics and pharmacodynamics of spinal opioids. In Sinatra RS, Hord AH, Ginsberg B, et al [eds]: Acute Pain: Mechanisms & Management, pp 102–111. St. Louis, Mosby–Year Book, 1992.)

in layer V of the dorsal horn and help modulate transmission of pain impulses to the thalamus.

Drugs can affect receptors in three ways: complete binding producing full activation, limited binding producing partial activation, and competitive binding blocking activation by other ligands. Agonists are agents that bind to and activate receptors in a dose-related manner. Partial agonists also bind and activate receptors but produce a submaximal response; less than 100% of the bound receptors are activated. These bound but nonactivated receptors are then unavailable for binding to other ligands. Partial μ agonists are agonists in small doses at the receptor, but in higher doses, they possess a competitive antagonistic effect because of their slow rate of dissociation from the μ receptor, which prevents other drugs from interacting at these sites. This also seems to be the cause of their ceiling effect in analgesic activity.[44] The third effect drugs can have is to antagonize the receptor. Antagonists bind to but do not activate receptors, thereby displacing agonists and making the receptors unavailable for binding to agonists or partial agonists.

Some opioids are agonists and antagonists, with a different action at two different receptors. These drugs are called agonists-antagonists. The ability of many opioids to bind at several different receptors may represent small differences in pharmacologic structure that allow preferential binding to one receptor rather than the other. Agonists-antagonists are usually antagonists at μ receptors and agonists at κ receptors. Butorphanol is an example of a mixed agonist-antagonist (Table 9–3).

The analgesia produced by opioid agonists may be produced spinally or supraspinally.[45] The combination of supraspinal and spinal activation by opioid is synergistic in providing analgesia.[31] Peripheral opioid receptors can also provide analgesia. In cases of inflammation, μ-, δ-, and κ-receptor activation have been shown to produce analgesia. Activation of μ receptors can prevent prostaglandin-mediated nociception sensitization by inhibiting the adenylate cyclase through which

prostaglandins act.[32] Although δ and κ agonists cannot prevent prostaglandin-induced hyperalgesia, they can prevent bradykinin-induced hyperalgesia.[32] These δ and κ receptors are thought to be located on sympathetic nerves.[46] Recognition that peripheral opioid receptors are present on primary afferent nerves and can provide analgesia has led to the use of opioids in regional blocks. The best results have been achieved when morphine was used intra-articularly for procedures on the knee.[47, 48]

Opioid receptors have also been detected on immune cells. Opioid modulation of chemotaxis, superoxide production, and mast cell degranulation has been reported.[49] These effects do not appear to be important in providing nociception.[50]

Pharmacology of Opioids Administered Spinally

The effects of opioids administered spinally are determined by the pharmacokinetics and pharmacodynamics of these drugs. Pharmacokinetics is the study of how various factors influence changes in the blood or tissue levels (or both) of a drug with time. Pharmacodynamics is the study of the relationship between drug tissue levels and their effects. For opioids administered spinally, pharmacokinetic factors influence how various drugs are distributed throughout the epidural and subarachnoid spaces, ultimately binding to opioid receptors in the dorsal horn. The dorsal horn is richly populated with opioid receptors, especially in layers II and III (i.e., substantia gelatinosa). The opioid receptors are protein complexes located within the bilayer lipid membrane of cell walls. These receptors are charged. Opioids are basic amines; the ionized form is favored for strong binding to the receptor.[51]

Table 9–3 Actions of Opioid Analgesics at Opioid Receptor Subtypes

| DRUG | ACTION AT RECEPTOR SUBTYPES | | | |
	μ	δ	κ	α
Agonists				
Morphine	Agonist	No effect	Weak agonist	No effect
Methadone	Agonist	No effect	Weak agonist	Unknown
Meperidine	Agonist	No effect	Agonist	Unknown
Fentanyl	Agonist	Weak agonist	Weak agonist	Unknown
Sufentanil	Agonist	Unknown	Unknown	Unknown
Hydromorphone	Agonist	Unknown	Unknown	Unknown
Partial agonists				
Buprenorphine	Partial agonist	Weak agonist	No effect	No effect
Agonist-antagonist				
Butorphanol	Weak antagonist	Unknown	Agonist	Agonist
Nalbuphine	Antagonist	Unknown	Partial agonist	Agonist
Antagonists				
Naloxone	Antagonist with low doses	Antagonist with medium doses	Antagonist with large doses	No effect

Modified from Ferrante FM: Opioids. In Ferrante FM, VadeBoncouer TR (eds): Postoperative Pain Management, pp 145–209. New York, Churchill Livingstone, 1993; and from Hedner T, Nordberg G: Opioid receptors: types, distribution, and pharmacological profiles. In Rawal N, Coombs DW (eds): Spinal Narcotics, pp 1–31. Reprinted by permission of Kluwer Academic Publishers, 1990.

Table 9–4 Opioid Pharmacokinetics

DRUG	PARTITION COEFFICIENT*	BINDING AFFINITY	RECEPTOR EFFICACY	DURATION EPIDURAL, h
Morphine	1.4	5.7	Moderate	8–22
Hydromorphone	1–2			8–10
Methadone	39		Moderate	4–10
Meperidine	116	193.0	Low	7–10
Alfentanil	126	19.0	Moderate	1–2
Fentanyl	813	1.6	High	2–4
Sufentanil	1778	0.1	Very high	4–6

*Octanol/pH 7.4 buffer partition coefficient.

Lipid Solubility

The onset and duration of spinal opioid analgesia is determined by pharmacokinetics, pharmacodynamics, receptor affinity, and intrinsic activity of each opioid administered. The primary pharmacokinetic determinant in predicting spinal opioid activity is lipid solubility. The partition coefficient, a measurement of how a drug is distributed between aqueous and lipid phases at a particular pH, describes that drug's lipophilic nature. Morphine, with a low partition coefficient of 1.4, is hydrophilic. Fentanyl, with a higher partition coefficient of 813, and sufentanil, with a partition coefficient of 1778, are lipophilic (Table 9–4). The lipophilic nature of a drug determines how far it spreads through the epidural space, dura, and cerebrospinal fluid; how quickly it enters the circulatory system; how much it binds to surrounding tissues; and how quickly clinical effects are seen.

Epidurally administered opioids must cross the dura and subarachnoid cerebrospinal fluid to bind to opiate receptors in the dorsal horn (Fig. 9–5). Opioids can bind to epidural fat and tissues; enter the epidural venous system and systemic circulation, creating measurable plasma concentrations; enter the posterior radicular spinal arteries and be delivered directly to the dorsal horn; and diffuse across the dura into the cerebrospinal fluid, spreading through the cerebrospinal fluid and binding to opioid receptors in the central nervous system.

Epidural and intraspinal administration of opioids for analgesia yields segmental analgesia, produced by binding to opioid receptors in the dorsal horn and resulting in analgesia at that level. Segmental analgesia requires a minimum concentration of the opioid in the cerebrospinal fluid and dorsal horn to provide analgesia compared with plasma levels producing the same amount of analgesia. However, epidurally administered opioids may produce analgesia through systemic absorption (i.e., plasma levels) and through segmental binding.

Highly lipophilic opioids, such as fentanyl, bind to epidural fat and lipid-rich tissues more than hydrophilic opioids, such as morphine. The amount bound

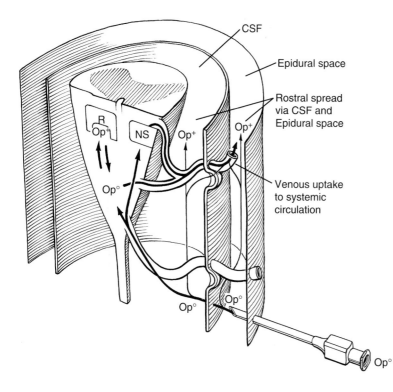

Figure 9–5 Distribution of opioid (Op) given epidurally. Drug diffuses along the epidural space, across the dura, through cerebrospinal fluid (CSF), and to the dorsal horn, where it binds to opioid receptors (R). Vascular uptake occurs in the epidural and subarachnoid spaces and in the spinal cord. NS, nonspecific lipid membrane binding sites.

varies, because the amount of epidural fat varies among patients. Lipophilic opioids also enter the venous circulation more quickly, with faster peak plasma levels. Hydrophilic drugs may have a more predictable but slower dural transfer, because they are not well absorbed by epidural fat or blood vessels.[52] Lipophilic opioids cross the dura quickly through arachnoid granulations, and they can enter the posterior radicular vessels faster, going directly to the dorsal horn. This may account for their faster clinical onset. However, because of their extensive uptake by tissues and vascular structures, lipophilic opioids have a more localized delivery; they do not spread as far through the cerebrospinal fluid (Fig. 9–6). Fentanyl, a highly lipophilic opioid, may spread only five to six dermatomes from the injection site, but morphine spreads throughout the cerebrospinal fluid. Because lipophilic opioids enter vascular space quickly, their duration of action is shorter.

Other Factors

Molecular size and weight correlate inversely with passage across the dura.[39] Protein binding, important in systemic administration, plays a minor role because the protein content of the cerebrospinal fluid is low.[53]

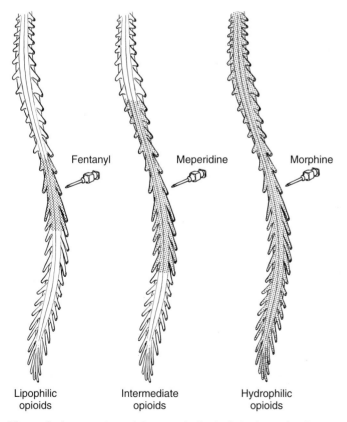

Fentanyl   Meperidine   Morphine

Lipophilic opioids   Intermediate opioids   Hydrophilic opioids

Figure 9–6 Comparison of the spread of opioids in the epidural space as determined by the lipophilic nature. (Modified from VadeBoncouer TR, Ferrante FM: Epidural and subarachnoid opioids. In Ferrante FM, VadeBoncouer TR [eds]: Postoperative Pain Management, pp 279–303. New York, Churchill Livingstone, 1993.)

The total dose of opioid administered influences the duration of activity and dermatomal spread, depending on the opioid given. A dose-dependent prolongation of effects has been observed with morphine[54]; with more lipophilic agents, little or no change in duration occurs when the epidural dose is increased above a critical amount (50–75 μg for fentanyl; 40–50 μg for sufentanil).[55, 56] For lipophilic agents, the volume of injectant is important. With larger volumes, the lipophilic opioid is distributed in a larger area, which may slightly increase the amount of dermatomal spread. The location of the epidural catheter is more important with lipophilic agents than hydrophilic agents in providing segmental analgesia, because lipophilic agents spread less.

Unlike systemically administered opioids, the termination of clinical action of spinally administered opioids results from vascular clearance from the spinal cord. Drug metabolism does not significantly influence the duration of action of spinally administered opioids. Peak plasma levels of fentanyl[57] and sufentanil[56] occur within 5 min after epidural administration. The vascular uptake of morphine is also rapid,[58] with peak plasma concentrations detected at 15 min. Conditions associated with epidural venous engorgement, such as pregnancy and portal hypertension, may further increase vascular uptake.[20]

Several early studies showed similar plasma levels for fentanyl given epidurally or by intravenous administration,[59, 60] suggesting that fentanyl given epidurally may be only a more expensive way of providing analgesia than intravenous administration. Other studies[61] with a larger sample size showed a definite spinal action of fentanyl and a decrease in plasma fentanyl levels with epidural administration compared with intravenous administration. Nonetheless, systemic plasma concentrations of fentanyl contribute to the segmental analgesia provided by its epidural administration. Hydrophilic opioids have a greater plasma-sparing effect than lipophilic drugs. Only 25% as much morphine is required epidurally as parenterally for equivalent pain relief. Meperidine, with a partition coefficient of 38.8, requires 70% of the intravenous dose when given epidurally.[62] Fentanyl, butorphanol, and alfentanil require almost 100% of the effective intravenous dose to provide epidural analgesia. The epidural doses of sufentanil are slightly larger than those required for intravenous analgesia.[63, 64]

Potency is defined by the ratio of analgesic response to the dose of drug required. It is influenced by several factors: ligand availability, receptor binding affinity, and intrinsic activity on the effector mechanism. Because spinal administration bypasses the blood-brain barrier, systemic and epidural potencies are not necessarily the same. Opioids with low lipid solubility have increased receptor accessibility with spinal administration and dramatic gains in potency relative to systemic administration.[65]

Efficacy is a measurement of the number of receptors that must be occupied to produce an effect, and it usually is equivalent to intrinsic activity. Sufentanil and naloxone have strong receptor affinities. However, naloxone has no efficacy, whereas sufentanil is a powerful μ-receptor activator. Opioid agonists with high receptor efficacy require fewer receptor sites to be occupied to achieve the desired analgesic effect. In this regard, a significantly greater number of receptors must be coupled with morphine than with an equal analgesic dose of the more potent opioid sufentanil.[66]

Dissociation kinetics of the receptor is an important determinant of duration, with a greater stability of the drug receptor complex providing a more prolonged duration of action. Of the opioids used clinically, alfentanil has the shortest receptor dissociation kinetics, followed by fentanyl, sufentanil, meperidine, and morphine[67] (see Table 9–4). Differences in the receptor kinetics for partial μ agonists and agonists-antagonists are not governed by lipophilic character or ionization. Instead, the analgesic response is dominated by the kinetics of dissociation from the receptors.

Tolerance is a pharmacodynamic mechanism that may decrease the effectiveness and analgesic duration of a given spinal opioid dose. Although tolerance develops more slowly with spinal administration than after parenteral dosing, it nevertheless is a commonly observed phenomenon, especially when opioids of lower efficacy are administered in doses larger than necessary to provide effective analgesia.[24, 68] Tolerance may result from desensitization when the receptor is uncoupled from its G protein; down-regulation when receptors are removed from the neuronal surface[57]; or a compensatory response (mediated by NMDA in the dorsal horn) that counteracts the effects of opiates, resulting in an enhanced nociceptive message.[69] Studies by Basbaum[69] suggest that spinal sensitization may be the best current explanation for tolerance, because NMDA antagonists can decrease the development of tolerance. Opioid agonists with high efficacy need to occupy fewer receptors to produce analgesia, and their use is less likely to lead to the rapid development of tolerance. These opioids may be more useful for chronic administration. Likewise, large intermittent boluses of opioids may lead to excessive receptor activation, with down-regulation of receptors. A continuous infusion with smaller doses may lead to less tolerance.

Hydrophilic Opioids: Morphine and Hydromorphone

Morphine is hydrophilic, with a partition coefficient of 1.4. Because morphine is not very lipophilic, it stays in the cerebrospinal fluid longer, slowly binding to the dorsal horn. This reservoir of drug provides a prolonged duration of action. Morphine also spreads throughout the cerebrospinal fluid, directly affecting the respiratory center (e.g., respiratory depression) and chemotactic zone (i.e., area postrema) in the brain stem (e.g., nausea and vomiting) (Fig. 9–7). The early risk of respiratory depression is related to the dose given and resultant plasma level. However, the delayed respiratory depression seen with morphine results from direct action on the respiratory center. The risk of delayed respiratory depression is increased with concomitant parenteral opioid administration.

Because of its wide rostral spread, morphine-induced analgesia can be provided to widely divergent anatomic areas, and the location of the catheter is less important. A lumbar catheter is as effective as a thoracic catheter in providing analgesia for post-thoracotomy patients when morphine is used.[70] Morphine has a slow onset but prolonged duration. Morphine-6-glucuronide, one of the principal metabolites of morphine, is also an effective spinal opioid.

Hydromorphone has become a common choice for epidural administration.[71, 72] No significant episodes of respiratory depression have occurred. Hydromorphone has a partition coefficient of 1.03, which is similar to that of morphine.[73] However, hydromorphone behaves more like meperidine clinically.

Intermediate Lipophilicity: Meperidine and Methadone

Opioids with intermediate lipophilic characteristics have partition coefficients ranging from 38 to 131 (Table 9–5). Because of their intermediate lipophilic nature, the onset of clinical activity is slower than with fentanyl but faster than with morphine. Intermediate agents spread over about 12 dermatomes, with less risk of respiratory depression than seen with morphine, and catheter placement near the painful area is less important. Meperidine has local anesthetic properties and activates μ receptors. This property can be used clinically. However, the accumulation of normeperidine, a major metabolite of meperidine, limits continuous clinical use, because normeperidine can cause central nervous system excitation and seizures, especially in patients with limited renal and hepatic function.[74] Methadone has produced fewer urinary and respiratory complications than morphine.

Lipophilic Agents: Fentanyl and Sufentanil

Lipophilic agents have a rapid analgesic onset of 5 to 10 min and last 2 to 5 h. Analgesia tends to be more regional, and catheter placement close to the spinal level corresponding to the pain is required because there is limited rostral spread. The incidence of delayed side effects is minimal.

Opioid Agonists-Antagonists

The epidural use of κ opiate agonists is associated with analgesia. Combined κ agonists and μ antagonists such as butorphanol and nalbuphine should provide segmental analgesia without as many μ receptor–mediated side effects (e.g., nausea, vomiting, pruritus, respiratory depression). Both agents have been used epidurally, along with buprenorphine, a partial μ agonist. These agents are relatively lipid soluble, with clinical onset of analgesia within 5 to 10 min and duration of analgesia of 4 to 6 h.[75, 76] Their use is associated with

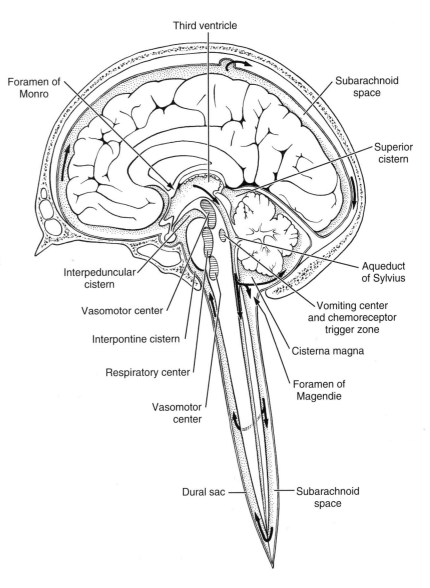

Figure 9–7 Spread of opioids to the brain through the subarachnoid space. (Modified from VadeBoncouer TR, Ferrante FM: Epidural and subarachnoid opioids. In Ferrante FM, VadeBoncouer TR [eds]: Postoperative Pain Management, pp 279–303. New York, Churchill Livingstone, 1993.)

fewer side effects, but the amount of analgesia is also limited (ceiling effect) compared with morphine.[59] In addition, epidural use of these drugs is associated with sedation in 50% to 90% of patients.[20, 77] Combinations of agonist and agonist-antagonist drugs may help control bothersome side effects. One study[78] showed that 3 mg of butorphanol combined with 4 mg of morphine had fewer side effects with analgesia similar to that of morphine alone.

Subarachnoid Administration of Opioids

The direct instillation of opioids into the cerebrospinal fluid produces potent analgesia. In general, segmental analgesia after subarachnoid administration requires smaller doses than epidural administration because the drug is delivered directly to the cerebrospinal fluid and because spinal cord competition for drug absorption by epidural fat and epidural blood vessels is

Table 9–5 Characteristics of Epidural Analgesia

	TYPE OF OPIOID			
CHARACTERISTIC	**Hydrophilic**	**Intermediate**	**Lipophilic**	**Agonist-Antagonist**
Onset, min	Slow, 60–120	Intermediate, 15–25	Fast, 5–10	Fast, 5–10
Duration, h	Long, 8–24	Intermediate, 6–10	Short, 2–6	Intermediate, 4–10
Dermatomal spread	Throughout CSF	10–12 Dermatomes	5–6 Dermatomes	
Respiratory depression	Early, systemic uptake; late, rostral flow	Early, systemic uptake	Early, systemic uptake	Early, systemic uptake

CSF, cerebrospinal fluid.

avoided. The onset of analgesia is usually faster because the drug is delivered closer to the receptor.[79] Lipid solubility is the primary factor determining the extent and duration of analgesia with subarachnoid administration (Fig. 9–8). In the past, microcatheters were used to deliver continuous spinal infusions, but since the safety alert issued by the Food and Drug Administration in 1992, they are rarely used. Most subarachnoid administration of opioids is accomplished as a single bolus.

Most clinical experience with subarachnoid administration of opioids has been with preservative-free morphine. Studies[80] looking at 0.1 and 0.25 mg of intrathecally administered morphine have shown no significant change in the carbon dioxide response curve, making the risk of respiratory depression minimal with these doses. More lipophilic agents have also been used spinally, but they have a much shorter duration. The ratio of effective subarachnoid doses of morphine (0.2–1.0 mg) compared with the epidural doses (2–5 mg) suggests that there is fairly reliable dural transfer of about 20% when morphine is administered epidurally.[81] Fentanyl in small doses (6.25 μg) has been recommended as a routine additive to bupivacaine given spinally for cesarean section. The combination has been shown to improve the quality of intraoperative analgesia while providing 3 h of postoperative analgesia.[82]

Other opioids have also been evaluated intrathecally. Meperidine given intrathecally possesses opioid and local anesthetic properties and has been used either with local anesthetics or as the sole agent in doses of 0.5 to 1.0 mg/kg for urologic procedures, cesarean section, and inguinal and perineal operations. It has provided excellent intraoperative and postoperative analgesia for 6 to 8 h without respiratory depression.[83–85]

Subarachnoid administration of sufentanil (10 μg) combined with hyperbaric bupivacaine has been shown[86] to provide postoperative analgesia similar to fentanyl (compared with morphine). Intrathecally administered methadone (1.0 mg) appears to afford analgesia lasting only about 6.5 h for orthopedic or urologic operations, which is inferior to analgesia provided by morphine.[87]

Intrathecally administered morphine has an onset time of 30 to 60 min and a duration of 18 to 24 h. Intrathecally administered fentanyl has an onset time of 5 min and a duration of 2 to 4 h. Efficacy and side effects appear to be dose related. The goal with intrathecal administration is to use the lowest effective dose to limit the risk of side effects. Dermatomal spread of intrathecally administered morphine appears to be unaffected by variations in the volume up to 2.5 mL. Dextrose and isotonic saline have been used as the diluent without a significant difference, although one study[88] reported slightly longer analgesia when isotonic saline was used as the diluent. Pharmacokinetics of morphine and fentanyl suggest that they may be combined effectively, producing a fast onset time (from fentanyl) and prolonged analgesia (from morphine). The addition of local anesthetic also helps decrease the nociceptive stimuli coming to the spinal cord and may improve efficacy.

There are few long-term studies of the histopathologic consequences of applying opioids to the neuraxis. In their review article, Cousins and Mather[20] found no supporting evidence for spinal cord pathology in animals or humans after spinal administration of morphine. Coombs and associates[89] reported posterior column degeneration in two of seven patients who had terminal cancer treated with chronic intrathecal ad-

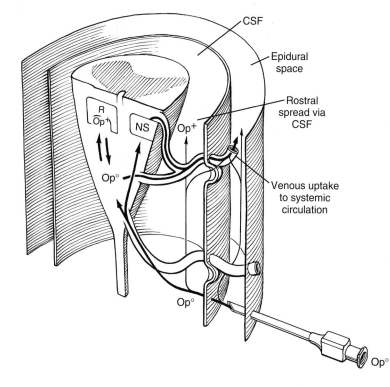

Figure 9–8 Distribution of opioids (Op) after subarachnoid administration. CSF, cerebrospinal fluid; NS, nonspecific lipid membrane binding sites; R, receptor. Vascular uptake occurs both in the subarachnoid space and on the spinal cord.

ministration of morphine. They concluded that the cause of these changes was obscure, but it seemed unlikely that the lesions were caused by the delivery system or spinal administration of morphine. The use of chronic intrathecal administration of opioids, although helpful in controlling severe chronic pain, must continue to be carefully evaluated.

Nonopioid Analgesics

Our understanding of nonopioid analgesia in the neuraxis is new and incomplete, but it is clear that there are several agents that can act additively or synergistically with opioids (Fig. 9–9). The α_2 agents, cyclooxygenase inhibitory compounds (nonsteroidal anti-inflammatory drugs), and local anesthetics have been shown to be synergistic when given with μ opioids. The δ and κ opioids are synergistic with α_2 agents. The κ opioids and cyclooxygenase inhibitors are additive.[34] There is no therapeutic cyclooxygenase inhibitory agent that can be given epidurally or intrathecally. However, studies by Yaksh and colleagues[90] have shown that nonsteroidal anti-inflammatory agents given orally, parenterally, or intravenously have activity at the spinal cord, where they help prevent prostaglandin-induced spinal sensitization.

Alpha₂-Adrenergic Agents

α_2-Adrenergic agents produce analgesia after spinal administration by presynaptic and postsynaptic mechanisms.[91, 92] Presynaptically, α_2 agonists release norepinephrine, which inhibits substance P release. Postsynaptically, they act directly to inhibit excitation of the substantia gelatinosa neurons. The primary analgesic site of α_2-adrenergic agonist activity appears to be spinal, because analgesia produced by clonidine, an α_2 agonist, is longer acting when injected epidurally than systemically. The α_2 agonists can cause cardiac depression and blood pressure changes. The hemodynamic

effects of α_2-adrenergic agonists are complex because of opposing effects at multiple sites; in the periphery, α_2-adrenergic agonists may increase blood pressure by direct postsynaptic vasoconstriction, and in the brain stem and spinal cord, they decrease blood pressure by decreasing sympathetic nervous system activity. As the dose of α_2 agonist increases, peripheral vasoconstriction eventually overwhelms the sympathetic effect, resulting in a biphasic response with decreased blood pressure at low doses and increased blood pressure at high ones.[93]

The site of injection of α_2 agents appears to be important. Spinal sympathetic effects are maximal at the anatomic sites of preganglionic sympathetic neurons. Consequently, α_2 agonists produce more hypotension when injected at thoracic dermatomes than at cervical or lower lumbar dermatomes. Blood pressure changes are more pronounced with spinal administration than with epidural administration. α_2-Adrenergic agonists act synergistically with opioids, and they enhance and prolong the action of local anesthetics.

α_2-Adrenergic receptors have been subdivided pharmacologically and genetically. At least three subtypes have been defined—α_{2A}, α_{2B}, and α_{2C}—but their anatomic and functional differences have not yet been determined.[94, 95] The α_2 receptors are coupled to G proteins and inhibit adenylate cyclase. α_2-Adrenoreceptor stimulation appears to affect potassium conductance and suppress calcium entry into nerve terminals.[93]

Clonidine and dexmedetomidine are two α_2 agonists that are undergoing clinical trials. Clonidine has a lipid solubility similar to meperidine. Analgesia after a bolus of clonidine given epidurally is brief, but continuous infusion can be used to prolong its effect. Clonidine has shown efficacy when combined with opioids in controlling neuropathic pain.[96]

Gamma-Aminobutyric Acid

Two forms of gamma-aminobutyric acid (GABA) receptors have been identified in the brain and spinal cord. $GABA_A$ consists of combinations of four types of subunits (α, β, σ, δ) and an active chloride ion channel. Clinical activity of the $GABA_A$ receptor depends on the various subunits that combine to form that particular receptor. The σ subunit is thought to confer benzodiazepine sensitivity. Barbiturates and propofol also interact with $GABA_A$, but the functional significance of $GABA_A$ subunit varieties has not been fully determined.[97]

$GABA_B$ is a transmembrane receptor that interacts with calcium. $GABA_B$ receptors have been located presynaptically on nerve terminals and postsynaptically in the brain and dorsal horn. Fifty percent of the spinal $GABA_B$ receptors have been associated with small diameter, primary afferent fibers. Baclofen, a drug used to treat spasticity, is active at $GABA_B$ receptors.

Midazolam can produce segmental spinal analgesia in rats and humans, probably by combining with a $GABA_A$ receptor complex in the spinal cord.[98] The use of midazolam to provide spinal analgesia is still limited,

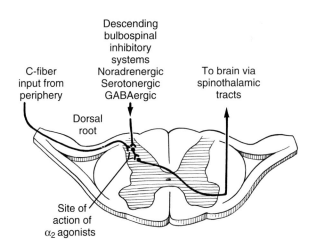

Figure 9–9 Cross section of spinal cord shows site of action of bulbospinal and α_2 systems.

and questions regarding the long-term safety of this drug in the neuraxis have not been answered. More studies are needed to assess the potentially efficacious interaction between spinally administered opiates and benzodiazepines.

N-*Methyl-D-Aspartate*

NMDA is a receptor linked to regulation of long-term neuronal potentiation in brain and spinal cord.[99] The NMDA receptor is a voltage-gated ion channel complex. When activated, Ca^{2+} enters the neuron, potentiating a host of possible interactions, including activation of nitric oxide synthetase. Nitric oxide has been suggested[100] to act as a retrograde neurotransmitter, modulating excitability and enhancing synaptic connection. NMDA is stimulated by excitatory amino acids, including glutamate. NMDA activation is linked to the production of hyperalgesia, allodynia, and long-term use-dependent changes in neuronal excitability, synaptic connectivity and strengthening, synaptic plasticity, and long-term potentiation.[101] NMDA involvement in multisynaptic nociceptive transmission and plasticity in the spinal cord leads to changes such as windup, facilitation, expansion of peripheral receptor fields, and central sensitization. NMDA antagonists, although not directly analgesic, may diminish postoperative pain by preventing the spinal sensitization and plasticity changes that can be produced after a noxious stimulus (e.g., operation) and that are thought to be NMDA mediated.

Ketamine is a clinically available NMDA antagonist, and other antagonists are being developed. Systemic administration of ketamine does diminish postoperative pain. There are concerns about the safety of ketamine for intraspinal use.

Summary

As our understanding of the various receptor interactions that modulate nociception grows, we can look forward to the development of more receptor-specific agents that minimize side effects. Toxicity issues are important, and much work still needs to be done before new therapeutic agents will be available.

References

1. Phelps R: Factors influencing perioperative parenteral narcotic analgesics. Probl Anesth 1988; 2: 362–375.
2. Pert CB, Snyder SH: Opiate receptor: demonstration in nervous tissue. Science 1973; 179: 1011–1014.
3. Behar M, Magora F, Olshwang D, et al: Epidural morphine in treatment of pain. Lancet 1979; 1: 527–529.
4. Wang JK, Nauss LA, Thomas JE: Pain relief by intrathecally applied morphine in man. Anesthesiology 1979; 50: 149–151.
5. Jaffe JH, Martin WR: Opioid analgesics and antagonists. In Gilman AG, Goodman LS, Rall TW, et al (eds): Goodman and Gilman's The Pharmacological Basis of Therapeutics, 7th ed, pp 491–531. New York, Macmillan Publishing, 1985.
6. Thorpe DH: Opiate structure and activity—a guide to understanding the receptor. Anesth Analg 1984; 63: 143–151.
7. Braenden OJ, Eddy NB, Halbach H: Synthetic substances with morphine-like effect: relationship between chemical structure and analgesic action. Bull World Health Organ 1955; 13: 937–998.
8. Kong H, Raynor K, Yasuda K, et al: A single residue, aspartic acid 95, in the δ opioid receptor specifies selective high affinity agonist binding. J Biol Chem 1993; 268: 23055–23058.
9. Fratta W, Yang HY, Majane B, et al: Distribution of beta-endorphin and related peptides in the hypothalamus and pituitary. Neuroscience 1979; 4: 1903–1908.
10. Rossier J, Vargo TM, Minick S, et al: Regional dissociation of beta-endorphin and enkephalin contents in rat brain and pituitary. Proc Natl Acad Sci U S A 1977; 74: 5162–5165.
11. Frederickson RCA: Endogenous opioids and related derivatives. In Kuhar MJ, Pasternak GW (eds): Analgesics: Neurochemical, Behavioral, and Clinical Perspectives, pp 9–68. New York, Raven Press, 1984.
12. Hedner T, Nordberg G: Opioid receptors: Types, distribution, and pharmacological profiles. In Rawal N, Coombs DW (eds): Spinal Narcotics, pp 1–31. Boston, Kluwer Academic Publishers, 1990.
13. Zamir N, Weber E, Palkovits M, et al: Differential processing of prodynorphin and proenkephalin in specific regions of the rat brain. Proc Natl Acad Sci U S A 1984; 81: 6886–6889.
14. Zamir N, Quirion R: Dynorphinergic pathways of Leu-enkephalin production in the rat brain. Neuropeptides 1985; 5: 441–444.
15. Zamir N, Palkovits M, Brownstein MJ: Distribution of immunoreactive dynorphin in the central nervous system of the rat. Brain Res 1983; 280: 81–93.
16. Yaksh TL: Multiple opioid receptor systems in brain and spinal cord: part 1. Eur J Anaesthesiol 1984; 1: 171–199.
17. Yaksh TL: Multiple opioid receptor systems in brain and spinal cord: part 2. Eur J Anaesthesiol 1984; 1: 201–243.
18. Basbaum AI: Endorphins and the control of pain: Anatomical studies of enkephalin and dynorphin. In Paton W, Mitchell J, Turner P (eds): IUPHAR 9th International Congress of Pharmacology, pp 359–365. London, Macmillan Press, 1984.
19. Martin WR, Eades CG, Thompson JA, et al: The effects of morphine- and nalorphine-like drugs in the nondependent and morphine-dependent chronic spinal dog. J Pharmacol Exp Ther 1976; 197: 517–532.
20. Cousins MJ, Mather LE: Intrathecal and epidural administration of opioids. Anesthesiology 1984; 61: 276–310.
21. Czlonkowski A, Costa T, Przewlocki R, et al: Opiate receptor binding sites in human spinal cord. Brain Res 1983; 267: 392–396.
22. Schmauss C, Yaksh TL: In vivo studies on spinal opiate receptor systems mediating antinociception: II. Pharmacological profiles suggesting a differential association of mu, delta and kappa receptors with visceral chemical and cutaneous thermal stimuli in the rat. J Pharmacol Exp Ther 1984; 228: 1–12.
23. Reisine T, Bell GI: Molecular biology of opioid receptors. Trends Neurosci 1993; 16: 506–510.
24. Yaksh TL: Spinal opiate analgesia: characteristics and principles of action. Pain 1981; 11: 293–346.
25. Zukin RS, Zukin SR: The case for multiple opiate receptors. Trends Neurosci 1984; 7: 160–164.
26. Bloor BC, Maze M, Segal I: Interaction between adrenergic and opioid pathways. In Estafanous FG (ed): Opioids in Anesthesia II, pp 34–46. Boston, Butterworth-Heinemann, 1991.
27. Yaksh TL: In vivo studies on spinal opiate receptor systems mediating antinociception: I. Mu and delta receptor profiles in the primate. J Pharmacol Exp Ther 1983; 226: 303–316.
28. Tung AS, Yaksh TL: In vivo evidence for multiple opiate receptors mediating analgesia in the rat spinal cord. Brain Res 1982; 247: 75–83.
29. Onofrio BM, Yaksh TL: Intrathecal delta-receptor ligand produces analgesia in man. (Letter to the editor.) Lancet 1983; 1: 1386–1387.
30. Vaught JL, Rothman RB, Westfall TC: Mu and delta receptors: Their role in analgesia in the differential effects of opioid peptides on analgesia. Life Sci 1982; 30: 1443–1455.

31. Yaksh TL, Malmberg AB: Interaction of spinal modulatory receptor systems. In Fields HL, Liebeskind JC (eds): Pharmacological Approaches to the Treatment of Chronic Pain: New Concepts and Critical Issues, pp 151–171. Seattle, IASP Press, 1994.

32. Mattia A, Vanderah T, Mosberg HI, et al: Lack of antinociceptive cross-tolerance between [D-Pen², D-Pen⁵]enkephalin and [D-Ala²]deltorphin II in mice: Evidence for delta receptor subtypes. J Pharmacol Exp Ther 1991; 258: 583–587.

33. Pasternak GW: Pharmacological mechanisms of opioid analgesics. Clin Neuropharmacol 1993; 16: 1–18.

34. Pleuvry BJ: Opioid receptors and their relevance to anaesthesia. Br J Anaesth 1993; 71: 119–126.

35. Schmauss C, Doherty C, Yaksh TL: The analgetic effects of an intrathecally administered partial opiate agonist, nalbuphine hydrochloride. Eur J Pharmacol 1982; 86: 1–7.

36. Ferrante FM: Opioids. In Ferrante FM, VadeBoncouer TR (eds): Postoperative Pain Management, pp 145–209. New York, Churchill Livingstone, 1993.

37. North RA: Opioid receptor types and membrane ion channels. TIPS 1986; 7: 114–115.

38. North RA: Membrane conductances and opioid receptor subtypes. NIDA Res Monogr 1986; 71: 81–88.

39. Zukin SR: Differing stereospecificities distinguish opiate receptor subtypes. Life Sci 1982; 31: 1307–1310.

40. Walker JM, Bowen WD, Walker FO, et al: Sigma receptors: biology and function. Pharmacol Rev 1990; 42: 355–402.

41. Su TP, Shukla K, Gund T: Steroid binding at sigma receptors: CNS and immunological implications. Ciba Found Symp 1990; 153: 107–113.

42. Grevel J, Sadée W: An opiate binding site in the rat brain is highly selective for 4,5-epoxymorphinans. Science 1983; 221: 1198–1201.

43. Aimone LD, Yaksh TL: Opioid modulation of capsaicin-evoked release of substance P from rat spinal cord in vivo. Peptides 1989; 10: 1127–1131.

44. Wood PL: Multiple opiate receptors: Support for unique mu, delta and kappa sites. Neuropharmacology 1982; 21: 487–497.

45. Roerig SC, Fujimoto JM: Multiplicative interaction between intrathecally and intracerebroventricularly administered mu opioid agonists but limited interactions between delta and kappa agonists for antinociception in mice. J Pharmacol Exp Ther 1989; 249: 762–768.

46. Taiwo YO, Levine JD: Kappa- and delta-opioids block sympathetically dependent hyperalgesia. J Neurosci 1991; 11: 928–932.

47. Stein C, Comisel K, Haimerl E, et al: Analgesic effect of intraarticular morphine after arthroscopic knee surgery. N Engl J Med 1991; 325: 1123–1126.

48. Khoury GF, Chen AC, Garland DE, et al: Intraarticular morphine, bupivacaine, and morphine/bupivacaine for pain control after knee videoarthroscopy. Anesthesiology 1992; 77: 263–266.

49. Sibinga NE, Goldstein A: Opioid peptides and opioid receptors in cells of the immune system. Annu Rev Immunol 1988; 6: 219–249.

50. Stein C: Peripheral mechanisms of opioid analgesia. Anesth Analg 1993; 76: 182–191.

51. Herz A, Teschemacher HJ: Activities and sites of antinociceptive action of morphine-like analgesics and kinetics of distribution following intravenous, intracerebral and intraventricular application. Adv Drug Res 1971; 6: 79–119.

52. Moore RA, Bullingham RE, McQuay HJ, et al: Dural permeability to narcotics: in vitro determination and application to extradural administration. Br J Anaesth 1982; 54: 1117–1128.

53. DeCastro J, Meynadier J, Zenz M: Regional Opioid Analgesia: Physiopharmacological Basis, Drugs, Equipment, and Clinical Application, pp 80-109. Boston, Kluwer Academic Publishers, 1991.

54. Nordberg G, Hedner T, Mellstrand T, et al: Pharmacokinetics of epidural morphine in man. Eur J Clin Pharmacol 1984; 26: 233–237.

55. Naulty JS, Datta S, Ostheimer GW, et al: Epidural fentanyl for postcesarean delivery pain management. Anesthesiology 1985; 63: 694–698.

56. Rosen MA, Dailey PA, Hughes SC, et al: Epidural sufentanil for postoperative analgesia after cesarean section. Anesthesiology 1988; 68: 448–454.

57. Bullingham RE, McQuay HJ, Moore RA: Unexpectedly high plasma fentanyl levels after epidural use. (Letter to the editor.) Lancet 1980; 1: 1361–1362.

58. Nordberg G, Hedner T, Mellstrand T, et al: Pharmacokinetic aspects of epidural morphine analgesia. Anesthesiology 1983; 58: 545–551.

59. Glass PS, Estok P, Ginsberg B, et al: Use of patient-controlled analgesia to compare the efficacy of epidural to intravenous fentanyl administration. Anesth Analg 1992; 74: 345–351.

60. Loper KA, Ready LB, Downey M, et al: Epidural and intravenous fentanyl infusions are clinically equivalent after knee surgery. Anesth Analg 1990; 70: 72–75.

61. Salomaki TE, Leppaluoto J, Laitinen JO, et al: Epidural versus intravenous fentanyl for reducing hormonal, metabolic, and physiologic responses after thoracotomy. Anesthesiology 1993; 79: 672–679.

62. Sjostrom S, Hartvig D, Tamsen A: Patient-controlled analgesia with extradural morphine or pethidine. Br J Anaesth 1988; 60: 358–366.

63. Eisenach JC: Epidural and spinal opioids. In Barash PG (ed): Refresher Courses in Anesthesiology, pp 65–79. Philadelphia, JB Lippincott, 1993.

64. Harbers JB, Hasenbos MA, Gort C, et al: Ventilatory function and continuous high thoracic epidural administration of bupivacaine with sufentanil intravenously or epidurally: a double-blind comparison. Reg Anesth 1991; 16: 65–71.

65. van den Hoogen RH, Colpaert FC: Epidural and subcutaneous morphine, meperidine (pethidine), fentanyl and sufentanil in the rat: Analgesia and other in vivo pharmacologic effects. Anesthesiology 1987; 66: 186–194.

66. Sosnowski M, Yaksh TL: Differential cross-tolerance between intrathecal morphine and sufentanil in the rat. Anesthesiology 1990; 73: 1141–1147.

67. Hug CC: Pharmacokinetics of new synthetic narcotic analgesics. In Estafanous FG (ed): Opioids in Anesthesia, pp 50–60. Boston, Butterworth, 1984.

68. Cousins MJ, Cherry DA, Gourlay GK: Acute and chronic pain: Use of spinal opioids. In Cousins MJ, Bridenbaugh PO (eds): Neural Blockade in Clinical Anesthesia and Management of Pain, 2nd ed, pp 955–1029. Philadelphia, JB Lippincott, 1988.

69. Basbaum AI: Mechanisms of substance P-mediated nociception and opioid-mediated antinociception. In Stanley TH, Ashburn MA (eds): Anesthesiology and Pain Management, pp 1–17. Dordrecht, Kluwer Academic Publishers, 1994.

70. Fromme GA, Steidl LJ, Danielson DR: Comparison of lumbar and thoracic epidural morphine for relief of postthoracotomy pain. Anesth Analg 1985; 64: 454–455.

71. Chaplan SR, Duncan SR, Brodsky JB, et al: Morphine and hydromorphone epidural analgesia: a prospective, randomized comparison. Anesthesiology 1992; 77: 1090–1094.

72. Brodsky JB, Chaplan SR, Brose WG, et al: Continuous epidural hydromorphone for postthoracotomy pain relief. Ann Thorac Surg 1990; 50: 888–893.

73. Coyle DE, Parab PV, Streng WH, et al: Is hydromorphone more lipid soluble than morphine? (Abstract.) Anesthesiology 1984; 61(Suppl): A240.

74. Kaiko RF, Foley KM, Grabinski PY, et al: Central nervous system excitatory effects of meperidine in cancer patients. Ann Neurol 1983; 13: 180–185.

75. Mok MS, Lippmann M, Wang JJ, et al: Efficacy of epidural nalbuphine in postoperative pain control. Anesthesiology 1984; 61(Suppl): A187.

76. Carl P, Crawford ME, Ravlo O, et al: Longterm treatment with epidural opioids: a retrospective study comprising 150 patients treated with morphine chloride and buprenorphine. Anaesthesia 1986; 41: 32–38.

77. Mok MS, Tsai YJ, Ho WM, et al: Efficacy of epidural butorphanol compared to morphine for the relief of postoperative pain. (Abstract.) Anesthesiology 1986; 65(Suppl): A175.

78. Lawhorn CD, McNitt JD, Fibuch EE, et al: Epidural morphine with butorphanol for postoperative analgesia after cesarean delivery. Anesth Analg 1991; 72: 53–57.

79. Chauvin M, Samii K, Schermann JM, et al: Plasma pharmacoki-

netics of morphine after I.M., extradural and intrathecal administration. Br J Anaesth 1982; 54: 843–847.

80. Abboud TK, Dror A, Mosaad P, et al: Mini-dose intrathecal morphine for the relief of post-cesarean section pain: safety, efficacy, and ventilatory responses to carbon dioxide. Anesth Analg 1988; 67: 137–143.

81. McQuay HJ, Sullivan AF, Smallman K, et al: Intrathecal opioids, potency and lipophilicity. Pain 1989; 36: 111–115.

82. Hunt CO, Naulty JS, Bader AM, et al: Perioperative analgesia with subarachnoid fentanyl-bupivacaine for cesarean delivery. Anesthesiology 1989; 71: 535–540.

83. Famewo CE, Naguib M: Spinal anaesthesia with meperidine as the sole agent. Can Anaesth Soc J 1985; 32: 533–537.

84. Patel D, Janardhan Y, Merai B, et al: Comparison of intrathecal meperidine and lidocaine in endoscopic urological procedures. Can J Anaesth 1990; 37: 567–570.

85. Tauzin-Fin P, Crozat P, Albin H, et al: Pharmacokinetics of pethidine after spinal anesthesia: clinical implications. (French.) Ann Fr Anesth Reanim 1987; 6: 33–37.

86. de Sousa H, de la Vega S: Spinal sufentanil. (Abstract.) Reg Anesth 1988; 13: 23.

87. Jacobson L, Chabal C, Brody MC, et al: Intrathecal methadone and morphine for postoperative analgesia: a comparison of the efficacy, duration, and side effects. Anesthesiology 1989; 70: 742–746.

88. Gray JR, Fromme GA, Nauss LA, et al: Intrathecal morphine for post-thoracotomy pain. Anesth Analg 1986; 65: 873–876.

89. Coombs DW, Fratkin JD, Meier FA, et al: Neuropathologic lesions and CSF morphine concentrations during chronic continuous intraspinal morphine infusion. A clinical and postmortem study. Pain 1985; 22: 337–351.

90. Yaksh TL, Vasco MR, Malmberg AB, et al: Central antinociception effects of nonsteroidal anti-inflammatory drugs. (Abstract.) Presented at the 7th World Congress on Pain, Paris, France, August 22–27, 1993.

91. Kuraishi Y, Hirota N, Sato Y, et al: Noradrenergic inhibition of the release of substance P from the primary afferents in the rabbit spinal dorsal horn. Brain Res 1985; 359: 177–182.

92. Post C, Arwestrom E, Minor BG, et al: Noradrenaline depletion increases noradrenaline-induced antinociception in mice. Neurosci Lett 1985; 59: 105–109.

93. Eisenach JC: Overview: first international symposium on alpha 2-adrenergic mechanisms of spinal anesthesia. Reg Anesth 1993; 18: 207–212.

94. Bylund DB: Subtypes of alpha 2-adrenoceptors: pharmacological and molecular biological evidence converge. Trends Pharmacol Sci 1988; 9: 356–361.

95. Harrison JK, Pearson WR, Lynch KR: Molecular characterization of alpha 1- and alpha 2-adrenoceptors. Trends Pharmacol Sci 1991; 12: 62–67.

96. Eisenach JC, Rauck RL, Buzzanell C, et al: Epidural clonidine analgesia for intractable cancer pain: phase I. Anesthesiology 1989; 71: 647–652.

97. Goodchild CS: GABA receptors and benzodiazepines. Br J Anaesth 1993; 71: 127–133.

98. Edwards M, Serrao JM, Gent JP, et al: On the mechanism by which midazolam causes spinally mediated analgesia. Anesthesiology 1990; 73: 273–277.

99. Collingridge GL, Singer W: Excitatory amino acid receptors and synaptic plasticity. Trends Pharmacol Sci 1990; 11: 290–296.

100. Lipton SA: Prospects for clinically tolerated NMDA antagonists: open-channel blockers and alternative redox states of nitric oxide. Trends Neurosci 1993; 16: 527–532.

101. Meller ST, Gebhart GF: Nitric oxide (NO) and nociceptive processing in the spinal cord. Pain 1993; 52: 127–136.

III

Induction of Regional Anesthesia

Equipment and Drugs

CHAPTER 10

Equipment

Joseph M. Neal, M.D., Dennis J. McMahon, B.S., C.B.E.T.

The practice of regional anesthesia is somewhat akin to great cooking. A successful recipe calls for equal parts art and science, a generous portion of patient- and surgeon-oriented finesse, a dash of good fortune, and effective regional anesthesia equipment and skills. This chapter addresses two aspects central to efficient performance of regional anesthesia—the induction room and the regional anesthesia equipment. The concept and design of induction rooms are discussed, along with monitoring issues and personnel requirements. The packaging and preparation of regional anesthesia equipment are explored, especially with reference to reusable versus disposable equipment, and specific concerns about needles, syringes, and nerve stimulators are addressed. Throughout the chapter, recommendations about specific products are avoided. If the anesthesiologist understands basic concepts of regional anesthesia equipment design, this knowledge enables the selection of quality equipment, regardless of the ever-changing world of manufacturers and new products.

The Induction Room

Concept of the Induction Room

Effective regional anesthesia practices most often designate an area within the surgical suite to prepare patients before entering the operating room (Fig. 10–1). This induction room markedly increases efficiency because it allows the patient to enter the operating room maximally prepared for completion of induction or start of positioning and skin preparation. Although not every hospital is able to have a designated induction room, almost all surgical suites have a holding area or some space that can be modified to facilitate

regional anesthesia. Besides block placement, a well-planned induction room serves other functions, including the early placement of intravenous access and invasive monitors. The induction room provides a central repository for anesthesia equipment and facilitates starting cases efficiently and minimizing operating room turnover.

The primary purpose of an induction room is to enable placement of regional blocks. A moderate amount of space, which is equipped with supplies and monitors, permits expeditious block placement in a relatively quiet, private atmosphere, away from the often frenetic pace of the surgical suite. Most regional blocks are safely performed in an induction room, although placement of hypobaric or hyperbaric spinal anesthetics is usually not advisable without extreme care during transport to the operating room.

A common criticism leveled at regional anesthesia, and therefore a frequent excuse not to use it in practice, is the time necessary to place a block. However, experienced practitioners perform blocks rapidly and efficiently, and anesthesiologists and surgeons often forget that time initially spent starting regional anesthetics is frequently compensated for at the end of the case, because the time necessary for emergence from general anesthesia may no longer be an issue. The induction room also can facilitate operating room turnover by enabling regional block placement while the operating room is being cleaned and restocked. Further advantage is gained by assessing block adequacy before the patient leaves the induction room, along with sufficient local anesthetic "soak time" while transferring the patient to the operating room. Significant psychologic advantage is realized by the anesthesiologist, patient, and surgical personnel when the patient arrives in the operating room sedated, anesthetized with a regional block, and ready for positioning or general

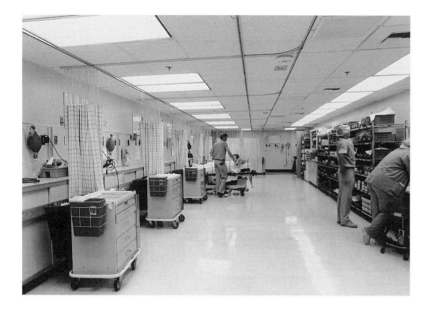

Figure 10–1 The Virginia Mason Clinic induction room.

anesthetic induction if a combined technique was prescribed.

Design of the Induction Room

Intelligent induction room design yields superior function, whether starting anew or modifying existing space. First, the strategically placed induction room is near the surgical suite's central command station and equipment storage. Second, induction room architecture should address workplace ergonomics, maintenance, patient care, and esthetic concerns. Third, well-planned storage provides immediate availability of essential supplies used on every case and intermediate availability of intermittently used supplies. Fourth, full resuscitation capability must be available.

Location Within the Surgical Suite

As patients enter a surgical suite, they often pass a central command station before being taken to a holding area or induction room. With the induction room nearby, clerical personnel can continue patient registration while the anesthesiologist or induction room personnel begin their preparations. The anesthesiologist can quickly access computer terminals for laboratory results or obtain controlled substances dispensed by the central command area. This convenient arrangement still affords patient observation. Information about the dynamics of case starts, completions, or changes is readily available to caregivers.

Proximity to equipment storage areas is essential. Commonly used supplies for intravenous access, monitoring, and regional anesthesia are readily available. Ideally, the induction room is also close to storage of equipment that, although not used routinely, still warrants easy access. For example, intravascular volume expanders, replacement batteries, or infrequently used airway items are not so far away as to create delay or inconvenience. Figure 10–2 illustrates the well-designed induction room's proximity to the central command area and storage.

Physical Design of the Induction Room

It is never possible to have a large enough induction room, but surgical suite floor space is valuable and scarce, and few areas have as much room as is desirable. Nevertheless, intelligent planning and use of the available space can result in smooth induction room dynamics. This section addresses issues of induction room design: space, storage, patient care, and maintenance.

The well-designed induction room meets three space needs: unobstructed to and fro movement of a patient's gurney; enough room to set up a regional block tray and minimal monitoring equipment; and space to permit unhindered movement of the anesthesiologist. As the floor plan enlarges, space considerations become

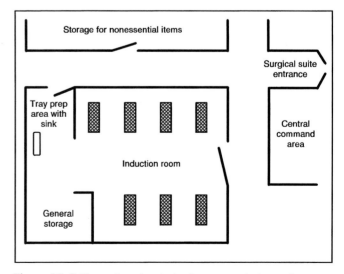

Figure 10–2 Illustration of an induction room relative to the overall surgical suite design.

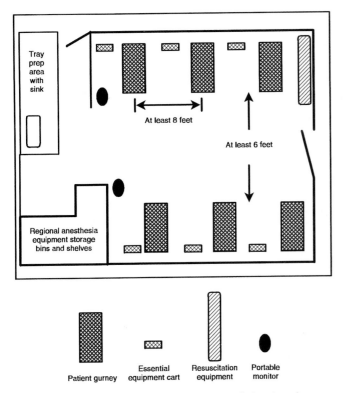

Figure 10–3 Illustration of an induction room design (not drawn to scale).

room design. First, essential equipment, such as intravenous access paraphernalia and basic monitors, is always stored near the patient (Fig. 10–4). Second, intermittently used equipment may be stored in the induction room but kept clear of patient stations and traffic patterns. Examples of general storage items include regional block trays, local anesthetics, and peripheral nerve stimulators (Fig. 10–5).

A well-designed induction room contains certain patient care items necessary for safety and comfort. Each patient station requires an immediately available oxygen source and suction equipment. Adequate electrical access must be properly modified to alleviate the risk of microshock. Each station and work area contains disposal bins for needles and sharp objects. Adequate illumination from overhead fixtures also features individual rheostat dimmer controls to avoid uncomfortable brightness in a supine patient's eyes. Also important is on-site, rapidly responsive temperature control. Care is taken to provide comfortable ambient temperature for surgical patients in gowns, not for scurrying anesthesia providers. To this end, warmed blankets are comforting to patients.

Hygienic functions, some essential and some merely convenient, must be provided. Essential equipment includes sterile and nonsterile gloves, protective masks and eye wear, and a lavatory used exclusively for hand washing. This sink must be separate from one designated for cleaning and maintenance, because splashing detergent may contaminate regional anesthesia equipment (Fig. 10–6). Facilities to package or sterilize (or both) nondisposable equipment may be located within the induction area.

Induction Room Esthetics

Preparation for an anesthetic and operation is stressful for the anesthesia personnel and patients. The induction room can be a safe haven or a house of horrors, depending on its design and especially on the attitudes and professionalism of those who work there.

more complicated. For example, if multiple gurneys are present, an individual patient station should be at least 8 ft wide with a 6-ft-wide aisle for unrestricted movement of personnel and other gurneys. Anesthesia carts on rollers fit between gurneys and are used for essential immediate storage and for a work top. Monitoring equipment is placed on portable carts or attached to the walls to save floor space. Figure 10–3 illustrates storage and space specifications of a typical induction room.

Two key concepts are important to overall induction

Figure 10–4 Essential equipment includes an anesthesia cart with a regional block tray on top, monitors, and resuscitation equipment. All equipment is at arm's length from the anesthesiologist.

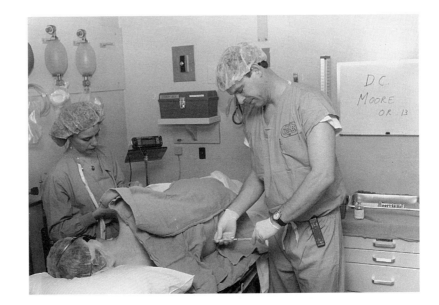

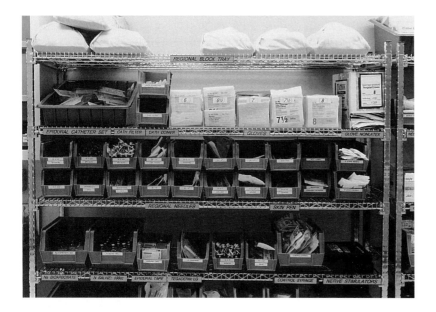

Figure 10–5 Storage for nonessential equipment is nearby but does not interfere with patient care. Shelves contain regional block trays, drugs, and bins with smaller items such as specific needles.

The ideal induction room provides the practitioner with a clean and efficient work area while allaying the patient's fear and trepidation.

If there is ever a place for genteel decorum in the surgical suite, it is the induction room. Respect for the patient's privacy and sensitivity to the patient's anxiety are crucial. The induction room experience is vastly improved by simple esthetics aimed at providing comfort, privacy, and freedom from experiencing unwanted and upsetting noise, conversation, and sights. All providers must exhibit their utmost professionalism in this setting. Loud talking, laughing, and "simply enjoying our jobs" may be interpreted by frightened patients as unnerving distraction generated by careless professionals. Recognizable conversation about patients or their conditions must never occur, and the patient's privacy is always protected. Pleasantly colored curtains, placed between gurneys and pulled, isolate patients from view. Cover patients' bodies for warmth and privacy,

especially during positioning for blocks. Dealing with partially uncovered patients receiving injections becomes so commonplace that we sometimes forget this is a scene infrequently encountered by the average patient. Calming posters of nature scenes or animals provide inexpensive diversion. These posters are best mounted on the ceiling, because patients are usually supine and staring upward.

Music has been a part of the surgical experience for nearly a century, beginning with live performances in dental and operating theaters.[1] Music exerts a calming or distracting influence on patients awaiting operation or undergoing medical procedures. A simple radio tuned to soothing music is inexpensive and readily available. Because tastes differ, patients may be encouraged to bring a cassette player and personal headphones for their own musical selections. Some institutions have installed individual audio systems that provide patients with their own volume-controlled

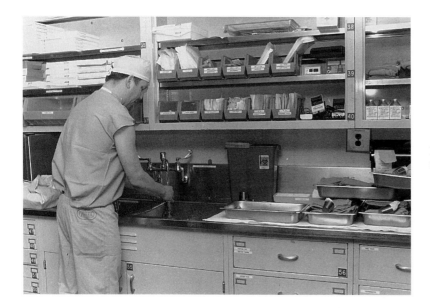

Figure 10–6 An anesthesia technician cleans reusable regional anesthesia trays.

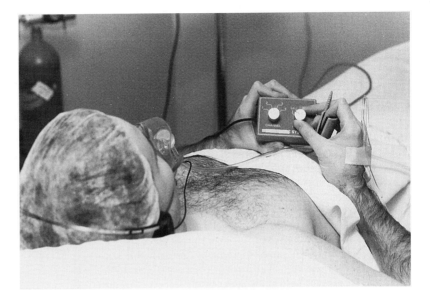

Figure 10–7 The music system allows each patient to select the musical style and control the volume.

headset. They can select from four or five general categories of music (e.g., classical, country, jazz, easy listening, top 40) from a centrally located continuous play compact disc player. Commercially available headsets can be wired into the induction room and individual operating rooms (Fig. 10–7). Proponents of surgical suite music, such as Thompson and colleagues at the Virginia Mason Clinic,[2] believe that music greatly alleviates anxiety during the entire perioperative period.

Place items within the induction room that enhance the practice of anesthesia providers. A telephone is especially useful if it has speakerphone capability. This feature allows the gloved anesthesiologist to depress the receiver button with an elbow, alleviating the necessity of regloving. A small library containing an atlas of regional anesthesia and a *Physicians' Desk Reference* is useful. Teaching and nonteaching settings benefit from skeletal models as guides for learning block placement. Charts detailing sensory dermatomes are also helpful if tastefully framed and out of the patient's line of sight.

Induction Room Storage

Each patient station requires an adjacent surface on which to prepare intravenous sets, to arrange a regional block tray, and to provide essential equipment for use in the induction room. Both of these needs are usually met by a mobile cart or cabinet, preferably with a series of drawers rather than open shelves. Shelves tend to collect dust and splashed liquid more readily than drawers, and drawers enable easier access to items commonly needed at each station. The induction room cart provides all essential equipment necessary for vascular access (i.e., intravenous, central, and arterial catheters), oxygen delivery, and delivery of a limited variety of medications and patient comfort items. Table 10–1 shows a representative inventory for an induction room cart.

For many years, carts for the induction room and anesthesia locations were purchased from the consumer market intended for general storage of tools and hard-

Table 10–1 Anesthesia Induction Room Cart Supply

SYRINGES, mL/G	**INTRAVENOUS SETS AND SOLUTIONS**
3/22	Standard set
5/21	Intravenous pump set
10/20	Lactated Ringer's
NEEDLES, G	Intravenous extension set
18	Intravenous plug
30	Stopcock, three-way
PHARMACEUTICALS	**OTHER**
Lidocaine, 1%	Alcohol wipes
INTRAVENOUS CATHETERS, in	Povidone-iodine solution
14 × 2	Povidone-iodine applicator
16 × 2	Benzoin tincture applicator
18 × 2	Towels
20 × 2	Emesis basins
18 × 1.25	O_2 masks
20 × 1.25	O_2 nasal cannulas
DRESSINGS AND MISCELLANEOUS	Needle recapper
Tape, 1 in	Sharps container
Gauze, 4 × 4 in	Syringe labels
Clear occlusive skin dressings	
Skin marker	
Tourniquets	

ware (e.g., Sears Craftsman carts). Various manufacturers have emerged during the past two decades who offer carts designed with the clinical setting in mind. These tend to have heavier-gauge metal, rounded corners and edges, more durable drawer support, replaceable plastic top surfaces, and various optional accessories including dividers, electrical power outlets, and monitor shelves. Different drawer sizes (i.e., 3-, 6-, and 12-in depths) can be mixed and matched to customize the cart to the user's needs. Most manufacturers also offer configurable drawer dividers that enable the user to customize each drawer to accommodate many small items. Although these carts tend to be more expensive initially, their added cost can be offset by longevity and flexibility. Appendix 10–1 provides a list of sources of carts for clinical settings.

Storage of general purpose regional anesthesia supplies is also an induction room function. Although the induction room should remain essentially a patient care setting, it often serves as a limited source of supplies for daily operations. It should not take on a warehouse atmosphere, and if possible, supplies should be deployed at one end or side of the room, out of view of patients. Good practice requires that medical supplies be removed from the external packaging in which they are shipped; bulk supplies of expendable items should be kept adjacent to, but not in, the surgical suite.[3] The same induction room standards apply to central supply departments. The area should have air circulation consistent with operating room standards, the temperature should not exceed 72° F, and the relative humidity should be no less than 35%. Sterile supplies should be stored a safe distance from the hazards of liquid splashes (i.e, sinks and any open containers of liquids), at least 8 in from the floor, and no closer than 18 in from the ceiling.[4] There should be no food or drink in the induction room. Realistic quantities of items should be stored in plastic or metal bins and replenished daily as needed. Regional anesthesia disposable items (e.g., trays, specialty needles, prepackaged sterile drugs) can be stocked on open shelves in appropriate quantities for average daily activity. Other items pertinent to an induction room are kept in designated spaces: disposable equipment for invasive monitoring techniques, accessories for difficult or unusual venous access, nerve stimulators and their associated needles, pulse counters, and patient comfort items.

Pharmaceuticals are stored in clean containers (i.e., metal or plastic cabinets or both) away from extremes of heat and moisture and in quantities realistic for weekly activity. Larger supplies of pharmaceutical items, such as bulk volumes of local anesthetics, can be kept in cabinets that ideally have doors to limit dust. All pharmaceuticals should be checked each month for out-of-date status. Because some drugs require storage at 2° to 8° C, a small (1.5 to 3 ft³) refrigerator is useful. It should be clearly identified for the storage of drugs only, to the exclusion of blood products and food. A thermometer is kept inside to monitor the temperature.

Emergency Equipment

Some anesthetic procedures performed in the induction room may be life threatening if complications oc-

cur. Rare complications of regional anesthesia include local anesthetic systemic toxicity, unintentionally high spinal anesthesia, and cardiac arrest. Any induction room must be equipped to provide resuscitation drugs and equipment on-site or readily available if there is an urgent need. Resuscitation capability requires oxygen, positive-pressure bag-valve masks, drugs for advanced cardiac life support, and equipment to secure an emergency airway (see Fig. 10–4). Drugs that may be considered unique to the induction room setting include barbiturates and benzodiazepines for local anesthetic-induced seizure control and succinylcholine for emergency airway control. Defibrillators and external pacemakers should be available within the surgical suite.

Induction Room Monitoring

Just as the induction room must be prepared for an unexpected anesthetic complication requiring patient resuscitation, it must also be equipped to monitor patients who are ill, sedated, or undergoing regional blocks. In large induction rooms, several patients may need to be monitored at once. This is accomplished cost effectively with portable monitoring devices, rather than equipping each patient station with expensive space-filling equipment.

Monitors may additionally serve a diagnostic role. Since Moore and Batra[5] first redefined the test dose to ascertain unintentional intravascular placement of an epidural needle or catheter, various devices have been used to determine beat-to-beat variation in the heart rate. Several options exist for this purpose. Portable battery-powered pulse counters that attach to a patient's finger or ear have largely replaced bulkier telemetry electrocardiogram monitors (Fig. 10–8). Pulse oximeters provide instantaneous pulse counting in addition to oxygen-saturation monitoring. The American Society of Anesthesiologists standards for basic intraoperative monitoring recommend pulse oximetry as routine monitoring during all anesthetics.[6] These guidelines extend to the sedated patient in the induction room who is undergoing regional anesthesia. If not available for every patient station, pulse oximeters can be mounted on movable stands and transferred from patient to patient. A few patients require more intensive monitoring in the induction room. For instance, patients undergoing epidural, celiac plexus, or other blocks that result in significant sympathectomy may require frequent blood pressure monitoring. Patients with cardiac disease benefit from continuous electrocardiogram monitoring. Rather than having these monitors available at each patient station, portable carts are available with equipment capable of monitoring blood pressure, pulse, oxygen saturation, and intravascular pressures (Fig. 10–9). This arrangement provides necessary services while conserving space and financial resources.

The Anesthesia Technician

The role of anesthesia technicians and technologists has gradually evolved to include various support func-

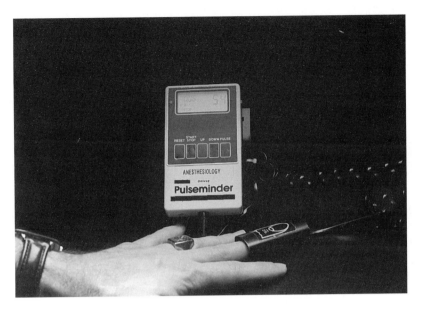

Figure 10–8 Pulse counter.

tions for safer and more efficient anesthesia practice. Although these functions are primarily focused at the anesthesia workstation, the anesthesia technician's duties in many settings include preoperative care of the patient, including checking in the patient on arrival, applying electrocardiogram electrodes and a blood pressure cuff, preparing the intravenous setup, assisting with invasive vascular techniques, positioning the patient during regional blocks, admixing medications under supervision, and assisting with transport of the patient to the operating room.[7] The anesthesia technician's presence adds a margin of safety and reassurance for the patient and expedites the preoperative stage of patient care for faster case turnover.

Anesthesia technicians have a wide spectrum of backgrounds and qualifications, and individual practices should decide the extent of anesthesia technicians' duties in the induction room. The training and certification of these allied health care personnel are being addressed by the American Society of Anesthesia Technicians and Technologists. Depending on resources and level of activity, the role of the anesthesia technician can be complementary to, but not in conflict with, the role of the induction room nurse.

The Induction Room Nurse

The induction room nurse markedly improves efficiency and cultivates good public relations in an active induction room. The induction room nurse is the primary facilitator and patient advocate. The nurse starts intravenous catheters, administers preoperative medications, fluffs pillows, and brings warm blankets. The nurse assists with regional block placement by positioning patients, administering sedative drugs under physician guidance, calming anxious patients, and helping the physician. The induction room nurse also keeps the room quiet and maintains the patient's privacy. Most importantly, the induction room nurse is the patient's advocate, allaying the patient's fears, explaining the reasons for surgical delay, and expertly handling any number of unanticipated events (Fig. 10–10).

Regional Anesthesia Equipment

The specialty of anesthesiology has always been concerned about safety, but little has been written specifically pertaining to regional anesthesia equipment. The

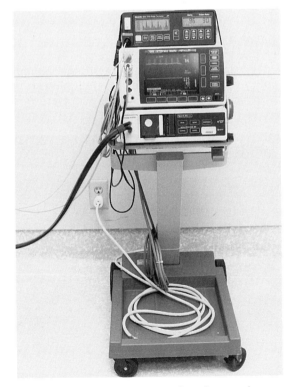

Figure 10–9 A portable monitoring pod can be moved among patients. (By permission of Spacelabs Corporation and Ohmeda Corporation, Division of BOC.)

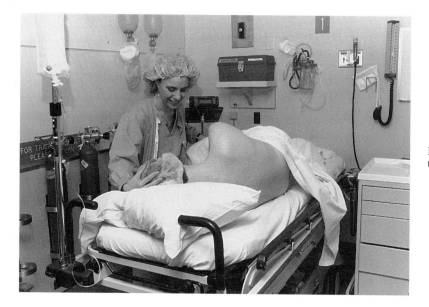

Figure 10–10 The induction room nurse is essential to efficiency and patient goodwill.

public may vaguely recall that spinal anesthesia was all but abandoned in the United Kingdom during the 1950s, but they may not be aware that this unfortunate occurrence was ultimately traceable to an equipment problem. The now-famous Woolley and Roe case was theorized to have resulted from chemically induced spinal cord injury secondary to mineral acids contaminating spinal anesthesia equipment.[8] Analysis of anesthetic accidents suggests that equipment failure is involved in only 4% of substantive negative outcomes and does not specifically incriminate regional anesthesia equipment as being a major contributor.[9] When the Canadian government tallied anesthesia-device alerts over a 5-year period, only one of six pertained to regional anesthesia equipment (i.e., small-bore catheters for continuous spinal anesthesia).[10]

After considering equipment safety, the anesthesiologist is presented with an array of choices for regional anesthesia equipment. Regional anesthesia can be elegant in its technical simplicity, but the manufacture, packaging, and maintenance of regional anesthesia equipment requires meticulous attention to detail. The selection of a particular piece of regional anesthetic equipment is often influenced more by advertising than literature-based evidence. This section discusses the setup and maintenance of regional anesthesia trays, especially regarding the choice between disposable and reusable options. Issues surrounding various needles, syringes, and peripheral nerve stimulators are presented, with practical emphasis on design controversies rather than a recommendation of specific products.

Regional Anesthesia Tray

Twenty years ago, regional anesthesia equipment was only available in single-item, multiple-use varieties. Disposable regional anesthesia sets were in their

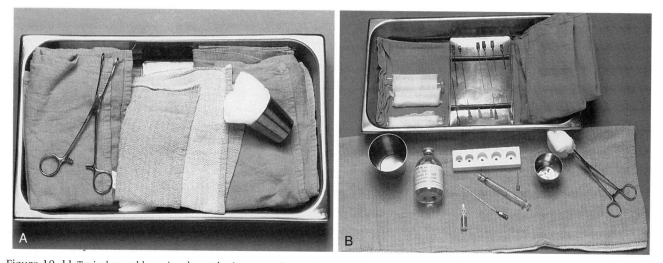

Figure 10–11 Typical reusable regional anesthesia tray. *A,* Top portion contains preparation and draping paraphernalia. *B,* Bottom portion contains assorted needles and syringes, saline for dilution or loss-of-resistance procedures, and epinephrine.

infancy and limited by questions of sterility, unacceptable variation in specifications and tolerances, and occasional problems with quality control.[11, 12] Disposable equipment is now manufactured to standards approaching those found with reusable options. For most practices, the choice becomes one of personal preference and cost. Reusable regional anesthesia trays offer the advantage of consistently excellent equipment that is customized to a particular practice's needs. Its disadvantages primarily pertain to the cost and quality issues of cleaning and sterilization. Practices that use regional anesthesia for 25% or more of their caseloads can usually justify reusable equipment.[13] Conversely, disposable regional anesthesia sets tend also to be expensive and to offer lesser-quality equipment, particularly glass "loss-of-resistance" syringes. However, the quality of disposable plastic syringes is constantly improving, and many manufacturers can customize disposable trays for an individual practice.

There is no evidence suggesting that disposable trays have fewer problems with sterility than reusable trays. One practice with a 65% regional anesthetic caseload performed an in-depth analysis of the options for anesthesia trays. The researchers determined that disposable trays and reusable trays were equally cost effective but that practitioners generally preferred the quality and customization of reusable equipment (Allen HW, Virginia Mason Medical Center, 1994: personal communication). Appendix 10–2 lists sources of reusable regional anesthesia tray components. Figure 10–11 illustrates a typical reusable regional anesthesia tray.

Components of reusable regional anesthesia trays are maintained and processed by anesthesia technicians or hospital central services. Cleaning occurs in an area designated for that purpose. Soaps, detergents, and chemical agents such as alcohol or phenol are not permitted in this area, because they may cause tissue damage if unintentionally left on equipment. Sterilization is best accomplished by steam autoclaving for 15 min at 121° C and 15 psi pressure.[14] Specific technical aspects of regional anesthesia equipment management have been addressed elsewhere.[13]

Needles and Catheters

Spinal Needles and Catheters

The anesthesiologist's choice of spinal needles is predicated on the following factors: disposable versus reusable, design of needle tip, needle diameter, and cost. Most available spinal needles are disposable and come in multiple gauges and tip designs, but their use is influenced by the inherent high cost of single-use equipment. The only commonly available reusable spinal needles are the 22- or 26-G Greene tips. This needle is three to five times more expensive than its disposable counterparts (1994 prices), but it generally lasts a year or longer and therefore is cost effective in busy regional anesthesia practices. Despite inherent concerns with sterilization, the Greene spinal needle was used for decades at the Virginia Mason Clinic without an adverse incident.

Developments in spinal needle technology have significantly changed the basic equipment for spinal anesthesia. The theory that noncutting-tip spinal needles spread rather than sever dural fibers, thereby decreasing the amount of cerebrospinal fluid leakage and decreasing the incidence of post–dural puncture headache, is not new. It was originally proposed in 1923 by H. M. Greene[15] and refined three decades later with the introduction of the pencil-point Whitacre needle.[16] However, not until the last decade did improvement in manufacturing enable mass production of relatively inexpensive needles with noncutting tips. Acceptance of these spinal needles, together with improved ability to produce smaller diameter needles, led to significant decreases in the incidence of post–dural puncture headache.[17]

Commonly used disposable Quincke, Whitacre, or Sprotte spinal needles are available in diameters from 22 to 29 G (Fig. 10–12). The Atraucan and Gertie Marx needles have undergone minimal peer-reviewed evaluation. The Quincke tip is the standard disposable

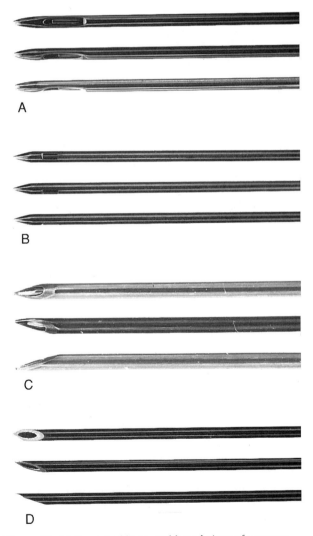

A

B

C

D

Figure 10–12 Frontal, oblique, and lateral views of common spinal needles. *A,* Sprotte needle. *B,* Whitacre needle. *C,* Greene needle. *D,* Quincke needle.

diamond-point needle found in most spinal anesthesia trays. Although inexpensive, even in smaller gauges, the needle may be associated with a relatively high incidence of post–dural puncture headache. The pencil-point Whitacre needle has a lateral orifice just proximal to the tip. The Sprotte needle is a modified Whitacre design with a more elongated pencil-point tip, larger lateral orifice, and larger internal diameter to promote the flow of cerebrospinal fluid.[18] Multiple studies comparing the Sprotte and Whitacre needles have demonstrated a similar incidence of post–dural puncture headache.[17] The Whitacre needle is one-half to one-third less expensive than the Sprotte (1994 prices).

Post–dural puncture headache develops in few children younger than 13 years of age, and the incidence in infants is unknown but believed to be small. Although noncutting-tip needles are available for pediatric patients, Quincke tips are recommended in newborns because the needles traverse dura smoothly with minimal bending.[19] Spinal introducer needles are also available in disposable and reusable forms (e.g., Pitkin introducer).

The technique of continuous spinal anesthesia with indwelling catheters has been used for decades. Tuohy[20] first reported the technique using ureteral catheters in 1944. Smaller-gauge catheters came into use in the 1960s,[21] and microcatheters (as small as 32 G) appeared in the late 1980s.[22] Two problems surfaced with continuous spinal catheters. First, microcatheters (27 G or smaller) were associated with frequent breakage, probably because their tensile strength is only 20% that of standard epidural catheters.[23] Second, episodes of cauda equina syndrome were reported[24] after some continuous spinal anesthetics with microcatheters. In these cases, the dose of local anesthetic given was larger than that normally used for routine spinal anesthesia, causing investigators to postulate that high concentrations of local anesthetic that pooled around nerves resulted in neurotoxicity.[25] The alleged association of spinal microcatheters with cauda equina syndrome led the Food and Drug Administration to prohibit their use in sizes of 27 G or smaller.[26] The use of larger catheters (e.g., 19- or 20-G epidural catheters) is still approved for continuous spinal anesthesia.

Epidural Needles and Catheters

Like spinal needles, epidural needles are available in reusable or disposable versions. The Crawford needle (Fig. 10–13) could be a component of reusable regional anesthesia trays and is most advantageous in practices that frequently perform single-shot epidural techniques, such as epidural injections of steroids. However, most practices exclusively use disposable epidural needles such as the sharp, curved-tip Tuohy or Hustead design. These often come prepackaged with compatible epidural catheters and skin dressing patches, may have etched gradations on the side for measurement of skin-to-epidural space distance, and may have fixed or disposable proximal flanges for improved grip. Sethna and Berde[19] reported favorable experience with 5-cm, 19-G epidural needles for infants and younger children.

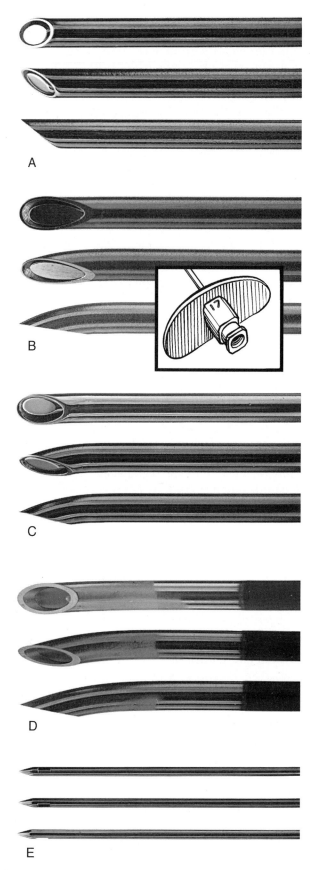

Figure 10–13 Frontal, oblique, and lateral views of common epidural needles. *A,* Crawford needle. *B,* Tuohy needle; the inset shows a winged hub assembly common to winged needles. *C,* Hustead needle. *D,* Curved, 18-G epidural needle. *E,* Whitacre, 27-G spinal needle.

Epidural catheters are made of nonreactive nylon, polyurethane, or silicone rubber materials. Available options vary in the number of distal orifices, presence or absence of a stylet, and catheter stiffness. Single, distal orifice catheters (Fig. 10–14) offer the advantage of placing all anesthetic solutions at the desired (and presumably known) location within the epidural space, but catheters with multiple side orifices (see Fig. 10–14) may result in greater anesthetic solution spread at the risk of injecting into areas other than the epidural space. No studies prove the advantage of one design over the other. Epidural catheters are available with or without a thin, metal wire stylet. Because the direction taken by soft catheters in the epidural space is unpredictable,[27] proponents of stylets claim improved directional control, although opponents are concerned with increased possibility of vascular or dural entry with a stiffer catheter. There is some evidence[28] that stiffer nylon catheters do result in more frequent epidural vein cannulation and dural puncture. Most epidural catheters are marked at centimeter intervals, enabling the anesthesiologist to ascertain depth of catheter placement initially and at follow-up examination. Pediatric epidural catheters are marked at 0.5-cm intervals.[19]

No convincing data are available to guide clinicians on when to remove an epidural catheter before risk of infection becomes significant.[29–34] Common practice suggests that 3 to 5 days is a standard, but many practices report leaving catheters in place as long as several weeks with daily follow-up. When even longer duration is desired for cancer patients, the Silastic Du Pen permanent epidural catheter is an example of a "permanent" catheter that can be used. It is tunneled through subcutaneous tissue from the epidural site to an injection port on the anterolateral abdominal wall.[35] Tunneled catheters decrease infection risk, improve patient comfort, and can remain in place for many months to more than a year.[32]

Specialized Regional Block Needles

The variety of peripheral nerve block needles is limited only by the imagination and budget of the anesthesiologists who promote their unique advantages. This section emphasizes the major attributes of regional block needles: tip design, length, gauge, and presence of a safety bead.

Perhaps the most commonly used selling point for block needles is the claim of decreased neural trauma,

even though the overall role of regional anesthesia in peripheral nerve injury is small.[36] Central to this argument is the theory that persistent nerve damage may occur during regional anesthesia from direct needle trauma or intraneural injection. Animal studies demonstrate anatomic damage to nerves traumatized by needles or injection of local anesthetics,[37, 38] although penetrating nerve with needle, even in a controlled setting, is difficult.[37] Human studies demonstrating nerve damage after intentional needle trauma[38] or axillary block technique[39] are less convincing, especially the often-quoted but statistically insignificant results reported by Selander and colleagues.[39] Moreover, no well-designed clinical outcome studies illuminate the possible association between injection trauma and perioperative nerve injury. Despite this general lack of understanding, manufacturers present arguments for choice between long-bevel (i.e., standard, sharp) needles and short-bevel (i.e., blunt, "B" bevel) needles.

Proponents of pencil-point[18, 37] or short-bevel designs[40] believe that blunt needles are less likely to injure and cut nerves. The direction a needle enters a nerve fascicle may also determine the extent of damage. Penetration with the bevel parallel to nerve fibers separates them and may cause less damage than transverse entry, which may cut fibers.[40] Short-bevel needles are often marketed specifically as safer instruments. Conversely, proponents of sharp-bevel needles think this design allows smoother passage through tissue planes and results in better control than the "popping" motion associated with blunt needles. They cite as supporting evidence difficulties with the study by Selander and colleagues[40] and animal data that suggest sharp needles may be less traumatic.

The report by Selander and colleagues[40] may be criticized on two points. First, although short-bevel needles were less likely to penetrate nerve fibers, when penetration did occur, the damage was more severe than with sharp needles. Second, Selander's group[40] evaluated only immediate changes in nerve fiber anatomy, although human electroneurographic signs of nerve damage are manifested not earlier than 1 week after injury.[38] Another animal study[41] suggested that sharp needles impale nerve fascicles less frequently than blunt needles, that the damage inflicted is less severe, and that reinnervation occurs more rapidly. One human study[38] suggested that delayed nerve damage is more likely to result from the chemical effects of intraneural local anesthetic injection than from mechanical needle damage. Neither side can point to outcome studies in humans that unequivocally implicate regional block needle design as a consistent factor in perioperative nerve injury.

The length and gauge of regional block needles are selected for the desired block. Deeper penetration, as for a celiac plexus or lumbar sympathetic block, requires longer (i.e., 5 or 6 in) and stiffer (i.e., 20- or 22-G) needles. Needles recommended for axillary block range from 5/8-in, 25-G standard needles to 1.5-in, 22-G short-bevel or pencil-point needles[18, 37] (Fig. 10–15). Some regional block needles have a safety bead integrated into the shaft design. This feature was originally

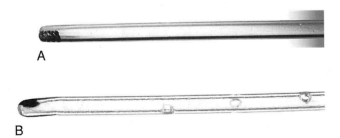

Figure 10–14 Epidural catheter designs. *A,* Single distal orifice. *B,* Closed tip with multiple side orifices.

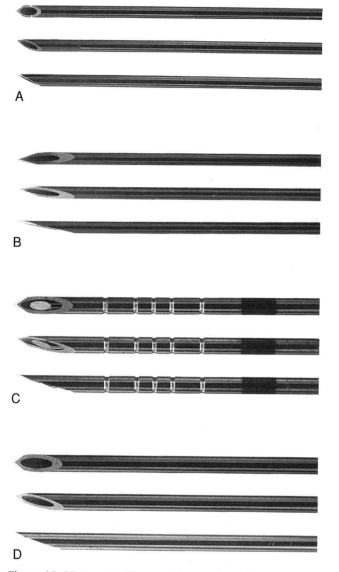

A

B

C

D

Figure 10–15 Frontal, oblique, and lateral views of regional block needles. *A,* Blunt-beveled, 25-G axillary block needle. *B,* Long-beveled, 25-G ("hypodermic") block needle. *C,* Ultrasound "imaging" needle. *D,* Short-beveled, 22-G regional block needle.

designed to ensure retrieval if the needle hub accidentally detached from the shaft. The protuberance also serves as a warning to proceed cautiously with blocks prone to contact vital structures, such as avoiding the pleural dome with supraclavicular blocks.

Syringes

The manufacture of syringes has improved in recent years, providing quality tools for regional anesthesia at reasonable cost. Precise-fitting, reusable glass syringes provide control and ease of operation which, until recently, were unattainable with disposable glass or plastic models. Although quite expensive, quality glass syringes are easy to clean and sterilize and provide years of service. Their smoothness of operation is unparal-

leled for loss-of-resistance techniques. Quality glass syringes consist of number-matched plungers and barrels with standardized Luer-Lok tip fittings for easy needle exchange. Their calibration markings are fused into the glass. Recently manufactured, single-use, plastic loss-of-resistance syringes perform nearly on par with their quality glass predecessors. The clinician may request that quality plastic syringes be included in customized disposable sets or may substitute them individually, as needed.

The well-stocked regional anesthesia tray should have at least four syringe models: a 1-mL tuberculin syringe for accurate measurement of epinephrine supplements, a 3-mL syringe for loss-of-resistance techniques, a 5- or 10-mL syringe (or both) for volume injections, and a 10-mL, three-ring control syringe (Fig. 10–16). The three-ring control syringe is extremely useful for the practice of regional anesthesia. It enables the clinician to function independently when performing blocks that require frequent aspiration. As with loss-of-resistance syringes, newer plastic versions exhibit quality and smoothness of operation comparable to more expensive glass models.

Peripheral Nerve Stimulators

The use of peripheral nerve stimulators in regional anesthesia is largely a matter of individual preference and is not consistently safer, faster, or more effective than paresthesia-seeking techniques. A peripheral nerve stimulator is never a substitute for proper anatomic block technique, but many anesthesiologists use peripheral nerve stimulators and find them valuable adjuncts to their practice. Proponents of peripheral

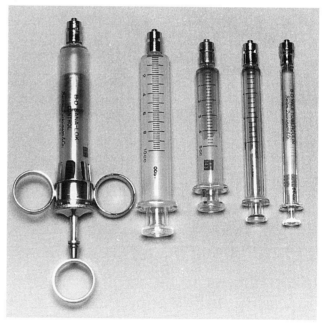

Figure 10–16 Reusable glass syringes. Left to right, Three-ring control syringe; 10-mL and 5-mL injection syringes; 3-mL loss-of-resistance syringe; 1-mL tuberculin syringe. (By permission of Becton Dickinson and Company.)

nerve stimulators claim more accurate placement of the needle, less risk of nerve damage, and enhanced ability to place a regional block in an uncooperative patient.[42, 43] In theory, the peripheral nerve stimulator facilitates the physician's ability to localize nerves,[43] but there are no data supporting improved outcome. Whether a peripheral nerve stimulator avoids paresthesia and decreases nerve injury is unknown, but the data reported by Selander and colleagues[39] suggest that, even when not being sought, paresthesia occurs in 40% of the cases when a needle is directed near a nerve. Peripheral nerve stimulators may offer an advantage in sedated patients, in patients impaired by drugs or alcohol, or in disease states such as uremia.[42] Although avoidance of intraneural injection is desirable because the resultant increases in intrafascicular pressure may cause neural ischemia,[44] use of a peripheral nerve stimulator does not guarantee protection from intraneural injection in the anesthetized patient.

Nerve stimulators designed for neuromuscular monitoring operate at currents much higher than necessary and are not recommended for peripheral nerve localization. Manufacturers market peripheral nerve stimulators that provide two separate ranges of current output and that can serve as a neuromuscular block monitor and for peripheral nerve location. Several models are designed solely for peripheral nerve stimulation. The ideal peripheral nerve stimulator should have the following characteristics: linear output; high and low outputs; a large, easily turned dial with digital display of actual current delivered; an identifiable polarity; a constant current output; a short stimulation pulse; and the ability to check the battery[45] (Fig. 10–17).

Insulated needles are preferred because they limit current output to the needle tip instead of along the entire needle shaft.[46] Insulated needles are available in various lengths, gauges, and bevel designs.[37, 43] Some incorporate tubing with a conventional Luer fitting to which a syringe can be connected. A list of sources for peripheral nerve stimulators is provided in Appendix 10–3.

The proper use of a peripheral nerve stimulator has been described elsewhere.[42, 43] Briefly, the anesthesiologist must check the battery and attach the negative electrode (usually black) to the needle. The positive electrode (usually red) is attached by an electrocardiograph electrode to the patient's body about 10 in from the area of stimulation.[47] Initially, the peripheral nerve stimulator is set at a 3-mA, 200-ms pulse duration and at one pulse per second. The needle is then slowly directed toward the peripheral nerve, using standard regional block anatomic guidelines. When contraction of the appropriate muscle is observed, the current is decreased to 0.5 to 0.1 mA, and the needle is adjusted to a point of maximum contraction with minimum current. A 1- to 2-mL injection of local anesthetic should result in a brief decrease in muscle contraction. The local anesthetic solution is injected to complete the process.

Conclusions

The well-designed induction room is close to the central command area and equipment storage areas of the surgical suite. All induction rooms require adequate space for the patient stretcher, essential equipment storage, and personnel movement. Essential equipment should be close to the patient, but less frequently used equipment is stored nearby without being in the way. Induction areas must be fitted with oxygen, suction, electrical, and climate-control facilities. Induction rooms also provide basic maintenance and hygiene functions, storage capability, monitoring, and necessary resuscitation equipment. The anesthesia technician and induction room nurse are invaluable members of the induction room team. The patient must have privacy and quiet, and professional decorum is expected from the staff.

Anesthesiologists in high-volume regional anesthesia practices often choose superior-quality, reusable equipment packaged in customized trays. However, the quality of some disposable equipment, particularly plastic loss-of-resistance and three-ring syringes, now rivals their expensive glass counterparts. The choice between reusable and disposable options is largely one of personal preference, because cost and quality are less difficult issues than in the past. Good-quality equipment may improve outcome. Noncutting-tip spinal needles have greatly decreased the incidence of post–dural puncture headache, but the contribution of regional block needle design to perioperative nerve injury or its prevention is less clear. Peripheral nerve stimulators are highly regarded by many anesthesiologists and offer advantages in selected settings, but no data are available that suggest their use improves outcome or limits complications.

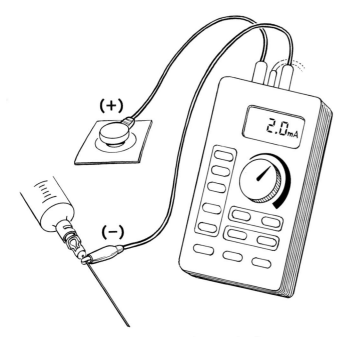

Figure 10–17 Peripheral nerve stimulator.

References

1. Podolsky E: Music as an anesthetic. Etude 1939; November: 706–707.

2. Thompson GE, McMahon DJ: Music and analgesia. In Kirby RR, Brown DL (eds): Problems in Anesthesia, vol 2, pp 376–385. Philadelphia, JB Lippincott, 1988.

3. Association of Operating Room Nurses: Standards and Recommended Practices for Perioperative Nursing, 1991; 3: 21–22.

4. International Association of Hospital Central Service Management: Central Service Technician Manual, 1986.

5. Moore DC, Batra MS: The components of an effective test dose prior to epidural block. Anesthesiology 1981; 55: 693–696.

6. American Society of Anesthesiologists: Standards for basic intraoperative monitoring, 1986, amended 1990; 1993. In 1994 Directory of Members, 59th ed, pp 735–736. Park Ridge, IL, American Society of Anesthesiologists, 1994.

7. McMahon DJ, Thompson GE: A survey of anesthesia support personnel in teaching programs. Med Instrum 1987; 21: 269–274.

8. Hutter CD: The Woolley and Roe case: a reassessment. Anaesthesia 1990; 45: 859–864.

9. Cooper JB, Newbower RS, Kitz RJ: An analysis of major errors and equipment failures in anesthesia management: considerations for prevention and detection. Anesthesiology 1984; 60: 34–42.

10. Gilron I: Anaesthesia equipment safety in Canada: the role of government regulation. Can J Anaesth 1993; 40: 987–992.

11. Eng M, Zorotovich RA: Broken-needle complication with a disposable spinal introducer. Anesthesiology 1977; 46: 147–148.

12. Seltzer JL, Porretta JC, Jackson BG: Plastic particulate contaminants in the medicine cups of disposable non-spinal regional anesthesia sets. Anesthesiology 1977; 47: 378–379.

13. McMahon D: Managing regional anesthesia equipment. In Kirby RR, Brown DL (eds): Problems in Anesthesia, vol 1, pp 592–601. Philadelphia, JB Lippincott, 1987.

14. Perkins JJ: Principles and Methods of Sterilization in Health Sciences, pp 163–166. Springfield, IL, Charles C Thomas, 1969.

15. Greene HM: Lumbar puncture and prevention of postpuncture headache. JAMA 1926; 86: 391–392.

16. Hart JR, Whitacre RJ: Pencil-point needle in prevention of postspinal headache. JAMA 1951; 147: 657–658.

17. Neal JM: Postdural puncture headache: prevention and treatment. In Eisenkraft JB (ed): Progress in Anesthesiology, vol VIII, pp 223–225. Philadelphia, WB Saunders, 1994.

18. Sprotte G, Schedel R, Pajunk H, et al: An "atraumatic" universal needle for single-shot regional anesthesia: clinical results and a 6 year trial in over 30,000 regional anesthesias. [German] Reg Anaesth 1987; 10: 104–108.

19. Sethna NF, Berde CB: Pediatric regional anesthesia equipment. Int Anesthesiol Clin 1992; 30: 163–176.

20. Tuohy EB: Continuous spinal anesthesia: its usefulness and technic involved. Anesthesiology 1944; 5: 142–148.

21. Bizzarri D, Giuffrida JG, Bandoc L, et al: Continuous spinal anesthesia using a special needle and catheter. Anesth Analg 1964; 43: 393–399.

22. Hurley RJ, Lambert DH: Continuous spinal anesthesia with a microcatheter technique: preliminary experience. Anesth Analg 1990; 70: 97–102.

23. Wissler RN, Blackshear RH, Bjoraker DG, et al: Tensile strength of spinal microcatheters. (Abstract) Anesthesiology 1990; 73: A505.

24. Rigler ML, Drasner K, Krejcie TC, et al: Cauda equina syndrome after continuous spinal anesthesia. Anesth Analg 1991; 72: 275–281.

25. Rigler ML, Drasner K: Distribution of catheter-injected local anesthetic in a model of the subarachnoid space. Anesthesiology 1991; 75: 684–692.

26. Benson JS: FDA safety alert: cauda equina syndrome with use of small-bone catheters in continuous spinal anesthesia. Rockville, MD, United States Food and Drug Administration, May 29, 1992.

27. Bridenbaugh LD, Moore DC, Bagdi P, et al: The position of plastic tubing in continuous-block techniques: an x-ray study of 552 patients. Anesthesiology 1968; 29: 1047–1049.

28. Rolbin SH, Hew E, Ogilvie G: A comparison of two types of epidural catheters. Can J Anaesth 1987; 34: 459–461.

29. Saady A: Epidural abscess complicating thoracic epidural analgesia. Anesthesiology 1976; 44: 244–246.

30. Strong WE: Epidural abscess associated with epidural catheterization: a rare event? Report of two cases with markedly delayed presentation. Anesthesiology 1991; 74: 943–946.

31. Fine PG, Hare BD, Zahniser JC: Epidural abscess following epidural catheterization in a chronic pain patient: a diagnostic dilemma. Anesthesiology 1988; 69: 422–424.

32. Du Pen SL, Peterson DG, Williams A, et al: Infection during chronic epidural catheterization: diagnosis and treatment. Anesthesiology 1990; 73: 905–909.

33. Hunt JR, Rigor BM Sr, Collins JR: The potential for contamination of continuous epidural catheters. Anesth Analg 1977; 56: 222–225.

34. Dawkins CJ: An analysis of the complications of extradural and caudal block. Anaesthesia 1969; 24: 554–563.

35. Du Pen SL, Peterson DG, Bogosian AC, et al: A new permanent exteriorized epidural catheter for narcotic self-administration to control cancer pain. Cancer 1987; 59: 986–993.

36. Kroll DA, Caplan RA, Posner K, et al: Nerve injury associated with anesthesia. Anesthesiology 1990; 73: 202–207.

37. Galindo A, Galindo A: Special needle for nerve blocks. Reg Anesth 1980; 5(2): 12–13.

38. Lofstrom B, Wennberg A, Wien L: Late disturbances in nerve function after block with local anaesthetic agents: an electroneurographic study. Acta Anaesthesiol Scand 1966; 10: 111–122.

39. Selander D, Edshage S, Wolff T: Paresthesiae or no paresthesiae? Nerve lesions after axillary blocks. Acta Anaesthesiol Scand 1979; 23: 27–33.

40. Selander D, Dhuner KG, Lundborg G: Peripheral nerve injury due to injection needles used for regional anesthesia: an experimental study of the acute effects of needle point trauma. Acta Anaesthesiol Scand 1977; 21: 182–188.

41. Rice AS, McMahon SB: Peripheral nerve injury caused by injection needles used in regional anaesthesia: influence of bevel configuration, studied in a rat model. Br J Anaesth 1992; 69: 433–438.

42. Horton WG: Use of peripheral nerve stimulator. In Kirby RR, Brown DL (eds): Problems in Anesthesia, vol 1, pp 588–591. Philadelphia, JB Lippincott, 1987.

43. Raj PP, Rosenblatt R, Montgomery SJ: Use of the nerve stimulator for peripheral blocks. Reg Anesth 1980; 5(2): 14–21.

44. Selander D, Sjostrand J: Longitudinal spread of intraneurally injected local anesthetics: an experimental study of the initial neural distribution following intraneural injections. Acta Anaesthesiol Scand 1978; 22: 622–634.

45. Ford DJ, Pither CE, Raj PP: Electrical characteristics of peripheral nerve stimulators: implications for nerve localization. Reg Anesth 1984; 9: 73–79.

46. Ford DJ, Pither C, Raj PP: Comparison of insulated and uninsulated needles for locating peripheral nerves with a peripheral nerve stimulator. Anesth Analg 1984; 63: 925–928.

47. Pither CE, Raj PP, Ford DJ: The use of nerve stimulators for regional anesthesia: a review of experimental characteristics, technique, and clinical applications. Reg Anesth 1985; 10: 49–58.

Sources of Medical Supply Carts

Armstrong Medical Industries, Inc.
Lincolnshire, IL 60069
(800) 323-4220

Blickman Health Industries
Fair Lawn, NJ 07410
(800) 247-5070

Blue Bell Bio-Medical
Blue Bell, PA 19422
(800) BLUEBELL

Harloff Manufacturing Co.
Colorado Springs, CO 80915
(800) 433-4064

Homak Manufacturing Co.
Chicago, IL 60632
(800) 874-6625

Lionville Systems, Inc.
Exton, PA 19341
(800) 523-7114

Milcare, Inc.
Zeeland, MI 49464
(616) 654-8000

Waterloo Industries, Inc.
Waterloo, IA 50704
(800) 833-4419

Sources of Reusable Regional Anesthesia Tray Components

Aesculap Instrument Co.
(forceps, needle holders)
Burlingame, CA 94010
(800) 258-1946

Baxter Healthcare *(trays, cups, forceps, needle holders)*
McGraw Park, IL 60085
(312) 473-0400

Becton Dickinson & Co.
(needles, syringes)
Rutherford, NJ 07070
(201) 460-2000

Havel's, Inc. *(needles)*
Cincinnati, OH 45227
(513) 271-2117

Popper & Sons, Inc.
(needles, syringes)
New Hyde Park, NY 11040
(516) 248-0300

Ranfac Corp. *(needles, syringes)*
Avon, MA 02322
(800) 272-6322

Vita Needle Co. *(needles)*
Needham, MA 02192
(617) 444-1780

APPENDIX 10–3
Sources of Peripheral Nerve Stimulators

B. Braun Medical, Inc.
Bethlehem, PA 18018
(800) 523-9695

HDC Corporation
San Jose, CA 95131
(800) 227-8162

Life Tech, Inc./Professional
Instruments
Houston, TX 77236
(800) 231-9841

Neuro Technology, Inc.
Houston, TX 77074
(800) 638-7689

CHAPTER 11

Intravenous and Inhaled Adjuncts

Ian Smith, F.R.C.A.,
Paul F. White, Ph.D., M.D., F.F.A.R.A.C.S.

Intravenous and inhaled adjuncts are frequently administered during local or regional anesthesia. The operating room environment may be frightening to patients, and many would prefer to be asleep or at least unaware of their surroundings. Adjunctive drugs can be administered to decrease anxiety, alleviate discomfort, improve hemodynamic stability, and induce a feeling of calmness. The use of a sedative medication allows patients to sleep through their operation, decreasing fatigue and boredom. Amnesia for the intraoperative period appears to be well received by most patients and many surgeons, while preventing unpleasant memories from influencing future behavior.

The injection of local anesthetic solutions is occasionally painful, especially when multiple injections are required into sensitive areas. Discomfort may also arise from traction on deeper structures and tissue planes as well as from the need for patients to remain immobile on a hard operating table. Finally, the surgical procedure may extend beyond the confines of the regional block or, with time, the effectiveness of the local anesthetic block may diminish. The use of supplemental, parenteral analgesics can prevent the initial pain of local anesthetic drug injection and may alleviate intraoperative discomfort unrelated to the surgical procedure.

It has become common practice to supplement local anesthetic techniques with various adjunctive medications to provide sedation, anxiolysis, and amnesia and to optimize patient comfort. These adjuvants can be delivered either intravenously or by inhalation. The degree of supplementation varies from case to case, depending on the needs and wishes of the individual patient and the nature of the particular surgical procedure. The level of sedation and analgesia may also need to be adjusted throughout the operation in response to changes in the degree of surgical stimulation. Adjusting the level of sedation to meet the current needs of the patient requires close contact between anesthesiologist and patient. Furthermore, many of the adjunctive sedative and analgesic medications are capable of producing profound cardiovascular and respiratory depression. When administered at higher doses, these drugs are capable of producing a state approaching general anesthesia. Careful monitoring and vigilance are required to prevent unintentional overdose. Because anesthesiologists are familiar with the titration of potent intravenous and inhaled drugs and are also skilled in patient monitoring, provision of analgesia, and airway management, they are ideally suited to provide patient care in these circumstances. The combination of patient monitoring and administration of adjunctive sedative-analgesic medications has become known as *monitored anesthesia care* in the United States and *sedoanalgesia* in the United Kingdom.

The American Society of Anesthesiologists has defined monitored anesthesia care as: "instances in which an anesthesiologist has been called upon to provide specific anesthesia services to a particular patient undergoing a planned procedure, in connection with which a patient receives local anesthesia or, in some cases, no anesthesia at all. In such a case, an anesthesiologist is providing specific services to the patient and is in control of his or her vital signs, and is available to administer anesthetics or provide other medical care as appropriate."

Although the systemic use of sedative and analgesic drugs in combination with local anesthesia is safe and effective, there is always the possibility of unanticipated complications and adverse drug interactions. As with general anesthetic techniques, preexisting medical conditions and chronic medication can influence the planned anesthetic technique and modify the individual patient's response to adjunctive medications during local and regional anesthesia. It is, therefore, the policy of the American Society of Anesthesiologists that any monitored anesthesia care procedure should include the following features:

1. Performance of a preoperative examination and evaluation
2. Prescription of the necessary anesthetic care
3. Personal participation in or medical direction of the plan of care
4. Continuous physical presence of the anesthesiologist or the resident or the nurse anesthetist being medically directed by an anesthesiologist
5. Proximate presence or immediate availability (in the case of medical direction) of the anesthesiologist for diagnosis or treatment of emergencies

Intravenous Medications

Intravenous injection is the most common route of administration of adjunctive sedative and analgesic medications. Intravenous administration results in a more predictable dose-effect relationship than intramuscular or oral administration. In contrast, delivery of drugs by inhalation requires a tight-fitting breathing circuit in order to deliver an effective concentration and to prevent pollution of the operating room environment. Furthermore, the pungent smell of volatile agents can irritate the airway and cause coughing.

The most popular intravenous adjuvants are the sedative-hypnotics (some of which also possess amnestic properties) and analgesics. Some drugs (e.g., ketamine, butorphanol) possess both sedative and analgesic-like properties. In addition, sympatholytic drugs are used as supplements to enhance sedation or to control hemodynamic responses. Finally, the benzodiazepine and opioid analgesic medications can have their effects terminated by specific competitive antagonists.

Sedative-Hypnotics: Benzodiazepines

The benzodiazepines are commonly used as sedative agents because of their wide spectrum of central nervous system activity, ease of administration, low incidence of side effects, and relatively high safety margin. All benzodiazepines possess similar pharmacologic properties, including anxiolysis, various degrees of amnesia, and dose-dependent sedation. Individual drugs in this class vary with respect to their potency as well as in their duration of action.

Diazepam is the prototypical compound and was previously popular as an oral or a parenteral sedative agent. However, diazepam has a prolonged duration of clinical effect, partially as a result of its slow metabolism and the presence of active metabolites (e.g., desmethyldiazepam) and enterohepatic recirculation. Even when patients appear to be awake after receiving diazepam, subclinical effects on subjective feelings and cognitive function may persist for several hours. Simulated driving skills have been shown to be impaired for up to 10 h after a single intravenous dose of diazepam (0.3 to 0.45 mg·kg^{-1}).[1] In elderly patients (diazepam is

often selected for local and regional anesthetic techniques because of concerns over recovery), the effects of diazepam may be even more prolonged. Diazepam is also insoluble in water, requiring an organic solvent (e.g., propylene glycol) to produce a stable intravenous solution. Such a solubilizing agent can produce a high incidence of venous irritation and phlebitis after intravenous injection. These undesirable properties are decreased if diazepam is solubilized in a lipid emulsion. This solution (Diazemuls) is commercially available in Europe but not in the United States.

Currently, midazolam is the benzodiazepine most frequently used for intravenous sedation. In contrast to diazepam, midazolam is water-soluble and does not cause pain on injection or venous irritation. Midazolam has a rapid onset of action and a short elimination half-life (2 to 4 h), and does not give rise to active metabolites. There is also no enterohepatic recirculation of the excreted drug, resulting in a predictable recovery after a single bolus dose of midazolam. Midazolam is more potent than diazepam and possesses a steeper dose-response curve (Fig. 11–1), so that the relative sedative potency of these two drugs varies depending on the clinical end point one is trying to achieve. Failure to recognize this difference in potency resulted in frequent overdosage when midazolam was first introduced. As with any potent drug, careful titration of midazolam to the desired clinical end point minimizes its side effects and decreases the likelihood of overdosage.

Midazolam also produces more profound perioperative amnesia and sedation than diazepam,[2] making it highly suitable for use as an adjuvant during local anesthesia. Despite the more rapid recovery from the sedative-hypnotic effects of midazolam (compared with diazepam), the use of higher doses of midazolam (e.g., ≥0.2 mg·kg^{-1}) or prolonged administration can still result in residual postoperative sedation and amnesia, thereby delaying recovery. Consequently, there has

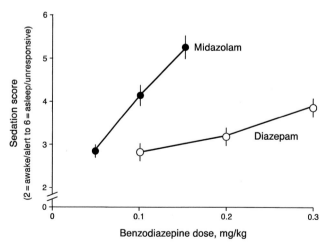

Figure 11–1 Relationship between the sedation score (2 = awake/alert to 6 = asleep/unresponsive) and the initial dose of midazolam or diazepam. Values represent mean ± standard error of the mean. (Data from White PF, Vasconez LO, Mathes SA, et al: Comparison of midazolam and diazepam for sedation during plastic surgery. Plast Reconstr Surg 1988; 81: 703–710.)

been considerable interest in finding alternative sedative agents that permit a rapid recovery after prolonged administration.

Intravenous Anesthetics

General Description

All intravenous anesthetic agents can be administered in low doses to provide sedation. The primary advantage in using decreased doses of the intravenous anesthetics is more rapid recovery from the residual sedative effects of these medications compared with the benzodiazepines. However, the therapeutic window between sedation and hypnosis (unconsciousness) is much smaller than with benzodiazepines, so that greater vigilance is required if intravenous anesthetics are to be administered safely for sedation.

The most useful anesthetic agents for providing sedation are those with a short duration of action. A continuous infusion of methohexital, 180 mg•h^{-1}, to supplement regional anesthesia produced acceptable intraoperative conditions with decreased postoperative impairment of psychomotor function compared with midazolam, 7.5 mg•h^{-1}. Methohexital was also associated with fewer intraoperative episodes of hemoglobin oxygen (O_2) desaturation than midazolam. In the same study population, etomidate, 32 mg•h^{-1}, also resulted in less psychomotor depression than midazolam, but it was associated with a higher incidence of pain on injection and postoperative nausea than either of the other two sedative-hypnotics.[3] Compared with the intravenous anesthetics, midazolam produced more reliable amnesia for intraoperative events. Despite poorer performance on postoperative paper and pencil tests as well as more residual sedation (as rated by an observer), the use of midazolam did not delay the dismissal of patients from the recovery area.

Propofol

Propofol has become popular as an intravenous anesthetic for brief outpatient procedures because of its favorable pharmacokinetic profile and low incidence of postoperative side effects. As a result of its rapid redistribution and high clearance rate, recovery from the sedative-hypnotic effects of propofol is rapid after single bolus doses as well as after more prolonged administration by continuous infusion. In addition to permitting rapid recovery after discontinuation of a propofol infusion, its pharmacokinetic and pharmacodynamic profile also allows for rapid responsiveness to changes in the rate of delivery. Finally, propofol is associated with a low incidence of perioperative side effects, particularly nausea and vomiting. These advantages of propofol are equally applicable when it is used in low doses to provide sedation or higher doses to produce hypnosis (or anesthesia).

During orthopedic surgery performed with regional anesthesia, a mean infusion rate of 3.8 mg•kg^{-1}•h^{-1} resulted in patients who were asleep but arousable to command.[4] The desired sedative level was reported to be easy to maintain by titrating the infusion rate, and recovery was rapid after completion of the operation. Within 4 min of discontinuing the propofol infusion, patients were awake and rapidly became clearheaded. Constant infusions of propofol, 0.5 to 4 mg•kg^{-1}•h^{-1}, produced dose-dependent increases in the level of sedation during urologic surgery with regional anesthesia (Fig. 11–2).[5] Recovery was rapid after each of the chosen doses. Optimal sedation in this elderly male population appeared to be achieved with a 2 mg•kg^{-1}•h^{-1} propofol infusion. However, titration is necessary because of the inherent pharmacokinetic and pharmacodynamic variability among patients.

Several investigators have compared propofol with midazolam for sedative use during local and regional anesthesia. Propofol, 3.7 mg•kg^{-1}•h^{-1}, and midazolam, 0.27 mg•kg^{-1}•h^{-1}, produced comparable levels of sedation during spinal anesthesia, but awakening was significantly faster after discontinuation of propofol (2 and 9 min, respectively).[6] Midazolam also resulted in impaired psychomotor function for up to 2 h postoperatively, whereas propofol produced no clinically demonstrable effect. Patients receiving midazolam, 0.04 mg•kg^{-1}•h^{-1}, required up to 2 h for full recovery, compared with 15 min after propofol, 2.65 mg•kg^{-1}•h^{-1}.[7] White and Negus[8] reported that titration of a sedative infusion was easier with propofol compared with midazolam and resulted in a lower incidence of oversedation. These authors also demonstrated decreased levels

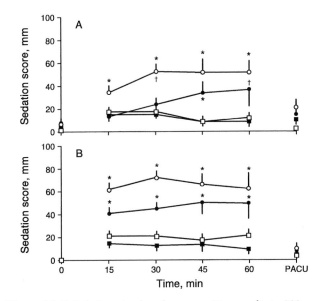

Figure 11–2 Sedation visual analog scores (0 = awake to 100 = almost asleep) recorded by patients (A) and by a blinded observer (B) before (time 0), during, and after postanesthesia care unit (PACU) sedation with propofol. Patients received propofol: 0.2 mg•kg^{-1} and 8 µg•kg^{-1}•min^{-1} (group 1, solid squares); 0.4 mg•kg^{-1} and 17 µg•kg^{-1}•min^{-1} (group 2, open squares); 0.5 mg•kg^{-1} and 33 µg•kg^{-1}•min^{-1} (group 3, solid circles); and 0.7 mg•kg^{-1} and 67 µg•kg^{-1}•min^{-1} (group 4, open circles). Values represent mean ± standard error of the mean. *$P < .05$ compared with group 1. †$P < .05$ compared with 15-min value in same group. (Data from Smith I, Monk TG, White PF, et al: Propofol infusion during regional anesthesia: sedative, amnestic, and anxiolytic properties. Anesth Analg 1994; 79: 313–319.)

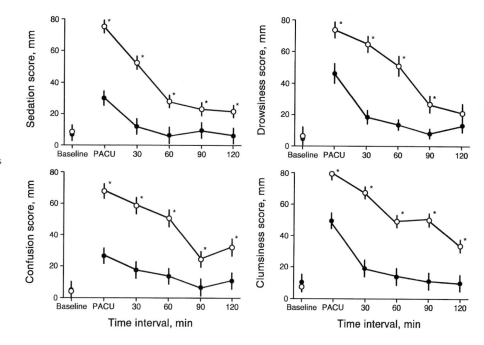

Figure 11–3 Perioperative sedation, drowsiness, confusion, and clumsiness visual analog scores (0 = minimal to 100 = maximal) for patients receiving either midazolam (open circles) or propofol (solid circles) during operation with local or regional anesthesia. Values represent median ± standard error of the mean. *P < .05 compared with propofol group. PACU, postanesthesia care unit. (Data from White PF, Negus JB: Sedative infusions during local and regional anesthesia: a comparison of midazolam and propofol. J Clin Anesth 1991; 3: 32–39.)

of postoperative sedation, drowsiness, confusion, clumsiness, and amnesia with propofol (Fig. 11–3).

Single bolus injections of propofol can also provide more satisfactory sedation during the injection of local anesthetic blocks compared with methohexital or midazolam.[9] Bolus doses of propofol, 0.5 mg•kg^{-1}, methohexital, 0.45 mg•kg^{-1}, and midazolam, 20 µg•kg^{-1}, all produced acceptable patient comfort during the injection of a retrobulbar or peribulbar block. However, propofol was most likely to prevent recall of the injection.[9] During upper gastrointestinal endoscopy, satisfactory conditions and complete amnesia for the diagnostic procedure were achieved with an average propofol infusion rate of 4.3 mg•kg^{-1}•h^{-1}.[10] Compared with midazolam, recovery was more rapid and fewer "hangover effects" were reported when propofol was used as the sole sedative agent for upper gastrointestinal endoscopy.[11] When propofol is used for endoscopy, it should be administered by an anesthesiologist (or someone under an anesthesiologist's direct supervision) and not by the surgeon or physician performing the endoscopy.

A further advantage resulting from the use of propofol for monitored anesthesia care is that it is associated with a low incidence of perioperative side effects. Low doses of propofol produce minimal depression of cardiovascular or respiratory systems, and involuntary movements and excitatory effects are rarely observed. The incidence of postoperative nausea is low after propofol sedation as a result of its antiemetic properties.[12] Low-dose infusions of propofol do not have any adverse subjective effects and can actually elevate the patient's mood (e.g., euphorigenic-like properties), which may be beneficial during the perioperative period.[13]

Compared with midazolam, amnesia for intraoperative events appears to be less marked with propofol.[5, 6, 8, 14] Amnesia does not appear to be reliably produced

by subhypnotic doses of propofol.[5] However, the incidence of intraoperative recall is decreased with increasing doses of propofol.[5] Nevertheless, the amnesia produced by propofol appears to be less profound than that achieved with midazolam and is less likely to persist into the early postoperative period. This has the advantage that patients are more likely to remember important postoperative information and instructions. For some patients, the transient memory loss in the postoperative period is very disturbing.

Analgesics

Although the local or regional anesthetic technique should provide pain relief for the surgical dissection, supplemental analgesia may be required for discomfort not directly related to the surgical incision. For example, during the initial injection of local anesthetic there may be discomfort related to the needle puncture(s) or injection of the local anesthetic solution. Although intravenous analgesia is not an acceptable alternative to an inadequate local anesthetic block, supplemental sedation and analgesia may be beneficial when the surgical field extends into deeper areas not anesthetized. There are also certain operations (e.g., transvaginal ovum retrieval) in which a local anesthetic block is impractical. Such procedures can be satisfactorily managed by a combination of systemic sedative and analgesic drugs. In addition, systemically acting analgesics may relieve the discomfort arising from pressure and traction on deep structures not directly affected by the local anesthetic solution. Analgesia may also be required to assist patients in remaining immobile for prolonged times on hard surfaces and to decrease the discomfort caused by the tourniquet required for intravenous regional anesthesia.

Ketamine

Ketamine is a phencyclidine derivative that can produce a dissociative anesthetic state characterized by profound analgesia. In lower (subanesthetic) doses, ketamine retains its analgesic properties and may also produce a useful degree of sedation without clinically significant respiratory depression. Ketamine, 0.25 to 0.75 mg•kg^{-1} given intravenously, produced satisfactory analgesia during the injection of large volumes of dilute local anesthetic solutions in the head and neck region in patients premedicated with midazolam.[2] The analgesia resulting from this dose of ketamine may also prove beneficial in the event of an incomplete local anesthetic block.

When administered alone, ketamine frequently produces unpleasant emergence phenomena and is also associated with a high incidence of other excitatory side effects. These undesirable properties can be prevented by the coadministration of benzodiazepines. In addition, this combination can result in enhanced sedation, amnesia, and improved cardiovascular stability. Propofol has also been reported to have a similar beneficial effect when coadministered with ketamine.[15] However, even when used as a supplement to other sedative-hypnotic drugs, ketamine still results in a high incidence of undesirable intraoperative movements, restlessness, dreaming, and postoperative confusion.[16] Furthermore, awakening and orientation may be delayed compared with alternative techniques.[15]

Opioid Analgesics

In isolation, the opioid analgesics do not produce reliable sedation in the absence of clinically significant ventilatory depression. However, these drugs are commonly used for the specific purpose of providing supplemental analgesia. Although analgesic doses of opioids alone produce minimal sedation, they are synergistic with sedative-hypnotics and can produce highly satisfactory conditions for surgery during local anesthesia. Furthermore, combinations of midazolam-alfentanil and fentanyl-propofol provided highly acceptable intraoperative conditions during extracorporeal shock wave lithotripsy for renal calculi compared with an epidural-based technique.[17] Postoperative recovery after these intravenous sedative-analgesic techniques was significantly faster compared with epidural anesthesia.

Opioid analgesics are associated with various well-known undesirable perioperative side effects, including respiratory depression, pruritus, and an increased incidence of nausea and vomiting. Respiratory depression is clearly the most dangerous of these adverse events. Administration of fentanyl, 2 μg•kg^{-1}, produced hypoxemia (defined as oxyhemoglobin saturation [Spo_2] <90%) in 50% of a group of healthy volunteers.[18] In contrast, no significant respiratory effects were observed with midazolam, 0.05 mg•kg^{-1}, in the same subjects. Combinations of opioid analgesics and benzodiazepines may be particularly dangerous because of their synergistic interactions. The combination of fentanyl, 2.0 μg•kg^{-1}, and midazolam, 0.05 mg•kg^{-1}, produced hypoxemia in 92% of the subjects and apnea (lasting at least 15 s) in 50%.[18] Similar synergistic interactions have been responsible for some fatalities reported after sedation techniques involving midazolam when it was initially introduced into clinical practice. The use of supplemental O_2 and adequate monitoring of respiratory function and hemoglobin O_2 saturation are clearly necessary when benzodiazepine-opioid combinations are administered during local and regional anesthesia.

There is much interest in the development of potent analgesics with fewer adverse side effects than the currently available opioid compounds. One of the more promising new opioids is remifentanil, a fentanyl derivative that is rapidly metabolized by nonspecific tissue esterases. The elimination half-life of remifentanil is only 8 to 10 min, and it has a short duration of clinical effect that is relatively independent of the duration of administration. Like other opioid analgesics, remifentanil produces various adverse side effects (including pruritus and respiratory depression). However, its brief duration of action decreases the clinical significance of these undesirable actions and virtually eliminates the need for antagonist drugs like naloxone. Preliminary studies suggest that an infusion of remifentanil, 0.05 to 0.1 μg•kg^{-1}•min^{-1}, provides satisfactory patient comfort and a significant degree of background analgesia (unpublished data). Remifentanil may be especially useful for procedures associated with considerable intraoperative discomfort but little postoperative pain (e.g., deep breast biopsies, transvaginal ovum retrieval), because its duration of action is too short to provide any residual analgesia. Further investigations are needed to determine how remifentanil interacts with commonly used sedative-hypnotic medications (e.g., midazolam, propofol) and whether these combinations offer any advantages over existing techniques.

Nonsteroidal Anti-inflammatory Drugs

Considerable interest has been focused on alternative analgesic drugs that do not possess opioid-related side effects. The nonsteroidal anti-inflammatory drugs (NSAIDs) are effective for treating moderate levels of pain and can decrease the dosage requirements for opioids when more profound analgesia is required. The parenterally administered NSAIDs, ketorolac and diclofenac, are most convenient to administer during the perioperative period. Compared with diclofenac, ketorolac causes less pain and inflammation after intramuscular administration and can also be administered intravenously.

Pretreatment with diclofenac, 75 mg intramuscularly, decreased the requirement for opioid supplementation during extracorporeal shock wave lithotripsy with midazolam sedation.[19] In addition, the use of diclofenac permitted slightly more rapid treatment of renal calculi. Ketorolac, 1 mg•kg^{-1} intravenously, produced a similar degree of intraoperative and postoperative analgesia as fentanyl, 3 μg•kg^{-1} intravenously, when these agents were used as the sole supplement to local anesthesia during minor operations.[20] In addition, substitution of ketorolac for fentanyl prevented pruritus and significantly decreased the incidence of postoperative nausea and vomiting. Other investigators[21] have failed to demonstrate a reduction in postoperative nausea when ketorolac was used in place of fentanyl. However, the overall incidence of nausea and vomiting was low in that investigation, in which patients received propofol for sedation. The use of ketorolac resulted in the requirement for higher doses of propofol to provide intraoperative sedation and an increased need for supplemental analgesia compared with patients receiving fentanyl.[21] Ketorolac also resulted in less postoperative sedation and permitted slightly earlier dismissal than fentanyl. However, ketorolac can occasionally produce severe side effects (e.g., prolonged bleeding time, hematoma formation, renal dysfunction), and its additional cost does not appear to be justified by the small benefits resulting from its use in many clinical situations.

Several investigators have found that oral premedication with NSAIDs can produce useful pain relief after operation, and this method of analgesia deserves further study during local and regional anesthesia. Administration of ibuprofen, 400 mg orally, before removal of impacted third molars during local anesthesia delayed the requirement for postoperative analgesia for 100 min compared with placebo.[22] However, the effects on intraoperative conditions and the requirement for supplemental medications were not reported. One significant advantage of orally administered NSAIDs is their low cost compared with parenterally administered NSAIDs.

Combined Techniques

Combinations of medications with sedative-hypnotic and analgesic properties are frequently used during monitored anesthesia care. Most of the analgesics do not produce reliable sedation, whereas the sedative-hypnotic medications are generally devoid of analgesic properties. Similarly, propofol provides highly satisfactory sedation, with a recovery more rapid than midazolam, but produces little or no intraoperative amnesia compared with the benzodiazepines. By combining medications with different properties, the desirable components of sedation, anxiolysis, amnesia, and analgesia can be provided with minimal side effects. Furthermore, the use of titratable drugs allows the balance of these features to be adjusted to the needs of the particular operation and the individual patient. For example, pretreatment with midazolam, 2 mg, significantly decreased patient anxiety, increased sedation scores, and enhanced amnesia for intraoperative events (Fig. 11–4) during operation performed with local anesthesia with propofol sedation compared with the use of propofol alone.[23] This small dose of midazolam did not increase postoperative sedation scores or result in prolonged amnesia and, more importantly, did not significantly delay recovery and dismissal.[23]

Combinations of propofol and opioid analgesics have been used to provide sedation during painful proce-

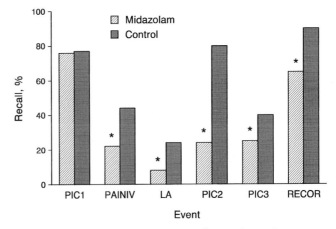

Figure 11–4 Percentage of patients recalling perioperative events after sedation with propofol (control) or propofol preceded by midazolam (midazolam). PIC1, picture preoperatively; PAINIV, pain from propofol injection; LA, pain from local anesthetic injection; PIC2, picture shown after midazolam/placebo; PIC3, picture shown at end of operation; RECOR, recall being in operating room. *$P <$ .05 compared with control group. (Data from Taylor E, Ghouri AF, White PF: Midazolam in combination with propofol for sedation during local anesthesia. J Clin Anesth 1992; 4: 213–216.)

dures for which local anesthetic infiltration is impractical. Transvaginal oocyte retrieval causes intermittent pain and may require a paracervical block for analgesia. Although propofol alone does not provide adequate patient comfort, a mixture of propofol and alfentanil provided satisfactory operating conditions and was well tolerated by the patients.[24] Although partial airway obstruction was observed in several patients, clinically significant decreases in Spo_2 did not occur. During extracorporeal shock wave lithotripsy therapy, a combination of propofol and fentanyl provided good operating conditions combined with hemodynamic stability, while permitting a more rapid recovery than an epidural-based anesthetic technique.[17]

Adjuvants

α_2-Adrenergic Receptor Agonists

Clonidine and dexmedetomidine are α_2-adrenergic receptor agonists with analgesic-sparing properties. Clonidine premedication given orally enhanced the onset and prolonged the duration of a neuraxial block.[25] However, the adjunctive use of the α_2 agonist increased the incidence of cardiovascular side effects. In addition, α_2 agonists interact with other centrally acting drugs to produce enhanced sedation and provide anxiolysis. In an animal model, both clonidine and morphine decreased the ED_{50} for the hypnotic effects of midazolam to a similar degree,[26] suggesting that clonidine may be useful during monitored anesthesia care. Compared with clonidine, dexmedetomidine is more selective for the α_2 receptor and is also more potent. Dexmedetomidine can significantly decrease the requirements for postoperative analgesia after operations with general anesthesia.[27] Compared with a placebo, pretreatment with dexmedetomidine, 1 $\mu g \cdot kg^{-1}$, decreased anxiety and the requirements for supplemental analgesia during hand surgery with intravenous regional anesthesia.[28] Compared with midazolam, 1.5 mg•kg^{-1}, dexmedetomidine, 2 μg•kg^{-1}, provided less satisfactory sedation for gynecologic surgery during paracervical block.[29] Dexmedetomidine had a slower onset of action, and a higher proportion of patients required supplemental propofol. However, complete awakening and recovery of psychomotor function was significantly more rapid after dexmedetomidine. In addition, the use of a specific α$_2$ antagonist, atipamezole, further improved recovery from dexmedetomidine.[29]

Although the sedative and analgesic properties of these α$_2$ agonists appear promising, they are not devoid of side effects. In particular, dexmedetomidine is associated with a high incidence of bradycardia, which may limit its clinical usefulness.[27, 28] Further investigations are required to determine the place of α$_2$ agonists in modern anesthetic practice.

β-Adrenergic Receptor Blockers

The use of β-adrenergic receptor antagonist drugs can prevent the acute cardiovascular and other somatic manifestations of situational anxiety, without producing sedation. Premedication with propranolol has been shown[30] to be as effective as diazepam for relieving acute anxiety, while decreasing the time to recovery. During arthroscopic surgery performed with general anesthesia, the short-acting β-blocker esmolol provided similar attenuation of the cardiovascular response to noxious stimuli as did alfentanil.[31] Although β-blockers modify cardiovascular responses to pain, they do not provide analgesia in awake patients. However, they may help to prevent serious cardiovascular disturbances in patients with hypertension.

Calcium Channel Antagonists

Although the calcium channel antagonists are not used as a routine component of monitored anesthesia care, they can be used to provide acute control of hypertensive episodes and may also be beneficial in treating acute myocardial ischemia. These agents may be administered intravenously; however, sublingual delivery also results in rapid absorption.

Antagonist Drugs

Flumazenil

Flumazenil is a specific benzodiazepine receptor antagonist that can rapidly reverse the amnestic and sedative properties of the benzodiazepines, without provoking a rebound increase in anxiety.[32] The availability of flumazenil might make it possible to administer higher doses of midazolam to achieve improved intraoperative sedation and amnesia, without delaying recovery. After 0.1 to 0.2 mg•min^{-1} of midazolam given intravenously (average of 10 mg over 60 to 70 min) during minor operations with local anesthesia, flumazenil, 1 mg intravenously, improved recovery and per-

mitted patients to be dismissed more than 20 min earlier than a placebo control group (Fig. 11–5).[33] Flumazenil was effective for decreasing the duration of postoperative amnesia but had no effect on amnesia during the operation.[33]

Compared with a propofol-based sedation technique, the combination of midazolam-flumazenil permitted similar recovery times (Fig. 11–5).[33] In addition, levels of intraoperative and postoperative amnesia were similar. However, patients receiving midazolam-flumazenil were more likely to report an increase in their level of sedation after their return home.[33] This resedation probably occurred because the half-life of flumazenil is significantly shorter than that of midazolam, allowing sedation to recur 1 to 2 h after the flumazenil was administered. The benefits of flumazenil do not appear to be sufficient to justify the routine use of this expensive antagonist during monitored anesthesia care. However, flumazenil is useful for treating residual benzodiazepine-induced sedation in patients who have increased sensitivity to the central nervous system effects of these drugs. Care must be taken to ensure that these patients are not dismissed prematurely, with the possibility of dangerous levels of sedation recurring outside the safety of the hospital or ambulatory surgery center environment.

Naloxone

Naloxone is a pure opioid receptor antagonist with no intrinsic analgesic properties. Its only indication is to antagonize undesirable side effects induced by the opioid analgesics (e.g., ventilatory depression, pruritus). Because it is difficult to antagonize opioid side effects without also reversing the analgesic properties, there is little to be gained from the routine administration of naloxone. Furthermore, this agent should be administered slowly and carefully titrated to effect, in order to prevent the reemergence of pain. Like flumazenil, the clinical duration of effect of naloxone is considerably shorter than that of most of the opioids, so care is needed to prevent a recurrence of the opioid-

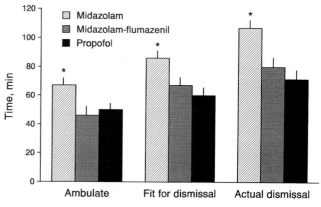

Figure 11–5 Recovery times after operation during local anesthesia in patients receiving midazolam, midazolam-flumazenil, or propofol for sedation. Mean values ± standard error of the mean. *$P < .05$ compared with other groups. (Data from Ghouri AF, Ramirez-Ruiz MA, White PF: Effect of flumazenil on recovery after midazolam and propofol sedation. Anesthesiology 1994; 81: 333–339.)

related side effects after dismissal. In the future, the availability of opioids, such as remifentanil, which have an extremely short duration of action, will further decrease the need for naloxone.

Inhaled Agents

Inhaled anesthetic agents can also be used to provide sedation for various surgical procedures, although this practice is currently most often used during dental surgery. The inhaled route for sedatives offers the advantage that intravenous injections are not required, which may be especially appealing to children and their parents. In addition, drugs may be rapidly eliminated from the lungs, so that recovery from sedation may be superior compared with intravenous administration. Low concentrations (30% to 50%) of nitrous oxide (N_2O) have been used to provide sedation for many years, and in addition, low concentrations of volatile anesthetic agents (e.g., 0.2 to 0.6 minimum alveolar concentration) can also be used during local or regional anesthesia.

Nitrous Oxide

N_2O is popular because it provides a significant degree of analgesia,[34] and its low anesthetic potency provides a considerable margin of safety. In a blind, crossover study in children, inhalation of 50% N_2O in O_2 prevented tachycardia and anxiety-induced vasoconstriction during outpatient dental treatment.[35] Inhalation of 50% to 70% N_2O also permitted the completion of various minor surgical procedures (including suturing, incision of abscesses, radial head fracture reduction) in children.[36] No major complications occurred, and only 0.3% of the children vomited. Because all of the patients remained awake, the authors[36] concluded that this low incidence of vomiting was not hazardous. However, in a group of volunteers who breathed 50% N_2O during simulated dental treatment, aspiration of radiopaque dye (placed on the back of the tongue) was demonstrated in 2 of 10 subjects.[37]

There are other problems associated with the use of N_2O during local or regional anesthesia. It is important to maintain an adequate inspired O_2 concentration. This can be achieved by the use of premixed gas cylinders (e.g., Nitronox, Entonox) that contain a fixed ratio of 1:1 N_2O and O_2. This also limits the maximum N_2O concentration to 50%, which avoids excessive sedation, but may also be inadequate if a loose-fitting mask allows excessive dilution with room air. Alternatively, an anesthetic delivery machine can be used to deliver a variable percentage of N_2O. For safety, this should be fitted with a mechanism to prevent delivery of a hypoxic mixture.[36] N_2O becomes less effective for producing sedation at higher altitudes,[34] as a result of the decreased partial pressure delivered. Finally, there is some evidence that chronic exposure to trace concentrations of N_2O from loose-fitting face masks may pose health hazards.[38]

Volatile Anesthetics

Low concentrations of volatile anesthetics can also be used to provide sedation and analgesia. In a crossover study,[39] isoflurane, 0.75%, provided analgesia superior to N_2O, 50%, and also produced more drowsiness when these agents were inhaled during labor. Patients undergoing extraction of impacted third molars reported greater relaxation when inhaling isoflurane, 0.5%, compared with N_2O, 33%.[40] In this crossover study design, patients expressed a preference for isoflurane, which was also associated with marginally more rapid recovery than N_2O. Most patients detected an odor when breathing either agent, and this was usually described as unpleasant.[40] However, the odor was not sufficiently unpleasant to cause patients to abandon the sedation technique, and most patients expressed a willingness to use isoflurane again.[40]

Compared with midazolam, 3 to 9 mg, given intravenously, inhalation of isoflurane, 0.4% to 1.2%, permitted faster recovery from sedation after oral surgery procedures that lasted 30 min.[41] However, midazolam permitted the desired sedative level to be achieved more rapidly and also provided better amnesia and improved surgical conditions during the initial injection of local anesthetic. Patients inhaling isoflurane had higher Spo_2 values than patients receiving midazolam, although only the isoflurane group received supplemental O_2. More isoflurane-sedated patients reported euphoria, but other perioperative side effects did not differ between the two treatment groups.[41] In a follow-up study,[42] these investigators confirmed the rapid recovery from isoflurane sedation and demonstrated significantly impaired memory function after midazolam sedation compared with the inhalation of isoflurane.

Because of the considerable potency of isoflurane, extreme vigilance is required in the administration of sedative doses of this agent. Specially designed vaporizers that limit the output concentration of isoflurane to 1.4% may increase safety.[41] However, even this concentration is sufficient to produce general anesthesia in certain patients and in the presence of adjunctive intravenously applied medications. In addition, isoflurane has a pungent odor and respiratory irritant properties, which can limit the rate at which adequate sedation is achieved[41] and may also be unacceptable to some patients. Finally, the safety of chronic exposure to trace concentrations of isoflurane is not known.

Monitoring Procedures During Monitored Anesthesia Care

Many of the sedative-hypnotic medications described have a narrow therapeutic range between sedative and general anesthetic doses. In addition, these agents may produce significant cardiovascular and respiratory depression and may impair airway reflexes. Furthermore, the responses of individual patients to similar doses (and even similar blood levels) of sedative-hypnotics vary considerably (Fig. 11–6).[5] It is, therefore, important that adequate means exist for monitoring the

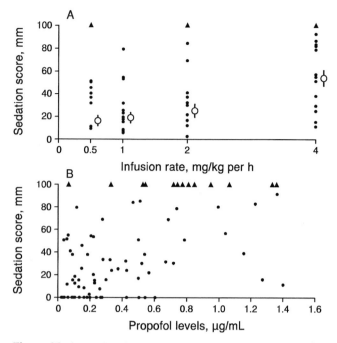

Figure 11–6 Visual analog scores for sedation (0 = awake to 100 = almost asleep) after 30 min of propofol infusion plotted against propofol infusion rate *(A)* or plasma propofol level at 30 min *(B)*. Circle and bar represent mean ± standard error of the mean, small dots represent individual patient values, and triangles represent patients who were too sedated to perform the evaluation. (Data from Smith I, Monk TG, White PF, et al: Propofol infusion during regional anesthesia: sedative, amnestic, and anxiolytic properties. Anesth Analg 1994; 79: 313–319.)

patient's responses to sedative medications and that facilities and equipment are available for airway support and resuscitation. The standard of monitoring during monitored anesthesia care procedures should be comparable with that for general anesthesia.

Effective monitoring of a patient undergoing monitored anesthesia care requires direct observation of the patient.[43] In addition to providing basic information on the rate, depth, and pattern of respiration, this permits an assessment of the patient's needs for adjunctive therapy. Verbal communication with the patient provides assurances that oxygenation and cerebral perfusion are adequate, while allowing the patient to express the desire for increased (or decreased) levels of sedation and supplemental analgesia. Although clinical monitoring is clearly the most important, there is also a need for electronic and electromechanical devices to provide additional information. Some of these devices can provide measurements that are not obtainable by simple observation (e.g., blood pressure, hemoglobin O_2 saturation). Other devices may increase the sensitivity of clinical observation—e.g., pulse oximetry provides an earlier warning of hypoxemia than visual perception of a change in skin or mucous membrane coloration. Monitoring devices may also allow information to be gathered when direct access to the patient is limited (e.g., during magnetic resonance imaging and computed tomographic scans, in the extracorporeal shock wave lithotripsy tank, or during radiography and radiotherapy procedures). The most common and most

severe potential problems during monitored anesthesia care procedures are hypotension, hypoxemia, and arrhythmias, which usually are detected by a combination of noninvasive blood pressure measurement and pulse oximetry. Nevertheless, these devices are prone to artifactual readings as a result of electrical interference and mechanical disturbances resulting from limb movements in awake patients.

The respiratory system can be monitored by a simple nonelectronic precordial stethoscope. The presence of clear breath sounds confirms airway patency, and the acoustic stethoscope is immune to electrical interference. Monitoring of the respiratory waveform is possible by attaching a capnograph catheter to the nasal prongs that are used to provide supplemental O_2.[44] In addition to providing an indication of the respiratory rate and pattern, the end-tidal carbon dioxide value obtained bears a reasonable relationship to arterial carbon dioxide levels.[45] Although simple and inexpensive modifications to nasal cannulae are effective,[44, 45] nasal cannulae with built-in carbon dioxide sampling lines are also commercially available (Salter Labs, Irvine, CA).

Intravenous Drug Delivery Methods

Syringe and Volumetric Pumps

Although sedative medications may be administered by intermittent boluses, there are advantages in the use of continuous infusions.[46, 47] In particular, the resultant level of sedation is more constant, whereas total drug doses and recovery times may be decreased. The use of continuous infusions requires an infusion pump, and a wide variety are available. The simplest devices are drip counters or flow regulators. However, these are not particularly accurate, which may be an important consideration when using potent sedative-hypnotic medications. In addition, these infusion controllers often require that a large fluid volume be administered.

Several syringe pumps are also available that allow more accurate dosing and more concentrated solutions to be infused. The simplest devices are calibrated to deliver a certain volume per unit time, so that the anesthesiologist has to calculate an appropriate infusion rate on the basis of drug concentration, desired dose, and patient weight. More sophisticated pumps allow input of the patient's weight and drug concentration, and built-in calculators allow drugs to be delivered in weight-specific doses and infusion rates. One pump, the Bard InfusOR, uses magnetic, drug-specific labels to adjust the drug concentration and select the appropriate range of infusion rates. Although these electronic infusion pumps make delivery of variable-rate infusions simpler, they represent a significant financial investment.

Pharmacokinetic-Based Pumps

To rapidly achieve a stable plasma concentration of an intravenously administered drug requires a three-stage delivery regimen. A bolus dose, or rapid loading infusion, is first administered to reach the target level. An infusion is then required to maintain this level as the drug rapidly redistributes, and subsequently the infusion rate needs to be decreased as the rate of drug redistribution decreases. Eventually, the rate of this maintenance infusion equals the rate of drug elimination. These dosage adjustments may be made manually,[48] but it is also possible to use population pharmacokinetic values to program a computer to make the alterations in infusion rate automatically.[49, 50] During lower limb surgery performed with regional anesthesia, the desired level of sedation was achieved 80% of the time when a computer-assisted continuous-infusion device was used to administer propofol.[51] However, because the optimal level of sedation may change rapidly during the operation, titration of sedative drugs to clinical end points may be more effective than the targeting of a specific plasma concentration. Furthermore, there may be a poor correlation between plasma drug concentrations and the resultant level of sedation (see Fig. 11–6).[5] In the limited comparisons conducted to date, the use of computer-assisted continuous-infusion devices for sedation does not appear to improve the quality of sedation or to permit more rapid recovery, compared with manual-infusion techniques.[52]

Patient-Controlled Sedation and Analgesia

Individual differences in sensitivity to sedative-hypnotic medications combined with variations in the degree of sedation that different patients desire make providing the optimum degree of sedation for every patient a challenge. In addition, the level of discomfort and surgical stimulation varies throughout the operative procedure, requiring adjustments in the degree of sedation and analgesia. Patient-controlled analgesia (PCA) has become popular because it allows patients to titrate pain-relieving medications to their individual needs. Several computerized infusion pumps are available for PCA. Because patients have to actively request each dose, excessive sedation results in a cessation of further demands, which should prevent serious overdosage.

PCA has been used to provide analgesia during operations. When PCA and anesthesiologist-administered analgesia were compared during transvaginal ovum retrieval, similar doses of alfentanil were required by both groups of patients, who also recorded similar pain and comfort scores.[53] Hemodynamic stability, perioperative side effects, and patient satisfaction were also similar in the two treatment groups.[53] In contrast, patients who self-administered a midazolam-fentanyl mixture as a supplement to epidural anesthesia for lower limb surgery reported improved intraoperative comfort compared with a group managed traditionally, despite the use of similar intravenous drug totals with the two methods.[54]

PCA pumps can also be used to administer sedative-hypnotic medications to provide patient-controlled sedation. Both propofol and midazolam, administered by patient-controlled methods, produced similar patient satisfaction to PCA with alfentanil used to supplement local infiltration anesthesia.[55] Recovery times were similar in all three groups; however, propofol was associated with a lower incidence of nausea than alfentanil.[55] In a crossover study design, patients undergoing repeat dental surgery required almost identical amounts of midazolam and reported equal satisfaction when sedation was administered either by an anesthesiologist or by patient-controlled methods.[56] However, it took longer to establish an adequate sedative level in the patient-controlled sedation group because of the lockout interval of the infusion pump. Even when a modified infusion pump with a lockout interval of only 1 min was used to deliver propofol, it was necessary for the anesthesiologist to administer an initial loading dose in order to achieve an adequate sedative level.[57] Subsequently, bolus doses of propofol, 0.7 mg•kg^{-1}, at a minimum of 1-min intervals provided highly satisfactory sedation during dental extractions.[57]

Further modifications to the infusion pump to completely eliminate the lockout interval and increase the rate of infusion to 3.3 mL•min^{-1} would allow for true patient-controlled sedation in which patients could rapidly establish the desired level of sedation themselves.[58] This technique has been successfully used during transvaginal oocyte retrieval, using either propofol or midazolam.[58] The infusion rate of the pump limited patients to a maximum of 33 mg•min^{-1} of propofol or 1.1 mg•min^{-1} alfentanil. Propofol permitted more rapid recovery of psychomotor function compared with midazolam and was also less likely to result in excessive sedation during the operation. Further studies are required to determine the optimal drugs and techniques for patient-controlled sedation. However, the greater patient participation, combined with the safety inherent in patients administering their own sedation, might lead to the increased use of patient-controlled sedation techniques in the future.

Summary

The use of sedative and analgesic adjuvants during local and regional anesthesia can enhance patient comfort and improve intraoperative conditions. This can increase the range of procedures that can safely and comfortably be performed without requiring general anesthesia. In addition, the same medications may be used when local anesthetics are either unnecessary or impractical. Although local anesthetic-based techniques are inherently safe, the use of potent sedative-hypnotic and analgesic drugs may cause significant depression of cardiovascular and respiratory function. This is particularly likely when drug combinations with additive or synergistic interactions are used. It is, therefore, essential that adequate monitoring and supplemental oxygen be used and that facilities for cardiopulmonary resuscitation be readily available. In all cases in which potent cardiorespiratory depressant drugs are administered, they should be given by personnel skilled in the management of unconscious patients. Although drugs like propofol can offer many advantages for procedures during monitored anesthesia care, the delivery of this potent intravenous anesthetic is also potentially more dangerous in unskilled hands. The involvement of anesthesiologists in the provision of monitored anesthesia care in all cases is crucial.

Sedative, hypnotic, and analgesic medications may be administered by intravenous or inhaled routes. Inhalation may be preferable in children, because it avoids the necessity for injections. However, the pungent odor and slow onset of inhaled agents as well as the bulky equipment for their administration limit the use of inhaled adjuvants. In contrast, intravenous administration is rapid and reliable, although recovery from the sedative effects may be prolonged. The availability of shorter-acting drugs and specific antagonists has decreased the significance of this problem. Whatever route of administration is chosen, careful titration of drugs to achieve the desired effect is vital, both to minimize the occurrence of undesirable side effects and to improve patient comfort. Allowing the patients to regulate their own level of sedation, either by intermittent inhalation (e.g., mini-inhaler) or by patient-controlled drug-delivery systems, may further enhance satisfaction and decrease side effects. Finally, the availability of agents with shorter and more specific actions as well as fewer adverse side effects will make monitored anesthesia care safer and more acceptable to patients (and surgeons) in the future.

References

1. Korttila K, Linnoila M: Recovery and skills related to driving after intravenous sedation: dose-response relationship with diazepam. Br J Anaesth 1975; 47: 457–463.
2. White PF, Vasconez LO, Mathes SA, et al: Comparison of midazolam and diazepam for sedation during plastic surgery. Plast Reconstr Surg 1988; 81: 703–712.
3. Urquhart ML, White PF: Comparison of sedative infusions during regional anesthesia—methohexital, etomidate, and midazolam. (Published erratum appears in Anesth Analg 1989; 68: 550.) Anesth Analg 1989; 68: 249–254.
4. Mackenzie N, Grant IS: Propofol for intravenous sedation. Anaesthesia 1987; 42: 3–6.
5. Smith I, Monk TG, White PF, et al: Propofol infusion during regional anesthesia: sedative, amnestic, and anxiolytic properties. Anesth Analg 1994; 79: 313–319.
6. Wilson E, Mackenzie N, Grant IS: A comparison of propofol and midazolam by infusion to provide sedation in patients who receive spinal anaesthesia. Anaesthesia 1988; 43 Suppl: 91–94.
7. Fanard L, Van Steenberge A, Demeire X, et al: Comparison between propofol and midazolam as sedative agents for surgery under regional anaesthesia. Anaesthesia 1988; 43 Suppl: 87–89.
8. White PF, Negus JB: Sedative infusions during local and regional anesthesia: a comparison of midazolam and propofol. J Clin Anesth 1991; 3: 32–39.
9. Ferrari LR, Donlon JV: A comparison of propofol, midazolam, and methohexital for sedation during retrobulbar and peribulbar block. J Clin Anesth 1992; 4: 93–96.
10. Dubois A, Balatoni E, Peeters JP, et al: Use of propofol for sedation during gastrointestinal endoscopies. Anaesthesia 1988; 43 Suppl: 75–80.
11. Patterson KW, Casey PB, Murray JP, et al: Propofol sedation for outpatient upper gastrointestinal endoscopy: comparison with midazolam. Br J Anaesth 1991; 67: 108–111.
12. Borgeat A, Wilder-Smith OH, Saiah M, et al: Subhypnotic doses of propofol possess direct antiemetic properties. Anesth Analg 1992; 74: 539–541.
13. Zacny JP, Lichtor JL, Coalson DW, et al: Subjective and psychomotor effects of subanesthetic doses of propofol in healthy volunteers. Anesthesiology 1992; 76: 696–702.
14. Pratila MG, Fischer ME, Alagesan R, et al: Propofol versus midazolam for monitored sedation: a comparison of intraoperative and recovery parameters. J Clin Anesth 1993; 5: 268–274.
15. Guit JB, Koning HM, Coster ML, et al: Ketamine as analgesic for total intravenous anaesthesia with propofol. Anaesthesia 1991; 46: 24–27.
16. Monk TG, Rater JM, White PF: Comparison of alfentanil and ketamine infusions in combination with midazolam for outpatient lithotripsy. Anesthesiology 1991; 74: 1023–1028.
17. Monk TG, Boure B, White PF, et al: Comparison of intravenous sedative-analgesic techniques for outpatient immersion lithotripsy. (Published erratum appears in Anesth Analg 1992; 74: 324.) Anesth Analg 1991; 72: 616–621.
18. Bailey PL, Pace NL, Ashburn MA, et al: Frequent hypoxemia and apnea after sedation with midazolam and fentanyl. Anesthesiology 1990; 73: 826–830.
19. Fredman B, Jedeikin R, Olsfanger D, et al: The opioid-sparing effect of diclofenac sodium in outpatient extracorporeal shock wave lithotripsy (ESWL). J Clin Anesth 1993; 5: 141–144.
20. Bosek V, Smith DB, Cox C: Ketorolac or fentanyl to supplement local anesthesia? J Clin Anesth 1992; 4: 480–483.
21. Ramirez-Ruiz M, Newson CD, White PF: Monitored anesthesia care: use of ketorolac, dezocine, and fentanyl. (Abstract.) Anesthesiology 1992; 77: a27.
22. Dionne RA, Cooper SA: Evaluation of preoperative ibuprofen for postoperative pain after removal of third molars. Oral Surg Oral Med Oral Pathol 1978; 45: 851–856.
23. Taylor E, Ghouri AF, White PF: Midazolam in combination with propofol for sedation during local anesthesia. J Clin Anesth 1992; 4: 213–216.
24. Sherry E: Admixture of propofol and alfentanil. Use for intravenous sedation and analgesia during transvaginal oocyte retrieval. Anaesthesia 1992; 47: 477–479.
25. Singh H, Liu J, Gaines GY, et al: Effect of oral clonidine and intrathecal fentanyl on tetracaine spinal block. Anesth Analg 1994; 79:1113–1116.
26. Kissin I, Brown PT, Bradley EL Jr: Additive clonidine-morphine interaction for enhancement of midazolam hypnotic effect. (Abstract.) Anesthesiology 1992; 77: a725.
27. Aho MS, Erkola OA, Scheinin H, et al: Effect of intravenously administered dexmedetomidine on pain after laparoscopic tubal ligation. Anesth Analg 1991; 73: 112–118.
28. Jaakola M-L, Scheinin H, Scheinin M, et al: Dexmedetomidine premedication before regional intravenous anesthesia in minor outpatient hand surgery. (Abstract.) Anesthesiology 1992; 77: a836.
29. Aho M, Erkola O, Kallio A, et al: Comparison of dexmedetomidine and midazolam sedation and antagonism of dexmedetomidine with atipamezole. J Clin Anesth 1993; 5: 194–203.
30. Dyck JB, Chung F: A comparison of propranolol and diazepam for preoperative anxiolysis. Can J Anaesth 1991; 38: 704–709.
31. Smith I, Van Hemelrijck J, White PF: Efficacy of esmolol versus alfentanil as a supplement to propofol–nitrous oxide anesthesia. Anesth Analg 1991; 73: 540–546.
32. White PF, Shafer A, Boyle WA III, et al: Benzodiazepine antagonism does not provoke a stress response. Anesthesiology 1989; 70: 636–639.
33. Ghouri AF, Ramirez-Ruiz MA, White PF: Effect of flumazenil on recovery after midazolam and propofol sedation. Anesthesiology 1994; 81: 333–339.
34. James MF, Manson ED, Dennett JE: Nitrous oxide analgesia and altitude. Anaesthesia 1982; 37: 285–288.
35. Brook AH, Major E, Winder M, et al: Inhalation sedation—an adjunct to improved dental care: preliminary communication. J R Soc Med 1979; 72: 756–760.
36. Griffin GC, Campbell VD, Jones R: Nitrous oxide–oxygen sedation for minor surgery. Experience in a pediatric setting. JAMA 1981; 245: 2411–2413.
37. Rubin J, Brock-Utne JG, Greenberg M, et al: Laryngeal incompetence during experimental "relative analgesia" using 50% nitrous oxide in oxygen. A preliminary report. Br J Anaesth 1977; 49: 1005–1008.

38. Sweeney B, Bingham RM, Amos RJ, et al: Toxicity of bone marrow in dentists exposed to nitrous oxide. Br Med J 1985; 291: 567–569.

39. McLeod DD, Ramayya GP, Tunstall ME: Self-administered isoflurane in labour. A comparative study with Entonox. Anaesthesia 1985; 40: 424–426.

40. Rodrigo MR, Rosenquist JB: Isoflurane for conscious sedation. Anaesthesia 1988; 43: 369–375.

41. Parbrook GD, Still DM, Parbrook EO: Comparison of i.v. sedation with midazolam and inhalation sedation with isoflurane in dental outpatients. Br J Anaesth 1989; 63: 81–86.

42. Ho ET, Parbrook GD, Still DM, et al: Memory function after i.v. midazolam or inhalation of isoflurane for sedation during dental surgery. Br J Anaesth 1990; 64: 337–340.

43. Vandam LD: The senses as monitors. In Blitt CD (ed): Monitoring in Anesthesia and Critical Care Medicine, pp 5–24. New York, Churchill Livingstone, 1985.

44. Goldman JM: A simple, easy, and inexpensive method for monitoring ETCO2 through nasal cannulae. (Letter to the editor.) Anesthesiology 1987; 67: 606.

45. Roy J, McNulty SE, Torjman MC: An improved nasal prong apparatus for end-tidal carbon dioxide monitoring in awake, sedated patients. J Clin Monit 1991; 7: 249–252.

46. White PF: Use of continuous infusion versus intermittent bolus administration of fentanyl or ketamine during outpatient anesthesia. Anesthesiology 1983; 59: 294–300.

47. Pace NA, Victory RA, White PF: Anesthetic infusion techniques—how to do it. J Clin Anesth 1992; 4(5 Suppl 1): 45s–52s.

48. Roberts FL, Dixon J, Lewis GT, et al: Induction and maintenance of propofol anaesthesia. A manual infusion scheme. Anaesthesia 1988; 43 Suppl: 14–17.

49. White M, Kenny GN: Intravenous propofol anaesthesia using a computerised infusion system. Anaesthesia 1990; 45: 204–209.

50. Kenny GN, White M: A portable computerised infusion system for propofol. (Letter to the editor.) Anaesthesia 1990; 45: 692–693.

51. Skipsey IG, Colvin JR, Mackenzie N, et al: Sedation with propofol during surgery under local blockade. Assessment of a target-controlled infusion system. Anaesthesia 1993; 48: 210–213.

52. Newson C, Victory R, Joshi G, et al: Propofol sedation: use of infusion pumps vs manual administration. (Abstract.) Anesthesiology 1993; 79: a3.

53. Zelcer J, White PF, Chester S, et al: Intraoperative patient-controlled analgesia: an alternative to physician administration during outpatient monitored anesthesia care. Anesth Analg 1992; 75: 41–44.

54. Park WY, Watkins PA: Patient-controlled sedation during epidural anesthesia. Anesth Analg 1991; 72: 304–307.

55. Ghouri AF, Taylor E, White PF: Patient-controlled drug administration during local anesthesia: a comparison of midazolam, propofol, and alfentanil. J Clin Anesth 1992; 4: 476–479.

56. Rodrigo MR, Tong CK: A comparison of patient and anaesthetist controlled midazolam sedation for dental surgery. Anaesthesia 1994; 49: 241–244.

57. Rudkin GE, Osborne GA, Curtis NJ: Intra-operative patient-controlled sedation. Anaesthesia 1991; 46: 90–92.

58. Cook LB, Lockwood GG, Moore CM, et al: True patient-controlled sedation. Anaesthesia 1993; 48: 1039–1044.

CHAPTER 12
Local Anesthetics

Bernadette Th. Veering, M.D., Ph.D.

Local anesthetic agents are among the most widely used drugs being administered in clinical practice to provide local or regional anesthesia. Because studies have shown some advantages of regional anesthesia over general anesthesia for certain surgical procedures, the use of regional anesthesia has regained popularity. Various local anesthetic agents are available with short-, medium-, or long-acting characteristics. The choice of a local anesthetic agent is governed by its primary characteristics and depends on factors such as the anesthetic procedure, surgical procedure, and physiologic status of the patient. Speed of onset, duration of action appropriate for surgery, and postoperative requirements for analgesia are the main clinical considerations. The local anesthesia should outlast the duration of the operation, and for prolonged operations, a repeated dose administration of a long-lasting local anesthetic or a continuous catheter technique is chosen. The potential for systemic toxicity should also be considered when choosing a local anesthetic.

Knowledge of the pharmacologic properties of local anesthetic agents is important in selecting the most appropriate agent in a specific clinical situation. The type of regional anesthetic procedure to be performed (e.g., sensory, sympathetic, motor) exerts a great influence on the type of agent to be used. The selection of local anesthetic agents depends also on the clinician's personal experience, practice style, and technical skill.

This chapter describes the characteristics of individual agents and the factors that direct the selection of the most appropriate local anesthetic agent for a specific surgical procedure.

Classification of Local Anesthetic Agents

Chemical Category

The clinically useful local anesthetic drugs belong to two chemical categories: agents with an ester link between the aromatic end of the molecule and the intermediate chain (i.e., amino-ester agents) and agents with an amide link between the aromatic portion and the intermediate group (i.e., amino-amide agents).

The chemical difference is reflected biologically in the site of metabolism: ester-type agents are mainly hydrolyzed by pseudocholinesterases in plasma and elsewhere, and amide compounds undergo enzymatic degradation predominantly in the liver. The chemical difference is also revealed in the allergic potential: a higher frequency of allergic reactions is observed with the ester-type agents that are derivatives of p-aminobenzoic acid.

Potency and Duration of Action

The clinically important properties of local anesthetic agents include speed of onset, potency, and duration of action. These clinical properties are partly related to the physicochemical properties of the agents, such as dissociation constant (pK_a), lipid solubility, and protein binding.[1, 2] These relationships are essentially what is observed in an isolated nerve, but in vivo, other actions of the local anesthetics may influence the anesthetic profile as well. The vasoactive properties of local anesthetics may influence their systemic absorption, resulting in more or fewer molecules available for regional block. The factors that increase the absorption decrease the apparent anesthetic potency and duration of action of a specific local anesthetic, and diffusion through nonnervous tissues and extraneural uptake also may play a role.

Another important clinical consideration is the ability to cause a differential block of sensory and motor fibers. For clinical use, it is common to divide local anesthetic agents into three groups on the basis of their inherent anesthetic potency and duration of regional block.[3] Group I includes procaine and chloroprocaine, which are agents with low anesthetic potency and short duration of action. Group II includes lidocaine, mepivacaine, and prilocaine, which are agents with intermediate anesthetic potency and duration of action. Group III includes tetracaine, bupivacaine, and etidocaine, which are agents with high intrinsic anesthetic potency and prolonged duration of action.

Local anesthetics also differ in their onset of action. Chloroprocaine, lidocaine, mepivacaine, prilocaine, and etidocaine have a relatively quick onset of action. Bupivacaine has an intermediate onset time, and procaine and tetracaine have a slow onset of action.

Specific Local Anesthetic Agents

Each of the local anesthetic agents has specific properties that render it valuable for the practitioner. The local anesthetic agents available for clinical use are summarized in Table 12–1.

Esters

Cocaine. Cocaine is an ester of benzoic acid. It provides excellent topical anesthesia, and it is the only local anesthetic that produces vasoconstriction at clinically useful concentrations. For this reason, it is commonly used in daily otolaryngologic practice in concentrations of 4% to 10%. Unfortunately, cocaine has highly addictive properties associated with a relatively high potential for systemic toxicity.[4] As a result, this agent is only for topical use.

Procaine. Procaine is a derivative of *p*-aminobenzoic acid. It is a relatively weak local anesthetic with a slow onset and short duration of action. It is used primarily for skin infiltration in concentrations of 0.5%, for diagnostic purposes, producing a differential spinal block at a concentration of 5%, and occasionally it is mixed with tetracaine for spinal anesthesia. The relatively low potency and rapid plasma hydrolysis of procaine contribute to its low potential for systemic toxicity. Procaine, however, is hydrolyzed to *p*-aminobenzoic acid, which may contribute to the rare allergic reactions associated with repeated use.

Chloroprocaine. Chloroprocaine is the 2-chloro derivative of procaine and has a rapid onset and a short duration of action. 2-Chloroprocaine is suitable for infiltration and epidural anesthesia in concentrations of 2% and 3%. This drug is useful when anesthesia is needed for procedures with a short duration. 2-Chloroprocaine is thought to have a low potential for systemic toxicity, because it is more rapidly hydrolyzed than procaine.[5] It is primarily used for epidural analgesia in obstetrics. The molecule, with its ester linkage, has a relatively high allergic potential. Older preparations of this drug contained sodium *m*-bisulfite as an antioxidant and occasionally were neurotoxic when large-volume, unintentional intrathecal injections resulted from epidural blocks. However, current preparations of chloroprocaine are free of *m*-bisulfite and are not considered neurotoxic. A clinical drawback with the new formulation of chloroprocaine is the persistent mild backache after epidural administration.[6]

Table 12–1 Suitable Local Anesthetics and Their Primary Clinical Uses

	MAXIMUM SINGLE DOSE, mg*		
AGENT	**Without Epinephrine**	**With Epinephrine**	**CLINICAL USE**
Ester-Linked			
Cocaine	150		Topical
Benzocaine	Unknown		Topical
Procaine	800	1000	Infiltration, spinal
Tetracaine	100		Topical, spinal
Chloroprocaine	800	1000	Infiltration, peripheral nerve blocks, obstetric epidural anesthesia
Amide-Linked			
Lidocaine	400	500	Topical, infiltration, IV regional, peripheral nerve blocks, epidural, spinal
Prilocaine	500	600	Infiltration, IV regional, surgical epidural anesthesia
Mepivacaine	300	500	Infiltration, peripheral nerve blocks, epidural
Bupivacaine	175	250	Infiltration, peripheral nerve blocks, epidural, spinal
Ropivacaine	250		Peripheral nerve blocks, surgical epidural anesthesia
Etidocaine	300	400	Infiltration, peripheral nerve blocks, surgical epidural anesthesia
Miscellaneous			
Dibucaine	50		Spinal
Articaine			Infiltration, epidural

*Recommended safe dose is influenced by many factors (see text) and should be adjusted for each site of injection. The total dose of epinephrine should not exceed 0.25 mg.
IV, intravenous.

Tetracaine. Tetracaine is the butyl-aminobenzoic acid derivative of procaine. It is a potent, long-acting local anesthetic that produces a high degree of motor block, with excellent qualities of sensory block. It is used primarily for spinal anesthesia in hyperbaric, hypobaric, or isobaric solutions. It undergoes hydrolysis by plasma cholinesterase, but the rate is slower than for procaine. Because the potential for systemic toxicity is relatively high, tetracaine is not used for other regional procedures requiring larger doses than those required for spinal anesthesia.

Amides

Lidocaine. Lidocaine is the most versatile and commonly used local anesthetic agent as a result of its rapid onset of action, inherent potency, and moderate duration of action. The limiting factor in clinical practice is its duration of action (up to 90 min). However, addition of epinephrine markedly prolongs its duration of action. Like most amino-amide compounds, lidocaine is metabolized primarily in the liver. The metabolites of lidocaine continue to have systemic pharmacologic activity.[7] The level of the principal pharmacologically active metabolites may play an additive role in the development of toxic reactions associated with repeated epidural administration of lidocaine.[8] Lidocaine is used in concentrations of 0.5% to 5.0%, depending on the mode of application. It has been used safely for all types of local anesthesia. The potential for systemic toxicity is intermediate, with lidocaine between procaine and bupivacaine.

Prilocaine. Prilocaine is an amino-amide local anesthetic derived from a toluidine derivative and a tertiary amine. Prilocaine has a clinical profile similar to that of lidocaine. It is characterized by a relatively rapid onset of action, a moderate duration of action, and a profound depth of regional block. Prilocaine is used in concentrations of 0.5% to 2%, depending on the mode of application. In Europe, it is used particularly for intravenous regional anesthesia, because central nervous system toxic effects are rarely seen after tourniquet deflation. Prilocaine is the least toxic among the amino-amide local anesthetics. Because clinically significant methemoglobinemia may occur after doses above 600 mg of prilocaine, this agent is not suitable for continuous analgesia.[9]

Mepivacaine. Mepivacaine is structurally related to lidocaine. It has a rapid onset of action, and its duration of action is somewhat longer than that of lidocaine when each agent is used without epinephrine. The addition of epinephrine prolongs the duration of action of mepivacaine by approximately 75%. Mepivacaine is not effective for topical anesthesia. It is used in concentrations of 0.5% to 2%, depending on the mode of application. The potential for systemic toxicity appears to be similar to that of lidocaine.

Bupivacaine. Bupivacaine, a homologue of mepivacaine, possesses a greater anesthetic potency and prolonged duration of action compared with mepivacaine. When used for peripheral nerve blocks, the onset of analgesia is relatively slow, but the duration of action is long. It is an ideal drug for several indications for which a long duration is desirable. The difference in the duration of analgesia between bupivacaine and bupivacaine with epinephrine is relatively small. Bupivacaine has the ability to provide separate blocks of sensory and motor fibers with changes in concentration. As a result, it is used successfully for obstetric anesthesia and postoperative pain management, for which analgesia without significant motor block is highly desirable. It is administered in concentrations of 0.06% to 0.75%, depending on the mode of administration. Bupivacaine is more cardiotoxic than equipotent concentrations of lidocaine.

Etidocaine. Etidocaine is structurally similar to lidocaine. Compared with bupivacaine, it is characterized by a faster onset of action and a similar duration of action. It produces a more profound effect on motor nerves than sensory ones. Addition of epinephrine to etidocaine solutions hardly prolongs the duration of action. Etidocaine is used in concentrations of 1% to 1.5%. The low concentrations are associated with a high degree of motor block and often with less sensory block. As a result, etidocaine is primarily useful for surgical procedures in which profound motor block is required. For surgical anesthesia, concentrations of 1.5% are used. Etidocaine is less toxic than the other long-acting local anesthetic, bupivacaine, because of its greater distribution and clearance, but it is not used widely in current practice.

Ropivacaine. Ropivacaine, a new long-acting amide-type local anesthetic is the *S* enantiomer of a chain-shortened homologue of bupivacaine (i.e., propyl instead of butyl side chain). Studies[10, 11] have shown ropivacaine to be a clinically effective local anesthetic for epidural and brachial plexus blocks, similar to bupivacaine in onset and the extent of sensory and motor blocks. Ropivacaine, like bupivacaine, has a dose-dependent duration of sensory and motor block; however, the duration of motor block is shorter with ropivacaine. The drug appears to be less arrhythmogenic and less potent than bupivacaine in depressing cardiac electrophysiologic variables.[12]

Miscellaneous

Articaine. Articaine belongs to the anilide group of local anesthetics, similar to lidocaine and mepivacaine, although it differs from these agents in that it has a thiophene ring instead of a benzene ring in its structure. No significant differences in clinical profile have been demonstrated between articaine and mepivacaine or lidocaine. However, there is evidence that a 4% solution of articaine with a 1:200,000 concentration of epinephrine provides a faster onset of action and better spreading than lidocaine in dental infiltration blocks.[13] Research[14] indicates that articaine is of similar potency to lidocaine but is much less potent than bupivacaine in depressing cardiac electrophysiologic variables.

Dibucaine. Dibucaine is a quinoline derivative with an amide bond in the intermediate chain. It is very toxic, and this limits its use to spinal anesthesia. Compared with tetracaine, the duration of regional block is slightly longer with dibucaine.[15]

Benzocaine. Benzocaine is an ester that does not contain the amino group common to other esters. For this reason, it is almost insoluble in water and is used exclusively and effectively for topical anesthesia.

Mixture of Local Anesthetics

The basis of mixing (i.e., compounding) local anesthetic is to obtain a block with a rapid onset and a long duration of action. 2-Chloroprocaine was used in combination with bupivacaine to produce a faster onset and prolonged sensory block after epidural administration.[16] Unfortunately, 2-chloroprocaine shortened the duration of bupivacaine's block. Isolated nerve studies[17] suggest that a metabolite of chloroprocaine may inhibit the binding of bupivacaine to the membrane site.

In contrast to epidural anesthesia, peripheral nerve blocks theoretically may benefit from mixtures of medium- and long-acting local anesthetics. Bupivacaine-prilocaine seems to be the most promising mixture because of the alkalinizing effect of this mixture on the final local anesthetic solution.[18] There do not appear to be any clinically significant advantages to the use of mixtures of local anesthetic agents. The use of continuous administration of the shorter-acting agents has considerable advantages in that duration is not a problem and a rapid effect can be obtained with a single drug.

Factors Influencing Anesthetic Activity

The essential qualities of regional anesthesia are onset, depth, and duration of sensory and motor blocks. These features are influenced primarily by the local anesthetic used, but several factors influence the quality of regional block as well.

Dose (Volume and Concentration)

The total dose (i.e., product of volume and concentration) is probably the main determinant of the pharmacodynamic profile of a local anesthetic agent. An increase in the dose of local anesthetic produces a faster onset and a longer duration of sensory block, and increasing the concentration results in a faster onset and a more profound motor block[19] (Fig. 12–1). The effective concentrations and volumes of local anesthetic agents vary with the type of regional anesthesia performed. Larger nerves are more difficult to anesthetize and require higher concentrations of local anesthetic than smaller nerve fibers.[20] For example, when lidocaine is used, satisfactory infiltration analgesia can be obtained at low concentrations (0.5%), but for an effective motor block during epidural analgesia, a higher concentration is needed.

The volume of anesthetic solutions may influence

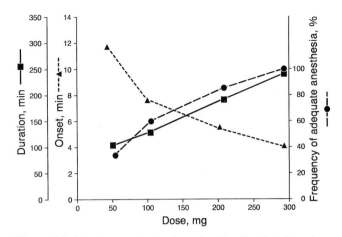

Figure 12–1 An increase in the dose of epidurally administered etidocaine produces a faster onset, a longer duration of sensory block, and improves the frequency of satisfactory anesthesia. (From Covino BG: Pharmacology of local anaesthetic agents. Br J Anaesth 1986; 58: 701–716. Published by the BMJ Publishing Group.)

the spread of anesthesia. Variations in volume (at a constant mass of drug) appear to have little influence on the spread of epidural anesthesia.[21] However, increasing the volume of a certain concentration of a local anesthetic solution injected into the epidural space usually results in a greater spread of anesthesia.

Addition of a Vasoconstrictor

The quality of a regional block may be improved by the concomitant use of vasoconstrictor agents, particularly epinephrine. This effect may be related to a decrease in the blood flow at the site of injection, leading to decreased vascular absorption and increased neuronal uptake of local anesthetic.[22] As a consequence, the depth and duration of neural blockade are increased. The effects of epinephrine on the quality of a regional block vary markedly with the site of injection and the type, dose, and concentration of the local anesthetic (Fig. 12–2).

For example, the addition of epinephrine to all local anesthetic solutions significantly prolongs the duration of action of infiltration anesthesia and peripheral nerve blocks, but the addition of epinephrine to prilocaine, etidocaine, and bupivacaine has little or no effect on the duration of action of epidural anesthesia.[23, 24] However, the addition of epinephrine to lidocaine and mepivacaine markedly prolongs the duration of action of epidural anesthesia.[25, 26] This differential effect may be related to the differences in physicochemical properties (e.g., local binding) and the intrinsic vasoactivity of the agents.[27] The intensity, but not the duration, of motor block is enhanced after the epidural administration of epinephrine-containing solutions of lidocaine, bupivacaine, and etidocaine and after subarachnoid administration of an epinephrine-containing hyperbaric bupivacaine solution[24, 28, 29] (Fig. 12–3). The effects of adding epinephrine are more important when the concentration of the local anesthetic solution is low than when it is high.

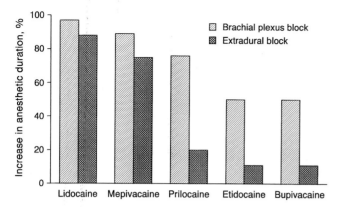

Figure 12–2 Percent increase in anesthetic duration of various local anesthetic agents resulting from the addition of epinephrine. The increase varies with the local anesthetic used and the regional block performed. (From Covino BG: Pharmacology of local anaesthetic agents. Br J Anaesth 1986; 58: 701–716. Published by the BMJ Publishing Group.)

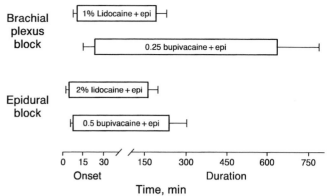

Figure 12–4 Comparative onset and duration of anesthesia of lidocaine and bupivacaine after epidural and brachial plexus block. epi, epinephrine. (Data from Covino BG: Clinical pharmacology of local anesthetic agents. In Cousins MJ, Bridenbaugh PO [eds]: Neural Blockade in Clinical Anesthesia and Management of Pain, 2nd ed, pp 111–144. Philadelphia, JB Lippincott, 1988.)

The optimal concentration of epinephrine is 1:200,000 (5 μg/mL), although lower concentrations are sometimes recommended in obstetrics. Its use may be contraindicated in patients taking tricyclic or related antidepressants because arrhythmias may result and is contraindicated in ring blocks and intravenous regional anesthesia because tissue ischemia may occur.[30]

Site of Injection

The onset and duration of action of a specific local anesthetic vary with the site of injection (Fig. 12–4). In general, the most rapid onset with the shortest duration of action follows subarachnoid or subcutaneous administration of local anesthetics, and the slowest onset times and longest durations are observed when major peripheral nerves are blocked, as in a brachial plexus block.[1] These differences in onset and duration

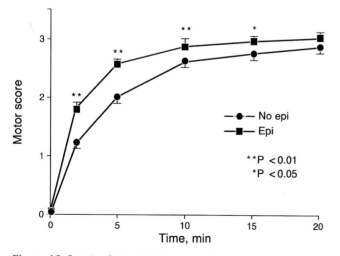

Figure 12–3 Epinephrine (Epi) improves the intensity of motor block when added to spinal hyperbaric bupivacaine. (From Abouleish EI: Epinephrine improves the quality of spinal hyperbaric bupivacaine for cesarean section. Anesth Analg 1987; 66: 395–400.)

of anesthesia can be attributed in part to particular anatomic aspects of the area of injection and variation in the rate of vascular absorption.

Selection of the Most Appropriate Agent

Maximum Dose

The dosage of local anesthetic administered must be tailored to where the drug is injected, because the toxic effects of a local anesthetic depend on the rapidity of absorption from the injection site and the total dose of the drug administered.

The peak plasma concentration after absorption of a local anesthetic from a correctly placed injection depends primarily on the site of injection. Independent of the local anesthetic used, the rate of absorption usually decreases in the following sequence: interpleural, intercostal, caudal, epidural, brachial plexus, subcutaneous, sciatic, and femoral blocks[31–33] (Fig. 12–5). This sequence is mainly related to the degree of vascularity and the local uptake into tissues and fat at the site of injection. Adding epinephrine decreases the peak plasma concentration of local anesthetic, but the degree of this reduction depends on the site of injection and the specific local anesthetic agent[32] (Fig. 12–6). In general, the greatest effects are seen after intercostal blocks and with short-acting agents. A recommended maximum safe dose should be related to the site of injection in addition to the presence or absence of epinephrine.[34]

Potential for Systemic Toxicity

The potential for systemic toxicity should be considered when choosing a local anesthetic. All local anesthetics are potentially toxic drugs, but some agents are more toxic than others. Systemic toxicity after the use of local anesthetic depends on a multiplicity of factors.

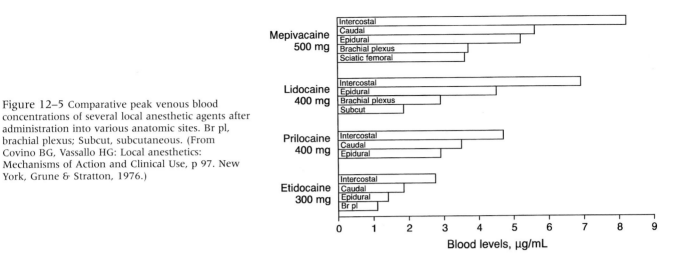

Figure 12–5 Comparative peak venous blood concentrations of several local anesthetic agents after administration into various anatomic sites. Br pl, brachial plexus; Subcut, subcutaneous. (From Covino BG, Vassallo HG: Local anesthetics: Mechanisms of Action and Clinical Use, p 97. New York, Grune & Stratton, 1976.)

It is directly related to the plasma concentrations of local anesthetic. Plasma concentration profiles and the potential risk of systemic toxicity after perineural administration of a local anesthetic depend on the administered dose and the balance between the rate processes involved in drug absorption and systemic disposition. The rate of metabolism varies markedly for different agents; chloroprocaine has the highest clearance of the ester-group compounds, and prilocaine has the highest clearance of the amide-group agents. The use of agents with high clearance rates should greatly decrease the potential for systemic toxicity, particularly during continued administration. In addition to intrinsic toxicity, the physician should consider the rate of administration, total amount administered, and admixture of a vasoconstrictor.

A compromise must be reached between dose and safety. The margin of safety of a local anesthetic lies in the difference between the maximum effective dose and the minimum toxic dose.[35] The safety and effectiveness of a local anesthetic depend on proper dosage

and on the technical competence of the anesthesiologist.

Use of Local Anesthetics for Regional Anesthesia Procedures

Topical Anesthesia

Topical anesthesia is achieved by application of local anesthetic agents to skin or mucous membrane. It blocks the touch sensation in skin or mucous membrane after penetrating the outer layers of the skin or mucosa. Topical anesthesia is used on the skin, conjunctiva, nasal passages, larynx, pharynx, tracheobronchial tree, rectum, and ureter. Application may be by means of direct instillation, soaked swabs, pastes, jellies, ointments, aerosol spray, or lozenges.

Some esters and amides are suitable for topical use. The speed of onset of anesthesia and its duration depend on the agent used, its vehicle, and the site to which it is applied. Higher doses and concentrations generally shorten the onset time and prolong the duration of anesthesia.

Cocaine, tetracaine, lidocaine, benzocaine, and dibucaine have been used mostly for topical anesthesia. These agents are prepared in various forms such as gel, aerosol spray, ointment, lozenges, drops, and cream. The preparation in which the drug is supplied depends on the intended site of application (Table 12–2). Adding epinephrine to local anesthetic solutions used for topical anesthesia does not affect the absorption of these agents.[36] Cornified skin is quite resistant to penetration of local anesthetic. This problem has been overcome by a cream preparation called a eutectic mixture of local anesthetics (EMLA). EMLA cream is a eutectic mixture of lidocaine base (2.5 g·dL[-1]) and prilocaine (2.5 g·dL[-1]) (Fig. 12–7). This preparation produces topical analgesia in normal skin within about 0.5 to 1 h and is especially useful in children before venous puncture and for dermatologic surgery.[37]

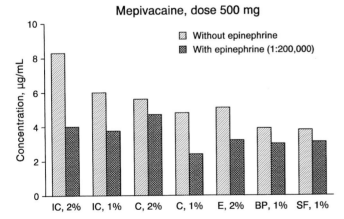

Figure 12–6 Mean peak plasma concentrations of mepivacaine after injection of 1% or 2% solutions with or without epinephrine for various regional block procedures. BP, brachial plexus block; C, caudal block; E, epidural block; IC, intercostal block; SF, sciatic and femoral block. (Modified from Tucker GT, Moore DC, Bridenbaugh PO, et al: Systemic absorption of mepivacaine in commonly used regional block procedures. Anesthesiology 1972; 37: 277–287.)

Table 12–2 Various Preparations Intended for Topical Anesthesia

ANESTHETIC INGREDIENT	CONCENTRATION, %	PHARMACEUTICAL APPLICATION FORM	INTENDED AREA OF USE
Benzocaine	1–5	Cream	Skin and mucous membrane
	20	Ointment	Skin and mucous membrane
	20	Aerosol	Skin and mucous membrane
Cocaine	4	Solution	Ear, nose, throat
Dibucaine	0.25–1	Cream	Skin
	0.25–1	Ointment	Skin
	0.25–1	Aerosol	Skin
	0.25	Solution	Ear
	2.5	Suppositories	Rectum
Dyclonine	0.5–1	Solution	Skin, oropharynx, tracheobronchial tree, urethra, rectum
Lidocaine	2.4	Solution	Oropharynx, tracheobronchial tree, nose
	2	Jelly	Urethra
	2.5–5	Ointment	Skin, mucous membrane, rectum
	2	Viscous	Oropharynx
	10	Suppositories	Rectum
	10	Aerosol	Gingival mucosa
Tetracaine	0.5–1	Ointment	Skin, rectum, mucous membrane
	0.5–1	Cream	Skin, rectum, mucous membrane
	0.25–1	Solution	Skin, rectum, mucous membrane

From Covino BG, Vassallo HG: Local Anesthetics: Mechanisms of Action and Clinical Use, p 93. New York, Grune & Stratton, 1976.

Infiltration Anesthesia

Local infiltration anesthesia is obtained by extravascular placement of local anesthetic in the area to be anesthetized. It is commonly performed for minor surgery. Subcutaneous and intradermal infiltration is performed around the lesion. The choice of local anesthetic agent depends on the size of the area to be anesthetized and on the desired duration of action. If a large surface is involved, large volumes of diluted agents should be used to avoid exceeding the maximum dosage limits of the various agents. Toxicity is not a high risk, especially if epinephrine is added.

The onset of action is almost immediate for all

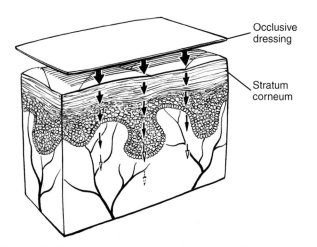

Figure 12–7 The barriers that a eutectic mixture of local anesthetics (EMLA) must penetrate to reach its site of action. (Redrawn from Local Anaesthetics in Theory and Practice. A short review, p 17. Astra Pain Control AB, Sweden, 1990.)

agents, but the various agents can be differentiated according to duration of infiltration anesthesia (Table 12–3). Effective infiltration anesthesia can be obtained with 0.25% to 1% solutions. The addition of epinephrine markedly prolongs the duration of action of all local anesthetics.[38] Concentrations of 1:200,000 to 1:500,000 are usual. Its use must be avoided when extremities such as fingers, toes, or penis are being anesthetized to avoid ischemic tissue damage.

Procaine and chloroprocaine have short durations; lidocaine, mepivacaine, and prilocaine demonstrate moderate durations; and bupivacaine and etidocaine exhibit long durations of action.

Intravenous Regional Anesthesia

With intravenous regional anesthesia, a local anesthetic solution is injected in a limb (usually arm) vein. The circulation of the limb is isolated from the rest of the circulation by a tourniquet. The mechanism by which local anesthetic produces intravenous regional anesthesia is complex and probably reflects action of the drug on nerve binding sites and on nerve trunks.[39] After injection of the solution, a rapid onset of analgesia and skeletal muscle relaxation usually occurs. In general, the use of large volumes of more dilute solutions offers the optimal conditions for satisfactory anesthesia and safety.

The amides lidocaine (0.25% to 0.5%) and prilocaine (0.5%) are most often used for this procedure.[40] In much of Europe, prilocaine is the drug of choice for intravenous regional anesthesia because of its relatively low potential for systemic toxicity.[41] A 0.5% solution provides excellent pain relief of long duration. Vasoconstrictors must not be added to the anesthetic solu-

Table 12–3 Local Anesthetic Concentration, Maximum Dose, and Duration of Infiltration Block Anesthesia

		PLAIN SOLUTION		EPINEPHRINE-CONTAINING SOLUTION	
AGENT	**CONCENTRATION, %**	**Maximum Dose, mg**	**Duration, min**	**Maximum Dose, mg**	**Duration, min**
Short Duration					
Procaine ⎫ Chloroprocaine ⎭	1.0–2.0	800	15–30	1000	30–90
Moderate Duration					
Lidocaine	0.5–1.0	300	30–60	500	120–360
Mepivacaine	0.5–1.0	300	45–90	500	120–360
Prilocaine	0.5–1.0	500	30–90	600	120–360
Long Duration					
Bupivacaine	0.25–0.5	175	120–240	225	180–420
Etidocaine	0.5–1.0	300	120–180	400	180–420

From Concepcion M, Covino BG: Rational use of local anaesthetics. Drugs 1984; 27: 256–270.

tion. Severe complications, including death, have been reported with the use of large doses of bupivacaine.[42] Sudden early tourniquet release may result in systemic toxicity when a relatively large dose enters into the systemic bloodstream.

Peripheral Nerve Block

Peripheral nerve block involves the inhibition of conduction in the nerve fibers of the peripheral nervous system. Peripheral nerve block is divided into minor and major nerve blocks. Minor nerve blocks involve a single nerve, such as the ulnar or radial nerve; major nerve blocks involve two or more nerves or a nerve plexus. In this section, the choice of local anesthetics is considered according to their duration of action.

Minor Nerve

The choice is based on the required duration of anesthesia. The duration of analgesia and motor block is prolonged significantly when epinephrine is added to the local anesthetic solutions. Procaine and chloroprocaine in concentrations of 1% exhibit a relatively short duration of action; lidocaine, mepivacaine, and prilocaine with concentrations of 0.5% to 1% have a relatively moderate duration, and 0.25% bupivacaine and 0.5% etidocaine are agents suitable for prolonged blocks.

Plexus and Major Nerve

The concentrations of local anesthetic solutions for a major nerve block depend on the degree of motor block desired. Epinephrine should be added to the appropriate solutions if large volumes are needed.

The solutions commonly used for major nerve blocks are lidocaine (1%), mepivacaine (1%), prilocaine (2%), bupivacaine (0.5%), and etidocaine (0.75% to 1%). The addition of epinephrine may prolong the action of local anesthetics by as much as 200% for short-acting agents, such as lidocaine, but by only 20% to 50% for longer-acting agents, such as bupivacaine and etidocaine.

Neuraxial Block

Epidural Anesthesia

Epidural anesthesia is achieved by administration of local anesthetic drugs into the epidural space. It is one of the most versatile regional blocks in use. The essential qualities of epidural anesthesia are the onset, spread, intensity, and duration of sensory and motor blocks. These features are influenced by the local anesthetic used. The larger the volume of a particular concentration of a local anesthetic solution injected into the epidural space, the greater is the spread of epidural anesthesia.[21] An increase in the mass of local anesthetic produces a faster onset and a longer duration of sensory block, and increasing the concentration results in a shorter onset time and increase in intensity of the motor block.[43] The dose of epidural local anesthetic agents is largely determined by the number of spinal segments to be blocked and the volume necessary to reach those segments. The ability of epinephrine to prolong the duration of action of regional block varies with the specific local anesthetic and its concentration. In general, the duration of shorter-acting agents, such as lidocaine and prilocaine, is markedly prolonged by the use of epinephrine (1:200,000), and the longer-acting agents, such as bupivacaine and etidocaine, are influenced less by the addition of epinephrine.[43]

Table 12–4 lists the agents and concentrations available, with their onset times and the quality of sensory and motor blocks.

2-Chloroprocaine is often selected when rapid onset and short duration of sensory anesthesia are appropriate. It results in dense sensory and motor block. Lidocaine is an excellent drug for epidural anesthesia and is characterized by a relatively rapid onset of action and short duration. The 1% solution is associated with minimal motor block, and the 2% solution of lidocaine with 1:200,000 epinephrine is associated with more profound motor block. Two percent solutions of mepivacaine and prilocaine are approximately similar to lidocaine with epinephrine in terms of clinical properties. Unlike lidocaine, the addition of epinephrine to

Table 12–4 Local Anesthetic Agents for Epidural Use

AGENT	CONCENTRATION, %	ONSET TO SURGICAL ANALGESIA, min	SENSORY BLOCK	MOTOR BLOCK
Chloroprocaine	2	10–15 7–10 (EPI)	Analgesic	Mild to moderate
	3	7–15 5–10 (EPI)	Analgesic	Dense
Lidocaine	1	15–30 10–20 (EPI)	Analgesic	Minimal
	2	10–20 7–15 (EPI)	Dense	Mild to moderate
Mepivacaine	1	15–30 10–20 (EPI)	Analgesic	Minimal
	2	10–20 7–15 (EPI)	Dense	Dense
Prilocaine	2	10–20 7–15 (EPI)	Dense	Minimal
	3	7–15 5–10 (EPI)	Dense	Dense
Bupivacaine	0.25	20–40 20–40 (EPI)	Analgesic	Minimal
	0.5	15–30 10–25 (EPI)	Dense	Mild to moderate
	0.75	15–30 10–20 (EPI)	Dense	Mild to moderate
Etidocaine	1	10–20 7–15 (EPI)	Moderate to dense	Moderate to dense
	1.5	7–15 5–10 (EPI)	Dense	Dense
Ropivacaine	0.5	20–40	Analgesic	Minimal
	0.75	15–30	Dense	Mild to moderate
	1	15–30	Dense	Moderate to dense

EPI, 1:200,000 concentration of epinephrine.

mepivacaine does not result in a marked prolongation of duration of epidural anesthesia.

Bupivacaine is commonly used for epidural anesthesia. With lower concentrations of bupivacaine, a significant separation of sensory anesthesia and motor block occurs.[44] As a result, 0.25% or even more diluted solutions are used in the management of obstetric analgesia and postoperative pain relief; in these situations, motor block is undesirable.[44, 45] With a 0.75% solution of bupivacaine, the onset time is shortened, the duration of neural block is prolonged, and the degree of motor block is more profound. With a 1% to 1.5% solution of etidocaine, no separation of sensory and motor blocks occurs. Etidocaine is characterized by rapid onset, prolonged duration of action, and profound motor block. As a result, it is suitable for procedures requiring dense motor block.

The long-acting, amide-type ropivacaine appears to be an effective long-acting local anesthetic when given epidurally.[46] A 0.5% solution of ropivacaine is less potent in producing a motor block than 0.5% bupivacaine[47] (Fig. 12–8).

Caudal Anesthesia

Caudal anesthesia is a form of epidural anesthesia. It is achieved by administration of local anesthetic drugs into the sacral canal through the sacral hiatus. When surgery is restricted to the perineum and surrounding tissues, a caudal block is a suitable technique. Analgesia of the lumbosacral spinal segments is often associated with minimal sympathetic block. Whether the single injection or continuous type of caudal anesthesia is used, the principles of administration are the same as for epidural anesthesia.

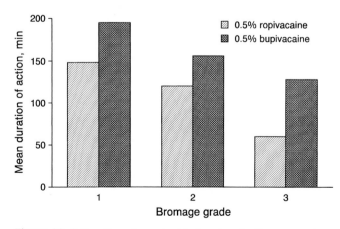

Figure 12–8 Duration of a motor block, using the Bromage scale, during epidural anesthesia with 0.5% ropivacaine and 0.5% bupivacaine solutions. (Data from Brockway MS, Bannister J, McClure JH, et al: Comparison of extradural ropivacaine and bupivacaine. Br J Anaesth 1991; 66: 31–37.)

Approximately twice the dose of local anesthetic drug is needed for caudal anesthesia than for lumbar epidural anesthesia because of the relatively large sacral canal and the free leakage of solution out of the large sacral foramina. Usually, 25 to 30 mL of lidocaine (2%) with epinephrine or bupivacaine (0.5%) provides adequate anesthesia.

Spinal Anesthesia

Spinal anesthesia is achieved by administration of local anesthetic drugs into the subarachnoid space. The most important clinical features of spinal anesthesia are the onset, spread (i.e., level), and duration of sensory analgesia and motor block. These qualities of the regional block may be influenced by the anesthetic solution, the anesthetic technique, and the patient.[48] The spread of analgesic solutions is determined by the baricity of the anesthetic solution, the position of the patient during and after the injection, and the concentration and volume to be injected. The main determinants of the duration of spinal anesthesia are the drug used and the total dose injected. The addition of epinephrine may prolong the duration of spinal anesthesia. Epinephrine consistently, although briefly, prolongs the duration of lidocaine- and bupivacaine-induced spinal anesthesia, particularly in the lumbar and sacral dermatomes.[49, 50] The greatest increase in duration occurs when epinephrine is added to tetracaine solutions.[51]

Spinal anesthesia has been attempted with many agents, but only a few remain in common use (Table 12–5). Among the amino-ester compounds, only two agents are prepared specifically for use in spinal anesthesia: procaine and tetracaine. Procaine (10%) is available as a hyperbaric, glucose-free solution and is characterized by a short onset time, a profound degree of sensory and motor block, and a relatively short duration. It is used primarily for diagnostic differential spinal blocks. Tetracaine may be used as a hyperbaric, isobaric, or hypobaric solution. The drug is available as freeze-dried (niphanoid) crystals or a 1% aqueous solution and is mixed with equal volumes of dextrose or isotonic saline to produce hyperbaric or isobaric 0.5% solutions of tetracaine. The hyperbaric solution is used most commonly. It provides a relatively rapid onset, excellent-quality sensory block, and profound motor block. Its duration of action is markedly prolonged by adding epinephrine.[51]

Of the amino amides, the most commonly used agents for spinal anesthesia are lidocaine and bupivacaine. Lidocaine is available as a hyperbaric solution in a concentration of 5%. It provides a rapid onset with a relatively short duration of action. A glucose-free 2% solution of lidocaine, which is essentially isobaric, provides a more intense motor block than a hyperbaric 5% solution of lidocaine.[52]

Bupivacaine has been widely used for spinal anesthesia in a glucose-free solution at a concentration of 0.5% or 0.75% or a hyperbaric solution at a concentration of 0.5% or 0.75% with dextrose.[53] The duration and quality of motor block of the lower limbs decrease with baricity. Glucose-free bupivacaine solutions provide a complete, profound, and long-lasting motor block of the lower limbs, and hyperbaric solutions of bupivacaine cause a profound motor block of the abdominal muscles of intermediate duration[54] (Fig. 12–9).

Dibucaine is available in isobaric, hypobaric, and hyperbaric solutions for spinal anesthesia, but its use is declining with the increasing use of bupivacaine. Dibucaine is more potent than tetracaine, although the onset of action of both agents is similar; the duration of spinal anesthesia is slightly longer with dibucaine.[15]

Subarachnoid injection of ropivacaine appears to result in a variable spread of analgesia with a good-quality motor block, in particular with the glucose-free 0.75% solution.[55]

Interpleural Regional Analgesia

Interpleural regional analgesia is achieved by the administration of local anesthetics into the pleural cavity by means of an interpleural catheter. This technique

Table 12–5 Spinal Anesthesia Agents

AGENT	USUAL CONCENTRATION, %	USUAL VOLUME, mL	TOTAL DOSE, mg	BARICITY	GLUCOSE CONCENTRATION, %	USUAL ANESTHETIC DURATION, min
Lidocaine	1.5–5.0	1–2	15–100	Hyperbaric	7.5	30–90
Mepivacaine	4	1–2	40–80	Hyperbaric	9.0	30–90
Tetracaine	0.25–1.0 0.1–0.3 0.5	1–4	5–20	Hyperbaric Hyperbaric* Isobaric†	5.0	75–150
Dibucaine	0.25 0.5 0.067	1–2 1–2 5–20	2.5–5.0 5–10 3–12	Hyperbaric Hyperbaric Hyperbaric	5.0	75–180
Bupivacaine	0.5 0.5–0.75	3–4 2–3	15–20 15–22.5	Isobaric‡ Hyperbaric	8.0	180–240 90–120

*Hyperbaric, 1% tetracaine in sterile water.
†Isobaric, 1% tetracaine in equal volume of cerebrospinal fluid.
‡Isobaric, glucose-free bupivacaine is slightly hypobaric.
From Concepcion M, Covino BG: Rational use of local anaesthetics. Drugs 1984; 27: 256–270.

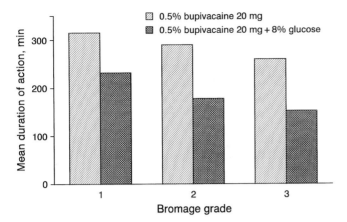

Figure 12–9 Duration of a motor block, using the Bromage scale, during spinal anesthesia with hyperbaric and glucose-free bupivacaine solutions. (Data from Axelsson KH, Widman GB, Sundberg AEA, et al: A double-blind study of motor blockade in the lower limbs: studies during spinal anaesthesia with hyperbaric and glucose-free 0.5% bupivacaine. Br J Anaesth 1985; 57: 960–970.)

provides analgesia but not anesthesia sufficient for the performance of surgery.[56] The mechanism of action appears to be, in part, diffusion of the local anesthetic from the pleural space into the intercostal muscles, resulting in multiple unilateral intercostal nerve blocks. Other analgesia mechanisms may include mediastinal splanchnic nerve block and systemic local anesthetic blood levels. This technique has been used successfully in patients after open cholecystectomy and in patients with multiple unilateral fractured ribs.

Bupivacaine is most often used. Large volumes (approximately 20 mL of a 0.5% solution) are needed to provide adequate analgesia. Relatively high plasma concentrations of bupivacaine have been reported after the interpleural administration of 100 mg of bupivacaine, indicating that the margin of safety may be small.[57] The addition of epinephrine lowered the plasma concentrations of bupivacaine. Continuous interpleural infusion of 0.25% solutions of bupivacaine provided adequate pain relief after cholecystectomy and was not associated with toxic levels of bupivacaine.[58]

Factors Influencing the Choice of Technique

Patient Characteristics

Patients may vary in their responses to the same dose of a local anesthetic. The physical status of the patient and several pathophysiologic conditions may modify the effects of local anesthetics. In principle, changes in the dose-response relationship can be accounted for by changes in pharmacodynamics, pharmacokinetics, or both. Careful evaluation of these factors is necessary in the choice of local anesthetic agents for the individual patient. The influence of some physical and pathophysiologic variables on the pharmacodynamics and pharmacokinetics of local anesthetic agents is summarized in Table 12–6.

Physiologic Factors

Age. Age has been associated with a higher upper level of analgesia after epidural administration of a fixed dose of bupivacaine[59, 60] (Fig. 12–10), and it has been reported[61] that the extent of analgesia increased with age after thoracic epidural administration of a fixed dose of mepivacaine. The increased spread is probably related to anatomic changes in the central nervous system and spinal canal (Fig. 12–11). Increased

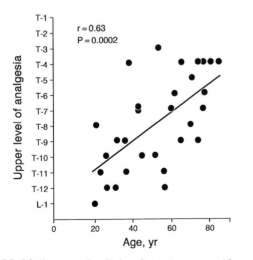

Figure 12–10 The upper level of analgesia increases with age after epidural administration of bupivacaine. (From Veering BTh, Burm AGL, van Kleef JW, et al: Epidural anesthesia with bupivacaine: effects of age on neural blockade and pharmacokinetics. Anesth Analg 1987; 66: 589–593.)

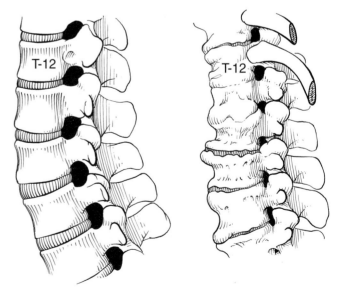

Figure 12–11 Blocking of the intervertebral foramina by osteoarthritic changes. On the left, part of the thoracolumbar spine is seen in the lateral view of a 32-year-old man and, on the right, of a 92-year-old man. Notice the disposition of the intervertebral foramina. (Redrawn from Bullough PG, Boachie-Adjei O: Atlas of Spinal Diseases. Philadelphia, JB Lippincott, 1988.)

Table 12–6 Influence of Some Physical and Pathophysiologic Variables on the Pharmacodynamics and Pharmacokinetics of Local Anesthetic Agents

VARIABLE	AGENT	ROUTE	CHANGE	CLINICAL IMPLICATION	REFERENCES
Physical					
Age					
Adults	B	Epi	Level of analgesia ↑	Injection at L4–5	59, 60
			Cl ↓	Dosage ↓	
	M	Epi-th	Level of analgesia ↑	Dosage ↓	61
	B-hyp	Sub	Level of analgesia ↑	Injection at L4–5	62, 63
				Sitting period ↑	
	B-plain	Sub	Duration of analgesia ↑	Dosage ↓	64
Infants	B	Caud	Duration of analgesia ↑	Dosage ↓	65, 66
	B	Caud	Cl ↑, Fu ↑	Caution	67, 68
Weight	B-plain	Sub	Level of analgesia ↑	Dosage ↓	69, 70
				Injection at L4–5	
Pregnancy	L	Epi	Level of analgesia ↑	Dosage ↓	71
	B-hyp	Sub	Level of analgesia ↑	Dosage ↓	72
Pathophysiologic					
Cardiovascular system					
Angina pectoris (unstable)	B	Epi-th	Major determinants of myocardial oxygen consumption ↓	Probably protective effects on ischemic myocardium	73
Arteriosclerosis	L, M, B	Epi	Level of analgesia ↑	Dosage ↓	74
Hepatic system					
Acute hepatitis	L	IV	$T_{1/2}$ ↑, V ↑	Reduce dose during continuous	75
Cirrhosis	L	IV	Cl ↓	administration	76
Renal system					
Renal failure	B-plain	Sub	Onset time ↓	Not suitable for renal transplantation	77
			Duration of analgesia ↓		
			Duration of motor block ↓		
	L, M, B	Brach	Duration of analgesia ↓	Administration long-acting agent (e.g., B)	78
			Onset time ↓		

B, bupivacaine; B-hyp, hyperbaric bupivacaine; Brach, brachial plexus; Caud, caudal; Cl, clearance; Epi, epidural; Epi-th, thoracic epidural; Fu, free fraction in plasma; IV, intravenous; L, lidocaine; M, mepivacaine; Sub, subarachnoid; $T_{1/2}$, terminal elimination half-life; V, volume of distribution; ↑, increase; ↓, decrease.

epidural resistance and decreased epidural compliance with advancing age may contribute to this enhanced spread in the elderly.[79]

Increasing age has been associated with a slightly higher spread of analgesia after subarachnoid administration of a hyperbaric bupivacaine solution[62, 63] and a prolonged duration of analgesia after subarachnoid administration of glucose-free bupivacaine solution.[64] Gradual degeneration of the central and peripheral nervous system may contribute to the increased sensitivity to local anesthetics in the elderly.

Increasing age has been associated with a decrease in the clearance of bupivacaine after epidural and subarachnoid administration.[59, 63, 64] Thus, plasma levels increase to higher levels with prolonged epidural infusion in older patients, and the infusion rates or top-up doses may need to be adjusted for older patients.

Weight and Height. Spinal and epidural anesthesia may be technically difficult in the obese patient, because bony landmarks are obscured. Increased pressure in the epidural space secondary to engorged veins may make predictability of the sensory anesthetic level difficult.[80]

The dose requirement for spinal anesthesia appears to be approximately 80% of normal and to have more variability than in nonobese patients.[69, 70] In obese patients, administration of glucose-free bupivacaine at L4-5 instead of L3-4 decreases the likelihood of exten-

sive spread.[70] However, with epidural anesthesia, the weight of patients appears to have little effect on the quality of a regional block.[21, 81] The use of epidural anesthesia intraoperatively and postoperatively is beneficial in morbidly obese patients, because it lowers the intrapulmonary shunt fraction and decreases the left ventricular work.[82]

With epidural and spinal anesthesia, the height of the patient can be ignored, except in extremely short or extremely tall individuals.[21, 83]

Pregnancy. Epidural and spinal anesthesia are often associated with high levels of analgesia in pregnant women. This exaggerated spread has been attributed to inferior vena caval compression in pregnancy, which results in a marked distension of the epidural venous plexus, decreasing the volume of the epidural space.[71] For these patients, the epidural and spinal dose requirements should be decreased. Increased susceptibility of nerves to local anesthetic or enhanced diffusion related to hormonal changes (or both) may also contribute to greater sensitivity in pregnant women.[72]

Pathophysiologic Factors

Regional anesthesia may benefit the compromised patient; minimal physiologic trespass often means fewer cardiac and pulmonary complications. However, emphasis should be placed on individualization, such as "matching the particular pathophysiology involved with the technique perceived to be least disruptive."[84]

Respiratory System. Patients with compromised respiratory function having peripheral surgery (not in abdomen or thorax) generally profit from the application of regional anesthetic techniques. The patients' ability to maintain appropriate ventilation is not distorted, and the patients can clear their own secretions. Spinal anesthesia does not adversely influence the partial pressure of arterial oxygen, intraoperatively or postoperatively, in patients undergoing hip surgery.[85] Epidural and spinal forms of anesthesia to thoracic levels are not associated with changes in minute ventilation, respiratory rate, and carbon dioxide sensitivity in patients free of clinically significant cardiac or pulmonary disease.[86, 87] Spinal or epidural anesthesia to midthoracic levels may seriously compromise ventilation in patients with severe pulmonary disease, who cannot afford impairment of any respiratory muscles.

Cardiovascular System. The potential risk of compromising the coronary circulation with sudden hypotension or of precipitating congestive cardiac failure with fluid preloading must be taken into account when making a decision about application of a spinal or epidural block in cardiac patients with compromised cardiac functions. Arteriosclerosis and occlusive arterial disease may lead to exaggerated spread of epidurally administered local anesthetic solutions.[74] Caution should be taken in determining the dosages for those patients.

High segmental epidural anesthesia in patients with unstable angina pectoris decreased the major indices of myocardial oxygen demand such as systolic blood pressure, pulmonary artery pressure, and heart rate without jeopardizing coronary perfusion pressure[73] (Fig. 12–12). However, it was demonstrated[88] that pa-

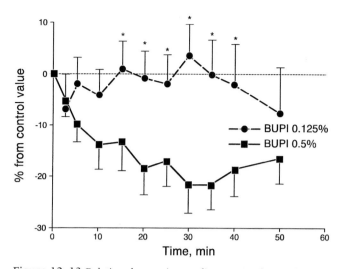

Figure 12–13 Relative changes in systolic pressure during the first 50 min after injection of a low and a high dose of bupivacaine (BUPI) through a spinal microcatheter. The anesthetic levels were the same in both groups; *$P < .05$. (From Labaille T, Benhamou D, Westermann J: Hemodynamic effects of continuous spinal anesthesia: a comparative study between low and high doses of bupivacaine. Reg Anesth 1992; 17: 193–196.)

tients with stable angina pectoris showed myocardial ischemia some hours after the application of spinal analgesia, probably because of increased cardiac preload and afterload, possibly further aggravated by the volume load. Thoracic epidural anesthesia with local anesthetics was effective in the treatment of severe, ischemic chest pain in patients with acute myocardial infarction.[89]

Continuous spinal anesthesia catheter techniques allow titration of small intermittent doses. The possibility of continuing the block step by step obviously decreases the risk of extensive hemodynamic effects[90] (Fig. 12–13). Patients with valvular heart diseases should maintain reasonable heart rate, preload, and contractility. High spinal or epidural anesthesia blocking the sympathetic cardiac innervation (T-1 to T-4) should be avoided in those patients.

Hepatic System. Because amide-type agents are predominantly metabolized in the liver, it is likely that hepatic diseases are associated with clinically more significant alterations in pharmacokinetics. Severe liver disease may decrease the detoxification processes of the amino amides (at the level of microsomal oxidation reactions within the liver) and amino esters (owing to decreased synthesis of plasma cholinesterase). Patients with acute hepatitis show increased elimination half-lives and distribution volumes of lidocaine.[75] In patients with severe liver cirrhosis, the clearance of lidocaine is markedly decreased.[76] As a consequence, systemic accumulation of the amino-amide agents is more extensive. This problem should be minimized by decreasing the dose.

Renal System. In chronic renal failure with the development of uremia, the clinical profile of bupivacaine changes after subarachnoid administration and brachial plexus blocks.[77, 78] After subarachnoid administration of glucose-free bupivacaine solution, the onset

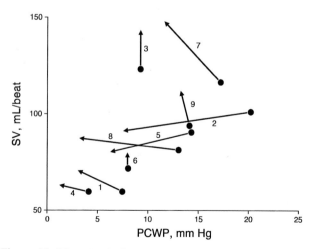

Figure 12–12 During high thoracic epidural anesthesia (TEA), the stroke volume (SV) increases, while the pulmonary wedge pressure (PCWP) decreases in patients with unstable angina pectoris. The circles indicate values before TEA, the arrows point to values during TEA, and the numbers indicate the individual patients. (From Blomberg S, Emanuelsson H, Ricksten S-E: Thoracic epidural anesthesia and central hemodynamics in patients with unstable angina pectoris. Anesth Analg 1989; 69: 558–562.)

of analgesia is more rapid and the duration of analgesia is shorter. This short duration in the abdominal area implies that it would not be possible to consistently perform renal transplantations during spinal anesthesia with bupivacaine. The main reason for these changes is probably the faster elimination from the site of action of local anesthetic into the hyperdynamic circulation observed in chronic renal failure.[91] Nevertheless, renal transplantation may effectively be performed with continuous epidural anesthesia.

Contraindications

Regional anesthesia is practiced with few absolute contraindications:

1. Active infection at the site of the puncture (i.e., skin infection), active septicemia (i.e., neuraxial or peripheral blocks), and meningitis (i.e., neuraxial blocks)
2. Allergy to local anesthetics
3. Use of anticoagulants (i.e., epidural and spinal blocks are contraindicated in patients within 24 h of receiving thrombolytic therapy, with known coagulopathies, or with significant thrombocytopenia,[92] although "individualization" of regional block must be kept in mind)
4. Uncorrected hypovolemia (i.e., contraindication to neuraxial blocks)
5. The patient's refusal or inability to cooperate with regional anesthesia.

Any plan for regional anesthesia is conditional on patient acceptance and cooperation.

Specialized Applications

The following sections address the application of local anesthetics within medical subspecialties.

Dentistry

For dental procedures, local anesthetic agents must be capable of diffusing through the outer bone lamina in the upper jaw. To achieve this, the concentrations of local anesthetics administered for dental use are much higher than for other clinical applications. Higher concentrations also are required because the volume injected cannot exceed a few milliliters to avoid the risk of tissue distension. Vasoconstrictive agents, such as epinephrine, are used mostly to maintain the high, localized concentration.

Solutions used commonly for infiltration and conduction anesthesia include 2% lidocaine with 1:80,000 epinephrine, 3% to 4% prilocaine with 1:200,000 epinephrine, 4% articaine with 1:200,000 epinephrine, 3% mepivacaine, and the longer-acting agents of 0.5% bupivacaine and 1.5% etidocaine, both with 1:200,000 epinephrine.[93]

Ophthalmology

Local infiltration with dilute solutions of tetracaine provides painless anesthesia of the cornea and conjunctiva. The use of local anesthesia for cataract surgery is increasing at the expense of general anesthesia. Retrobulbar and peribulbar techniques are effective in achieving analgesia, akinesis of the globe and orbicularis oculi, and low intraocular pressure.

A short-onset drug, such as lidocaine or mepivacaine, is usually mixed with a long-duration local anesthetic, such as bupivacaine or etidocaine. The adjuvant hyaluronidase helps decrease onset time in retrobulbar anesthesia when used with a mixture of lidocaine and bupivacaine.[94]

Adding fresh epinephrine to the local anesthetic solution with hyaluronidase results in a higher pH, shortening the onset and prolonging the duration of the peribulbar block[95] (Fig. 12–14).

Otorhinolaryngology

Topical anesthesia, often in combination with infiltration anesthesia of specific nerves, can be an excellent choice for certain otorhinolaryngologic procedures. Topical anesthesia is often advantageous to shrink mucous membranes by vasoconstriction.

Cotton swabs soaked in a 4% solution of lidocaine with 1:200,000 epinephrine or 4% to 5% cocaine and aerosol sprays with 4% to 10% cocaine or 10% lidocaine are used for topical anesthesia.

Lidocaine (0.5% to 1%), prilocaine (1%), and bupivacaine (0.5%), all with epinephrine, are most often used for infiltration. Preincisional infiltration of the tonsils with a 0.25% solution of bupivacaine with 1:200,000 epinephrine markedly decreased the intensity of pain after tonsillectomy well beyond the immediate postoperative period[96] (Fig. 12–15).

Obstetrics

The goal of labor analgesia is to provide optimal pain relief with minimal risk to mother and fetus. Continuous lumbar epidural anesthesia is the most versatile technique, because it can be used for pain relief

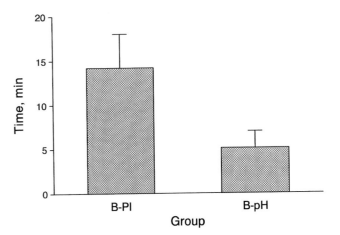

Figure 12–14 Peribulbar block with pH-adjusted bupivacaine (B-pH) results in faster onset times to complete akinesia compared with injections with plain bupivacaine (B-Pl). (From Zahl K, Jordan A, McGroarty J, et al: pH-Adjusted bupivacaine and hyaluronidase for peribulbar block. Anesthesiology 1990; 72: 230–232.)

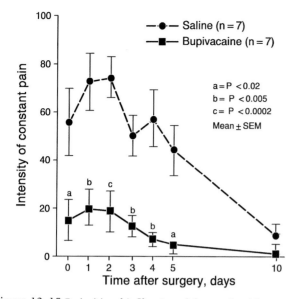

Figure 12–15 Preincisional infiltration of the tonsils with bupivacaine 0.25% with epinephrine markedly decreases the intensity of pain in the postoperative period after tonsillectomy. (From Jebeles JA, Reilly JS, Gutierrez JF, et al: The effect of preincisional infiltration of tonsils with bupivacaine on the pain following tonsillectomy under general anesthesia. Pain 1991; 47: 305–308.)

for the first stage of labor and as anesthesia for subsequent vaginal delivery or cesarean section, if necessary.

A combination of low concentrations of local anesthetic with opioids has become popular for labor and delivery. It offers excellent analgesia with a minimum of side effects.[97] This section, however, considers the use of local anesthetic solutions without opioids in obstetrics.

Labor. With chloroprocaine, placental transfer is small, and toxic reactions in the mother are unlikely. Chloroprocaine produces intense motor and sensory block rapidly, but because it has a short duration and rapid offset, many anesthesiologists find it unsuitable for use throughout labor. It can be used to initiate a block when rapid pain relief is required before continuing with a longer-acting agent. Lidocaine (1.5%) provides effective pain relief with moderate motor block.[98] In labor analgesia, it is used to provide rapidly profound motor and sensory block (e.g., emergency forceps delivery).

Bupivacaine remains the most popular local anesthetic used for labor pain relief because of the differential nerve block. When used as a 0.25% or even more diluted solution, it provides adequate sensory analgesia with minimal motor block. Epinephrine added to dilute solutions of bupivacaine for epidural block in laboring parturients improves the speed of action and duration of sensory analgesia.[99]

Although limited experience is available with ropivacaine in pregnancy, the first study comparing bupivacaine with ropivacaine showed no major differences regarding the characteristics of pain relief in labor.[100]

Cesarean Section. Analgesic requirements for cesarean section are different from those of vaginal delivery. The block height must reach as far as T-4, and preservation of motor power is unnecessary for delivery.

Epidural Anesthesia. Because of its extremely rapid onset and metabolism and its low risk of systemic toxicity, chloroprocaine (3%) is a useful drug for cesarean delivery.[101] Lidocaine (2%) is suitable but requires the addition of epinephrine to ensure adequate lumbosacral anesthesia.[102]

Mepivacaine (2%) has been used successfully in volumes of 15 to 20 mL.[103] Bupivacaine (0.5%) produces good operating conditions for cesarean section. Adequate anesthesia is usually achieved with 15 to 25 mL of the solution, given in divided doses through an epidural catheter.

Spinal Anesthesia. Spinal anesthesia is becoming increasingly popular in obstetric practice because it provides rapid onset, excellent-quality sensory block, and profound motor block. Hyperbaric solutions of lidocaine (5.0%) and tetracaine (0.5%) have been used for spinal anesthesia for cesarean section. The major drawback with lidocaine is its short duration of action. Hyperbaric 0.5% tetracaine has, however, a less predictable onset of action and duration. Bupivacaine has gained popularity as a glucose-free solution or a hyperbaric solution.[104]

Pediatrics

Regional anesthetic techniques performed immediately after the induction of general anesthesia may decrease the anesthetic requirements during surgery and provide excellent, profound postoperative analgesia in infants and children.[105] Caudal anesthesia is the most widely used block, but the epidural block has gained popularity. Children vary in size, and aspects of their anatomy change as they grow. As a consequence, pharmacokinetic and physiologic differences between children and adults contribute to the use of regional anesthesia in children. From a pharmacodynamic point of view, it appears that local anesthetics act more rapidly, their effects lasts longer, and lower concentrations are needed to block nerve conduction in infants and young children than in adults.[65, 66] The addition of epinephrine increases the duration of action of bupivacaine after caudal administration by 50% to 100% in infants[65] (Fig. 12–16).

Bupivacaine is the most commonly used agent in caudal anesthesia. The multiple dosage regimens are based on patient age, height, and weight and on pharmacodynamic and pharmacokinetic studies. Peak plasma concentrations in infants and children after caudal injection of lidocaine, mepivacaine, or bupivacaine appear to be broadly comparable to those in adults, given a similar dose on a mg/kg basis.[106] The clearance of bupivacaine is consistently higher in infants and children compared with adults.[67, 68] Because the free fraction of bupivacaine is markedly increased in young infants (1 to 6 mo),[68] caution must be exercised in the use of bupivacaine in infants younger than 6 mo of age. Continuous epidural infusions of bupivacaine have been shown to be safe and effective for managing postoperative pain in pediatric patients.[107]

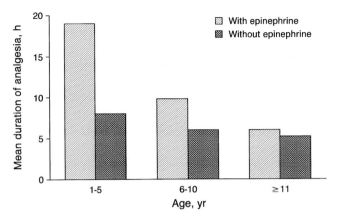

Figure 12–16 Addition of epinephrine increases the duration of action of bupivacaine after caudal administration by 50% to 100% in infants. (Data from Warner MA, Kunkel SE, Offord KO, et al: The effects of age, epinephrine, and operative site on duration of caudal analgesia in pediatric patients. Anesth Analg 1987; 66: 995–998.)

The concentration should not exceed 0.25% if the motor block is to be minimized.

Tetracaine has been the most popular local anesthetic used for spinal anesthesia in infants and children. The dose of a hyperbaric tetracaine solution may be roughly estimated at 0.4 mg/kg.[108] No data are available on the use of ropivacaine in children.

Surgery

The decision to use a regional anesthetic technique for a surgical procedure depends on the nature of the operation, the site of the operation, and the need for postoperative pain treatment. Suggested techniques of regional anesthesia according to surgical procedures are summarized in Table 12–7.

Major procedures often require the addition of a light general anesthetic to the regional technique. However, deep anesthesia is not required, and consciousness is often rapidly recovered.

Regional anesthesia has its limitations. It is not applicable to all kinds of operations and often it requires more skill than general anesthesia. However, epidural and spinal anesthesia appear to decrease the endocrine-metabolic stress response to surgery.[109] This effect applies mostly to lower abdominal, perineal, and lower limb surgery. There is also evidence that hip operations are associated with fewer short-term complications when performed under epidural and spinal anesthesia.[110]

By using epidural catheter techniques, a limited number of dermatomes can be blocked at the appropriate level for operation. The choice between the single-shot and the catheter technique largely depends on the estimated duration of operation and the need for postoperative pain relief. Subarachnoid block is a most useful anesthetic for lower body operations. Compared with epidural or spinal anesthesia, peripheral nerve blocks are not associated with the hypotension resulting from a sympathetic block. However, peripheral nerve blocks may require more technical skills.

The local anesthetic agent and dosage must be selected on the basis of the expected duration of surgery and the degree of motor block required. If minimal motor block is required for the surgical procedure, low concentrations of local anesthetic (e.g., 0.25% bupivacaine, 1% lidocaine, 1% prilocaine) should be chosen. However, for more profound motor block, 2% lidocaine or 2% mepivacaine or the long-acting agents such as 0.75% bupivacaine or 1.5% etidocaine are recommended. When epinephrine is used as an adjuvant to the local anesthetic solution, the quality of neural block is improved, particularly with lidocaine.

Spinal anesthesia with a glucose-free bupivacaine solution is characterized by a complete, profound, and long-lasting motor block of the lower limbs and is suitable for operation on a lower limb.[54]

Outpatients

The most useful regional techniques for outpatients are those that involve a rapid onset and have a high degree of reliability and predictability. Intravenous regional anesthesia and spinal anesthesia are highly efficacious in the outpatient setting. Brachial plexus blocks have been used successfully for prolonged operations on upper limbs in outpatient settings.[111]

Outpatient surgery necessitates careful selection of shorter-acting agents, such as chloroprocaine or lidocaine. Lidocaine (0.5%) and prilocaine (0.5%) are the drugs of choice for intravenous regional anesthesia. For spinal anesthesia, the agent most frequently used is hyperbaric 5% or isobaric 2% lidocaine. Epidural use of the short- and intermediate-acting local anesthetics 2-chloroprocaine and lidocaine is safe and effective for outpatient procedures.[112]

The major drawback with chloroprocaine given epidurally appears to be backache.[113] Local infiltration of the surgical wound with dilute solutions of the long-acting local anesthetic bupivacaine (0.25%) or etidocaine (1%) provides prolonged postoperative analgesia.

Postoperative Pain

Regional anesthesia techniques are effective for providing pain relief. Single-injection techniques and continuous-catheter techniques may be useful in the management of postoperative pain after minor and major surgical procedures, respectively. Wound infiltration with local anesthetic, peripheral nerve blocks, intercostal blocks, interpleural blocks, intra-articular regional injection with local anesthetic, and spinal anesthesia are suitable methods of regional anesthesia to provide postoperative pain relief after a wide variety of surgical procedures.[114] Use of the combination of local anesthetics and intraspinal opioids has increased in the management of postoperative pain.[115]

Bupivacaine is usually the preferred local anesthetic because of its prolonged duration of action and its ability to provide separation of sensory and motor fiber effect. An epidural infusion with a local anesthetic can create a localized band of analgesia at the site of incision without sedation. A potential problem associated with continuous epidural anesthesia provided by inter-

Table 12–7 Suggested Techniques of Regional Anesthesia According to Surgical Procedure

REGIONAL ANESTHETIC TECHNIQUE	REQUIRED DERMATOMAL INNERVATION	TYPE OF SURGERY
		Upper extremity
Interscalene block	C-3 to T-1	Shoulder
Brachial plexus block	C-5 to T-2	Elbow, forearm, wrist, hand
Intravenous regional anesthesia	C-5 to T-1	Forearm, wrist, hand
Peripheral n blocks		
Ulnar n, median n, radial n	C-5 to T-1	Wrist, hand
	T-2 to T-6	Thoracic
Epidural block*		
Intercostal block		
Interpleural block		Unilateral
	T-4 to L-1	Upper abdominal
Epidural block*		Gastric, bowel, cholecystectomy, liver, abdominal aortic aneurysm
Celiac plexus block with intercostal block	T-4 to T-11	Upper abdominal
		Gastric, bowel, cholecystectomy, liver
		Lower abdominal
Epidural block or subarachnoid block	T-10 to L-1	Inguinal
	T-6 to L-1	Intestine, pelvis
	S-2 to S-5	Perineal, rectal
Caudal block	S-2 to S-5	Perineal, rectal
Ilioinguinal n block with iliohypogastric n block	T-10 to L-1	Inguinal
		Genitourinary
Epidural block*	T-4 to T-12	Nephrectomy
Epidural block or subarachnoid block	T-6 to S-5	TUR bladder
	T-9 to S-5	TUR prostate
	T-6 to S-5	Testis and ovary
	T-10 to S-5	Vagina and uterus
Caudal block	S-1 to S-5	Hypospadias
Penile block	S-1 to S-5	Circumcision
		Lower extremity
Epidural block or subarachnoid block	T-10 to S-2	Hip
	L-1 to S-2	Entire leg
3-in-1 Block with sciatic n block	L-1 to S-2	Entire leg
Psoas compartment block with sciatic n block	L-1 to S-2	Entire leg
Sciatic-femoral-lateral femoral cutaneous, obturator n block	L-1 to S-2	Upper leg, knee, lower leg
Intra-articular injection	L-3 to L-4	Knee
Ankle block	L-3 to S-2	Foot

*Epidural block, continuous epidural or single-shot epidural.
n, nerve; TUR, transurethral resection.

mittent or continuous infusions of local anesthetic agents is accumulation of the agent, which sometimes leads to systemic toxic effects.[116, 117] This course is probably more extensive and faster with the shorter-acting agents lidocaine and mepivacaine than with the longer-acting agents etidocaine and bupivacaine.[117] Toxic reactions after long-term epidural infusion of bupivacaine have been observed rarely despite relatively high plasma concentrations of the drug.[118] This may be related to alterations in the plasma protein binding of bupivacaine, resulting in increased total plasma concentrations without a concomitant increase in the free bupivacaine concentration.

Summary

The choice of a local anesthetic drug must be individualized to each clinical situation. It varies as a function of the regional anesthetic procedure and the clinical status of the patient. It is important to know how much of which drug is to be injected. The volume to be injected depends on the particular technique. Increasing the dosage of a local anesthetic agent, achieved by an increase in concentration or volume of the local anesthetic solution or both, usually results in a shorter latency, a longer duration of action, and a more dense block.

Bupivacaine and lidocaine can be used for all regional anesthetic techniques.

Epinephrine is frequently added to local anesthetic solutions to improve the quality of regional block. This effect varies with the site of injection and the type, dose, and concentration of the individual local anesthetic drug. Adding epinephrine to a local anesthetic solution is more important when the concentration of the local anesthetic solution is low. The longer-acting agents are influenced less by the addition of epinephrine, particularly when such agents are used for epidural anesthesia.

A test dose of a local anesthetic containing epinephrine is commonly administered to detect an uninten-

Table 12–8 Factors Influencing the Choice of Local
Anesthetic Agents

Specific nerves to be blocked
Onset time (e.g., rapid for acute pain, urgent operation)
Required duration of effect
Need for postoperative treatment
Likely rate of vascular absorption
Potential for systemic toxicity
Clinical status and characteristics of the patient
Skills of the anesthesiologist

tional intravascular injection. Elderly patients may have a decreased response to a given dose of epinephrine, because the sensitivity to β-agonists decreases with advancing age. The anesthesiologist may consider increasing the concentration of epinephrine up to 10 to 15 μg/mL in elderly patients.

Because elderly patients are more sensitive to local anesthetic agents than younger patients, several recommendations can be made for the safe administration of epidural and spinal anesthesia in older patients. It is important to limit the amount of sympathetic block associated with increased levels of analgesia in older patients after epidural administration of a local anesthetic solution and subarachnoid administration of a hyperbaric local anesthetic solution. With epidural anesthesia, the dose should be decreased or the local anesthetic should be injected at a lower interspace. Injection at the L4-5 or L5-S1 interspace probably decreases the cephalad spread by approximately two to four segments and thereby the potential sequelae of high thoracic block in older patients.

For spinal anesthesia using a hyperbaric solution, the sitting period may be lengthened for 10 to 15 min. Another possibility is to inject the solution at a lower intervertebral interspace, such as L4-5 or L5-S1. Plain 0.5% bupivacaine administered through a spinal catheter in titrated low doses, with the patient in a slight Trendelenburg position, offers considerable advantages. The possibility of continuing the block step by step decreases the risk of extensive hemodynamic effects.

An improved understanding of the physiologic changes resulting from regional anesthesia in patients has led to increased use of regional anesthetic procedures during the past decade. Local anesthetic agents are safe and effective drugs with known predictable toxicity when used properly. Prudent use of local anesthetic agents requires knowledge of their pharmacokinetics, pharmacodynamics, and toxicity as well as an estimation of surgical requirements and duration and postoperative analgesia requirements (Table 12–8). The appropriate local anesthetic agent must be matched to patient, procedure, regional technique, and physician. Whatever drug is chosen, the total dosage should be calculated for each patient and kept within acceptable limits.

References

1. Covino BG: Pharmacology of local anaesthetic agents. Br J Anaesth 1986; 58: 701–716.

2. Tucker GT, Mather LE: Properties, absorption, and disposition of local anesthetic agents. In Cousins MJ, Bridenbaugh PO (eds): Neural Blockade in Clinical Anesthesia and Management of Pain, 2nd ed, pp 47–110. Philadelphia, JB Lippincott, 1988.

3. Concepcion M, Covino BG: Rational use of local anaesthetics. Drugs 1984; 27: 256–270.

4. Fleming JA, Byck R, Barash PG: Pharmacology and therapeutic applications of cocaine. Anesthesiology 1990; 73: 518–531.

5. Foldes FF, Davidson GM, Duncalf D, et al: The intravenous toxicity of local anesthetic agents in man. Clin Pharmacol Ther 1965; 6: 328–335.

6. Stevens RA, Chester WL, Artuso JD, et al: Back pain after epidural anesthesia with chloroprocaine in volunteers: preliminary report. Reg Anesth 1991; 16: 199–203.

7. Narang PK, Crouthamel WG, Carliner NH, et al: Lidocaine and its active metabolites. Clin Pharmacol Ther 1978; 24: 654–662.

8. Inoue R, Suganuma T, Echizen H, et al: Plasma concentrations of lidocaine and its principal metabolites during intermittent epidural anesthesia. Anesthesiology 1985; 63: 304–310.

9. Hjelm M, Holmdahl MH: Biochemical effects of aromatic amines. II. Cyanosis, methaemoglobinaemia and Heinz-body formation induced by a local anaesthetic agent (prilocaine). Acta Anaesthesiol Scand 1965; 9: 99–120.

10. Brown DL, Carpenter RL, Thompson GE: Comparison of 0.5% ropivacaine and 0.5% bupivacaine for epidural anesthesia in patients undergoing lower-extremity surgery. Anesthesiology 1990; 72: 633–636.

11. Hickey R, Hoffman J, Ramamurthy S: A comparison of ropivacaine 0.5% and bupivacaine 0.5% for brachial plexus block. Anesthesiology 1991; 74: 639–642.

12. Moller R, Covino BG: Cardiac electrophysiologic properties of bupivacaine and lidocaine compared with those of ropivacaine, a new amide local anesthetic. Anesthesiology 1990; 72: 322–329.

13. Cowan A: Clinical assessment of a new local anesthetic agent—carticaine. Oral Surg Oral Med Oral Pathol 1977; 43: 174–180.

14. Moller RA, Covino BG: Cardiac electrophysiologic effects of articaine compared with bupivacaine and lidocaine. Anesth Analg 1993; 76: 1266–1273.

15. Rocco AG, Francis DM, Wark JA, et al: A clinical double-blind study of dibucaine and tetracaine in spinal anesthesia. Anesth Analg 1982; 61: 133–137.

16. Cohen SE, Thurlow A: Comparison of a chloroprocaine–bupivacaine mixture with chloroprocaine and bupivacaine used individually for obstetric epidural analgesia. Anesthesiology 1979; 51: 288–292.

17. Corke BC, Carlson CG, Dettbarn WD: The influence of 2-chloroprocaine on the subsequent analgesic potency of bupivacaine. Anesthesiology 1984; 60: 25–27.

18. Tryba M, Borner P: Clinical effectiveness and systemic toxicity of various mixtures of prilocaine and bupivacaine in axillary plexus block. (German.) Reg Anaesth 1988; 11: 40–49.

19. Scott DB, McClure JH, Giasi RM, et al: Effects of concentration of local anaesthetic drugs in extradural block. Br J Anaesth 1980; 52: 1033–1037.

20. Galindo A, Hernandez J, Benavides O, et al: Quality of spinal extradural anaesthesia: the influence of spinal nerve root diameter. Br J Anaesth 1975; 47: 41–47.

21. Duggan J, Bowler GM, McClure JH, et al: Extradural block with bupivacaine: influence of dose, volume, concentration and patient characteristics. Br J Anaesth 1988; 61: 324–331.

22. Tucker GT: Pharmacokinetics of local anaesthetics. Br J Anaesth 1986; 58: 717–731.

23. Bridenbaugh PO, Tucker GT, Moore DC, et al: Role of epinephrine in regional block anesthesia with etidocaine: a double-blind study. Anesth Analg 1974; 53: 430–436.

24. Sinclair CJ, Scott DB: Comparison of bupivacaine and etidocaine in extradural blockade. Br J Anaesth 1984; 56: 147–153.

25. Murphy TM, Mather LE, Stanton-Hicks MDA, et al: The effects of adding adrenaline to etidocaine and lignocaine in extradural anaesthesia. I: Block characteristics and cardiovascular effects. Br J Anaesth 1976; 48: 893–897.

26. Swerdlow M, Jones R: The duration of action of bupivacaine, prilocaine and lignocaine. Br J Anaesth 1970; 42: 335–339.

27. Covino BG, Vassallo HG: Local Anesthetics: Mechanisms of Action and Clinical Use, p 95. New York, Grune & Stratton, 1976.

28. Burm AG, van Kleef JW, Gladines MP, et al: Epidural anesthesia with lidocaine and bupivacaine: effects of epinephrine on the plasma concentration profiles. Anesth Analg 1986; 65: 1281–1284.

29. Abouleish EI: Epinephrine improves the quality of spinal hyperbaric bupivacaine for cesarean section. Anesth Analg 1987; 66: 395–400.

30. Boakes AJ, Laurence DR, Teoh PC, et al: Interactions between sympathomimetic amines and antidepressant agents in man. Br Med J 1973; 1: 311–315.

31. Scott DB, Jebson PJ, Braid DP, et al: Factors affecting plasma levels of lignocaine and prilocaine. Br J Anaesth 1972; 44: 1040–1049.

32. Tucker GT, Mather LE: Clinical pharmacokinetics of local anaesthetics. Clin Pharmacokinet 1979; 4: 241–278.

33. Safran D, Kuhlman G, Orhant EE, et al: Continuous intercostal blockade with lidocaine after thoracic surgery. Clinical and pharmacokinetic study. Anesth Analg 1990; 70: 345–349.

34. Scott DB: "Maximum recommended doses" of local anaesthetic drugs. (Editorial.) Br J Anaesth 1989; 63: 373–374.

35. Reynolds F: Adverse effects of local anaesthetics. Br J Anaesth 1987; 59: 78–95.

36. Adriani J, Campbell D: Fatalities following topical application of local anesthetics to mucous membranes. J Am Med Assoc 1956; 162: 1527–1530.

37. Buckley MM, Benfield P: Eutectic lidocaine/prilocaine cream. A review of the topical anaesthetic/analgesic efficacy of a eutectic mixture of local anaesthetics (EMLA). Drugs 1993; 46: 126–151.

38. Hassan HG, Renck H, Lindberg B, et al: Effects of adjuvants to local anaesthetics on their duration. I. Studies of dextrans of widely varying molecular weight and adrenaline in rat infraorbital nerve block. Acta Anaesthesiol Scand 1985; 29: 375–379.

39. Rosenberg PH: 1992 ASRA Lecture. Intravenous regional anesthesia: nerve block by multiple mechanisms. Reg Anesth 1993; 18: 1–5.

40. Bader AM, Concepcion M, Hurley RJ, et al: Comparison of lidocaine and prilocaine for intravenous regional anesthesia. Anesthesiology 1988; 69: 409–412.

41. Tryba M, Zenz M, Hausmann E: Prolonged analgesia after cuff release following i.v. regional analgesia with prilocaine. Br J Anaesth 1983; 55: 631–634.

42. Reynolds F: Bupivacaine and intravenous regional anaesthesia. (Editorial.) Anaesthesia 1984; 39: 105–107.

43. Cousins MJ, Bromage PR: Epidural neural blockade. In Cousins MJ, Bridenbaugh PO (eds): Neural Blockade in Clinical Anesthesia and Management of Pain, 2nd ed, pp 253–360. Philadelphia, JB Lippincott, 1988.

44. Bromage PR: An evaluation of bupivacaine in epidural analgesia for obstetrics. Can Anaesth Soc J 1969; 16: 46–56.

45. Prithvi RP, Denson DD, Joyce TH III, et al: Evaluation of continuous extravascular infusion of bupivacaine for prolonged pain relief. (Abstract.) Pain 1981; 11: S251.

46. Concepcion M, Arthur GR, Steele SM, et al: A new local anesthetic, ropivacaine. Its epidural effects in humans. Anesth Analg 1990; 70: 80–85.

47. Brockway MS, Bannister J, McClure JH, et al: Comparison of extradural ropivacaine and bupivacaine. Br J Anaesth 1991; 66: 31–37.

48. Greene NM: Distribution of local anesthetic solutions within the subarachnoid space. Anesth Analg 1985; 64: 715–730.

49. Chambers WA, Littlewood DG, Logan MR, et al: Effect of added epinephrine on spinal anesthesia with lidocaine. Anesth Analg 1981; 60: 417–420.

50. Chambers WA, Littlewood DG, Scott DB: Spinal anesthesia with hyperbaric bupivacaine: effect of added vasoconstrictors. Anesth Analg 1982; 61: 49–52.

51. Concepcion M, Maddi R, Francis D, et al: Vasoconstrictors in spinal anesthesia with tetracaine—a comparison of epinephrine and phenylephrine. Anesth Analg 1984; 63: 134–138.

52. Toft P, Bruun-Mogensen C, Kristensen J, et al: A comparison of glucose-free 2% lidocaine and hyperbaric 5% lidocaine for spinal anaesthesia. Acta Anaesthesiol Scand 1990; 34: 109–113.

53. Tuominen M: Bupivacaine spinal anaesthesia. Acta Anaesthesiol Scand 1991; 35: 1–10.

54. Axelsson KH, Widman GB, Sundberg AE, et al: A double-blind study of motor blockade in the lower limbs. Studies during spinal anaesthesia with hyperbaric and glucose-free 0.5% bupivacaine. Br J Anaesth 1985; 57: 960–970.

55. van Kleef JW, Veering BT, Burm AG: Spinal anesthesia with ropivacaine: a double-blind study on the efficacy and safety of 0.5% and 0.75% solutions in patients undergoing minor lower limb surgery. Anesth Analg 1994; 78: 1125–1130.

56. Murphy DF: Interpleural analgesia. Br J Anaesth 1993; 71: 426–434.

57. Gin T, Chan K, Kan AF, et al: Effect of adrenaline on venous plasma concentrations of bupivacaine after interpleural administration. Br J Anaesth 1990; 64: 662–666.

58. van Kleef JW, Logeman EA, Burm AG, et al: Continuous interpleural infusion of bupivacaine for postoperative analgesia after surgery with flank incisions: a double-blind comparison of 0.25% and 0.5% solutions. Anesth Analg 1992; 75: 268–274.

59. Veering BT, Burm AG, van Kleef JW, et al: Epidural anesthesia with bupivacaine: effects of age on neural blockade and pharmacokinetics. Anesth Analg 1987; 66: 589–593.

60. Nydahl PA, Philipson L, Axelsson K, et al: Epidural anesthesia with 0.5% bupivacaine: influence of age on sensory and motor blockade. Anesth Analg 1991; 73: 780–786.

61. Hirabayashi Y, Shimizu R: Effect of age on extradural dose requirement in thoracic extradural anaesthesia. Br J Anaesth 1993; 71: 445–446.

62. Racle JP, Benkhadra A, Poy JY, et al: Spinal analgesia with hyperbaric bupivacaine: influence of age. Br J Anaesth 1988; 60: 508–514.

63. Veering BT, Burm AG, Spierdijk J: Spinal anaesthesia with hyperbaric bupivacaine. Effects of age on neural blockade and pharmacokinetics. Br J Anaesth 1988; 60: 187–194.

64. Veering BT, Burm AG, van Kleef JW, et al: Spinal anesthesia with glucose-free bupivacaine: effects of age on neural blockade and pharmacokinetics. Anesth Analg 1987; 66: 965–970.

65. Warner MA, Kunkel SE, Offord KO, et al: The effects of age, epinephrine, and operative site on duration of caudal analgesia in pediatric patients. Anesth Analg 1987; 66: 995–998.

66. Wolf AR, Valley RD, Fear DW, et al: Bupivacaine for caudal analgesia in infants and children: the optimal effective concentration. Anesthesiology 1988; 69: 102–106.

67. Ecoffey C, Desparmet J, Maury M, et al: Bupivacaine in children: pharmacokinetics following caudal anesthesia. Anesthesiology 1985; 63: 447–448.

68. Mazoit JX, Denson DD, Samii K: Pharmacokinetics of bupivacaine following caudal anesthesia in infants. Anesthesiology 1988; 68: 387–391.

69. Pitkanen MT: Body mass and spread of spinal anesthesia with bupivacaine. Anesth Analg 1987; 66: 127–131.

70. Taivainen T, Tuominen M, Rosenberg PH: Influence of obesity on the spread of spinal analgesia after injection of plain 0.5% bupivacaine at the L3-4 or L4-5 interspace. Br J Anaesth 1990; 64: 542–546.

71. Fagraeus L, Urban BJ, Bromage PR: Spread of epidural analgesia in early pregnancy. Anesthesiology 1983; 58: 184–187.

72. Datta S, Lambert DH, Gregus J, et al: Differential sensitivities of mammalian nerve fibers during pregnancy. Anesth Analg 1983; 62: 1070–1072.

73. Blomberg S, Emanuelsson H, Ricksten SE: Thoracic epidural anesthesia and central hemodynamics in patients with unstable angina pectoris. Anesth Analg 1989; 69: 558–562.

74. Bromage PR: Exaggerated spread of epidural analgesia in arteriosclerotic patients: dosage in relation to biological and chronological ageing. Br Med J 1962; 2: 1634–1638.

75. Williams RL, Blaschke TF, Meffin PJ, et al: Influence of viral hepatitis on the disposition of two compounds with high hepatic clearance: lidocaine and indocyanine green. Clin Pharmacol Ther 1976; 20: 290–299.

76. Thomson PD, Melmon KL, Richardson JA, et al: Lidocaine pharmacokinetics in advanced heart failure, liver disease, and renal failure in humans. Ann Intern Med 1973; 78: 499–508.

77. Orko R, Pitkanen M, Rosenberg PH: Subarachnoid anaesthesia with 0.75% bupivacaine in patients with chronic renal failure. Br J Anaesth 1986; 58: 605–609.

78. Bromage PR, Gertel M: Brachial plexus anesthesia in chronic renal failure. Anesthesiology 1972; 36: 488–493.
79. Hirabayashi Y, Shimizu R, Matsuda I, et al: Effect of extradural compliance and resistance on spread of extradural analgesia. Br J Anaesth 1990; 65: 508–513.
80. Buckley FP, Robinson NB, Simonowitz DA, et al: Anaesthesia in the morbidly obese. A comparison of anaesthetic and analgesic regimens for upper abdominal surgery. Anaesthesia 1983; 38: 840–851.
81. Milligan KR, Cramp P, Schatz L, et al: The effect of positioning and obesity on epidural analgesic spread. (Abstract.) Anesth Analg 1991; 72: S185.
82. Gelman S, Laws HL, Potzick J, et al: Thoracic epidural vs balanced anesthesia in morbid obesity: an intraoperative and postoperative hemodynamic study. Anesth Analg 1980; 59: 902–908.
83. Norris MC: Patient variables and the subarachnoid spread of hyperbaric bupivacaine in the term parturient. Anesthesiology 1990; 72: 478–482.
84. Sullivan DR, Siker ES: The pros and cons of regional anesthesia. In Stephen CR, Assaf RAE (eds): Geriatric Anesthesia: Principles and Practice, pp 277–290. Boston, Butterworths, 1986.
85. McKenzie PJ, Wishart HY, Dewar KM, et al: Comparison of the effects of spinal anaesthesia and general anaesthesia on postoperative oxygenation and perioperative mortality. Br J Anaesth 1980; 52: 49–54.
86. Sundberg A, Wattwil M, Arvill A: Respiratory effects of high thoracic epidural anaesthesia. Acta Anaesthesiol Scand 1986; 30: 215–217.
87. Steinbrook RA, Concepcion M: Respiratory effects of spinal anesthesia: resting ventilation and single-breath CO_2 response. Anesth Analg 1991; 72: 182–186.
88. Christensen EF, Sogaard P, Egebo K, et al: Myocardial ischaemia and spinal analgesia in patients with angina pectoris. Br J Anaesth 1993; 71: 472–475.
89. Toft P, Jorgensen A: Continuous thoracic epidural analgesia for the control of pain in myocardial infarction. Intensive Care Med 1987; 13: 388–389.
90. Labaille T, Benhamou D, Westermann J: Hemodynamic effects of continuous spinal anesthesia: a comparative study between low and high doses of bupivacaine. Reg Anesth 1992; 17: 193–196.
91. Mostert JW, Evers JL, Hobika GH, et al: The haemodynamic response to chronic renal failure as studied in the azotaemic state. Br J Anaesth 1970; 42: 397–411.
92. Horlocker TT, Wedel DJ: Anticoagulants, antiplatelet therapy, and neuraxis blockade. Anesth Clin North Am 1992; 10: 1–11.
93. Yagiela JA: Regional anesthesia for dental procedures. Int Anesthesiol Clin 1989; 27: 68–82.
94. Nicoll JM, Treuren B, Acharya PA, et al: Retrobulbar anesthesia: the role of hyaluronidase. Anesth Analg 1986; 65: 1324–1328.
95. Zahl K, Jordan A, McGroarty J, et al: pH-adjusted bupivacaine and hyaluronidase for peribulbar block. Anesthesiology 1990; 72: 230–232.
96. Jebeles JA, Reilly JS, Gutierrez JF, et al: The effect of pre-incisional infiltration of tonsils with bupivacaine on the pain following tonsillectomy under general anesthesia. Pain 1991; 47: 305–308.
97. Reynolds F: Extradural opioids in labour. Br J Anaesth 1989; 63: 251–253.
98. Abboud TK, Afrasiabi A, Sarkis F, et al: Continuous infusion epidural analgesia in parturients receiving bupivacaine, chloroprocaine, or lidocaine—maternal, fetal, and neonatal effects. Anesth Analg 1984; 63: 421–428.
99. Eisenach JC, Grice SC, Dewan DM: Epinephrine enhances analgesia produced by epidural bupivacaine during labor. Anesth Analg 1987; 66: 447–451.
100. McCrae AG, Jozwiak H, McClure JH: Bupivacaine v ropivacaine in obstetric epidural analgesia. (Abstract.) Reg Anesth 1993; 18(Suppl): 64.
101. de Leon-Casasola OA, Lema MJ, Emrich L, et al: Continuous 2-chloroprocaine infusion versus intermittent bolus injections of bupivacaine or 2-chloroprocaine for epidural anesthesia in cesarean delivery. Reg Anesth 1991; 16: 154–160.
102. Norton AC, Davis AG, Spicer RJ: Lignocaine 2% with adrenaline for epidural caesarean section. A comparison with 0.5% bupivacaine. Anaesthesia 1988; 43: 844–849.
103. Abboud TK, Moore MJ, Jacobs J, et al: Epidural mepivacaine for cesarean section: maternal and neonatal effect. Reg Anesth 1987; 12: 76–79.
104. Kestin IG: Spinal anaesthesia in obstetrics. Br J Anaesth 1991; 66: 596–607.
105. Dalens B: Regional anesthesia in children. Anesth Analg 1989; 68: 654–672.
106. Takasaki M: Blood concentrations of lidocaine, mepivacaine and bupivacaine during caudal analgesia in children. Acta Anaesthesiol Scand 1984; 28: 211–214.
107. Desparmet J, Meistelman C, Barre J, et al: Continuous epidural infusion of bupivacaine for postoperative pain relief in children. Anesthesiology 1987; 67: 108–110.
108. Abajian JC, Mellish RW, Browne AF, et al: Spinal anesthesia for surgery in the high-risk infant. Anesth Analg 1984; 63: 359–362.
109. Kehlet H: Modification of responses to surgery by neural blockade: clinical implications. In Cousins MJ, Bridenbaugh PO (eds): Neural Blockade in Clinical Anesthesia and Management of Pain, 2nd ed, pp 145–188. Philadelphia, JB Lippincott, 1988.
110. Davis FM, Woolner DF, Frampton C, et al: Prospective, multi-centre trial of mortality following general or spinal anaesthesia for hip fracture surgery in the elderly. Br J Anaesth 1987; 59: 1080–1088.
111. Baysinger CL, Bowe EA, Bowe LS, et al: Brachial plexus blockade versus general anesthesia for orthopedic operation on the upper extremity in outpatients. (Abstract.) Anesthesiology 1990; 73: A43.
112. Kopacz DJ, Mulroy MF: Chloroprocaine and lidocaine decrease hospital stay and admission rate after outpatient epidural anesthesia. Reg Anesth 1990; 15: 19–25.
113. Allen RW, Fee JP, Moore J: A preliminary assessment of epidural chloroprocaine for day procedures. Anaesthesia 1993; 48: 773–775.
114. Rosenberg PH: Local anaesthesia techniques. Acta Anaesthesiol Scand Suppl 1993; 100: 132–134.
115. Ready LB: Intraspinal opioid analgesia in the perioperative period. Anesth Clin North Am 1992; 10: 145–159.
116. Takasaki M, Oh-oka T, Doi K, et al: Blood levels of mepivacaine during continuous epidural anesthesia. Anesth Analg 1987; 66: 337–340.
117. Tucker GT, Cooper S, Littlewood D, et al: Observed and predicted accumulation of local anaesthetic agents during continuous extradural analgesia. Br J Anaesth 1977; 49: 237–242.
118. Ross RA, Clarke JE, Armitage EN: Postoperative pain prevention by continuous epidural infusion. A study of the clinical effects and the plasma concentrations obtained. Anaesthesia 1980; 35: 663–668.

CHAPTER 13

Neuraxial Administration of Opioids and Nonopioids

Narinder Rawal, M.D., Ph.D.

The identification of opioid receptors has opened new horizons in pain management. By bypassing blood and blood-brain barrier, small doses of opioids administered in the subarachnoid or the epidural space provide profound and prolonged segmental analgesia. This undoubtedly represents a major breakthrough in pain management.

Since their introduction into clinical practice in 1979, opioids given spinally have achieved international popularity in various clinical settings, as the sole analgesic agent or in combination with low-dose local anesthetic. Numerous studies have shown that spinal administration of opioids provides profound postoperative analgesia with fewer central and systemic adverse effects than opioids administered systemically. Segmental analgesia induced by spinal administration of opioids has a role in the management of a wide variety of surgical and nonsurgical painful conditions. The technique has been used successfully to treat intraoperative, postoperative, traumatic, obstetric, chronic, and cancer pain. Several reviews have appeared in the literature.[1–6]

Neuraxial Administration of Opioids for Postoperative Pain

The unique feature of opioids given neuraxially for analgesia is the lack of sensory, sympathetic, or motor block, which allows patients to ambulate without the risk of orthostatic hypotension or motor incoordination usually associated with local anesthetics administered epidurally or opioids administered parenterally. These advantages of neuraxial administration of opioids are particularly beneficial for high-risk patients undergoing major operation, patients with compromised pulmonary or cardiovascular function, grossly obese patients, and elderly patients.[7–10] There is no conclusive evidence that opioids injected epidurally or intrathecally provide "at-rest" analgesia of better quality than that provided by opioids given parenterally. What is beyond doubt is the ability of epidurally administered morphine to produce more prolonged analgesia at doses that are far less than usual intramuscular or intravenous doses. For intrathecal administration, the analgesic doses of morphine are only 2% to 5% of parenteral doses of morphine, and these patients are expected to be less drowsy, more cooperative, and more mobile.

Management of postoperative pain is the most frequent indication for analgesia produced by neuraxial administration of opioids. The technique has been used to provide pain relief after a wide variety of surgical procedures, such as upper and lower abdominal and thoracic operations, including cardiac, perineal, and orthopedic operations. Neuraxial administration of opioids has also been used to provide analgesia in different age groups, including children, and is considered particularly beneficial in elderly high-risk patients.[1, 2, 11–14] Many controlled studies have documented the efficacy of the technique for postoperative pain. In terms of analgesia and restoration of postoperative pulmonary function after abdominal or thoracic operation, the technique has been superior to alternative methods such as intermittent intramuscular injection of opioids,[7, 8, 11, 15, 16] patient-controlled analgesia (PCA) with opioids given intravenously,[17, 18] intercostal block,[7] and epidural block with local anesthetics.[15, 16, 19, 20] Neuraxial administration of opioids has been used for treating pain from fractured ribs and in patients with multiple injuries in an intensive care unit (ICU). In the ICU patient with multiple injuries for whom frequent assessment of level of consciousness is important, analgesia produced by neuraxial administration of opioids appears superior to a parenteral analgesic-sedative combination.[21] Most of these impressive results are seen when the opioid used is morphine.

The enormous international literature shows that pain management by opioids given neuraxially is well accepted worldwide. Several years ago, a nationwide Swedish survey[11] showed that all anesthesia departments in the country routinely used the technique. A later 17-nation European survey showed that all the hospitals surveyed used epidural administration of opioids for management of acute pain, and the use was increasing.[22] However, there was a great difference among the countries. As a percentage of all surgical procedures (including outpatient surgery), use of opioids given epidurally ranged from 0.7% (Ireland) to 19.3% (Denmark) (Fig. 13–1). Intrathecal administration of opioids is used far less frequently in Europe (Fig 13–2).

Combination of Opioids and Local Anesthetics

The rationale for the combination technique is that these two types of drugs eliminate pain by acting at two distinct sites: the local anesthetic at the nerve axon and the opioid at the receptor site in the spinal cord. Local anesthetic and opioid combination techniques have been studied extensively in the obstetric population. If even an extremely low concentration of local anesthetic is added to the opioid, the quality of analgesia may be superior.[23] As expected, pain relief at rest is better than during movement. Neuraxial administration of opioids alone provides good pain relief at rest but may not be adequate during physiotherapy and mobilization. This need prompted the increased use of combination therapy.

Fentanyl was the first opioid widely used as an adjunct to local anesthetics for labor. Patients receiving epidural injections of local anesthetics combined with opioids report more rapid onset of analgesia, more profound and long-lasting relief of labor pain, and less motor block than patients receiving either drug alone. The addition of fentanyl or sufentanil to local anesthetics for epidural anesthesia is becoming routine in many institutions.

Because patients undergoing knee replacement are not immediately ambulatory in the early postoperative period, they are uniquely suited for an analgesic regimen that includes some degree of regional block that facilitates vigorous physical therapy and continuous passive motion of the operated knee. Epidural local anesthetics alone are incapable of maintaining a level of sensory anesthesia for a prolonged period because of tachyphylaxis. Coadministration of morphine[20] and fentanyl[24] has been shown to delay the regression of sensory anesthesia in postoperative patients receiving bupivacaine epidurally. In a controlled study of patients undergoing total knee replacement, Ferrante and colleagues[25] demonstrated that a bupivacaine-meperidine combination was associated with a significantly slower regression of sensory block compared with a fentanyl-bupivacaine combination. There was no difference in the rate of regression of sensory anesthesia among patients receiving bupivacaine alone or a fentanyl-bupivacaine combination.

Although combination therapy is used for postoperative and labor pain, the results are more impressive in labor pain, because labor pain is not relieved by opioids alone given epidurally. After a bolus of 10 mL of 0.25% bupivacaine combined with 50 μg of fentanyl, a contin-

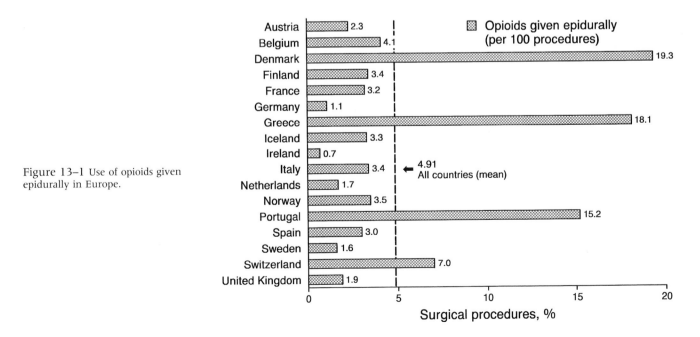

Figure 13–1 Use of opioids given epidurally in Europe.

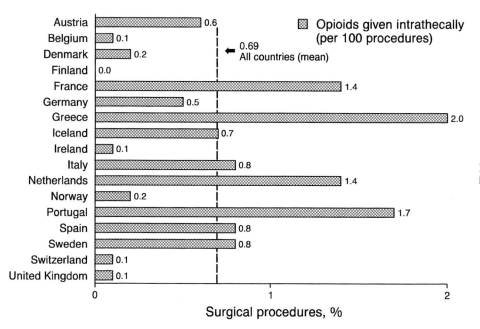

Figure 13-2 Use of opioids given intrathecally in Europe.

uous infusion of subanalgesic doses of bupivacaine (0.0625%) and fentanyl (1 to 2 μg/mL) at a rate of 10 mL/h provides effective analgesia without motor block. Many anesthesiologists have demonstrated that combined with opioid the dose of local anesthetic required can be decreased by one half to two thirds and still provide excellent analgesia throughout labor.

In general, no adverse effects on the mother or neonate have been associated with the combination technique. However, neonatal respiratory depression has been reported after 20 μg sufentanil.[26] Large doses of fentanyl (150 to 200 μg) given epidurally, when used as the sole analgesic during labor, have resulted in severe neonatal respiratory depression requiring intubation and naloxone.[27] Caution should be exercised when using large doses of opioids until their safety in neonates has been established. When sufentanil is selected, the local anesthetic concentration can be decreased further. Naulty[28] demonstrated that a 10-mL bolus of 0.0625% or 0.125% bupivacaine combined with 1 to 2 μg/mL of sufentanil, followed by 0.031% bupivacaine combined with 0.2 to 0.3 μg/mL of sufentanil delivered at a rate of 6 to 10 mL/h, provides excellent analgesia with minimal maternal motor weakness.

The choice of local anesthetic also appears to play a role. Fentanyl added to bupivacaine accelerates the onset of the epidural block and decreases the requirement for local anesthetic; however, these advantages of fentanyl are lost if the local anesthetic is lidocaine.[29] The role of volume of injectant (i.e., whether fentanyl should be diluted for improvement of analgesia) is unclear.[5] For example, improved analgesia has been reported with undiluted[30] and with diluted[31] fentanyl.

Epidural infusion of fentanyl (10 μg/mL) provided as effective postoperative analgesia after abdominal or thoracic operations as epidural administration of the same dose of fentanyl combined with 0.1% bupivacaine. This lack of synergy is thought to be a result of

the low concentration of local anesthetic. It appears that the type of pain is an important factor for analgesic effects of combination therapy with low-dose local anesthetic drugs. Bupivacaine given epidurally in concentrations of 0.1% or less has provided effective labor analgesia in several studies, but the postoperative analgesic effects of such combinations have been disappointing after various types of operations.[32-34]

Despite convincing animal data and human clinical data, several controlled studies[32-35] comparing combination therapy with opioids alone have questioned the practice of adding bupivacaine to opioid. Bupivacaine has the potential to cause local anesthetic–related side effects such as hypotension, motor weakness, urinary retention, and pressure sores from skin sensory loss. The use of bupivacaine may delay mobilization in some patients.[36] The optimum combination that has opioid-sparing synergistic effect without delaying mobilization is yet to be established. In some studies, the combination of local anesthetic drugs and opioids did not improve analgesia and was instead associated with increased morbidity. This effect has been reported for a fentanyl-bupivacaine combination after orthopedic surgery[32] and after abdominal or thoracic surgery[35] and for a hydromorphone-bupivacaine combination after cesarean section.[37] Similarly, when morphine alone was compared with a morphine-bupivacaine combination after thoracotomy[30] or after abdominal surgery,[31] no difference in analgesia or adverse effects was found.

The factors that influence the rate of epidural infusion of opioid that is necessary for effective analgesia include the site and type of operation, type of pain (labor versus after surgery), choice of opioid and its loading dose, volume of injectant, concentration of local anesthetic, and patient characteristics that influence epidural pharmacokinetics and pharmacodynamics of the given opioid.[38] The location of the catheter tip in the epidural space is also important; bupivacaine (0.1%) with fentanyl given through a lumbar catheter was associated with a high incidence of lower limb weakness,[39] but motor weakness was insignificant when local anesthetic (0.1% to 0.2% bupivacaine) was administered at the thoracic level.[40, 41]

Patient-Controlled Epidural Analgesia

The increasing popularity of the intravenous PCA technique in pain management has generated interest in the use of opioids delivered epidurally using a PCA pump. This technique allows the patient to self–titrate epidural administration of opioid or an opioid–local anesthetic combination to the desired level of analgesia. Epidural PCA (PCEA) can be expected to combine the flexibility and convenience of PCA with the superior analgesia of epidural administration of opioids.[18, 37, 42] PCEA can be used as an investigational tool to eliminate bias regarding appropriate dose of opioid administration. This was done in a study to compare the lumbar and the thoracic routes of sufentanil administration for post-thoracotomy pain.[43] In a comparison[44] between continuous epidural administration of opioid and PCEA techniques, the latter was shown to result in a significant decrease in total dose requirement to achieve similar level of analgesia. In a randomized study[45] of PCEA using fentanyl, bupivacaine, or their combination for pain management after orthopedic surgery, it was shown that combining the two drugs reduced the requirements for each drug by 20% to 25%. The patients received 0.125% bupivacaine, fentanyl (5 μg/mL), or their combination as a 4-mL bolus with a 10-min lock-out time. Hypotension was observed in 33% of patients. The researchers speculated that this effect could result from the administration of bupivacaine boluses. However, in a study[46] of patients undergoing posttraumatic pelvic reconstruction, PCEA was no better than continuous epidural technique for postoperative analgesia.

It has been suggested that PCEA with opioids results in a more rapid recovery and shorter hospitalization than intravenous PCA or opioids given intramuscularly.[47, 48] Because of high lipophilicity and consequent rapid onset, drugs such as fentanyl, sufentanil, and alfentanil have been studied for PCEA.[49–52] A bolus of 10 to 30 μg of sufentanil followed by a basal infusion rate of 5 μg/h with a 5-μg demand dose and a 10- to 20-min lock-out interval have been recommended.[38, 53] However, major problems are the lack of any advantages in terms of analgesia, adverse-effect profile, and blood levels when these drugs are administered epidurally compared with intravenous administration. No differences in analgesia were found between PCEA and intravenous PCA with fentanyl[54] or with alfentanil.[51] In the latter study, 10 of 13 patients had oxygen desaturation (oxygen saturation < 85%) in the PCEA group compared with 4 of 13 patients in the intravenous PCA group. Another study demonstrated[37] that hydromorphone with PCEA was superior to intravenous PCA because effective analgesia is provided by a lower dose of opioid, which leads to a more rapid recovery in patients undergoing cesarean section.

However, results from other studies of PCEA are less impressive. A high incidence of numbness and leg weakness has been reported during epidural infusion of 0.1% bupivacaine with opioid (fentanyl or morphine). In one controlled study[55] of cesarean section patients, PCEA with fentanyl and a single dose of morphine given epidurally were compared for postoperative analgesia. Pain relief, satisfaction with pain relief, and use of supplemental analgesics were similar in both groups. The mean 24-h dose of fentanyl given epidurally was 680 μg. Pruritus was less common in the fentanyl group; the incidence of nausea was similar. The researchers concluded that PCEA with fentanyl did not provide any advantage over a single dose of morphine given epidurally. In this study, the cost of PCEA with fentanyl ($57.15) was seven times more than that for morphine given epidurally ($7.57). Another study[53] concluded that the considerably simpler and cheaper technique of injecting 4 to 5 mg of morphine every 12 h provided analgesia as effective as PCEA with sufentanil. The cost of PCEA was also reported in a comparative study[55] of PCEA with fentanyl or sufentanil for postcesarean pain relief. In this masked (double-blind) study, both opioids provided a high level of patient satisfaction, although dizziness and vomiting were more frequent after sufentanil. The average hospital drug cost for sufentanil ($120.40) was about 27 times higher than for fentanyl ($4.50). Not surprisingly, the researchers concluded that epidural administration of sufentanil offered no advantages over epidural administration of fentanyl combined with bupivacaine.

Although the concept of PCA ensures adequate analgesia, the selection of drug concentrations, combinations, bolus doses, lock-out intervals, and basal infusion rates is often arbitrary, making comparisons between different studies difficult. It is also difficult to draw meaningful conclusions because of factors such as small populations of patients with multiple surgical procedures, comparisons of different drugs and modes of delivery, and use of combinations consisting of a large variety of local anesthetic concentrations and opioid drugs and dosages.[49–52, 54, 56] The issues become more complicated because of techniques in which the added drug may be a low-dose local anesthetic given to patients receiving continuous infusion of opioids or vice versa (e.g., PCEA with opioid to supplement a continuous infusion of local anesthetic).[57]

Another problem with PCEA is the role of basal infusion mode. This has been questioned on the grounds that basal infusion leads to higher drug use without decreasing pain scores or the number of patient demands for analgesic medication.[37] It has also been suggested that a programming error may have more serious consequences with a basal infusion mode than with the conventional intermittent-dosing technique.

There are no randomized studies to identify the ideal lipophilic opioid. Appropriate dosage regimens for PCEA after different types of operations also should be defined. Studies are needed to evaluate the cost-benefit ratio of this technique. These issues must be addressed before the role of PCEA in pain management can be established.

Route Selection: Epidural or Intrathecal?

The efficacy, optimal dose, duration of analgesia, and adverse-effect profile of opioids given epidurally have been extensively documented, but there is a paucity of similar information for opioids given intrathecally. The intrathecal route is a direct one because there is no dura to be penetrated and the drug is deposited close to its site of action—the opioid receptors. Compared with the intrathecal route, epidural administration is complicated by pharmacokinetics of dural penetration, epidural fat deposition, and systemic absorption of opioids. Moreover, it is thought that the analgesia after intrathecal administration of morphine is more predictable, more intense, and longer lasting than that after epidural administration of morphine. This is particularly valid in multitrauma patients in the ICU[21] and in laboring parturients.[58] Intrathecal administration of sufentanil has been shown[59] to provide better and longer-lasting analgesia than epidural administration of sufentanil for labor pain. Numerous reports have documented the excellent and prolonged analgesia after intrathecal administration of morphine.

Intrathecal administration of opioids has the advantages of simplicity, reliability, and low-dose requirements. To compensate for the effects of systemic uptake and fat sequestration, the epidural dose of morphine is about 10 to 20 times greater than that required for intrathecal injection.[60] Because excellent analgesia is achieved by a small dose, the patients can be expected to be less sedated, more cooperative, and more mobile, with all the attendant advantages.[2]

Morphine was the first opioid administered intrathecally and remains the most commonly used drug worldwide. Morphine is usually injected before the surgical procedure. Intrathecal administration of 0.8 mg of morphine has been shown to provide effective analgesia after cholecystectomy[61] and after aortic aneurysm surgery.[62] Morphine in 1-mg doses given intrathecally provides good analgesia after spinal operation.[63] In another study,[64] 0.5 to 1 mg of morphine given intrathecally resulted in shorter hospitalization after aortic operation. Earlier studies used intrathecal administration of morphine in doses up to 100 times larger than those currently being used. More recent experience[18, 65–68] suggests that doses as low as 0.1 to 0.5 mg may provide adequate analgesia after abdominal, orthopedic, and thoracic surgery. There is convincing evidence that doses lower than 0.5 mg provide excellent postoperative analgesia. Our controlled study[19] showed that 0.2 mg of morphine combined with bupivacaine given intrathecally for cesarean section provided good to excellent intraoperative and postoperative analgesia. No serious adverse effects occurred. However, these doses are not adequate for labor pain. Our study[69] showed that neither intrathecal administration of morphine 0.2 mg nor epidural administration of 0.125% bupivacaine alone reliably relieved labor

pain, although the combination of the two was effective. Similarly, intrathecal injection of a combination of 0.25 mg morphine and 25 μg fentanyl was ineffective for labor analgesia.[70]

Even low doses of morphine given intrathecally may be associated with delayed respiratory depression, especially in high-risk patients. Two Swedish surveys[11, 71] showed that the risk of delayed respiratory depression may be considerably higher if morphine is injected intrathecally rather than epidurally. In the follow-up survey,[11] delayed respiratory depression was observed in three patients after 0.3 mg of morphine given intrathecally. However, there are data to show that morphine (0.1 to 0.4 mg) given intrathecally can be used safely on regular wards of a community hospital if the floor nurses are properly trained.[72] There is a need for prospective studies to determine the safety aspects of intrathecal versus epidural administration of opioids.

Several reports of intrathecal administration of nonmorphine opioids have appeared in the literature. A technique that is simple and quick and provides reliable and prolonged postoperative pain relief has obvious attraction. Milligan and Fogarty[73] demonstrated that the concomitant administration of diacetylmorphine (heroin) while inducing anesthesia with bupivacaine given spinally provided significantly improved analgesia after hip replacement. It has been claimed[59, 74] that sufentanil given intrathecally provides rapid and effective pain relief during labor. In a controlled study[75] in which 10 μg of sufentanil was administered intrathecally, epidurally, or intravenously for management of labor pain, sufentanil given intrathecally provided rapid and effective analgesia of 1 to 2 h, but the drug was unsatisfactory by the other two routes, suggesting that the site of action is primarily neuraxial rather than systemic. This is consistent with the pharmacokinetic data on sufentanil. The concentration of sufentanil in the cerebrospinal fluid after a bolus dose of 75 μg administered epidurally is similar to cerebrospinal fluid levels after 15 μg given intrathecally.[76] In another study,[77] 10 μg of sufentanil given intrathecally added to bupivacaine significantly prolonged duration of perioperative and postoperative analgesia. Increasing the dose of sufentanil resulted in significantly increased incidence of pruritus without any advantage in terms of analgesia. Fentanyl has also been studied for postoperative analgesia after hip surgery[78] and thoracotomy.[79] Owing to its short duration of analgesia, this opioid was administered by a continuous intrathecal infusion.[78, 79]

In a controlled comparison of intrathecal administration of fentanyl and morphine in patients undergoing hip arthroplasty, Niemi and colleagues[78] demonstrated that intrathecal administration of morphine analgesia was superior, that there was no difference between analgesia provided by 200 μg of morphine given as a single bolus or the same dose given as a continuous infusion over a 24-h period, and that the risk of adverse effects such as pruritus and nausea was similar with both drugs. However, the frequency of urinary retention was higher in patients who received morphine intrathecally as a bolus injection.

Some studies have reported unusual effects, such as

sensory and autonomic changes and limb rigidity, after intrathecal administration of sufentanil. Cohen and associates[80] have demonstrated that 10 μg of sufentanil administered intrathecally for labor analgesia may be associated with sensory and autonomic changes. Fetal heart rate changes occurred in 15% of cases but were not associated with adverse neonatal outcome. Segmental sensory changes and hypotension suggest that analgesia may result from local anesthetic effect in addition to activity at spinal cord opioid receptors. The researchers recommended careful monitoring of maternal blood pressure and fetal heart rate after intrathecal administration of sufentanil. They also recommended that patients with marked sensory changes should not ambulate. A high incidence of hypotension (50%) has been reported[81] after epidural administration of fentanyl.

Newman and colleagues[82] described seven cases of transient lower limb rigidity in laboring patients after intrathecal administration of 10 μg of sufentanil combined with epinephrine. The phenomenon was unilateral in two patients and bilateral in five patients.

A retrospective review[83] demonstrated that kidney donors who received opioids intrathecally had less long-term residual pain for up to 1 year after the operation than patients managed with PCA alone. It was speculated that perioperative intrathecal analgesia may preemptively interfere with central sensitization and may provide lasting benefits far beyond the immediate perioperative period.

The reasons for the limited popularity of the intrathecal compared with the epidural route (see Fig. 13–2) may be the unreliability of catheter technology at present, the risk of post–dural puncture headache, less prolonged analgesia with lipid-soluble opioids than with hydrophilic morphine (more than 20 h) after a single injection, a greater risk of adverse effects including late-onset respiratory depression, and a greater risk of spinal cord neurotoxicity.

Drug Selection: Opioids

The European survey showed that various opioids are being used epidurally and intrathecally. Morphine and fentanyl are the most frequently used opioids in Europe (Table 13–1).

On the basis of pharmacologic models proposed for spinal opioid transport, the risk of late-onset respiratory depression is higher with hydrophilic morphine than with lipophilic opioids such as fentanyl, sufentanil, and meperidine. These lipophilic drugs are considered safe because of segmental localization that minimizes drug availability for rostral migration through the cerebrospinal fluid to reach the medullary respiratory centers by diffusion and bulk flow. This circumstance has led to the widespread use of fentanyl as a "safe" opioid for epidural administration. However, the earlier belief that continuous epidural infusions of fentanyl do not cause late-onset respiratory depression has been shown to be incorrect[84, 85] (see Table 13–7). In a study[14] of patients undergoing urologic surgery, 50 μg of fentanyl

given intrathecally caused apnea and periodic breathing in two of seven patients. In this study, respiratory depression, as assessed by ventilatory response to carbon dioxide (CO_2), occurred in all patients. The depression persisted for 300 min, but the changes were significant for 150 min. Lower doses (25 μg and 12.5 μg) were not associated with respiratory depression. These cases demonstrated that respiratory depression may occur with opioids previously considered safe.

The potency of opioids given epidurally is thought to be inversely related to lipophilicity. Opioids such as fentanyl, sufentanil, meperidine, and buprenorphine are more lipophilic than morphine and so less potent. In a study[86] comparing 100 μg/h of fentanyl given epidurally or intravenously for postoperative analgesia after knee surgery, pain scores at rest and with movement, adverse effects, and plasma fentanyl levels were identical in the two groups. Patient-controlled titration of PCEA or intravenous PCA for fentanyl administration did not demonstrate any significant difference in the quality of postoperative analgesia.[54] Similar results have been reported after intravenous versus epidural administration of other lipophilic opioids such as sufentanil,[87–89] alfentanil,[90] meperidine,[91] diacetylmorphine,[92] and butorphanol.[93]

In a review of the literature, Chrubasik and coworkers[6] concluded that there were no arguments that could justify the placement of an epidural catheter if lipophilic opioids such as sufentanil, buprenorphine, or methadone are to be used postoperatively. Dosage requirements and quality of analgesia are similar whether these drugs are administered intravenously or epidurally. The plasma or serum concentrations during continuous epidural administration of these opioids are indistinguishable from those during continuous intravenous infusion. The researchers concluded that the risk of respiratory depression might be higher during continuous epidural than continuous intravenous treatment because of the dual distribution of epidural opioids to the brain stem through blood and cerebrospinal fluid. However, in one study[94] of patients undergoing thoracotomy, plasma fentanyl levels after epidural administration of fentanyl were lower than the levels after intravenous infusion. For thoracotomy pain, a reduction of lumbar epidural versus intravenous dose of fentanyl has been claimed[95] and denied.[96]

Despite the proximity of these drugs to opioid receptors in the spinal cord, the analgesic effect of many dose regimens for lipophilic opioids is achieved predominantly through systemic uptake rather than through spinal mechanisms. This is supported by data showing that the site of catheter placement (lumbar versus thoracic) does not affect the quality of analgesia. Coe and colleagues[97] demonstrated that, in patients who have undergone thoracic operations, continuous infusion of fentanyl through an epidural catheter placed in the lumbar or thoracic space resulted in similar analgesic effects, dosage requirements, and incidence of adverse effects. It seems that the early onset of analgesia after lipophilic opioids may not be enough to justify the risks, inconvenience, and additional cost of the epidural compared with the parenteral route.[90, 91]

Table 13–1 Choice of Opioids for Epidural or Intrathecal Administration in Europe*

| | CHOICE, % | | | |
| | Epidural | | Intrathecal | |
OPIOID	Mean	Range	Mean	Range
Morphine	81.2	20–100	54.9	20–100
Fentanyl	59.5	0–100	14.7	0–57
Sufentanil	22.2	0–80	7.1	0–40
Buprenorphine	14.9	0–71.4	1.7	0–28†
Meperidine	9.6	0–33	2.3	0–20†
Diacetylmorphine	4.7	0–80‡	2.3	0–20†
Alfentanil	3.5	0–20‡		
Nicomorphine	2.3	0–40‡		
Piritramide	1.8	0–20‡	1.2	0–20†
Oxycodone	1.2	0–20‡		
Methadone	1.0	0–16.7‡		

*Data from Rawal N: Epidural and intrathecal opioids for postoperative pain management in Europe: a 17-nation survey. (Abstract.) Reg Anesth 1995; 20: A45.
†These opioids are used intrathecally in only the following countries: buprenorphine (Italy), pethidine (France, Portugal), diamorphine (Ireland, UK), and piritramide (Austria).
‡These opioids are used epidurally in only the following countries: diamorphine (UK), alfentanil (Belgium, Ireland, Norway), nicomorphine (Netherlands), piritramide (Austria, Germany), oxycodone (Finland), and methadone (Spain, UK).
UK, United Kingdom.

It appears that morphine is the only opioid that fulfills the requirements of prolonged, sedation-free segmental analgesia. A few studies have shown that morphine is cost effective in high-risk patients. There is a need for similar, controlled outcome studies using lipophilic opioids.

The choice of opioid may also depend on hospital or state nursing regulations regarding the administration of opioids in epidural or intrathecal catheters (Table 13–2). This may be one reason why intermittent administration of morphine in epidural catheters is common in countries where nurses are allowed to inject drugs. Conversely, continuous epidural infusion techniques are popular in countries where nurses are not allowed to inject drugs in epidural or intrathecal catheters.

Neuraxial Administration of Nonopioids

In the last two decades, there has been a tremendous advancement in our knowledge about the role of the spinal cord in nociceptive transmission and the various pharmacologic systems that are involved in modulating such transmission. Broadly, the three main classes of agents available for pain management by the epidural or intrathecal route are local anesthetics, opioids, and selected nonopioids. Local anesthetics, although effective, produce motor and orthostatic side effects because of the nonselective nature of neural block. Opioids, such as morphine, are widely used but may occasionally produce side effects, including respiratory depression. Lipophilic opioids, such as fentanyl or sufentanil, may or may not be associated with decreased risk of respiratory depression; current evidence is inconclusive. Combinations of opioids and local anesthetics may provide excellent analgesia, but the optimal concentrations and doses for different drug combinations have not been determined. Epidural and intrathecal administration of nonopioids such as clonidine, alone or as adjuvants to local anesthetics or opioids, have the potential of providing effective analgesia with minimal side effects.

Inhibition of afferent nociceptive transmission by mechanisms other than those acting on spinal opioid receptors has been demonstrated in several neurophysiologic studies. Agents that are not selective for opioid receptors, such as serotonergic, muscarinic, adenosinergic, γ-aminobutyric acid, somatostatin agonists, and substance P antagonists, are thought to inhibit pain modulation at the spinal level. However, in animal studies, the spinal administration of some of these agents has been associated with motor dysfunction or neurotoxicity. In clinical practice, analgesic effects have been demonstrated after epidural or intrathecal administration of nonopioid drugs such as clonidine,[98–100] somatostatin,[101, 102] octreotide,[103] ketamine,[104, 105] calcitonin,[106] midazolam,[107] and droperidol.[108] Table 13–3 delineates the use of nonopioid analgesic drugs by the epidural or the intrathecal route.

Although there is ample evidence that the administration of these drugs in the epidural or subarachnoid space provides analgesia, many of these drugs are still experimental. The exception is the α_2-adrenergic ago-

Table 13–2 17-Nation European Survey on Acute Pain Management: Nursing Regulations Regarding Use of Drugs Through Catheters

| | NURSES ALLOWED TO ADMINISTER DRUGS, % OF HOSPITALS | | | |
| | Yes | | No | |
CATHETER	Mean	Range	Mean	Range
Intravenous	80	60–100	20	14–60
Epidural	49	20–100	51*	0–100
Intrathecal	6	10–40	82	60–100

*In Belgium, the Netherlands, Ireland, and The United Kingdom, nurses are not allowed to inject drugs through epidural catheters in 80% to 100% of hospitals.[22]

Table 13–3 Spinal Administration of Nonopioid Analgesics Postoperatively in Europe*

| | FREQUENCY OF ADMINISTRATION, % | | | |
| | Epidural | | Intrathecal | |
DRUG	Mean	Range	Mean	Range
Bupivacaine	53	20–80	21.2	0–50
Clonidine	26.8	0–80	8.2	0–40†
Lidocaine	11.7	0–50	9.9	0–33
Steroids (e.g., prednisolone)	6.7	0–33.3‡		
Mepivacaine	4.0	0–33‡		
Ketamine	3.5	0–20‡		
Tenoxicam	1.2	0–20‡		
Somatostatin	1.2	0–20‡	1.2	0–20†
Droperidol	1.0	0–16.7‡		
Tetracaine			2.1	0–25
Prilocaine			0.6	
Midazolam			0.6	0–10†

*Data from Rawal N: Epidural and intrathecal opioids for postoperative pain management in Europe: a 17-nation survey. (Abstract.) Reg Anesth 1995; 20: A45.
†These nonopioids were used intrathecally in the following countries: clonidine (Austria, Finland, France, Norway, Sweden), somatostatin (Sweden), and midazolam (United Kingdom).
‡These nonopioids were used epidurally in the following countries: mepivacaine (Iceland, Italy, Sweden), steroids (Finland, Iceland, Norway, Portugal), ketamine (Austria, Norway, Portugal), tenoxicam (Portugal), somatostatin (Sweden), and droperidol (Greece).

nist clonidine, which is the nonopioid that has been studied most extensively.

α_2-Adrenergic Agonist Clonidine

Clonidine is a selective α_2-adrenergic agonist that produces analgesia in animals and humans by a nonopioid mechanism.[98] It is thought to inhibit nociceptive impulses by activating postjunctional α_2-adrenoceptors in the dorsal horn of the spinal cord. Yohimbine, a selective α_2-adrenergic antagonist, effectively reverses clonidine-induced analgesia, but α_1- or β-adrenergic antagonists have no significant effects. Clonidine was studied systematically in different animal models for possible neurotoxicity before its clinical use.[109]

There are widely conflicting reports of the efficacy, duration, and potency of epidurally compared with systemically administered clonidine.[11, 12] It has been investigated in postoperative pain studies as the sole agent and in combination with other analgesia techniques, such as epidural administration of opioids or local anesthetics. Conflicting findings for the postoperative analgesic efficacy of epidural administration of clonidine have resulted. In one controlled study,[110] the effect of 3 μg/kg of clonidine given epidurally did not differ from saline placebo. Similarly, in a study of patients undergoing knee surgery,[111] clonidine (75 μg) given epidurally failed to demonstrate any potentiation of analgesia when added to morphine (3 mg) given epidurally; the latter drug provided significantly more effective analgesia. However, in other studies, doses of approximately 2 μg/kg have provided adequate postoperative analgesia after thoracotomy,[112] knee surgery,[100] and hysterectomy.[113]

In most studies, clonidine has been administered by bolus injection, resulting in analgesia lasting from 2 to 5 h.[114] In one study,[98] clonidine analgesia was dose-related. In patients undergoing knee or abdominal operation, doses of 700 to 900 μg provided better and longer-lasting analgesia than 100- to 300-μg and 400- to 600-μg doses. In another study,[115] 150 μg of clonidine given intrathecally provided effective analgesia after cesarean section. The analgesia lasted 5 to 9 h. Unexpectedly, the frequency of adverse effects was less in the higher-dose groups.[98] As with lipophilic opioids, the analgesia and serum levels are similar whether clonidine (2 μg/kg) is administered epidurally or intramuscularly, suggesting a systemic effect.

In volunteers, Eisenach[106] demonstrated that clonidine given epidurally provided a similar degree of analgesia but less respiratory depression than alfentanil given intravenously. The researchers also reported that analgesia correlated better with clonidine levels in cerebrospinal fluid than in plasma and that lower extremity analgesia was superior to upper extremity analgesia, convincingly demonstrating a spinal site of analgesia. The minimum effective analgesic concentration in cerebrospinal fluid was 76 μg/mL $\pm$ 15.

In a masked (double-blind), placebo-controlled study, Fogarty and associates[116] compared the analgesic effects of intrathecal administration of 75 to 100 μg of clonidine or 1 mg of morphine after spinal anesthesia in patients undergoing total hip replacement. Clonidine given intrathecally prolonged the duration of spinal analgesia but was markedly inferior to morphine given intrathecally in providing subsequent postoperative analgesia. The side effects were similar in all groups. The researchers[116] concluded that 75 to 100 μg of clonidine given intrathecally conferred little advantage in terms of postoperative analgesia or side effects.

The reason for the discrepancy in postoperative analgesic effects of spinal administration of clonidine remains unclear. It appears that doses considerably larger than those used in early studies may be necessary for effective analgesia, but large doses may be associated with a higher risk of side effects such as sedation, bradycardia, hypotension, and dry mouth. The hypotensive effect of systemic clonidine is primarily a supraspinal effect of the drug on brain stem receptors.

Neuraxial administration of clonidine also has a local effect on sympathetic nerves in the spinal cord. α_2-Depressor effects predominate at lower plasma concentrations, and α_1-pressor effects are seen with large doses. The hypotensive effect is exaggerated in hypertensive patients and when clonidine is administered in the thoracic region rather than the lumbar region.[115]

Combination of α_2-Adrenergic Agonists and Other Drugs

α_2-Adrenergic agents are useful adjuncts to local anesthetic solutions. Clonidine prolongs the duration of a local anesthetic block in laboratory animals[117, 118] and in humans.[119, 120] The intensity of a sensory and motor block is unaffected by subarachnoid administration of clonidine. These effects are dose-related; the type of local anesthetic does not seem to be important.[121] The prolongation of local anesthetic block is more pronounced after 150 μg of clonidine than after 200 μg of epinephrine.[119, 120] Prolongation of the sensory and motor block also occurs after clonidine-containing local anesthetic solutions are injected epidurally.[122, 123] Data on the effect of epidural administration of clonidine on local anesthetic kinetics are conflicting: an increase[124] and a decrease[123] in plasma lidocaine levels have been reported.

As with subarachnoid administration, epidural administration of clonidine may cause bradycardia, hypotension, and sedation. These effects are explained by rapid absorption and elimination. The hemodynamic effects result from action at spinal sites and sedation from action at central sites.

Epidural administration of clonidine in doses ranging from 3 to 10 μg/kg may prolong postoperative analgesia by 4 to 7 h when added to local anesthetics.[98] It has also been shown that oral administration of clonidine prolongs tetracaine spinal anesthesia.[125]

A synergism between α-adrenergic and opioid systems has been proposed.[126] The obvious benefit of such an interaction may lie in the potential to treat pain by manipulation of different receptors to achieve good-quality analgesia with a minimum of adverse effects.[127] Epidural administration of clonidine decreases postoperative requirements for opioids.[121, 128] It also prolongs the duration of analgesia achieved by epidural administration of opioids such as morphine, fentanyl, and sufentanil.[121, 129, 130] A controlled trial conducted by Mogensen and colleagues[114] showed that epidural administration of clonidine enhanced the postoperative analgesia obtained from a combination of low-dose epidural bupivacaine and morphine, but hypotension was a problem.

Somatostatin and Octreotide

There are several groups of regulatory peptides that affect transmission or inhibition of nociceptive pathways. One such neuropeptide that has been studied in humans is somatostatin.

The rationale for using somatostatin given neuraxially was the localization of specific somatostatin receptors in the spinal cord and the demonstration of an inhibitory effect of somatostatin on nociceptive neurons. The first clinical use of somatostatin given intrathecally was reported in 1984. Effective analgesia was achieved in cancer patients who were tolerant to opioids. The analgesia was not reversed by naloxone, suggesting a nonopioid mechanism of analgesia.[101] Subsequent studies[131] in patients with postoperative pain confirmed the capability of somatostatin to induce potent and sedation-free analgesia.

The main problem with somatostatin is the risk of neurotoxicity, which appears to be dose and species related.[132, 133] Another difficulty is that somatostatin is an unstable peptide, which makes long-term infusion impractical.

Octreotide is a stable analogue of somatostatin. It was demonstrated[103] to be a potent analgesic for cancer pain. The role of this potent, nonopioid analgesic in the management of acute and chronic pain needs further investigation.

Ketamine

Ketamine is a phencyclidine derivative with analgesic properties that are thought to be mediated by multiple mechanisms, including central and peripheral sites of action. Ketamine binds stereospecifically to opioid receptors, but a significant contribution to its analgesic efficacy may come from interaction with cholinergic, adrenergic, and serotonergic systems.[134–137] An opioid mechanism of ketamine analgesia has been disputed by Tung and Yaksh,[138] who found that analgesia was reversed by methysergide but not by naloxone, suggesting a serotonergic mechanism. Ketamine and phencyclidine selectively decreased responses of central neurons to N-methyl-D-aspartate, but this effect is not known to mediate analgesia.[139, 140]

Ketamine has local anesthetic action when given by intravenous regional techniques.[141] In animal studies, the direct action of ketamine on the spinal cord is controversial. Mori and Shingu[142] demonstrated that ketamine analgesia was not mediated by a direct action on the dorsal horn.

In clinical practice, conflicting results have been reported when epidural administration of ketamine was used for pain management. There are several reports claiming[105, 140] and denying[137, 142–144] the analgesic efficacy of epidural administration of ketamine. It has been reported[105] that 4 mg of ketamine given epidurally provided effective analgesia after lower abdominal, perineal, or lower extremity surgical procedures. Similar results were demonstrated by Naguib and coworkers[104] at an epidural dose of 30 mg. The onset of analgesia occurs in about 20 min, and the duration of pain relief after a single injection is about 3 to 4 h. In one study,[140] the addition of ketamine (0.5 mg/kg) to bupivacaine for caudal analgesia in children significantly improved the quality and duration of analgesia compared with administration of bupivacaine alone.

However, the results from other studies[145–147] were less impressive, even when large doses of ketamine given epidurally were used. Ivankovich and McCarthy[146] demonstrated that 7 mg of ketamine given epidurally, followed by a continuous infusion of 10 mg/h, provided inadequate analgesia in patients undergoing thoracotomies and hip replacements. In one masked (double-blind) study,[144] ketamine (4 to 8 mg) given epidurally was inadequate for pain relief after gynecologic operations.

In another masked (double-blind) study[137] in which epidural administration of ketamine and diamorphine was compared, 5 mg of diamorphine was superior to 30 mg of ketamine in terms of duration and quality of analgesia. Two studies[145, 146] were terminated because of inadequate analgesia after ketamine given epidurally. Adverse effects such as sedation, blurred vision, tachycardia, hypertension, and hallucinations have been associated with epidural administration of ketamine.[143, 145, 147, 148]

Another problem is the lack of consensus regarding the neurotoxic potential of the drug. Intrathecal administration of ketamine was not neurotoxic in baboons.[149] However, focal degeneration with loss of myelin and axoplasm has been observed[150] in spinal nerve roots of monkeys after ketamine given intrathecally. Histopathologic changes in the spinal cord have also been reported[151] in rats receiving ketamine intrathecally. The usefulness of epidural administration of ketamine alone for postoperative pain appears to be quite limited. Large doses of ketamine given intrathecally may have neurotoxic potential in humans.

Summary

Research has demonstrated the increasing importance of the spinal cord in processing and modulating nociceptive input. Different groups of drugs, each acting by a unique mechanism, have been shown to block nociceptive afferent transmission. None of the neuraxially administered local anesthetics, opioids, or nonopioids produce analgesia without side effects. Nonopioids such as α_2 agonists may be more suited as adjuvants rather than sole analgesic agents, and their main role lies in decreasing the dose requirements of other analgesics. Neuraxial administration of somatostatin and ketamine may have neurotoxic potential. The role of these drugs and of midazolam in pain management appears to be limited. Preliminary results suggest that the neuropeptide octreotide has potent analgesic effects. Balanced neuraxial analgesia using a combination of low doses of drugs, with separate but synergistic mechanisms of analgesia, may produce the best results.

Neurotoxic Potential of Drugs Given Neuraxially

A wide range of opioids has been studied in an effort to achieve analgesia without respiratory depression. Fentanyl, sufentanil, and meperidine are used routinely in many hospitals. Other opioids that have been studied are buprenorphine, diamorphine, alfentanil, lofentanil, butorphanol, hydromorphone, nalbuphine, methadone, nicomorphine, pentazocine, phenoperidine, meptazinol, and tramadol.[91, 152–163] There is a general lack of comparative data for these drugs. The major differences among opioids are latency of onset, duration of analgesia, and adverse effects. The quality of analgesia appears to be similar for all drugs.

The introduction of new neuraxially administered analgesic drugs should be approached with caution because administration of drugs into the subarachnoid or epidural space is potentially dangerous.[164] The debate related to cauda equina syndrome has highlighted the advisability of limiting concentration and dose of drugs administered in the subarachnoid space. Histologic examination of spinal cords in animals and humans after prolonged epidural administration of morphine did not reveal any abnormalities. Similar results were reported[165] for large doses of morphine injected intrathecally in monkeys. Even unintentional massive doses of 50 to 100 mg of morphine given epidurally[166, 167] produced no serious physiologic effects other than predictable naloxone-reversible respiratory depression. Patients with cancer pain receiving daily doses of 480 mg of morphine epidurally or 60 mg intrathecally showed no evidence of any physiologic or neurologic changes.[168] No other opioid has been studied as extensively as morphine with regard to safety for epidural or intrathecal administration. Although neurotoxic data are not available for meperidine or fentanyl, these drugs have a good safety record; no neurologic complications have been reported despite use of thousands of doses of these drugs.

Neurotoxicity of opioids may be route dependent. In sheep studies,[169] large doses of sufentanil and butorphanol that are safe epidurally resulted in major histopathologic changes in the spinal cord when administered intrathecally. However, the doses studied were far larger than recommended clinical doses. This suggests that some of the opioids that are intended for the epidural space may have neurotoxic potential if unintentionally deposited in the subarachnoid space. This probably results from the proximity of the drug to the spinal cord, because the dura is known to be an effective barrier to the harmful effect of drugs. It is therefore important to perform animal neurotoxicity studies followed by controlled clinical trials before widespread use of new drugs. Coombs[164] remarked that "the list of spinal agents currently in clinical use or under clinical study that have yet to undergo even rudimentary testing is truly remarkable."

Site of Epidural Catheter Placement: Lumbar or Thoracic?

The exact mechanism of action of epidurally administered lipid-soluble opioids is controversial. Some data suggest that lipid-soluble opioids provide pain relief predominantly as a result of systemic absorption rather than by a direct effect on spinal cord opioid receptors.

Theoretically, this makes location of epidural catheters important. Several studies[170-172] reported that epidural infusion of opioids through lumbar catheters provided adequate post-thoracotomy analgesia. Other studies[94, 173] demonstrated superior analgesia when the opioid was administered in the thoracic rather than the lumbar region.

Salomäki and colleagues[94] and Bodily and associates[173] found that the doses of fentanyl given epidurally for post-thoracotomy pain were considerably lower when the catheter was in the thoracic rather than the lumbar epidural space. This was disputed by Coe and colleagues[97] and Swenson and coworkers,[43] who were unable to show any clinical advantage (with respect to quality of analgesia, severity of side effects, amount of opioid used, or postoperative pulmonary function) of thoracic over lumbar administration of fentanyl and sufentanil, respectively, in the thoracotomy patient. Similar conclusions were drawn by Haak-van der Lely and colleagues[174] when they compared lumbar with thoracic administration of sufentanil for intraoperative analgesia for thoracotomy. Guinard and associates[175] showed that patients undergoing thoracotomy with fentanyl given epidurally for analgesia had shorter hospital stays with thoracic than lumbar administration.

In contrast, morphine spreads easily through cerebrospinal fluid; this explains why morphine is capable of providing analgesia after thoracic operation even if the drug is administered in the caudal epidural space.[176] Several studies[177-180] showed that lumbar epidural administration of morphine was as effective as thoracic administration for pain relief after thoracotomy or upper abdominal operation. However, in one study,[180] a decreased dose requirement was demonstrated for thoracic administration of morphine after thoracotomy.

Additional studies of fentanyl and other lipid-soluble opioids are necessary to establish the importance of catheter location.

Neuraxial Administration of Opioids and Outcome Studies

Evidence suggests that the technique of pain control does have a significant influence on the incidence of postoperative complications. In patients undergoing thoracic or major abdominal operation, epidural technique using local anesthetics or opioids or their combination can be expected to improve postoperative pulmonary function considerably and to decrease the risk of pulmonary and thromboembolic complications.[8-10] After gallbladder surgery, similar results can be achieved by using intercostal block instead of opioids given intramuscularly.[7]

These techniques may be particularly useful for the high-risk patient and the patient with compromised pulmonary function preoperatively.[7-10] This was demonstrated in a masked (double-blind) study in which the effects of morphine given intramuscularly and epidurally on early and late pulmonary function were compared in grossly obese patients undergoing gastroplasty for weight reduction. Patients receiving mor-

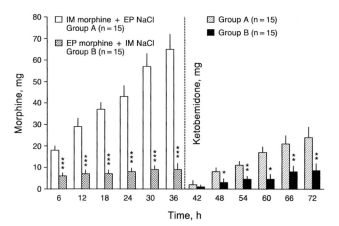

Figure 13–3 Comparison between intramuscular (IM) and epidural (EP) administration of morphine for postgastroplasty analgesia in grossly obese patients. Equianalgesic doses of morphine given intramuscularly were up to 7 times larger. * $P < .05$, ** $P < .01$, *** $P < .001$. (Redrawn from Rawal N, Sjöstrand U, Christoffersson E, et al: Comparison of intramuscular and epidural morphine for postoperative analgesia in the grossly obese: influence on postoperative ambulation and pulmonary function. Anesth Analg 1984; 63: 583–592.)

phine epidurally were more alert and mobile. Equianalgesic doses of morphine given intramuscularly were as much as seven times larger during the first 36 h; in the remaining 36 h of the study, the dosage of ketobemidone (opioid) to achieve effective analgesia was also significantly higher (Fig. 13–3). Significantly earlier recovery of peak expiratory flow rate (Fig. 13–4), decreased incidence of pulmonary complications such as atelectasis and parenchymal infiltrations, and briefer hospitalization (Table 13–4) were also seen in patients receiving morphine epidurally.[8]

The effects of epidural anesthesia and postoperative

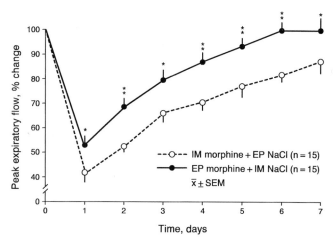

Figure 13–4 Influence of intramuscular (IM) and epidural (EP) administration of morphine analgesia on postoperative peak expiratory flow changes in grossly obese patients. Recovery took 7 d in the epidural group and 9 d in the intramuscular group. * $P < .05$ and ** $P < .01$. (Redrawn from Rawal N, Sjöstrand U, Christoffersson E, et al: Comparison of intramuscular and epidural morphine for postoperative analgesia in the grossly obese: influence on postoperative ambulation and pulmonary function. Anesth Analg 1984; 63: 583–592.)

Table 13–4 Influence of Epidural or Intramuscular Administration of Morphine Analgesia on Postoperative Gastrointestinal Motility and Hospitalization Time

VARIABLE	INTRAMUSCULAR MORPHINE AND EPIDURAL SALINE, MEAN ± SEM	EPIDURAL MORPHINE AND INTRAMUSCULAR SALINE, MEAN ± SEM	PROBABILITY
Postoperative hospitalization time, d	9.0 ± 0.60	7.1 ± 0.30	<0.05
Flatus, h	75.1 ± 3.08	56.7 ± 3.06	<0.05
Feces, h	92.7 ± 2.92	68.4 ± 3.51	<0.05
Postoperative gastric aspirate, mL/day			
Day 1	211 ± 43.9	227 ± 44 (n = 12)	NS
Day 2	192 ± 43.2	351 ± 57.9 (n = 12)	<0.05
Day 3	243 ± 62.8	422 ± 53.8 (n = 12)	<0.05

From Rawal N, Sjöstrand U, Christoffersson E, et al: Comparison of intramuscular and epidural morphine for postoperative analgesia in the grossly obese: influence on postoperative ambulation and pulmonary function. Anesth Analg 1984; 63: 583–592.

analgesia on postoperative morbidity were evaluated in a group of high-risk patients undergoing major abdominal, thoracic, or vascular surgery.[9] Patients receiving intraoperative epidural block and postoperative epidural local anesthetics or opioids (or both) had decreased postoperative morbidity and improved operative outcome compared with their counterparts receiving intraoperative general anesthesia and postoperative opioid analgesia parenterally. Patients in the epidural group had a lower incidence of postoperative respiratory and cardiovascular complications, decreased stress response, briefer hospitalization, decreased costs, and lower mortality rates.

In a study[10] of patients with arteriosclerotic vascular disease undergoing aortic bypass, postoperative analgesia was provided with epidural analgesia or on-demand opioids. Among patients receiving epidural analgesia, the incidence of thrombotic, infectious, and cardiovascular complications and the duration of stay in the ICU were significantly decreased.

For high-risk patients undergoing major operation, epidural analgesia using local anesthetics or opioids (or both) is the method of choice and is cost effective. The only alternative for many patients is prolonged postoperative ventilator treatment. However, the postoperative outcome benefits of epidural technique using local anesthetics, opioids, or their combination in low-risk patients are not as impressive. In a retrospective study[17] of 684 patients receiving opioid analgesia by five different techniques (i.e., epidural morphine, epidural morphine plus fentanyl, intrathecal morphine, intramuscular opioids, PCA) for analgesia after cesarean section, accelerated recovery or improved outcome was not demonstrated with use of newer techniques, such as spinal administration of opioids or PCA, compared with conventional opioid therapy given intramuscularly. Similarly, in a controlled study,[181] epidural analgesia with bupivacaine and opioid combination failed to show any decrease in the incidence of postoperative pulmonary complications or decrease in the length of hospital stay in patients undergoing abdominal procedures.

The 17-nation European survey showed that most anesthesiologists thought that spinal administration of opioids affects postoperative outcome, decreases hospitalization time, and decreases morbidity.[22] In this respect, morphine was considered superior to other opioids (Table 13–5).

Side Effects of Neuraxial Administration of Opioids

Some of the reported side effects of spinal administration of opioids, such as nausea, vomiting, hypotension, somnolence, and early respiratory depression, are dose–related and are thought to result from the vascular uptake of opioids. The effects of neuraxial administration of opioids on gastrointestinal function have also received attention.[182, 183] The nonsystemic and characteristic adverse effects are pruritus, urinary retention, and late-onset respiratory depression.

Pruritus

The reported incidence of itching varies after opioids given neuraxially. Figures ranging from 0% to 100% have been published. The probable reason is that, if not asked specifically, most patients do not complain about this complication because of its mild nature. In large series,[1] the incidence of pruritus after epidural administration of up to 5 mg of morphine is less than 10%, and the risk of severe, distressing itching is about 1%.

Morphine injected into the medullary dorsal horn of

Table 13–5 Opinion of European Anesthesiologists Regarding the Role of Opioids Given Epidurally in Decreasing Postoperative Morbidity and Hospitalization Time

ROLE OF OPIOID	OPINION OF ANALGESIA GIVEN EPIDURALLY, %	
	Morphine	Nonmorphine Opioids*
Affect outcome	61	39
Decrease hospitalization time	48	34
Decrease morbidity†	68	42

*Fentanyl, sufentanil, and meperidine.
†Major operation, high-risk patients, trauma patients, and old patients.
Data from Rawal N: Epidural and intrathecal opioids for postoperative pain management in Europe: a 17-nation survey. (Abstract.) Reg Anesth 1995; 20: A45.

monkeys produces pronounced facial scratching. This effect is dose dependent and naloxone reversible. Interestingly, morphine given intramuscularly produced a substantial reduction in scratching behavior in monkeys.[184] The researchers speculated that morphine has pruritus-provoking and -modulating activity, depending on the site of action.

Pruritus has been associated with almost all opioids. Pregnant patients appear more at risk, regardless of the opioid administered. The addition of epinephrine to the opioid given epidurally appears to increase the risk of pruritus. Patients treated for cancer pain with epidural or intrathecal administration of opioids for weeks or months do not experience pruritus after the first or second day, presumably because of the rapid development of tolerance.[1] In a controlled study[185] of a post–cesarean section population, the incidence of pruritus was compared after epidural administration of four different opioids. The patients received the following doses: morphine, 5 mg; fentanyl, 50 μg; buprenorphine, 0.3 mg; or butorphanol, 1 mg. The incidence of pruritus was highest among patients receiving morphine or fentanyl (Table 13–6). The incidence was low after butorphanol and zero after buprenorphine. The researchers speculated that the occurrence of pruritus may be related to opioid receptor affinity. The incidence is high after μ-receptor agonist opioids (morphine and fentanyl) and low after κ-receptor agonists (butorphanol).

Localization of pruritus may vary with the opioid used. In one study,[186] fentanyl given epidurally caused segmental pruritus whereas morphine given epidurally was associated with generalized pruritus.

The epidural administration of morphine may reactivate herpes simplex in pregnant patients. Epidural administration of meperidine and fentanyl has also reactivated herpes.[187, 188] In a retrospective survey of 5000 patients who received morphine epidurally for pain relief after cesarean section, pruritus affected 60% of patients. In this study, oral herpes simplex lesions were reactivated in 3% to 5% of patients; this is far lower than the 15% incidence reported in other studies. The cause of herpes simplex after epidural administration of morphine is unclear. Because most cases occur around the nose and mouth, it is presumed that the viral agents are latent in the neuronal pathway of the trigeminal nerve. The virus is theorized to be reactivated by mechanical irritation of sensory nerves in response to facial itching. Alternatively, herpes simplex reactivation may be related to the rostral spread in cerebrospinal fluid of morphine given spinally and consequent high concentrations of morphine in the substantia gelatinosa of the trigeminal nerve.[189] It has been speculated that herpes simplex after delivery may cause herpes encephalitis in the infant. However, the role of spinal administration of morphine as a cause of herpes simplex reactivation has been questioned.[190] As many as 84% of pregnant women previously infected with herpes simplex have peripartum recurrences whether or not opioids are used neuraxially.[191]

Antihistaminic drugs and naloxone have been used successfully to manage pruritus. Prophylactic intravenous infusion of naloxone at the rate of 5 μg/kg/h can decrease the frequency of pruritus induced by morphine given epidurally without reversing analgesia.[192] Subhypnotic doses (10 mg) of propofol have relieved pruritus induced by the spinal administration of morphine.[193] The antipruritic action lasted more than 60 min in 85% of patients. The effective use of droperidol given intravenously to treat pruritus induced by epidural administration of morphine has been reported[194] and denied.[195]

Prophylactic administration of opioid antagonists such as naloxone,[192, 196, 197] naltrexone,[198, 199] nalbuphine,[196, 200] and butorphanol[199, 201] has been recommended for prevention of pruritus, nausea, vomiting, and other adverse effects of spinal administration of opioids. However, because of the mild nature of some side effects and rarity of others, few patients require treatment; many patients would receive drug therapy unnecessarily. Meticulous dose titration may be necessary to avoid reversal of analgesia, and antagonist drugs have side effects of their own. The routine use of opioid antagonists would also result in increased costs and added nursing workloads.[200]

Most of the studies on prophylactic opioid antagonist administration are of patients undergoing cesarean section. In one study,[196] intravenous therapy with nalbuphine was superior to that with naloxone. In another study,[199] 3 mg of butorphanol given epidurally was better than 3 mg of nalbuphine given epidurally or 6 mg of naltrexone given orally.

Urinary Retention

The reported incidence[1, 202] of urinary retention after epidural or intrathecal administration of opioids varies

Table 13–6 Incidence of Pruritus After Epidural Administration of Opioids

		INCIDENCE*		
OPIOID	**DOSE**	**Patients, no.**	**%**	**DURATION OF ANALGESIA, min**
Morphine	5 mg	9	60	932 ± 87
Fentanyl	50 μg	7	47	145 ± 38
Buprenorphine	0.3 mg	0	0	388 ± 55
Butorphanol	1 mg	1	7	97 ± 23

*Fifteen patients were in each group.
Modified from Ackerman WE, Juneja MM, Kaczorowski DM, et al: A comparison of the incidence of pruritus following epidural opioid administration in the parturient. Can J Anaesth 1989; 36:388–391.

considerably. It is difficult to establish the incidence of urinary retention because most patients who received opioids epidurally or intrathecally are high-risk patients undergoing major operations who are usually catheterized.

Cystometric studies of volunteers injected epidurally with 2, 4, or 10 mg of morphine demonstrated a decrease in the strength of the detrusor contraction, which leads to a corresponding increase in bladder capacity. These urodynamic changes are noticed within 15 to 30 min, last an average of 15 h after epidural injection, and are unrelated to the morphine dose. Intramuscular or intravenous injection of morphine had no effect on the detrusor contraction, suggesting that urinary retention is not a systemic effect (Fig. 13–5). Because analgesia and detrusor changes occur about 15 to 30 min after epidural injection of opioids and because the cystometric changes are naloxone reversible (Fig. 13–6), the site of action must be at opioid receptors in the spinal cord.[192, 202]

Some workers have speculated that urinary retention may be less likely if agonist-antagonist opioids are used. Urodynamic studies[203, 204] using dogs have shown that the effects of intrathecal administration of fentanyl, alfentanil, and buprenorphine on the urinary bladder are different. Intrathecal administration of fentanyl is associated with decreased detrusor tone whereas intrathecal administration of buprenorphine or alfentanil had no effect on the detrusor.

Intrathecal injection of μ- and δ-receptor agonist drugs causes bladder relaxation, but κ-receptor agonists do not affect vesical muscles.[205] This suggests that opioids with more κ-receptor properties would probably be associated with a lower incidence of and less severe urinary retention. In one report,[161] epidural injection of a κ-agonist opioid, pentazocine, caused no urinary retention. A similar result was reported for buprenorphine given epidurally. Another study[163] comparing

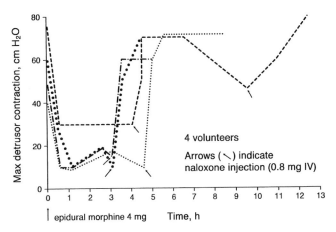

Figure 13–6 Influence of a single intravenous (IV) injection of naloxone on the decreased strength of detrusor contraction. Detrusor strength and bladder capacity were restored, and volunteers could micturate. Max, maximum. (Redrawn from Rawal N, Möllefors K, Axelsson K, et al: An experimental study of urodynamic effects of epidural morphine and of naloxone reversal. Anesth Analg 1983; 62: 641–647.)

epidural administration of morphine and methadone for analgesia after cesarean section showed that urinary retention is less frequent and of shorter duration after methadone given epidurally. However, these results were not confirmed by Jacobson and colleagues,[206] who compared intrathecal administration of methadone (5 mg) with morphine (0.5 mg) for analgesia after total knee or hip replacement. Urinary retention, although less frequent after methadone given intrathecally, was nevertheless noted in more than 50% of patients.

Studies of volunteers and patients showed that naloxone given intravenously could prevent or reverse the urodynamic changes after morphine given epidurally. However, the usual doses of naloxone that reverse respiratory depression were inadequate to reverse urinary bladder changes. Larger doses of naloxone (e.g., 0.4 mg intravenous bolus injection followed by 10 μg/kg/h) usually reverse the urodynamic changes but also may partially or completely reverse analgesia.[192] Naloxone infused at a low dose (e.g., 1 μg/kg/h) has been shown[32] to decrease the risk of urinary retention after diamorphine given intrathecally. However, this advantage was achieved at the price of decreased analgesia. An inability to void in the postoperative period is also seen in patients not receiving neuraxial opioids. Voiding is also influenced by factors such as increased antidiuretic hormone, type and anatomic site of the operation, supine position, perioperative and postoperative hypovolemia, and deep sedation. In some cases, the failure of naloxone to reverse urinary retention may be related to these factors. If patients are unable to void 6 h after surgery and naloxone is ineffective, a single in-and-out catheterization is indicated to prevent myogenic bladder dysfunction because of prolonged overdistension.

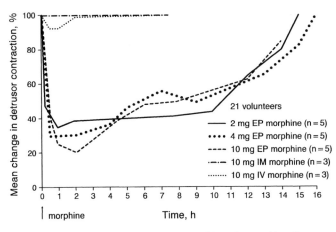

Figure 13–5 Irrespective of dosage, morphine given epidurally (EP) decreases the strength of detrusor contraction, resulting in increased bladder capacity and urinary retention in volunteers. Detrusor function and micturition are unaffected by 10 mg of morphine given intramuscularly (IM) or intravenously (IV). (Redrawn from Rawal N, Möllefors K, Axelsson K, et al: An experimental study of urodynamic effects of epidural morphine and of naloxone reversal. Anesth Analg 1983; 62: 641–647.)

Respiratory Depression

The true incidence of clinically significant respiratory depression with perioperative analgesia is unknown.

Data from anecdotal case reports, prospective controlled studies, and retrospective nationwide surveys show wide variations in the incidence of respiratory depression because of factors such as differences in patient populations, type of operations, and pain scores among groups. Other factors may be the use of sedatives and opioids given parenterally, use of epidural local anesthetics, intermittent rather than continuous respiratory monitoring, and different respiratory parameters monitored in different studies.[2, 11, 12, 207] Because of the rarity of late-onset respiratory depression, small sample sizes, and invasive respiratory measurement techniques, most prospective studies[12] of epidural administration of morphine have not detected clinically significant respiratory depression.

Respiratory depression after neuraxial administration of opioids has been studied in far greater detail than for any other opioid delivery route. One of the purported advantages of neuraxial compared with parenteral administration of opioids is the lack of respiratory depression. Patients with compromised respiratory and cardiac function often benefit from opioid analgesia given neuraxially rather than intramuscularly. The most frequent indication for using epidural administration of opioids in the Swedish survey[11] was the management of postoperative pain in high-risk patients undergoing major thoracic, abdominal, or orthopedic operations.

Respiratory depression continues to be the most feared side effect. After epidural administration of morphine, respiratory depression may occur within 1 h; if lipophilic opioids are used, onset of this complication may be noted within minutes. In general, early-onset respiratory depression is a minor problem of opioid analgesia given epidurally, and late-onset respiratory depression is potentially more problematic because it may occur hours after injection of the opioid.

Delayed respiratory depression is thought to result from the rostral spread of opioids in the cerebrospinal fluid. The plasma levels after morphine given epidurally are relatively low, but cerebrospinal fluid concentrations are several hundred times higher.[208] This morphine-laden cerebrospinal fluid reaches medullary respiratory centers by diffusion and bulk flow. There is no evidence, from laboratory or clinical experiments, that has confirmed the hypothesis of sudden respiratory depression because of arrival intracranially of large boluses of opioid at some distant time. Respiratory depression progresses slowly rather than occurring suddenly.[5]

The CO_2 response studies of volunteers that I did with Wattwil[209] demonstrated a dose-dependent depression of ventilatory control. After 2 mg and 4 mg of morphine given epidurally, respiratory depression was mild to moderate, respectively, and similar to that after 10 mg of morphine given intravenously. However, 10 mg of morphine given epidurally was associated with a significant and prolonged respiratory depression for as long as 22 h. In patients who received 4 mg of morphine epidurally for postcholecystectomy pain, the CO_2 response was depressed despite a normal respiratory rate. Respiratory rate alone is not a good indicator of respiratory depression. Similar results have been reported by others. In a controlled study,[210] respiratory depression was studied by inductive plethysmography after epidural or intravenous administration of morphine for post-thoracotomy pain. In the epidural group, respiratory rates were lower and values for partial pressure of arterial CO_2 were higher for 2 to 12 h after 5-mg doses. Periods of hypopnea or apnea were observed in six of eight patients, all of whom received at least 10 mg of morphine epidurally. In contrast, only one of five patients receiving morphine intravenously had apneic periods.

Are Lipophilic Opioids Safer?

On the basis of pharmacologic models proposed for epidural and intrathecal transport of opioids, the risk of late-onset respiratory depression is higher with morphine than with lipophilic opioids (i.e., meperidine, fentanyl, and sufentanil). Lipophilic opioids are considered safer because of segmental localization after injection such that, theoretically, minimal agent is available for rostral migration in the cerebrospinal fluid. However, some data suggest that this may not be true. Gourlay and coworkers[211] demonstrated rapid cephalad flow of meperidine injected in the lumbar epidural space. A prolonged depression of the CO_2 response curve after epidural and intrathecal administration of fentanyl[14, 212] and epidural administration of sufentanil[213] also suggests cephalad migration of the drug. Despite high lipid solubility and strong μ-receptor affinity, these drugs are not restricted to the spinal cord. Rostral spread through cerebrospinal fluid and by direct transit in epidural veins may be significant.[212]

Although the risk of respiratory depression appears to be lower after epidural administration of lipophilic opioids, these drugs are not completely risk free. Early- and late-onset respiratory depression have been reported[1, 2, 12, 84, 85, 213–218] after epidural administration of fentanyl, meperidine, diamorphine, hydromorphone, methadone, and sufentanil. Buprenorphine given epidurally in 0.15-mg doses produced prolonged and biphasic depression of the CO_2 response that lasted 8 to 12 h. A similar depression of ventilatory response to CO_2 that lasted 12 h was noted after 2 to 4 mg of butorphanol given epidurally.[219] Epidural administration of fentanyl has also been associated with a decrease in the CO_2 response curve that lasted 30 to 120 min after a single injection of 200 μg in healthy volunteers and throughout the 18-h study period in patients undergoing orthopedic procedures who received a 1-μg/kg bolus followed by 1 μg/kg/h. In one report,[85] three patients who received a combination of bupivacaine and fentanyl as a continuous infusion became unconscious after 3 to 26 h; one patient had to be tracheally intubated. All three responded to naloxone given intravenously (Table 13–7). There are several reports of severe respiratory depression after sufentanil given epidurally. This is usually early in onset[220, 221]; however, severe bradypnea and respiratory arrest after 50-μg and 75-μg doses have been reported.[217, 222]

There is considerable evidence that a healthy obstet-

Table 13–7 Respiratory Arrest During Epidural Infusion of Bupivacaine and Fentanyl

AGE, yr	ASA PS	EPIDURAL CATHETER LEVEL	DOSE	COMMENTS
64	III	T6–7	Bupivacaine (0.2%) + fentanyl (100 mg/h)	Unconscious (17 h) Naloxone reversal Cardiac arrest team called
70	II	T4–5	Bupivacaine (0.2%) + fentanyl (60 mg/h)	Unconscious (3 h) Apnea Naloxone (0.4 mg) two times Cardiac arrest team called
53	III	T4–5	Bupivacaine (0.2 %) + fentanyl (100 mg/h)	Unconscious (26 h) Apnea Intubated (no response) Ephedrine Naloxone reversal Cardiac arrest team called

ASA, American Society of Anesthesiologists; PS, physical status.
Data from Weightman WM: Respiratory arrest during epidural infusion of bupivacaine and fentanyl. Anaesth Intensive Care 1991; 19: 282–284.

ric population is not at high risk for respiratory depression. In a large retrospective survey involving almost 5000 subjects who received morphine epidurally for analgesia after cesarean section, Fuller and colleagues[223] emphasized that routine nursing observations of the postpartum patients sufficed to detect respiratory depression. The researchers thought that all mothers who receive morphine, by whatever route, may experience transient desaturation. However, there was no evidence to indicate that these episodes are more severe than those encountered in sleep.[224] It has been hypothesized that the respiratory changes of pregnancy confer some protection against opioid-induced hypopnea. Pregnant women are thought to be at low risk for respiratory depression.[18, 224] In one editorial,[224] it was suggested that after cesarean section women can safely receive morphine epidurally and be transferred to routine postpartum care. However, hourly nursing observation of respiratory rate and somnolence is necessary for at least 12 h.

The use of opioids by any route is always associated with the risk of respiratory depression. There is evidence[225] to suggest that the degree of respiratory depression with opioids given intramuscularly is significant and usually goes unnoticed. It has been demonstrated[76] that 0.1 to 0.25 mg of morphine given intrathecally does not depress the response to CO_2, but 8 mg of morphine given intramuscularly was associated with a 40% decrease in the CO_2 response slope. The low prevalence of respiratory depression after morphine given epidurally compares favorably with the suggested prevalence[226] of 0.9% of serious respiratory depression after the systemic use of opioids. Some physicians[225] think that opioids given epidurally with good monitoring are safer than opioids given intramuscularly with routine casual or no monitoring. Table 13–8 shows the opinion of European anesthesiologists regarding the safety of different routes of opioid administration. Most anesthesiologists considered intrathecal and epidural routes most dangerous. As many as 25% of anesthesiologists considered PCA and up to 16% considered intramuscular and subcutaneous administration of opioids most dangerous (see Table 13–8).

In a study[227] in which oxygen saturation was compared after PCA and intramuscular administration of meperidine and epidural administration of morphine after cesarean section, decreases in oxygen saturation occurred in all groups but were most marked in patients treated with PCA with meperidine. The researchers concluded that all postoperative patients receiving opioid analgesia, irrespective of route, merit observation for respiratory depression.

In a retrospective study,[228] eight cases of respiratory depression were detected from the charts of about 1600 patients who had received PCA. These patients were drowsy or unarousable, with low oxygen saturation and respiratory rates of 4 to 7/min. Two patients were found obstructed and cyanotic. All patients required naloxone given intravenously and oxygen. The following risk factors were identified: concurrent use of background infusion, advanced age, concomitant administration of sedatives, and preexisting sleep apnea syndrome. No cases were attributed to anesthesiologist error or equipment malfunction. The researcher concluded that the risk of respiratory depression after PCA is similar to that after opioids given intramuscularly or neuraxially. Knowledgeable medical and nursing staff, appropriate protocols, and frequent patient follow-up are essential for safe use of PCA. Available data[229] suggest that the overall risk of severe respiratory depression from appropriate doses of opioids is similar regardless of the route of administration.

Evidence suggests that the lipophilic opioids may be somewhat safer than hydrophilic morphine, but data from large series are necessary for every lipophilic opioid before its safety is established. Close monitoring of patients for several hours is advisable after giving drugs like fentanyl and sufentanil, and supplemental opioids should be administered with caution.[212, 215]

Neuraxial Administration of Opioids and Monitoring Routines

It is generally agreed that all patients who are treated with opioids given neuraxially should be observed

Table 13–8 Opinion of European Anesthesiologists Regarding Safety of Opioids by Different Routes

| ROUTE | BELIEVE MOST DANGEROUS, % OF ANESTHESIOLOGISTS | | COUNTRIES |
	Mean	Range	
Intramuscular	2	0–10	France, UK
Subcutaneous (e.g., morphine)	4	0–16	Germany, Greece, Italy, UK
Patient-controlled analgesia	8	0–25	Denmark, Ireland, Netherlands, Switzerland, UK
Epidural	27	20–80	Belgium, Finland, France, Germany, Iceland, Ireland, Portugal, Sweden, UK
Intrathecal	68	20–90	Every country

UK, United Kingdom.
Data from Rawal N: Epidural and intrathecal opioids for postoperative pain management in Europe: a 17-nation survey. (Abstract.) Reg Anesth 1995; 20:A45.

carefully because of the risk of late-onset respiratory depression. However, there is no consensus regarding the duration, the technique, or the level of monitoring. Many anesthesiologists have recommended an observation period of 12 to 24 h when morphine is administered epidurally or intrathecally. This appears to be derived from CO_2 response studies[2, 209] showing a depression of ventilatory drive over 22 h. However, in clinical practice, respiratory depression occurring more than 12 h after epidural administration of therapeutic doses of morphine (up to 5 mg) is extremely rare. This is probably because CO_2 response studies are performed in volunteers, and the potent respiratory stimulant effect of surgical pain is missing. Etches[230] maintained that the risk of respiratory depression after opioids given neuraxially has to be kept in the right perspective. Opioids by any route of administration can cause potentially life-threatening respiratory depression. For morphine given parenterally, this risk is thought to be about 0.9%. Etches estimated that about 1% of patients require naloxone for management of hypoventilation after PCA. Similarly, data from several large studies[11, 71, 223, 231] show that the risk of respiratory depression after morphine given neuraxially is less than 1% (Table 13–9). The reports of serious respiratory depression induced by opioids given spinally have decreased in the last decade, presumably because of the use of smaller doses and greater appreciation of risk factors.

Since the introduction of neuraxial administration of opioids for pain management in 1979, the technique has been used in hundreds of thousands of patients worldwide. Several anecdotal reports of late-onset respiratory depression and near misses have been published, but no death has been reported so far. However,

the European survey showed that one anesthesiologist in Belgium and one in the United Kingdom were aware of death after respiratory arrest induced by opioids given epidurally.[22] The death in Belgium occurred in 1985 and was caused by morphine given epidurally. The death in the United Kingdom was caused by diamorphine given epidurally; no anesthesiologist was available to resuscitate the patient. Further details about these cases are not available (Table 13–10).

The results from large surveys involving thousands of patients suggest that the risk of late-onset respiratory depression after morphine given epidurally is less than 1%; this can be decreased further if certain risk factors are avoided (Table 13–11). The risk of respiratory depression after other opioids may or may not be less; current data are inconclusive. What is clear is that respiratory depression after neuraxial administration of opioids is unpredictable and may be associated with any opioid.

Respiratory rate alone is inadequate to establish the presence or absence of respiratory depression.[209] Short periods of apnea are common during sleep or in patients receiving opioids by any route. Monitoring of level of consciousness is important because increasing sedation is associated[5] with increasing respiratory depression. Simple bedside assessment of level of consciousness may be superior to sophisticated apnea-monitoring devices.[232–234] Although the risk should not be underestimated, it is also clear that it is not necessary to monitor most patients in an ICU or a postanesthesia care unit.[3, 72, 232–235] About 70% of respondents in the European survey considered neuraxial administration of opioids safe on surgical wards if the patients were in American Society of Anesthesiologists class I–II.[22] However, about 60% actually monitored such

Table 13–9 Incidence of Respiratory Depression After Epidural Administration of Morphine

PATIENTS, no.	DOSE, mg	CASES, no.*	INCIDENCE, %	REFERENCE
6,000–9,000	2–4	23	0.25–0.4	Gustafsson et al[71]
1,085	4–6	10	0.9	Stenseth et al[231]
14,000	4	13	0.09	Rawal et al[11]
4,880	2–5	12	0.25	Fuller et al[223]

*Respiratory depression.

Table 13–10 Serious Complications After Neuraxial Administration of Opioids for Postoperative Pain*

COUNTRY	COMPLICATION	OPIOID	DOSE	ROUTE	YEAR	COMMENTS
Austria	Resp. arrest	Sufentanil	30 μg	IT	1991	
Belgium	Resp. dep.	Morphine		Ep	1985	Respiratory depression in 2 cases
	Death	Morphine		Ep		Patient intubated and ventilated
Denmark	Resp. dep.					
Finland	CNS damage	Morphine and scopolamine		Ep	1986	Accidental overdose (10 times normal dose) of wrong drug
	Resp. dep.	Morphine		Ep	"Years ago"	Accidental overdose (10 times normal dose)
France	Meningitis					
	Resp. dep.					
Germany	Resp. dep.				1985–1986	Respiratory depression in 2 cases
Ireland	Ep hematoma					Two cases, permanent paraplegia developed in 1 patient
Italy	Resp. dep.	Morphine	2 mg	Ep and IT		Inadvertent subarachnoid injection of Ep dose
	Resp. dep.	Morphine		Ep PCA		
Netherlands	Resp. dep.					
Spain	Resp. dep.					
	Ep hematoma					
	Arachnoiditis					
	"Infection"					
Sweden	Resp. dep.	Morphine	4 mg	IT	1981	Old patient (> 80 yr) required assisted ventilation for several hours
United Kingdom	Resp. dep. (2–3 cases)					
	Resp. arrest—death	Diamorphine				Anesthesiologist unavailable to resuscitate patient
	Resp. dep.	Diamorphine				Subarachnoid migration of epidural catheter

*These incidents occurred during a 14-year period. These imprecise data are in response to the question, "Are you aware of any death or other serious complication of epidural/intrathecal opioid therapy?"

CNS, central nervous system; dep., depression; Ep, epidural; IT, intrathecal; PCA, patient-controlled analgesia; Resp., respiratory.

patients on the wards (Table 13–12). There is increasing evidence that most patients can be safely monitored on regular wards if personnel are trained and preprinted guidelines for potential emergencies are provided, patient selection and opioid dosing are appropriate, and the respiratory rate and level of sedation are checked every hour. Since 1992, these guidelines have been accepted by the Swedish Society of Anesthesiology and Intensive Care. Patients of any age who receive opioids neuraxially can now be nursed on regular wards. This approval is for the use of morphine; the observation time is 12 h after every injection.

Table 13–11 Predisposing Factors for Development of Late-Onset Respiratory Depression After Spinal Administration of Opioids

Advanced age
High-risk patients
Large doses of opioids
Use of water-soluble opioids
Intrathecal administration of opioids (compared with epidural)
Concomitant use of parenteral administration of opioids or sedatives or both
Opioid-naive patient (lack of tolerance to opioids)
Thoracic epidural administration of opioids

Data from two Swedish nationwide studies, Gustafsson LL, Schildt B, Jacobsen K: Adverse effects of extradural and intrathecal opiates: report of a nationwide survey in Sweden. Br J Anaesth 1982; 54: 479–486; Rawal N, Arnér S, Gustafsson LL, et al: Present state of extradural and intrathecal opioid analgesia in Sweden. A nationwide follow-up survey. Br J Anaesth 1987; 59: 791–799), comprising more than 20,000 patients and data from Etches RC: Complications of acute pain management. Anesthesiol Clin North Am 1992; 10: 417–433 and Morgan M: The rational use of intrathecal and extradural opioids. Br J Anaesth 1989; 63: 165–188.

Data from more than 20,000 patients from the Swedish surveys and from other large studies[2, 11, 71] show that respiratory depression, if it occurs, is manifest within 12 h after injection of morphine. At my institution, the 12-h observation routine has been used for thousands of patients without any major problems. For lipophilic opioids, the observation period can be decreased (e.g., to 4 to 6 h after fentanyl and sufentanil). However, more data are necessary before observation routines for lipophilic opioids can be established. The cumulative effects of repeated doses or of continuous infusions on respiration are also unclear at present.

Results from the European survey show that the monitoring routines and surveillance times after epidural administration of morphine (Fig. 13–7) and nonmorphine opioids (Table 13–13) vary greatly among different countries. There seems to be a definite need

Table 13–12 European Surveillance Routines After Spinal Administration of Opioids

SETTING	PATIENTS NURSED, %	
	ASA Class I–II	ASA Class III–IV
Intensive care unit	22	43
Postanesthesia care unit	55	63
Surgical ward*	59	26

*70% of anesthesiologists consider spinal administration of opioids safe on surgical wards.

ASA, American Society of Anesthesiologists.

Data from Rawal N: Epidural and intrathecal opioids for postoperative pain management in Europe: a 17-nation survey. (Abstract.) Reg Anesth 1995; 20: A45.

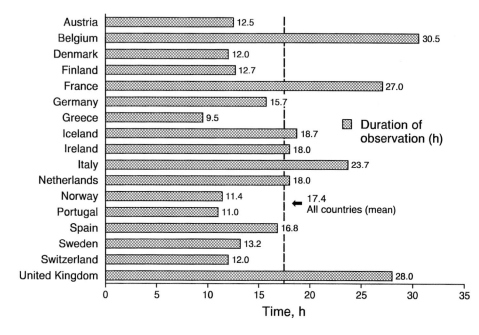

Figure 13–7 Duration of surveillance after an epidural administration of morphine.

for guidelines and surveillance recommendations from organizations such as the International Association for Study of Pain.

Prophylactic Antagonist Administration

The potential advantage of prophylactic opioid antagonists for patients receiving opioids neuraxially is that they may prevent respiratory depression that might otherwise go unnoticed if patients are monitored intermittently. This would increase the safety of opioids given neuraxially and allow their use beyond the confines of the ICU and postanesthesia care unit. Naloxone is effective in reversing respiratory depression associated with neuraxial administration of opioids, but its

action is of shorter duration than that of most opioids and there is a risk of recurrence of respiratory depression after a single dose. Its short elimination half-life necessitates repeated intravenous injections. This can be overcome by administration of continuous infusion of low-dose naloxone.[192, 236] A continuous intravenous infusion of 0.4 to 0.6 mg/h decreased the incidence of pruritus in patients who had received 0.5 to 1 mg of morphine intrathecally for labor pain. The umbilical vein plasma level of naloxone was low (1.92 ng/mL ± 0.28). This study[236] demonstrated that low-dose morphine given intrathecally or naloxone given intravenously during labor had no effect on the newborn.

Mixed agonist-antagonist drugs such as nalbuphine or butorphanol have also been used. Because nalbuphine has analgesic properties, it may attenuate the hemodynamic consequences of analgesia reversal associated with the administration of large doses of naloxone. Naloxone and nalbuphine require careful dose titration to achieve satisfactory reversal of respiratory depression without reversal of analgesia or precipitation of adverse hemodynamic effects. The analgesia-reducing effects of naloxone may be different for different opioids. A dose of 5 μg/kg/h did not affect analgesia produced by morphine given epidurally,[192] whereas a much lower dose (1 μg/kg/h) of naloxone was associated with a decrease of analgesia produced by diamorphine given intrathecally.[237] The results with nalbuphine pretreatment have been contradictory.[203, 238] Synthetic analogues of naloxone such as naltrexone and nalmefene have been developed.[239] Nalmefene has a considerably longer elimination half-life than naloxone, so its reversal effects after a single injection can be expected to outlast the analgesic effects of most opioids. Increasing the dose of nalmefene from 0.5 to 2 mg resulted in a fourfold prolongation of the antagonist effect. In contrast, increasing the usual 0.4-mg dose of naloxone has little effect on its duration of action.

Table 13–13 European Monitoring Routines After Epidural Administration of Opioid

OPIOID	DURATION OF POSTOPERATIVE SURVEILLANCE, h	
	Mean	Range
Morphine	17.4	1–72
Fentanyl	9.5	3–24
Sufentanil	6.5	1–24
Buprenorphine	10.5	2–48
Meperidine	5	4–6
Diacetylmorphine	NA	NA
Alfentanil	24*	24*
Nicomorphine	NA	NA
Piritramide	24*	24*
Methadone	8*	8*

*Response received from only one hospital.
NA = no answer.
Data from Rawal N: Epidural and intrathecal opioids for postoperative pain management in Europe: a 17-nation survey. (Abstract.) Reg Anesth 1995; 20: A45.

References

1. Cousins MJ, Mather LE: Intrathecal and epidural administration of opioids. Anesthesiology 1984; 61: 276–310.
2. Morgan M: The rational use of intrathecal and extradural opioids. Br J Anaesth 1989; 63: 165–188.
3. Rawal N: Spinal opioids. In Raj PP (ed): Practical Management of Pain, 2nd ed, pp 829–850. St. Louis, Mosby–Year Book, 1992.
4. Shnider SM: Epidural and subarachnoid opiates—with and without local anesthetics for pain management in obstetrics. ASA Refresher Course Lectures 1991; 125: 1–7.
5. Vercauteren MP: The role of perispinal route for postsurgical pain relief. Baillieres Clin Anaesth 1993; 7: 769–792.
6. Chrubasik J, Chrubasik S, Martin E: Benefits and risks of epidural opioids in the treatment of postoperative pain. In Chrubasik J, Cousins M, Martin E (eds): Advances in Pain Therapy II, pp 94–113. New York, Springer-Verlag, 1993.
7. Rawal N, Sjöstrand UH, Dahlstrom B, et al: Epidural morphine for postoperative pain relief: a comparative study with intramuscular narcotic and intercostal nerve block. Anesth Analg 1982; 61: 93–98.
8. Rawal N, Sjöstrand U, Christoffersson E, et al: Comparison of intramuscular and epidural morphine for postoperative analgesia in the grossly obese: influence on postoperative ambulation and pulmonary function. Anesth Analg 1984; 63: 583–592.
9. Yeager MP, Glass DD, Neff RK, et al: Epidural anesthesia and analgesia in high-risk surgical patients. Anesthesiology 1987; 66: 729–736.
10. Tuman KJ, McCarthy RJ, March RJ, et al: Effects of epidural anesthesia and analgesia on coagulation and outcome after major vascular surgery. Anesth Analg 1991; 73: 696–704.
11. Rawal N, Arner S, Gustafsson LL, et al: Present state of extradural and intrathecal opioid analgesia in Sweden. A nationwide follow-up survey. Br J Anaesth 1987; 59: 791–799.
12. Etches RC, Sandler AN, Daley MD: Respiratory depression and spinal opioids. Can J Anaesth 1989; 36: 165–185.
13. Capogna G, Celleno D, Tagariello V, et al: Intrathecal buprenorphine for postoperative analgesia in the elderly patient. Anaesthesia 1988; 43: 128–130.
14. Varrassi G, Celleno D, Capogna G, et al: Ventilatory effects of subarachnoid fentanyl in the elderly. Anaesthesia 1992; 47: 558–562.
15. Brownridge P, Frewin DB: A comparative study of techniques of postoperative analgesia following caesarean section and lower abdominal surgery. Anaesth Intensive Care 1985; 13: 123–130.
16. Kilbride MJ, Senagore AJ, Mazier WP, et al: Epidural analgesia. Surg Gynecol Obstet 1992; 174: 137–140.
17. Cohen SE, Subak LL, Brose WG, et al: Analgesia after cesarean delivery: patient evaluations and costs of five opioid techniques. Reg Anesth 1991; 16: 141–149.
18. Egan KJ, Ready LB: Patient satisfaction with intravenous PCA or epidural morphine. Can J Anaesth 1994; 41: 6–11.
19. Abouleish E, Rawal N, Fallon K, et al: Combined intrathecal morphine and bupivacaine for cesarean section. Anesth Analg 1988; 67: 370–374.
20. Hjortsø N-C, Lund C, Mogensen T, et al: Epidural morphine improves pain relief and maintains sensory analgesia during continuous epidural bupivacaine after abdominal surgery. Anesth Analg 1986; 65: 1033–1036.
21. Rawal N, Tandon B: Epidural and intrathecal morphine in ICUs. Intensive Care Med 1985; 11: 129–133.
22. Rawal N: Epidural and intrathecal opioids for postoperative pain management in Europe: A 17-nation survey. (Abstract.) Reg Anesth 1995; 20: A45.
23. Naulty JS: Cesarean delivery analgesia with subarachnoid bupivacaine, fentanyl and morphine. (Abstract.) Anesthesiology 1989; 71: a864.
24. Rucci FS, Cardamone M, Migliori P: Fentanyl and bupivacaine mixtures for extradural blockade. Br J Anaesth 1985; 57: 275–284.
25. Ferrante FM, Fanciullo GJ, Grichnik KP, et al: Regression of sensory anesthesia during continuous epidural infusions of bupivacaine and opioid for total knee replacement. Anesth Analg 1993; 77: 1179–1184.
26. Van Steenberge A, Debroux HC, Noorduin H: Extradural bupivacaine with sufentanil for vaginal delivery. A double-blind trial. Br J Anaesth 1987; 59: 1518–1522.
27. Carrie LES, O'Sullivan GM, Seegobin R: Epidural fentanyl in labour. Anaesthesia 1981; 36: 965–969.
28. Naulty JS: Continuous infusions of local anesthetics and narcotics for epidural analgesia in the management of labor. Int Anesthesiol Clin 1990; 28: 17–24.
29. Breen TW, Janzen JA: Epidural fentanyl and caesarean section: when should fentanyl be given? Can J Anaesth 1992; 39: 317–322.
30. Gaffud MP, Bansal P, Lawton C, et al: Surgical analgesia for cesarean delivery with epidural bupivacaine and fentanyl. Anesthesiology 1986; 65: 331–334.
31. Birnbach DJ, Johnson MD, Arcario T, et al: Effect of diluent volume on analgesia produced by epidural fentanyl. Anesth Analg 1989; 68: 808–810.
32. Badner NH, Reimer EJ, Komar WE, et al: Low-dose bupivacaine does not improve postoperative epidural fentanyl analgesia in orthopedic patients. Anesth Analg 1991; 72: 337–341.
33. Logas WG, el-Baz N, el-Ganzouri A, et al: Continuous thoracic epidural analgesia for postoperative pain relief following thoracotomy: a randomized prospective study. Anesthesiology 1987; 67: 787–791.
34. Cullen ML, Staren ED, el-Ganzouri A, et al: Continuous epidural infusion for analgesia after major abdominal operations: a randomized, prospective, double-blind study. Surgery 1985; 98: 718–728.
35. Badner NH, Komar WE: Bupivacaine 0.1% does not improve post-operative epidural fentanyl analgesia after abdominal or thoracic surgery. Can J Anaesth 1992; 39: 330–336.
36. Paech MJ, Westmore MD: Postoperative epidural fentanyl infusion—is the addition of 0.1% bupivacaine of benefit? Anaesth Intensive Care 1994; 22: 9–14.
37. Parker RK, White PF: Epidural patient-controlled analgesia: an alternative to intravenous patient-controlled analgesia for pain relief after cesarean delivery. Anesth Analg 1992; 75: 245–251.
38. Grass JA: Sufentanil: clinical use as postoperative analgesic—epidural/intrathecal route. J Pain Symptom Manage 1992; 7: 271–286.
39. Fischer RL, Lubenow TR, Liceaga A, et al: Comparison of continuous epidural infusion of fentanyl-bupivacaine and morphine-bupivacaine in management of postoperative pain. Anesth Analg 1988; 67: 559–563.
40. Dahl JB, Rosenberg J, Hansen BL, et al: Differential analgesic effects of low-dose epidural morphine and morphine-bupivacaine at rest and during mobilization after major abdominal surgery. Anesth Analg 1992; 74: 362–365.
41. George KA, Wright PM, Chisakuta A: Continuous thoracic epidural fentanyl for post-thoracotomy pain relief: with or without bupivacaine? Anaesthesia 1991; 46: 732–736.
42. Curry PD, Pacsoo C, Heap DG: Patient-controlled epidural analgesia in obstetric anaesthetic practice. Pain 1994; 57: 125–127.
43. Swenson JD, Hullander RM, Bready RJ, et al: A comparison of patient controlled epidural analgesia with sufentanil by the lumbar versus thoracic route after thoracotomy. Anesth Analg 1994; 78: 215–218.
44. Marlowe S, Engstrom R, White PF: Epidural patient-controlled analgesia (PCA): an alternative to continuous epidural infusions. Pain 1989; 37: 97–101.
45. Cooper DW, Turner G: Patient-controlled extradural analgesia to compare bupivacaine, fentanyl and bupivacaine with fentanyl in the treatment of postoperative pain. Br J Anaesth 1993; 70: 503–507.
46. Nolan JP, Dow AA, Parr MJ, et al: Patient-controlled epidural analgesia following post-traumatic pelvic reconstruction. A comparison with continuous epidural analgesia. Anaesthesia 1992; 47: 1037–1041.
47. Bellamy CD, McDonnell FJ, Colclough GW: Postoperative epidural pain management results in shorter hospital stay than IV PCA morphine: a comparison in anterior cruciate ligament repair. (Abstract.) Anesthesiology 1989; 71: a686.
48. Lamer TJ: Postoperative pain management with epidural narcotics results in shorter hospital stay than IV or IM narcotics. (Abstract.) Reg Anesth 1990; 15: 83.

49. Boudreault D, Brasseur L, Samii K, et al: Comparison of continuous epidural bupivacaine infusion plus either continuous epidural infusion or patient-controlled epidural injection of fentanyl for postoperative analgesia. Anesth Analg 1991; 73: 132–137.

50. Ferrante FM, Lu L, Jamison SB, et al: Patient-controlled epidural analgesia: demand dosing. Anesth Analg 1991; 73: 547–552.

51. Hongnat JM, Bellenfant F, Levy R, et al: Epidural versus intravenous alfentanil by PCA in postoperative patients. (Abstract.) Anesthesiology 1991; 75: a754.

52. Chrubasik J, Geller E, Graf R, et al: A double-blind comparison of epidural fentanyl and sufentanil with intravenous sufentanil for abdominal surgery pain management. (Abstract.) Anesthesiology 1991; 75: a752.

53. Miguel R, Timble G: Patient-controlled epidural sufentanil. Reg Anesth 1990; 15: 35.

54. Glass PS, Estok P, Ginsberg B, et al: Use of patient-controlled analgesia to compare the efficacy of epidural to intravenous fentanyl administration. Anesth Analg 1992; 74: 345–351.

55. Yu PY, Gambling DR: A comparative study of patient-controlled epidural fentanyl and single dose epidural morphine for postcaesarean analgesia. Can J Anaesth 1993; 40: 416–420.

56. Cohen S, Amar D, Pantuck CB, et al: Postcesarean delivery epidural patient-controlled analgesia. Fentanyl or sufentanil? Anesthesiology 1993; 78: 486–491.

57. Bisgaard C, Mouridsen P, Dahl JB: Continuous lumbar epidural bupivacaine plus morphine versus epidural morphine after major abdominal surgery. Eur J Anaesthesiol 1990; 7: 219–225.

58. Abboud TK, Shnider SM, Dailey PA, et al: Intrathecal administration of hyperbaric morphine for the relief of pain in labour. Br J Anaesth 1984; 56: 1351–1360.

59. Camann WR, Minzter BH, Denney RA, et al: Intrathecal sufentanil for labor analgesia. Effects of added epinephrine. Anesthesiology 1993; 78: 870–874.

60. Stoelting RK: Intrathecal morphine—an underused combination for postoperative pain management. Anesth Analg 1989; 68: 707–709.

61. Downing R, Davis I, Black J, et al: When do patients given intrathecal morphine need postoperative systemic opiates? Ann R Coll Surg Engl 1985; 67: 251–253.

62. Davis I: Intrathecal morphine in aortic aneurysm surgery. Anaesthesia 1987; 42: 491–497.

63. O'Neill P, Knickenberg C, Bogahalanda S, et al: Use of intrathecal morphine for postoperative pain relief following lumber spine surgery. J Neurosurg 1985; 63: 413–416.

64. Isaacson IJ, Weitz FI, Berry AJ, et al: Intrathecal morphine's effect on the postoperative course of patients undergoing abdominal aortic surgery. (Abstract.) Anesth Analg 1987; 66: s86.

65. Abboud TK, Dror A, Mosaad P, et al: Mini-dose intrathecal morphine for the relief of post-cesarean section pain: safety, efficacy, and ventilatory responses to carbon dioxide. Anesth Analg 1988; 67: 137–143.

66. Holmström B, Laugaland K, Rawal N, et al: Combined spinal epidural block versus spinal and epidural block for orthopaedic surgery. Can J Anaesth 1993; 40: 601–606.

67. Vanstrum GS, Bjornson KM, Ilko R: Postoperative effects of intrathecal morphine in coronary artery bypass surgery. Anesth Analg 1988; 67: 261–267.

68. Sarma VJ, Bostrom UV: Intrathecal morphine for the relief of post-hysterectomy pain—a double-blind, dose-response study. Acta Anaesthesiol Scand 1993; 37: 223–227.

69. Abouleish E, Rawal N, Shaw J, et al: Intrathecal morphine 0.2 mg versus epidural bupivacaine 0.125% or their combination: effects on parturients. Anesthesiology 1991; 74: 711–716.

70. Caldwell LE, Rosen MA, Shnider SM: Subarachnoid morphine and fentanyl for labor analgesia. Efficacy and adverse effects. Reg Anesth 1994; 19: 2–8.

71. Gustafsson LL, Schildt B, Jacobsen K: Adverse effects of extradural and intrathecal opiates: report of a nationwide survey in Sweden. Br J Anaesth 1982; 54: 479–486.

72. Domsky M, Kwartowitz J: Efficacy of subarachnoid morphine in a community hospital. Reg Anesth 1992; 17: 279–282.

73. Milligan KR, Fogarty DJ: The characteristics of analgesic requirements following subarachnoid diamorphine in patients undergoing total hip replacement. Reg Anesth 1993; 18: 114–117.

74. Honet JE, Arkoosh VA, Huffnagle HJ, et al: Comparison of fentanyl, meperidine, and sufentanil for intrathecal labor analgesia. (Abstract.) Anesthesiology 1991; 75: a839.

75. Camann WR, Denney RA, Holby ED, et al: A comparison of intrathecal, epidural, and intravenous sufentanil for labor analgesia. Anesthesiology 1992; 77: 884–887.

76. Hansdottir V, Hedner T, Woestenborghs R, et al: The CSF and plasma pharmacokinetics of sufentanil after intrathecal administration. Anesthesiology 1991; 74: 264–269.

77. Courtney MA, Bader AM, Hartwell B, et al: Perioperative analgesia with subarachnoid sufentanil administration. Reg Anesth 1992; 17: 274–278.

78. Niemi L, Pitkanen MT, Tuominen MK, et al: Comparison of intrathecal fentanyl infusion with intrathecal morphine infusion or bolus for postoperative pain relief after hip arthroplasty. Anesth Analg 1993; 77: 126–130.

79. Guinard JP, Chiolero R, Mavrocordatos P, et al: Prolonged intrathecal fentanyl analgesia via 32-gauge catheters after thoracotomy. Anesth Analg 1993; 77: 936–941.

80. Cohen SE, Cherry CM, Holbrook RH Jr, et al: Intrathecal sufentanil for labor analgesia—sensory changes, side effects, and fetal heart rate changes. Anesth Analg 1993; 77: 1155–1160.

81. Haak-van der Lely F, van Kleef JW, Gesink-van der Veer BJ, et al: Efficacy of epidurally administered sufentanil versus bupivacaine during thoracic surgery. A randomised placebo-controlled double-blind study. Anaesthesia 1994; 49: 116–118.

82. Newman LM, Patel RV, Krolick T, et al: Muscular spasm in the lower limbs of laboring patients after intrathecal administration of epinephrine and sufentanil. Anesthesiology 1994; 80: 468–471.

83. Gwirtz KH, Beckes KA, Maddock RP, et al: Subarachnoid opioid analgesia reduces long-term post-surgical pain after nephrectomy. Reg Anesth 1994; 19: 98–103.

84. Brockway MS, Noble DW, Sharwood-Smith GH, et al: Profound respiratory depression after extradural fentanyl. Br J Anaesth 1990; 64: 243–245.

85. Weightman WM: Respiratory arrest during epidural infusion of bupivacaine and fentanyl. Anaesth Intensive Care 1991; 19: 282–284.

86. Loper KA, Ready LB, Downey M, et al: Epidural and intravenous fentanyl infusions are clinically equivalent after knee surgery. Anesth Analg 1990; 70: 72–75.

87. Cohen SE, Tan S, White PF: Sufentanil analgesia following cesarean section: epidural versus intravenous administration. Anesthesiology 1988; 68: 129–134.

88. Harbers JB, Hasenbos MA, Gort C, et al: Ventilatory function and continuous high thoracic epidural administration of bupivacaine with sufentanil intravenously or epidurally: a double-blind comparison. Reg Anesth 1991; 16: 65–71.

89. Geller E, Chrubasik J, Graf R, et al: A randomized double-blind comparison of epidural sufentanil versus intravenous sufentanil or epidural fentanyl analgesia after major abdominal surgery. Anesth Analg 1993; 76: 1243–1250.

90. Camu F, Debucquoy F: Alfentanil infusion for postoperative pain: a comparison of epidural and intravenous routes. Anesthesiology 1991; 75: 171–178.

91. Nagle CJ, McQuay HJ: Extradural pethidine. (Letter to the editor.) Br J Anaesth 1990; 65: 730–731.

92. Jacobson L, Phillips PD, Hull CJ, et al: Extradural versus intramuscular diamorphine. A controlled study of analgesic and adverse effects in the postoperative period. Anaesthesia 1983; 38: 10–18.

93. Camann WR, Loferski BL, Fanciullo GJ, et al: Does epidural administration of butorphanol offer any clinical advantage over the intravenous route? A double-blind, placebo-controlled trial. Anesthesiology 1992; 76: 216–220.

94. Salomäki TE, Laitinen JO, Nuutinen LS: A randomized double-blind comparison of epidural versus intravenous fentanyl infusion for analgesia after thoracotomy. Anesthesiology 1991; 75: 790–795.

95. Grant RP, Dolman JF, Harper JA, et al: Patient-controlled lumbar epidural fentanyl compared with patient-controlled intravenous fentanyl for post-thoracotomy pain. Can J Anaesth 1992; 39: 214–219.

96. Sandler AN, Stringer D, Panos L, et al: A randomized, double-blind comparison of lumbar epidural and intravenous fentanyl infusions for postthoracotomy pain relief. Analgesic, pharmacokinetic, and respiratory effects. Anesthesiology 1992; 77: 626–634.

97. Coe A, Sarginson R, Smith MW, et al: Pain following thoracotomy. A randomised, double-blind comparison of lumbar versus thoracic epidural fentanyl. Anaesthesia 1991; 46: 918–921.

98. Eisenach JC, Lysak SZ, Viscomi CM: Epidural clonidine analgesia following surgery: phase I. Anesthesiology 1989; 71: 640–646.

99. Kalia PK, Madan R, Batra RK, et al: Clinical study on epidural clonidine for postoperative analgesia. Indian J Med Res 1986; 83: 550–552.

100. Bonnet F, Boico O, Rostaing S, et al: Postoperative analgesia with extradural clonidine. Br J Anaesth 1989; 63: 465–469.

101. Chrubasik J, Meynadier J, Blond S, et al: Somatostatin, a potent analgesic. (Letter to the editor.) Lancet 1984; 2: 1208–1209.

102. Mollenholt P, Rawal N, Gordh T, et al: Analgesic and histopathological effects of intrathecal and epidural somatostatin in cancer patients. Reg Anesth 1991; 15: s21.

103. Penn RD, Paice JA, Kroin JS: Octreotide: a potent new nonopiate analgesic for intrathecal infusion. Pain 1992; 49: 13–19.

104. Naguib M, Adu-Gyamfi Y, Absood GH, et al: Epidural ketamine for postoperative analgesia. Can Anaesth Soc J 1986; 33: 16–21.

105. Islas JA, Astorga J, Laredo M: Epidural ketamine for control of postoperative pain. Anesth Analg 1985; 64: 1161–1162.

106. Eisenach JC: Demonstrating safety of subarachnoid calcitonin: patients or animals? (Abstract.) Anesth Analg 1988; 67: 298.

107. Serrao JM, Marks RL, Morley SJ, et al: Intrathecal midazolam for the treatment of chronic mechanical low back pain: a controlled comparison with epidural steroid in a pilot study. Pain 1992; 48: 5–12.

108. Bach V, Carl P, Ravlo O, et al: Potentiation of epidural opioids with epidural droperidol. A one year retrospective study. Anaesthesia 1986; 41: 1116–1119.

109. Gordh T Jr, Post C, Olsson Y: Evaluation of the toxicity of subarachnoid clonidine, guanfacine, and a substance P-antagonist on rat spinal cord and nerve roots: light and electron microscopic observations after chronic intrathecal administration. Anesth Analg 1986; 65: 1303–1311.

110. Gordh T Jr: Epidural clonidine for treatment of postoperative pain after thoracotomy. A double-blind placebo-controlled study. Acta Anaesthesiol Scand 1988; 32: 702–709.

111. Van Essen EJ, Bovill JG, Ploeger EJ: Extradural clonidine does not potentiate analgesia produced by extradural morphine after meniscectomy. Br J Anaesth 1991; 66: 237–241.

112. Petit J, Oksenhendler G, Colas G, et al: Pharmacokinetics and effects of epidural clonidine in acute postoperative pain. Reg Anesth 1989; 14: s2–s43.

113. Lund C, Qvitzau S, Greulich A, et al: Comparison of the effects of extradural clonidine with those of morphine on postoperative pain, stress responses, cardiopulmonary function and motor and sensory block. Br J Anaesth 1989; 63: 516–519.

114. Mogensen T, Eliasen K, Ejlersen E, et al: Epidural clonidine enhances postoperative analgesia from a combined low-dose epidural bupivacaine and morphine regimen. Anesth Analg 1992; 75: 607–610.

115. Rauck RL: Current concepts in the role of clonidine for the management of pain. Postgraduate course, pp 417–430. New York, Memorial Sloan-Kettering Cancer Center, 1992.

116. Fogarty DJ, Carabine UA, Milligan KR: Comparison of the analgesic effects of intrathecal clonidine and intrathecal morphine after spinal anaesthesia in patients undergoing total hip replacement. Br J Anaesth 1993; 71: 661–664.

117. Bedder MD, Kozody R, Palahniuk RJ, et al: Clonidine prolongs canine tetracaine spinal anaesthesia. Can Anaesth Soc J 1986; 33: 591–596.

118. Mensink FJ, Kozody R, Kehler CH, et al: Dose-response relationship of clonidine in tetracaine spinal anaesthesia. Anesthesiology 1987; 67: 717–721.

119. Racle JP, Benkhadra A, Poy JY, et al: Prolongation of isobaric bupivacaine spinal anaesthesia with epinephrine and clonidine for hip surgery in the elderly. Anesth Analg 1987; 66: 442–446.

120. Racle JP, Poy JY, Benkhadra A, et al: Prolongation of spinal anesthesia with hyperbaric bupivacaine by adrenaline and clonidine in the elderly (French). Ann Fr Anesth Reanim 1988; 7: 139–144.

121. Bonnet F, Liu N, Delaunay L: Combination of α-adrenergic agonists and local anesthetics. Proceedings of the Third Joint ESRA-ASRA Congress, 1992, pp 201–210.

122. Tzeng JI, Wang JJ, Mok MS, et al: Clonidine potentiates lidocaine-induced epidural anesthesia. (Abstract.) Anesth Analg 1989; 68: s298.

123. Veillette Y, Orhant E, Benhamou D, et al: Addition of clonidine decreases lidocaine absorption after epidural injection. (Abstract.) Anesthesiology 1989; 71: a267.

124. Nishikawa T, Dohi S: Clinical evaluation of clonidine added to lidocaine solution for epidural anesthesia. Anesthesiology 1990; 73: 853–859.

125. Ota K, Namiki A, Iwasaki H, et al: Dosing interval for prolongation of tetracaine spinal anesthesia by oral clonidine in humans. Anesth Analg 1994; 79: 1117–1120.

126. Spaulding TC, Fielding S, Venafro JJ, et al: Antinociceptive activity of clonidine and its potentiation of morphine analgesia. Eur J Pharmacol 1979; 58: 19–25.

127. Carabine UA, Milligan KR, Mulholland D, et al: Extradural clonidine infusions for analgesia after total hip replacement. Br J Anaesth 1992; 68: 338–343.

128. Crosby G, Russo MA: Spinal blood flow during tetracaine spinal anesthesia in conscious rats. (Abstract.) Anesth Analg 1989; 68: s64.

129. Motsch J, Graber E, Ludwig K: Addition of clonidine enhances postoperative analgesia from epidural morphine: a double-blind study. Anesthesiology 1990; 73: 1067–1073.

130. Rostaing S, Bonnet F, Levron JC, et al: Effect of epidural clonidine on analgesia and pharmacokinetics of epidural fentanyl in postoperative patients. Anesthesiology 1991; 75: 420–425.

131. Chrubasik J, Meynadier J, Scherpereel P, et al: The effect of epidural somatostatin on postoperative pain. Anesth Analg 1985; 64: 1085–1088.

132. Mollenholt P, Post C, Paulsson I, et al: Intrathecal somatostatin in the guinea pig: effects on spinal cord blood flow, histopathology and motor function. Pain 1992; 51: 343–347.

133. Gaumann DM, Yaksh TL, Post C, et al: Intrathecal somatostatin in cat and mouse studies on pain, motor behavior, and histopathology. Anesth Analg 1989; 68: 623–632.

134. Finck AD, Ngai SH: Opiate receptor mediation of ketamine analgesia. Anesthesiology 1982; 56: 291–297.

135. Wachtel RE: Ketamine decreases the open time of single-channel currents activated by acetylcholine. Anesthesiology 1988; 68: 563–570.

136. Pekoe GM, Smith DJ: Ketamine analgesia: mediation by biogenic amine and endogenous opiate processes. (Abstract.) Anesthesiology 1979; 51: s36.

137. Peat SJ, Bras P, Hanna MH: A double-blind comparison of epidural ketamine and diamorphine for postoperative analgesia. Anaesthesia 1989; 44: 555–558.

138. Tung AS, Yaksh TL: Analgesic effect of intrathecal ketamine in the rat. Reg Anesth 1981; 6: 91–94.

139. Anis NA, Berry SC, Burton NR, et al: The dissociative anaesthetics, ketamine and phencyclidine, selectively reduce excitation of central mammalian neurones by N-methyl-aspartate. Br J Pharmacol 1983; 79: 565–575.

140. Naguib M, Sharif AM, Seraj M, et al: Ketamine for caudal analgesia in children: comparison with caudal bupivacaine. Br J Anaesth 1991; 67: 559–564.

141. Amiot JF, Bouju P, Palacci JH, et al: Intravenous regional anaesthesia with ketamine. Anaesthesia 1985; 40: 899–901.

142. Mori K, Shingu K: Epidural ketamine does not produce analgesia. (Letter to the editor.) Anesthesiology 1988; 68: 296–298.

143. Ravat F, Dorne R, Baechle JP, et al: Epidural ketamine or morphine for postoperative analgesia. Anesthesiology 1987; 66: 819–822.

144. Kawana Y, Sato H, Shimada H, et al: Epidural ketamine for postoperative pain relief after gynecologic operations: a double-blind study and comparison with epidural morphine. Anesth Analg 1987; 66: 735–738.

145. Van der Auwera D, Verborgh C, Camu F: Epidural ketamine for postoperative analgesia. (Letter to the editor.) Anesth Analg 1987; 66: 1340.

146. Ivankovich AD, McCarthy RJ: Epidural ketamine for control of postoperative pain: two comments. (Letter to the editor.) Anesth Analg 1986; 65: 989–990.

147. Brock-Utne JG, Rubin J, Mankowitz E: Epidural ketamine for control of postoperative pain: two comments. (Letter to the editor.) Anesth Analg 1986; 65: 990.

148. Schneider I, Diltoer M: Continuous epidural infusion of ketamine during labour. (Letter to the editor.) Can J Anaesth 1987; 34: 657–658.

149. Brock-Utne JG, Kallichurum S, Mankowitz E, et al: Intrathecal ketamine with preservative—histological effects on spinal nerve roots of baboons. S Afr Med J 1982; 61: 440–441.

150. Brock-Utne JG, Mankowitz E, Kallichurum S, et al: Effects of intrathecal saline and ketamine with and without preservative on the spinal nerve roots of monkeys. S Afr Med J 1982; 61: 360–361.

151. Ahuja BR: Analgesic effect of intrathecal ketamine in rats. Br J Anaesth 1983; 55: 991–995.

152. Abboud TK, Moore M, Zhu J, et al: Epidural butorphanol or morphine for the relief of post-cesarean section pain: ventilatory responses to carbon dioxide. Anesth Analg 1987; 66: 887–893.

153. Macrae DJ, Munishankrappa S, Burrow LM, et al: Double-blind comparison of the efficacy of extradural diamorphine, extradural phenoperidine and i.m. diamorphine following caesarean section. Br J Anaesth 1987; 59: 354–359.

154. Dougherty TB, Baysinger CL, Gooding DJ: Epidural hydromorphone for postoperative analgesia after delivery by cesarean section. Reg Anesth 1986; 11: 118–122.

155. Henderson SK, Matthew EB, Cohen H, et al: Epidural hydromorphone: a double-blind comparison with intramuscular hydromorphone for postcesarean section analgesia. Anesthesiology 1987; 66: 825–830.

156. Bilsback P, Rolly G, Tampubolon O: Efficacy of the extradural administration of lofentanil, buprenorphine or saline in the management of postoperative pain. A double-blind study. Br J Anaesth 1985; 57: 943–948.

157. Rao U, Campbell IT, Catley DM, et al: Epidural meptazinol for pain relief after lower abdominal surgery. Anaesthesia 1985; 40: 754–758.

158. Kalia PK, Madan R, Saksena R, et al: Epidural pentazocine for postoperative pain relief. Anesth Analg 1983; 62: 949–950.

159. Paterson GM, McQuay HJ, Bullingham RE, et al: Intradural morphine and diamorphine. Dose response studies. Anaesthesia 1984; 39: 113–117.

160. Evron S, Samueloff A, Simon A, et al: Urinary function during epidural analgesia with methadone and morphine in postcesarean section patients. Pain 1985; 23: 135–144.

161. Knape JT: Early respiratory depression resistant to naloxone following epidural buprenorphine. Anesthesiology 1986; 64: 382–384.

162. Matthew EB, Henderson SK, Avram MJ, et al: Epidural hydromorphone versus epidural morphine for postcesarean section analgesia. (Abstract.) Anesth Analg 1987; 66: s112.

163. Baraka A, Jabbour S, Ghabash M, et al: A comparison of epidural tramadol and epidural morphine for postoperative analgesia. Can J Anaesth 1993; 40: 308–313.

164. Coombs DW: Neurotoxicity of spinally used drugs. Proceedings of 2nd International Symposium on the Management of Acute and Cancer Pain. Paris, May, 1992.

165. Abouleish E, Barmada MA, Nemoto EM, et al: Acute and chronic effects of intrathecal morphine in monkeys. Br J Anaesth 1981; 53: 1027–1032.

166. Robinson RJ, Lenis S, Elliot M: Accidental epidural narcotic overdose. (Letter to the editor.) Can Anaesth Soc J 1984; 31: 594–595.

167. Rawal N, Sjöstrand U, Dahlstrom B: Postoperative pain relief by epidural morphine. Anesth Analg 1981; 60: 726–731.

168. Arnér S, Rawal N, Gustafsson LL: Clinical experience of long-term treatment with epidural and intrathecal opioids—a nationwide survey. Acta Anaesthesiol Scand 1988; 32: 253–259.

169. Rawal N, Nuutinen L, Raj PP, et al: Behavioral and histopathologic effects following intrathecal administration of butorphanol, sufentanil, and nalbuphine in sheep. Anesthesiology 1991; 75: 1025–1034.

170. Badner NH, Sandler AN, Koren G, et al: Lumbar epidural fentanyl infusions for post-thoracotomy patients: analgesic, respiratory, and pharmacokinetic effects. J Cardiothorac Anesth 1990; 4: 543–551.

171. Melendez JA, Cirella VN, Delphin ES: Lumbar epidural fentanyl analgesia after thoracic surgery. J Cardiothorac Anesth 1989; 3: 150–153.

172. Hurford WE, Dutton RP, Alfille PH, et al: Comparison of thoracic and lumbar epidural infusions of bupivacaine and fentanyl for post-thoracotomy analgesia. J Cardiothorac Vasc Anesth 1993; 7: 521–525.

173. Bodily MN, Chamberlain DP, Ramsey DH, et al: Lumbar versus thoracic epidural catheter for post-thoracotomy analgesia. (Abstract.) Anesthesiology 1989; 71: a1146.

174. Haak-van der Lely F, van Kleef JW, Burm AG, et al: An intraoperative comparison of lumbar with thoracic epidural sufentanil for thoracotomy. Anaesthesia 1994; 49: 119–121.

175. Guinard JP, Mavrocordatos P, Chiolero R, et al: A randomized comparison of intravenous versus lumbar and thoracic epidural fentanyl for analgesia after thoracotomy. Anesthesiology 1992; 77: 1108–1115.

176. Brodsky JB, Kretzschmar KM, Mark JB: Caudal epidural morphine for post-thoracotomy pain. Anesth Analg 1988; 67: 409–410.

177. Fromme GA, Steidl LJ, Danielson DR: Comparison of lumbar and thoracic epidural morphine for relief of postthoracotomy pain. Anesth Analg 1985; 64: 454–455.

178. Wang BC, Hiller JM, Simon EJ, et al: Distribution of ^{3}H-morphine following lumbar subarachnoid injection in unanesthetized rabbits. Anesthesiology 1989; 70: 817–824.

179. Hakanson E, Bengtsson M, Rutberg H, et al: Epidural morphine by the thoracic or lumbar routes in cholecystectomy. Effect on postoperative pain and respiratory variables. Anaesth Intensive Care 1989; 17: 166–169.

180. Grant GJ, Zakowski M, Ramanathan S, et al: Thoracic versus lumbar administration of epidural morphine for postoperative analgesia after thoracotomy. Reg Anesth 1993; 18: 351–355.

181. Jayr C, Thomas H, Rey A, et al: Postoperative pulmonary complications. Epidural analgesia using bupivacaine and opioids versus parenteral opioids. Anesthesiology 1993; 78: 666–676.

182. Thorén T, Wattwil M: Effects on gastric emptying of thoracic epidural analgesia with morphine or bupivacaine. Anesth Analg 1988; 67: 687–694.

183. Geddes SM, Thorburn J, Logan RW: Gastric emptying following caesarean section and the effect of epidural fentanyl. Anaesthesia 1991; 46: 1016–1018.

184. Thomas DA, Williams GM, Iwata K, et al: Multiple effects of morphine on facial scratching in monkeys. Anesth Analg 1993; 77: 933–935.

185. Ackerman WE, Juneja MM, Kaczorowski DM, et al: A comparison of the incidence of pruritus following epidural opioid administration in the parturient. Can J Anaesth 1989; 36: 388–391.

186. White MJ, Berghausen EJ, Dumont SW, et al: Side effects during continuous epidural infusion of morphine and fentanyl. Can J Anaesth 1992; 39: 576–582.

187. Acalovschi I, Ene V, Lorinczi E, et al: Saddle block with pethidine for perineal operations. Br J Anaesth 1986; 58: 1012–1016.

188. Valley MA, Bourke DL, McKenzie AM: Recurrence of thoracic and labial herpes simplex virus infection in a patient receiving epidural fentanyl. Anesthesiology 1992; 76: 1056–1057.

189. Gieraerts R, Navalgund A, Vaes L, et al: Increased incidence of itching and herpes simplex in patients given epidural morphine after cesarean section. Anesth Analg 1987; 66: 1321–1324.

190. Abouleish E: Intrathecal morphine as a cause for herpes simplex should be scratched out. (Letter to the editor.) Anesthesiology 1991; 75: 919–920.

191. Stagno S, Whitley RJ: Herpesvirus infections of pregnancy. Part II: Herpes simplex virus and varicella-zoster virus infections. N Engl J Med 1985; 313: 1327–1330.

192. Rawal N, Schott U, Dahlstrom B, et al: Influence of naloxone infusion on analgesia and respiratory depression following epidural morphine. Anesthesiology 1986; 64: 194–201.

193. Borgeat A, Wilder-Smith OH, Saiah M, et al: Subhypnotic doses

of propofol relieve pruritus induced by epidural and intrathecal morphine. Anesthesiology 1992; 76: 510–512.

194. Horta ML, Horta BL: Inhibition of epidural morphine-induced pruritus by intravenous droperidol. Reg Anesth 1993; 18: 118–120.

195. Carvalho JC, Mathias RS, Senra WG, et al: Systemic droperidol and epidural morphine in the management of postoperative pain. (Letter to the editor.) Anesth Analg 1991; 72: 416.

196. Cohen SE, Ratner EF, Kreitzman TR, et al: Nalbuphine is better than naloxone for treatment of side effects after epidural morphine. Anesth Analg 1992; 75: 747–752.

197. Korbon GA, James DJ, Verlander M, et al: Intramuscular naloxone reverses the side effects of epidural morphine while preserving analgesia. Reg Anesth 1985; 10: 16–20.

198. Abboud TK, Lee K, Zhu J, et al: Prophylactic oral naltrexone with intrathecal morphine for cesarean section: effects on adverse reactions and analgesia. Anesth Analg 1990; 71: 367–370.

199. Wittels B, Glosten B, Faure EA, et al: Opioid antagonist adjuncts to epidural morphine for postcesarean analgesia: maternal outcomes. Anesth Analg 1993; 77: 925–932.

200. Penning JP, Samson B, Baxter AD: Reversal of epidural morphine-induced respiratory depression and pruritus with nalbuphine. Can J Anaesth 1988; 35: 599–604.

201. Lawhorn CD, McNitt JD, Fibuch EE, et al: Epidural morphine with butorphanol for postoperative analgesia after cesarean delivery. Anesth Analg 1991; 72: 53–57.

202. Rawal N, Möllefors K, Axelsson K, et al: An experimental study of urodynamic effects of epidural morphine and of naloxone reversal. Anesth Analg 1983; 62: 641–647.

203. Drenger B, Magora F: Urodynamic studies after intrathecal fentanyl and buprenorphine in the dog. Anesth Analg 1989; 69: 348–353.

204. Drenger B, Sughayer H, Chrubasik J, et al: Dose-response effect of intrathecal alfentanil on canine lower urinary tract dynamics. Anesth Analg 1993; 76: 786–790.

205. Dray A: Epidural opiates and urinary retention: new models provide new insights. (Editorial.) Anesthesiology 1988; 68: 323–324.

206. Jacobson L, Chabal C, Brody MC, et al: Intrathecal methadone 5 mg and morphine 0.5 mg for postoperative analgesia: a comparison of the efficacy, duration and side effects. (Abstract.) Anesth Analg 1989; 68: s132.

207. Gregg R: Spinal analgesia. Anesth Clin North Am 1989; 7: 79–100.

208. Nordberg G, Hedner T, Mellstrand T, et al: Pharmacokinetics of epidural morphine in man. Eur J Clin Pharmacol 1984; 26: 233–237.

209. Rawal N, Wattwil M: Respiratory depression after epidural morphine—an experimental and clinical study. Anesth Analg 1984; 63: 8–14.

210. Sandler AN, Chovaz P, Whiting W: Respiratory depression following epidural morphine: a clinical study. Can Anaesth Soc J 1986; 33: 542–549.

211. Gourlay GK, Cherry DA, Cousins MJ: Cephalad migration of morphine in CSF following lumbar epidural administration in patients with cancer pain. Pain 1985; 23: 317–326.

212. Renaud B, Brichant JF, Clergue F, et al: Continuous epidural fentanyl: ventilatory effects and plasma kinetics. (Abstract.) Anesthesiology 1985; 63: a234.

213. Cohen SE, Labaille T, Benhamou D, et al: Respiratory effects of epidural sufentanil after cesarean section. Anesth Analg 1992; 74: 677–682.

214. Dyer RA, Camden-Smith K, James MF: Epidural lidocaine with sufentanil and epinephrine for abdominal hysterectomy under general anaesthesia: respiratory depression and postoperative analgesia. Can J Anaesth 1992; 39: 220–225.

215. Wang CY: Respiratory depression after extradural fentanyl. (Letter to the editor.) Br J Anaesth 1992; 69: 544.

216. Chrubasik J, Chrubasik S, Black A: Respiratory depression after extradural fentanyl. (Letter to the editor.) Br J Anaesth 1993; 71: 164–166.

217. Stienstra R, Pannekoek BJ: Respiratory arrest following extradural sufentanil. Anaesthesia 1993; 48: 1055–1056.

218. Noble DW, Morrison LM, Brockway MS, et al: Respiratory depression after extradural fentanyl. (Letter to the editor.) Br J Anaesth 1994; 72: 251–252.

219. Murphy DF, MacEvilly M: Pain relief with epidural buprenorphine after spinal fusion: a comparison with intramuscular morphine. Acta Anaesthesiol Scand 1984; 28: 144–146.

220. Steinstra R, van Poorten F: Immediate respiratory arrest after caudal epidural sufentanil. (Letter to the editor.) Anesthesiology 1989; 71: 993–994.

221. Blackburn C: Respiratory arrest after epidural sufentanil. (Letter to the editor.) Anaesthesia 1987; 42: 665–666.

222. Whiting WC, Sandler AN, Lau LC, et al: Analgesic and respiratory effects of epidural sufentanil in patients following thoracotomy. Anesthesiology 1988; 69: 36–43.

223. Fuller JG, McMorland GH, Douglas MJ: Epidural morphine for analgesia after caesarean section: a report of 4880 patients. Can J Anaesth 1990; 37: 636–640.

224. Writer WD: Epidural morphine for post-caesarean analgesia. (Editorial.) Can J Anaesth 1990; 37: 608–612.

225. Hughes SC: The safety of intraspinal narcotics in the obstetric patient. Surv Anesth 1989; 33: 261–264.

226. Miller RR, Greenblatt DJ: Drug effects in hospitalized patients. In Miller RR, Greenblatt DJ (eds): Experiences of the Boston Collaborative Drug Surveillance Program 1966–1975. New York, Biomedical Publications, 1976.

227. Brose WG, Cohen SE: Oxyhemoglobin saturation following cesarean section in patients receiving epidural morphine, PCA, or im meperidine analgesia. Anesthesiology 1989; 70: 948–953.

228. Etches RC: Respiratory depression associated with patient-controlled analgesia: a review of eight cases. Can J Anaesth 1994; 41: 125–132.

229. Baxter AD: Respiratory depression with patient-controlled analgesia. (Editorial.) Can J Anaesth 1994; 41: 87–90.

230. Etches RC: Complications of acute pain management. Anesthesiol Clin North Am 1992; 10: 417–433.

231. Stenseth R, Sellevold O, Breivik H: Epidural morphine for postoperative pain: experience with 1085 patients. Acta Anaesthesiol Scand 1985; 29: 148–156.

232. Cross DA, Hunt JB: Feasibility of epidural morphine for postoperative analgesia in a small community hospital. Anesth Analg 1991; 72: 765–768.

233. Ready LB, Loper KA, Nessly M, et al: Postoperative epidural morphine is safe on surgical wards. Anesthesiology 1991; 75: 452–456.

234. Cross DA, Hunt JB: Epidural morphine in a small community hospital: a false sense of security. (Response to letter.) Anesth Analg 1992; 74: 469–470.

235. Young T, McDonnell FJ: Treatment of pain on the surgical ward using epidural morphine. (Letter to the editor.) Anesthesiology 1992; 76: 155–156.

236. Dailey PA, Brookshire GL, Shnider SM, et al: Naloxone decreases side effects after intrathecal morphine for labor. Anesth Analg 1985; 64: 658–666.

237. Wright PM, O'Toole DP, Barron DW: The influence of naloxone infusion on the action of intrathecal diamorphine: low-dose naloxone and neuroendocrine responses. Acta Anaesthesiol Scand 1992; 36: 230–233.

238. Morgan PJ, Mehta S, Kapala DM: Nalbuphine pretreatment in cesarean section patients receiving epidural morphine. Reg Anesth 1991; 16: 84–88.

239. Gal TJ, DiFazio CA: Prolonged antagonism of opioid action with intravenous nalmefene in man. Anesthesiology 1986; 64: 175–180.

CHAPTER 14

Additives to Local Anesthetic Solutions

Cosmo A. DiFazio, M.D., Ph.D.
John C. Rowlingson, M.D.

Shorten Onset Time
Limit the Absorption of Local
   Anesthetic
Increase the Intensity of Anesthetic
   Action

Preserve the Stability of Local
   Anesthetic Drugs in Solution
   p-Aminobenzoic Acid
   Metabisulfite
   Ethylenediaminetetraacetate

The local anesthetic solutions used to produce regional anesthesia are manufactured containing one or more additives, and the clinician planning to use them also frequently uses other additives to achieve specific goals. The additives commonly used are placed in the local anesthetic solutions to accomplish one of the following goals:

1. Shorten the onset time of local anesthetic action.
2. Increase the duration of action of local anesthesia by decreasing systemic absorption, thus also decreasing the potential for systemic toxicity.
3. Increase the intensity of anesthetic block.
4. Stabilize the local anesthetic drug in solution.

Shorten Onset Time

The clinician using regional anesthesia is faced with the need to produce an adequate intensity and duration of block in an acceptable time and frequently must do so with a single dose of local anesthetic. Conceptually, for any local anesthetic, the production (onset) of a regional block is a function of how much and how soon the drug enters the nerve and produces anesthetic concentrations at the receptor site. The goal of achieving a rapid onset of regional block has centered on increasing the concentration of the active form of the local anesthetic that reaches the receptor site in the sodium channel of the nerve. The local anesthetics exist in solution as a mixture of two forms: the base and the cationic forms (Fig. 14–1). The amount of each form present depends on the pH of the solution and the pK_a of the drug, i.e., the Henderson-Hasselbalch equation:

$$pK_a = pH - \log \frac{cation}{base}$$

The drugs are thought to penetrate the nerve membrane in their lipid-soluble, uncharged base form and then reequilibrate in the axoplasm of the nerve into the charged cationic and uncharged base forms (Fig. 14–2) in accord with the Henderson-Hasselbalch equa-

tion. The concentration of the base form then becomes equal outside the nerve membrane and in the nerve axoplasm. The cationic form, the active form of the drug, enters the sodium channel from the axoplasmic side of the nerve membrane and binds to an anionic site within the sodium channel that ionically or physically blocks sodium ion movements.

Contemporary approaches used to speed the onset of action of the local anesthetic drugs depend on increasing the rate of formation of the cationic form in the axoplasm. The two most commonly used specific approaches to achieve this goal have been (1) increasing the pH of the local anesthetic solution injected and (2) using the carbonated local anesthetic solutions. In the technique of acute pH adjustment, the addition of sodium bicarbonate solutions has raised the pH of the commercially available local anesthetic solutions. These solutions are all acidic, having a pH ranging from 3.0 to 6.5.[1] The pK_a of the local anesthetic drugs in common use ranges from 7.6 to 8.9. According to the Henderson-Hasselbalch equation, the commercially available local anesthetic solutions for injection will be almost entirely in the cationic form, and only an exceedingly small amount of drug will be present in the nonionized, lipid-soluble base form. The cationic drug form placed outside of the nerve membrane will not cross the membrane. In order to increase the amount of the lipid-soluble base form present in solution and needed to cross the nerve membrane, one can increase the pH of the solution, decrease the pK_a of the drug being injected, or increase the concentration of the local anesthetic drug used. Increasing the drug concentration is limited by the increased potential for local anesthetic systemic toxicity because peak drug plasma concentrations achieved as a result of absorption are directly related to the amount of drug injected.[2] Also, the higher local anesthetic concentration might injure nerves directly.

Use of pH adjustment of the local anesthetic solution is an old technique first reported in 1910 by Gros and recently repopularized following in vitro and in vivo observations by Galindo.[3] Several subsequent human studies demonstrated that marked decreases in onset

232

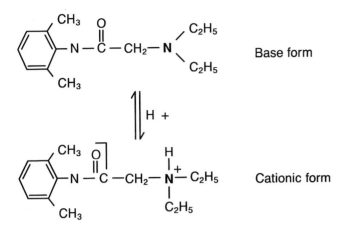

Figure 14–1 The cationic and base forms of lidocaine.

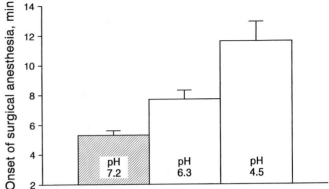

Figure 14–3 The onset time for surgical epidural anesthesia with lidocaine pH adjustment and after acute addition of epinephrine to plain lidocaine compared with pH-stabilized epinephrine-containing lidocaine. (Modified from DiFazio CA, Carron H, Grosslight KR, et al: Comparison of pH-adjusted lidocaine solutions for epidural anesthesia. Anesth Analg 1986; 65: 760–764.)

time were achievable when major changes were made in the pH of the local anesthetic solution being injected, and that this could be accomplished without precipitation of the drug from solution. Major pH adjustments are frequently accomplished with the commercially prepared local anesthetic solutions that contain epinephrine. These are very acidic in order to maintain stability of the epinephrine in solution. The limiting factors in pH adjustment of any local anesthetic solution are the solubility of the local anesthetic base in solution and the amount of local anesthetic base produced by pH adjustment.

Clinically, DiFazio et al[4] demonstrated that a greater than 50% decrease in onset time for epidural anesthesia occurred when the pH of commercially available lidocaine with epinephrine (pH = 4.5) was raised to 7.2 by the addition of bicarbonate (Fig. 14–3). Similarly, acutely adding epinephrine to a plain lidocaine solution (pH = 6.35), rather than using lidocaine already having epinephrine added (pH = 4.5), produces a shorter onset time that is midway between commercial lidocaine adjusted with bicarbonate and the commercially prepared epinephrine-lidocaine solutions. Hilgier[5] reported approximately 50% shortening in onset time for brachial plexus anesthesia when bupiva-

caine with epinephrine (pH = 3.9) was pH adjusted to a level of 6.4 immediately before injection. These large changes in pH reported by both DiFazio et al[4] and Hilgier[5] resulted in a major increase in the amount of free-base local anesthetic available in solution for nerve penetration and thus in similar marked decreases (approximately 50%) in the onset time for anesthesia. Smaller changes in pH and decreases in onset time using pH-adjusted bupivacaine solutions without epinephrine for epidural anesthesia in pregnant patients have been reported by McMorland et al[6] using 0.25% bupivacaine. Multiple other studies of pH-adjusted bupivacaine in epidural and other block models have shown an inconsistent effect in shortening onset time (Table 14–1). In other studies, improved onset time with pH-adjusted mepivacaine[11] has been reported with brachial plexus anesthesia.

Studies with pH adjustment of commercially available local anesthetic solutions containing epinephrine are consistent and indicate a shortening of anesthetic onset time after pH adjustment. However, other studies using pH adjustment of non–epinephrine-containing solutions of lidocaine, bupivacaine, and mepivacaine (Tables 14–1 and 14–2) have produced less consistent results. In one report,[17] the solubility of the local anesthetic bases was determined for multiple local anesthetics, hence defining the maximum amount of base that can be in solution with pH adjustment for each local anesthetic (Fig. 14–4). The amount of base produced was directly related to the total concentration of the drug in solution and to the pH of the resultant solution. The concentration of base and cation was assumed to follow the Henderson-Hasselbalch equation. As the pH of the solution is increased further, a greater amount of base will be produced than is soluble in the (saturated) solution. At this point, the local anesthetic base precipitates out of solution, and the total amount of drug remaining in solution is decreased. If it is correct that base penetration of the nerve membrane is the rate-limiting step for onset time, then because the base solubility of lidocaine and

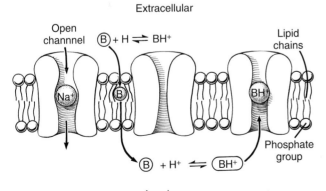

Figure 14–2 The penetration of local anesthetic base (B) and equilibration in axoplasm with cationic form (BH⁺) and block of the sodium channel. (Modified from de Jong RH: Local Anesthetics, p 49. St Louis, Mosby–Year Book, 1994.)

Table 14–1 pH Adjustment: Bupivacaine

REFERENCE	BUPIVACAINE, %	BLOCK	ONSET TIME, min Control → pH Adjusted	pH Control → pH Adjusted
Hilgier[5]	0.5 with epi	Brachial plexus	24.3 → 9.8	3.9 → 6.4
McMorland et al[6]	0.5 plain	Epidural	24.8 → 18.1 peak	5.5 → 7.0
McMorland et al[6]	0.5 with epi	Epidural	26.0 → 18.5	5.5 → 7.0
Bedder et al[7]	0.5 plain	Brachial plexus	17.7 → 16.3	5.5 → 7.1
Coventry and Todd[8]	0.5 with epi	Sciatic nerve	25.0 → 12.5	3.9 → 6.4
Tackley and Coe[9]	0.5 plain	Epidural	45.0 → 30.0	5.1 → 6.3
Stevens et al[10]	0.5 with epi freshly added	Epidural	No change (mean 28 → 30)	5.3 → 7.0

epi, epinephrine.

mepivacaine is the greatest, these local anesthetics should have the highest potential for significant shortening of their onset time with pH changes of acidic solutions. Furthermore, from this study, it was evident that increasing the pH of the local anesthetic solution beyond the saturation point cannot cause a further decrease in onset time for block because further increases in base concentration in solution cannot occur.

The pH adjustment of 2-chloroprocaine solutions has also been evaluated. Commercial solutions of this drug are very acidic (pH = 3) in order to maintain the drug's stability in solution. With pH adjustment, the changes in 2-chloroprocaine onset are small and difficult to document, if present at all. Undoubtedly, this is related to the fact that the onset time for 2-chloroprocaine is already short. As an aside, because the best results of decreasing onset time have been achieved by pH adjustment of the very acidic, epinephrine-containing local anesthetic solutions, one should also consider if the changes produced in pH are also affecting the amount of cationic and base forms of epinephrine present in solution. This may also cause a change in the pharmacologic activity of the epinephrine (pK$_a$ = 8.6) and the amount of active form of epinephrine present to produce the desired vasoconstrictive effect that allows for a longer duration of contact of the local anesthetic with the nerve. If, like local anesthetics, the amount of base form present is the limiting factor for epinephrine activity, increasing the pH with bicarbonate should also improve the vasoconstriction produced by epinephrine.

Another approach to shortening onset time of surgical anesthesia with regional blocks has been the use of carbonated local anesthetic solutions. With these solutions, the local anesthetic cation is the carbonate rather than the hydrochloride salt available in other commercial local anesthetic solutions, and CO_2 is added to the solution in order to maintain a high concentration of the carbonate anion. At this time, carbonated local anesthetics are available in other parts of the world but are not available in the United States. Several studies by Bromage et al[18, 19] found that onset time was shortened (on average by 40%), the spread of anesthesia was more extensive, and a better quality of regional block was achieved when carbonated rather than an uncarbonated lidocaine solution was used. Although not universally observed clinically, numerous animal studies[20] using carbonated lidocaine have demonstrated shortened onset time and improved regional block. In a more recent clinical study by Sukhani and Winnie,[21] carbonated lidocaine with epinephrine produced more rapid and more complete anesthesia of the brachial plexus than the lidocaine hydrochloride solution. The use of other carbonated local anesthetics, however, has not produced the significant improvement seen with lidocaine. For instance, studies using carbonated bupivacaine epidurally have not consistently found shortened onset time.[22]

Several explanations have been put forth to explain how a carbonated local anesthetic improves anesthetic activity, and the most likely follow:

1. The increased CO_2 in the local anesthetic solution

Table 14–2 pH Adjustment: Lidocaine or Mepivacaine

REFERENCE	DRUG	CONC, %	BLOCK	ONSET TIME, min Control → pH Adjusted	pH Control → pH Adjusted
DiFazio et al[4]	Commercial lidocaine	1.5 with epi	Epidural	11 → 5	4.6 → 7.2
	Commercial lidocaine	1.5 with epi freshly added	Epidural	11 → 8	6.35 → 7.2
Liepert et al[12]	Lidocaine	2.0 plain	Epidural	10.4 → 9.3	6.5 → 7.0
Fukuda et al[13]	Lidocaine	1.0 plain	Epidural	11 → 7.5	6.68 → 7.40
Candido et al[14]	Mepivacaine	1.5 plain	Brachial plexus	No change	5.7 → 7.5
Tetzlaff et al[11]	Mepivacaine	1.5 plain	Interscalene	3 → 1	5.6 → 7.3
Quinlan et al[15]	Mepivacaine	1.25 plain	Axillary	17 → 10	5.6 → 7.3
Capogna et al[16]	Mepivacaine	2.0 plain	Epidural	16.5 → 9	5.85 → 7.3

Conc, concentration; epi, epinephrine.

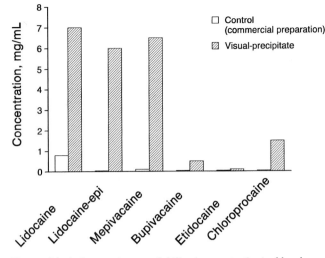

Figure 14–4 The maximum solubility (concentration) of local anesthetic base and that found in commercially available solutions at 37° C. epi, epinephrine. (From DiFazio CA, Rowlingson JC, Moscicki JC: Ph adjustment of local anesthetics. [Abstract.] Reg Anesth 1994; 19[Suppl 2]: 70.)

placed around the nerve penetrates the nerve membrane and enters the nerve axoplasm. This, in turn, produces a decrease in the pH of the axoplasm and causes an increase in the cationic form of the local anesthetic present in the axoplasm. Because this is the active form of the local anesthetic drug, it follows that increasing the concentration of the cationic form in the axoplasm and thus at the receptor site produces a greater degree of block of the sodium channel and does it sooner. Furthermore, high concentrations of the cationic form in the axoplasm cannot cross the nerve membrane and thus remain in the axoplasm to exert a clinical effect. This is similar to "ion trapping" of local anesthetics described in acidic conditions in a fetus.

2. Carbon dioxide may cause some degree of direct neural blockade.

3. A further contribution to shortened onset time may also be the result of an increased pH of the solution injected around the nerve that occurs with CO_2 loss. Solutions of carbonated lidocaine have a pH of 6.5 and a Pco_2 of 700 mm Hg. As carbon dioxide is lost on opening the vial, the pH of the solution can increase to around 7 and, thus, the pH change can modestly increase the fraction of drug base in solution available for nerve penetration.

A further consideration in the use of pH-adjusted solutions is that the addition of bicarbonate to local anesthetic solutions not only produces a change in pH of the solution but also causes a small increase in Pco_2 in solution. For lidocaine with epinephrine solutions that have been pH adjusted with bicarbonate, a Pco_2 of approximately 100 mm Hg is achieved. This is considerably less than the Pco_2 of 700 mm Hg that is present in the carbonated local anesthetic solutions; however, the modest increase in Pco_2 produced by the addition of bicarbonate may also contribute to a decrease in the onset time of the local anesthetic by one of the mechanisms described for the carbonated solutions.

Another way to modify the onset time of local anesthetic action is to warm the solution. Although the exact mechanism for this effect is not entirely clear, it is likely to be related to a decrease in the pK_a of the local anesthetic that results from increasing temperature.[23] For example, the pK_a of lidocaine at 25° C is 7.91, whereas the pK_a at 38° is 7.25. Therefore, a decrease in the pK_a of lidocaine at constant pH increases the amount of base present in solution. Faster onset of action of anesthesia with bupivacaine was seen in women having vaginal or cesarean deliveries when bupivacaine solutions were warmed to 37.7° C before epidural injection.[24] The duration of anesthesia was unchanged, as was the subsequent degree of motor block when the warmed bupivacaine solutions were used.

Limit the Absorption of Local Anesthetic

Additives that have vasoconstrictive properties are added to local anesthetic solutions to decrease the rate of vascular absorption of the local anesthetic. A decrease in absorption of the local anesthetic from the site injected has several beneficial effects. For example, it allows more anesthetic molecules to diffuse to the nerve membrane and, thus, improves the intensity and duration of anesthetic effect.[25] Several vasoconstrictors have been used, including epinephrine, norepinephrine, and phenylephrine. None appear to be superior to epinephrine in decreasing local anesthetic absorption. Epinephrine in a concentration of 1:200,000 has been reported[26] to be optimal for delaying absorption and prolonging the duration of lidocaine for epidural or intercostal use. However, this was questioned in a study in which epinephrine 1:400,000 and 1:600,000 appeared to delay the absorption of lidocaine in a manner similar to the 1:200,000 concentration.[27] All of these epinephrine-containing solutions had considerably less lidocaine absorption than the control lidocaine solution not containing epinephrine. Peak blood levels of lidocaine achieved with all epinephrine-containing lidocaine solutions were similar and not significantly different from one another. This suggests that when the epinephrine-containing local anesthetic solutions are used to treat patients who may also have an increased sensitivity to epinephrine, as has been postulated for example in the preeclamptic patient, a solution containing 1:600,000 epinephrine is a better alternative than the conventional 1:200,000 solution.

The ability of epinephrine to prolong the duration of anesthesia also depends on the local anesthetic used and the site injected. For infiltration anesthesia or for peripheral nerve blocks, epinephrine significantly extends the duration of almost all agents. However, for epidural anesthesia, the duration is prolonged by epinephrine for drugs of low to moderate lipid solubility, e.g., lidocaine and mepivacaine, but it is not prolonged when epinephrine is combined with lipid-soluble local anesthetic agents such as bupivacaine and etidocaine.[25] In areas such as the epidural space, the compartment contains a significant amount of lipid (fat). Therefore, the local anesthetic will be partitioned between the nerve membrane and the fat within the epidural space or be undergoing systemic absorption. For a lipid-soluble agent, decreasing the amount of drug undergoing vascular absorption has a minimal effect on the amount of drug available for nerve penetration because most of the drug leaving the epidural space does so by absorption into fat (Fig. 14–5). In contrast, for local anesthetic drugs with low lipid solubility, absorption or removal into the fat compartment is small whereas removal from the epidural space by vascular absorption is a major component. In this circumstance, decreasing vascular absorption by the addition of epinephrine allows for greater nerve penetration by the drug.

In Figures 14–5 and 14–6, the effect of epinephrine on the diffusion of the local anesthetic into blood vessels, nerves, and fat is depicted for local anesthetics with high and low lipid solubility. Physical constants, including lipid solubility of local anesthetics, are indicated in Table 14–3. It is apparent that increasing vasoconstriction, thereby delaying vascular absorption, by epinephrine addition allows for more local anesthetic to diffuse to the nerve membrane for the local anesthetic drugs with lower lipid solubilities. The addition of epinephrine to such local anesthetic solutions then has the advantage of increasing the duration of epidural local anesthetic action by apparently increasing the concentration of the local anesthetic achieved within the nerves and thus increasing the intensity of

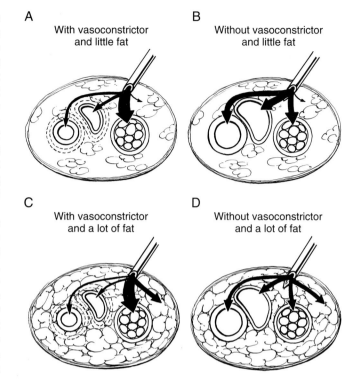

Figure 14–6 Vasoconstrictors and local anesthetics with low to moderate lipid solubility (lidocaine/mepivacaine). *A* and *B* represent injection into a site with little fat such as brachial plexus or peripheral nerve block. *C* and *D* represent an epidural injection, i.e., a site with considerable fat.

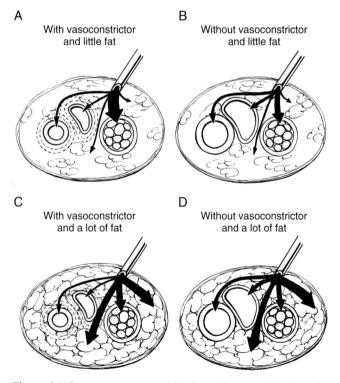

Figure 14–5 Vasoconstrictors and local anesthetics with high lipid solubility (bupivacaine/etidocaine). *A* and *B* represent injection into a site with little fat such as brachial plexus or peripheral nerve block. *C* and *D* represent an epidural injection, i.e., a site with considerable fat.

neural blockade. In addition, the local anesthetic peak serum concentration is also decreased as a result of decreased vascular absorption after epidural administration of such drugs.

When local anesthetics are used for epidural anesthesia, epinephrine decreases the absorption and prolongs the block of the local anesthetics for all except those with higher lipid solubility such as bupivacaine and etidocaine. In contrast, an increase in duration of all local anesthetics is achieved when they are injected into areas having little fat, e.g., peripheral nerve blocks such as brachial plexus blocks. The increase in duration of brachial plexus anesthesia with lidocaine and mepivacaine caused by the addition of epinephrine is 75% to 90%, and with bupivacaine and etidocaine, approximately 50%. In contrast, an increase in duration of only 10% to 15% occurs when epinephrine is added to these lipid-soluble drugs and they are used in the epidural space where significant amounts of fat are present.

When local anesthetics are injected at the neural site, the local anesthetics themselves, as a secondary effect, are vasoconstrictors at low concentrations, whereas at higher concentrations the drugs tend to be vasodilators. Clinically useful blood concentrations of local anesthetic, e.g., for lidocaine a 2 to 5 μg/mL blood level, have only minor if any vasoconstrictive effect. Further increases in serum lidocaine concentration cause an increase in vasoconstriction until a concentra-

Table 14–3 Physical Properties of Local Anesthetics

PROPERTY	PROCAINE	LIDOCAINE	MEPIVACAINE	BUPIVACAINE	ETIDOCAINE	ROPIVACAINE
Molecular weight	236	234	246	288	276	274
pK$_a$	8.9	7.7	7.6	8.1	7.7	8.0
Lipid solubility	1	4	1	30	140	2.8

tion is reached that produces vasodilation.[28] Concentrations achieved after local injection around a nerve are considerably higher and exert a vasodilatory effect. Bupivacaine produced progressive vasoconstriction of cremaster arterioles up to concentrations of 0.1%, and concentrations of bupivacaine of 0.25% produced minimal to slight vasodilation (Fig. 14–7). When local anesthetics are injected in concentrations producing anesthesia of the skin, another variable affecting duration appears to be present. For example, 1% plain lidocaine produces vasodilation, whereas cocaine and ropivacaine, on the basis of the skin blanching seen clinically, appear to continue to produce vasoconstriction.

Increase the Intensity of Anesthetic Action

In addition to the effects of epinephrine, increased intensity and duration of local anesthetic action have also been achieved by the use of adjunct drugs such as opioids or α_2-adrenergic agonists mixed with the local anesthetic solutions for spinal or epidural anesthesia. These drugs combined with local anesthetics decrease sensory input to the central nervous system by action at a site different from the site of action of the local anesthetics. Opioids such as fentanyl, sufentanil, and morphine, most commonly used with local anesthetics, are thought to act by suppression of sensory input at Rexed laminae II and V of the dorsal horn of the spinal cord. In early studies, Justins and coworkers[29] combined fentanyl with local anesthetics and produced more complete anesthesia with the epidural application of the mixture than when the local anesthetics were used alone. The local anesthetic activity of opioids has

also been evaluated, and of the opioids in common use, only meperidine has local anesthetic properties such that it can be used without other local anesthetics. A study by Sangarlangkarn and associates,[30] for example, demonstrated that spinal anesthesia of surgical intensity in patients undergoing lower abdominal or lower extremity surgical procedures could be obtained by the subarachnoid injection of meperidine. Increased intraoperative nausea, vomiting, and drowsiness along with postoperative itching and urinary retention occurred as side effects of using meperidine as the sole local anesthetic. The combination of opioids with local anesthetics for epidural use is widespread in obstetrics and in postoperative pain management. This combination has been observed to increase the analgesic activity more than would occur from the use of either of the drugs given individually. Chestnut et al,[31] for example, demonstrated that low concentrations of fentanyl (1 μg/mL) added to extremely dilute solutions of bupivacaine (0.0625%) produced effective analgesia without the production of motor block in laboring patients. The addition of other opioids to local anesthetics has produced similar results.

Monoamines other than epinephrine have likewise been used to improve analgesia. This has been shown with α_2-adrenergic agonists such as clonidine combined with minimal doses of local anesthetic or opioids and applied spinally. Mensink et al[32] studied the use of graduated doses of clonidine as an adjunct to tetracaine spinal anesthesia in dogs and found that an increase in sensory and motor block occurred with a dose of clonidine between 50 and 150 μg. Racle and coworkers[33] also reported that 150 μg of clonidine added to 3 mL of 0.5% bupivacaine resulted in a significant increase in the duration of both motor and sensory anesthesia that was considerably greater than that produced by the addition of 0.2 mg of epinephrine to bupivacaine. The improved duration of spinal anesthesia in these elderly patients undergoing hip surgery was achieved without any significant increase in the incidence or degree of hypotension related to the primary anesthetic. Although clonidine can produce analgesia directly when given systemically, the doses used for potentiating local anesthetics are much smaller and would not be adequate to produce analgesia by a systemic effect. It appears that clonidine is a useful monoamine adjunct when added to local anesthetics for improving intensity and duration of regional anesthesia and analgesia.

The analgesic effect of epinephrine and clonidine is believed to be mediated at the spinal cord through α_2-adrenoreceptors and the inhibition of substance P release at the dorsal horn. Other α_2-adrenergic agents

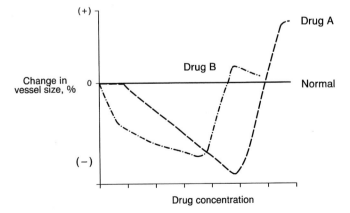

Figure 14–7 Vascular effects of lidocaine (Drug A) and bupivacaine (Drug B) on rat cremaster arteriolar size with topical drug application.

have likewise been used to improve analgesia produced by local anesthetic administration.

Preserve the Stability of Local Anesthetic Drugs in Solution

Preservatives added to local anesthetic solutions include (1) p-aminobenzoic acid (PABA) derivatives such as methylparaben, ethylparaben, or propylparaben; (2) sodium bisulfite (or metabisulfite); and (3) ethylenediaminetetraacetate (EDTA).

p-Aminobenzoic Acid

PABA derivatives are consistently added to multidose vials as an antibacterial agent to inhibit growth of any contaminant entering the vial with repeated use. This chemical, however, is known to be allergenic and is likely to have been the causative agent in many cases of suspected local anesthetic allergies in the past. Likewise, ester-based local anesthetics such as procaine, 2-chloroprocaine, or tetracaine are all structurally related to PABA and all can be metabolized to PABA derivatives. Intradermal injection of these ester-based local anesthetics has been reported to have a 30% incidence of positive skin reactions, even in patients without a history of local anesthetic allergy. In contrast, positive allergic reactions are extremely rare with the amide local anesthetics. Therefore, whenever a multidose vial of ester or amide local anesthetic is used, one should always be prepared for an allergic reaction after injection of the local anesthetic solution. All parabens have been removed from the contemporary formulations of epidural or spinal local anesthetic solutions. These are currently packaged as single-dose vials.

Metabisulfite

Usually the sodium salt of metabisulfite or bisulfite is added to local anesthetic solutions containing epinephrine to act mainly as an antioxidant to prevent the breakdown of epinephrine. This addition results in a greater stability and shelf life of the product. The pH of the solution is usually adjusted to be 4.5 or less. Wang and colleagues[34] and subsequently Gissen and associates[35] investigated the role of bisulfite in producing prolonged sensory-motor dysfunction after the use of 2-chloroprocaine solutions containing high concentrations of bisulfite, e.g., 0.2% bisulfite as was present in Nesacaine CE. In their investigations, Gissen et al[35] identified the role of bisulfite in producing the neurotoxicity after the use of this 2-chloroprocaine (Nesacaine CE) solution. They concluded that in the presence of a low pH (Nesacaine CE has a pH of 3.2), this preservative leads to the formation of SO_2 and sulfurous acid, with the latter being neurotoxic. Essential to this concept is that SO_2 and sulfurous acid are formed in an acid medium and that prolonged exposure to high concentrations of the drug solution that contains bisulfite in an acid solution leads to the formation of these substances. The reaction of bisulfite and an acid solution is shown by the following equation:

$$Na_2SO_3 + H_2O \rightleftharpoons NaHSO_3 + H^+ \rightleftharpoons H_2SO_3 \rightleftharpoons SO_2 + H_2O$$

(sodium metabisulfite) (sodium bisulfite) (sulfurous acid)

The damage (prolonged paralysis) produced by sodium bisulfite in such a solution appears to be concentration dependent. If this drug solution is injected into the subarachnoid space where minimal buffering is available, the acidic bisulfite solution remains localized and thus can cause damage because it can be absorbed or eliminated only minimally. Wang and coworkers[34] and other researchers such as Ready et al[36] have also found that sodium metabisulfite caused extensive and irreversible damage when administered in high concentrations into the subarachnoid space in rabbits. Thus, local anesthetic solutions planned for epidural or spinal anesthesia should contain only low bisulfite concentrations (0.1%). When a low pH is essential, i.e., epinephrine-containing solutions, the pH of the solution should be 4.5 or greater. Under these conditions, use of these solutions should minimize neurotoxicity.

Ethylenediaminetetraacetate

Because of the potential toxicity of metabisulfite (bisulfite), a new formulation of 2-chloroprocaine was prepared that contained EDTA as a preservative instead of metabisulfite. The potential neurotoxic effects of EDTA were investigated by Wang et al,[37] who administered subarachnoid doses of this chemical and demonstrated that tetanic contractions of the hind limbs occurred after a brief period of hind limb paralysis. Epidural administration of EDTA-containing solutions has also been associated with the development of significant back pain.[38] This is probably secondary to chelation of calcium ions of paraspinous muscles, causing severe muscle spasm in these patients. Postoperative pain after epidural administration of 2-chloroprocaine in patients has been severe enough to require hospitalization for opioid administration for 24 h. Current work on 2-chloroprocaine formulations centers on total removal of both bisulfite and EDTA.

References

1. Moore DC: The pH of local anesthetic solutions. Anesth Analg 1981; 60: 833–834.
2. Covino BG: Pharmacology of local anaesthetic agents. Br J Anaesth 1986; 58: 701–716.
3. Galindo A: pH adjusted local anesthetics: clinical experience. Reg Anesth 1983; 8: 35–36.
4. DiFazio CA, Carron H, Grosslight KR, et al: Comparison of pH-adjusted lidocaine solutions for epidural anesthesia. Anesth Analg 1986; 65: 760–764.
5. Hilgier M: Alkalinization of bupivacaine for brachial plexus block. Reg Anesth 1985; 10: 59–61.
6. McMorland GH, Douglas MJ, Jeffery WK, et al: Effect of pH-

adjustment of bupivacaine on onset and duration of epidural analgesia in parturients. Can Anaesth Soc J 1986; 33: 537–541.

7. Bedder MD, Kozody R, Craig DB: Comparison of bupivacaine and alkalinized bupivacaine in brachial plexus anesthesia. Anesth Analg 1988; 67: 48–52.

8. Coventry DM, Todd JG: Alkalinisation of bupivacaine for sciatic nerve blockade. Anaesthesia 1989; 44: 467–470.

9. Tackley RM, Coe AJ: Alkalinized bupivacaine and adrenaline for epidural caesarean section. A comparison with 0.5% bupivacaine. Anaesthesia 1988; 43: 1019–1021.

10. Stevens RA, Chester WL, Grueter JA, et al: The effect of pH adjustment of 0.5% bupivacaine on the latency of epidural anesthesia. Reg Anesth 1989; 14: 236–239.

11. Tetzlaff JE, Yoon HJ, O'Hara J, et al: Alkalinization of mepivacaine accelerates onset of interscalene block for shoulder surgery. Reg Anesth 1990; 15: 242–244.

12. Liepert DJ, Douglas MJ, McMorland GH, et al: Comparison of lidocaine CO_2, two per cent lidocaine hydrochloride and pH adjusted lidocaine hydrochloride for caesarean section anesthesia. Can J Anaesth 1990; 37: 333–336.

13. Fukuda T, Sato S, Okubo N, et al: Effect of pH-adjustment and concentration of local anesthetics on the onset of epidural anesthesia. Masui 1988; 37: 809–814.

14. Candido KD, Raza SM, Vasireddy AR: pH adjusted mepivacaine for upper extremity conduction anesthesia. (Abstract.) Reg Anesth 1989; 14(Suppl): 93.

15. Quinlan JJ, Oleksey K, Murphy FL: Alkalinization of mepivacaine for axillary block. Anesth Analg 1992; 74: 371–374.

16. Capogna G, Celleno D, Tagariello V: The effect of pH adjustment of 2% mepivacaine on epidural anesthesia. Reg Anesth 1989; 14: 121–123.

17. DiFazio CA, Rowlingson JC, Moscicki JC: Ph adjustment of local anesthetics. (Abstract.) Reg Anesth 1994; 19(Suppl 2): 70.

18. Bromage PR: A comparison of the hydrochloride and carbon dioxide salts of lidocaine and prilocaine in epidural analgesia. Acta Anaesthesiol Scand Suppl 1965; 16: 55–69.

19. Bromage PR, Burfoot MF, Crowell DE, et al: Quality of epidural blockade. 3. Carbonated local anaesthetic solutions. Br J Anaesth 1967; 39: 197–209.

20. Condouris GA, Shakalis A: Potentiation of the nerve-depressant effect of local anaesthetics by carbon dioxide. Nature 1964; 204: 57–59.

21. Sukhani R, Winnie AP: Clinical pharmacokinetics of carbonated local anesthetics. II: Interscalene brachial block model. Anesth Analg 1987; 66: 1245–1250.

22. Brown DT, Morison DH, Covino BG, et al: Comparison of carbonated bupivacaine and bupivacaine hydrochloride for extradural anaesthesia. Br J Anaesth 1980; 52: 419–422.

23. Kamaya H, Hayes JJ Jr, Ueda I: Dissociation constants of local anesthetics and their temperature dependence. Anesth Analg 1983; 62: 1025–1030.

24. Mehta PM, Theriot E, Mehrotra D, et al: A simple technique to make bupivacaine a rapid-acting epidural anesthetic. Reg Anesth 1987; 12: 135–138.

25. Tucker GT, Mather LE: Absorption and disposition of local anesthetics: pharmacokinetics. In Cousins MJ, Bridenbaugh PO (eds): Neural Blockade in Clinical Anesthesia and Management of Pain, pp 45–85. Philadelphia, JB Lippincott, 1980.

26. Braid DP, Scott DB: The systemic absorption of local analgesic drugs. Br J Anaesth 1965; 37: 394–404.

27. Ohno H, Watanabe M, Saitoh J, et al: Effect of epinephrine concentration on lidocaine disposition during epidural anesthesia. Anesthesiology 1988; 68: 625–628.

28. Johns RA, DiFazio CA, Longnecker DE: Lidocaine constricts or dilates rat arterioles in a dose-dependent manner. Anesthesiology 1985; 62: 141–144.

29. Justins DM, Knott C, Luthman J, et al: Epidural versus intramuscular fentanyl. Analgesia and pharmacokinetics in labour. Anaesthesia 1983; 38: 937–942.

30. Sangarlangkarn S, Klaewtanong V, Jonglerttrakool P, et al: Meperidine as a spinal anesthetic agent: a comparison with lidocaine-glucose. Anesth Analg 1987; 66: 235–240.

31. Chestnut DH, Owen CL, Bates JN, et al: Continuous infusion epidural analgesia during labor: a randomized, double-blind comparison of 0.0625% bupivacaine/0.0002% fentanyl versus 0.125% bupivacaine. Anesthesiology 1988; 68: 754–759.

32. Mensink FJ, Kozody R, Kehler CH, et al: Dose-response relationship of clonidine in tetracaine spinal anesthesia. Anesthesiology 1987; 67: 717–721.

33. Racle JP, Benkhadra A, Poy JY, et al: Prolongation of isobaric bupivacaine spinal anesthesia with epinephrine and clonidine for hip surgery in the elderly. Anesth Analg 1987; 66: 442–446.

34. Wang BC, Hillman DE, Spielholz NI, et al: Chronic neurological deficits and Nesacaine-CE—an effect of the anesthetic, 2-chloroprocaine, or the antioxidant, sodium bisulfite? Anesth Analg 1984; 63: 445–447.

35. Gissen AJ, Datta S, Lambert D: The chloroprocaine controversy. II. Is chloroprocaine neurotoxic? Reg Anesth 1984; 9: 134–145.

36. Ready LB, Plumer MH, Haschke RH, et al: Neurotoxicity of intrathecal local anesthetics in rabbits. Anesthesiology 1985; 63: 364–370.

37. Wang BC, Li D, Hiller JM, et al: Lumbar subarachnoid ethylenediaminetetraacetate induces hindlimb tetanic contractions in rats: prevention by $CaCl_2$ pretreatment; observation of spinal nerve root degeneration. Anesth Analg 1992; 75: 895–899.

38. Fibuch EE, Opper SE: Back pain following epidurally administered Nesacaine-MPF. Anesth Analg 1989; 69: 113–115.

Block Technique

CHAPTER 15

Head and Neck Regional Blocks

John H. Tucker, M.D., F.R.C.P.C.,

James F. Flynn, M.D., F.R.C.P.C.

Before widespread acceptance of tracheal intubation for general anesthesia, nerve blocks were a preferred method of providing surgical anesthesia. Early developments in the field of regional anesthesia can be attributed to nonanesthesiologists. The role of the anesthesiologist grew to the point at which regional anesthesia primarily was in the domain of the anesthesiologist, although certain head and neck blocks remain exceptions.

Despite this change, blocks of the head and neck lend themselves to a regional anesthesia technique that also provides postoperative analgesia. With a proliferation of interest in diagnosis and management of acute and chronic pain syndromes, regional block in this area serves a diagnostic and therapeutic purpose. The use of fiberoptic aids to intubation is an important skill for the management of the airway.

In this anatomic region more than any other, small doses of local anesthetic provide effective neural block, but these same small doses may produce systemic toxicity, with volumes as low as 0.5 mL causing convulsion related to intravascular injection into cerebral blood vessels.[1] The incidence of systemic toxicity may differ for certain types of regional block,[2] and appropriate measures should be immediately available to treat potential complications[3] (Table 15–1). Clinical judgment of the anesthesiologist with a thorough understanding of the local anatomy reinforces the concept that patients undergoing head and neck regional block require the same level of monitoring as patients undergoing general anesthesia.

Innervation of the head and neck is through the 12 cranial and upper 4 cervical nerves. The majority of these nerves serve specialized functions and have specific clinical relevance. Sensory innervation of the face (Fig. 15–1) is from the trigeminal nerve, and its gasserian ganglion is located on the floor of the middle cranial fossa and there divides into three branches: ophthalmic (V1), maxillary (V2), and mandibular (V3). The only motor function is to the muscles of mastication. Cutaneous innervation of the posterior areas of the head and neck is from the cervical nerves. The dorsal branch of the second cervical nerve terminates in the greater occipital nerve, providing cutaneous innervation to the posterior scalp region. The lesser occipital nerve, from C-2 and C-3, supplies the lateral aspect of the head. The ventral rami of the second, third, and fourth cervical rami provide innervation to the arteries and lateral neck region.

Regional anesthesia for ophthalmologic surgery most often is performed by ophthalmologists; however, this tends to be an institutional decision. Hamilton and colleagues[4] described more than 12,000 cases performed by one anesthesiologist during a 5-year period.

Interventional skills and mastery of the airway are crucial for the anesthesiologist. Airway block may be the most important regional block to master. Anatomic deformities, facial trauma, and unstable cervical verte-

Table 15–1. Specific Complications of Head and Neck Blocks

Brain-stem anesthesia
Convulsions (small volume, 0.5 mL)
Hematoma
Respiratory distress
　Recurrent laryngeal
　Phrenic
　Pneumothorax
　Sensory and motor nerves to airway
Systemic toxicity (topical)
Subarachnoid or epidural block (unintended)

brae may require that the patient is awake during tracheal intubation. A more detailed anatomic discussion is available elsewhere.[5, 6]

Trigeminal Nerve Blocks

Central

Gasserian Ganglion

The largest of the cranial nerves, the trigeminal nerve, is a mixed somatic nerve with principally sensory function. It arises from the base of the pons and sends sensory fibers to the crescent-shaped gasserian ganglion on the petrous bone above the foramen ovale. It separates into its three divisions (Table 15–2) in the middle cranial fossa. The trigeminal (gasserian) ganglion is partly contained within a reflection of dura mater (Meckel's cave) covering the posterior two thirds of the ganglion and bathing it in cerebrospinal fluid.

The ganglion is bordered medially by the cavernous sinus and internal carotid artery, inferiorly by the greater petrosal nerve and apex of petrous part of the temporal bone, and superiorly by the temporal lobe of the brain. The mandibular branch leaves through the foramen ovale, and access to the ganglion is via this opening.[7]

Block of the gasserian ganglion is rarely used now for operation, and its main use is in diagnostic and therapeutic maneuvers for trigeminal neuralgia (tic douloureux). Patients with this condition are managed medically with carbamazepine or occasionally clonazepam or baclofen. Patients who fail to respond to medical treatment are treated with radiofrequency gangliolysis or microvascular decompression.[8] The principal use of gasserian ganglion block is as a diagnostic block before neurolysis. Gangliolysis has replaced injection of neurolytic agents.[9] For most patients, loss of facial sensation is an acceptable trade-off for relief of pain, but some find it disturbing, and a diagnostic procedure gives the patient a trial.

A small volume of anesthetic, 1 to 3 mL, produces satisfactory anesthesia. Apart from the risk of damage to the surrounding structures, the ganglion is partially bathed in cerebrospinal fluid and direct injection into the cerebrospinal fluid is possible. Fluoroscopic guidance facilitates passage through the foramen ovale.[8] The patient is supine, and the anesthesiologist is at the patient's side. A 22-G, 10-cm needle is inserted at a point medial to the clenched masseter muscle, 3 cm lateral to the corner of the mouth. Plane of insertion is in line with the pupil (Fig. 15–2), and the needle is inserted contacting the infratemporal surface of the greater wing of the sphenoid bone, anterior to the foramen ovale (at a depth of 4 to 6 cm) (if the oral cavity is entered, a new needle is used). The needle is withdrawn and redirected, entering the foramen ovale an additional 1 to 1.5 cm.

As the foramen is entered, mandibular paresthesia is usually elicited. Paresthesias from the ophthalmic nerve (V1) or the maxillary nerve (V2) should also be achieved. Absence of V1 or V2 paresthesia may mean the foramen has not been entered. A local anesthetic vol-

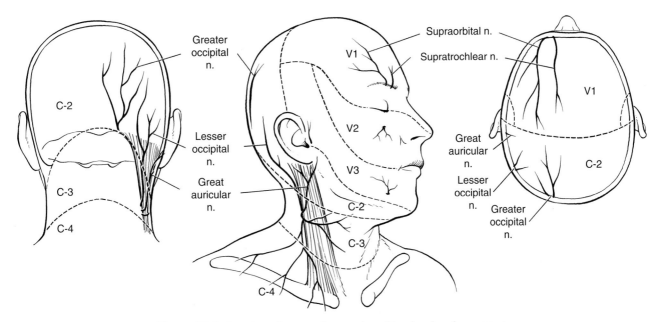

Figure 15–1 Overview of sensory innervation of head and neck. n., nerve.

Table 15–2. Simplified Guide to the Trigeminal Nerve and Its Divisions

VARIABLE	DIVISIONS		
	Ophthalmic (V1)	Maxillary (V2)	Mandibular (V3)
Function	Sensory	Sensory	Sensory
			Muscles of mastication
Exit skull	Superior orbital fissure	Foramen rotundum	Foramen ovale
Parasympathetic ganglion	Ciliary	Sphenopalatine	Submandibular
			Otic
Terminal branches	Lacrimal	Zygomatic	Inferior alveolar (mental)
	Nasociliary	Infraorbital	Anterior branch (motor)
	Frontal (supraorbital)	Superior alveolar nerves	Lingual
	(supratrochlear)	Sphenopalatine branches	Posterior branch: auriculotemporal, buccal
Cutaneous distribution	Eye	Midface	Lower jaw
	Forehead	Upper jaw	

ume of 1.0 mL produces anesthesia in 5 to 10 min, and a 1.0-mL injection is repeated if the block is incomplete.

Passage through the foramen is painful, so sedation is generally needed. Monitoring should be vigilant because profound bradycardia has been described,[8] and there are potential risks of intravascular or subarachnoid injection.

Maxillary Nerve

Maxillary nerve (V2) block in the pterygopalatine fossa is used in the assessment of facial neuralgia and for specific surgical procedures in its distribution[10] (Fig. 15–3). Entirely sensory, the maxillary nerve exits the middle cranial fossa via foramen rotundum, crosses the pterygopalatine fossa medial to the lateral pterygoid plate, and enters the orbit through the inferior orbital fissure.

With the patient supine, mouth closed, and head rotated away from the anesthesiologist, a 22-G, 8-cm needle is inserted below the zygomatic arch overlying the coronoid notch of the mandible. (Subcutaneous infiltration may block branches of the facial nerve supplying the orbicularis oculi muscles.) The needle is advanced in a slightly cephalomedial direction (Fig. 15–3), striking the lateral surface of the lateral pterygoid plate at a depth of about 5 cm. The needle is withdrawn and advanced cephaloanteriorly in a stepwise fashion no more than an additional 1 cm, thus entering the pterygopalatine fossa. A local anesthetic volume of 5.0 mL produces adequate anesthesia.

The pterygopalatine fossa is highly vascular, so care must be exercised to prevent intravascular injection, and hematoma formation is common. Spillage of local anesthetic into the orbit may affect the ocular muscles or the optic nerve.

Mandibular Nerve

Mandibular nerve (V3) block is used in the assessment of facial neuralgias and for surgical procedures in

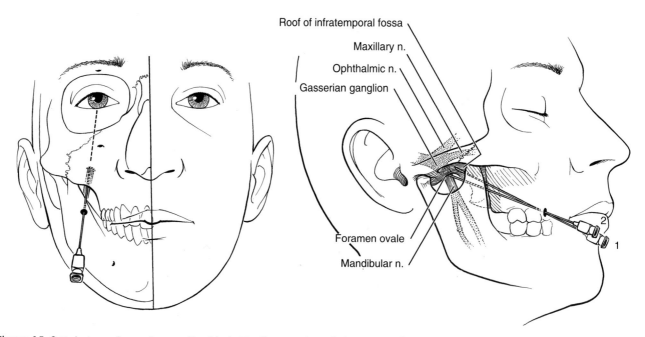

Figure 15–2 Technique of gasserian ganglion block. Needle entry through foramen ovale into gasserian ganglion: (1) needle is withdrawn and redirected in a stepwise manner until foramen ovale is entered, and (2) if too medial, needle may meet resistance from pterygoid plate. If too posterior, needle may penetrate branch of external carotid artery. n., nerve.

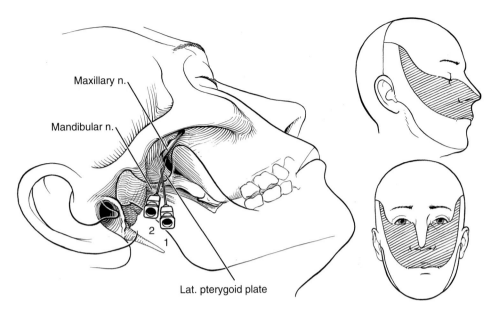

Figure 15–3 Maxillary nerve (n.) block. (1) Initial advancement to lateral (lat.) pterygoid plate. (2) *Anterior* advancement 1 cm to pterygopalatine fossa. On right, the cutaneous distribution of the maxillary nerve (V2) is shown.

its distribution (Fig. 15–4). Dental procedures on the lower jaw may be performed, although an intraoral approach[11] tends to be the preferred dental method. A mixed motor sensory nerve with its anterior divisions supplying the muscles of mastication, the mandibular nerve is primarily sensory. It exits the cranium through the foramen ovale and parallels the posterior aspects of the lateral pterygoid plate, descending toward the mandible (see Fig. 15–2).

The initial technique simulates maxillary nerve block. With the patient supine, mouth closed, and head rotated away from the anesthesiologist, a 22-G, 8-cm needle is advanced from a point below the zygomatic arch overlying the coronoid notch of the mandible. Advancing in a cephalomedial direction (see Fig. 15–4), the needle contacts the lateral surface of the lateral pterygoid plate at a depth of 5 cm, and the needle is systematically redirected and walked posteriorly in a horizontal plane (Fig. 15–4) until a paresthesia to the lower jaw or teeth is attained. The needle should be advanced less than an additional 1.0 cm; otherwise, the pharynx may be entered. As in V2 block, 5.0 mL of anesthetic is injected and should produce satisfactory anesthesia. Precautions as for the V2 block should be exercised.

Terminal Branches

The terminal sensory branches of the trigeminal nerve supplying the face-ophthalmic (supraorbital and supratrochlear), maxillary (infraorbital), and mandibular (mental) regions may be blocked to provide surgical anesthesia for superficial procedures, postoperative analgesia (Fig. 15–5), as a means of temporary pain relief in intractable facial pain, or as a prognostic maneuver

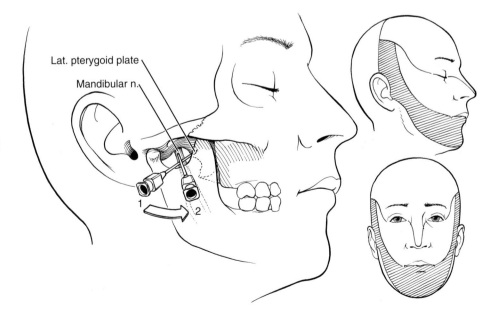

Figure 15–4 Mandibular nerve (n.) block. Needle placement is shown on left. (1) Initial advancement to lateral (lat.) pterygoid plate. (2) Needle is walked posteriorly in a horizontal plane, advancing less than 1.0 cm. Cutaneous distribution of the mandibular nerve is shown on right.

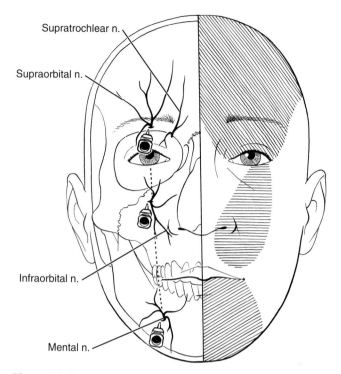

Figure 15–5 Technique of distal trigeminal nerve (n.) block. Note the location of the foramen in the vertical plane through the corner of the mouth and pupil. Innervation of branches of distal trigeminal nerve is shown on right side of face.

before peripheral neurectomy. Peripheral neurectomy is not the primary surgical approach in trigeminal neuralgia; however, it may have a role in patients too ill for the central approach or with a failed central approach.[12] The authors' experience for selected patients who have a positive peripheral diagnostic block has been reasonable relief of their pain.

Small volumes (2 to 4 mL) of local anesthetic will block the individual nerves, and a small-gauge (23 to 25) short needle will suffice. Care should be taken not to inject into the foramen.

Neurolytic block of these and other peripheral nerves is controversial. There is the potential for neuralgias and skin sloughing or necrosis, and the long-term success is not certain.[13] If neurolytic block is attempted, small volumes (1.0 mL) are used. Patient selection is important, as is a frank discussion of the risks and benefits.[14] The authors' personal bias is against neurolytic peripheral nerve blocks for benign conditions.

With the patient supine and pupils midline, the supraorbital, infraorbital, and mental nerves lie along a vertical line drawn through the corner of the mouth and the pupil (see Fig. 15–5).

Supraorbital Nerve

The supraorbital nerve is found along the vertical line (Fig. 15–5) at the level of the supraorbital notch. With needle insertion in a cephalomedial direction, 2 to 4 mL of anesthetic is infiltrated between the skin and frontal bone.

Supratrochlear Nerve

The supratrochlear nerve (Fig. 15–5) supplies the skin of the medial forehead and upper eyelid. It is easily blocked with superficial infiltration by a medial extension at the site of supraorbital nerve block.

Infraorbital Nerve

Exiting through the infraorbital foramen, the infraorbital nerve may be found about 1 cm below the orbital rim and 1 cm from the lateral wall of the nose along the vertical plane through the eye (Fig. 15–5). The needle is inserted from a point slightly below and medial to the foramen. Care should be exercised to not approach from the lateral side because the needle may be inserted in the canal, causing injury to the nerve or accompanying artery or puncturing the floor of the orbit.

Mental Nerve

Innervating the lower lip and corresponding gingival surface from the corner of the mouth to the midline, the mental nerve exits through the mental foramen (Fig. 15–5). With advancing age, resorption of the mandibular bone brings the foramen relatively nearer the alveolar surface of the mandible. The foramen is approached anteriorly, and infiltration is performed close to the bone. Care should be exercised to not enter the foramen.

Cervical Plexus Blocks

Cervical plexus block can be used in various surgical procedures, including superficial operations on the neck and shoulders, thyroid operations, and, particularly, carotid endarterectomies in which awake neurologic monitoring is a simple and reliable method of neurologic assessment.[15–20]

The sensory innervation of the cervical plexus is derived from C-2, C-3, and C-4.[21] Branches are divided into superficial and deep. The superficial branches pierce the deep cervical fascia just posterior to the sternocleidomastoid muscle as four distinct branches: the lesser occipital, great auricular, transverse cervical, and supraclavicular nerves (Fig. 15–6). These branches supply the skin over the neck from the mandible to the clavicle anteriorly and laterally. The deep branches of the cervical plexus provide motor innervation to most of the neck and the diaphragm via the phrenic nerve, and they contribute to the axillary nerve.

Superficial Cervical Plexus Block

The supine patient turns the head slightly opposite the side to be blocked and lifts the head off the table to bring the sternocleidomastoid muscle into prominence. At the midpoint along the posterior border of the sternocleidomastoid, a 22-G, 4-cm needle is inserted subcutaneously, posterior and immediately deep

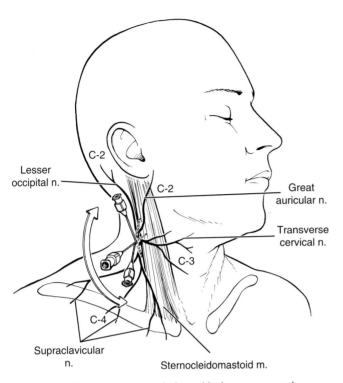

Figure 15–6 Superficial cervical plexus block: anatomy and technique. m., muscle; n., nerve.

Deep Cervical Plexus Block

The patient is placed supine with the head turned slightly away from the side to be blocked. A line is drawn between the mastoid process and Chassaignac's tubercle (the anterior tubercle of the transverse process of C-6). A second line is drawn parallel to and 1 cm posterior to the first (Fig. 15–7). The transverse process of C-4 is then located by first identifying the C-2 transverse process (1 to 2 cm caudal to the mastoid process) and palpating caudally to the C-4 transverse process (about 3 cm). A 22-G, 4-cm needle is inserted on this line and advanced toward the C-4 transverse process until bony contact is made at a depth of 1.5 to 3 cm. It is useful to achieve a paresthesia, which may require needle redirection anteriorly or posteriorly. Local anesthetic (10 to 12 mL of 1.5% lidocaine) is deposited after aspiration.

Significant complications are rare with the superficial technique but can occur with both blocks. Injection into the vertebral arteries can cause seizures with very small volumes. Phrenic nerve paresis is a frequent side effect, and bilateral cervical plexus blocks are usually avoided for this reason. Epidural or subarachnoid injection is also a potential problem. Cervical sympathetic block producing Horner's syndrome or laryngeal nerve block with hoarseness is also a possible result. If the block is incomplete, it can be supplemented with injection of 0.5% lidocaine in the carotid sheath by the surgeon.

to the muscle, and 5 mL of local anesthetic is injected (see Fig. 15–6). The needle is then redirected both superiorly and inferiorly along the posterior border of the sternocleidomastoid muscle, and an additional 5 mL is injected along each of these sites. Effective superficial cervical plexus block depends on a large volume of local anesthetic, and 15 mL is required. Although 1.5% lidocaine is frequently used, superficial cervical plexus block does not involve motor relaxation, and 0.5% or 0.75% lidocaine is more appropriate, with epinephrine 1:200,000 added for prolongation.

Ophthalmic Blocks

If anesthesiologists provide this service, they must still rely on ophthalmologists to detect and manage complications that may arise such as retrobulbar hemorrhage, scleral perforation, and optic nerve damage.

Because regional anesthesia for eye surgery involves

Figure 15–7 Deep cervical plexus block: anatomy and technique.

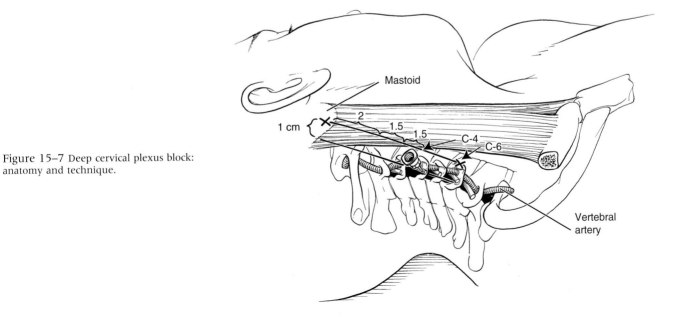

the placement of a needle in close proximity to several important structures, knowledge of orbital anatomy is essential to performing these blocks safely. The orbit is a pear-shaped bony cavity measuring 4 to 5 cm from orbital rim to apex. The medial walls are parallel to the sagittal plane, and the lateral walls are angled 45° from the sagittal plane. The globe lies within the orbit and is 2 to 2.5 cm long.[22-24] Movement of the globe is accomplished by four rectus muscles (superior, inferior, medial, and lateral) and two oblique muscles (superior and inferior). The rectus muscles form a cone from their anterior insertions on the globe to their posterior termination at the orbital apex. This muscle cone defines the intraconal space (into which the retrobulbar block is directed) and the extraconal space (into which the peribulbar block is directed). Because most of the structural contents of the orbit, including the globe, optic nerve, ciliary ganglion, and major vessels, are contained within the muscle cone, the retrobulbar approach is associated with a higher complication rate.

Sensory supply to the orbit is provided by branches of the ophthalmic division of the trigeminal nerve (V1). This also supplies the upper lid, whereas the lower lid is supplied by the maxillary division (V2). Motor supply to the extraocular muscles is provided by cranial nerve III (superior rectus, medial rectus, inferior rectus, and inferior oblique), cranial nerve IV (superior oblique), and cranial nerve VI (lateral rectus). Parasympathetic and sympathetic supply passes through the ciliary ganglion. The levator muscle is innervated by cranial nerve III. The orbicularis oculi is the major protractor of the eyelids and is supplied by cranial nerve VII.

Selected intraocular surgical procedures can be performed with topical anesthetic alone, but regional anesthesia is preferred. The goals of anesthesia for intraocular operation are globe anesthesia, extraocular muscle akinesis, and orbicularis akinesis. Absence of eye movement during operation allows controlled insertion and manipulation of intraocular instruments. Eye muscle and lid akinesis is important to avoid unwanted pressure on the eye, particularly when intraocular operation is complicated by vitreous loss. These requirements are met by retrobulbar block in combination with orbicularis regional anesthesia or by peribulbar block alone.

Retrobulbar Block

Ophthalmic blocks should be undertaken with patient monitoring, intravenous access, and ability to manage the airway. Before administration of the block, the axial length of the eye should be checked, because the technique is varied slightly when there is significant axial myopia in order to avoid globe perforation. The supine patient is instructed to look straight up at the ceiling. Although a superomedial direction of gaze was traditionally preferred, this position rotates the optic nerve and vessels into the path of the needle and may increase the risk of complications.[25-27]

There are two major choices of needles for retrobulbar block: the standard sharp 25-G, 3.0-cm needle or a short-beveled needle such as the Atkinson. The short-beveled needle may decrease the risk of scleral perforation and nerve and vessel damage.[22] After palpation of the globe, the retrobulbar needle is inserted transcutaneously immediately above the inferior orbital rim at the junction of the lateral and middle thirds of the margin (Fig. 15-8). A skin wheal is raised, and after allowing time for dermal anesthesia, the needle is directed posteriorly to avoid globe penetration. Once the needle tip is beyond the globe, it is pointed upward toward the apex of the orbit in order to enter the muscle cone. A slight resistance can often be felt as the needle enters the intraconal space. In patients with axial length greater than 24 mm, care is taken to avoid

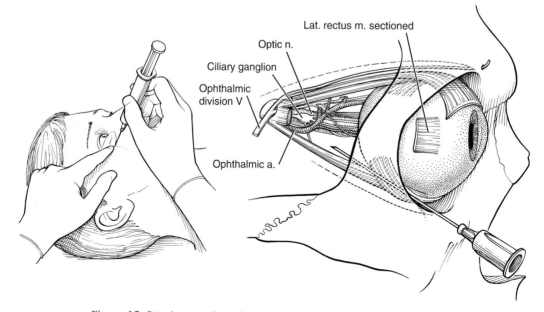

Lat. rectus m. sectioned

Optic n.

Ciliary ganglion

Ophthalmic division V

Ophthalmic a.

Figure 15-8 Technique of retrobulbar block. a., artery; m., muscle; n., nerve.

directing the needle toward the apex prematurely. A final depth of 2.5 to 3 cm is adequate; advancing the needle beyond this point increases the risk of optic nerve trauma or intraoptic sheath injection of anesthetic.

Various local anesthetic solutions have been used for retrobulbar block, and a volume of 2 to 4 mL is sufficient. A 1:1 or 2:1 mixture of bupivacaine 0.75% and lidocaine 2% with 1/100,000 epinephrine produces adequate anesthesia. Alkalinization and hyaluronidase may improve efficacy.[28–30] After aspiration, local anesthetic is deposited over 1 min, and gentle pressure is then applied to the globe. The early onset of ptosis is a good indicator of a successful block. Paralysis of eye movement occurs within 5 min of injection. If significant eye movement is present after this, the retrobulbar injection can be repeated with an additional 2 to 3 mL, or, alternatively, a peribulbar block can be used. If there is movement in only one or two fields of gaze, local injection of 1 to 2 mL can be done just outside the muscle in this region.

Because retrobulbar blocks do not provide eyelid akinesia, a separate facial nerve block is needed to prevent patients from squeezing the eyelids during operation. This can be accomplished by blocking cranial nerve VII at its exit from the stylomastoid foramen (Nadbath block), at the condyle of the mandible (O'Brien block), or at the level of the orbicularis oculi muscle (Van Lint block).[22] Unfortunately, all three techniques are somewhat uncomfortable for the patient. The Van Lint block is administered by inserting a 25-G, 4-cm needle at the lower inferolateral orbital rim, and after injection of 1 mL, further local anesthetic is directed subcutaneously along the lateral and inferior margins of the rim (Fig. 15–9).

Peribulbar Block

Modifications of the classic retrobulbar technique have been made to decrease the risk of complications

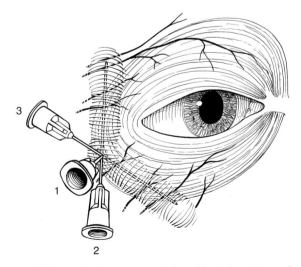

Figure 15–9 Regional anesthesia of the orbicularis oculi muscle: Van Lint method. (1) Local anesthetic (1 mL) is injected subcutaneously at the inferolateral orbital rim. (2 and 3) The needle is repositioned, and local anesthetic is deposited along the lateral superior and inferior margins of the rim.

and minimize patient discomfort. In 1986, Davis and Mandel[31] reported on the use of peribulbar anesthesia, and since that time it has become an increasingly popular approach. The technique involves injection of a larger volume (4 to 6 mL) of local anesthetic into the extraconal space. Peribulbar anesthesia relies on bulk spread of local anesthetic, and a longer time (up to 15 min) is required to produce anesthesia. Also, until this newer technique is mastered, initial attempts may result in incomplete akinesis of the lid and extraocular muscles. However, the advantages are several and include decreased risks of retrobulbar hemorrhage, globe penetration, optic nerve trauma, and intraoptic sheath injection with resultant brain stem anesthesia. The discomfort of the facial block is also avoided.

Peribulbar block can be performed by single- or dual-needle injections.[22, 31–33] Patient positioning, direction of gaze, and injection site are similar to those of the retrobulbar block. The needle is inserted though the skin or inferotemporal conjunctiva, and a wheal is raised. The needle is advanced along the direction of the floor of the orbit, outside the muscle cone to a depth of no more than 2.5 cm, and 4 to 6 mL of local anesthetic is injected over 1 to 2 min. A further 1 mL of local anesthetic is deposited in the orbicularis oculi muscle on withdrawal of the needle in the single-injection technique. The dual-needle approach includes a second injection given through the skin midway between the medial canthus and supraorbital notch. The needle is directed posteriorly to a maximum depth of 2.5 cm, and infiltration is continued as the needle is slowly withdrawn. Firm downward pressure is applied to the globe so that the anesthetic permeates upward to gain access to the preseptal orbicularis. Periorbital blanching of the skin is often seen if epinephrine is used, and this reliably predicts block of the orbicularis oculi muscle.

Although complications of retrobulbar block are rare and risks are decreased in peribulbar block, potentially disastrous outcomes can occur (Table 15–3). Immediately after retrobulbar or peribulbar injection, firm pressure should be placed on the eye to decrease the risk of significant retrobulbar hemorrhage. Massage, either manually or by using a mechanical device such as a Honan balloon at 30 mm Hg, is applied to decrease intraocular pressure and promote spread of local anesthetic. Severe hemorrhage is recognized by increasing proptosis, subconjunctival heme, globe immobility, and increased intraocular pressure. Extreme pain may be a sign of globe penetration and should be evaluated. Vigilance is required to allow early detection of intra-arterial or brain-stem anesthesia and timely resuscitation.

Airway Blocks

All anesthesiologists will at times be required to manage patients with difficult airways, airway trauma, airway compromise, or unstable cervical spines. Regional airway blocks are an essential component of managing these situations, and if there is one group of

Table 15–3. Complications of Retrobulbar or Peribulbar Block

COMPLICATION	INCIDENCE, %	TIME FROM INJECTION TO DIAGNOSIS	CLINICAL NOTES
Eyelid, conjunctival and peribulbar ecchymosis	3	Minutes	Frequent complication
Globe perforation	<0.1*	Immediate to several days	Associated with severe pain and loss of vision
Retrobulbar hemorrhage	1*	Seconds to minutes	Signs include proptosis and globe immobility
Intravascular injection	Rare*	Immediate	Can result in a seizure 2° to retrograde flow
Brain-stem anesthesia	0.2*	Usually within 2 min	Severe shaking is an early warning symptom, and contralateral extraocular partial akinesia is pathognomonic
Temporary vision loss	Expected*	5–10 min	Transient, lasting about 60 min, not total blindness
Permanent loss of vision	Rare*	Variable	May result from trauma to globe, optic nerve, or central retinal artery or from retrobulbar hemorrhage
Diplopia	0.5	Variable	Results from intramuscular injection and is usually temporary
Ptosis	Expected	Seconds	Often takes 4 days or longer to resolve
Vasovagal problems	0.5–1	Immediate	Oculocardiac reflex
Cardiopulmonary arrest	Rare	Immediate to several minutes	May be vasovagal, 2° to intra-arterial injection or brain-stem anesthesia
Infection and abscesses	Rare	Several days	Can occur if the medial orbital wall is punctured

*Risk probably decreased in peribulbar compared to retrobulbar block. 2°, secondary.

Data from Meyers EF, Ramirez RC, Boniuk I: Grand mal seizures after retrobulbar block. Arch Ophthalmol 1978; 96: 847; Ramsay RC, Knobloch WH: Ocular perforation following retrobulbar anesthesia for retinal detachment surgery. Am J Ophthalmol 1978; 86: 61–64; Rosenblatt RM, May DR, Barsoumian K: Cardiopulmonary arrest after retrobulbar block. Am J Ophthalmol 1980; 90: 425–427; Hamilton RC, Gimbel HV, Strunin L: Regional anaesthesia for 12,000 cataract extraction and intraocular lens implantation procedures. Can J Anaesth 1988; 35: 615–623; Lee DS, Kwon NJ: Shivering following retrobulbar block. Can J Anaesth 1988; 35: 294–296; Hay A, Flynn HW Jr, Hoffman JI, et al.: Needle penetration of the globe during retrobulbar and peribulbar injections. Ophthalmology 1991; 98: 1017–1024; and Wong DHW: Regional anaesthesia for intraocular surgery. Can J Anaesth 1993; 40: 635–657.

regional blocks with which all anesthesiologists should be familiar, this is the one.

Airway Anatomy

An understanding of the anatomy and sensory innervation of the airway is critical for performing these blocks. Sensory innervation of the airway is derived from four sources (Fig. 15–10). The maxillary branch of the trigeminal nerve (V2) supplies the upper teeth and gums, vestibule of the nose, upper lip, nasal cavity, palate, and the anterior roof of the pharynx (Fig. 15–10). The mandibular branch (V3) supplies the anterior two thirds of the tongue (Fig. 15–10). Branches of the glossopharyngeal nerve (IX) include (1) the pharyngeal nerves that are sensory to the pharyngeal wall and oropharyngeal isthmus; (2) the tonsillar nerves that are sensory to the soft palate, tonsils, and pharyngeal arches; and (3) sensory branches to the posterior third of the tongue and roof of the pharynx (Fig. 15–10). The vagus nerve (X) supplies the airway mucosa from the level of the epiglottis to the distal airways (Fig. 15–10). The internal laryngeal nerve, a branch of the superior laryngeal nerve, supplies the larynx above the vocal cords and the lower part of the pharynx. The external laryngeal branch of the superior laryngeal nerve provides motor innervation to the cricothyroid muscle. The recurrent laryngeal nerve supplies the larynx below the vocal folds and the upper part of the esophagus. The vagus nerve is primarily parasympathetic but also contains some cervical sympathetic fibers and motor fibers to laryngeal muscles.

Superior Laryngeal Block

Although a separate superior laryngeal nerve block is usually not required with translaryngeal block, it can be used to provide anesthesia above the vocal cords. The superior laryngeal nerve leaves the main trunk of the vagus to course through the neck and pass inferior to the greater cornu of the hyoid bone. With the patient supine and the neck extended, the hyoid bone is displaced toward the side to be blocked (Fig. 15–11). A 25-G, 2.5-cm needle is walked off the inferior border of the greater cornu of the hyoid, and 3 mL of local anesthetic (1% lidocaine) is infiltrated superficial and deep to the thyrohyoid membrane.

Translaryngeal Block

Translaryngeal nerve block provides anesthesia of the airway mucosa below the cords. Laryngeal mucosa above the vocal cord and the epiglottis is also blocked as local anesthetic is coughed onto superior laryngeal structures (Fig. 15–12). The patient is supine with the neck extended. The cricothyroid membrane between the thyroid and cricoid cartilages is palpated (Fig. 15–12), and a 22-G or 25-G needle is inserted in the midline, aspirating as the needle is advanced. Once air is freely aspirated, 3 to 4 mL of 4% lidocaine is injected rapidly and the needle is withdrawn. This usually produces a bout of coughing, which is a consideration for patients in whom coughing is undesirable. A separate superior laryngeal block is generally not necessary be-

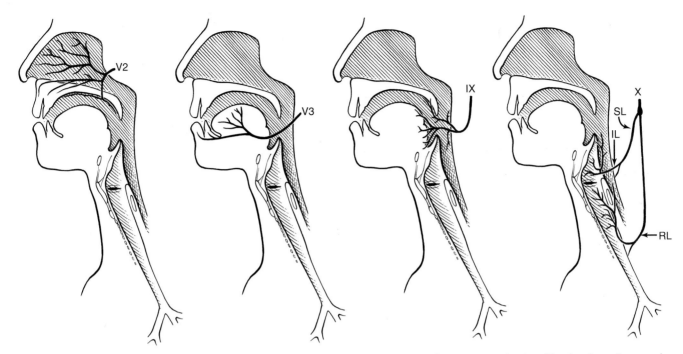

Figure 15–10 Sensory innervation of the airway. Structures innervated by the trigeminal nerve (V2 and V3) and by the glossopharyngeal nerve (IX). Sensory distribution of the vagus nerve (X) is also depicted. IL, internal laryngeal nerve; RL, recurrent laryngeal nerve; SL, superior laryngeal nerve.

cause coughing spreads the anesthetic above the vocal cords. Many anesthesiologists are reluctant to use this block in patients at high risk of gastric aspiration. However, in situations in which fiberoptic intubation is

required, some method of blocking the trachea is essential to provide adequate airway anesthesia before proceeding.

Glossopharyngeal Block

Glossopharyngeal block provides anesthesia of the mucosa of the pharynx, soft palate, and posterior third of the tongue, and it abolishes the gag reflex. The glossopharyngeal nerve exits from the jugular foramen at the base of the skull in close association with other nerves and vessels of the carotid sheath (Fig. 15–13). It can be blocked as it leaves the jugular foramen in association with the styloid process or intraorally. For the peristyloid approach, the patient is supine with the head in the neutral position. The styloid process is identified by deep palpation midway between the mastoid process and the angle of the jaw (Fig. 15–13). A short 22-G needle is inserted and advanced until it impinges on the styloid process. The needle is walked posteriorly until bony contact is lost. After aspiration for blood, 5 to 7 mL of 0.5% lidocaine is injected.

The intraoral approach requires adequate mouth opening, and a laryngoscope blade is used to depress the tongue. An angled 22-G, 9-cm needle is inserted submucosally at the caudad portion of the posterior tonsillar pillar, and, after aspiration, 5 mL of local anesthetic is injected (Fig. 15–14) and this is repeated on the opposite side. An appropriate needle for the intraoral approach is not readily available but can be created by taking a spinal needle and putting a bend at the distal 1-cm tip. The major potential side effect from either technique is intravascular injection, and careful

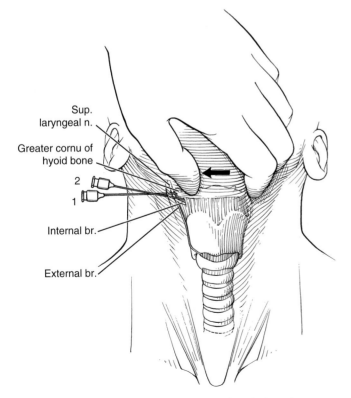

Figure 15–11 Superior (sup.) laryngeal block technique. br., branch; n., nerve.

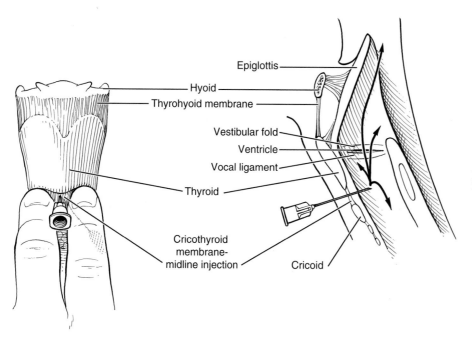

Figure 15–12 Translaryngeal block: local anesthetic spread and technique.

aspiration is essential. This block can be used for post-tonsillectomy pain, but its main use is for anesthesia for airway endoscopy.[34] It is expected that the 10th and 11th cranial nerves are blocked along with the 9th cranial nerve with the peristyloid technique.

Topical Anesthesia of the Airway

It is possible to provide effective topical airway anesthesia. The following is a description of a technique that the authors use. After administration of nebulized lidocaine (2 to 3 mL of 2%) over 15 min, the patient is given a mixture of 2% viscous lidocaine 15 mL and 4% lidocaine 15 mL to gargle and swish around the mouth several times without swallowing. The posterior portion of the tongue and the pharynx are then sprayed with lidocaine (10 mg per spray, 4 to 5 times). If nasal intubation is planned, 3 to 4 mL of 4% cocaine is delivered to the nares and nasal cavities by a de Vilbiss atomizer. The superior laryngeal and glossopharyngeal nerves are anesthetized by sliding cotton pledgets held in Krause forceps and soaked in 4% lidocaine along the posterior portion of the tongue to rest in the pyriform fossa on each side: pledgets are held in place

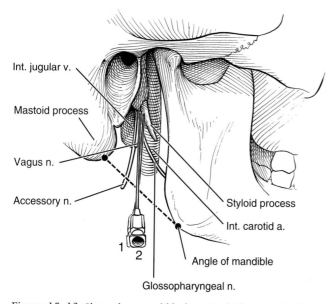

Figure 15–13 Glossopharyngeal block: peristyloid approach. (1) Initial needle position, (2) Final needle position, after bony contact is lost. a., artery; int., internal; n., nerve; v., vein.

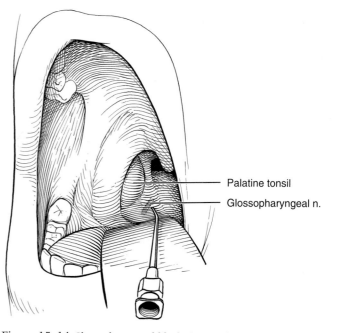

Figure 15–14 Glossopharyngeal block: intraoral anatomy and technique. n., nerve.

for 3 min, and elimination of the gag reflex indicates adequate block. Another pledget is applied to the uvula and posterior pharynx to ensure adequate anesthesia of these structures. Finally, with the tongue retracted, lidocaine spray (4 to 5 times) is directed toward the trachea as the patient inhales to provide anesthesia of the vocal cords and below. At least 15 min is required to provide topical anesthesia for fiberoptic intubation, and rushing results only in inadequate anesthesia. Although large amounts of local anesthetics are given, systemic toxicity is seldom seen, possibly because much of the anesthetic is discarded and does not reach the systemic circulation.[35] Small doses of intravenously administered benzodiazepines at the time of topical application may also serve to decrease systemic toxicity.

Many alternate forms of topical anesthesia have been described,[35-37] and it is important to become familiar with one method that works. Premedication with a drying agent (glycopyrrolate 0.2 to 0.4 mg) is helpful. Patient cooperation is important; excessive sedation is not a substitute for adequate anesthesia and should be avoided.

Miscellaneous Blocks

Accessory Nerve (11th Cranial) Block

Few indications exist for block of the accessory nerve, and it may be unintentionally blocked during superficial cervical plexus block. The nerve passes obliquely caudad and laterally, piercing the deep surface of the sternocleidomastoid muscle. At the posterior border of the sternocleidomastoid muscle at the junction of the upper and middle third, the nerve is superficial in the fascial roof of the posterior triangle, reaching the anterior border of the trapezius muscle, which it supplies. The posterior triangle forms inferiorly by the middle third of the clavicle, anteriorly by the posterior border of the sternocleidomastoid, and laterally by the anterior border of trapezius. At its superficial location in the posterior triangle, the nerve is readily blocked with 10 mL of local anesthetic (1% lidocaine) at the posterior border of the sternocleidomastoid muscle. The principal indication is as an adjunct to interscalene brachial plexus block to prevent trapezius movement.

Several other sensory nerves—the lesser occipital (C-2 to C-3), great auricular (C-2 to C-3), anterior cutaneous (C-2 to C-3), and supraclavicular nerves (C-3 to C-4)—are also found in the posterior triangle[38] and may also be blocked along with the accessory nerve.

Field Block of the Ear

The ear is supplied by cutaneous branches of the spinal and cranial nerves.[39] The auricle is innervated by the great auricular and the lesser occipital nerves, supplying the posterior surface of the ear and a variable portion of the anterior surface, and by the auriculotemporal branch of the mandibular nerve, supplying

the remainder of the anterior surface. The external auditory canal may also be supplied by terminal branches of the facial and glossopharyngeal nerves.

The posterior aspect of the ear may be anesthetized by infiltration close to the posterior aspect of the auricle over the mastoid process with 6 to 10 mL of local anesthetic (Fig. 15–15). The auriculotemporal nerve is blocked by infiltration of 6 to 10 mL of local anesthetic anterior to the ear, beginning at the zygoma. Clinically, this infiltration provides adequate anesthesia for procedures such as otoplasty, reconstruction of the pinna, and excision of cysts. Occasionally, anesthesia of the concha may be inadequate, but it can be blocked with subcutaneous infiltration of 2 to 3 mL of local anesthetic posteriorly through the conchal cartilage.

Sphenopalatine Ganglion Block

The sphenopalatine (pterygopalatine) ganglion located superficially in the pterygopalatine fossa is at a crossroad of structures involved in pain perception and affective components of pain. It receives branches of the petrosal nerves, cervical sympathetic chain, afferent trigeminothalamic fibers, autonomic fibers to the carotid plexus and hypophysis, and neuropeptide-containing neurons to the cerebral vasculature.[40]

Block of the sphenopalatine ganglion may be accomplished by injection, topical anesthesia, or aerosol spray. Injection is with a fine-tipped, 120°-angled needle inserted through the greater palatine foramen at the posterior edge of the hard palate medial to the third molar. The needle is advanced 3 to 5 cm through the foramen, and 2 mL of local anesthetic solution is injected.[41]

A simpler method involves soaking a cotton-tip applicator with a 4% lidocaine solution (Fig. 15–16). The first applicator is passed along the upper border of the

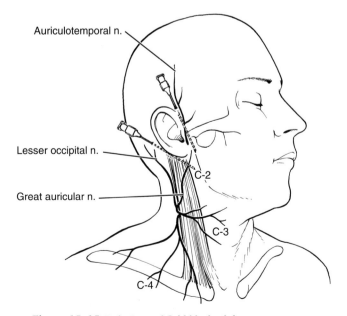

Figure 15–15 Technique of field block of the ear. n., nerve.

inferior turbinate bone to the posterior wall of the pharynx. The second applicator is passed along the upper border of the middle turbinate. Solution (1.0 mL) is deposited along the shaft and left in place for 20 min.[42, 43]

Popularized by Sluder[44] in the early 1900s to treat sphenopalatine ganglion neuralgia, sphenopalatine ganglion block is being promoted as a simple, safe, and effective means of dealing with an assortment of chronic pain problems.[42, 43, 45] Personal experience supports these observations, but controlled studies are lacking.

Occipital Nerve Block

The greater occipital nerve arises from the dorsal rami of the second cervical nerve together with a smaller branch of the third cervical nerve. The nerve supplies the skin over the medial portion of the posterior scalp to the vertex.

The block is performed with the patient sitting and the chin flexed on the chest. The nerve emerges from the cervical musculature, becoming subcutaneous inferior to the superior nuchal line. Local anesthetic (5 mL) is injected at the level of the superior nuchal line one third of the way between the external occipital protuberance and mastoid process. The occipital artery may serve as a landmark, and if paresthesia is encountered, the needle should be withdrawn slightly and the local anesthetic injected in a fanwise distribution (Fig. 15–17).

The block is useful for scalp anesthesia, but its principal use is in the diagnosis and treatment of occipital neuralgia. Occipital block is generally reserved for patients with characteristic pain and headache in the

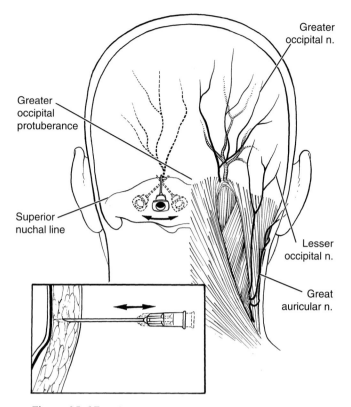

Figure 15–17 Technique of occipital nerve block. n., nerve.

suboccipital region with radiation over the posterior scalp. It is effective in relieving acute headaches, and pain outside the blocked area may also be abolished.[46] Long-term treatment with repeated injection of local anesthetics and corticosteroids has been advocated.[47] In patients receiving temporary benefit, neurosurgeons have advocated sectioning of the second and third cranial roots or the occipital nerves, but controversy exists as to whether neurolysis has long-term benefits.[48]

Conclusion

Many anesthesiologists are reluctant to undertake nerve blocks in the region of the head and neck, but techniques can be mastered with a knowledge of the anatomy. Blocks of the sphenopalatine, occipital, and trigeminal nerve and its branches are useful in pain management. Psychologic aspects of these chronic pain syndromes are important considerations. Each anesthesiologist must develop a personal method of airway block that produces consistently adequate intubating conditions. Thorough preparation is critical for all head and neck blocks because potential complications can occur suddenly and include injection of small volumes of local anesthetic that causes seizures.

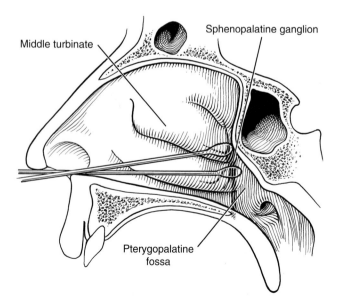

Figure 15–16 Simplified technique of sphenopalatine ganglion block. (Modified from Waldman SD: Evaluation and treatment of common headache and facial pain syndrome. In Raj PP: Practical Management of Pain, 2nd ed, pp 198–218. St. Louis, Mosby–Year Book, 1992.)

References

1. Kozody R, Ready LB, Barsa JE, et al: Dose requirement of local anaesthetic to produce grand mal seizure during stellate ganglion block. Can Anaesth Soc J 1982; 29: 489–491.

2. Brown DL, Hall JA, Ransom DM, et al: Local anesthetic–induced seizures and regional anesthesia: incidence and the absence of bupivacaine-induced cardiovascular collapse. Reg Anesth 1994; 19: 13.

3. Cousins MJ, Bridenbaugh PO (eds): Neural Blockade in Clinical Anesthesia and Management of Pain, 2nd ed. Philadelphia, JB Lippincott, 1988.

4. Hamilton RC, Gimbel HV, Strunin L: Regional anaesthesia for 12,000 cataract extraction and intraocular lens implantation procedures. Can J Anaesth 1988; 35: 615–623.

5. Clemente CD (ed): Gray's Anatomy. Anatomy of the Human Body, 30th American ed. Philadelphia, Lea & Febiger, 1985.

6. Brown DL: Atlas of Regional Anesthesia, pp 121–128. Philadelphia, WB Saunders Co, 1992.

7. Snell RS, Katz J: Clinical Anatomy for Anesthesiologists, pp 233–239. Norwalk, CT, Appleton & Lange, 1988.

8. Rovit RL, Murali R, Jannetta PJ (eds): Trigeminal Neuralgia. Baltimore, Williams & Wilkins, 1990.

9. Loeser JD: What to do about tic douloureux. JAMA 1978; 239: 1153–1155.

10. Taylor WE Jr, Donovan MG: An alternative to the transpalatal maxillary nerve block. Laryngoscope 1989; 99: 109–110.

11. Malamed SF: The Gow-Gates mandibular block. Evaluation after 4,275 cases. Oral Surg Oral Med Oral Pathol 1981; 51: 463–467.

12. Loeser JD, Sweet WH, Tew JM Jr, et al: Neurosurgical operations involving peripheral nerves. In Bonica JJ (ed): The Management of Pain, 2nd ed, vol II, pp 2044–2066. Philadelphia, Lea & Febiger, 1990.

13. Ramamurthy S, Walsh NE, Schoenfeld LS, et al: Evaluation of neurolytic blocks using phenol and cryogenic block in the management of chronic pain. J Pain Symptom Manage 1989; 4: 72–75.

14. Swerdlow M: Complications of neurolytic blockade. In Cousins MJ, Bridenbaugh PO (eds): Neural Blockade in Clinical Anesthesia and Management of Pain, 2nd ed, pp 719–735. Philadelphia, JB Lippincott, 1988.

15. Davies MJ, Mooney PH, Scott DA, et al: Neurologic changes during carotid endarterectomy under cervical block predict a high risk of postoperative stroke. Anesthesiology 1993; 78: 829–833.

16. Davies MJ, Murrell GC, Cronin KD, et al: Carotid endarterectomy under cervical plexus block—a prospective clinical audit. Anaesth Intensive Care 1990; 18: 219–223.

17. Peitzman AB, Webster MW, Loubeau JM, et al: Carotid endarterectomy under regional (conductive) anesthesia. Ann Surg 1982; 196: 59–64.

18. Silbert BS, Koumoundouros E, Davies MJ, et al: Comparison of the processed electroencephalogram and awake neurological assessment during carotid endarterectomy. Anaesth Intensive Care 1989; 17: 298–304.

19. Prough DS, Scuderi PE, Stullken E, et al: Myocardial infarction following regional anaesthesia for carotid endarterectomy. Can Anaesth Soc J 1984; 31: 192–196.

20. Cirone R, Sullivan P, Posner M, et al: Regional vs general anaesthesia for carotid endarterectomy surgery. (Abstract.) Can Anaesth 1994; May; 41: A37.

21. Winnie AP, Ramamurthy S, Durrani Z, et al: Interscalene cervical plexus block: a single-injection technic. Anesth Analg 1975; 54: 370–375.

22. Wong DHW: Regional anaesthesia for intraocular surgery. Can J Anaesth 1993; 40: 635–657.

23. Doxanas MT, Anderson RL: Clinical Orbital Anatomy. Baltimore, Williams & Wilkins, 1984.

24. Feitl ME, Krupin T: Neural blockade for ophthalmologic surgery. In Cousins MJ, Bridenbaugh PO (eds): Neural Blockade in Clinical Anesthesia and Management of Pain, 2nd ed, pp 577–592. Philadelphia, JB Lippincott, 1988.

25. Unsold R, Stanley JA, DeGroot J: The CT-topography of retrobulbar anesthesia. Anatomic-clinical correlation of complications and suggestion of a modified technique. Albrecht Von Graefes Arch Klin Exp Ophthalmol 1981; 217: 125–136.

26. Liu C, Youl B, Moseley I: Magnetic resonance imaging of the optic nerve in extremes of gaze. Implications for the positioning of the globe for retrobulbar anaesthesia. Br J Ophthalmol 1992; 76: 728–733.

27. Katsev DA, Drews RC, Rose BT: An anatomic study of retrobulbar needle path length. Ophthalmology 1989; 96: 1221–1224.

28. Sarvela J, Nikki P: Hyaluronidase improves regional ophthalmic anaesthesia with etidocaine. Can J Anaesth 1992; 39: 920–924.

29. Lewis P, Hamilton RC, Loken RG, et al: Comparison of plain with pH-adjusted bupivacaine with hyaluronidase for peribulbar block. Can J Anaesth 1992; 39: 555–558.

30. Roberts JE, MacLeod BA, Hollands RH: Improved peribulbar anaesthesia with alkalinization and hyaluronidase. Can J Anaesth 1993; 40: 835–838.

31. Davis DB II, Mandel MR: Posterior peribulbar anesthesia: an alternative to retrobulbar anesthesia. J Cataract Refract Surg 1986; 12: 182–184.

32. Loots JH, Venter JA: Posterior peribulbar anaesthesia for intraocular surgery. S Afr Med J 1988; 74: 507–509.

33. Donlon JR: Anesthesia for ophthalmic surgery: an update. Curr Rev Clin Anesth 1989; 9: 114–119.

34. Barton S, Williams JD: Glossopharyngeal nerve block. Arch Otolaryngol 1971; 93: 186–188.

35. Berger R, McConnell JW, Phillips B, et al: Safety and efficacy of using high-dose topical and nebulized anesthesia to obtain endobronchial cultures. Chest 1989; 95: 299–303.

36. Randell T, Yli-Hankala A, Valli H, et al: Topical anaesthesia of the nasal mucosa for fibreoptic airway endoscopy. Br J Anaesth 1992; 68: 164–167.

37. Graham DR, Hay JG, Clague J, et al: Comparison of three different methods used to achieve local anesthesia for fiberoptic bronchoscopy. Chest 1992; 102: 704–707.

38. Berry H, MacDonald EA, Mrazek AC: Accessory nerve palsy: a review of 23 cases. Can J Neurol 1991; 18: 337–341.

39. Kaplan JN, Cummings CW: Pain in the ear, midface, and aerodigestive tract. In Bonica JJ (ed): The Management of Pain, 2nd ed, vol I, pp 769–783. Philadelphia, Lea & Febiger, 1990.

40. Silverman DG, Spencer RF, Kitahata LM, et al: Lack of effect of sphenopalatine ganglion block with intranasal lidocaine on submaximal effort tourniquet test pain. Reg Anesth 1993; 18: 356–360.

41. Katz J: Atlas of Regional Anesthesia, pp 16–17. Norwalk, CT, Appleton-Century-Crofts, 1985.

42. Lebovits AH, Alfred H, Lefkowitz M: Sphenopalatine ganglion block: clinical use in the pain management clinic. Clin J Pain 1990; 6: 131–136.

43. Russell AV: Sphenopalatine ganglion block: the final gate to switching off pain. Pain Monitor 1992; 3(4): 3–4.

44. Sluder G: Etiology, diagnosis, prognosis and treatment of sphenopalatine ganglion neuralgia. JAMA 1913; 61: 1201–1205.

45. Russell AL: Sphenopalatine block—the cheapest technique in the management of chronic pain. (Letter to the editor.) Clin J Pain 1991; 7: 256–257.

46. Sjaastad O: The headache of challenge in our time: cervicogenic headache. Funct Neurol 1990; 5: 155–158.

47. Anthony M: Headache and the greater occipital nerve. Clin Neurol Neurosurg 1992; 94: 297–301.

48. Bovim G, Fredriksen TA, Stolt-Nielsen A, et al: Neurolysis of the greater occipital nerve in cervicogenic headache. A follow up study. Headache 1992; 32: 175–179.

CHAPTER 16
Upper Extremity Blocks

William F. Urmey, M.D.

Regional anesthesia, if performed properly, offers many advantages over general anesthesia for operation on the upper extremity. This chapter focuses on techniques for regional block of the entire upper extremity at the level of the brachial plexus. In addition, descriptions of techniques that are often used clinically for blocking isolated peripheral nerves at the arm, wrist, or hand are included.

Methods of brachial plexus block with local anesthetics have been described since the 19th century. Brachial plexus block can be applied to produce surgical anesthesia, pain relief, or sympathectomy that can, with appropriate technique, cover any site within the entire length of the upper extremity. This includes the skin, subcutaneous tissues, underlying muscles, joints, and bones from the shoulder to the fingertips (with the exception of the small area of skin that is innervated by nerves from the T-2 nerve root).

Numerous clinical studies support local anesthetic block of the brachial plexus as an effective method of providing reliable anesthesia or analgesia of the upper extremity. Some studies have reported success rates approaching 100%,[1, 2] whereas other reports[3] showed failure rates of up to 30%. At the author's institution, more than 1500 brachial plexus blocks are performed annually, representing approximately 20% of the total anesthetic procedures. With success rates in the 97% range,[4] this anesthetic has served as a reliable workhorse. In this chapter, some possible reasons are presented for the large discrepancies in success rates reported for brachial plexus block by various investigators. Only from a thorough understanding of the relevant functional anatomy as well as adherence to some basic principles of proper technique can one achieve excellent success rates with minimal complications.

Anatomy

The brachial plexus arises from the C-5 to T-1 nerve roots (Fig. 16–1). In addition, the plexus infrequently has contributions from either C-4 or T-2. The nerve roots that form the brachial plexus are encased by a layer of fascia that arises from the prevertebral fascia and muscular fascia surrounding the anterior scalene and middle scalene muscles.[5] This fascia is continuous with the fascia that encompasses the cervical plexus.[6] Thus, the cervical and brachial plexuses are continuous, i.e., there is no fascial or fibrous separation between the cervical and brachial plexuses.

The C-5 through T-1 nerve roots fuse to form three distinct trunks: superior, middle, and inferior. The superior trunk is formed from C-5 and C-6. The middle trunk is formed from C-7 alone, and the inferior trunk is formed from the joining together of the C-8 and the T-1 nerve roots.

It is at this level that the tubular neural bundle passes under the clavicle and over the first rib, both important relations of the brachial plexus, and is joined by the subclavian artery to become a neurovascular bundle (Fig. 16–2). It is the fact that the subclavian artery and more distally the axillary artery are so intimately related to the nerves in this neurovascular bundle that allows the anesthesiologist to use the artery as

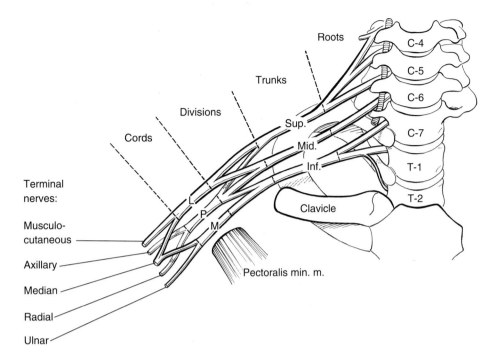

Figure 16–1 Brachial plexus. Inf., inferior; L, lateral; M, medial; m., muscle; Mid., middle; min., minor; P, posterior; Sup., superior.

an important landmark in blocking the plexus. It is these neurovascular anatomic relationships that Winnie[7] has taken advantage of in popularizing the perivascular techniques of brachial plexus block.

Each trunk divides into anterior and posterior divisions. The divisions go on to change orientation and mingle to form three cords, now oriented as the lateral, medial, and posterior cords. These were named to describe their anatomic relationship to the artery. The cords now form, at the level of the axilla, the terminal nerves. These include the musculocutaneous nerve,

which arises from the lateral cord; the median nerve, the lateral root of which comes from the lateral cord and the medial root from the medial cord; the ulnar nerve, the medial brachiocutaneous nerve, and the medial antebrachial cutaneous nerve, all of which arise from the medial cord; and the axillary and radial nerves, which are the terminal nerves of the posterior cord.

The musculocutaneous nerve has motor and sensory fibers. The motor innervation is to the coracobrachialis, brachialis, and biceps muscles. The sensory branch of

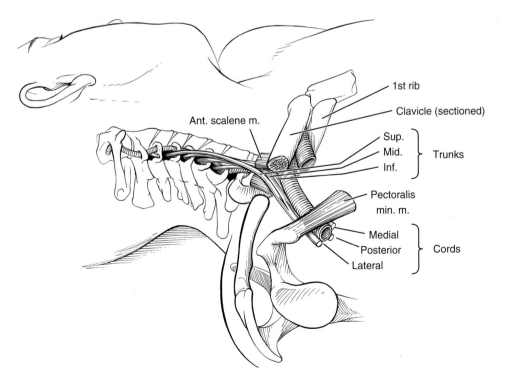

Figure 16–2 Skeletal anatomy of brachial plexus in relation to artery, clavicle, and first rib shows how neural bundle becomes neurovascular bundle. Ant., anterior; Inf., inferior; m., muscle, Mid., middle; min., minor; Sup., superior.

this nerve is the lateral antebrachial cutaneous nerve, which provides sensory innervation to the lateral, mostly flexor, surface of the forearm (Fig. 16–3). Thus, the musculocutaneous nerve arises from the C-5 and C-6 nerve roots, the most cephalad nerve roots in the plexus, but it supplies sensory innervation to the lower forearm. It also exits the plexus proximally, at the level of the coracobrachialis muscle. It is for these anatomic reasons that high incidences of failure to block the musculocutaneous nerve during axillary block have been reported,[8–10] whereas the nerve is reliably blocked by the interscalene route.

The median nerve originates from the C-5 to T-1 nerve roots and has motor and sensory branches. It forms from a joining of the lateral and medial cords and runs in close apposition to the brachial artery. The sensory fibers arise from C-6 to C-8 and supply the palmar surface of the hand, the first three fingers, and half of the fourth finger. The motor fibers arise from C-5 to T-1 and supply the flexor muscles of the hand. Block of the median nerve results in inability to appose the thumb.

The ulnar nerve originates from the C-8 and T-1 nerve roots. It is the major nerve that arises from the medial cord. The ulnar nerve supplies sensory innervation to the medial half of the hand, the fifth finger, and half of the fourth finger. The ulnar nerve gives motor innervation to the interosseous muscles of the hand and to hand flexors in the forearm.

The axillary nerve originates from the posterior cord: the C-5 and C-6 nerve roots. Therefore, it is more reliably blocked by the interscalene route than other brachial techniques. The motor fibers from the axillary nerve innervate the deltoid muscle. Inability to abduct the arm against gravity is an early finding after interscalene brachial plexus block due to block of the axillary nerve. Sensory fibers supply the posterior shoulder and arm.

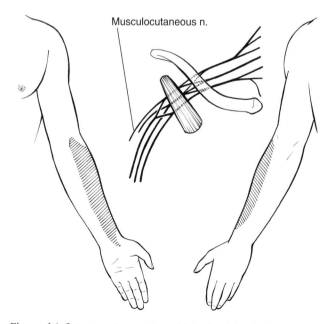

Musculocutaneous n.

Figure 16–3 Sensory innervation of lateral antebrachial cutaneous nerve (n.), which is derived from the musculocutaneous nerve.

The terminal branch of the posterior cord is the radial nerve, which originates from the C-5 to T-1 nerve root. The sensory innervation from this nerve is to the posterior regions of the forearm and hand. The motor innervation supplies the triceps muscle, the extensor muscles of the thumb and fingers, and the brachioradialis muscle. An early sign of axillary brachial plexus block is the inability to extend the arm at the elbow as a result of radial nerve block.

Sympathetic Innervation to the Upper Extremity

The middle and inferior cervical ganglia are closely related to the cervical and brachial plexuses. They are also related to the superior cervical ganglion as well as to each other. Branches from the middle cervical ganglion are associated with the first four spinal nerves.[11] Branches from this ganglion are anatomically related to and receive fibers from the recurrent laryngeal nerve. The inferior cervical ganglion is located between the transverse process of the last cervical vertebra and the neck of the first rib. It sends sympathetic branches anterior to and posterior to the subclavian artery. Thus, the cervical and brachial plexuses of somatic nerves are closely related anatomically to the cervical sympathetics. The inferior cervical sympathetic ganglion is frequently fused with the first thoracic sympathetic ganglion to form the stellate ganglion. The cervical sympathetic chain also has contributions from the upper thoracic nerves that supply preganglionic fibers. Any of these ganglia, therefore, can be blocked by brachial plexus block performed above the clavicle, especially when the block extends into the cervical plexus.

In addition, postganglionic sympathetic fibers associated with somatic nerves from the brachial plexus[12] supply the upper extremity. Therefore, block of the somatic nerves results in sympathetic block to a significant degree. For this reason, brachial or brachial-cervical plexus block causes effective vasodilation of the entire upper extremity. In fact, the sympathetic block that accompanies the somatic nerve block is often used clinically as an early indicator of success. Changes in skin electrical resistance, a secondary phenomenon owing to sympathetic block, have been measured by an ohmmeter.[13] The change in resistance occurred early and was a reliable indicator of subsequent sensory block. The coupling of sympathetic and somatic nerve blocks also explains why a sympathetic block occurs after a wrist block or any block of the peripheral nerves of the arm or hand. Brachial plexus block or peripheral nerve blocks can, therefore, be used for diagnostic or therapeutic vasodilation, including perioperative therapy (e.g., reflex sympathetic dystrophy or post-traumatic reimplantation in the upper extremity).[14, 15]

Anatomic Relations of the Brachial Plexus

It is helpful for the anesthesiologist to have a detailed understanding of the anatomic relationships of the brachial plexus. Success or failure of routine brachial plexus blocks as well as ability to minimize undesired side effects and complications depends on an appreciation of the relevant anatomy. The common approaches to the brachial plexus above or below the clavicle come close to important anatomic structures in the neck, chest, and axilla. Further, many common side effects of the block simply reflect extension of the local anesthetic block to these nearby structures. This, for example, may explain the superior laryngeal nerve block seen after interscalene block. Less frequent side effects as well as the correlation between a specific approach to blocking the plexus and the incidence of a side effect can be readily explained once the anatomy is known.

The brachial plexus can be conceived of as being surrounded by a fibrous sheath[7, 8] that, after injection of local anesthetic distends it, becomes tubular, elongated, or sausage shaped (Fig. 16–4). This fibrous sheath limits flow of the injectant out of what is thought of as the confines of the brachial plexus. This idea has been studied and developed by Winnie and associates,[16] who used this concept to explain and promote efficacy of a single injection into the sheath causing anesthesia of the entire brachial plexus. Although it may not be the tough fibrous sheath that Winnie has proposed, it still forms the basis for a useful model.[17]

The sheath itself arises from the muscular fascia that invests the anterior and middle scalene muscles. Thus, the plexus of nerves must lie between these two mus-

cles. On this basis, the anterior and middle scalene muscles and the subtle groove between them form a reliable landmark. This landmark forms the basis for interscalene block and aids with the subclavian perivascular approach.

Again, the brachial plexus is continuous with the cervical plexus; therefore, an injection of sufficient volume may extend cephalad into the cervical plexus. The cervical plexus gives rise to the phrenic nerve, an important portion of the plexus, which is formed from the C-3 to C-5 nerve roots. Most phrenic fibers are from the fourth cervical nerve. After leaving the cervical plexus, the phrenic nerve is found on the anterior surface of the anterior scalene muscle. It is, therefore, in close proximity to the brachial plexus even after it exits the cervical plexus.

At the level of the first rib, the subclavian artery joins the brachial plexus within the confines of a fascial sheath and thus begins the neurovascular bundle that extends caudad into the axilla. The relationship of the plexus to the subclavian artery, which more distally becomes the axillary artery, forms the basis of the perivascular techniques for anesthetizing the brachial plexus. The subclavian artery lies just inferior and anterior to the plexus immediately superior to the first rib. The first rib is another important landmark that is used in supraclavicular block and forms a backstop to prevent the needle from entering the lung.

The recurrent laryngeal nerve is closely apposed and

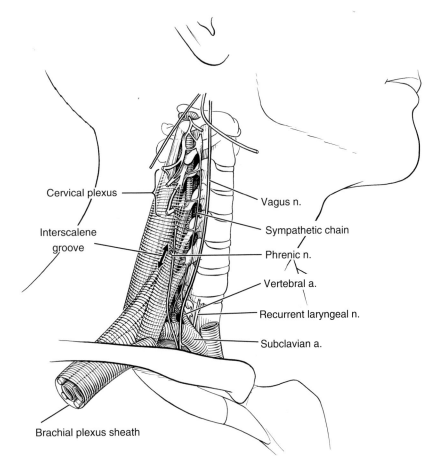

Figure 16–4 Elongated tubular brachial plexus is surrounded by sheath underlying scalene groove and communicating with cervical plexus. a., artery; n., nerve.

Cervical plexus

Interscalene groove

Vagus n.

Sympathetic chain

Phrenic n.

Vertebral a.

Recurrent laryngeal n.

Subclavian a.

Brachial plexus sheath

immediately anterior to the subclavian artery. It may, therefore, be blocked during brachial plexus block.

The vertebral artery is a branch of the subclavian artery. The vertebral artery enters the vertebral foramen at the level of C-6. It is closely related to the brachial plexus, and an injection can unintentionally enter this artery.

Because the nerve roots of the brachial plexus exit from the vertebral transverse processes, rarely, unintentional needle direction can result in an epidural or an intrathecal injection. This may be more likely if the needle is directed too medially or if the needle angle is oriented too horizontally.

Applied Anatomy of the Brachial Plexus

Careful application of knowledge of the anatomy of the brachial plexus and its immediate relations allows the anesthesiologist to maximize brachial plexus block performance and success while minimizing side effects and complications.

The brachial plexus is an elongated anatomic structure that typically extends 6 to 8 cm in the adult from the nerve roots to the terminal nerves in the axilla. As shown in Figure 16–5, injections at different points along the plexus produce different patterns of sensory (and motor) anesthesia. The goal is to target the entry point in the plexus where a single injection produces the desired pattern of anesthesia. The plexus is confined by an outer fascial sheath that has been described as tough and fibrous.[7, 8] Although this may not be entirely true,[17] the idea of an outer limiting sheath has been supported by radiographic contrast studies,[16] methylene blue injection,[17] latex injection,[17] gelatin injection,[18] and anatomic dissection.[17]

Thompson and Rorie[19] described the occurrence of septa—thin connective tissue sheaths in the brachial plexus. Each terminal nerve had its own fascial compartment within the brachial plexus outer sheath. The authors used these findings to help explain the clinical phenomenon of anesthetic sparing in the distribution of a single terminal nerve. On the basis of this study, some have advocated several separate injections and individual nerve location by paresthesia or stimulator. Other investigators[17] studied the anatomy of 18 cadavers and believed they clarified the apparent discrepancy between Thompson and Rorie's findings and the success rate of single-injection techniques. The septa were identified by Partridge and associates,[17] but the nerves were found to communicate at the level of the cords. Further, these septa were thin and appeared to pose only a minimal impediment to spread of dye after single injection.

On the basis of the experience at the author's institution as well as that of others,[1] a single perivascular injection of adequate volume produces anesthesia at a success rate approaching 100%. In the infrequent case in which a single nerve is spared, the septa or the proximity of the nerve to the injection needle may be the explanation.

It is also important to recognize which nerves outside of the brachial plexus are and are not anesthetized by brachial plexus injection. The brachial plexus is in anatomic continuity with the cervical plexus above it (see Fig. 16–4). There is no anatomic "stop sign" that prevents flow upward into the cervical plexus. The author and his colleagues[20] take advantage of this fact when administering anesthesia for shoulder surgery; interscalene block usually anesthetizes C-4 and C-3 nerve roots as well. On the other hand, the T-2 nerve root that forms the intercostobrachial nerve is not included in the brachial plexus. It supplies the skin over the anterior and posterior region of the shoulder (Fig. 16–6). This nerve must be blocked separately or local skin infiltration must be used during most surgical procedures on the shoulder.

Distribution of Local Anesthetic Injected Near the Brachial Plexus

Many factors can influence the distribution of local anesthetic injected near the brachial plexus[16]: point or points of injection, volume, arm position, digital pressure, and use of a tourniquet. Spread of local anesthetic has been measured by radiologic studies of contrast-labeled local anesthetic,[16] by ultrasonography,[21] and by resulting sensory-motor block.[10, 22] The goal of the anesthesiologist is to make maximal use of these factors to promote more complete spread throughout the plexus. More proximal spread is often desired with distal (i.e., axillary) injection, and more distal spread is the goal for proximal (i.e., interscalene) injection. Each of these factors is considered separately below.

Point of Injection

The point of injection along the brachial plexus clearly affects anesthetic distribution within the sheath more than any other factor[10] (see Fig. 16–5). This is most evident when a proximal injection in the plexus sheath, e.g., interscalene block, is compared with distal injection, e.g., axillary block (Fig. 16–7). However, even with the same approach, needle position can affect the resulting block. For example, during axillary block, if the needle is placed high in the proximal axilla, a different distribution of anesthetic is achieved than if injection is made more distally in the axilla.[16] Blocks above the clavicle cause preferential block of the upper brachial and lower cervical portions of the respective plexuses. The axillary and infraclavicular blocks, by contrast, seldom affect the cervical plexus, preferentially blocking the distal portion of the plexus. Supraclavicular and subclavian perivascular blocks anesthetize the middle of the brachial plexus and are probably characterized by the most homogeneous spread of anesthetic throughout the plexus with a single injection point.[10]

Figure 16–5 shows typical sensory distributions of anesthesia after interscalene, subclavian perivascular, axillary, and combined axillary and interscalene blocks. Approaches above the clavicle result in some degree of

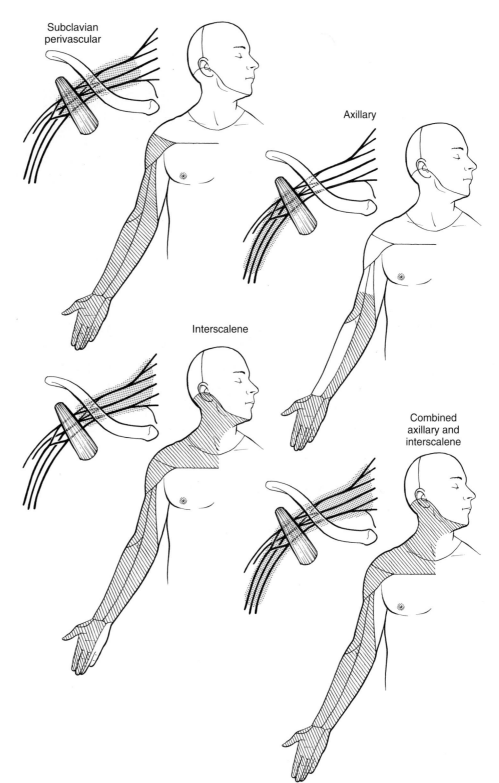

Figure 16–5 Typical distribution of local anesthetic solution in brachial plexus after injection at various points and corresponding typical sensory block patterns are shown.

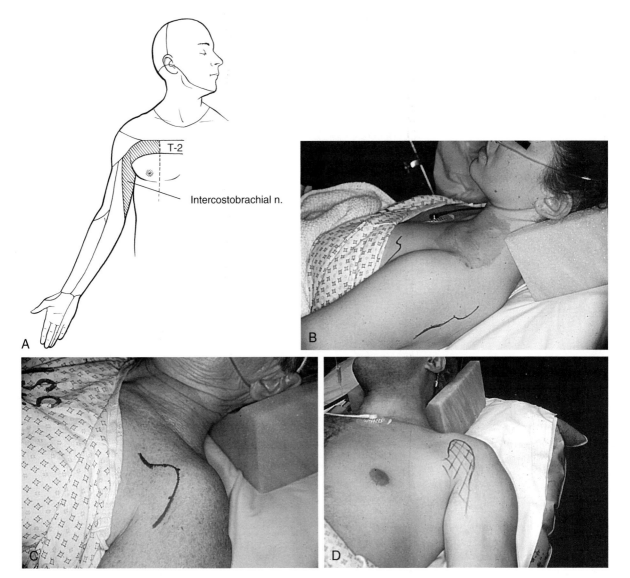

Figure 16–6 *A*, Sensory innervation and course of intercostobrachial nerve (n.) (T-2). Three photographs show real sensory distribution in patients: *B*, no tongue; *C*, small tongue; *D*, large tongue.

cervical sensory anesthesia as well as brachial plexus anesthesia.

The author[23] described a technique in which two injections are made to achieve more complete spread. This technique, called combined axillary/interscalene block, is used routinely by the author for procedures on the elbow to avoid the incidence of pneumothorax associated, albeit rarely, with subclavian perivascular block. This technique typically results in early onset of anesthesia and resulted in ulnar and musculocutaneous nerve block in every case studied in this series. Thus, a complete spread to both ends of the plexus was inferred.

Volume

From measurements in fresh cadavers, de Jong[8] estimated that 42 mL of anesthetic is needed to anesthetize the musculocutaneous nerve during axillary block.

Winnie and colleagues[16] compared spread of radiographic contrast–labeled anesthetic and found more complete spread with 40 mL in interscalene, subclavian perivascular, and axillary blocks compared with blocks with 20 mL. The author and associates[22] noted somewhat less cervical spread when a 25-mL injection for interscalene block was compared with a 45-mL injection. Lanz and coworkers[10] demonstrated that, even with 50-mL injections, the plexus sheath was not completely filled. As a generalization, 40 to 50 mL is necessary to ensure reliable spread if a single-injection technique is chosen. Data from the author and his colleagues[24] showed that higher volumes resulted in an increased success rate during interscalene block.

Digital Pressure

Winnie[25] has advocated the use of digital pressure above the injection site to inhibit cephalad spread of

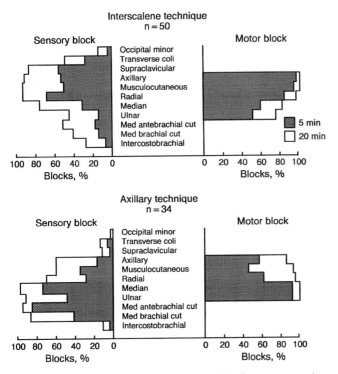

Figure 16–7 Interscalene block and axillary block success rates in providing sensory and motor anesthesia of separate peripheral nerve distributions of the upper extremity. cut, cutaneous; Med., medial. (From Lanz E, Theiss D, Jankovic D: The extent of blockade following various techniques of brachial plexus block. Anesth Analg 1983; 62: 55–58.)

local anesthetic solution during interscalene block. This was supported by radiographic contrast studies in which photographs were taken immediately after injection. The author and colleagues[22] made clinical measurements that showed no difference in several variables indicating block extent and success between groups randomly assigned to interscalene block with or without digital pressure (Fig. 16–8). There was an early delayed onset in high cervical sensory anesthesia to pinprick in the digital pressure group, but there was no significant difference between the groups by 5 min after injection. Thus, the ability to manipulate the distribution of local anesthetic in the brachial plexus by digital pressure appears to be transient, with eventual spread occurring after withdrawal of the pressure, at least with higher volumes (45 mL). Further, vagal reactions may be precipitated by digital pressure on the neck. Bradycardia and asystole have occurred during interscalene block[26] (author's unpublished observations). For this reason, the author advocates the use of digital pressure only with axillary block where pressure against the humerus may be used to limit caudad spread of anesthetic solution.

Applications of Brachial Plexus Block

Brachial plexus block is a versatile and reliable regional anesthetic technique with multiple applications. Advantages of brachial plexus block compared with

general anesthesia are listed in Table 16–1. These include early dismissal of the patient from the recovery room (or to home for the outpatient[27]). With appropriate postanesthetic instructions and in the absence of surgical contraindications, the patient can be dismissed from the ambulatory unit while the upper extremity remains anesthetized. Brachial plexus block promotes a smooth transition to pain control by regional, parenteral, or oral administration of analgesics.

Brandl and Taeger[28] compared interscalene block combined with general anesthesia to general anesthesia alone in patients undergoing shoulder surgery. They noted that 35% of patients with the interscalene block did not require additional analgesics in the first 24 h postoperatively and that only 32% needed opioids. This contrasted with the patients who received general anesthesia alone: 95% required analgesics in the first 24 h, and 86% needed opioids. This may be attributed, in part, to a preemptive analgesic effect similar to that measured after other regional anesthesia techniques.[29]

An exciting new concept and application of this preemptive analgesia by using a nerve sheath or plexus block may be taken advantage of after extremity amputation. Fisher and Meller[30] showed that postoperative continuous regional analgesia administered by a catheter, which had been directly placed in a transected nerve sheath, resulted in complete absence of phantom limb pain in 11 patients during a 12-month period. This occurred despite the presence of preoperative limb pain. This study involved lower limb amputees. However, the implications for brachial plexus infusions of local anesthetic in upper limb amputees and reflex sympathetic dystrophy patients are obvious.

Brachial plexus infusions are often used to increase upper extremity blood flow,[31] e.g., for hand reimplantation procedures. Brachial plexus infusion of local anesthetic has been used to reverse vascular insufficiency in exacerbations of Raynaud's disease (author's unpublished information) and after hand surgery.[32] Although it is difficult to study, it may be theorized that brachial plexus block decreases the incidence of reflex sympathetic dystrophy after hand or arm surgery.

Continuous brachial plexus block is used frequently at the author's institution to allow patients to undergo continuous passive motion at the elbow joint by machine (Fig. 16–9). Early postoperative continuous motion helps to minimize the formation of intra-articular adhesions and thereby maximizes postoperative function.

Interscalene block has many applications (Table

Table 16–1 Advantages of Brachial Plexus Block Compared With General Anesthesia

Early dismissal for outpatients
Smooth transition to pain control
Increased blood flow to extremity
Theoretic decrease in incidence of reflex sympathetic dystrophy
Less nausea and vomiting
Less drowsiness
Less urinary retention
Tracheal intubation not required

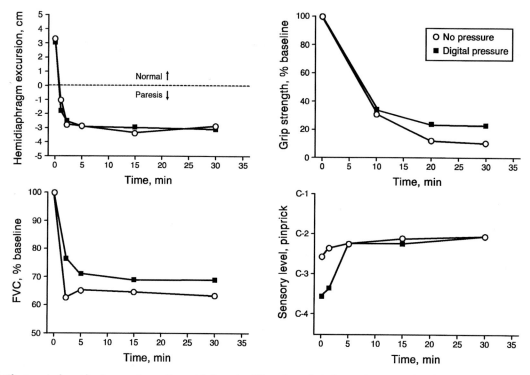

Figure 16–8 Changes in hemidiaphragmatic motion with forced sniffing, forced vital capacity (FVC), hand grip strength (dynamometry), and sensory anesthesia (pinprick) as a function of time from interscalene block (time zero). Digital pressure resulted in no significant clinical differences after 5 min. (Data from Urmey WF, Gloeggler PJ, Parab S, et al: Does a digital pressure technique for interscalene block alter measurable sensory, motor, or diaphragm effects? [Abstract.] Anesth Analg 1992; 74: S327.)

16–2) but is used mostly to provide excellent anesthesia for shoulder operation.[24] It offers some advantages over general anesthesia. These include easy patient positioning and maintenance of intraoperative position, because shoulder surgery is being performed increasingly in the "beach chair" or sitting position[33] (Fig. 16–10). Newer applications of interscalene block include a report on its use for pacemaker insertion[34] and its use for carotid endarterectomy.

Axillary block has many uses and is preferable for distal upper extremity procedures. Axillary block allows the use of an occlusive tourniquet on the arm for bloodless hand surgery. Supraclavicular or subcla-vian perivascular block is ideal for elbow surgery but is associated with a small but finite incidence of pneumothorax. As more and more upper extremity operations are performed in the outpatient setting, an alternative to subclavian perivascular or supraclavicular block that is as effective for elbow surgery is combined axillary and interscalene block.[23] This technique divides a large (50 to 55 mL) dose of local anesthetic solution between these conventional injection sites. Another modification of supraclavicular block that may decrease the incidence of pneumothorax has been developed by Brown and colleagues.[35]

The infraclavicular approach has been used for postoperative analgesia after modified radical mastectomy and upper extremity surgery.[36]

Approaches to Anesthetizing the Brachial Plexus

There have been many approaches to the brachial plexus described in the literature. Historically, various

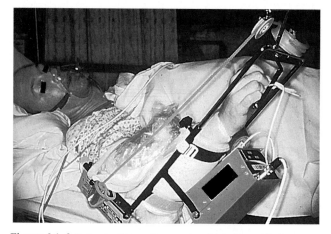

Figure 16–9 Patient with continuous brachial plexus block undergoing continuous passive motion at the elbow by machine.

Table 16–2 Interscalene Block Applications

Shoulder surgery
Humeral fractures
Elbow surgery
Neck surgery—carotid endarterectomy
Brachial plexus exploration
Cervical sympathetic block
Phrenic nerve block
Postoperative analgesia

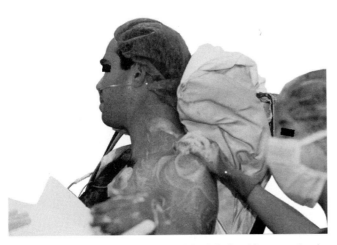

Figure 16–10 Patient being prepared for left shoulder operation in the sitting or beach chair position.

approaches were made at different levels, often with multiple injections or fanning of the injection needle. These approaches evolved through the work of many regional anesthesiologists (many of whom were surgeons) during the past century. Today, four major techniques are used routinely: (1) interscalene block, (2) supraclavicular or subclavian perivascular block, (3) infraclavicular block, and (4) axillary block.

Interscalene Block

The interscalene block was first described by Winnie in 1970.[5] There have been only minor modifications in the technique since its first description. This approach takes advantage of the relatively constant anatomic relationship between the brachial plexus and the anterior and middle scalene muscles. Because the fascia surrounding the brachial plexus originates from the muscular fascia of the anterior and middle scalene muscles, the nerves must lie between the two muscles in the interscalene groove.

This technique can be performed with paresthesia or nerve stimulator to determine needle position near the plexus. However, the author prefers the single paresthesia technique originally described by Winnie because of the high success rate.

To elicit paresthesia, it is important that the patient not be overly sedated. A clouded sensorium can often interfere with the perception of paresthesias or with communication between the patient and the anesthesiologist. The anesthesiologist should give clear instructions to the patient that a small pinch will be felt as the needle passes through skin. After that, a small tingle or dull ache or pain in the shoulder, arm, or hand will be felt. The patient is instructed to immediately notify the anesthesiologist when this feeling occurs by saying "Now" or "Stop" and then describing the location verbally without moving, looking, or pointing to the spot where it is felt. The patient should be warned that the feeling may intensify with injection and there may be a transient perception of burning or tingling down the arm.

After appropriate monitoring, including the electrocardiogram and pulse oximetry, the patient is placed in the supine position. The patient's head and shoulders should be at the same level, i.e., pillows should be removed and the operating room table straightened. The patient's neck is cleansed with an antiseptic. A 23-G, 2.5-cm needle can be used in most patients. Occasionally, a 3.7-cm needle is needed in large or obese patients. A needle longer than 3.7 cm has never been needed in the author's experience. The patient's head should be turned away from the side of the block at an approximately 45° angle with the table or bed surface. The interscalene groove is located by palpation (Fig. 16–11). The posterior border of the lateral head (clavicular head) of the sternocleidomastoid muscle is palpated at the approximate level of the cricoid cartilage (C-6). It is usually necessary to have the patient raise the head a few inches off the bed or table for the anesthesiologist to adequately feel the posterior border of the sternocleidomastoid muscle. The fingers are then rolled laterally over the anterior scalene muscle (which usually lies partly under the sternocleidomastoid). A subtle narrow groove is identified just lateral to that. If the scalene muscles cannot be appreciated, have the patient take a slow, deep breath through the nose. This may help to accentuate the muscles by giving them increased tone.[37] The reason for this is that the scalene muscles are respiratory muscles and have been found by electromyographic studies to be active with every inspiration.[38] Once classified as accessory muscles of respiration, they have since been reclassified by respiratory physiologists as a result of these electromyographic data.

The needle is introduced slowly, moving millimeter by millimeter in a dorsal, medial, and caudal direction. This direction is not necessary for entering the sheath, but it helps to avoid unintentional entry into the vertebral artery, epidural space, or subarachnoid space.[5] Thus, the direction is chosen to be the opposite of the strategy used to deliberately enter the epidural space, where a cephalad and ventral direction is used.

As stated previously, the patient identifies when a paresthesia is felt. The paresthesia may be to the shoulder, arm, or hand. Shoulder paresthesias, once thought to be inadequate (for fear of misinterpreting stimulation of the suprascapular nerve during its course outside of the plexus), have been found to be as reliable as more distal paresthesias[39] and are routinely accepted at the author's institution. Shoulder paresthesias occur as the first perceived paresthesia in approximately 50% of patients. Increased success as well as less patient discomfort and, theoretically, less potential for neurapraxia may be attained through acceptance of the shoulder paresthesia.

If the presence of a paresthesia is reliably articulated by the patient, after a negative result of aspiration for blood, 40 to 50 mL of local anesthetic is injected in approximately 5-mL divided doses by using an immobile needle technique with extension tubing.

With larger volumes, a visible swelling appears in most patients, defining the inferior portion of the supraclavicular brachial plexus (Fig. 16–12). Onset of

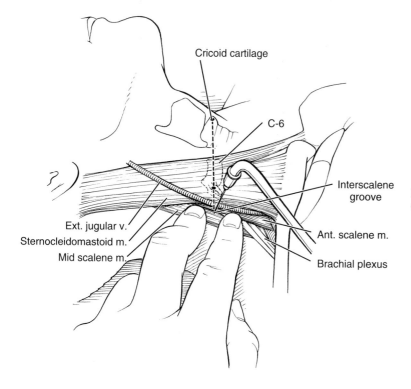

Figure 16–11 Interscalene block. Ant., anterior; Ext., external; m., muscle; v., vein.

block sufficient for operation usually takes approximately 15 min. However, early signs can be used to predict block success. Pinprick testing within 2 min shows decreased sensation on the superior aspect of the shoulder or the C-5 or the C-6 dermatome. This occurs earliest because the block is performed at this level. Inability to raise or abduct the straightened arm against gravity follows within a few minutes (the deltoid sign). A perceptible decrease in handgrip strength may be seen, and pronation of the hand during maximal grip is usually noted. Horner's syndrome on the side of the block can be used for confirmation of the accompanying sympathetic block. However, the appearance of Horner's syndrome does not necessarily indicate successful interscalene block, because the stel-

late ganglion can be blocked without blocking the plexus.

The intercostobrachial nerve (T-2 dermatome) is typically outside of the brachial plexus. Although the T-2 dermatome is usually illustrated in textbooks as in Figure 16–6A, a variable "tongue" or "tail" of T-2 may be present (see Fig. 16–6B to D). This is often in the incision line of an anterior shoulder procedure. Surgeons must be encouraged to infiltrate the T-2 dermatome with local anesthetic. Similarly, a posterior area for posterior incisions or arthroscopy portals may require subcutaneous infiltration with local anesthetic. The underlying joint, bone, and muscles of the shoulder are innervated by the brachial plexus.

Supraclavicular or Subclavian Perivascular Block

The supraclavicular approach to the brachial plexus was first described by Kulenkampff in 1911.[40] This was the first technique described for percutaneous infiltration of the brachial plexus.[41] Because of its simplicity and efficacy, supraclavicular block was the most popular method of anesthetizing the brachial plexus for decades.[42] Kulenkampff's technique, with minor variations, has been termed the "classic or traditional"[43] method of supraclavicular block. This block is characterized by a typically fast onset and complete block with local anesthetic.[10] This occurs because the plexus is blocked where it is most compact. The classic supraclavicular block is avoided by some investigators, owing to reports[35, 44] of the incidence of pneumothorax, ranging from 2% to 6%.

In part because of the association with pneumotho-

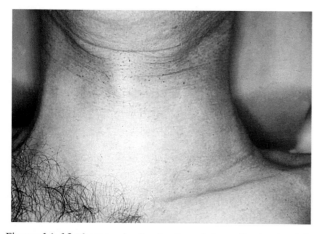

Figure 16–12 Photograph of patient's neck immediately after left interscalene block. Note swelling and loss of landmarks on the side of the block.

rax and after careful reevaluation of brachial plexus anatomy, the subclavian perivascular technique was developed by Winnie and Collins in 1964.[45] This technique uses the presence of the subclavian artery in the neurovascular bundle as the main landmark and avoids "walking" the needle over the first rib in search of multiple paresthesias and multiple injections (Fig. 16–13). The needle is directed away from the cupula of the lung and theoretically is associated with a lower incidence of pneumothorax. However, pneumothorax is still reported, and the needle tip is in close proximity to the lung's apex. Another problem with the technique is unintentional arterial puncture, which has been reported[46] in up to 25% of cases by anesthesiologists experienced with the technique. In this anatomic area, compression of the subclavian artery in an attempt to stop bleeding after puncture is not always effective. Hematoma formation has been reported[47] up to 20% of the time after arterial puncture.

Other modifications of the traditional supraclavicular technique designed to increase success while minimizing the incidence of pneumothorax have been described. Korbon and colleagues[48] advocated first rib palpation to improve the ease of performance while theoretically decreasing the chance of pneumothorax. Brown and associates[35] devised an anatomically sound approach to supraclavicular block that was designed to minimize pneumothorax. This technique uses a 5- to 6-cm needle on the lateral border of the sternocleidomastoid at the clavicle. A "plumb bob" parasagittal orientation of the needle is used to seek a paresthesia. Moorthy and coworkers[49] proposed a new modification, the supraclavicular lateral perivascular approach. This may be safer, but Moorthy et al reported a success rate of only 72% despite the necessity of a nerve stimulator and Doppler probe to perform the technique as described.

Classic Technique of Supraclavicular Block

A skin wheal is made over the midclavicle posterior to the subclavian artery. A 3.7-cm, 22-G needle is introduced caudally until bone is encountered. The needle is then walked over the first rib until a paresthesia is obtained. The site of paresthesia may correlate with success.[46] Middle or inferior trunk paresthesias may be preferable. The patient notifies the anesthesiologist, as during interscalene block. After a negative result of aspiration, 40 mL of local anesthetic solution is injected in increments.

Technique of Subclavian Perivascular Block

The subclavian artery is palpated immediately lateral to the clavicular head of the sternocleidomastoid muscle at the C-6 (cricoid cartilage) level in the interscalene groove. A 3.7-cm needle is inserted directly caudally immediately posterior to the palpated subclavian arterial pulse. The patient communicates when a paresthesia is felt. The first rib provides a backstop that prevents unintentional entry into the pleural space. Injection of 40 mL is made after a negative result of aspiration.

Infraclavicular Block

The infraclavicular block was described by Raj and colleagues[50] in 1973. It is rarely used for surgical anesthesia, but it is useful when several days of continuous analgesia are needed for acute or chronic pain treatment. Its advantages here are similar to those cited for a subclavian central venous catheter, i.e., the catheter is relatively immobile and easily dressed. The problem with the block is that the needle is introduced in a location distant from the brachial plexus and therefore requires a long needle.

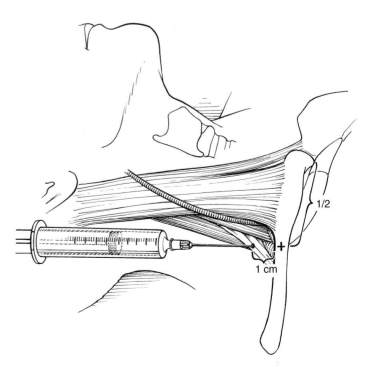

Figure 16–13 Supraclavicular block (classic technique).

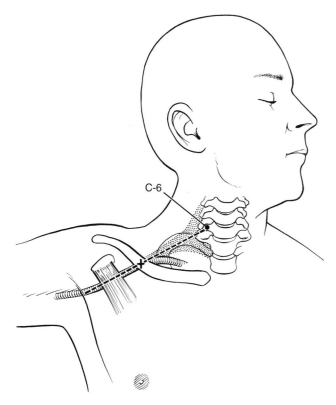

Figure 16–14 Reference line connecting C-6 tubercle and brachial artery through midclavicle for the infraclavicular technique of Raj et al.[50]

A line is determined between the C-6 tubercle and the brachial artery through the midclavicle (Fig. 16–14). After local infiltration, a needle at least 8.7 cm long is attached to a variable nerve stimulator and introduced at a point approximately 2.5 cm below the midclavicle and directed toward the brachial artery. Muscular twitching at the wrist or hand is sought. The point of maximal twitching with minimal current <1 mA is determined. Local anesthetic (1 mL) is injected. If this stops the twitching, the remainder of the dose is injected in aliquots after negative results of frequent aspirations for blood. A catheter is then threaded either through the needle or over the needle if an extracatheter system is used.

Axillary Block

Axillary block was first described by Hirschel in 1911.[51] It is at present the most popular of brachial plexus block techniques. Axillary block differs from approaches to the plexus above the clavicle in that it is performed at the level of the terminal nerves of the plexus. The resulting pattern of anesthesia, therefore, is not dermatomal, as it is after interscalene block. For this reason, it is not unusual for a single nerve to be spared with this approach. Sparing of single nerves may occur in part because of the presence of the septa, but usually only a single injection is necessary for complete brachial plexus block.

The axillary approach is unique in that any one of three techniques—transarterial, paresthesia, or nerve stimulator—can achieve high success rates. Attempts have been made to compare these three techniques during axillary block.[52, 53] Goldberg and associates[3] most recently compared all three techniques in 59 patients. However, the highest success rate they reported was only 80%. These investigators reported no difference in success among techniques, but this information is of doubtful significance considering their low overall success. The highest success rate in a large series has been reported with the transarterial technique by Cockings et al.[1] In this study, supervised residents achieved a 99% success rate. This author's experience agrees with these findings. At The Hospital for Special Surgery, the transarterial technique is the preferred method of axillary block, with success rates approaching 100%. A transarterial technique often yields a paresthesia,[54] although it is not deliberately elicited. The technique can be converted easily to another technique if this happens.

Although the nerves are frequently illustrated in textbooks as surrounding the axillary artery in a standard fashion, there is some variability in location[17] (Fig. 16–15). Similarly, the vein may be located outside the neurovascular bundle in a small percentage of patients. For this reason and because of the frequent inability to aspirate blood with a small needle in a vein, a transvenous technique for axillary block cannot be recommended. If venous blood is encountered, it is best to remove the needle and begin again.

The patient may be lightly sedated for a transarterial technique. If the anesthesiologist is seeking a paresthesia, it is necessary to ensure the patient is not oversedated. With the patient in the supine position, the arm is elevated to 90° (Fig. 16–16). The patient's artery is located between the index and middle fingers of the anesthesiologist. A 23-G, 2.5-cm needle is adequate except for obese patients, in which case a 22-G, 3.7-

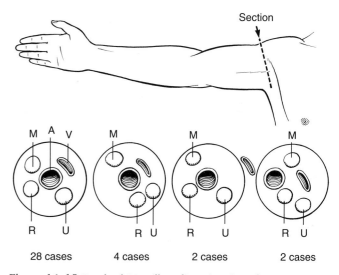

Figure 16–15 Result of 36 axillary dissections in cadavers. Note variable anatomy. A, artery; M, median nerve; R, radial nerve; U, ulnar nerve; V, vein. (Redrawn from Partridge BL, Katz J, Benirschke K: Functional anatomy of the brachial plexus sheath: implications for anesthesia. Anesthesiology 1987; 66: 743–747.)

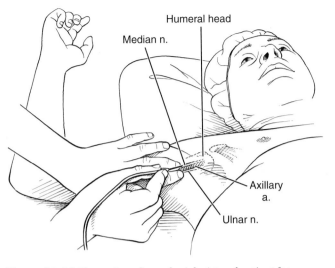

Figure 16–16 Illustration of anesthesiologist and patient for axillary block. Patient's arm bent at 90°. Anesthesiologist's fingers straddle artery (a.); humeral head is shown and facilitates plexus fixation. n., nerve.

cm needle suffices. With light digital pressure, with the nondominant hand, the artery is fixed against the humeral head high in the axilla. The needle is advanced slowly until blood is aspirated or paresthesia is reported. If a paresthesia is obtained, after negative aspiration for blood, the total volume of 40 to 50 mL of local anesthetic solution is injected in 5-mL increments with aspiration between injections. If arterial blood is obtained, the needle is continued slowly forward. The tendency of most novices is to plunge through the artery. This practice defeats the aim of ensuring that the needle tip is stationed as close as possible to the deep aspect of the axillary artery. When blood is no longer aspirated, the local anesthetic is injected, in increments, all behind the artery. After approximately 20-mL total injection volume, and again after 35-mL injection (or any time when needle or patient movement is suspected), the needle can be brought slowly back with continued aspiration until arterial blood is aspirated again. This reconfirms proper position in the plexus. The needle is advanced about 1 mm until blood can no longer be aspirated, and then the injection is completed.

After completion of the injection, the arm is lowered to the side. This may decrease impingement of the humeral head on the plexus and help promote cephalad spread of anesthetic solution in the sheath.[7] Firm digital pressure is applied over the injection site for a few minutes if a transarterial technique is used.

An early sign of block success is loss of ability to extend the arm against gravity at the elbow as a result of radial nerve block.

Techniques for Identifying the Brachial Plexus

Because the brachial plexus is confined by a fascial sheath, injection within the limits of the sheath pro-

duces plexus anesthesia in most cases. Therefore, accuracy in determining entry into the sheath correlates with success rate. Analogous to epidural anesthesia, there are different methods for determining entry into the sheath. Some generalizations and guidelines apply to these methods, independent of the brachial plexus approach.

The plexus is surrounded by fascia. Some advocate using tactile feedback when the needle passes through this fascia[41] to determine that the needle is within the sheath. The feeling of a "pop" or "fascial click" (especially with the use of a short-bevel needle) can sometimes be used. Partridge and coworkers[17] found that in fresh cadavers when needles were placed by experienced anesthesiologists using this method, subsequent dissection revealed a poor correlation with sheath entry. There are other anatomic structures that can simulate this click, and therefore this technique is not recommended.

Paresthesia Technique

Deliberate search for a paresthesia is a long-standing, tried and true method of determining position within the brachial plexus. Some authors have advised seeking multiple paresthesias.[55] Winnie's[25] concept of a single fascial injection decreased this practice, although considerable debate continues about these varied techniques.

The most important concern with the paresthesia technique is the rare occurrence of nerve damage from the needle or intraneural injection.[56] This is largely theoretic, however. No well-controlled study has demonstrated a significant increase in postoperative neurapraxia with a paresthesia technique. Selander et al[54] compared the paresthesia technique with the transarterial technique during axillary block. There was an insignificant increase in postoperative neurapraxias in the paresthesia group. These were transient sequelae, however, and any clinical significance is doubtful. Considering all these data, the author believes it is best to use a small needle, minimize multiple painful paresthesias, and keep patients lightly sedated during brachial plexus block.

Transarterial Technique

The transarterial technique takes advantage of the fact that the sheath is a neurovascular sheath and uses a periarterial position to ensure needle position within the sheath. Because the neural sheath becomes a neurovascular sheath at the level of the subclavian artery, a transarterial technique can only be used at this level or distal to this level, i.e., not for interscalene block. It is not the recommended technique, however, for subclavian perivascular or supraclavicular injection for two reasons. First, it is not always effective,[47] with only a 37% to 40% success rate in one study. Second and more importantly, it is difficult to apply effective compression of the subclavian artery, and therefore the risk of hematoma makes this approach inadvisable. In the study by Hickey and associates,[47] a 12% to 20% hematoma rate was encountered.

The transarterial approach is not contraindicated in the axilla, where, by contrast, it has perhaps the highest reported success rate[1] and an acceptable rate of side effects. Lower success rates have also been reported, which may illustrate the importance of the anesthesiologist in any anesthesia technique.[3, 9] The transarterial technique may be associated with a different distribution of anesthetic,[52] and this may explain the possible high success rate. Axillary hematoma may occur and may cause nerve compression,[54] but this is exceedingly rare, easily diagnosed, and should be easily treated in this accessible anatomic area.

Nerve Stimulator Technique

The nerve stimulator assists in positioning the needle tip near the brachial plexus, with reported high success rates.[53, 57] Success rates as low as 79% have also been reported.[58] Success is maximized if certain principles are followed for nerve stimulator use. These include use of an insulated needle[59] and negative polarity for the needle, which has been shown to decrease the amount of current necessary for stimulation. Use of an uninsulated needle has been shown[59] to lead to errors in placement of up to 0.8 cm. In addition, attention to the motor response itself may alter success. For instance, with axillary block, eliciting elbow flexion is not as effective as wrist flexion.[58] Stimulation should begin in the 3- to 5-mA range and be decreased until less than 1 mA produces the characteristic motor response. The lowest current should be sought that results in appropriate motor response. Once this is achieved, 1 mL of local anesthetic solution should be injected. If twitching does not stop abruptly, it may indicate that the needle is outside the plexus and the anesthesiologist should reposition the needle. This small injection to inhibit stimulation presumably works as a test not by causing instant anesthesia of the stimulated nerve (saline or air injection produces the same effect) but rather by altering the internal milieu that allows for minimal current to elicit motor contractions. The presumed reason for failure with this technique is either direct muscle stimulation or needle stimulation of peripheral nerves through the fascia in some cases.

In conclusion, there are many ways to determine proper position of the injection needle in the plexus. Some methods have higher success rates for a given brachial plexus block approach. More important than the technique used, however, is the experience of the anesthesiologist. Success achieved with any of these techniques improves with increased clinical experience.

Continuous Brachial Plexus Block

Continuous brachial plexus block was first described by Ansbro,[60] who used a catheter technique in 1946. It has increased in popularity because of the development of lengthy microvascular techniques for limb reimplantation[15] and the more widespread use of postoperative analgesia by infusion techniques. The continuous technique finds frequent use at the author's institution for patients undergoing elbow surgery who benefit from continuous passive motion (see Fig. 16–9). Compass-hinge procedures to increase range of motion of the elbow joint, thereby preventing ankylosis (Fig. 16–17), are excellent applications of the technique.

Extracatheter techniques[14, 61] as well as various techniques for placing catheters through the needle[15, 26] have been used. Success rates close to 95% have been reported.[15] Large doses of anesthetic have been used without reported toxic reactions.[62–64] However, the accumulation of local anesthetic active metabolites may present a new problem after prolonged infusion.[65] Rosenberg and colleagues[26] found that systemic bupivacaine concentration increased between 12 and 24 h after start of infusion. The concentrations of its metabolites, desbutylbupivacaine and 4-hydroxybupivacaine, continued to increase and were at their peak levels at the end of a 48-h infusion of 0.25% bupivacaine.[66] This has important implications for any prolonged infusions of bupivacaine.

When continuous brachial plexus block is performed, a nerve stimulator technique is most often used. The interscalene, subclavian perivascular, or axillary approach can be used. The interscalene and subclavian perivascular routes are more stable and the catheter site is more easily dressed than with the axillary route. However, the axillary route is used by many for elbow, forearm, or hand analgesia. To ensure anesthesia, an initial dose of 40 to 50 mL of local anesthetic is administered. After the procedure, a continuous infusion of a more dilute solution (e.g., bupivacaine 0.25%) is started at a rate of 6 to 10 mL/h, depending on patient size and comfort. With proper nursing care, patients can be dismissed from the recovery room to a postsurgical care floor. The catheter should be free of injection ports and carefully labeled to avoid unintentional injections that may be intended as intravenous.

Local Anesthetic Choice

The ideal local anesthetic for brachial plexus block, independent of approach, combines several properties. It should have (1) rapid onset characteristics, (2) adequate potency to ensure complete sensory and motor nerve block, (3) adequate duration for the planned procedure, and (4) low toxicity. Mepivacaine or lidocaine 1.5% with freshly added epinephrine (unless contraindicated) provides excellent anesthesia for most routine procedures. Bupivacaine (and now ropivacaine) or a continuous technique can be used for longer procedures or to offer postoperative analgesia. Longer-acting local anesthetics may not be suitable for shorter procedures for two primary reasons. First, if a long duration of anesthesia is not needed, long-acting local anesthetics make it difficult to assess return of nerve function. Second, prolonged regional block may put

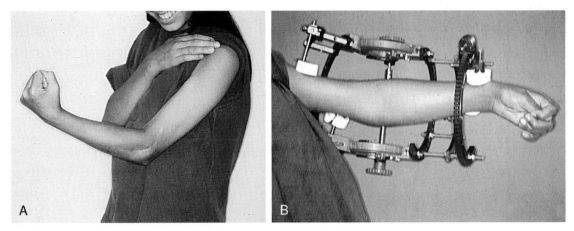

Figure 16–17 *A*, Patient with ankylosed elbow joint after fracture. *B*, Compass hinge allows flexion and extension for months postoperatively, preventing recurrence of ankylosis after open reduction.

patients at risk of postoperative nerve injuries from unrecognized pressure on upper extremity nerves or stretching from malpositioning.

Typical durations of the local anesthetics commonly used for brachial plexus block are shown in Table 16–3. Lidocaine and mepivacaine are of intermediate duration. Another intermediate-duration local anesthetic that is associated with lower toxicity is prilocaine. This drug has been shown to have similar blocking properties in 1.5% concentration as lidocaine. Prilocaine is characterized by shorter duration (2.3 h versus 3.9 h in one study[67]) compared with lidocaine, when both drugs have epinephrine added. Methemoglobinemia is almost nonexistent as a problem with the usual doses used for brachial plexus block. This issue appears to have been overstated in the literature and in physician education in general. In view of the newer data on systemic accumulation of local anesthetics or their metabolites (or both), prilocaine, by virtue of its rapid metabolism and low toxicity,[67] may prove more advantageous than other local anesthetics. Its shorter duration may be beneficial for shorter outpatient procedures, where it should result in quicker recovery. Nevertheless, prilocaine is no longer commercially available in the United States.

Bupivacaine and ropivacaine with epinephrine have been shown to provide profound sensory-motor anesthesia of 9 to 11 h duration[68, 69] and analgesia persisting up to 24 h. Ropivacaine has anesthetic characteristics similar to those of bupivacaine, but it is associated with less cardiotoxicity. It will soon be available for routine clinical use in the United States.

As important as the choice of agent is the concentration used, because the number of milligrams of local anesthetic as well as the volume of injectant contributes to the ultimate success of the block. At present, the author uses mepivacaine or lidocaine in 1.5% to 2% concentrations. Bupivacaine can be used in the 0.5% or 0.75% concentration[66] when the injection is above the clavicle. Bupivacaine 0.5% allows for an adequate volume to be used without significantly exceeding suggested toxic limits. Although 0.25% bupivacaine has been used by many anesthesiologists, there is evidence that this may result in an unacceptable degree of block failure. In a study by Hickey and coworkers,[70] there was a 41% failure rate for bupivacaine 0.25% and a 36% failure rate for ropivacaine 0.25%. Hickey et al[69] have published data with only a 9% failure rate for bupivacaine or ropivacaine in 0.5% concentration.

Pharmacologic agents have been added to local anesthetics in attempts to improve onset, quality, and duration of local anesthetic effect in brachial plexus block. Epinephrine is widely used in regional anesthesia to prolong duration and quality of nerve blocks. Epinephrine's mechanism of action is believed to be mostly through its α-receptor blocking properties. This action decreases systemic absorption and thereby allows additional local anesthetic to remain in the plexus. Epinephrine is used routinely at the author's institution for this reason as well as to detect unintentional intravascular injection. Epinephrine is usually added to the local anesthetic to achieve an approximate 5 μg/mL final concentration. Epinephrine also allows

Table 16–3 Typical Duration of Local Anesthetics for Brachial Plexus Block

LOCAL ANESTHETIC	DOSE, mL	DURATION OF SURGICAL ANESTHESIA, h
Prilocaine 1.5%	40–55	1.5–3
Lidocaine 1.5% with epinephrine	40–55	2–4
Mepivacaine 1.5% with epinephrine	40–55	3–5
Bupivacaine 0.5%	40	9–11
Ropivacaine 0.5%	40	9–11

larger doses of local anesthetic to be injected into the plexus without producing toxic systemic levels.[17, 24, 62]

Another α-receptor blocking drug that has been found to extend the duration of brachial plexus block is clonidine.[71, 72] In a study comparing the effects of clonidine with those of epinephrine, Gaumann and associates[72] found that clonidine offered no advantages compared with epinephrine. They discovered that peak local anesthetic concentrations were higher when clonidine was used than with epinephrine added. It appears, therefore, that as an α_2-receptor blocker, clonidine does not exert its effect through local vasoconstriction and decreased systemic absorption. It is possible that clonidine may have some degree of local anesthetic activity. The authors concluded that clonidine may have some use as an additive in patients in whom epinephrine is contraindicated. Tryba et al[73] found a longer anesthetic duration with prilocaine plus clonidine compared with clonidine alone.

Another commonly used additive agent with a well-documented effect in improving onset and quality of brachial plexus block is sodium bicarbonate. This effect has been demonstrated in vitro and in clinical studies.[74, 75] Quinlan and colleagues[76] found that alkalinizing mepivacaine, in a study of axillary block patients, decreased onset time. More importantly, they demonstrated improved quality of clinically measured regional block in several terminal nerve distributions (Fig. 16–18). This improved block quality may represent better spread of the drug through membranes and better penetration of septa at this level of the plexus. It may also reflect the local anesthetic properties that bicarbonate itself may possess.[77] Although bicarbonate exerts a measurable effect when added to lidocaine, mepivacaine, or prilocaine, it has not been shown to augment bupivacaine significantly.[78]

One additive that has been shown to have no effect is morphine. It has been experimented with on the basis of evidence of opioid receptors located perineurally.[79] Despite evidence that morphine may have effects on peripheral nerves,[80–83] Racz et al[79] found no differences in onset time, duration, or degree of postoperative analgesia in a randomized masked (double-blind) study. No effect was found by James and associates[84] when they studied the effect on tourniquet pain during axillary block. Thus, it appears that any effects of opioids at the level of the brachial plexus are clinically insignificant.

Another additive that was experimented with in an attempt to promote diffusion of local anesthetic throughout the plexus is hyaluronidase.[85] Study of its effects showed no difference in anesthesia onset or block characteristics[86, 87] for brachial block.

Plasma Concentrations of Local Anesthetic After Brachial Plexus Block

Two generalizations can be made with regard to measured plasma local anesthetic levels after brachial plexus injection. First, plasma concentrations are relatively low compared with those measured with other regional anesthesia techniques.[88] Second, plasma concentrations are independent of approach: interscalene, subclavian perivascular, or axillary.[89] Lower systemic levels that have been measured with other regional anesthetics may result because, although larger volumes and total doses are usually used during brachial plexus block, the solution is largely limited to the brachial plexus sheath,[16] which has a limited vascular surface area for absorption. This is in complete contrast to anesthetic techniques such as interpleural, epidural, or intercostal, in which the drug is spread widely in a thin potential space with a high vascular surface area for absorption. Therefore, the same milligram per kilogram doses should not be applied to the brachial plexus, where larger total doses have been well tolerated. There have been many reports of higher doses used without toxic reactions.[1, 2, 20, 22, 39, 62, 66, 68, 90, 91]

In a study of rhesus monkeys in which intravenous infusion of mepivacaine was given to induce seizures, the mean plasma concentration at the onset of seizures

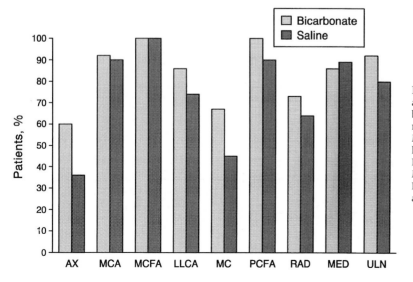

Figure 16–18 Percentage of patients in whom anesthesia developed during study period after axillary block with and without bicarbonate for each terminal nerve. AX, axillary; MCA, medial cutaneous of arm; MCFA, medial cutaneous of forearm; LLCA, lower lateral cutaneous of arm; MC, musculocutaneous; PCFA, posterior cutaneous of forearm; RAD, radial; MED, median; ULN, ulnar. (From Quinlan JJ, Oleksey K, Murphy FL: Alkalinization of mepivacaine for axillary block. Anesth Analg 1992; 74: 371–374.)

was 22.4 μg/mL ± 4.2 (Table 16–4).[92] A typical concentration profile from arterial plasma samples after injection of 53 mL (800 mg) 1.5% mepivacaine with epinephrine is shown in Figure 16–19. In this study by the author and his coworkers,[24] systemic absorption was higher with an 800-mg dose compared with a 400-mg dose of mepivacaine 1.5% in an interscalene block, but no toxic reactions or symptoms occurred despite patients not being premedicated or sedated. Mean arterial peak plasma level was 4.94 μg/mL ± 1.15 for the higher dose, far below what would be expected to cause seizures. Similar findings have been reported for venous plasma levels by Finucane and Yilling[62] after 10.5 mg/kg mepivacaine with epinephrine administered for axillary blocks. In several studies,[24, 62, 64, 93] rare peak mepivacaine concentrations greater than 6 μg/mL have been reported but without toxic symptoms. Buettner et al[64] used a continuous axillary technique to administer a total of 1600 mg mepivacaine in 8 h, without signs of toxicity.

Bupivacaine concentrations between 0.8 and 4.3 μg/mL have been reported[91] after brachial plexus blocks with injections of 200 mg of 0.5% bupivacaine. Doses in the same range with added epinephrine resulted in mean plasma concentrations of 1.63 μg/mL and 1.49 μg/mL in two different studies.[26, 65] Thus, epinephrine is recommended with larger bupivacaine doses. Bupivacaine concentrations less than 4.0 μg/mL are considered to be below the typical toxic range.[92, 94, 95]

The author and his colleagues[24] have found that arterial plasma levels are independent of body mass, height, or surface area (Fig. 16–20) after interscalene injection of mepivacaine.

When continuous techniques are used for extended periods, larger cumulative doses of local anesthetic may be administered.[64, 96] During continuous techniques, bupivacaine may accumulate in the circulation, although this is of doubtful clinical significance if appropriate doses and rates of infusion are used.

Table 16–4 Local Anesthetic–Induced Seizures: Dosage and Plasma Levels

ANESTHETIC	ANIMAL NUMBER	WEIGHT, kg	INFUSION RATE, mg/kg/min	DOSE, mg/kg	PLASMA CONCENTRATION, μg/mL Onset	PLASMA CONCENTRATION, μg/mL Arrest	PREVIOUS DRUGS
Lidocaine	1	6.7	3.1	12.7(5)*			
	2	4.8	4.3	11.7(3)	24.8	6.5	L(2)*
	3	5.3	3.9	11.2(4)	23.6	3.6	L(3)
	4	5.0	4.1	15.8			M
	5	4.9	4.2	11.6	33.1	<9.1†	P
	6	5.0	4.1	19.0			M,P
	8	8.4	2.5	17.1(3)			
	9	4.1	5.0	14.7	21.4	<4.3‡	
	10	7.7	2.7	12.5(3)			
	11	7.1	2.9	18.5(2)	23.5	<9.3‡	
	12	4.6	4.5	17.0(3)			
	13	4.9	4.2	8.9	20.6	7.1	
Mean		5.7	3.8	14.2	24.5	5.7	
SD		1.4	0.8	3.2	4.5	1.9	
Prilocaine	1	7.5	2.8	16.5(2)	18.6	7.9	L(5),M,L(2)
	2	5.1	4.0	14.6(2)	14	7.5	L(3),P,M(2)
	3	5.8	3.5	18.2			L(5)
	4	5.3	3.9	24.0	27.5	12.3	M,L
	5	4.9	4.2	15.4	23.2	8.4	
	6	4.4	4.7	20.4			
	7	6.7	3.1		16	9.9	
	14	5.3	3.9	17.4	23.7	9.3	
Mean		5.6	3.8	18.1	20.5	9.2	
SD		1.0	0.6	3.2	5.2	1.8	
Mepivacaine	1	7.6	2.7	13.3			L(5)
	2	5.1	4.0	15.3(2)	18	5.1	L(3),P
	3	5.8	3.5	13.9(2)	24	2.8	L(5),P
	4	4.5	4.6	24.0	20.3	<7.6†	
	5	5.0	4.1	13.4	27.3		P,L
	6	4.7	4.4	28.9(2)			P
	7	7.7	2.7	15.8	17.8	10.8	P
	15	4.7	4.4	25.4	26.7	10.5	
Mean		5.6	3.8	18.8	22.4	7.3	
SD		1.3	0.8	6.3	4.2	4	

*Figures in parentheses indicate number of determinations; corresponding doses are mean values.
†Seizures terminated with thiamylal; corresponding data are not included in calculations.
‡Seizures continued; animal died.
L, lidocaine; M, mepivacaine; P, prilocaine.
From Munson ES, Gutnick MJ, Wagman IH: Local anesthetic drug–induced seizures in rhesus monkeys. Anesth Analg 1970; 49: 986–994.

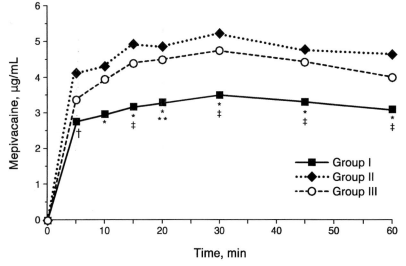

Figure 16–19 Arterial plasma mepivacaine concentration as a function of time (injection = time zero) for interscalene block. Group I = 30 mL 1.5% mepivacaine (400 mg), group II = 40 mL 2% mepivacaine (800 mg), and group III = 53 mL 1.5% mepivacaine (800 mg). No patient demonstrated toxic signs or symptoms. $*P < .01$ compared with group II, $†P < .05$ compared with group II, $‡P < .05$ compared with group III, $**P < .01$ compared with group III.

Side Effects of Brachial Plexus Block

Whereas side effects that are common to all regional local anesthetic techniques may occur during brachial plexus block, this section addresses those that are more specifically associated with brachial plexus block and those side effects that occur most frequently. Most side effects can be explained by the anatomic relationships of the brachial plexus in the neck and thorax. Of the common approaches to the plexus, only axillary block is sufficiently remote from the neck and thorax to avoid most of these side effects (Table 16–5).

Ipsilateral sympathetic block occurs with great frequency with blocks performed above the clavicle—in more than 50% in patients who have interscalene or subclavian perivascular blocks. Therefore, a high incidence of Horner's syndrome[97, 98] should be anticipated and explained to the patient. This can be regarded as a benign side effect. The basis for this is cervical extension of the injected local anesthetic and the close proximity of the stellate ganglion to the plexus. Hoarseness,[98] possibly secondary to recurrent laryngeal nerve block, may be explained by the proximity of the recurrent laryngeal nerve[7] to the brachial plexus and diffusion of drug to block this nerve. Hoarseness, in the author's experience and opinion, is more likely to result from cervical sympathetic block and secondary injection of laryngeal and pharyngeal blood vessels, resulting in a "heavier" vocal cord on the side of the block. The result of either mechanism is usually only transient hoarseness accompanying the anesthesia. However, hoarseness and vocal cord function are rarely of clinical significance. The author and his colleagues have observed patients with severe paroxysms of coughing after interscalene block presumably as a result of aspiration of small amounts of saliva or ingested fluid and a block-induced inability to completely protect the airway. Reports of bronchospasm[99] and precipitation of an asthmatic attack[100] have been associated with interscalene block. Although the authors of these reports ascribed the symptoms to sympathetic block, this author believes that small degrees of aspiration (due to cord paresis) of saliva in patients with reactive airways is a more likely explanation for this bronchospasm during brachial plexus block. Coughing can be treated with an opioid such as fentanyl with antitussive effects.

Unintentional injection of local anesthetic into the

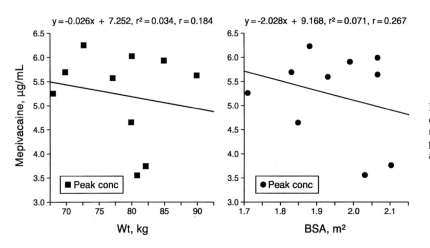

Figure 16–20 Peak mepivacaine arterial plasma concentration after interscalene blocks with fixed mepivacaine dose (800 mg). No correlation of plasma concentration with patient body surface area (BSA) or patient weight (Wt) was found.

Table 16–5 Possible Side Effects of Brachial Plexus Block

COMMON TO ALL REGIONAL ANESTHESIA	PARTICULAR TO BRACHIAL PLEXUS BLOCK
Unintentional intravascular injection	Ipsilateral sympathetic block
Trauma to nerves	Horner's syndrome
Hematoma	Recurrent laryngeal nerve block
Anesthetic overdose	Hoarseness
True allergy to local anesthetic or preservative	Unintentional injection of local anesthetic into epidural or subarachnoid spaces
	Phrenic nerve paralysis
	Ipsilateral hemidiaphragmatic paralysis
	Pneumothorax

epidural or subarachnoid space during interscalene block can occur but should be extremely rare if proper needle length (usually 2.5 cm) is used and the anatomy is understood. There have been reports of unintentional epidural anesthesia[101, 102] during attempted interscalene block, including epidural catheter placement with an attempted continuous interscalene technique.[103] Total spinal anesthesia has also been reported.[104]

The fascial compartment may be continuous between left and right cervicobrachial plexuses and result in unintentional spread of local anesthetic from one brachial plexus to the other.[6] This can result, rarely, in some degree of bilateral upper extremity anesthesia or analgesia.[105, 106] Bilateral brachial plexus block can be clinically distinguished from unintentional cervical epidural injection by pinprick evaluation of upper thoracic dermatomes, which are usually blocked to some extent by epidural injection but spared by bilateral brachial plexus block.

Phrenic nerve paresis has been reported as a possible complication of supraclavicular block, with incidences varying from 28% to 80%.[107–109] The author and colleagues[90] noted that ipsilateral hemidiaphragmatic paresis occurred in 100% of patients who had interscalene block. These investigators used ultrasonography to make the diagnosis. This has been substantiated by other studies[2, 20, 110] reporting an incidence of diaphragmatic paresis of 100%. Therefore, phrenic nerve paresis should be thought of as an expected side effect rather than a complication of interscalene block, much as a sympathetic block during spinal anesthesia.

Interscalene block can be expected to decrease pulmonary function, as a result of unilateral phrenic nerve block, approximately 25%, according to a study by Urmey and McDonald.[2] Interscalene block leads to characteristic changes in chest wall mechanics. It should, therefore, be avoided in patients unable to tolerate these consistent side effects. A decrease in the concentration of the local anesthetic mixture to 0.125% bupivacaine did not prevent deterioration of diaphragmatic motility and ventilatory function[111] during continuous interscalene block. A decrease of the volume to 20 mL of 1.5% mepivacaine also did not avoid diaphragm paresis.[20] Single-injection interscalene block with 0.5% bupivacaine caused hemidiaphragmatic paresis of greater than 9 h duration.[68]

Paresis of the phrenic nerve occurs rapidly after interscalene block, with all pulmonary function changes essentially complete by 15 min. If respiratory problems occur, they can be expected to occur early, while the patient is receiving care from the anesthesiologist. Respiratory failure has been reported[44] after combined general and interscalene block anesthesia in the lateral position with the unblocked side dependent. One must take care with this position because the functional hemidiaphragm may be restricted in the dependent position. This may lead to intraoperative ventilatory insufficiency and decreases in oxygen saturation. These effects are temporary and recede as the block wears off. Persistent phrenic nerve paresis has also been reported after interscalene block,[112] most likely from direct phrenic nerve injury by needle contact outside of the plexus.

As with any regional anesthetic technique, there is always a rare possibility of neural trauma and resulting nerve injury with brachial plexus block.[113] This risk has not been shown to depend on techniques or needle selection, and neurapraxia is usually only transient in nature.[54, 114] In a review[115] of closed claims for upper extremity neurapraxias, more were associated with general than regional anesthesia.

Neurapraxias are not limited to the duration of the surgical procedure. Improper positioning postoperatively while the block is still in effect must be carefully avoided. This is especially true for patients with longer-acting local anesthetic, brachial plexus blocks and those with continuous blocks.

Another position-related complication results from the beach chair or sitting position for shoulder operation.[33] This position optimizes diaphragmatic geometry and improves pulmonary function during interscalene block. However, it has been associated with an approximately 30% incidence of hypotension,[24, 116, 117] which may be associated with bradycardia. This syncopal reaction may be similar to what occurs in the dental chair. It may be precipitated by β_2-adrenergic agents[118] or possibly by a β_2 effect of epinephrine in the local anesthetic that is systemically absorbed. Hypotension is reliably produced after prolonged passive head-up tilt[119, 120] and has been attributed to the Bezold-Jarisch reflex during shoulder operation in the sitting position.[120] Patients must be carefully monitored with continuous electrocardiogram and frequent blood pressure determinations when in the sitting position (see Fig. 16–10), irrespective of type of anesthesia administered.

A more serious, albeit infrequent, complication—pneumothorax—has been associated with interscalene,

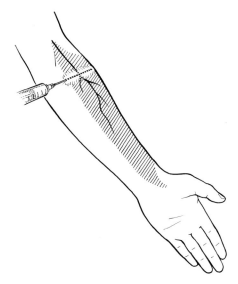

Figure 16–21 Lateral antebrachial cutaneous nerve block.

supraclavicular, and infraclavicular techniques. The subclavian perivascular technique decreases the incidence but is still associated with a finite incidence of pneumothorax of approximately 1%.

The axillary technique has been associated with hematoma formation, false aneurysm,[121, 122] and unintentional arterial catheterization during continuous blocks.[123]

Peripheral Nerve Blocks of the Upper Extremity

The most useful distal peripheral nerve block for routine operation is the wrist block. This block is composed principally of separate blocks of the median, radial, and ulnar nerves, with subcutaneous ring injection, similar to ankle block. The wrist block is used for procedures on the hand when no arm tourniquet is needed or when it is surgically indicated to allow the extrinsic muscles to the hand, located in the forearm, to have motor function remain intact. For example, this situation occurs with trigger finger repair; the wrist block allows the surgeon to check for triggering during the operative procedure. Wrist blocks with longer-act-

ing local anesthetics can be used for prolonged postoperative analgesia after hand operation. There are diagnostic and therapeutic uses of this block as well. Wrist block produces a reliable sympathetic block of the hand. This can be used for diagnosis of vasospasm or therapy for patients with Raynaud's disease.

Other approaches to peripheral nerve block of the upper extremity have been described[124] but have little clinical practical utility. Blocks of the ulnar, median, or radial nerves at the elbow, for example, can be performed to supplement incomplete brachial plexus blocks. The author prefers to supplement by reinjecting the brachial plexus, usually via another approach. For example, if an axillary block is incomplete, one can perform an interscalene block with decreased local anesthetic dose. Blocks of the ulnar nerve, at the elbow in particular, should be performed carefully and with adequate indication. Many patients have subclinical ulnar neuropathies in this area, and this nerve is occasionally injured at the exposed elbow location during operation.

One peripheral nerve block at the forearm that is an exception to this generalization is lateral antebrachial cutaneous nerve block (Fig. 16–21). This nerve is the terminal sensory branch of the musculocutaneous nerve. The musculocutaneous nerve is formed from the C-5 and C-6 nerve roots and exits the plexus proximally. As a result of this proximal location, this nerve may be missed by routine axillary block. Sometimes isolated lateral antebrachial cutaneous nerve sparing occurs after an otherwise completely successful axillary block. This nerve can be easily and quickly blocked.

Median Nerve

The median nerve lies deep to the palmaris longus tendon. It is superficial, as are the other nerves at the wrist. A common mistake is to insert the needle too deep. Although paresthesia can be sought,[125] it is not necessary and perhaps should be avoided.[126, 127] A 25- or 27-G needle is used to block the nerve with approximately 7 mL of local anesthetic. The median nerve is subfascial, as is the ulnar nerve. The radial nerve is more superficial. With regard to this aspect of the anatomy, wrist block is analogous to ankle block. The palmar cutaneous branch of the median nerve as well as

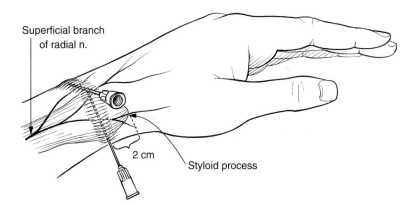

Figure 16–22 Radial nerve (n.) block. See text.

Superficial branch
of radial n.

2 cm

Styloid process

other more superficial cutaneous branches of the radial and ulnar nerves can be blocked by subcutaneous ring infiltration with a 27- or 30-G needle.

Ulnar Nerve

The ulnar nerve lies just medial to the ulnar artery and immediately lateral to the tendon of the flexor carpi ulnaris. It is superficial and is blocked, preferably without obtaining paresthesia, by 5 mL of local anesthetic injected 1 to 2 cm proximal to the distal palmar crease.

Radial Nerve

The radial nerve is blocked approximately 2 cm proximal to the radial styloid process at the wrist. By blocking at this point, the dorsal branch of the radial nerve can be blocked by a single needle entry. The radial nerve lies just lateral to the radial artery. It is superficial and can be blocked by injecting 5 mL of local anesthetic with a 27-G needle. After injection, the needle is located subcutaneously (without removing the needle) and injection is made over a 2-cm distance projecting laterally and dorsally (Fig. 16–22). This maneuver blocks the dorsal branch of the radial nerve.

Ring Block

After the major nerve blocks, minor branches can be anesthetized by partial ring subcutaneous infiltration over the palmar surface of the wrist with a 27-G needle.

Lateral Antebrachial Cutaneous Nerve Block Technique

The lateral antebrachial cutaneous nerve is anesthetized in the palmar region of the forearm (see Fig. 16–21). The nerve is blocked superficially one third of the total distance from the antecubital fossa to the palmar crease at the wrist. A 27-G needle is inserted where an imaginary axial line bisects the forearm, and local anesthetic is infiltrated 3 to 4 cm laterally in the subcutaneous tissue. This block is used to supplement lateral antebrachial cutaneous nerve sparing after incomplete axillary brachial plexus block.

Conclusion

Brachial plexus block has evolved into a reliable method of providing anesthesia or analgesia to the upper extremity. The applications for this useful block are expanding to meet the demands of changing intraoperative and postoperative patient care. Attention to

the principles discussed may help to increase success and satisfaction with this form of regional anesthesia.

Clinical Notes:

1. *When learning the transarterial axillary block, anesthesiologists have a tendency to advance rapidly through the axillary artery once blood is encountered. This may result in a less exact position of the needle tip behind the artery. It is important to advance slowly through the artery, allowing blood to back up in the extension tubing during aspiration. It also improves success to reenter the artery one or two times during the procedure.*
2. *When the onset of axillary block is assessed (especially after the transarterial technique), an early sign that has a high correlation with block success is the inability to extend the forearm at the elbow. This results from radial nerve block.*
3. *For any axillary block technique, the axillary artery forms a reliable landmark to the plexus location. When not palpable in the axilla, it may often be palpated more distally (as the brachial artery) and followed proximally to the axilla. If this fails, Doppler imaging or ultrasound may be used to determine the artery's location.*
4. *If a patient has a contraindication to brachial plexus block above the clavicle (e.g., local infection or neoplasm), an alternative may be used to block the upper brachial and lower cervical plexuses. A continuous axillary brachial plexus block with the needle aimed proximally often allows the catheter to be threaded to a position above the clavicle or first rib.*
5. *Part of the art of regional anesthesia is the ability to judge the quality of regional block after a regional technique. This allows the anesthesiologist to proceed with the procedure with confidence. There are several signs that can be elicited after interscalene block. Because the injection is performed at the C-6 level, pinprick testing at C-5 and C-6 reveals rapid loss of sensation (usually within 2 to 5 min). Inability to lift the arm against gravity at the shoulder (only later at the elbow) soon follows. Within about 10 min, a decrease in handgrip strength is usually demonstrable and in most cases is accompanied by unintentional pronation of the forearm.*
6. *In patients in whom the interscalene groove is difficult to palpate, percutaneous stimulation with a nerve stimulator and coupling gel may help to determine its location. Use of an exploring lead to find the point of maximal motor response is not uncomfortable for most patients and may help one to detect the groove.*
7. *Dyspnea after interscalene block or subclavian perivascular block of the brachial plexus is rare. Despite the large reductions in pulmonary function that occur during interscalene block, only the occasional patient complains of*

dyspnea. If dyspnea occurs, the following guidelines may be helpful in alleviating the symptoms or treating respiratory compromise:
a. Observe and reassure patient.
b. Place patient in sitting position, as tolerated. This optimizes diaphragmatic mechanics, increases functional residual capacity, and has been shown to significantly increase forced vital capacity.
c. Auscultate the contralateral lung to eliminate the possibility of contralateral abnormality. Auscultation of the ipsilateral lung field often reveals diminished breath sound as a result of hemidiaphragmatic paresis. Although pneumothorax is possible, it is highly unlikely if the technique is performed correctly. Nevertheless, a chest radiograph may be indicated if pneumothorax is suspected.
d. Positive pressure ventilation or assistance with a face mask or tracheal intubation should be performed if clinically indicated (although this is rare).

8. The T-2 dermatome (intercostobrachial nerve) is not blocked when one blocks the brachial plexus. Infiltration of the skin with bupivacaine lasts until the closure is completed for most shoulder operations. Infiltration with lidocaine or mepivacaine most often dissipates well before the brachial plexus block does when these same agents are used for brachial plexus anesthesia.

References

1. Cockings E, Moore PL, Lewis RC: Transarterial brachial plexus blockade using high doses of 1.5% mepivacaine. Reg Anesth 1987; 12: 159–164.
2. Urmey WF, McDonald M: Hemidiaphragmatic paresis during interscalene brachial plexus block: effects on pulmonary function and chest wall mechanics. Anesth Analg 1992; 74: 352–357.
3. Goldberg ME, Gregg C, Larijani GE, et al: A comparison of three methods of axillary approach to brachial plexus blockade for upper extremity surgery. Anesthesiology 1987; 66: 814–816.
4. King RS, Urquhart BL, Urquhart BJ, et al: Factors influencing the success of brachial plexus block. (Abstract.) Reg Anesth 1991; 16: 63.
5. Winnie AP: Interscalene brachial plexus block. Anesth Analg 1970; 49: 455–466.
6. Ward ME: The interscalene approach to the brachial plexus. Anaesthesia 1974; 29: 147–157.
7. Winnie AP: Plexus Anesthesia: Perivascular Techniques of Brachial Plexus Block, 2nd ed, p 117. Philadelphia, WB Saunders Co, 1990.
8. de Jong RH: Axillary block of the brachial plexus. Anesthesiology 1961; 22: 215–225.
9. Youssef MS, Desgrand DA: Comparison of two methods of axillary brachial plexus anaesthesia. Br J Anaesth 1988; 60: 841–844.
10. Lanz E, Theiss D, Jankovic D: The extent of blockade following various techniques of brachial plexus block. Anesth Analg 1983; 62: 55–58.
11. Clemente CD: Gray's Anatomy of the Human Body, 30th American ed. Philadelphia, Lea & Febiger, 1985.
12. Winnie AP: Plexus Anesthesia: Perivascular Techniques of Brachial Plexus Block, 2nd ed, p 44. Philadelphia, WB Saunders Co, 1990.
13. Smith GB, Wilson GR, Curry CH, et al: Predicting successful brachial plexus block using changes in skin electrical resistance. Br J Anaesth 1988; 60: 703–708.
14. Vatashsky E, Aronson HB: Continuous interscalene brachial plexus block for surgical operations on the hand. (Letter to the editor.) Anesthesiology 1980; 53: 356.
15. Matsuda M, Kato N, Hosoi M: Continuous brachial plexus block for replantation in the upper extremity. Hand 1982; 14: 129–134.
16. Winnie AP, Radonjic R, Akkineni SR, et al: Factors influencing distribution of local anesthetic injected into the brachial plexus sheath. Anesth Analg 1979; 58: 225–234.
17. Partridge BL, Katz J, Benirschke K: Functional anatomy of the brachial plexus sheath: implications for anesthesia. Anesthesiology 1987; 66: 743–747.
18. Vester-Andersen T, Broby-Johansen U, Bro-Rasmussen F: Perivascular axillary block VI: the distribution of gelatine solution injected into the axillary neurovascular sheath of cadavers. Acta Anaesthesiol Scand 1986; 30: 18–22.
19. Thompson GE, Rorie DK: Functional anatomy of the brachial plexus sheaths. Anesthesiology 1983; 59: 117–122.
20. Urmey WF, Gloeggler PJ: Pulmonary function changes during interscalene brachial plexus block: effects of decreasing local anesthetic injection volume. Reg Anesth 1993; 18: 244–249.
21. Ting PL, Sivagnanaratnam V: Ultrasonographic study of the spread of local anaesthetic during axillary brachial plexus block. Br J Anaesth 1989; 63: 326–329.
22. Urmey WF, Gloeggler PJ, Parab S, et al: Does a digital pressure technique alter measurable sensory, motor, or diaphragm effects? (Abstract.) Anesth Analg 1992; 74: s327.
23. Urmey WF: Combined axillary-interscalene (axis) brachial plexus block for elbow surgery. (Abstract.) Reg Anesth 1993; 18: 88.
24. Urmey WF, Stanton J, Sharrock NE: Interscalene block: effects of dose, volume, and mepivacaine concentration on anesthesia and plasma levels. (Abstract.) Reg Anesth 1994; 19: 34.
25. Winnie AP: Plexus Anesthesia: Perivascular Techniques of Brachial Plexus Block, 2nd ed, p 185. Philadelphia, WB Saunders Co, 1990.
26. Rosenberg PH, Pere P, Hekali R, et al: Plasma concentrations of bupivacaine and two of its metabolites during continuous interscalene brachial plexus block. Br J Anaesth 1991; 66: 25–30.
27. Davis WJ, Lennon RL, Wedel DJ: Brachial plexus anesthesia for outpatient surgical procedures on an upper extremity. Mayo Clin Proc 1991; 66: 470–473.
28. Brandl F, Taeger K: The combination of general anesthesia and interscalene block in shoulder surgery. (German.) Anaesthesist 1991; 40: 537–542.
29. McQuay H, Weir L, Porter B, et al: A model for comparison of local anesthetics in man. Anesth Analg 1982; 61: 418–422.
30. Fisher A, Meller Y: Continuous postoperative regional analgesia by nerve sheath block for amputation surgery—a pilot study. Anesth Analg 1991; 72: 300–303.
31. Wenger CB, Stephenson LA, Durkin MA: Effect of nerve block on response of forearm blood flow to local temperature. J Appl Physiol 1986; 61: 227–232.
32. Audenaert SM, Vickers H, Burgess RC: Axillary block for vascular insufficiency after repair of radial club hands in an infant. Anesthesiology 1991; 74: 368–370.
33. Skyhar MJ, Altchek DW, Warren RF, et al: Shoulder arthroscopy with the patient in the beach-chair position. Arthroscopy 1988; 4: 256–259.
34. Martin R, Dupuis JY, Tetrault JP: Regional anesthesia for pacemaker insertion. Reg Anesth 1989; 14: 81–84.
35. Brown DL, Cahill DR, Bridenbaugh LD: Supraclavicular nerve block: anatomic analysis of a method to prevent pneumothorax. Anesth Analg 1993; 76: 530–534.
36. Fassoulaki A: Brachial plexus block for pain relief after modified radical mastectomy. Anesth Analg 1982; 61: 986–987.
37. Sharrock NE, Bruce G: An improved technique for locating the interscalene groove. Anesthesiology 1976; 44: 431–433.
38. Loring SH, DeTroyer A: Actions of the respiratory muscles. Lung Biol Health Dis 1985; 29: 327–349.
39. Roch JJ, Sharrock NE, Neudachin L: Interscalene brachial

plexus block for shoulder surgery: a proximal paresthesia is effective. Anesth Analg 1992; 75: 386–388.

40. Kulenkampff D: Die Anästhesia des Plexus brachialis. Zentralbl Chir 1911; 38: 1337–1340.

41. Bonica JJ, Moore DC, Orlov M: Brachial plexus block anesthesia. Am J Surg 1949; 78: 65–79.

42. Brand L, Papper EM: A comparison of supraclavicular and axillary techniques for brachial plexus blocks. Anesthesiology 1961; 22: 226–229.

43. Winnie AP: Regional anesthesia. Surg Clin North Am 1975; 55: 861–892.

44. Gentili M, Lefoulon-Gourves M, Mamelle JC, et al: Acute respiratory failure following interscalene block: a pitfall of combined general and regional anesthesia. (Letter to the editor.) Reg Anesth 1994; 19: 292.

45. Winnie AP, Collins VJ: The subclavian perivascular technique of brachial plexus anesthesia. Anesthesiology 1964; 25: 353–363.

46. Hickey R, Garland TA, Ramamurthy S: Subclavian perivascular block: influence of location of paresthesia. Anesth Analg 1989; 68: 767–771.

47. Hickey R, Hoffman J, Ramamurthy S: Transarterial techniques are not effective for subclavian perivascular block. Reg Anesth 1990; 15: 245–249.

48. Korbon GA, Carron H, Lander CJ: First rib palpation: a safer, easier technique for supraclavicular brachial plexus block. Anesth Analg 1989; 68: 682–685.

49. Moorthy SS, Schmidt SI, Dierdorf SF, et al: A supraclavicular lateral paravascular approach for brachial plexus regional anesthesia. Anesth Analg 1991; 72: 241–244.

50. Raj PP, Montgomery SJ, Nettles D, et al: Infraclavicular brachial plexus block—a new approach. Anesth Analg 1973; 52: 897–904.

51. Hirschel G: Die Anästhesierung des Plexus brachialis bei Operationen an der oberen Extremität. Munch Med Wochenschr 1911; 43: 1555.

52. Pere P, Pitkänen M, Tuominen M, et al: Clinical and radiological comparison of perivascular and transarterial techniques of axillary brachial plexus block. Br J Anaesth 1993; 70: 276–279.

53. Tuominen MK, Pitkänen MT, Numminen MK, et al: Quality of axillary brachial plexus block: comparison of success rate using perivascular and nerve stimulator techniques. Anaesthesia 1987; 42: 20–22.

54. Selander D, Edshage S, Wolff T: Paresthesiae or no paresthesiae? Nerve lesions after axillary blocks. Acta Anaesthesiol Scand 1979; 23: 27–33.

55. Murphy TM: Nerve blocks in anesthesia. In Miller RD (ed): Anesthesia, pp 608–634. New York, Churchill Livingstone, 1981.

56. Plevak DJ, Linstromberg JW, Danielson DR: Paresthesia vs nonparesthesia—the axillary block. (Abstract.) Anesthesiology 1983; 59: a216.

57. Fleck JW, Moorthy SS, Daniel J, et al: Brachial plexus block: a comparison of the supraclavicular lateral paravascular and axillary approaches. Reg Anesth 1994; 19: 14–17.

58. Riegler FX: Brachial plexus block with the nerve stimulator: motor response characteristics at three sites. Reg Anesth 1992; 17: 295–299.

59. Ford DJ, Pither C, Raj PP: Comparison of insulated and uninsulated needles for locating peripheral nerves with a peripheral nerve stimulator. Anesth Analg 1984; 63: 925–928.

60. Ansbro FP: A method of continuous brachial plexus block. Am J Surg 1946; 71: 716–722.

61. Selander D: Catheter technique in axillary plexus block: presentation of a new method. Acta Anaesthesiol Scand 1977; 21: 324–329.

62. Finucane BT, Yilling F: Safety of supplementing axillary brachial plexus blocks. Anesthesiology 1989; 70: 401–403.

63. Tuominen M, Haasio J, Hekali R, et al: Continuous interscalene brachial plexus block: clinical efficacy, technical problems and bupivacaine plasma concentrations. Acta Anaesthesiol Scand 1989; 33: 84–88.

64. Buettner J, Klose R, Hoppe U, et al: Serum levels of mepivacaine-HCl during continuous axillary brachial plexus block. Reg Anesth 1989; 14: 124–127.

65. Pihlajamaki KK, Lindberg RL: Bupivacaine with and without

adrenaline in interscalene brachial plexus blockade: studies in patients with rheumatoid arthritis. Br J Anaesth 1987; 59: 1420–1424.

66. Pere P, Tuominen M, Rosenberg PH: Cumulation of bupivacaine, desbutylbupivacaine and 4-hydroxybupivacaine during and after continuous interscalene brachial plexus block. Acta Anaesthesiol Scand 1991; 35: 647–650.

67. Arthur GR, Scott DH, Boyes RN, et al: Pharmacokinetic and clinical pharmacological studies with mepivacaine and prilocaine. Br J Anaesth 1979; 51: 481–485.

68. Urmey WF, Gloeggler PJ: Effects of bupivacaine 0.5% compared with mepivacaine 1.5% used for interscalene brachial plexus block. (Abstract.) Reg Anesth 1992; 17: 13.

69. Hickey R, Hoffman J, Ramamurthy S: A comparison of ropivacaine 0.5% and bupivacaine 0.5% for brachial plexus block. Anesthesiology 1991; 74: 639–642.

70. Hickey R, Rowley CL, Candido KD, et al: A comparative study of 0.25% ropivacaine and 0.25% bupivacaine for brachial plexus block. Anesth Analg 1992; 75: 602–606.

71. Singelyn FJ, Dangoisse M, Bartholomee S, et al: Adding clonidine to mepivacaine prolongs the duration of anesthesia and analgesia after axillary brachial plexus block. Reg Anesth 1992; 17: 148–150.

72. Gaumann D, Forster A, Griessen M, et al: Comparison between clonidine and epinephrine admixture to lidocaine in brachial plexus block. Anesth Analg 1992; 75: 69–74.

73. Tryba M, Lammers A, Zenz M: Clonidine prolongs the duration of analgesia after prilocaine for axillary plexus block: a randomized controlled double-blind study. (Abstract.) Reg Anesth 1992; 17: 16.

74. Tetzlaff JE, Yoon HJ, O'Hara J, et al: Alkalinization of mepivacaine accelerates onset of interscalene block for shoulder surgery. Reg Anesth 1990; 15: 242–244.

75. DiOrio S, Ellis R: Comparison of pH-adjusted and plain solutions of mepivacaine for brachial plexus anesthesia. (Abstract.) Reg Anesth 1988; 13: 3.

76. Quinlan JJ, Oleksey K, Murphy FL: Alkalinization of mepivacaine for axillary block. Anesth Analg 1992; 74: 371–374.

77. Raymond S, Wong K, Strichartz G: Mechanisms for potentiation of local anesthetic action by CO_2: bicarbonate solutions. (Abstract.) Anesthesiology 1989; 71: a711.

78. Bedder MD, Kozody R, Craig DB: Comparison of bupivacaine and alkalinized bupivacaine in brachial plexus anesthesia. Anesth Analg 1988; 67: 48–52.

79. Racz H, Gunning K, Della Santa D, et al: Evaluation of the effect of perineuronal morphine on the quality of postoperative analgesia after axillary plexus block: a randomized double-blind study. Anesth Analg 1991; 72: 769–772.

80. Mays KS, Lipman JJ, Schnapp M: Local analgesia without anesthesia using peripheral perineural morphine injections. Anesth Analg 1987; 66: 417–420.

81. Sanchez R, Nielsen H, Heslet L, et al: Neuronal blockade with morphine: a hypothesis. Anaesthesia 1984; 39: 788–789.

82. Gissen AJ, Gugino LD, Datta S, et al: Effects of fentanyl and sufentanil on peripheral mammalian nerves. Anesth Analg 1987; 66: 1272–1276.

83. Stein C, Comisel K, Haimerl E, et al: Analgesic effect of intraarticular morphine after arthroscopic knee surgery. N Engl J Med 1991; 325: 1123–1126.

84. James M, Lamer TJ, Lennon RL, et al: Axillary block anesthesia using mepivacaine plus morphine during upper extremity surgery: effects on tourniquet related hemodynamic changes. (Abstract.) Reg Anesth 1992; 17: 73.

85. Moore DC: Regional Block: A Handbook for Use in the Clinical Practice of Medicine and Surgery, 4th ed. Springfield, IL, Charles C Thomas, 1965.

86. Harley N, Gjessing J: A critical assessment of supraclavicular brachial plexus block. Anaesthesia 1969; 24: 564–570.

87. Rosenquist RW, Finucane BT, Berman S: Hyaluronidase and axillary brachial plexus block: Effect on latency and plasma levels of mepivacaine. (Abstract.) Reg Anesth 1989; 14: 50.

88. Scott DB: "Maximum recommended doses" of local anaesthetic drugs. (Editorial.) Br J Anaesth 1989; 63: 373–374.

89. Maclean D, Chambers WA, Tucker GT, et al: Plasma prilocaine concentrations after three techniques of brachial plexus blockade. Br J Anaesth 1988; 60: 136–139.

90. Urmey WF, Talts KH, Sharrock NE: One hundred percent incidence of hemidiaphragmatic paresis associated with interscalene brachial plexus anesthesia as diagnosed by ultrasonography. Anesth Analg 1991; 72: 498–503.

91. Pihlajamaki KK: Inverse correlation between the peak venous serum concentration of bupivacaine and the weight of the patient during interscalene brachial plexus block. Br J Anaesth 1991; 67: 621–622.

92. Munson ES, Gutnick MJ, Wagman IH: Local anesthetic drug-induced seizures in rhesus monkeys. Anesth Analg 1970; 49: 986–997.

93. Wildsmith JA, Tucker GT, Cooper S, et al: Plasma concentrations of local anaesthetics after interscalene brachial plexus block. Br J Anaesth 1977; 49: 461–466.

94. Denson DD, Myers JA, Hartrick CT, et al: The relationship between free bupivacaine concentration and central nervous system toxicity. (Abstract.) Anesthesiology 1984; 61: a211.

95. Scott DB: Evaluation of the toxicity of local anaesthetic agents in man. Br J Anaesth 1975; 47: 56–61.

96. Tuominen M, Pitkänen M, Rosenberg PH: Postoperative pain relief and bupivacaine plasma levels during continuous interscalene brachial plexus block. Acta Anaesthesiol Scand 1987; 31: 276–278.

97. Al-Khafaji JM, Ellias MA: Incidence of Horner syndrome with interscalene brachial plexus block and its importance in the management of head injury. (Letter to the editor.) Anesthesiology 1986; 64: 127.

98. Seltzer JL: Hoarseness and Horner's syndrome after interscalene brachial plexus block. Anesth Analg 1977; 56: 585–586.

99. Thiagarajah S, Lear E, Azar I, et al: Bronchospasm following interscalene brachial plexus block. Anesthesiology 1984; 61: 759–761.

100. Lim EK: Inter-scalene brachial plexus block in the asthmatic patient. (Letter to the editor.) Anaesthesia 1979; 34: 370.

101. Scammell SJ: Case report: inadvertent epidural anaesthesia as a complication of interscalene brachial plexus block. Anaesth Intensive Care 1979; 7: 56–57.

102. Kumar A, Battit GE, Froese AB, et al: Bilateral cervical and thoracic epidural blockade complicating interscalene brachial plexus block: report of two cases. Anesthesiology 1971; 35: 650–652.

103. Cook LB: Unsuspected extradural catheterization in an interscalene block. Br J Anaesth 1991; 67: 473–475.

104. Ross S, Scarborough CD: Total spinal anesthesia following brachial-plexus block. Anesthesiology 1973; 39: 458.

105. Lombard TP, Couper JL: Bilateral spread of analgesia following interscalene brachial plexus block. Anesthesiology 1983; 58: 472–473.

106. Cobcroft MD: Letter: bilateral spread of analgesia with interscalene brachial plexus block. Anaesth Intensive Care 1976; 4: 73.

107. Dhuner K-G, Moberg E, Önne L: Paresis of the phrenic nerve during brachial plexus block analgesia and its importance. Acta Chir Scand 1955; 109: 53–57.

108. Knoblanche GE: The incidence and aetiology of phrenic nerve blockade associated with supraclavicular brachial plexus block. Anaesth Intensive Care 1979; 7: 346–349.

109. Shaw WM: Paralysis of the phrenic nerve during brachial plexus anesthesia. Anesthesiology 1949; 10: 627–628.

110. Pere P, Pitkänen M, Rosenberg PH, et al: Effect of continuous interscalene brachial plexus block on diaphragm motion and on ventilatory function. Acta Anaesthesiol Scand 1992; 36: 53–57.

111. Pere P: The effect of continuous interscalene brachial plexus block with 0.125% bupivacaine plus fentanyl on diaphragmatic motility and ventilatory function. Reg Anesth 1993; 18: 93–97.

112. Bashein G, Robertson HT, Kennedy WF Jr: Persistent phrenic nerve paresis following interscalene brachial plexus block. Anesthesiology 1985; 63: 102–104.

113. Barutell C, Vidal F, Raich M, et al: A neurological complication following interscalene brachial plexus block. Anaesthesia 1980; 35: 365–367.

114. Woolley EJ, Vandam LD: Neurological sequelae of brachial plexus nerve block. Ann Surg 1959; 149: 53–60.

115. Kroll DA, Caplan RA, Posner K, et al: Nerve injury associated with anesthesia. Anesthesiology 1990; 73: 202–207.

116. Tetzlaff JE, Yoon HJ, Reaney J, et al: Shoulder surgery under regional anesthesia may be associated with lower blood loss than general anesthesia. (Abstract.) Reg Anesth 1991; 15: 41.

117. Roch J, Sharrock NE: Hypotension during shoulder arthroscopy in the sitting position under interscalene block. (Abstract.) Reg Anesth 1991; 15: 64.

118. Almquist A, Goldenberg IF, Milstein S, et al: Provocation of bradycardia and hypotension by isoproterenol and upright posture in patients with unexplained syncope. N Engl J Med 1989; 320: 346–351.

119. Sander-Jensen K, Secher NH, Astrup A, et al: Hypotension induced by passive head-up tilt: endocrine and circulatory mechanisms. Am J Physiol 1986; 251: r742–r748.

120. Gold BS, Weitz SR, Lurie KG: Intraoperative "syncope": evaluation with tilt-table testing. Anesthesiology 1992; 76: 635–637.

121. Zipkin M, Backus WW, Scott B, et al: False aneurysm of the axillary artery following brachial plexus block. J Clin Anesth 1991; 3: 143–145.

122. Groh GI, Gainor BJ, Jeffries JT, et al: Pseudoaneurysm of the axillary artery with median-nerve deficit after axillary block anesthesia: a case report. J Bone Joint Surg Am 1990; 72: 1407–1408.

123. Tuominen MK, Pere P, Rosenberg PH: Unintentional arterial catheterization and bupivacaine toxicity associated with continuous interscalene brachial plexus block. Anesthesiology 1991; 75: 356–358.

124. Hoerster W, Kreuscher H, Niesel HC, et al: Regional Anesthesia, 2nd ed. St. Louis, Mosby–Year Book, 1990.

125. Abadir A: Anesthesia for hand surgery. Orthop Clin North Am 1970; 1: 205–212.

126. Wilson KM: Distal forearm regional block anesthesia for carpal tunnel release. J Hand Surg (Am) 1993; 18: 438–440.

127. Winnie AP: Plexus Anesthesia: Perivascular Techniques of Brachial Plexus Block, 2nd ed, p 56. Philadelphia, WB Saunders Co, 1990.

CHAPTER 17

Lower Extremity Blocks

James N. Rogers, M.D., Somayaji Ramamurthy, M.D.

Spinal, epidural, or caudal anesthesia provides practical and consistent somatic block of the lower extremities. There are patients, however, such as those with head injury or cardiovascular instability, in whom general or neuraxial anesthesia may not be ideal. In these instances, specific, unilateral, peripheral, lower extremity nerve blocks provide significant advantages over the more common neuraxial block techniques.

Technical expertise with lower extremity nerve blocks appears more difficult to develop compared with the brachial plexus blocks. Unlike the upper extremity, the nerve supply to the lower extremity is widely separated, originating from both the lumbar plexus and the sacral plexus, and is located deep under thick muscles. In addition, for most surgical procedures, at least two of the widely separated nerves must be blocked. If a pneumatic tourniquet is used on the thigh for a surgical procedure on a leg or foot, all nerves innervating the thigh must be blocked as well as the sciatic and saphenous nerves supplying the leg and foot. Patients will still have the ability to use truncal and contralateral lower extremity muscles to move about, possibly disrupting the surgical procedure, if they become uncooperative.

Lower extremity, peripheral nerve blocks can provide distinct advantages in healthy patients as well. Unilateral lower extremity blocks with long-acting local anesthetics can be especially helpful in the outpatient setting, allowing the patient to ambulate with crutches with little to no pain.[1, 2] Techniques for continuous infusion via a catheter can provide long-lasting postoperative analgesia.[3, 4] Peripheral blocks can be used in patients with localized back infections. In patients who have compromised or unstable cardiovascular function, the likelihood of hypotension is decreased because the sympathetic block can be limited to one lower extremity.

Tverskoy and colleagues[5] and others have also suggested that peripheral neural block may decrease postoperative pain to a greater extent than epidural or subarachnoid local anesthetics alone. Woolf and Chong[6] suggested that this occurs by prevention of central sensitization of low-threshold mechanoreceptors and nociceptors at the level of the spinal cord by blocking the transmission of impulses to the dorsal horn.

Preparation

All patients scheduled for lower extremity operation should be considered candidates for a regional anesthetic technique. A regional anesthetic technique can be used as the only anesthetic, as a supplement to general anesthesia, or as part of the postoperative pain management plan. Patient refusal is an absolute contraindication to regional anesthesia, although a calm, rational attempt at patient education should be made. A careful history and especially a complete neurologic examination should be undertaken before any regional block to document possible preexisting neurologic disease processes.

Patient education is an important aspect of preblock preparation and decreases most patient anxiety. The explanation should be simple to understand but thorough in detail. A description of the procedure, expected sensations, and results as well as a discussion of the risks and benefits of the procedure should be reviewed with the patient. Supplemental medications such as a mild dose of opioid or an anxiolytic-amnestic such as midazolam can decrease the discomfort from the needle and provide amnesia while still allowing the patient to cooperate with the procedure.

Monitoring should be provided at the same level as

279

for any other anesthetic during placement of the block as well as during the surgical procedure, because patients undergoing any regional technique may develop life-threatening cardiovascular or respiratory depression. Careful attention to the patient's mental status should be maintained through verbal contact throughout the procedure. Changes in the mental status may be an early warning sign of clinical events needing treatment.

Nerve Supply

The lower extremity is supplied by anterior rami of the five lumbar nerves and the first two or three sacral nerves. These form the lumbar and sacral plexuses.

The upper portion of the lumbar plexus primarily provides innervation to the anterior abdominal wall. The iliohypogastric nerve (L-1) provides innervation to the skin of the buttock and the abdominal wall muscles. The ilioinguinal nerve (L-1) provides cutaneous innervation to the perineum and the adjoining portion of the medial thigh. The genitofemoral nerve (L-1 to L-2) supplies a portion of the genital area and provides a lumboinguinal branch that supplies the skin over the femoral triangle.

The five major nerves of the lower extremity are located distal to the iliohypogastric, ilioinguinal, and genitofemoral nerves. Three nerves, the lateral femoral cutaneous nerve (L-2 to L-3), the femoral nerve (L-2 to L-4), and the obturator nerve (L-2 to L-4), are derived from the lumbar plexus. The other two nerves are the posterior cutaneous nerve of the thigh (S-1 to S-3) and the sciatic nerve (L-4 to S-3). The posterior cutaneous nerve of the thigh is derived from the sacral plexus and courses with the sciatic nerve through the pelvis and exits via the greater sciatic foramen. The posterior cutaneous nerve of the thigh is considered together with the sciatic nerve when discussing the various sciatic nerve block techniques.

Lateral Femoral Cutaneous Nerve Block

The lateral femoral cutaneous nerve block can be useful for anesthetizing small skin graft donor sites on the lateral aspect of the thigh. It may be necessary as a supplement to the femoral, obturator, and sciatic nerve blocks for operations on the lower extremity, particularly when a thigh tourniquet is used.

The lateral femoral cutaneous nerve (L-2 to L-3) emerges along the lateral border of the psoas muscle caudal to the ilioinguinal nerve. It courses obliquely deep to the iliac fascia across the iliac muscle and enters the thigh by passing posterior to the inguinal ligament, just medial to the anterior superior iliac spine. It provides cutaneous innervation to the lateral aspect of the thigh to the knee. A large area over the lateral aspect of the thigh can be effectively blocked with this procedure.

Technique

The block is performed by placing the patient in the supine position and palpating the anterior superior iliac spine. A needle is inserted at a point 1 cm medial and caudal to the anterior superior iliac spine and advanced deep to the fascia lata. Local anesthetic (5 to 10 mL) is injected in a fanwise manner (Fig. 17–1).

The nerve can also be blocked by directing the needle superiorly beneath the inguinal ligament into the facial compartment containing the nerve cephalad to the level of the inguinal ligament. This fascial compartment can be identified by directing a short-bevel needle medial to the anterior superior iliac spine and advancing it through the external oblique aponeurosis, the internal oblique muscle, and the iliac fascia. The short-bevel needle allows the anesthesiologist to feel a distinct loss of resistance or "pop" as the two fascial layers are penetrated. The authors believe this technique is reliable.

It is possible to unintentionally block the femoral nerve when large amounts of local anesthetics are injected using this technique. This occurs because of the spread of local anesthetic medially beneath the iliac fascia.

Complications

The lateral femoral cutaneous nerve block poses no significant risks, with the exception of a rare dysesthesia if the nerve is injured during the injection.

Femoral Nerve Block

In order to provide complete anesthesia for the lower extremity, a femoral nerve block is usually combined with a sciatic block as well as lateral femoral cutaneous and obturator nerve blocks. Alone, the femoral nerve block can be used in operations on the anterior portion of the thigh. It can be particularly effective in providing analgesia in patients with a femoral fracture[7, 8] and as an adjunct to general anesthesia in patients undergoing knee surgery. Blocks performed before operation have been shown[9] to decrease postoperative opioid requirements by as much as 80% in the recovery room and by 40% during the first 24 h postoperatively.

The femoral nerve (L-2 to L-4) lies in a groove formed between the psoas major and the iliac muscles, entering the thigh deep to the inguinal ligament (Fig. 17–2). It provides sensation over the anteromedial aspect of the thigh and the medial aspect of the leg. The nerve also supplies the quadriceps, sartorius, and pectineal muscles.

At the level of the inguinal ligament, the femoral nerve lies anterior to the iliopsoas muscle and slightly lateral to the femoral artery. It does not lie within the femoral vascular sheath. The nerve lies deep to the fascia lata and iliac fascia and lies within its own sheath. At the level of the inguinal ligament, the femoral nerve divides into anterior (superficial) and poste-

A

B

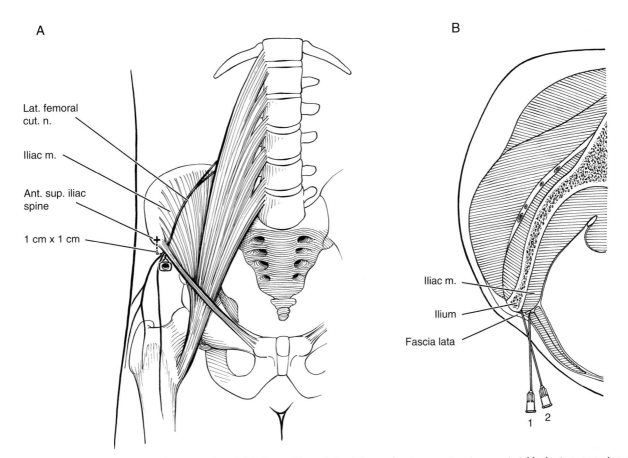

Lat. femoral
cut. n.

Iliac m.

Ant. sup. iliac
spine

1 cm x 1 cm

Iliac m.

Ilium

Fascia lata

1 2

Figure 17–1 Anteroposterior *(A)* and cross-sectional *(B)* views of lateral (Lat.) femoral cutaneous (cut.) nerve (n.) block. Ant., anterior; m., muscle; sup., superior.

rior (deep) bundles. The anterior bundle provides cutaneous innervation of the skin overlying the anterior surface of the thigh as well as providing motor innervation to the sartorius muscle. The posterior bundle provides innervation to the quadriceps muscles and the knee joint with its medial ligament. It also gives rise to the saphenous nerve, which supplies cutaneous innervation to the medial aspect of the calf to the level of the medial malleolus.

Technique

The most important landmark for performing a femoral nerve block is the femoral artery (Fig. 17–3). The needle is inserted 1 to 2 cm caudal to the inguinal ligament and lateral to the femoral artery. The needle is advanced in a lateral and posterior direction just distal to the inguinal ligament. A short-bevel needle, and the characteristic "pop," can be used to identify penetration of the fascia lata and the iliac fascia. Remember that the femoral nerve lies deep to both. When a nerve stimulator is used, contraction of the quadriceps muscle confirms correct placement of the needle. A local anesthetic agent (10 to 15 mL) is usually adequate to block the femoral nerve.

The proximal portion of the anterior thigh is innervated by the ilioinguinal and genitofemoral nerves and is not blocked by a femoral nerve block.

A catheter can also be placed within the femoral nerve sheath. This allows the continuous infusion of local anesthetics. This continuous block theoretically allows operation of any duration to be performed and can be especially useful in providing postoperative analgesia to patients.[10]

Complications

Complications associated with femoral nerve block are rare. Hematoma at the site is a possibility but is usually not clinically significant. If an arterial puncture is achieved, direct pressure is usually adequate to prevent the development of a hematoma. The presence of a femoral artery vascular graft is a relative contraindication to femoral nerve block. As in the case of the sciatic nerve block, residual dysesthesias are rare.

Obturator Nerve Block

The obturator nerve block by itself can be extremely useful as a diagnostic, prognostic, or therapeutic procedure in patients with adductor spasm. Adductor spasm can occur as a complication of stroke, spinal cord injury, multiple sclerosis, and other neuromuscular disorders. Adductor spasm is a major cause of disability,

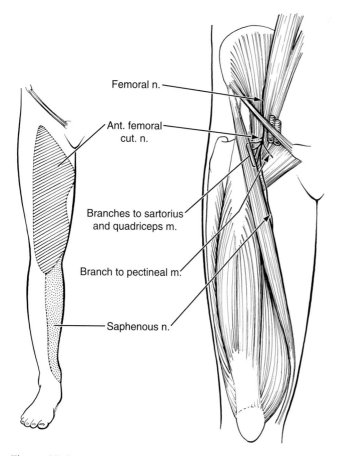

Figure 17–2 Femoral nerve (n.). Anterior view. Ant., anterior; cut., cutaneous; m., muscle.

be blocked is placed in slight abduction. It is usually not necessary to shave the pubic area. With aseptic technique, a 22-G, 8-cm needle is inserted in the horizontal plane at a point 1.5 cm lateral and 1.5 cm inferior to the pubic tubercle. The needle is advanced until the inferior ramus of the pubis is contacted. The needle depth at which the bone is contacted should be noted. The needle is withdrawn and redirected in a lateral and slightly superior direction parallel to the superior ramus of the pubis. The needle is advanced 2 to 3 cm beyond the previously noted depth until a paresthesia is elicited (Fig. 17–4). If a nerve stimulator is used, adductor muscle contraction should be used to correctly locate the obturator nerve. A nerve stimulator may facilitate identification of the obturator nerve. Local anesthetic (10 mL) is injected to block the nerve.

Confirmation of a successful obturator nerve block is demonstrated by paresis of the adductor muscles, because the cutaneous contribution of the obturator nerve is inconsistent.

An alternative approach using the femoral artery and adductor longus tendon as landmarks has been described by Wassef.[12] A mark is made on the skin 1 to 2 cm medial to the femoral artery just caudad to the inguinal ligament. This mark is used to indicate the ultimate needle direction toward the obturator canal. The adductor longus tendon is then identified near its insertion site at the pubis. A 22-G, 8-cm insulated

making physical therapy, hygienic care, and walking difficult. An obturator nerve block is also necessary for patients undergoing operation at the level of or proximal to the knee.

The obturator nerve is formed by the union of the ventral branches of the anterior primary rami of L-2, L-3, and L-4 within the substance of the psoas muscle. It emerges from the medial border of the psoas muscle at the brim of the pelvis. The nerve courses caudad and anteriorly along the lateral wall of the pelvis along the obturator vessels to the obturator foramen. There it enters the thigh, supplying the adductor muscles and providing innervation to the hip and knee joints.

As the nerve passes through the obturator canal, it divides into anterior and posterior branches. The anterior branch supplies the hip joint, the anterior adductor muscles, and cutaneous branches to the medial aspect of the thigh. The cutaneous innervation of the obturator nerve can be extremely variable and can be nonexistent in some people. The posterior branch supplies the deep adductor muscles and frequently sends a branch to the knee joint.

Technique

The traditional approach was first described by Labat.[11] The patient is asked to lie supine, and the leg to

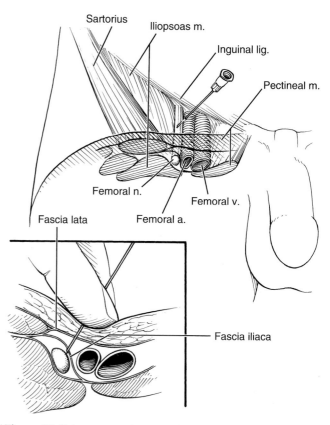

Figure 17–3 Anteroposterior *(A)* and cross-sectional *(B)* views of the femoral nerve (n.), which lies between the fascia lata and the iliac fascia, lateral to the femoral artery (a.) and vein (v.). lig., ligament; m, muscle.

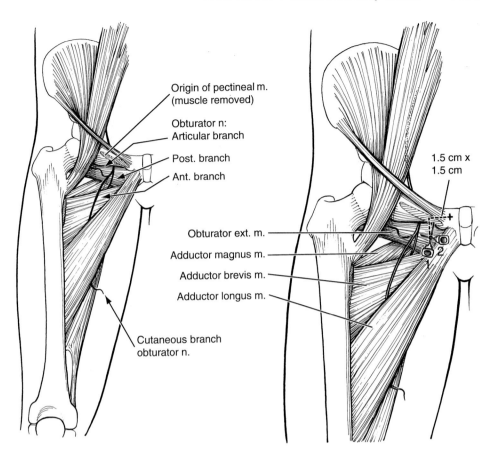

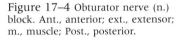

Figure 17–4 Obturator nerve (n.) block. Ant., anterior; ext., extensor; m., muscle; Post., posterior.

needle is introduced posterior to the adductor longus tendon and directed laterally, with a slight posterior and cephalad inclination toward the skin mark. Again, the needle is advanced until adductor muscle contraction is elicited with a nerve stimulator.

Complications

The obturator nerve block has side effects and complications similar to those of the femoral nerve block.

Three-in-One Block

The goal of the three-in-one block described by Winnie and coworkers[13] is to block three nerves with a single injection similar to the brachial plexus technique. Although the lateral femoral nerve is easily blocked alone, the obturator nerve can be difficult to block and the procedure can be quite uncomfortable for the patient. By slightly modifying the femoral nerve block technique and increasing the volume of the local anesthetic used, all three nerves may be blocked.

The three-in-one block technique is performed by inserting the needle at the same point as for an inguinal femoral nerve block but with the needle directed in a slightly cephalad direction (Fig. 17–5). After localization of the femoral nerve by either paresthesia or nerve stimulator, digital pressure is applied distal to the nee-

dle entry site. Then 30 mL of local anesthetic is injected after a negative result of aspiration for blood. A continuous block can be achieved by threading a catheter 15 to 20 cm cephalad within the femoral nerve sheath.[14]

Whether all three nerves are reliably blocked by this technique is somewhat controversial, and the mechanism of block is unclear. It was originally thought that

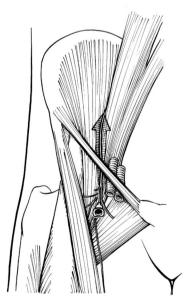

Figure 17–5 Three-in-one block.

the large volume of local anesthetic spread transversely or subfascially between the iliac and psoas muscles and blocked the nerves at the level of the lumbar plexus. Confirmation of local anesthetic spread cephalad to the level of the lumbar plexus has been confirmed by only one study—that by Lonsdale.[15] Clinically, the femoral and lateral femoral nerves are easily blocked with this technique, but that may occur by diffusion of the local anesthetic beneath the iliac fascia.

A major point of contention has been whether the obturator nerve is really blocked with a three-in-one block. Many of the studies have looked at only the loss of cutaneous sensation in the distribution of the obturator nerve as an indication of successful obturator block. The cutaneous distribution of the obturator nerve can, however, be inconsistent and may even be absent in some patients.

Motor block of the thigh adductor muscles is the best way to identify a successful obturator nerve block, but motor evaluation has rarely been used to identify successful obturator nerve block. Further substantiation is needed to confirm the mechanism of local anesthetic block and clarify which of the three nerves are blocked reliably.

Sciatic Nerve Block

A sciatic nerve block can be a useful technique for providing surgical anesthesia as well as postoperative analgesia of the lower leg and foot. Some consider a sciatic nerve block unreliable, technically difficult, and uncomfortable for the patient. Nevertheless, with appropriate sedation, most patients are able to provide an accurate verbal report of paresthesia. Reported rates of success have been as high as 95% with paresthesia techniques. Insulated needles and nerve stimulators make it easier for some to perform this block in sedated or even anesthetized patients with a high rate of success.

The sciatic nerve is the largest nerve in the body. It originates from both the lumbar and sacral plexuses. The sciatic nerve really consists of two major nerve trunks anatomically: the tibial and common peroneal nerves. The tibial nerve is derived from the anterior rami of L-4 to S-3. The common peroneal nerve is derived from the dorsal branches of the anterior rami of the same nerve roots.

The sciatic nerve exits the pelvis along with the posterior cutaneous nerve of the thigh through the sciatic foramen deep to the piriform muscle. It passes between the greater trochanter and the ischial tuberosity. It becomes superficial at the inferior border of the gluteus maximus muscle and courses down the posterior aspect of the thigh. At the cephalad aspect of the popliteal fossa, the sciatic nerve separates into the tibial and common peroneal nerves.

The sciatic nerve provides sensory innervation to most of the lower leg and foot from distal to the knee and motor innervation to the plantar and dorsiflexor muscles of the foot.

A regional block of the sciatic nerve can be achieved anywhere along the course of the nerve. Most of the approaches have been developed mainly to avoid positioning problems that may be present in trauma patients or in the elderly. The sciatic nerve can be blocked at the sciatic notch, at the level of the ischial tuberosity, at the greater trochanter, or in the proximal popliteal fossa.

Classic Approach

The classic technique described by Labat[11] blocks the nerve at the level of the greater sciatic notch, using the piriform muscle as a landmark. At this level, the sciatic nerve is accompanied by the posterior femoral cutaneous and pudendal nerves. The patient is placed in the lateral Sims position with the side to be blocked uppermost. The upper knee is flexed to place the heel of this extremity in position to abut the knee of the contralateral leg. Some patients may find this position uncomfortable, particularly those with orthopedic problems.

The landmarks are the cephalad aspect of the greater trochanter and the posterior superior iliac spine. A line is drawn connecting these two points, corresponding approximately to the superior border of the piriform muscle and the upper border of the sciatic notch. A perpendicular line is extended caudomedially from the midpoint of the first line. The point of injection is 3 to 5 cm distal on this perpendicular line. Verification of the insertion point can be made by drawing a third line connecting the cephalad portion of the greater trochanter and the sacral hiatus. This third line compensates for the height of the patient. The intersection of lines 2 and 3 is the point of needle insertion (Fig. 17–6).

A 22-G, 10- to 12-cm spinal needle is introduced at an angle so that if the needle was long enough, it would contact the pubic symphysis, and advanced to a depth of 6 to 10 cm until a paresthesia is reported in the distribution of the sciatic nerve, preferably in the foot. If periosteum is contacted, the needle is systematically redirected medially or laterally. Contact with the periosteum may produce a local paresthesia that may be mistaken for a true sciatic nerve paresthesia. A nerve stimulator can be helpful in locating the nerve, particularly in unresponsive patients.[16]

Doppler ultrasonography can also be used to locate the dominant arterial structure within the sciatic notch.[17] The needle is then advanced in the same orientation as the probe until a paresthesia is obtained. Successful block has been reported in one or two attempts in 70% of patients. After a negative result of aspiration for blood, 20 to 30 mL of a local anesthetic is injected.

A continuous sciatic nerve block can be performed by using a standard 16-G intravenous infusion cannula attached to a nerve stimulator. After obtaining muscle contraction in the lower leg, preferably dorsiflexion or plantar flexion of the foot, an epidural catheter is advanced through the catheter (after removal of the needle stylet), about 6 cm into the neurovascular

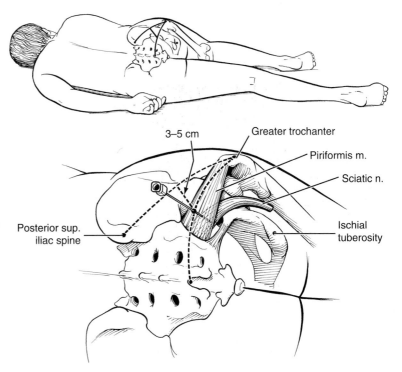

Figure 17–6 Classic sciatic nerve (n.) block. Piriformis muscle (m.) injection. Needle insertion site 3 to 5 cm below midpoint of line connecting posterior superior iliac spine and greater trochanter. sup., superior. (Modified from Brown DL: Atlas of Regional Anesthesia, p 84. Philadelphia, WB Saunders Co, 1992.)

space. Continuous infusion of a local anesthetic with an infusion pump can provide continuous analgesia.[3]

The advantage of the classic approach is that both the posterior femoral cutaneous and pudendal nerves are usually blocked at the same time as the sciatic nerve. This is especially important if a thigh tourniquet is used during operation.

Posterior Approach

A more distal posterior approach can also be used, with the patient in the Sims position or prone. The ischial tuberosity and the greater trochanter are identified, and a line is drawn connecting these two points. A 22-G, 10- to 12-cm subarachnoid needle is inserted at the midpoint of the line and redirected if necessary until a paresthesia is elicited in the lower leg. The posterior femoral cutaneous nerve is often blocked as well at this level, but the pudendal nerve is missed frequently.

Anterior Approach

The anterior approach allows the sciatic nerve to be blocked without moving the patient from a supine position.[11, 18] The anterior approach is especially helpful in trauma patients with a painful leg. However, the anterior approach can be painful and sedation is often necessary. The nerve is deep at this point and difficult to locate. A nerve stimulator may be helpful in identifying the nerve. The posterior cutaneous nerve of the thigh may not be blocked with this approach, resulting in tourniquet pain if a thigh tourniquet is used during operation.

The patient is placed in the supine position, with the leg in a neutral position. The anterior superior iliac spine and the pubic tubercle are identified and marked. A line is then drawn connecting these two points. The line should overlie the inguinal ligament. The line is divided into three equal parts.

A perpendicular line is drawn distally (caudolaterally) from the junction of the medial and middle thirds. A third line is drawn parallel to the first line starting from the cephalad portion of the greater trochanter. The point of intersection of this third line and the perpendicular line is the insertion point of the needle (Fig. 17–7).

A 22-G, 15-cm spinal needle is inserted and directed slightly laterally from a parasagittal plane and advanced until periosteum is contacted (usually the lesser trochanter). The needle is partially withdrawn and redirected medially and posteriorly to pass beyond the femur until a paresthesia is elicited. After a negative result of aspiration for blood, 20 to 25 mL of a local anesthetic agent is injected.

In supine adults, the sciatic neurovascular compartment is usually 4.5 to 6 cm beyond the anterior surface of the femur. In children, however, the distance varies according to age and size of the child. In children, a loss of resistance technique using a 16-G needle has been described with a high success rate (95%) by McNicol.[19] A 10-mL syringe is attached to the needle and inserted through a skin wheal by using the traditional anterior approach technique. Continuous pressure is applied on the syringe plunger as the needle is advanced past the femur. As the needle enters the neurovascular compartment, a sudden loss of resistance is encountered. Smaller-gauge needles are not used because they may have too much internal resistance to allow clear identification of the loss of resis-

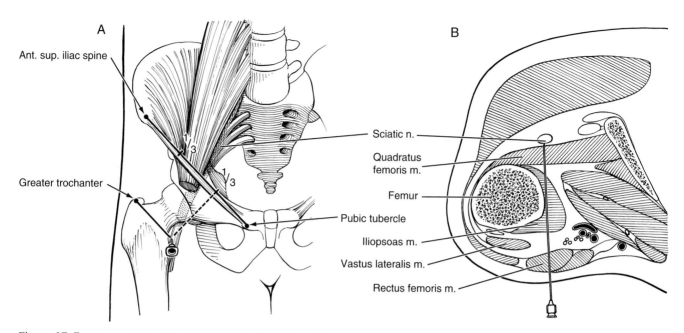

Figure 17–7 Anteroposterior *(A)* and cross-sectional *(B)* views of anterior sciatic nerve (n.) block. Ant., anterior; m., muscle; sup., superior.

tance on entering the neurovascular compartment. After aspirating to minimize the possibility of intravascular position, the local anesthetic agent is injected.

Lithotomy Approach

In this sciatic nerve block technique, the leg to be blocked is held in the lithotomy position by stirrups, mechanical devices, an assistant, or even over the shoulder of the anesthesiologist.[20, 21] This technique allows the patient to remain in a more comfortable supine position, but movement of the leg may prove prohibitively painful in patients with a traumatic leg injury. The point of needle insertion is the midpoint of a line drawn between the greater trochanter and the ischial tuberosity (Fig. 17–8). A 10- to 12-cm needle is directed posteromedially until a paresthesia is obtained.

A nerve stimulator can be helpful in localizing the nerve, particularly in a patient who is unable to report a paresthesia. Local anesthetic (20 to 25 mL) is injected.

Lateral Approach

The lateral approach, initially described by Ichiyanagi,[22] was difficult and never became popular. A new lateral approach described by Guardini et al[23] seems easier. It blocks the sciatic nerve just posterior to the quadrate muscle of the thigh in the subgluteal space.

In this newer approach, the greater trochanter is identified and a 22-G, 12- to 15-cm needle is inserted 3 cm distal to the maximum lateral prominence of the trochanter, close to its posterior margin. The needle is inserted until the periosteum is contacted. The needle is then partially withdrawn and redirected posteriorly

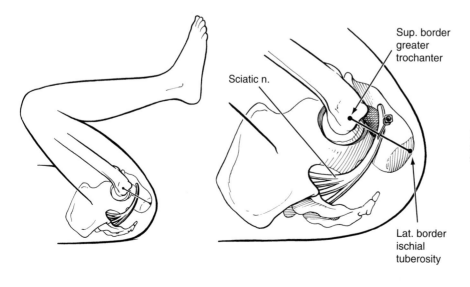

Figure 17–8 Lithotomy position for sciatic nerve (n.) block. Lat., lateral; sup., superior.

and medially to slide posterior to the femoral shaft until a paresthesia or a contraction of the calf muscles or the anterior compartment muscles occurs with the use of a nerve stimulator. The local anesthetic is then injected (Fig. 17–9).

The main advantage of this technique is that the patient can remain in the supine position and the leg need not be manipulated. When using a nerve stimulator, it is important to make sure that the muscle contractions occur in the calf muscles or in the muscles of the anterior compartment. It is possible, using this technique, to stimulate the nerve branch supplying the two heads of the biceps muscle of the thigh. Elicitation of thigh muscle contraction could result in misidentification of the nerve and misplacement of the local anesthetic.

Complications

Although the sciatic nerve is mostly somatic in function, there are sympathetic fibers included. The resulting sympathetic block may allow some mild venous pooling, but this is usually insufficient to cause clinically significant hypotension. Residual dysesthesias have been reported but usually improve in 1 to 3 days.

Nerve Blocks at the Knee

It is possible to block the saphenous, common peroneal, and tibial nerves at the level of the knee. Regional blocks at the level of the knee have been used successfully to provide anesthesia for a wide variety of surgical procedures, including synovectomies, toe amputations, ligament and tendon repairs, and hallux valgus proce-

dures.[24] Kempthorne and Brown[25] have shown these blocks to be useful in children as an adjunct to general anesthesia as well as for postoperative analgesia. Diagnostic tibial nerve blocks can also be helpful in evaluating patients with spastic hemiparesis or myotonic disorders.[26]

Some textbooks of regional anesthesia were less than enthusiastic in encouraging individual nerve blocks at the knee because knee blocks were thought to be difficult to perform and there was a possibility of a postanesthetic neuritis.[27] Studies[24, 25] have shown these nerve blocks can be performed safely and successfully at the level of the knee, even in children.

The common peroneal and tibial nerves are extensions of the sciatic nerve. The sciatic nerve bifurcates at the cephalad aspect of the popliteal fossa bordered by the biceps muscle of the thigh laterally and the semimembranous and semitendinous muscles medially. The caudad half of the popliteal fossa is bordered by the two heads of the gastrocnemius muscle. Techniques have been described[28] in which the tibial and common peroneal nerves are blocked with one injection, but it is possible to miss one of the branches. Identifying the two nerves separately and performing individual nerve blocks may increase the likelihood of success.

Tibial Nerve Block

The tibial nerve is the larger of the two branches of the sciatic nerve and supplies motor innervation to the flexor muscles at the back of the knee joint and calf. The cutaneous innervation supplies the skin overlying the popliteal fossa and along the posterior portion of the leg to the ankle. It courses through the center of the popliteal fossa as it proceeds distally down the leg.

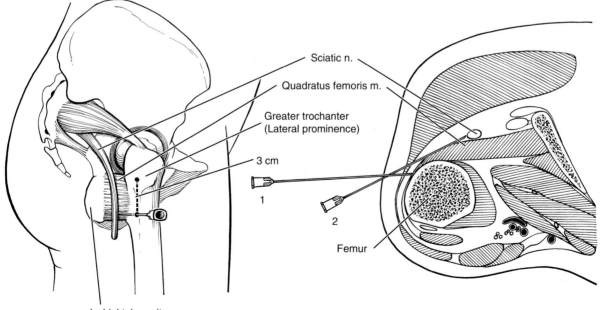

Figure 17–9 Lateral sciatic nerve (n.) block. (1) Initial needle position. (2) Final needle position. m., muscle.

The tibial nerve is blocked at the level of the knee by having the patient in the prone position. The knee is flexed to allow palpation of the proximal popliteal fossa borders and identification of the skin crease behind the knee joint. Once these structures are outlined, a needle is inserted approximately 5 cm cephalad to the crease line and just lateral to the line bisecting the popliteal fossa. A nerve stimulator may be used to identify the tibial nerve by eliciting plantar flexion of the foot. The average depth from skin to nerve in adults is 1.5 to 2.0 cm.[28] Local anesthetic (5 mL) is injected to block the tibial nerve (Fig. 17–10).

Common Peroneal Nerve Block

The common peroneal nerve is about half the size of the tibial nerve. It contains articular branches to the knee joint and provides motor innervation to the extensor muscles of the foot and cutaneous nerves to the lateral aspect of the leg, heel, and ankle. It separates from the tibial nerve at the superior aspect of the popliteal fossa and courses laterally around the fibular head. There it divides into the deep and superficial peroneal nerves.

The common peroneal nerve can be palpated easily as it crosses the neck of the fibula. A 25-G needle is inserted next to the nerve and allowed to contact the periosteum, taking care to avoid an intraneural injection. The needle is withdrawn slightly, and 5 mL of a local anesthetic agent is injected (Fig. 17–11). A nerve stimulator may be used to identify the nerve by eliciting contraction of the anterior compartment muscles.

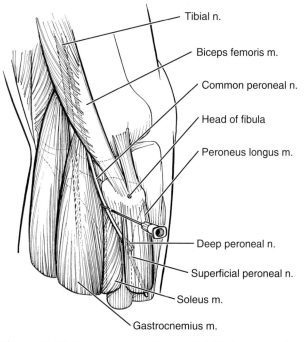

Figure 17–11 Common peroneal nerve (n.) block. m., muscle.

Saphenous Nerve Block

The saphenous nerve (L-3 to L-4) is the terminal branch of the femoral nerve. It provides cutaneous innervation to the skin overlying the medial, anteromedial, and posteromedial aspects of the leg from just cephalad to the knee to the level of the medial

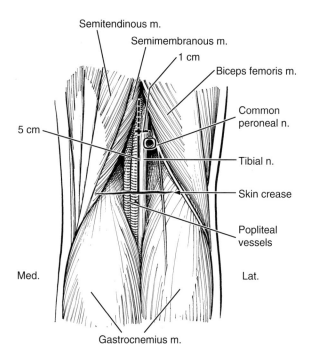

Figure 17–10 Tibial nerve (n.) block. Lat., lateral; m., muscle; Med., medial.

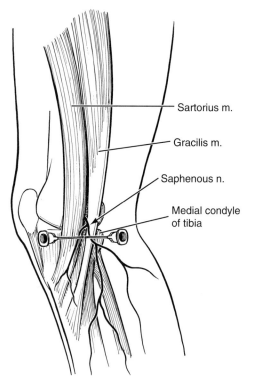

Figure 17–12 Saphenous nerve (n.) block. m., muscle.

malleolus (and in some patients to the medial aspect at the base of the great toe). There is no motor component.

The saphenous nerve is blocked by subcutaneous infiltration of 5 to 10 mL of a local anesthetic in a 5-cm area just distal to the medial surface of the tibial condyle. Because the saphenous nerve may accompany the saphenous vein, the patient should be made aware of the possibility of a hematoma from venous puncture (Fig. 17–12).

Complications

Complications from regional blocks at the knee are rare. Severe, crampy pain on injection suggests the possibility of an intraneural injection, and the injection should be stopped and the needle repositioned before continuing.

Ankle Blocks

Ankle blocks can be used to provide anesthesia for nearly all surgical procedures performed on the foot.[24, 29] These procedures include Morton's neuroma resection; operations on the great toe, including bunionectomy and amputation; amputation of midfoot or other toes; metatarsal osteotomy; incision and drainage; and débridement procedures. The ankle block, however, does not provide anesthesia for tourniquet pain and does not provide a complete motor block of the foot.

There are five terminal branches of the tibial, common peroneal, and femoral nerves that supply the ankle and foot and must be blocked to provide comprehensive foot anesthesia. These include the posterior tibial, sural, superficial peroneal, deep peroneal, and saphenous nerves. These nerves are easily blocked at the level of the ankle (Fig. 17–13).

Posterior Tibial Nerve Block

The posterior tibial nerve (L-4 to S-3) is located along the medial aspect of the Achilles tendon, lying just posterior to the posterior tibial artery. The nerve gives off a medial calcaneal branch to the medial aspect of the heel, dividing behind the medial malleolus into the medial and lateral plantar nerves. The medial plantar nerve supplies the medial two thirds of the sole of the foot as well as the plantar portion of the medial three

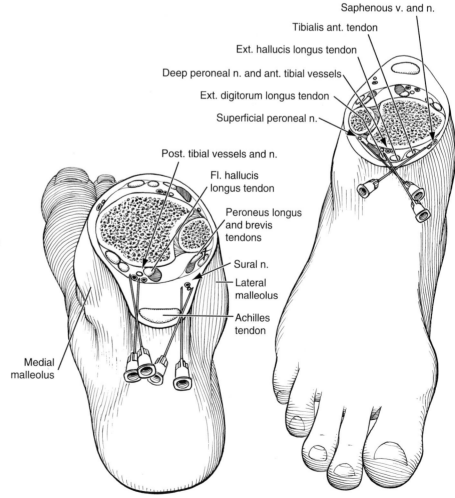

Figure 17–13 Ankle block. ant., anterior; Ext., extensor; Fl., flexor; n., nerve; Post., posterior; v., vein.

Saphenous v. and n.
Tibialis ant. tendon
Ext. hallucis longus tendon
Deep peroneal n. and ant. tibial vessels
Ext. digitorum longus tendon
Superficial peroneal n.
Post. tibial vessels and n.
Fl. hallucis longus tendon
Peroneus longus and brevis tendons
Sural n.
Lateral malleolus
Achilles tendon
Medial malleolus

and one-half toes. The lateral plantar nerve supplies the lateral one third of the sole and the plantar portion of the lateral one and one-half toes.

The posterior tibial nerve is easily blocked with the patient in the prone position with the foot supported by a pillow. A skin wheal is raised along the medial aspect of the Achilles tendon at the level of the superior border of the medial malleolus. A 3-cm needle is then advanced via the wheal toward the posterior aspect of the tibia, posterior to the artery. If a paresthesia is elicited, 3 to 5 mL of local anesthetic is injected after a negative result of aspiration for blood. If a paresthesia is not elicited, the needle is advanced until the tibial periosteum is contacted. The needle is withdrawn 0.5 cm, and 5 to 7 mL of local anesthetic is injected.

Sural Nerve Block

The sural nerve is a cutaneous nerve that consists of fibers from both the tibial and common peroneal nerves. It lies subcutaneously somewhat distal to the middle of the leg and lies near the short saphenous vein behind and distal to the lateral malleolus. It supplies the posterolateral surface of the leg, the lateral side of the foot, and the lateral aspect of the fifth toe.

The patient remains in the same position as for the posterior tibial nerve block. A skin wheal is raised lateral to the Achilles tendon at the level of the lateral malleolus. A 3-cm needle is inserted to a depth of 1 cm and directed toward the lateral border of the fibula. If a paresthesia cannot be elicited, 3 to 5 mL of a local anesthetic can be injected subcutaneously in a fanwise manner from the lateral border of the Achilles tendon to the lateral border of the fibula.

Superficial Peroneal Nerve Block

The superficial peroneal nerve (L-4 to S-2) exits the deep fascia of the leg at the anterior aspect of the distal two thirds of the lower leg. From that point, the superficial peroneal nerve lies subcutaneously and supplies the dorsum of the foot and toes, with the exception of the contiguous surfaces of the great and second toes.

The superficial peroneal nerve is blocked by subcutaneous infiltration of 5 mL of a local anesthetic agent from the anterior border of the tibia to the superior aspect of the lateral malleolus.

Deep Peroneal Nerve Block

The deep peroneal nerve (L-4 to S-2) courses down the anterior portion of the interosseous membrane of the leg and extends midway between the malleoli on to the dorsum of the foot. At this point, the nerve lies lateral to the tendon of the extensor hallucis longus muscle and the anterior tibial artery. It supplies motor innervation to the short extensors of the toes and

cutaneous innervation to adjacent areas of the first and second toes.

The deep peroneal nerve is blocked by placing the needle between the tendon of the extensor hallucis longus muscle and the anterior tibial tendon just superior to the level of the malleoli. The tendon of the extensor hallucis longus muscle can be identified by having the patient extend the great toe. If the artery can be palpated, the needle is placed just lateral to the artery. The needle is advanced toward the tibia, and 3 to 5 mL of local anesthetic is injected deep to the fascia.

Saphenous Nerve Block

The saphenous nerve is the terminal branch of the femoral nerve. It reaches its cutaneous course at the medial aspect of the knee joint and follows the great saphenous vein to the medial malleolus. It supplies cutaneous innervation to the medial aspect of the lower leg anterior to the medial malleolus and the medial aspect of the foot. It may extend as far anterior as the metatarsophalangeal joint of the great toe.

The saphenous nerve is blocked by subcutaneously injecting 3 to 5 mL of local anesthetic immediately proximal and anterior to the medial malleolus to the anterior border of the tibia. This skin wheal completes a semicircle extending from both malleoli, blocking the saphenous and superficial peroneal nerves.

In general, all five nerve blocks at the ankle form a ring of infiltration around the ankle at the level of the malleoli. Large volumes of local anesthetic, especially those containing epinephrine, may cause vascular occlusion. Otherwise, regional block at the ankle is a highly successful means of providing surgical anesthesia to the foot.

Summary

Lower extremity regional block can be an important tool in the hands of the anesthesiologist, especially in cases in which a major conduction block such as a spinal or epidural block is not in the patient's best interest. Precise regional block also enables the anesthesiologist to provide postoperative analgesia with minimal interruption of the patient's physiologic processes. Unilateral lower extremity blocks often allow the patient to ambulate with only the aid of crutches.

Lower extremity regional block, like all regional techniques, requires extensive knowledge of the anatomy of the nervous system in order to be successful. Labat[11] said it best: "Anatomy is the foundation upon which the entire concept of regional anesthesia is built." The knowledge of superficial landmarks, bony prominences, tendons, blood vessels, and the course of the nerves serves as a guide for advancing the needle toward its target.

The placement of a catheter for continuous infusion along an individual nerve such as the sciatic or femoral nerve can provide prolonged analgesia without the bothersome side effects of opioid medications.[3, 10] The sympathetic block enhances delivery of oxygen-rich blood to the tissues and aids in wound healing and early mobilization. The risk of a deep venous thrombosis developing may also be decreased.

When lower extremity block is indicated in a critically ill patient, it would be best if the anesthesiologist was not trying the block for the first time. Expertise in these blocks is best achieved when they are routinely used in healthy patients. Only when they are a part of the anesthesiologist's routine practice can confidence be developed in these blocks.

References

1. Patel NJ, Flashburg MH, Paskin S, et al: A regional anesthetic technique compared to general anesthesia for outpatient knee arthroscopy. Anesth Analg 1986; 65: 185–187.
2. McQuay HJ, Carroll D, Moore RA: Postoperative orthopaedic pain—the effect of opiate premedication and local anaesthetic blocks. Pain 1988; 33: 291–295.
3. Smith BE, Fischer HB, Scott PV: Continuous sciatic nerve block. Anaesthesia 1984; 39: 155–157.
4. Edwards ND, Wright EM: Continuous low-dose 3-in-1 nerve blockade for postoperative pain relief after total knee replacement. Anesth Analg 1992; 75: 265–267.
5. Tverskoy M, Cozacov C, Ayache M, et al: Postoperative pain after inguinal herniorrhaphy with different types of anesthesia. Anesth Analg 1990; 70: 29–35.
6. Woolf CJ, Chong MS: Preemptive analgesia—treating postoperative pain by preventing the establishment of central sensitization. Anesth Analg 1993; 77: 362–379.
7. Berry FR: Analgesia in patients with fractured shaft of femur. Anaesthesia 1977; 32: 576–577.
8. Howard CB, Mackie IG, Fairclough J, et al: Femoral neck surgery using a local anaesthetic technique. Anaesthesia 1983; 38: 993–994.
9. Ringrose NH, Cross MJ: Femoral nerve block in knee joint surgery. Am J Sports Med 1984; 12: 398–402.
10. Rosenblatt RM: Continuous femoral anesthesia for lower extremity surgery. Anesth Analg 1980; 59: 631–632.
11. Labat G: Regional Anesthesia: Its Technic and Clinical Application. Philadelphia, WB Saunders Co, 1922.
12. Wassef MR: Interadductor approach to obturator nerve blockade for spastic conditions of adductor thigh muscles. Reg Anesth 1993; 18: 13–17.
13. Winnie AP, Ramamurthy S, Durrani Z: The inguinal paravascular technic of lumbar plexus anesthesia: the "3-in-1 block." Anesth Analg 1973; 52: 989–996.
14. Dahl JB, Christiansen CL, Daugaard JJ, et al: Continuous blockade of the lumbar plexus after knee surgery—postoperative analgesia and bupivacaine plasma concentrations. A controlled clinical trial. Anaesthesia 1988; 43: 1015–1018.
15. Lonsdale M: 3-in-1 block: confirmation of Winnie's anatomical hypothesis. (Letter to the editor.) Anesth Analg 1988; 67: 601–602.
16. Pither CE, Raj PP, Ford DJ: The use of peripheral nerve stimulators for regional anesthesia: a review of experimental characteristics, techniques, and clinical applications. Reg Anesth 1985; 10: 49–58.
17. Hullander M, Spillane W, Leivers D, et al: The use of Doppler ultrasound to assist with sciatic nerve blocks. Reg Anesth 1991; 16: 282–284.
18. Beck GP: Anterior approach to sciatic nerve block. Anesthesiology 1963; 24: 222–224.
19. McNicol LR: Anterior approach to sciatic nerve block in children: loss of resistance or nerve stimulator for identifying the neurovascular compartment. (Letter to the editor.) Anesth Analg 1987; 66: 1199–1200.
20. Raj PP, Parks RI, Watson TD, et al: New single-position supine approach to sciatic-femoral nerve block. Anesth Analg 1975; 54: 489–493.
21. Winnie AP, Ramamurthy S, Durrani Z, et al: Plexus blocks for lower extremity surgery: new answers to old problems. Anesthesiol Rev 1974; 1: 11–16.
22. Ichiyanagi K: Sciatic nerve block: lateral approach with the patient supine. Anesthesiology 1959; 20: 601–604.
23. Guardini R, Waldron BA, Wallace WA: Sciatic nerve block: a new lateral approach. Acta Anaesthsiol Scand 1985; 29: 515–519.
24. Kofoed H: Peripheral nerve blocks at the knee and ankle in operations for common foot disorders. Clin Orthop 1982; 168: 97–101.
25. Kempthorne PM, Brown TC: Nerve blocks around the knee in children. Anaesth Intensive Care 1984; 12: 14–17.
26. Arendzen JH, van Duijn H, Beckmann MK, et al: Diagnostic blocks of the tibial nerve in spastic hemiparesis. Effects on clinical, electrophysiological and gait parameters. Scand J Rehabil Med 1992; 24: 75–81.
27. Lofstrom B: Block at the knee-joint. In Eriksson E (ed): Illustrated Handbook in Local Anaesthesia, 2nd ed, p 111. London, Lloyd-Luke (Medical Books) Ltd, 1979.
28. Rorie DK, Byer DE, Nelson DO, et al: Assessment of block of the sciatic nerve in the popliteal fossa. Anesth Analg 1980; 59: 371–376.
29. Sarrafian SK, Ibrahim IN, Breihan JH: Ankle-foot peripheral nerve block for mid and forefoot surgery. Foot Ankle 1983; 4: 86–90.

CHAPTER 18

Regional Anesthesia of the Trunk

Dan J. Kopacz, M.D.

Because the trunk makes up a large proportion of the body, by necessity, regional anesthesia in this area encompasses a wide variety of block techniques. Similarly, with the wide variety of existing anatomic relationships, block techniques span a broad spectrum. Straightforward infiltration of local anesthetic solution is performed with minimal regard for needle placement relative to individual anatomic features. In contrast, the far more complex techniques of depositing solution in the proximity of specific nerves, while avoiding nearby structures that could potentially lead to adverse consequences (blood vessels, dural sac, lung parenchyma), can also be required in this area of the body (Fig. 18–1). Although these blocks are never all used simultaneously in any one patient, it is often desirable to use several of these blocks together (e.g., intercostal block of T-4 to T-12 and paravertebral lumbar somatic block of L-1 to L-3 for aortobifemoral bypass grafting) or in combination with blocks described in other chapters (e.g., breast block for mastectomy and brachial plexus block for axillary node dissection). Not surprisingly, the decision of which block(s) to use in a given instance is governed by many factors (patient attributes, anesthesiologist experience, surgical necessities). Frequently, many options exist to attain the same result—a successful block and a comfortable patient. It is suggested that the practitioner choose one technique and use it repeatedly until it is mastered, rather than alternating between techniques, which is likely to be less successful and more frustrating for all involved. Too often these techniques are used only when they are really needed (i.e., when general anesthesia is contraindicated), and failure frequently results. For one to become proficient, it is necessary to use these techniques often so that one will have enough experience to attain a successful block when it is really needed.

In general, only superficial surgical procedures can be performed with these blocks alone. With the avail-

ability of modern intravenous and inhalational anesthetic agents and neuromuscular relaxants, attempts to perform major explorative intra-abdominal procedures with a regional anesthetic alone are generally unwarranted. Although there may be no response to skin incision or dissection through the anterior abdominal wall, because there are often partially blocked or additional unblocked pathways over which pain can be transmitted (vagus and phrenic nerves, autonomic fibers), once the peritoneal cavity is entered, patient discomfort frequently follows. However, combining regional and general anesthesia can offer multiple advantages over a general anesthetic alone. The amount of general anesthetic agent (inhalational or intravenous), opioids, and neuromuscular blocking agent is drastically reduced, often resulting in a rapidly awakening, comfortable patient at the end of the operation. A clear patient sensorium and an improved level of comfort often lead to swift tracheal extubation and transport from the operating suite to the recovery area. Although not specifically proved, the decreased costs from the reduction in amount of other drugs used and the patient's expeditious course from the operating suite through the recovery room likely more than offset the cost, in time and money, required to institute the regional anesthetic before the operation begins.

In this chapter, each nerve block section describes the pertinent anatomy, the technical details of the block itself, any options that can be used during its performance, and many of the clinical situations in which the block can be used in the management of surgical or chronic pain. Physiologic effects and resultant local anesthetic levels of these blocks, when available, are outlined. Obviously, the list of clinical situations cannot be all-inclusive, and many unique situations will arise in which the judicious application of one or more of these blocks is of value. Because many of these techniques can be performed in slightly

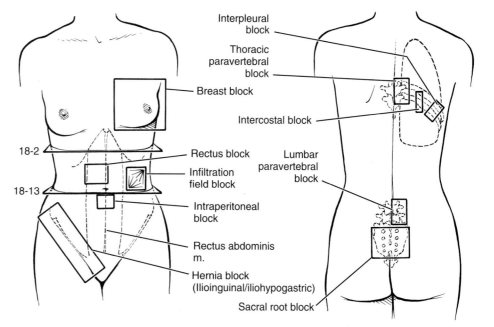

Figure 18–1 Blocks included in this chapter range from straightforward techniques with simple anatomic concepts and mechanisms of action (infiltration or field block) to techniques encompassing complex anatomy and physiology and requiring highly specific placement of needles if success is to be attained and complications avoided (paravertebral, intercostal, and interpleural). Areas from which cross sections in Figures 18–2 and 18–13 have been cut are shown.

different ways and can be instituted at several different times (preoperatively, intraoperatively, postoperatively) during the perioperative period, comparative studies among techniques or with other techniques that can be used to anesthetize the trunk (epidural or spinal) are difficult to control and perform. As such, their results are frequently difficult to interpret and are open to criticism, as evidenced by an extensive review of the possible modalities for managing post-thoracotomy pain.[1] Most sections conclude with clinical notes that may help in the performance of a block or its use in patient care.

Each block should start with the anesthesiologist developing an anatomic mental image, marking surface landmarks, careful positioning of both patient and physician, aseptic skin preparation, and draping. Many of the blocks in this section require a large number of injections. For maximum patient comfort, the practitioner will be best aided by the generous use of sedatives when these blocks are performed in the preoperative period. During this process, ensuring an adequate airway, providing supplemental oxygen, and continuous patient monitoring are ideal for patient safety. Depending on the clinical scenario, variable and often large volumes of a local anesthetic agent may be used (Table 18–1), and one should be constantly aware of the maximum recommended doses of the agents. The lower concentration shown for each block is the minimum that is clinically effective and can be arrived at by diluting a higher concentration of drug with saline to increase the available amount, in situations in which large volumes are necessary. If the higher concentration is used without dilution, the total mass of agent would exceed the recommended maximum.

Each section describes the needle(s), syringe, and local anesthetic agent most frequently used, but modifications may always be made to fit the situation (e.g., patient size) and availability. For instance, many operating suites are not stocked with varying lengths of reusable short-beveled peripheral nerve block needles. Often, a standard length (3.5 in, 9 cm) 22-G spinal needle can be used with little difficulty in situations in which an 8- or 10-cm needle is described.

Anatomic Overview

Most regional block techniques are percutaneous procedures, and a clear mental image of the three-dimensional anatomy of the area is necessary. The "shotgun" approach to regional block is seldom successful and (like the nerve stimulator) is no substitute for knowledge of the anatomy. Use your fingertips to palpate superficial structures and extensions of your fingers (finder needle) to feel the deeper structures so

Table 18–1 Volume and Concentration Required for Regional Anesthetic Techniques

| REGIONAL TECHNIQUE | LOCAL ANESTHETIC | | INJECTED VOLUME RANGE, mL | REMARKS |
	Lidocaine, %	Bupivacaine, %		
Infiltration or field or rectus block	0.25–1.0	0.125–0.25	20–120	Addition of epinephrine decreases surgical bleeding and prolongs duration of block; primarily a sensory block
Breast block	0.25–1.0	0.125–0.25	40–120	Epinephrine decreases bleeding and prolongs duration; higher concentration is necessary if brachial plexus and intercostal block included
Intercostal nerve block	1.0–1.5	0.25–0.5	3–60	Use 3–5 mL/rib; if multiple intercostal nerves blocked, epinephrine required to minimize systemic absorption
Interpleural block	1.0–1.5	0.25–0.5	20–30	Patient positioning main determinant of extent of block and must be maintained for 15–20 min; higher concentrations increase duration only
Thoracic paravertebral block	1.0–1.5	0.25–0.5	6–60	Single injection of 20 mL covers four dermatomes; if more than four dermatomes desired, second injection required; 6–8 mL for single nerve root
Lumbar paravertebral block	1.0–1.5	0.25–0.5	6–60	Unlike thoracic paravertebral block, spread of solution is limited; individual block of each nerve (dermatome) is recommended
Hernia block	0.25–1.0	0.125–0.25	40–120	Sensory block only; addition of epinephrine decreases surgical bleeding and prolongs duration of block
Intraperitoneal block	0.15–0.5	0.1–0.25	100–300	Large dilute volumes necessary to spread to all surfaces of peritoneum; residual should be removed by suctioning after 10–15 min
Cave of Retzius block	1.0–1.5	0.25–0.5	20–30	Use two to three passes, 8–10 mL/injection; addition of epinephrine decreases surgical bleeding and prolongs duration of block
Sacral root block	1.0–1.5	0.25–0.5	20–40	Use 4–8 mL/root; solution may spread to neighboring roots, so a small volume (1 mL) should be used for diagnostic (or neurolytic) blocks

that you can ascertain the anatomy of the region before depositing anesthetic solution to produce blocks.

Bones

It is necessary to understand the anatomy of only two bones to successfully perform peripheral nerve block in the trunk: the vertebra and the rib. Yet, the differences between a thoracic and a lumbar vertebra are significant, and the novice will benefit greatly from the meticulous study of a model of the human spine. The transverse processes of the lumbar vertebrae (L-1 to L-5) and the midthoracic vertebrae (T-4 to T-8) are located directly lateral from the superior edge of spinous processes. In the lumbar region, the transverse process and the spinous process are of the same vertebra. In the midthoracic region, owing to the exaggerated angulation of the spinous processes, the transverse process of a lower vertebra is lateral to the spinous process of a higher vertebra. The transverse processes of the intervening vertebrae (T-9 to T-12) are lateral to the interspaces between the spinous processes of two vertebrae. From the posterior view, the ribs appear as extensions of the thoracic transverse processes. A needle placed too far laterally contacts the rib and gives the operator a false sense of being in contact with the transverse process.

Ribs articulate with the superior and inferior demifacets of two adjacent vertebrae at their most medial point. Just lateral, the rib again articulates at its tubercle with the anterior surface of the transverse process of its own (the lower of these two) vertebra as it starts its caudally inclined course around the trunk. On its anterior (intrathoracic) surface, the rib acquires a groove along its inferior edge, which gradually disappears as the rib flattens along the lateral chest wall. The intercostal nerve and vessels reside within this costal groove.

Nerves

The intercostal nerves are the primary rami of T-1 through T-11. Many fibers from T-1 unite with fibers from C-8 to form the lowest trunk of the brachial plexus. These fibers leave the intercostal space by crossing the neck of the first rib, while a smaller bundle continues on a genuine intercostal course. The only other notable variation in intercostal nerves is the distribution of some fibers from T-2 and T-3 to form the intercostobrachial nerve. Terminal distribution of this nerve is to the skin of the medial aspect of the upper arm. Somatic innervation of the area from the nipples to below the umbilicus is provided by segmental spinal nerves from T-4 to T-11. The portion of chest wall cephalad to the nipples has overlapping innervation from the segmental spinal nerves of T-2 and T-3 and from peripheral branches from the cervical plexus (supraclavicular nerves, C-3 to C-4). Because incisions for most thoracic and upper abdominal procedures generally do not extend above the T-4 dermatome, anesthetizing these nerves is not necessary. The intercostal

nerve of T-12 is not a true intercostal nerve because it does not course between two ribs or between layers of intercostal muscles. It is sometimes termed a "subcostal nerve." Some of its fibers unite with fibers from the first lumbar nerve and are terminally represented as the iliohypogastric and ilioinguinal nerves.

The typical segmental intercostal nerve has five important branches (Fig. 18–2). The first two are the paired gray and white rami communicantes, which pass anteriorly to and from the sympathetic ganglion and chain. The third branch arises as the posterior cutaneous branch and supplies the skin and muscles in the paravertebral region and the articulation of the ribs and vertebrae. The fourth branch is the lateral cutaneous division, which arises just anterior to the midaxillary line, immediately sending subcutaneous fibers both posteriorly and anteriorly to supply skin of much of the chest and abdominal wall. The final branch of an intercostal nerve is the anterior cutaneous branch. In the upper five nerves, this branch terminates after penetrating the external intercostal and pectoralis major muscles to innervate the breast and front of the thorax. The lower six anterior cutaneous nerves terminate after piercing the sheath of the rectus abdominis muscle to which they supply motor branches. Terminal fibers continue anteriorly and become superficial near the linea alba, providing cutaneous innervation to the midline of the abdomen.

Regional block techniques for the trunk are similar in that they all anesthetize these same nerves. What distinguishes the different techniques is the location along these nerves at which local anesthetic solution is deposited (see Fig. 18–2). When paravertebral (lumbar or thoracic, sacral root) blocks are performed, solution is deposited in the region just lateral to the intervertebral foramen, where the rami communicantes and posterior cutaneous branches are emanating. Further lateral, intercostal and interpleural blocks anesthetize the nerve between the takeoff of the posterior and lateral cutaneous branches. The remaining blocks (infiltration, field block, rectus block, breast block, intraperitoneal block, hernia block) anesthetize the nerve at or anterior to this lateral branch or anesthetize the terminal endings of the nerves themselves. There is substantial overlap between nerves, both horizontally (across the midline, anterior cutaneous nerve overlapping lateral cutaneous nerve) and vertically between intercostal nerves. Because of this, the more distal the attempt at anesthetizing a peripheral nerve, the greater the chance for incomplete block and the greater the need to anesthetize neighboring nerves with overlapping distribution.

Muscles

The presence and orientation of muscles of the thorax are nearly identical to corresponding muscles of the abdomen (see Figs. 18–2 and 18–13). Along the lateral wall, segmental nerves (and vessels) are separated from the visceral compartments only by the peritoneum or pleura and a single muscle layer (innermost intercostal muscle in the chest, transverse abdominal

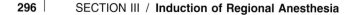

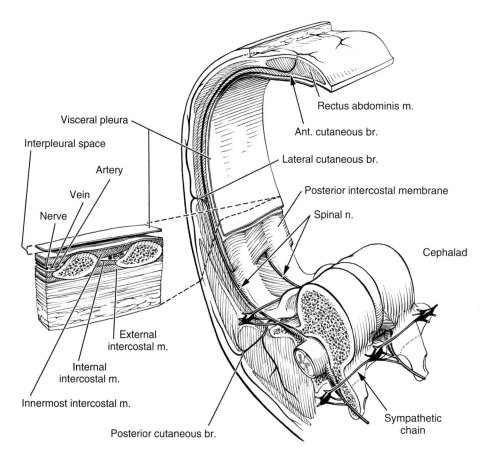

Figure 18–2 Intercostal, thoracic paravertebral, and interpleural blocks all involve interruption of transmission through the same spinal nerves but at different distances after their emergence from the dural sheath. Because of significant overlap between levels, all of these techniques require blocks of several (at least three) adjacent nerves or injection of large volumes of local anesthetic to attain successful anesthesia or analgesia in the perioperative period. br., branch; m., muscle; n., nerve.

muscle in the abdomen). More superficially, the internal intercostal muscle (and internal abdominal muscle) is oriented with fibers extending from its lateral origins on an inferior rib to its medial attachments to the next superior rib. The most superficial muscles (external intercostal in the thorax, external abdominal oblique in the abdomen) are oriented perpendicular to these previous internal layers, coursing from lateral and superior origins to medial and inferior attachments (terminations).

In the anterior part of the abdomen, the external and internal oblique muscles terminate and are replaced by the thick vertical rectus abdominal muscle. The internal oblique fascia splits, fusing with the external abdominal oblique fascia to form the anterior rectus sheath and fusing with the transverse abdominal fascia to form the posterior rectus sheath. In the lower third of the abdomen, this posterior sheath dissipates, leaving little more than peritoneum separating the rectus muscle from the peritoneal cavity. The rectus abdominal muscle attaches superiorly to the anterior xiphoid and the fifth, sixth, and seventh costal cartilages. No corresponding muscle continues into the thorax. In the abdomen, all fascial layers fuse in the midline to form the tough linea alba.

Infiltration, Field Block, or Rectus Block

Pertinent Anatomy

As the lower five intercostal nerves course anteriorly from beneath the costal cartilages, they take up posi-

tion between the transverse abdominal and internal abdominal oblique muscles, giving off branches to all layers of the abdominal wall: skin, subcutaneous tissue, muscle fasciae, and the muscles themselves. The main nerve trunks eventually surface and terminate after penetrating the rectus abdominal muscle at its posterolateral border. Tendinous intersections exist within the rectus muscle, which tend to create segmental distribution of these intercostal nerve terminals. Anteriorly, the rectus sheath (muscle fascia) is tough and fibrous from pubis to xiphoid. Posteriorly, it is strong and readily identifiable only down to the level of the umbilicus.

Technique Options

Unfortunately, emphasis on the teaching and use of field block has largely disappeared since the advent of safer general anesthetic and neuromuscular blocking agents. Infiltration anesthesia, commonly used by surgeons without assistance from anesthesiology personnel, is often thought of as being identical to field block anesthesia. Although both are commonly lumped together under the term "local anesthesia," substantial differences exist between these techniques.

During infiltration, local anesthetic solution is injected directly into the line of incision and nearby tissues, effectively flooding the individual local nerve endings to produce anesthesia (Fig. 18–3A). Infiltration often is performed randomly, using large volumes of

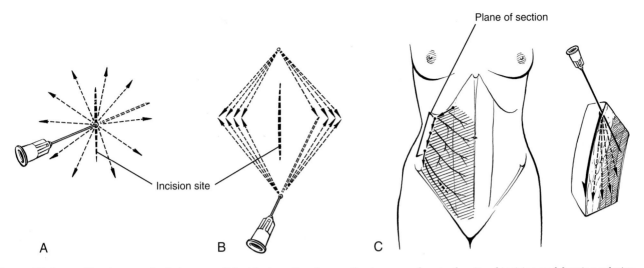

Figure 18–3 *A,* Infiltration anesthesia is accomplished by inserting the needle at or very close to the site of incision and fanning solution through multiple redirections of the needle. Solution should be deposited as far down as the anticipated depth of the procedure (i.e., for superficial incisions, only the skin and subcutaneous tissues are infiltrated; for deeper incisions, the muscles of the abdominal wall and their fasciae must be anesthetized as well). *B,* Field block is accomplished by surrounding the incision with walls of anesthetic solution. Like infiltration anesthesia, depth of block depends on the anticipated depth of the surgical procedure. Often, the needle may need to be introduced through several points, and compared with infiltration anesthesia, less solution is used, and less anatomic distortion and perhaps less inhibition of wound healing occur. *C,* For abdominal field block, the terminal branches of the intercostal nerves can be best anesthetized as they emerge from behind the costal cartilages to distribute between the transverse abdominal and internal abdominal oblique muscles. Below the costal margin, the block can be extended along the anterior axillary line until the anterior superior iliac spine is contacted.

solution to cover wide areas. In contrast, field blocks produce an encircling of the site of incision with walls of local anesthetic solution through which nerve trunks must pass before branching into terminal nerve endings (Fig. 18–3*B*). Although discrete nerves are not specifically blocked, less solution tends to be necessary. Because solution is not injected directly into the wound, no anatomic distortion is produced at the surgical site, and better muscle relaxation may be attained. Wound healing is unaffected by field block, but it may be from the local edema of infiltration. For abdominal field block, this technique primarily involves the final branchings of the intercostal nerves at the points where they pass the costal margins of the anterior and lateral abdominal walls (Fig. 18–3*C*; see also Fig. 18–13). Below the costal margin, it is easiest to extend the field block along the anterior axillary line until the anterior superior iliac spine of the iliac bone is encountered (so-called costoiliac block).[2]

The tough fibrous nature of the anterior and posterior rectus sheaths allows for a more specialized rectus field block for midline incisions (see Fig. 18–2). Because of tendinous intersections within the rectus muscle itself, two to six sites may need to be injected, depending on the location and size of the surgical incision. With the patient lying supine, at points 3 cm from the midline bilaterally, a short-bevel 5-cm, 22-G needle is passed posteriorly through the skin and subcutaneous tissue until the firm resistance of the anterior rectus sheath is encountered. If this sheath is not convincingly demonstrated, the block should be discontinued. With controlled steady pressure, a definitive pop is felt as the needle penetrates this sheath. As the needle is advanced further through the softer belly of the muscle, it approaches the posterior rectus sheath,

which is apparent as a second firm resistance. At this point, 10 mL of local anesthetic solution is injected. Blocks above the umbilicus should be performed first and needle depth should be noted before attempting blocks below the umbilicus, where injection just after the loss of first resistance (anterior sheath) is sufficient.

Use in Surgery, Postoperative Analgesia, and Pain Management

In general, infiltration and field block techniques alone are satisfactory only for superficial procedures. Although they will not provide sufficient anesthesia for most deep surgical procedures, particularly if the abdominal cavity is explored, a decrease in anesthetic requirements can be achieved. Rectus block has proved useful in the management of surgical pain after incisional and umbilical hernias, postpartum and laparoscopic tubal ligation, cesarean section when a midline incision is used,[3] and outpatient laparoscopy.[4] Infiltration and field blocks can be useful in diagnosing abdominal nerve entrapment syndromes or localized myofascial problems.

Physiologic Effects, Resultant Local Anesthetic Levels, and Comparison With Other Techniques

Few studies have directly evaluated the physiologic effects of these techniques or compared them with other available techniques. Studies have produced controversial results, but often an improvement in immediate postoperative analgesia is attained when bupivacaine is infiltrated compared with no infiltration or to a saline control. A decrease in pulmonary complications (atelectasis on chest radiograph, pulmonary function test measurements) and a reduction in postoperative opioid requirements have also been shown.[5–9] When properly performed, no sympathetic block and a limited degree of muscle relaxation are produced, so few physiologic alterations would be suspected.

If large areas are to be anesthetized, local anesthetic systemic toxicity is possible, because large volumes of agent (up to 120 mL) can be necessary. However, lower concentrations of drug can be used, and in general, local anesthetic absorption from skin and subcutaneous tissue is much lower than after other regional block techniques. Scott et al[10] have shown that the absorption of 400 mg of lidocaine after subcutaneous abdominal infiltration produces plasma lidocaine levels that are 30% of those resulting from intercostal block and 50% of those produced by lumbar epidural injection. The decrease in plasma local anesthetic levels by the addition of epinephrine is also greater for infiltration compared with the other nerve block techniques.

Clinical Note: *The benefit of a short-bevel (or reusable) needle is no more obvious than when performing a field block of the abdomen, where the blunt bevel provides useful feedback on the exact location of the needle tip as it passes fascial layers. Excessive penetration and resultant perforation of the peritoneum and underlying organs such as liver, intestine, bladder, or uterus are the chief concerns. When a rectus block is performed, a visible bulge in the abdominal wall on injection indicates that the needle is too superficial. These blocks may be difficult, if not contraindicated, in the obese or cachectic patient, the patient with a distended abdomen (ascites), or the elderly patient with poor abdominal muscle tone in whom fascial layers are not apparent.*

Breast Block

Pertinent Anatomy

The breast and axillary nodes derive their innervation from multiple sources. The majority of the glandular breast tissue and overlying skin is innervated by branches from the lateral and anterior cutaneous divisions of the first to sixth intercostal nerves. These branches approach the breast from the medial, lateral, and inferior directions, with additional branches coming deep from beneath the pectoralis muscles. Skin overlying the superior portion of the breast is innervated by the supraclavicular nerves from the superficial cervical plexus. The axilla and the pectoral muscles are innervated by the brachial plexus (C-5 to T-1) and the intercostobrachial nerve (T2-3).

Technique Options

Depending on the planned operative procedure, the required regional anesthetic may range from infiltration of small amounts of local anesthetic solution to a complex combination of several of the techniques (intercostal block, brachial plexus block). The appropriate level of sedation is dictated by the clinical situation. In instances when multiple injections are planned, patient comfort is enhanced by moderately heavy sedation.

Biopsy of small masses in the breast can normally be accomplished with infiltration alone. Deep or larger lesions (including simple mastectomy, breast augmentation, and breast reduction) require field blocks. The large numbers of cutaneous branches essentially require that the breast be completely encircled with local anesthetic solution. Nerves penetrating the lateral and inferior margins of the breast can be anesthetized by blocking the second to sixth intercostal nerves (Fig. 18–4A). Thoracic epidural or paravertebral block can be performed to cover these same dermatomes. Medial branches, overlapping from the opposite side, require skin infiltration along the entire sternum, from its notch to the xiphoid process (Fig. 18–4B). Superior branches, from the supraclavicular nerves of the superficial cervical plexus, require infiltration along the inferior edge of the clavicle from acromion to sternal notch. Branches arising from deep tissues can be anesthetized by infiltration into the retromammary space between the pectoralis major muscle and the breast and by infiltration posterior to the pectoral muscles where they are innervated by the medial and lateral pectoral nerves.

In this process, large volumes (40 to 120 mL) of dilute (0.25% to 1.0% lidocaine, 0.125% to 0.25% bupivacaine) local anesthetic solution may be required. For this reason, if bilateral simple mastectomy (or reduction mammoplasty) is to be performed, thoracic paravertebral or thoracic epidural anesthesia is more appropriate to avoid local anesthetic systemic toxicity.

Use in Surgery, Postoperative Analgesia, and Pain Management

Because of the increased complexity of the procedure and for emotional and psychologic reasons, radical mastectomy is most appropriately accomplished with general anesthesia. If general anesthesia is strongly contraindicated, the breast itself can be anesthetized as described above for simple mastectomy. In addition, it will be necessary to perform a supraclavicular brachial plexus block to anesthetize the axilla and the innervation of the pectoral muscles. It should be discussed with the surgeon preoperatively that solution may spread distally and that the motor fibers of the brachial plexus will be anesthetized. Efforts to avoid trauma to the brachial plexus by detecting it with direct electrical stimulation in the axilla may be ineffective. Because the overlying skin is undermined and denervated dur-

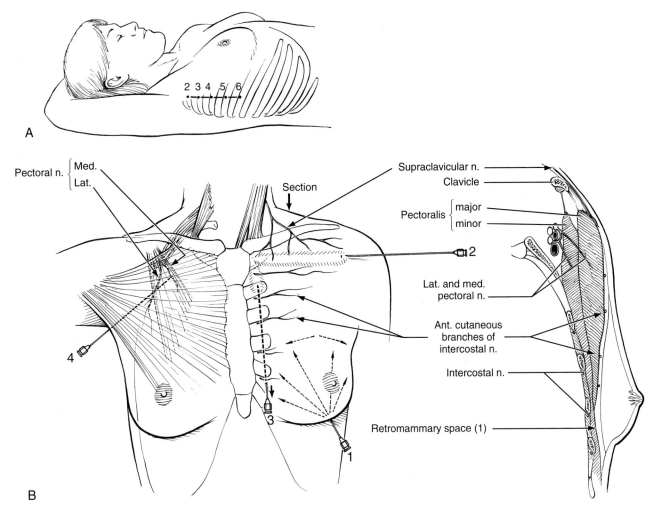

Figure 18–4 Breast block can be accomplished two ways, depending on the magnitude of the planned operation. For small procedures (biopsy, lumpectomy), infiltration field block or infiltration of the retromammary space (*B1*) where the innervation of the breast emerges through or from behind the pectoralis muscle is frequently sufficient. For extensive procedures (reduction or augmentation mammoplasty, mastectomy with or without axillary dissection), better anesthesia is attained by addressing all points of innervation: *A*, anesthetizing intercostal nerves T-3 to T-7 using either lateral or posterior approach; *B2*, infiltrating subcutaneously along the inferior edge of the clavicle to anesthetize the supraclavicular branches of the cervical plexus; *B3*, infiltrating subcutaneously along the lateral sternal border to anesthetize terminal branches crossing the midline; and *B4*, performing a supraclavicular brachial plexus block or infiltrating beneath the pectoralis muscle to anesthetize the medial and lateral pectoral nerves. Ant., anterior; Lat., lateral; Med., medial; n., nerve.

ing radical mastectomy, postoperative pain is not severe.

Although postmastectomy pain is most often seen weeks to months later as a chronic, perhaps sympathetically mediated pain syndrome, it may also be seen in the immediate postoperative period. It is not known whether regional anesthetic techniques minimize its incidence or severity. Like other sympathetically mediated pain, opioids are relatively ineffective and early treatment with sympathetic block (stellate ganglion block) seems most efficacious.

Physiologic Effects, Resultant Local Anesthetic Levels, and Comparison With Other Techniques

No studies have been performed to look at the physiologic effects of breast block or to directly compare it with other anesthetic techniques. Surgical blood loss is decreased when cervical epidural anesthesia is used in conjunction with general anesthesia for radical mastectomy.[11] This same beneficial effect is also thought to occur with field block of the breast, either alone or in combination with general anesthesia.

Clinical Note: *Except when infiltrating at the incision itself, injection into glandular breast tissue is of little value. Infiltration over long distances is required for field block of the breast, so a 10- to 12-cm needle (a disposable spinal needle works well) decreases the number of painful skin wheals that are required. If radical mastectomy is performed with regional block, immediate reconstruction with tissue implants can be performed without any additional anesthesia. Newer reconstructive techniques using transverse abdominal muscle* *flaps (TRAM flap) require additional regional anesthesia of the abdomen. Because this also significantly increases the operative duration, supplementation with general anesthesia will most likely be necessary.*

Intercostal Nerve Block

Pertinent Anatomy

As the thoracic paravertebral space extends laterally, it is in continuity with the intercostal spaces. In the paravertebral region, there is only fatty connective tissue between nerve and pleura. Medial to the angles of the ribs, the intercostal nerves lie between the pleura and the fascia of the internal intercostal muscle (also called the posterior intercostal membrane) (see Fig. 18–2). At the angle of the rib (6 to 8 cm from the spinous processes), the nerve comes to lie between the internal intercostal muscle and the innermost intercostal muscle. At this position, the costal groove of the rib is broadest and deepest. A cadaver study[12] has shown that the nerve remains subcostal only 17% of the time, has most frequently (73%) moved inferiorly into the midzone between ribs, and is often branching. The nerve is accompanied by intercostal veins and an artery, which lie superior to the nerve in the inferior groove of each rib, which accounts for the high plasma local anesthetic levels after intercostal block. About 5 to 8 cm further lateral, the costal groove ceases to exist and becomes the sharp inferior edge of the rib; the lateral cutaneous branch of the intercostal nerve takes off. This branch is of significance to the anesthesiologist, because it immediately sends off branches in both the anterior and posterior directions. If local anesthetic is deposited anterior to the takeoff of the lateral cutaneous nerve, complete truncal anesthesia is unlikely to develop.

Technique Options

Bilateral intercostal block is most easily performed with the patient in the full prone position, but it can also be successfully accomplished with the patient supine (Fig. 18–5A and C). The prone and lateral positions allow for block of the nerves at the angle of the ribs, where a larger margin of safety is present before pleura is encountered and block of the nerve occurs before the takeoff of the lateral cutaneous branch. When performing the block with the patient prone, positioning a pillow under the patient's upper abdomen widens the intercostal spaces. Allowing the patient's arms to dangle over the sides of the anesthetic table (Fig. 18–5A) allows the scapulae to move laterally, facilitating block of the upper intercostal nerves.

Although the lateral decubitus position can also be used, because it is technically difficult to manipulate the needle and syringe on the dependent side, only the top intercostal nerves can be safely blocked. After block

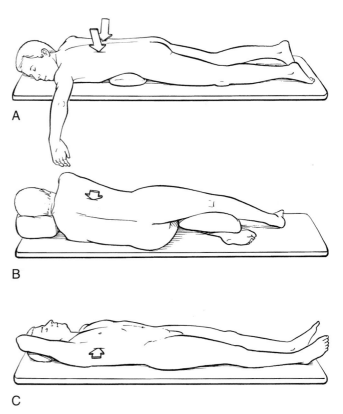

Figure 18–5 Intercostal block can be performed with the patient in any of three positions. *A,* The prone position allows (1) injection further posterior; (2) better retraction of the scapulae to allow better access to the second to sixth ribs; and (3) bilateral intercostal block to be performed without repositioning, as is necessary with positioning shown in *B* with patient in the lateral decubitus position (for unilateral block of the nondependent nerves), if bilateral blocks are to be performed. *C,* The supine position is the easiest to use if a patient is still receiving general anesthesia at the end of operation, but the lateral cutaneous branch (see Fig. 18–2) may not be anesthetized if injection is performed too far anterior.

of one side, the patient can be repositioned in the opposite decubitus position to perform intercostal block of the remaining side (Fig. 18–5B).

After proper positioning, it is best to first mark the planned injection sites; it is easy to become confused if multiple sites are to be injected. An initial line (two lines if bilateral blocks are being performed) should be drawn parallel and lateral to the spine, at the point where the ribs can be most easily palpated. Palpation of the ribs is difficult immediately adjacent to the spine, where they are covered by the thick paraspinal muscles. As palpation is performed beyond the lateral margins of these muscles, the ribs can be easily felt 6 to 9 cm from the midline. The tip of the 12th rib should be distinctly felt near the caudal end of this line. Because the fusiform-shaped paraspinal muscle group tapers cephalad and to best avoid the scapula, the cephalad end of this line may be only 4 to 5 cm from the midline. Starting from the 12th rib, which is the easiest to feel, and working cephalad, the intercostal spaces are palpated along this line and marks are made at the inferior edge of each rib. For abdominal surgery, six or seven (T-5 to T-11 or T-12) pairs of ribs are marked. For thoracic or other unilateral chest wall surgery, only the appropriate side and ribs are marked. The distance between ribs gradually decreases as one moves cephalad, so these marks should get progressively closer together (Fig. 18–6A).

After intravenous cannulation, mild sedation, and assurance of adequate ventilation and oxygenation, skin wheals are raised at all of these marked sites. It is most comfortable for a right-handed anesthesiologist to stand at the patient's left side. The technical performance of an intercostal nerve block is a sequence of alternating hand motions. Beginning at the lowest rib to be anesthetized, the anesthesiologist's left hand (closest to the patient's head) first palpates the skin wheal and stretches it from its initial position at the inferior edge of the rib over the middle of the rib, intentionally forming a small mound of skin in advance of the finger (Fig. 18–6B). The right hand next places a 3- to 4-cm, 22-G short-bevel needle, with a syringe attached containing local anesthetic, immediately off the tip of the retracting finger and through the skin wheal onto the middle of the rib (Fig. 18–6C). Although the next step is awkward and often neglected, it is the most important step to ensure that the needle is being safely controlled by a hand in close contact with the patient's body. The thumb and first two fingers of the left hand, which were previously retracting skin, shift to firmly grasp the needle shaft at the point where it enters the skin (Fig. 18–6D). This left hand then walks the needle caudad, with the right hand doing nothing more than supporting the syringe. The slight tension of the retracted skin is often enough to allow a passive walking of the needle to the inferior edge of the rib. When one feels the needle slip off the inferior edge of the rib, it is advanced 2 to 3 mm further, where a subtle give or pop of the fascia of the internal intercostal muscle may be felt. The right hand now slowly injects 3 to 5 mL of local anesthetic solution (Fig. 18–6E). Using the left hand to slowly move the needle in and out 1 mm decreases the risk of significant intravascular injection and helps ensure proper spread of solution into the fascial plane containing the nerve (Fig. 18–6H). To accomplish these same goals, an alternative method is to deposit half of the solution (1 to 2 mL) without needle motion and briefly bring the needle tip back up onto the rib with the left hand (Fig. 18–6F). The needle is then walked back off the rib to deposit the remaining solution at a slightly different spot (Fig. 18–6G). After injection, the needle is removed to the subcutaneous tissue (Fig. 18–6I), the next higher rib is palpated with the left hand, and this process is repeated for each of the nerves to be blocked (Fig. 18–6J).

Although this alternating sequence initially seems tedious, it is rapidly learned. At all times when the needle is not in contact with a rib, it is being controlled by the hand that is in close contact with the patient's body. If the patient moves suddenly, the entire hand–needle–patient body will move as a unit, preventing further penetration of the needle and minimizing complications.

Catheters can be placed in both the intercostal and thoracic paravertebral spaces and repeat injection can be used as an effective means of providing postoperative analgesia. It is difficult to comment on the relative effectiveness, owing to the differences in technique (percutaneous versus internal placement intraoperatively, the distance the catheter is passed, and an inability to be certain of the final catheter tip location).

Use in Surgery, Postoperative Analgesia, and Pain Management

Small umbilical and incisional hernias, minor breast surgery,[13] extracorporeal lithotripsy,[14] and cardiac pacemaker insertion[15] using intercostal block have been described. Block of two or three nerves is a simple way to prepare for insertion of thoracostomy or feeding gastrostomy tubes. In general, some degree of supplemental anesthesia must complement the block for most other surgical procedures. Intercostal block may also be combined with brachial plexus block for more extensive operations on the breast, upper extremities, and axilla. For intra-abdominal procedures, celiac plexus block may be added to provide visceral anesthesia. Pain from pelvic structures is not relieved by intercostal block, and operations in that region are better performed with spinal, caudal, or lumbar epidural techniques.

The most effective but least exploited use of this block is for postoperative control of pain. Perhaps the simplest demonstration of this technique is the amount of benefit derived from simply blocking the right 10th, 11th, and 12th intercostal nerves in patients having an appendectomy.[16] Intercostal nerve block is extremely effective in providing pain relief for fractured ribs. Herpes zoster pain may be relieved and even treated in this way. Intercostal nerve block can also be helpful in the differential diagnosis of visceral versus abdominal wall pain.

Physiologic Effects, Resultant Local Anesthetic Levels, and Comparison With Other Techniques

Three studies have examined the effects of intercostal blocks on lung volumes and gas flow rates in healthy volunteers.[17–19] Statistically insignificant decreases are detected in most of the lung capacities and flows (total lung capacity 1% to 4%, forced vital capacity 4% to 7%, peak expiratory flow 4% to 18%, functional residual capacity 0% to 8%, and peak expiratory airway pressure 7%). Furthermore, these changes appear to be entirely due to alterations in extrapulmonary chest wall mechanics. Elastic recoil and measurements of intrinsic pulmonary (Pa_{O_2}, Pa_{CO_2}, and ventilatory response to Pa_{CO_2}) and bronchial (ratio of dead space gas volume to tidal gas volume, mid-peak expiratory flow) function are unaltered. Interestingly, there was also no difference among 0.25% bupivacaine, 1.0% lidocaine, and 0.5% etidocaine, although one would have expected a more potent motor block

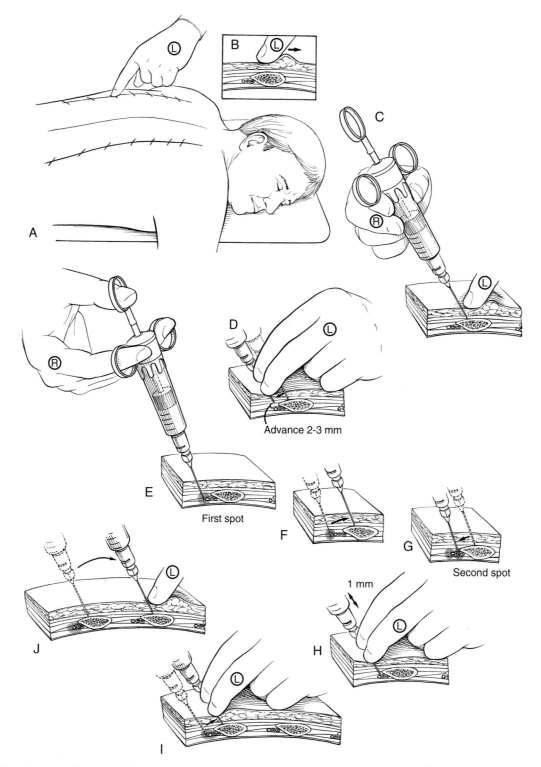

Figure 18–6 Performance of intercostal block involves a sequence of steps alternating between each of the anesthesiologist's hands. *A,* The anesthesiologist's hand closest to the patient's head (cephalic) first locates the target interspace and then *(B)* retracts the skin over the rib above. *C,* The hand closest to the patient's feet (caudad) places the needle (and attached syringe containing local anesthetic) through the skin onto the rib at about a 30° angle, with the needle bevel directed cephalad. *D,* The cephalic hand then grasps the needle, while maintaining contact with the patient, and allows the tension of the retracted skin to walk the needle off the inferior edge of the rib and advance 2 to 3 mm. *E,* The caudad hand then injects 3 to 5 mL of solution (the left hand holding the needle has been removed from *E* through *G* for illustrative purposes—it should *not* let go of the needle during injection). *F,* The cephalic hand places the needle back on the rib after injection (or alternatively it may be removed entirely, *I*), and immediately the sequence is started again at the next highest interspace *(J)*. During the actual injection, aspiration is unnecessary (and because of the small size of these vessels, not helpful) if the needle is placed back on the inferior edge of the rib and walked off a second time *(G)* to deposit solution in a slightly different location. *H,* Alternatively, the needle may be moved in and out 1 mm during injection. These actions ensure that all of the solution is not injected into an artery or vein, which lies in close proximity to the nerve. L, left; R, right.

from etidocaine. Ventilatory function was well maintained in subjects, even at extremes in demand imposed by graded increases in exercise on a cycle ergometer.

Numerous studies have evaluated the pulmonary changes after thoracic and upper abdominal surgery by comparing the analgesia from intercostal block, parenteral opioids, and epidural morphine.[20-24] Although it is difficult to compare these studies directly because of the many methodologic differences (timing and dose of analgesics, site of incision [midline versus subcostal], timing of pulmonary measurements), in general, epidural morphine and intercostal block offer significant improvement over parenteral opioids in overall analgesia and in preserving pulmonary function. Pulmonary measurements (peak expiratory flow rate, forced expiratory volume in 1 s, forced vital capacity) tend to decrease to only 60% to 90% of baseline preoperative levels, compared with 40% to 60% when parenteral opioids are used. More importantly, effective analgesia with intercostal block has been shown to decrease the incidence of postoperative pulmonary complications (atelectasis, pneumonia).[25]

The actual incidence of pneumothorax is extremely low, but many physicians avoid this block because of purported high frequency. The incidence of clinically significant pneumothorax was only 0.073% when physicians in all stages of training performed more than 10,000 individual intercostal nerve blocks.[26] The incidence of radiographically detectable pneumothorax was 0.42% in a second study in which preoperative and postoperative chest films were taken in 200 consecutive patients. The one pneumothorax detected was entirely asymptomatic (silent) and would not have been detected had the chest radiographs not been taken as a part of the study.[27] Although one attempts to avoid parietal pleural penetration, pneumothorax will not result unless the visceral pleura is also pierced. Treatment of pneumothorax by careful observation is usually all that is needed. Reabsorption of a small pneumothorax is also aided by administration of oxygen. Needle aspiration or chest tube drainage, each with their own possible complications, should be performed only if the pneumothorax is symptomatic or if there is failure to reexpand the lung with these preliminary maneuvers.

The possibility of local anesthetic systemic toxicity exists, because blood levels after intercostal and interpleural block are higher than after other regional anesthetic procedures. Systemic toxic reactions rarely occur in patients having diagnostic or therapeutic blocks because smaller volumes of more dilute solutions of drug are used. Greater amounts of more concentrated drug are injected to provide complete motor and sensory block in surgical patients. These greater doses may result in delayed systemic toxicity, so that patients should be monitored for 15 to 20 min after completion of the block.

Peak plasma concentrations after intercostal block depend on the local anesthetic agent used, the concentration and volume injected, and whether or not epinephrine is added. Epinephrine seems to decrease plasma concentrations 30% to 50% for mepivacaine and bupivacaine, but it does not influence the concentrations of etidocaine when it is used for intercostal block.[28] As a general rule, a plasma concentration of 0.1 μg/mL is produced by the injection of every 10 mg of bupivacaine with epinephrine.

Performance of intraoperative intercostal injection appears to be associated with a higher incidence of complications. Multiple cases of total spinal anesthesia, manifesting as hypotension and bradycardia, dilated pupils, and prolonged anesthesia and paralysis, have been reported after intrathoracic intercostal block at the end of surgery during general anesthesia.[29, 30] In most of these instances, the blocks were performed under direct vision, at a site more medial than would be chosen for the percutaneous approach. Injection of local anesthetic into a dural root cuff or directly into nerve tissue itself with extensive intrafascicular spread is the proposed mechanism for the resultant widespread block.

Clinical Note: *If one wants to combine celiac plexus or lumbar somatic nerve blocks with intercostal block, it is technically easiest to perform all blocks with the patient in the prone position.*

Special attention is needed so that a given rib is not palpated, marked, and its nerve blocked twice (proximal superiorly and distal laterally) while another is being missed entirely. Because the ribs are symmetric, markings should line up with those of the opposite side when bilateral blocks are being performed. In thin patients, the ribs may take a deceptively steep course. In these patients, it may be easier to walk the needle off the rib by taking a slightly medial path, which is more perpendicular (shortest distance) to the long axis.

Careful attention to several details while walking the needle off the rib improves patient comfort and block success. Dragging the needle across the sensitive periosteum is painful; lifting the needle slightly with each little walk causes substantially less pain, even if it is necessary to recontact the rib several times. Although the nerve may have already descended into a midposition between the ribs, because the distance between the fasciae of the internal intercostal and innermost intercostal muscles is greatest at the intercostal groove, maintenance of a slight cephalad tilt (15° to 20°, up into the groove) increases the success of injecting into this narrow intercostal target space. If the needle is allowed to pivot while it is walked off the rib, resulting in the needle pointing caudad, the chance of a successful block is decreased.

Interpleural Block

Pertinent Anatomy

The visceral pleura tightly envelops the lung, following its fissures and indentations. At the chest wall, diaphragm, and mediastinal margins of the lung, the pleura reflects back onto itself to form the parietal pleura, which follows the contours of the chest wall. Projected to the chest wall, anteriorly these lines of reflection emerge near the xiphoid, pass laterally to reach the midaxillary line at its intersection with the 10th rib, and cross the neck of the 12th rib to reach its posterior reflection about 4 cm from the midline. Interpleural anesthesia can technically be accomplished anywhere within these fixed boundaries.

Anesthesia is attained by topical contact of free nerve ending in the pleural surfaces and by diffusion of local anesthetic solution to nerves in proximity to the pleural surfaces (Fig. 18–7). Anteriorly, laterally, and posteriorly, the parietal pleura is in close approximation to the intercostal nerves. Medially, the sympathetic chain and splanchnic, phrenic, and vagus nerves are adjacent. The epidural and subarachnoid spaces are at a greater distance and are generally not believed to be a site of local anesthetic action during interpleural anesthesia. However, these structures are separated from the parietal pleura only by the fat and loose connective tissues of the epidural and paravertebral spaces, and if there is a significant breach of the parietal pleura (e.g., posterior thoracotomy), tracking of anesthetic solution to these structures is also possible. Superiorly, the inferior roots of the brachial plexus pass a short distance over the cupula, where they may be anesthetized by interpleural solution before reaching the first rib and continuing into the axilla.

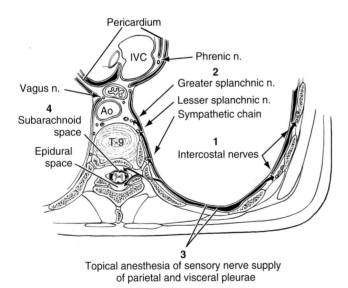

3
Topical anesthesia of sensory nerve supply
of parietal and visceral pleurae

Figure 18–7 Local anesthetic instilled into the pleural space has several probable mechanisms of action: (1) Local anesthetic crosses the parietal pleura (posteriorly and laterally) to cause block of intercostal nerves. (2) Local anesthetic causes sympathetic block by crossing the parietal pleura medially to anesthetize the lesser (anteriorly) and greater splanchnic nerves and the sympathetic chain (posteriorly). (3) Sensory nerve endings in the visceral and parietal pleurae are topically anesthetized. (4) Additionally, some local anesthetic may diffuse across the dural root sleeve (particularly if the posterior pleura has been incised) into the epidural or subarachnoid space. Ao, aorta; IVC, inferior vena cava; n., nerve.

Technique Options

Interpleural catheters are most commonly placed posteriorly with the patient in the lateral or semiprone position. In patients unable to assume this position, the technique can also be performed laterally at the midaxillary line or anteriorly at the midclavicular line with the patient in the supine position. The hallmark of this technique is detection of the negative interpleural pressure, so placement of the catheter should be performed either preoperatively or postoperatively in the awake patient or during general anesthesia with the patient breathing spontaneously. Placement should be avoided during positive pressure ventilation, because the interpleural pressure is no longer negative and the risk of pneumothorax, and the subsequent possibility of a tension pneumothorax, is increased.[31]

When using the posterior approach, with the patient in either the lateral or the prone position, the ipsilateral arm should be allowed to dangle in front of the body or off the table to retract the scapula as far anterolaterally as possible (Fig. 18–8A). After aseptic skin preparation and draping, the skin is first anesthetized at a point 8 to 10 cm lateral from the midline, overlying the top edge of a rib. Infiltration is carried deeper with a 2- or 3-cm, 22-G needle, until the rib is contacted. Because the periosteum is quite sensitive, additional injection of local anesthetic at this point minimizes discomfort. This finder needle is removed and replaced with a 16- or 18-G Tuohy needle. After recontacting the rib, and with the hand controlling the needle in firm contact with the patient's back, the needle is gently walked cephalad until it slides off the superior edge of the rib (Fig. 18–8B). The bevel should be aimed in the direction in which the catheter eventually is passed.

At this stage, one of two methods may be safely used. In the first option, the stylet is removed and replaced with a frictionless (saline lubricated or polished dry), glass 10-mL syringe containing 3 to 5 mL of air (Fig. 18–8C).[32] The needle-syringe unit is then slowly advanced until entrance into the interpleural space is detected when the plunger is pulled in to evacuate the syringe by the negative interpleural pressure (Fig. 18–8D). If awake, the patient should be warned that a brief twinge may be felt as the parietal pleura is penetrated. Gentle intermittent tapping of the plunger can ensure that the needle is not being plugged and that the plunger is not sticking in the barrel of the syringe. Both of these situations could result in the needle being advanced too far, because no movement of the plunger would occur. Generation of a true continuous positive pressure within the syringe should be avoided. If this technique is used preoperatively, avoidance of nitrous oxide should be considered during subsequent general anesthesia, because a significant expansion of the small pneumothorax that is created could occur.

Once the tip of the needle is safely within the interpleural space, the syringe is removed and the interpleural catheter is passed 5 to 6 cm into the space. The needle is removed, and an occlusive dressing is applied.

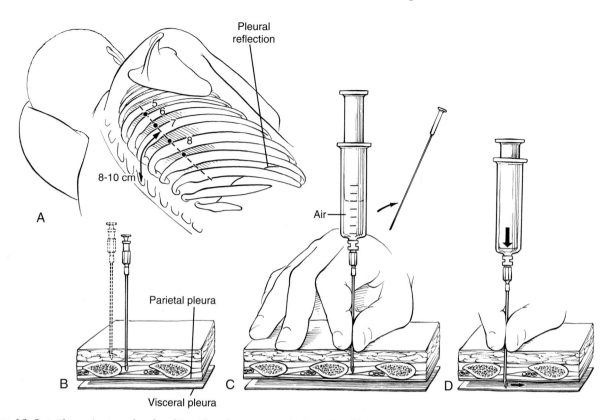

Figure 18–8 *A,* The patient can be placed in either the prone or the lateral position (operative side up) for interpleural block. The ipsilateral arm is allowed to dangle off the table, moving the scapula forward. The site of interpleural catheter placement is chosen from the fifth to the eighth intercostal space, 8 to 10 cm lateral (posterior axillary line). *B,* After aseptic skin preparation and skin and periosteal infiltration, an 18-G Tuohy needle is placed on the superior edge of the rib with the bevel directed in the cephalad direction. The needle is walked cephalad just until contact with the superior edge of the rib is lost. *C,* At this point, while the needle is carefully held with one hand braced against the patient's back, the stylet is removed and replaced with a moistened, 10-mL glass syringe containing approximately 5 mL of air. *D,* The needle and syringe are slowly advanced as a unit until identification of the pleural space occurs when the plunger of the syringe and the contained air are pulled down by the negative interpleural pressure. An epidural catheter is advanced 5 to 6 cm into the pleural space and, after negative aspiration, is secured in place.

Aspiration of the catheter may produce a small amount (<20 mL) of air or fluid. If blood or large amounts of air or fluid are obtained, the catheter should be removed and replaced or the technique should be abandoned. Spread of local anesthetic solution within the interpleural space is primarily dominated by gravity, but to a lesser degree it is also influenced by the volume and the location of the catheter.[33] These factors must be taken into account before placement of the catheter and injection of solution.

The second option necessitates the removal of the plunger from a saline-containing syringe.[34] Once connected, close attention is directed to the meniscus at the saline-air interface. During slow advancement of the needle-syringe unit, entrance into the interpleural space is heralded by the falling column of saline, which is now open to the atmosphere. A catheter can be passed into the open-ended syringe barrel, through the saline and needle, and into the interpleural space. The advantage of this technique is that no air is introduced or allowed to entrain the interpleural space.

The use of loss of resistance to positive pressure should be avoided. Unlike the dense ligamentum flavum during epidural placement, the resistances offered by various tissues during interpleural catheter place-

ment are subtle and inconsistent. One cannot be certain whether the loss of resistance is from the interpleural space itself or from a false loss of resistance, which can occur between intercostal muscles or when the catheter is advanced too far into lung parenchyma.

Before local anesthetic injection, the patient should be placed in a position to maximize the desired effect. Because solution movement is governed by gravity, the block is greatest at the most dependent point.[35] Positioning the patient with the operative side up causes solution to pool medially, maximizing the amount of subsequent sympathetic block. The supine and operative side down positions cause solution to accumulate near the intercostal nerves, minimizing the amount of sympathetic block. A head down position can increase the amount of cervical and upper thoracic sympathetic block and, in some instances, produce anesthesia of the inferior roots of the brachial plexus.

As in epidural anesthesia, a small epinephrine-containing test dose should be initially administered to detect inadvertent intravascular placement. The total dose (20 to 30 mL) should be given by intermittent injection over 2 to 3 min, and the position should be maintained for 20 to 30 min to allow the anesthetic to set. Bupivacaine has been used most often, although any local anesthetic agent can be used. Bupivacaine 0.25% appears to have an onset and duration of action nearly identical to those of the 0.5% concentration. In fact, the duration of action appears to be proportional to the mass of drug given (100 mg produces 8 h of analgesia), not the concentration or volume.[36] Less lipid-soluble agents would be expected to produce block of proportionately shorter duration.

Use in Surgery, Postoperative Analgesia, and Pain Management

Although fear of pneumothorax and high serum local anesthetic levels have attenuated the initial enthusiasm, interpleural block remains a valuable anesthetic and analgesia option in selected clinical situations. Combination with light general anesthesia is often necessary. Interpleural analgesia is perhaps best used for open cholecystectomy, renal surgery, and unilateral breast procedures. After cholecystectomy, opioid requirements and visual analogue pain scores (VAS) are decreased and pulmonary variables are improved when interpleural analgesia is used.[37, 38]

Usefulness of interpleural block during thoracotomy is controversial, because the duration of block appears to be significantly decreased when the parietal pleura is interrupted and a thoracostomy drainage tube is present.[39, 40] However, instillation of local anesthetic through a chest tube (used as an interpleural catheter) may be a beneficial adjunct in the treatment of post-thoracotomy pain, if adequate analgesia is difficult to attain by other means and the tube can be clamped for 20 min without patient hazard.

Bilateral interpleural catheters have been reported[41] for upper abdominal surgery and bilateral pulmonary surgery through sternotomy. The consequences of bilateral pneumothoraces and the vigilance necessary to rapidly detect and treat them if they occur are obvious.

When interpleural block is used to provide analgesia for multiple rib fractures, dramatic improvement of pulmonary function can be attained.[42] Treatment of upper limb ischemia, reflex sympathetic dystrophy, and pain of acute and chronic pancreatitis has been described.[43–46] Interpleural catheters have been used to treat spontaneous and iatrogenic pneumothoraces. Preliminary reports were optimistic about the use of interpleural block in patients who previously have been resistant to treatment, including those with tumor invasion of the brachial plexus, vertebral metastases, and severe postherpetic neuralgia.[47, 48] Catheters have been tunneled subcutaneously for the long-term management of thoracic pain in cancer patients.[49] Injection of phenol into the interpleural space was beneficial in managing a patient with esophageal cancer in whom other means of analgesia had been tried and found to be ineffective.[50] Although interpleural analgesia may not be a first choice in the treatment of many of these pathologic situations, its use may be beneficial in providing an opioid or treatment holiday, which some advocate in these circumstances.

Physiologic Effects, Resultant Local Anesthetic Levels, and Comparison With Other Techniques

The complications of interpleural injection of local anesthetic have been extensively reviewed. Initial estimates of the incidence of pneumothorax are approximately 2%.[51] Most reported cases have occurred when patients were being mechanically ventilated, an active loss of resistance technique was used, there was unanticipated patient movement, or the needle was unintentionally occluded. The true incidence of pneumothorax, with proper indications and use of sound technique, is most likely even less.

Serum local anesthetic levels reach a peak in 20 to 30 min and tend to be higher than when equal amounts are injected for multiple intercostal nerve blocks. The analgesia also tends to be less intense and of shorter duration.[52] The addition of epinephrine does not decrease serum bupivacaine levels, nor does it appear to increase the duration or intensity of block.

The concurrent sympathetic block often produces Horner's syndrome, which should be anticipated and can be used as a sign of successful catheter placement if it is detected. Ipsilateral bronchospasm has been reported,[53] theoretically owing to the unilateral sympathetic block. Phrenic nerve paresis does occur in some instances, but its incidence and clinical significance remain to be elucidated.[54, 55] Cholestasis, documented by clinical and laboratory findings, has been described in three patients with right interpleural catheters used to treat upper extremity reflex sympathetic dystrophy.[56]

Clinical Note: *Like intercostal and thoracic paravertebral block, fear of pneumothorax deters many clinicians from using interpleural block. Patient selection is of utmost importance during the initial learning of this technique. When first learning and attempting this technique, one should consider choosing patients in whom the chest will be surgically opened and in whom a thoracostomy tube is planned postoperatively. In these patients, if pneumothorax occurs during interpleural placement, its immediate treatment is ensured.*

Thoracic Paravertebral (Somatic) Nerve Block

Pertinent Anatomy

Many similarities exist between thoracic paravertebral nerve block and lumbar paravertebral nerve block. In essence, a bony landmark is used in both to position the needle in proximity to the segmental spinal nerve. However, the differences that do exist are of paramount importance and must be thoroughly understood before attempting this technique (Fig. 18–9). Most importantly, during thoracic paravertebral block the lung

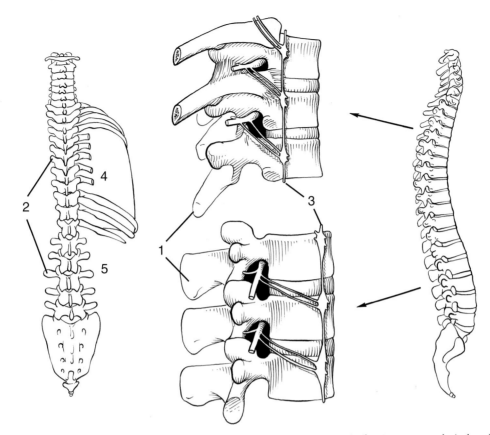

Figure 18–9 Thoracic paravertebral block and lumbar paravertebral block initially appear similar. However, technical performance of the blocks, resultant anesthesia, and potential complications are significantly different because of anatomic differences between these regions: (1) angulation of the spinous processes (which makes the technical performance of epidural anesthesia as well as paravertebral block distinctly different in the thoracic compared with the lumbar region), (2) size of vertebral body and transverse processes (and proximity to neighboring dural sleeve), (3) proximity of sympathetic chain, (4) presence of pleura and lung in the thoracic region, and (5) absence of ribs in the lumbar region.

and pleura are in close proximity, making pneumothorax a possible risk. Second, the ribs, which are not present in the lumbar region, can occasionally cause confusion when one attempts to identify the appropriate bony landmark (vertebral transverse process) in the thoracic region. Third, during performance of a lumbar paravertebral block, the injection is into the body of the psoas muscle where the nerve roots are reorganizing to form the lumbar plexus. This muscle has been demonstrated to confine thoracic paravertebral block to the thoracic region, and one would likewise expect it to confine lumbar injections to the lumbar region.[57] No analogous muscle exists in the thorax, and paravertebral injections are made into the loose connective tissue that separates the parietal pleura from the bony boundaries of the thoracic paravertebral space (rib, vertebral transverse process, and vertebral body), allowing easier spread of thoracic paravertebral injections. Finally, because of the smaller size of the thoracic vertebrae, the sympathetic chain and splanchnic nerves are closer to the injection site. The psoas muscle effectively contains the somatic nerves, and a lumbar paravertebral injection within its fascia segregates them from the sympathetic chain. Because no such fascial layers separate the sympathetic chain in the thoracic region, ipsilateral sympathetic block can be anticipated.

Technique Options

The classic technique of performing thoracic paravertebral block requires localization of the thoracic vertebral transverse process. The block can be performed with the patient in the prone, lateral, or sitting position. A skin wheal is raised 3 cm lateral to the cephalad edge of the spinous process of the vertebra above the desired level (Fig. 18–10A). Because of the extreme angulation of the spinous processes in the thoracic region, when a 6- to 8-cm needle is inserted through this wheal, parallel to the midline plane, the transverse process of the next lower vertebra is normally contacted at a depth of 2 to 5 cm.

The needle can then be walked off either the cephalad or caudad edge of the transverse process and advanced 1 to 2 cm further (Fig. 18–10B). Walking off the cephalad edge of the transverse process puts the needle tip in proximity to the nerve root of the vertebra above as it courses inferiorly to enter the intercostal groove (Fig. 18–10C, needle 2); walking off the inferior edge places the needle tip near the nerve root of the corresponding vertebra as it emerges from beneath the transverse process (Fig. 18–10C, needle 1). After careful aspiration, 6 to 8 mL of anesthetic solution is injected.

A loss of resistance can be felt as the needle penetrates the costotransverse ligament to enter the para-

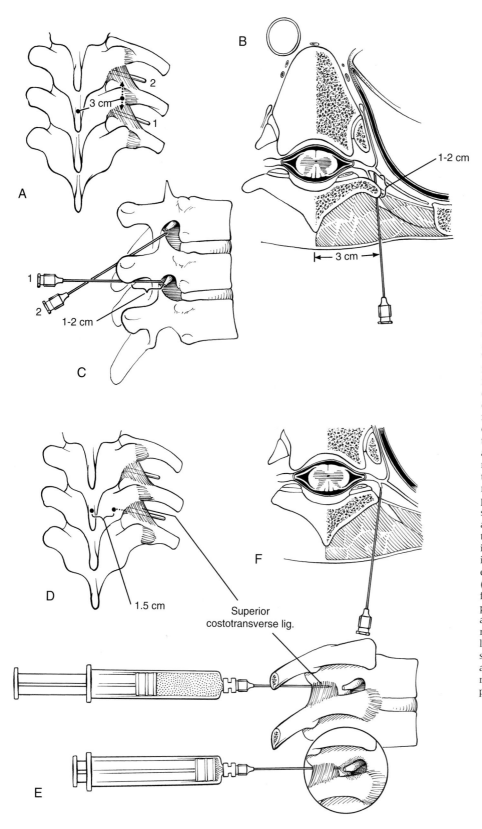

Figure 18–10 Two distinctly different techniques exist for performing a thoracic paravertebral (somatic) nerve block. In both, because of the greater angulation of the spinous process in the thoracic region, the superior edge of the spinous process of the vertebrae above that to be blocked is used as the starting point. *A,* In the classic approach, the transverse process is located 3 cm below a point 3 cm lateral to the superior edge of the spinous process. As in the lumbar region, the needle is walked off the inferior edge of the transverse process *(C1)* with a slight medial inclination, but it is advanced only 1 to 2 cm further *(B).* This approach has the advantage of the needle being directed medially away from the pleura, but this medial direction also makes it more likely to enter the epidural space. Because the nerve roots in the thoracic region emerge at the midpoint between transverse processes, this block can just as easily be performed by walking the needle off the superior edge of the transverse process to anesthetize the root one level above *(C2).* In the paralaminar approach, the needle is started more medial (1.5 cm) and advanced directly perpendicular until the lamina is contacted. *D,* The needle is directed laterally to walk off the inferior edge of the lamina where it enters the costotransverse ligament (lig.) and resistance is felt. *E,* A fluid-filled syringe is attached, and with its plunger compressed, the unit is advanced slowly until a loss of resistance occurs after leaving the ligament and entering the paravertebral space *(F).* At this point, no further advancement is made, because the needle is directed lateral toward the parietal pleura.

vertebral space. In addition, the needle may be directed 20° to 30° medial to avoid pleura if the skin wheal had initially been placed too far lateral and the rib has been mistakenly contacted instead of the transverse process. In this circumstance, lateral deviation of the needle tip may result in pleural penetration and possible pneumothorax (Fig. 18–11). A medial inclination also places the needle tip closer to the nerve root as it emerges from the intervertebral foramen, such that occasionally the vertebra itself is contacted. If this occurs, the needle can be withdrawn 0.5 cm, and after negative aspiration, local anesthetic solution can be injected. Although the intentional locating of the vertebral body has been used, it is generally not recommended, because it is possible to enter the epidural or subarachnoid space through the intervertebral foramen.

A final modification involves first locating the lamina instead of the transverse process, by starting at a more medial point—1.5 cm lateral to the cephalad edge of the spinous process—and walking the needle caudad and lateral off the lamina into the costotransverse ligament (Fig. 18–10D). With this approach, a loss of resistance technique is used while the needle passes through this ligament (Fig. 18–10E). Once the loss occurs, solution is injected without any further advancement, because the direction of the needle is lateral toward the pleura (Fig. 18–10F).

A catheter can be positioned in the thoracic paravertebral space by first entering the intercostal space at the angle of the rib with a Tuohy needle, using otherwise standard intercostal technique. By orienting the needle with its bevel medial, a catheter passed 3 to 5 cm will be consistently positioned in or near the paravertebral space.[58] The final position of the tip of the catheter is normally 2 to 3 cm medial to the medial border of the innermost intercostal muscle where subsequent doses of solution are free to spread up and down the paravertebral space. Unfortunately, this method of placing paravertebral catheters has a failure rate of 20% to 30%, and the occurrence of a temporary neuritis is of concern.[59, 60] It may also be helpful to angle the needle slightly toward the midline to facilitate passage of the catheter, which also directs the needle tangential to the parietal pleura. A slight pop or loss of resistance may be felt as the blunt Tuohy needle penetrates the posterior intercostal membrane (see Fig. 18–2).

Use in Surgery, Postoperative Analgesia, and Pain Management

When combined with light general anesthesia, thoracic paravertebral nerve block can be substituted for intercostal block for intra-abdominal operations and thoracic procedures. Except for superficial operations, it generally cannot be used as the sole anesthetic for operation.

Thoracic paravertebral block has been used effectively in the treatment of chronic post-thoracotomy pain, with relief from a single injection of local anesthetic lasting more than 1 month in 60% of patients. Theoretically, the pain from damage to the costovertebral ligaments, muscles, and posterior cutaneous nerve can be relieved with a paravertebral block but not with an intercostal block. Treatment of chronic postmastectomy pain and postherpetic neuralgia is less successful.[61] Acute herpes zoster has been treated with thoracic paravertebral catheterization and continuous infusion of 0.25% bupivacaine at 5 mL/h for 4 days.[62]

Like lumbar paravertebral somatic block, when thoracic paravertebral nerve block is used for diagnostic purposes, it is preferable to use only small volumes of local anesthetic solution in order to limit spread centrally or to adjacent lumbar nerves. Injection should be limited to 0.5 to 1 mL of drug at each site to attain the best diagnostic information. One should look for a specific paresthesia to the involved area or use fluoroscopy for precise needle positioning.

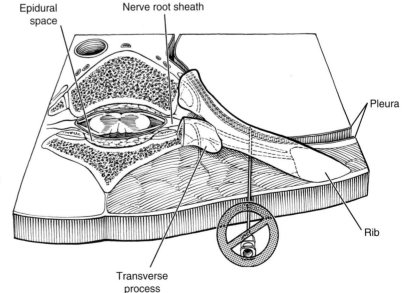

Figure 18–11 Thoracic somatic (paravertebral) nerve block is similar in concept to lumbar somatic block, but care must be taken because of anatomic differences in the thoracic region. (1) The presence of pleura and lung necessitates that needles not be directed laterally. (2) The presence of ribs may complicate the picture. If they are mistaken for transverse processes, advancing a needle any significant distance beyond them will most certainly result in a pneumothorax. (3) Because the dimensions of the thoracic vertebrae are smaller than those in the lumbar region and nerve root sheaths may extend beyond the intervertebral foramen, care must be taken to avoid unintentional intrathecal or epidural injection.

Epidural space

Nerve root sheath

Pleura

Rib

Transverse process

Physiologic Effects, Resultant Local Anesthetic Levels, and Comparison With Other Techniques

Because of the proximity of the sympathetic chain and splanchnic nerves, ipsilateral sympathetic block can be expected. However, if thoracic paravertebral block (or catheterization) is performed on only one side, minimal hemodynamic changes occur. Hypotension occurred significantly less often with unilateral thoracic paravertebral block compared with thoracic epidural bupivacaine 0.25% in post-thoracotomy patients.[63] A comparison with patients receiving a low concentration of epidural bupivacaine combined with opioids has not been done. If bilateral paravertebral block is performed, sympathetic block equivalent to spinal or epidural anesthesia to the thoracic region and the possibility of hypotension can be anticipated. Paravertebral injections, even when performed properly, may not be entirely restricted to the paravertebral space. Solution can track through the intervertebral foramina, where it enters the epidural space and is free to course up and down the space, or across the midline.[64] The incidence of solution tracking into the ipsilateral epidural space is as high as 70%, with bilateral epidural spread occurring in 7% of injections. For these reasons, thoracic paravertebral block is sometimes referred to as a "partial epidural."[64]

Pneumothorax has been reported, but its incidence is unknown. Furthermore, the safety of the different techniques for performing thoracic paravertebral block with respect to risk of pneumothorax is also unknown. Penetration of the parietal pleura with subsequent interpleural injection, without attendant puncture of the visceral pleura, occurred in 7% of injections in one study.[64] Intravascular and subarachnoid injections are possible.

Clinical Note: *To avoid accidental puncture of the pleura, it is imperative that the transverse process be found without passing the needle any deeper than necessary. Because of minor anatomic differences between patients, the transverse process may not always be directly lateral to the cephalad aspect of the spinous process. If the transverse process is initially not contacted at a depth of 3 cm, the needle should be withdrawn, redirected slightly caudad, and reinserted 3 cm. If the transverse process is still not contacted, the needle should be withdrawn again, redirected slightly cephalad, and advanced 3 cm. Only then should the needle be advanced deeper in search of the transverse process.*

Lumbar Paravertebral (Somatic) Nerve Block

Pertinent Anatomy

Lumbar paravertebral somatic nerve block has many similarities to both thoracic paravertebral block and intercostal nerve block. Instead of using ribs as bony landmarks, as in intercostal block, the primary bony guide becomes the transverse process of the lumbar vertebral body. The lumbar nerve roots exit their respective intervertebral foramina just inferior to the caudad edge of each transverse process. In doing so, they tend to course anterior to the tips of the transverse processes of the next lower vertebrae. These nerves divide immediately into anterior and posterior branches. The small posterior branches supply the skin of the lower back and the paravertebral muscles. Of primary interest, however, are the anterior branches of the first four lumbar nerves. These nerves, together with a small branch from the 12th thoracic nerve, form the lumbar plexus. This plexus is largely contained within the substance of the psoas major muscle, and most of the peripheral branches exit laterally in a plane between the psoas and quadratus lumborum muscles.

Many of the major branches of the lumbar plexus (i.e., the iliohypogastric [T-12 to L-1], ilioinguinal [L-1], and lateral femoral cutaneous nerves [L-2 to L-3]) continue laterally around the rim of the pelvis, where their terminal branches approach and pass near the anterior superior iliac spine. The genitofemoral (L-1 to L-2), obturator (L-2 to L-4), and femoral nerves (L-2 to L-4) emerge to surround the psoas major muscle by lying along its anterior, medial, and lateral surfaces, respectively. They then pass caudad into the groin, pelvis, and lower extremity. There is considerable overlap of cutaneous branches of individual nerves. Paravertebral nerve block of L-1 to L-4 results in sensory and motor block of the groin and much of the upper leg. For intra-abdominal, pelvic, or groin operations, it is necessary to block only the upper two lumbar segments.

Technique Options

As in thoracic paravertebral block, locating the transverse process is fundamental to a successful block. The patient's prone position is identical to that described for intercostal block. Injection sites are marked 3 to 4 cm lateral to the cephalad edge of the spinous processes of the corresponding vertebrae, and skin wheals are raised (Fig. 18–12A). The distance between any two lumbar transverse processes is about 2 cm. In surgical patients, the block can be performed with the same sedation used for intercostal block. An 8-cm, 22-G needle is inserted anteriorly in a parasagittal plane until it contacts the transverse process at a depth of 3 to 5 cm. The needle should then be withdrawn to a subcutaneous level and redirected to slide off the caudad edge of the transverse process. The needle is advanced another 3 to 4 cm beyond the point where it previously made contact with bone, and 6 to 8 mL of local anesthetic solution is injected as the needle is withdrawn 2 to 3 cm (Fig. 18–12C and D). Success can be improved by first injecting half of the solution, redirecting the needle slightly medial or lateral, and reinserting the needle through a different path to inject the remaining solution (Fig. 18–12B). A small field block is thereby created in the area through which the nerve must pass.

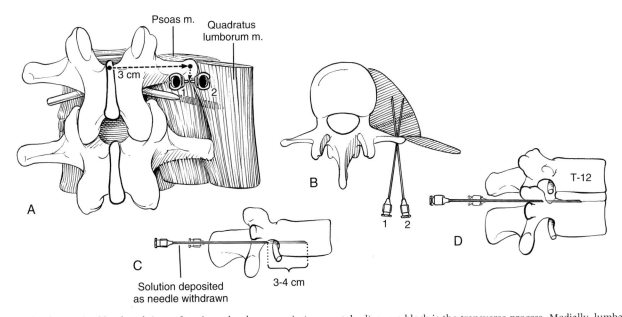

Figure 18–12 The chief landmark in performing a lumbar somatic (paravertebral) nerve block is the transverse process. Medially, lumbar nerves leave the intervertebral foramen just caudad to the corresponding transverse process. After entering the psoas muscle (m.), they slope caudally to pass just superior to transverse processes of the next caudad vertebra. To perform a lumbar somatic (paravertebral) nerve block, the transverse process is first located approximately 3 to 5 cm deep to a point 3 cm directly lateral from the cephalad edge of the spinous process (A). The needle is gently walked off the inferior edge of the transverse process and advanced 3 to 4 cm beyond (B). C, Solution (6 to 8 mL) is slowly injected as the needle is withdrawn 2 to 3 cm (B1). Once above the plane of the transverse process, further injection is of no value. However, success can be improved by relocating the transverse process, again walking the needle off it, this time slightly more medial, and reinfiltrating in a second path (B2). D, An alternative method, which is particularly useful for anesthetizing the nerve root of T-12, is to walk the needle off the superior edge of the transverse process of the vertebra below (L-1 for anesthesia of T-12), taking a slightly lateral angulation.

Paresthesia is not sought unless the block is being performed to isolate a single nerve for diagnostic purposes. This process is repeated at each of the lumbar levels at which anesthesia is desired. A needle placed at the inferior edge of a transverse process will be close to nerves from two lumbar segments. Medially, it will be close to the nerve exiting the vertebral foramen; laterally, it will be near the nerve from the next most cephalad vertebral level. Hence, local anesthetic solution injected at the proper depth inferior to one lumbar vertebral process can result in nerve block of two or more root segments. The useful concentrations of local anesthetic are the same as those used for intercostal block.

Use in Surgery, Postoperative Analgesia, and Pain Management

Lumbar paravertebral nerve block can occasionally be used as the sole anesthetic for operation. Groin operations such as herniorrhaphy or femoral pseudoaneurysm repair or embolectomy can be performed with lumbar block (particularly in patients who have received anticoagulants in whom neuraxial block is best avoided), but supplementation with local infiltration or intravenously administered drugs is usually necessary. Block of T-12 to L-2 effectively complements intercostal (T-6 to T-11) block for intra-abdominal and pelvic procedures, particularly when the incision extends to the pubis.

When the block is used for diagnostic purposes, it is preferable to use only small volumes of local anesthetic solution to limit spread centrally or to adjacent lumbar nerves. Fluoroscopy or a nerve stimulator can be used to position the needle precisely before injecting only a small amount (0.5 to 1 mL) of drug. Lumbar somatic block can be useful in the differential diagnosis of groin or genital pain, such as the nerve entrapment syndromes that sometimes follow herniorrhaphy.

Physiologic Effects, Resultant Local Anesthetic Levels, and Comparison With Other Techniques

It is possible to inject into intravascular, epidural, or subarachnoid spaces during performance of this block. If the needle is inserted too far medially, it could enter a vertebral foramen or penetrate a dural sleeve to produce spinal anesthesia. Likewise, spread of solution into the epidural space or within the psoas muscle can produce anesthesia over the lower extremities. The risk of intravascular injection can be minimized by aspiration and by avoiding injection of large volumes. The lumbar sympathetic chain may be anesthetized from either local block of gray and white rami communicantes or deeper penetration of local anesthetic drug to the sympathetic chain itself. The limited degree of sympathetic block does not usually produce noticeable hemodynamic changes.

Clinical Note: *It is fairly easy to slip off the inferior edges of the transverse processes of L-1 to L-4. Paravertebral block of L-5 is substantially more difficult, if not impossible, because of obstruction by the pelvic brim. The subcostal nerve (T-12) is only variably blocked by the intercostal approach, because there are no intercostal muscles, fascia, or space to receive and channel anesthetic solution. Greater success in blocking this nerve can be accomplished by treating it as a lumbar nerve and using a paravertebral block. However, instead of contacting T-12 and walking the needle off it inferiorly, one can contact the transverse process of L-1 and walk the needle off its superior edge. Therefore, T-12 and L-1 are both blocked through the same skin site.*

Ilioinguinal, Iliohypogastric, or Hernia (Iliac Crest) Block

Pertinent Anatomy

The primary peripheral nerves of the groin region, the ilioinguinal and iliohypogastric, follow a course around the abdominal wall that is roughly parallel to the intercostal nerves and in close approximation to the iliac crest. Like the intercostal nerves, they initially are located between the fasciae of the inner two layers of muscle (the transverse abdominal and the internal abdominal oblique muscles). The iliohypogastric nerve (T-12 to L-1) penetrates the internal abdominal oblique muscle in the vicinity of the anterior superior iliac spine to lie between it and the external abdominal oblique muscle (Fig. 18–13). The ilioinguinal nerve (L-1) does not penetrate the internal abdominal oblique muscle until it has passed a variable distance medial to the anterior superior iliac spine to traverse the inguinal canal. Further anterior, both nerves become superficial as they terminate in branches to skin and muscles of the inguinal and scrotal regions. The genitofemoral nerve (L-1 to L-2) divides near where it emerges from the psoas muscle. Its genital branch enters the deep inguinal ring and continues with the structures of the spermatic cord, passing just lateral to the pubic tubercle, to innervate the cremaster muscle and the skin and fascia of the scrotum. The femoral branch continues under the inguinal ligament to innervate a variable amount of skin over the femoral triangle and anterior thigh.

Technique Options

In blocking the inguinal region, two requirements must be fulfilled. First, the ilioinguinal and iliohypogastric nerves must be blocked. Second, a field block or infiltration is necessary to anesthetize terminal nerve fibers that overlap from adjacent regions. The primary landmark in performing a hernia block is the anterior

superior iliac spine, which is prominent even in an obese patient.

Ilioinguinal and iliohypogastric nerve blocks can be performed in two ways. The patient lies in the supine position. First, from a point 2 to 3 cm medially along a line connecting the anterior superior iliac spine and the umbilicus (approximately 2 cm medial and 2 cm cephalad to the anterior superior iliac spine), a total of approximately 10 mL of solution is infiltrated by using a 5-cm, 22-G needle (Fig. 18–13A). As the needle is inserted in an anteroposterior orientation to a depth of 2 to 4 cm, the resistance of the layers of muscle fasciae should be appreciated. Because the ilioinguinal nerve is most likely located between the transverse abdominal and the internal abdominal oblique muscles and the iliohypogastric nerve is located between the internal abdominal oblique and external abdominal oblique muscles at this point, it is important to infiltrate at all depths and for several centimeters along this line to ensure adequate spread of solution to these nerves.

In the second option, a point is marked on the skin roughly 3 cm medial and 3 cm inferior to the anterior superior iliac spine. A skin wheal is raised, and an 8-cm, 22-G needle is inserted in a cephalolateral direction to contact the inner surface of the ilium (Fig. 18–13B). Ten milliliters of local anesthetic solution is injected as the needle is slowly withdrawn. The needle is then reinserted at a somewhat steeper angle to ensure penetration of all three lateral abdominal muscles. The injection is repeated as the needle is withdrawn. In an obese or heavily muscled patient, a third injection may be necessary at an even steeper angle.

Infiltration of the remainder of the inguinal region can be accomplished in one of two ways. A field block can be performed to enclose the area bounded by the umbilicus, the anterior superior iliac spine (or the point used for ilioinguinal or iliohypogastric block), and the pubic tubercle (Fig. 18–14A). This serves to anesthetize the terminal branches of the ipsilateral T-10 to T-12 intercostal nerves coming from the cephalolateral margin, the contralateral intercostal nerves overlapping the midline, and the femoral branches of the genitofemoral nerve entering from the region of the inguinal ligament. Alternatively, because it will still be necessary for the surgeon to infiltrate the line of incision, this infiltration can be extended outward in all directions to accomplish the same objective (Fig. 18–14B).

Although these injections may be adequate for herniorrhaphy, additional direct local infiltration may be needed to have a completely pain-free operation. Because it is especially difficult to atraumatically anesthetize all the structures in the internal ring with a percutaneous injection, it is preferable for the surgeon to inject 2 to 3 mL of local anesthetic directly into the covering of the spermatic cord (and into muscle if a relaxing incision is to be made) as soon as it is exposed.

Use in Surgery, Postoperative Analgesia, and Pain Management

The issue of the clinical importance of preemptive analgesia is particularly controversial in studies of in-

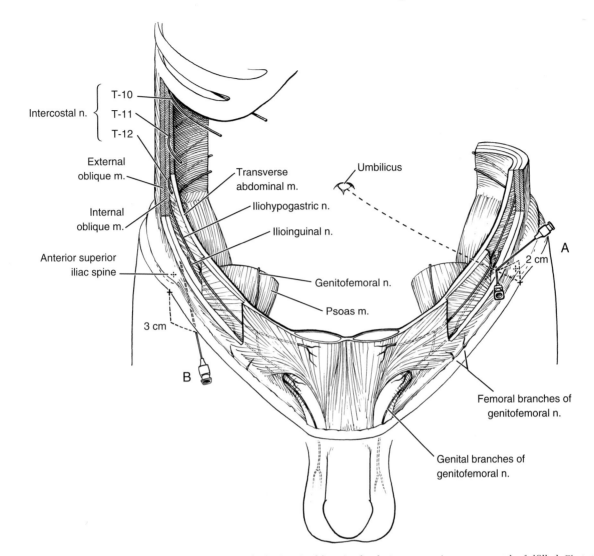

Figure 18–13 To block the inguinal region (most frequently for inguinal herniorrhaphy), two requirements must be fulfilled. First, the primary peripheral nerves of the region (ilioinguinal and iliohypogastric nerves) must be blocked. Second, a field block or infiltration to anesthetize terminal nerve (n.) fibers that overlap from adjacent regions is necessary. Ilioinguinal and iliohypogastric nerve blocks can be performed two ways. *A*, From a point 2 to 3 cm cephalad along the line connecting the anterior superior iliac spine and the umbilicus (approximately 2 cm medial and 2 cm cephalad to the anterior superior iliac spine), a total of approximately 10 mL of solution is infiltrated. As the needle is inserted to a depth of 2 to 4 cm, the resistance of several layers of muscle (m.) fasciae should be appreciated. Because the ilioinguinal nerve is emerging through the internal oblique muscle or coursing between the external and internal oblique muscles and the iliohypogastric nerve is emerging through the transverse abdominal muscle or coursing between the transverse abdominal and internal oblique muscles near this point, it is important to infiltrate at all depths and for several centimeters along this line to ensure adequate spread of solution to these nerves. *B*, Alternatively, an iliac crest block can be performed. From a point 3 cm medial and 3 cm caudad to the anterior iliac spine, the needle is advanced lateral and slightly cephalad to contact the interior of the iliac crest. Again, approximately 10 mL of solution is infiltrated as this needle is withdrawn. The needle is redirected medial and reinserted to the same depth several times.

guinal hernia repair. Tverskoy and coworkers[65] first demonstrated, at 1, 2, and 10 days after operation, marked decreases in analgesic requirements and in pain measurements at rest, during movement, and with pressure applied to the incision when spinal anesthesia or general anesthesia with presurgical wound infiltration was compared with general anesthesia alone. The differences between spinal anesthesia and general anesthesia alone were less prominent than in those receiving general anesthesia and local infiltration, who had less pain with pressure applied to their incisions even at 10 days after operation. When they specifically evaluated the timing of wound infiltration for

the management of postoperative inguinal hernia pain, Ejlersen and associates[66] showed that the first demand for additional analgesics was significantly later (165 min versus 225 min) and the percentage of patients not requiring analgesics at all was significantly greater (42% versus 6%) in patients receiving preincisional local anesthetic infiltration (1% lidocaine plain) compared with infiltration at the end of operation. However, Dierking and colleagues[67] were unable to demonstrate these differences in a study of nearly identical design.

Hernia block can be used successfully for repair of recurrent hernia; however, the scar tissue and unpre-

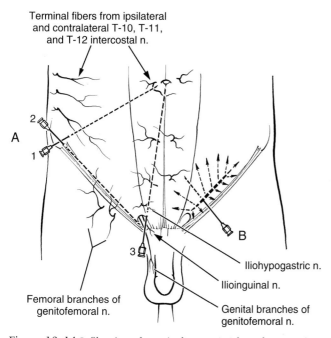

Terminal fibers from ipsilateral
and contralateral T-10, T-11,
and T-12 intercostal n.

A

B

Iliohypogastric n.

Ilioinguinal n.

Femoral branches of
genitofemoral n.

Genital branches of
genitofemoral n.

Figure 18–14 Infiltration of terminal nerve (n.) branches entering the inguinal region from adjacent areas can be accomplished in one of two ways. *A1, 2, 3, A* field block can be performed to anesthetize the area bounded by the umbilicus, the anterior superior iliac spine (or the point used for ilioinguinal and iliohypogastric or iliac crest block), and the pubic tubercle. *B,* Alternatively, the surgeon can infiltrate the line of incision and outward from it in all directions. Infiltration of the femoral branches of the genitofemoral nerve and the recurrent branches from the femoral nerve (or the femoral nerve itself) is not necessary for inguinal herniorrhaphy if a field block has been performed. Infiltration of the genital branches of the genitofemoral nerve, just lateral to the pubic tubercle, may be useful to identify the source of scrotal or inguinal pain, but it is, likewise, not necessary for inguinal herniorrhaphy. n., nerve.

dictable anatomic distortion from the previous operation may cause poor diffusion of the local anesthetic solution. If difficulties or mesh reinforcement of the repair are anticipated, neuraxial blocks (spinal or epidural) may produce a more satisfactory anesthesia for all involved.

Bilateral ilioinguinal nerve block, 10 mL of plain 0.5% bupivacaine per side, during general anesthesia for cesarean section has also been shown to significantly decrease pain scores and opioid requirements in the first 24 h after operation.[68] Ilioinguinal or iliohypogastric nerve block may be useful in diagnosing nerve entrapment syndromes after herniorrhaphy; infiltration of the genital branches of the genitofemoral nerve, just lateral to the pubic tubercle, may be useful to identify the etiology of scrotal pain. A series of blocks may be necessary to treat chronic pain syndromes in this region, and a technique of placing a catheter between the layers of abdominal muscles for repeated injection has been described.[69]

Physiologic Effects, Resultant Local Anesthetic Levels, and Comparison With Other Techniques

Fairly large volumes of local anesthetic solution can be injected with this block, and the anesthesiologist

must use lower concentrations of drug (0.25% to 1.0% lidocaine or 0.125% to 0.25% bupivacaine with epinephrine) as well as watch for signs and symptoms of systemic toxic reactions. It is possible to penetrate peritoneum, intestine, or blood vessels. Aspiration should be performed before each injection. The solution can spread to produce anesthesia of the lateral buttock, thigh, and front of the leg in the distribution of the femoral or lateral femoral cutaneous nerves. This can interfere with ambulation and complicate an anticipated outpatient procedure.

Clinical Note: *Like other field block techniques, success depends on spreading a large volume of anesthetic solution between all abdominal wall muscle layers. Inadequate block is most often the result of injections being made too superficially, into just the skin and the subcutaneous tissues, without anesthetizing the iliohypogastric and ilioinguinal nerves, which lie below one and two layers of muscle, respectively. Careful titration of the level of sedation is important. Near the end of the procedure, the patient should be alert enough to bear down and test the adequacy of the surgical repair.*

Intraperitoneal (Peritoneal Lavage) Block

Pertinent Anatomy

Analogous to the pleura in the thorax, the peritoneum surrounds the organs of the abdomen. Solution instilled into the peritoneal cavity is free to pass throughout this space. Unlike the pleural space, where the intercostal nerves are only minimally separated from the pleural surfaces, several layers of abdominal muscle tissue may separate the peritoneal surface from large somatic nerves. Intraperitoneal local anesthetic primarily produces visceral and autonomic block by anesthetizing nerves within superficial layers of the abdominal organs and free nerve endings within the peritoneum.

Technique Options

Peritoneal block is easily performed after surgical opening of the peritoneum, by simply pouring solution into the incision. The laparoscope can also be used as a port of entry for the lavage solution. Large volumes of dilute local anesthetic solution are necessary to produce effective anesthesia. One hundred to three hundred milliliters of solution (e.g., 0.15% to 0.5% lidocaine or 0.10% to 0.25% bupivacaine) is instilled and left in the abdomen for 10 min, and then any residual is removed by suctioning. The Trendelenburg position aids the spread of solution to the upper abdomen (celiac plexus) and the inferior surface of the diaphragm, often improving analgesia. The technique is generally ineffective in patients who have had multiple previous abdominal procedures, because free flow through the peritoneal cavity may be limited by adhesions or other anatomic changes.

Use in Surgery, Postoperative Analgesia, and Pain Management

Peritoneal instillation is satisfactory as the sole anesthetic for laparoscopic tubal ligation,[70] if surgical manipulation is consciously gentle and overdistension of the pneumoperitoneum is avoided. The incidence and severity of referred shoulder pain are decreased,[71] and combined with wound infiltration (or rectus sheath block), one can often provide an extensive pain-free period for patients after laparoscopic procedures.[72] A marked shrinking of the intestine, which benefits surgical exposure, is occasionally observed.

In contrast to laparoscopic procedures, the benefit of intraperitoneal local anesthetic after open laparotomy is controversial. Although some studies have demonstrated improvements in analgesia, decreased hyperglycemic (stress) response, and improved colonic motility,[73] others have not shown these benefits,[74] even when the anesthetic is infused continuously through an intraperitoneal catheter.[75]

Physiologic Effects, Resultant Local Anesthetic Levels, and Comparison With Other Techniques

Although local anesthetic solutions are readily absorbed from mucosal surfaces, serum local anesthetic levels are surprisingly low after interperitoneal block (highest level, 2.2 μg/mL after 500 mg of 0.5% lidocaine).[70] No comparative studies have been reported. Because of the large volumes used, local anesthetic systemic toxicity is possible. The technique should be avoided in situations of excessive inflammation, where greater local anesthetic uptake is anticipated.

Clinical Note: *Intraperitoneal block can provide a brief extension of other regional anesthetic techniques used for the abdomen, or a filling in of an otherwise patchy block, when repeating (or redosing) the initial block is undesirable. Because lavage of all peritoneal surfaces may be difficult, a jostling of the abdomen and tilting of the operating table may aid distribution. Effectiveness is improved if the solution can be left undisturbed for 5 to 10 min before suctioning of residual solution.*

Cave of Retzius Block

Pertinent Anatomy

The variable space located between the urinary bladder and symphysis pubis is known as the cave of Retzius. This space contains a great venous plexus as well as many terminating nerve fibers of the sacral plexus, which can be blocked at this location.

Technique Options

With the patient supine, a skin wheal is raised 2 to 3 cm cephalad to the pubic symphysis. Subcutaneous infiltration can be performed laterally in the line of skin incision for retropubic prostatectomy. An 8-cm needle is then directed to the posterior aspect of the os pubis and anterior to the bladder. If bone is encountered, the needle is walked posteriorly, maintaining the same caudal angle, until it is felt to slide off the back of the pubis, where it is advanced an additional 2 cm (Fig. 18–15A). Care should be taken to not change the angle of needle insertion in order to avoid bladder penetration (Fig. 18–15B). Ten milliliters of local anesthetic solution is injected as the needle reaches its maximum depth and is slowly withdrawn. This process is repeated with two lateral injections made through the same skin wheal.

Use in Surgery, Postoperative Analgesia, and Pain Management

Cave of Retzius block can be a useful adjunct to anesthesia for prostatectomy or bladder procedures, when other techniques are contraindicated. It provides analgesia, decreases bleeding if vasoconstrictors are used, and facilitates the surgical dissection. The block may be combined with intercostal, or lumbar somatic, or rectus block. The block is occasionally useful in patients who have severe pain as a result of bladder spasm after transurethral prostatectomy. There are few other useful nonsurgical applications for cave of Retzius block.

Physiologic Effects, Resultant Local Anesthetic Levels, and Comparison With Other Techniques

The chief concern is for excessive intravascular injection, owing to the nearby plexus of veins. Bladder puncture may occur, but it is unlikely unless the block is attempted in a patient with a distended bladder. Urinary retention is a theoretic concern, because this block is usually performed only in patients who already or will soon have indwelling catheters.

Sacral Root (Transsacral) Block

Pertinent Anatomy

Sacral root block is technically a paravertebral block, analogous to that in the thoracic and lumbar regions. However, unlike these higher regions, where segmen-

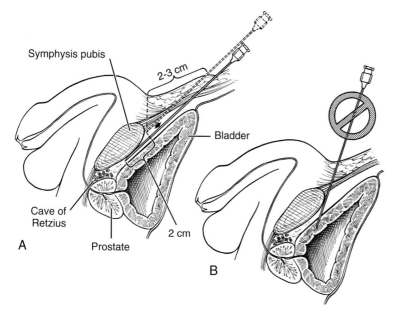

Symphysis pubis

2-3 cm

Bladder

Cave of
Retzius

Prostate

2 cm

A

B

Figure 18–15 *A,* Cave of Retzius block is most effective if two or three injections are made. From a point 2 to 3 cm cephalad to the pubic symphysis, the needle is directed immediately posterior to the pubic bone to pass between it and the urinary bladder. If bone is encountered, the needle is walked posteriorly, maintaining the same caudal angle, until it is noted to slide off the back of the pubis and then advanced an additional 2 to 3 cm. Solution is injected as the needle is withdrawn, and this is repeated one or two more times with the needle redirected slightly lateral. *B,* Care should be taken not to change the angle of needle insertion so as to avoid bladder penetration.

tal nerves initially course through soft tissue spaces, the initial courses of the segmental sacral nerves are within the bony sacrum. Nerve roots divide into anterior and posterior divisions that exit the sacrum through their respective sacral foramina (S-1 to S-4). The fifth sacral nerve and the coccygeal nerve exit inferiorly through the sacral hiatus.

Posterior divisions supply the skin and musculature of the gluteal region. Anterior divisions, with the anterior divisions of L-4 and L-5, form the sacral plexus, which innervates the pelvic structures, perineum, and much of the lower extremity, mostly through its large sciatic nerve (L-4 to S-3).

Technique Options

The posterior sacral foramina are found on a line from 2 to 3 cm medial to the posterior superior iliac spine (between S-1 and S-2) to 1 to 2 cm lateral to the sacral cornu. Depending on patient size, the S-2 and S-4 foramina are found about 2 cm caudad from the line intersecting the posterior superior iliac spine and 1 to 2 cm cephalad of the sacral cornu, respectively. The S-3 foramen is equidistant between the two, and S-1 is equidistant above S-2 (Fig. 18–16).

To perform this block, the patient is placed prone with a pillow beneath the hips. If more than one foramen is to be located, the S-2 foramen is easiest and should be done first. The tissue overlying S-1 and S-2 is thicker; thus, an 8-cm needle should be used, whereas a 6-cm needle is sufficient at lower levels. The depth of the posterior bony plate of the sacrum should first be determined by aiming slightly above the intended target foramen. The needle is then walked into the appropriate foramen and advanced an additional 1 to 2 cm to lie close to the anterior primary ramus before injection of 4 to 8 mL of solution. Paresthesia may be encountered at any time but is not specifically

sought. The S-5 (and coccygeal) root can be anesthetized just lateral to the cornua by walking the needle off the inferior edge of the sacrum and injecting solution after advancing the needle 0.5 to 1 cm further. If difficulties are encountered during needle placement, radiographic guidance may be beneficial.

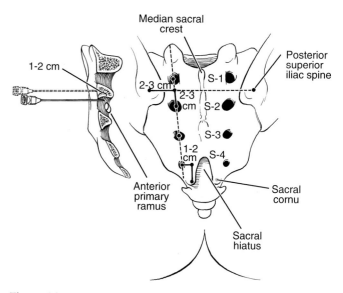

Median sacral
crest

1-2 cm

2-3 cm

2-3
cm

1-2
cm

S-1

S-2

S-3

S-4

Posterior
superior
iliac spine

Anterior
primary
ramus

Sacral
cornu

Sacral
hiatus

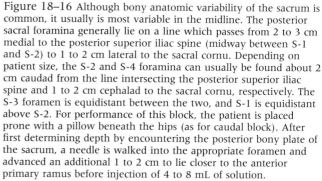

Figure 18–16 Although bony anatomic variability of the sacrum is common, it usually is most variable in the midline. The posterior sacral foramina generally lie on a line which passes from 2 to 3 cm medial to the posterior superior iliac spine (midway between S-1 and S-2) to 1 to 2 cm lateral to the sacral cornu. Depending on patient size, the S-2 and S-4 foramina can usually be found about 2 cm caudad from the line intersecting the posterior superior iliac spine and 1 to 2 cm cephalad to the sacral cornu, respectively. The S-3 foramen is equidistant between the two, and S-1 is equidistant above S-2. For performance of this block, the patient is placed prone with a pillow beneath the hips (as for caudal block). After first determining depth by encountering the posterior bony plate of the sacrum, a needle is walked into the appropriate foramen and advanced an additional 1 to 2 cm to lie closer to the anterior primary ramus before injection of 4 to 8 mL of solution.

Use in Surgery, Postoperative Analgesia, and Pain Management

Although sacral root block could be used for anesthesia and analgesia of surgical procedures of the pelvis, rectum, and perineum, spinal or epidural (caudal) anesthesia is more comfortable for the patient and technically easier to perform. The main indications for sacral root block are in the management of malignant and chronic pain and in the diagnosis and possible treatment of patients with dysfunctional bladders.[76] The bladder is usually innervated by a single dominant nerve, which is most often a third sacral nerve but can also be a second sacral nerve. For diagnostic procedures, when one is trying to selectively block a single root, the volume should be limited to 1 mL, particularly if neurolysis is being considered, because greater volumes have been shown to spread to more than one nerve root.[77] Intravenous and intrathecal injections are remotely possible, and perforation of pelvic organs can occur with excessive (>2.5 cm) needle advancement after entering the posterior foramen.

Conclusion

Regional anesthesia, alone or combined with light general anesthesia, is justifiable and beneficial in almost every thoracic or abdominal operation. A wide variety of techniques are available to render the patient insensible to surgical manipulations and to provide a solid foundation of postoperative analgesia after thoracic and abdominal procedures. To use these techniques successfully, the anesthesiologist must be of the mind-set that inability to provide complete anesthesia with regional techniques alone does not mean that he or she has failed. To gain the greatest experience, training in the use of these techniques must begin early.[78] Thereafter, their use must be frequent, and once proficiency in these skills is attained, they will be invaluable.

References

1. Kavanagh BP, Katz J, Sandler AN: Pain control after thoracic surgery: a review of current techniques. Anesthesiology 1994; 81: 737–759.
2. Adriani J: Labat's Regional Anesthesia: Techniques and Clinical Applications. St. Louis, Warren H Green, 1985.
3. Templeton T: Rectus block for postoperative pain relief. Reg Anesth 1993; 18: 258–260.
4. Smith BE, Suchak M, Siggins D, et al: Rectus sheath block for diagnostic laparoscopy. Anaesthesia 1988; 43: 947–948.
5. Partridge BL, Stabile BE: The effects of incisional bupivacaine on postoperative narcotic requirements, oxygen saturation and length of stay in the post-anesthesia care unit. Acta Anaesthesiol Scand 1990; 34: 486–491.
6. Patel JM, Lanzafame RJ, Williams JS, et al: The effect of incisional infiltration of bupivacaine hydrochloride upon pulmonary functions, atelectasis and narcotic need following elective cholecystectomy. Surg Gynecol Obstet 1983; 157: 338–340.
7. Moss G, Regal ME, Lichtig L: Reducing postoperative pain, narcotics, and length of hospitalization. Surgery 1986; 99: 206–210.
8. van Raay JJ, Roukema JA, Lenderink BW: Intraoperative wound infiltration with bupivacaine in patients undergoing elective cholecystectomy. Arch Surg 1992; 127: 457–459.
9. Egan TM, Herman SJ, Doucette EJ, et al: A randomized, controlled trial to determine the effectiveness of fascial infiltration of bupivacaine in preventing respiratory complications after elective abdominal surgery. Surgery 1988; 104: 734–740.
10. Scott DB, Jebson PJ, Braid DP, et al: Factors affecting plasma levels of lignocaine and prilocaine. Br J Anaesth 1972; 44: 1040–1049.
11. Takeshima R, Dohi S: Cervical epidural anesthesia and surgical blood loss in radical mastectomy. Reg Anesth 1986; 11: 171–175.
12. Hardy PA: Anatomical variation in the position of the proximal intercostal nerve. Br J Anaesth 1988; 61: 338–339.
13. Atanassoff PG, Alon E, Pasch T, et al: Intercostal nerve block for minor breast surgery. Reg Anesth 1991; 16: 23–27.
14. Malhotra V, Long CW, Meister MJ: Intercostal blocks with local infiltration anesthesia for extracorporeal shock wave lithotripsy. Anesth Analg 1987; 66: 85–88.
15. Raza SM, Vasireddy AR, Candido KD, et al: A complete regional anesthesia technique for cardiac pacemaker insertion. J Cardiothorac Vasc Anesth 1991; 5: 54–56.
16. Bunting P, McGeachie JF: Intercostal nerve blockade producing analgesia after appendectomy. Br J Anaesth 1988; 61: 169–172.
17. Jakobson S, Ivarsson I: Effects of intercostal nerve blocks (bupivacaine 0.25% and etidocaine 0.5%) on chest wall mechanics in healthy men. Acta Anaesthesiol Scand 1977; 21: 489–496.
18. Jakobson S, Fridriksson H, Hedenstrom H, et al: Effects of intercostal nerve blocks on pulmonary mechanics in healthy men. Acta Anaesthesiol Scand 1980; 24: 482–486.
19. Hecker BR, Bjurstrom R, Schoene RB: Effect of intercostal nerve blockade on respiratory mechanics and CO_2 chemosensitivity at rest and exercise. Anesthesiology 1989; 70: 13–18.
20. Faust RJ, Nauss LA: Post-thoracotomy intercostal block: comparison of its effects on pulmonary function with those of intramuscular meperidine. Anesth Analg 1976; 55: 542–546.
21. Engberg G: Respiratory performance after upper abdominal surgery. A comparison of pain relief with intercostal blocks and centrally acting analgesics. Acta Anaesthesiol Scand 1985; 29: 427–433.
22. Engberg G: Factors influencing the respiratory capacity after upper abdominal surgery. Acta Anaesthesiol Scand 1985; 29: 434–445.
23. Rawal N, Sjostrand UH, Dahlstrom B, et al: Epidural morphine for postoperative pain relief: a comparative study with intramuscular narcotic and intercostal nerve block. Anesth Analg 1982; 61: 93–98.
24. Richardson J, Sabanathan S, Eng J, et al: Continuous intercostal nerve block versus epidural morphine for postthoracotomy analgesia. Ann Thorac Surg 1993; 55: 377–380.
25. Engberg G, Wiklund L: Pulmonary complications after upper abdominal surgery: their prevention with intercostal blocks. Acta Anaesthesiol Scand 1988; 32: 1–9.
26. Moore DC, Bridenbaugh LD: Oxygen: the antidote for systemic toxic reactions from local anesthetic drugs. JAMA 1960; 174: 842–847.
27. Moore DC, Bridenbaugh LD: Pneumothorax: its incidence following intercostal nerve block. JAMA 1962; 182: 1005–1008.
28. Johnson MD, Mickler T, Arthur GR, et al: Bupivacaine with and without epinephrine for intercostal nerve block. J Cardiothorac Anesth 1990; 4: 200–203.
29. Gauntlett IS: Total spinal anesthesia following intercostal nerve block. (Published erratum appears in Anesthesiology 1987; 66: 97.) Anesthesiology 1986; 65: 82–84.
30. Sury MR, Bingham RM: Accidental spinal anaesthesia following intrathoracic intercostal nerve blockade. A case report. Anaesthesia 1986; 41: 401–403.
31. Symreng T, Gomez MN, Johnson B, et al: Intrapleural bupivacaine—technical considerations and intraoperative use. J Cardiothorac Anesth 1989; 3: 139–143.
32. Reiestad F, Strømskag KE: Interpleural catheter in the management of postoperative pain: a preliminary report. Reg Anesth 1986; 11: 89–91.
33. Iwama H, Tase C, Kawamae K, et al: Catheter location and patient position affect spread of interpleural regional analgesia. (Letter to the editor.) Anesthesiology 1993; 79: 1153–1154.
34. Ben-David B, Lee E: The falling column: a new technique for interpleural catheter placement. (Letter to the editor.) Anesth Analg 1990; 71: 212.

35. Riegler FX, VadeBoncouer TR, Pelligrino DA: Interpleural anesthetics in the dog: differential somatic neural blockade. Anesthesiology 1989; 71: 744–750.

36. Strømskag KE, Reiestad F, Holmqvist EL, et al: Intrapleural administration of 0.25%, 0.375%, and 0.5% bupivacaine with epinephrine after cholecystectomy. Anesth Analg 1988; 67: 430–434.

37. Rademaker BM, Sih IL, Kalkman CJ, et al: Effects of interpleurally administered bupivacaine 0.5% on opioid analgesic requirements and endocrine response during and after cholecystectomy: a randomized double-blind controlled study. Acta Anaesthesiol Scand 1991; 35: 108–112.

38. Frenette L, Boudreault D, Guay J: Interpleural analgesia improves pulmonary function after cholecystectomy. Can J Anaesth 1991; 38: 71–74.

39. Ferrante FM, Chan VW, Arthur GR, et al: Interpleural analgesia after thoracotomy. Anesth Analg 1991; 72: 105–109.

40. Symreng T, Gomez MN, Rossi N: Intrapleural bupivacaine v saline after thoracotomy—effects on pain and lung function—a double-blind study. J Cardiothorac Anesth 1989; 3: 144–149.

41. Lee E, Ben-David B: Bilateral interpleural block for midline upper abdominal surgery. (Letter to the editor.) Can J Anaesth 1991; 38: 683–684.

42. Rocco A, Reiestad F, Gudman J, et al: Intrapleural administration of local anesthetics for pain relief in patients with multiple rib fractures. Reg Anesth 1987; 12: 10–14.

43. Perkins G: Interpleural anaesthesia in the management of upper limb ischaemia. A report of three cases. Anaesth Intensive Care 1991; 19: 575–578.

44. Reiestad F, McIlvaine WB, Kvalheim L, et al: Interpleural analgesia in treatment of upper extremity reflex sympathetic dystrophy. Anesth Analg 1989; 69: 671–673.

45. Reiestad F, McIlvaine WB, Kvalheim L, et al: Successful treatment of chronic pancreatitis pain with interpleural analgesia. Can J Anaesth 1989; 36: 713–716.

46. Ahlburg P, Noreng M, Molgaard J, et al: Treatment of pancreatic pain with interpleural bupivacaine: an open trial. Acta Anaesthesiol Scand 1990; 34: 156–157.

47. Dionne C: Tumour invasion of the brachial plexus: management of pain with intrapleural analgesia. (Letter to the editor.) Can J Anaesth 1992; 39: 520–521.

48. Reiestad F, McIlvaine WB, Barnes M, et al: Interpleural analgesia in the treatment of severe thoracic postherpetic neuralgia. Reg Anesth 1990; 15: 113–117.

49. Vaghadia H, Jenkins LC: Use of a Doppler ultrasound stethoscope for intercostal nerve block. Can J Anaesth 1988; 35: 86–89.

50. Lema MJ, Myers DP, De Leon-Casasola O, et al: Pleural phenol therapy for the treatment of chronic esophageal cancer pain. Reg Anesth 1992; 17: 166–170.

51. Strømskag KE, Minor B, Steen PA: Side effects and complications related to interpleural analgesia: an update. Acta Anaesthesiol Scand 1990; 34: 473–477.

52. van Kleef JW, Burm AG, Vletter AA: Single-dose interpleural versus intercostal blockade: nerve block characteristics and plasma concentration profiles after administration of 0.5% bupivacaine with epinephrine. Anesth Analg 1990; 70: 484–488.

53. Shantha TR: Unilateral bronchospasm after interpleural analgesia. Anesth Analg 1992; 74: 291–293.

54. Lauder GR: Interpleural analgesia and phrenic nerve paralysis. Anaesthesia 1993; 48: 315–316.

55. Kowalski SE, Bradley BD, Greengrass RA, et al: Effects of interpleural bupivacaine (0.5%) on canine diaphragmatic function. Anesth Analg 1992; 75: 400–404.

56. Billstrom R, Blomberg HM: Cholestasis after interpleural bupivacaine for chronic upper limb pain. Anesth Analg 1993; 76: 1158–1159.

57. Lonnqvist PA, Hildingsson U: The caudal boundary of the thoracic paravertebral space. A study in human cadavers. Anaesthesia 1992; 47: 1051–1052.

58. Hord AH, Wang JM, Pai UT, et al: Anatomic spread of India ink in the human intercostal space with radiographic correlation. Reg Anesth 1991; 16: 13–16.

59. Conacher ID, Kokri M: Postoperative paravertebral blocks for thoracic surgery. A radiological appraisal. Br J Anaesth 1987; 59: 155–161.

60. Crossley AW, Hosie HE: Radiographic study of intercostal nerve blockade in healthy volunteers. Br J Anaesth 1987; 59: 149–154.

61. Kirvela O, Antila H: Thoracic paravertebral block in chronic postoperative pain. Reg Anesth 1992; 17: 348–350.

62. Johnson LR, Rocco AG, Ferrante FM: Continuous subpleural-paravertebral block in acute thoracic herpes zoster. Anesth Analg 1988; 67: 1105–1108.

63. Matthews PJ, Govenden V: Comparison of continuous paravertebral and extradural infusions of bupivacaine for pain relief after thoracotomy. Br J Anaesth 1989; 62: 204–205.

64. Purcell-Jones G, Pither CE, Justins DM: Paravertebral somatic nerve block: a clinical, radiographic, and computed tomographic study in chronic pain patients. Anesth Analg 1989; 68: 32–39.

65. Tverskoy M, Cozacov C, Ayache M, et al: Postoperative pain after inguinal herniorrhaphy with different types of anesthesia. Anesth Analg 1990; 70: 29–35.

66. Ejlersen E, Andersen HB, Eliasen K, et al: A comparison between preincisional and postincisional lidocaine infiltration and postoperative pain. Anesth Analg 1992; 74: 495–498.

67. Dierking GW, Dahl JB, Kanstrup J, et al: Effect of pre- vs postoperative inguinal field block on postoperative pain after herniorrhaphy. Br J Anaesth 1992; 68: 344–348.

68. Bunting P, McConachie I: Ilioinguinal nerve blockade for analgesia after caesarean section. Br J Anaesth 1988; 61: 773–775.

69. Ghia JN, Blank JW, McAdams CG: A new interabdominis approach to inguinal region block for the management of chronic pain. Reg Anesth 1991; 16: 72–78.

70. Deeb R, Viechnicki M: Laparoscopic tubal ligation under peritoneal lavage anesthesia. Reg Anesth 1985; 10: 24–27.

71. Narchi P, Benhamou D, Fernandez H: Intraperitoneal local anaesthetic for shoulder pain after day-case laparoscopy. Lancet 1991; 338: 1569–1570.

72. Helvacioglu A, Weis R: Operative laparoscopy and postoperative pain relief. Fertil Steril 1992; 57: 548–552.

73. Rimback G, Cassuto J, Faxen A, et al: Effect of inter-abdominal bupivacaine instillation on postoperative colonic motility. Gut 1986; 27: 170–175.

74. Wallin G, Cassuto J, Hogstrom S, et al: Influence of intraperitoneal anesthesia on pain and the sympathoadrenal response to abdominal surgery. Acta Anaesthesiol Scand 1988; 32: 553–558.

75. Scott NB, Mogensen T, Greulich A, et al: No effect of continuous i.p. infusion of bupivacaine on postoperative analgesia, pulmonary function and the stress response to surgery. Br J Anaesth 1988; 61: 165–168.

76. Simon DL, Carron H, Rowlingson JC: Treatment of bladder pain with transsacral nerve block. Anesth Analg 1982; 61: 46–48.

77. Clark AJ, Awad SA: Selective transsacral nerve root blocks. Reg Anesth 1990; 15: 125–129.

78. Kopacz DJ, Bridenbaugh LD: Are anesthesia residency programs failing regional anesthesia? The past, present, and future. Reg Anesth 1993; 18: 84–87.

CHAPTER 19

Neuraxial Blocks

Rom A. Stevens, M.D.

Spinal Anesthesia

History

Spinal anesthesia is the introduction of a local anesthetic into the spinal intrathecal space to produce anesthesia (loss of sensation) and motor block. This form of anesthesia is unique in the sense that a small dose of local anesthetic, too small to have any systemic toxic effects, can produce profound surgical anesthesia. By slightly altering the solution containing this drug, different effects can be produced. For example, a block confined to the sacral dermatomes (saddle block) for perianal surgery or a block providing anesthesia and profound muscle relaxation of the lower abdomen for herniorrhaphy can be achieved. This anesthetic is quite versatile, indeed.

Spinal anesthesia is one of the oldest forms of regional anesthesia, with its clinical use for surgery by August Bier of the University of Berlin[1] dating to 1898. Before using spinal anesthesia on their patients, Professor Bier and an assistant first subjected themselves to spinal anesthesia. Bier and his assistant thereby became the first to report post–dural puncture headache (PDPH). Spinal anesthesia grew in popularity in Europe and North America until the late 1940s, when advances in general anesthesia techniques (mainly introduction of curare for neuromuscular block and widespread use of tracheal intubation) and two widely publicized cases in the United Kingdom of paralysis after spinal anesthesia led to a decline in its use.[2] Since the 1970s, owing in part to the halothane hepatitis issue as well as to increased use in obstetric anesthesia, and later in the 1980s owing to interest in providing postoperative analgesia, the popularity of both spinal and epidural techniques has again been on the rise. However, only in recent years have the scientific principles behind epidural and spinal anesthesia been rigorously researched. Clinical studies aimed at expanding the understanding of these principles have dominated the regional anesthesia literature in the past decade.

In this chapter, the term "epidural" should be taken as synonymous with the terms "spinal epidural," "extradural," and "peridural." The reader will find much of the information on spinal anesthesia also applies to epidural anesthesia. Epidural anesthesia was

319

used clinically in the first decade of the 20th century, shortly after Professor Bier developed spinal anesthesia.[3] However, it was not until the 1930s that Dogliotti,[4] and Gutiérrez[5] (in Argentina) first published textbooks on the subject in an attempt to bring together some of the qualitative measurements and systematic observations, rather than rely on only clinical impressions, that had guided anesthesiologists up to that time. During and shortly after the Second World War, German anesthesiologists[6, 7] published accounts of their experiences of using tetracaine dissolved in a viscous solution (plombe technique) to achieve restricted epidural blocks of long duration. Although this experience encompassed several thousand cases, this technique never became popular worldwide. A major technologic breakthrough in the technique of epidural anesthesia occurred when Tuohy's needle and catheter technique, originally developed for continuous spinal anesthesia,[8] made continuous epidural anesthesia more practical.

Despite a hiatus in interest after introduction of curare, epidural anesthesia survived, primarily as a result of use of continuous caudal analgesia in labor. During the 1960s, Professor Philip Bromage, at McGill University, and Professor John Bonica, at the University of Washington, began investigating the physiology and pharmacology of epidural anesthesia. It is because of these two individuals and their coworkers that today we have a body of expanding scientific knowledge of epidural anesthesia. During the 1970s and 1980s, the increasing popularity of continuous epidural blocks for labor analgesia led to a renaissance of interest in this technique among anesthesiologists and surgeons. In the last 10 years, research on the topic of epidural anesthesia has been focused primarily on the advantages of epidural anesthesia vis-à-vis general anesthesia with respect to attenuation of the stress hormone response to surgery,[9] decreasing blood loss,[10] deep venous thrombosis prophylaxis,[11] increased patency of vascular grafts,[12] and improvements in postoperative pain therapy.[13]

Patient Selection and Preparation

There are many factors influencing the success of regional anesthesia, which precede the patient's arrival in the operating suite. Many of these factors (surgeon's, nurses', and patient's cooperation) are addressed in Chapter 1. Therefore, this discussion concentrates on patient selection. This is an important step in the success of spinal or epidural anesthesia. First, it is necessary to obtain the patient's informed consent, explain major and minor complications, and give the patient a reasonable idea of what to expect. This is preferably done the day before operation, when the anesthesiologist will not be stressed trying to answer all the patient's questions and at the same time trying to get the patient ready for operation. During this preoperative conversation, the anesthesiologist must attempt to gauge the patient's emotional state and level of maturity. An unreasonably anxious or immature patient may not hold still long enough for a block to be placed, despite prior

consent and judicious sedation, or may be too worried the block will not provide adequate analgesia. A patient may also be overly concerned with possible complications of anesthesia—e.g., paralysis. All of these subjects are best addressed before the arrival of the patient in the operating theater.

Additionally, one must choose the proper anesthetic for the planned surgical procedure. A hypobaric spinal anesthetic is practical for a total hip arthroplasty in the lateral decubitus position or for perianal surgery, if the patient will be in the jackknife position. An isobaric spinal anesthetic may be just right for a surgical procedure on the knee but not on the abdomen. A hyperbaric spinal anesthetic would be appropriate for a lower abdominal operation; an upper abdominal operation would probably require the addition of a light general anesthetic because of the difficulty in blocking all nociceptive input from the upper abdomen with contemporary spinal or epidural anesthesia. Therefore, some thought must go into the planning of any regional anesthetic if one wishes to keep both patient and surgeon coadvocates of regional anesthesia.

Patient selection is also important when teaching trainees. A morbidly obese patient is probably unsuitable for a junior resident to try learning spinal anesthesia. This patient (and the resident) would be better served by having the anesthetic administered by a more experienced anesthesiologist. A thin patient with easily palpable spinous processes would provide a better teaching model for the resident. Additionally, the patient must be free of absolute contraindications to neuraxial block. These include patient refusal, increased intracranial pressure, infection at the site of needle puncture, uncorrected hypovolemia, and significant coagulopathy. Relative contraindications may include sepsis or unstable neurologic diseases.[2] Thus, common sense must be applied in choosing the patient. This is the first step to ensure success with any regional anesthetic.

Anatomy

As with any regional anesthetic technique, a good understanding of anatomy is essential to success. The anatomy of the spinal canal and surrounding structures is presented in detail in Chapters 3 and 4, so it is reviewed only briefly here. The vertebral column is made up of 7 cervical, 12 thoracic, 5 lumbar, 5 fused sacral, and 4 coccygeal vertebrae. There are four curves in this column: cervical and lumbar, which are anteriorly convex; and thoracic and sacral curves, which are anteriorly concave (Fig. 19–1). There are several ligaments, which bind the column together and provide stability: supraspinous ligament, interspinous ligament, ligamentum flavum (yellow ligament), and two longitudinal ligaments—anterior and posterior (Fig. 19–2).

The spinal canal extends from the foramen magnum of the cranium to the sacrococcygeal ligament at the termination of the vertebral column. Enclosed in this canal are, among many other structures, three spaces

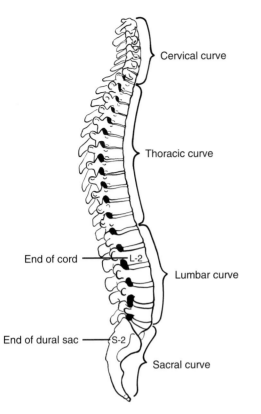

Figure 19–1 Vertebral column. Note termination of spinal cord at L1-2; termination of dural sac at S-2. There are four curves of the vertebral column: the cervical and lumbar curves are convex anteriorly; the thoracic and sacral are concave anteriorly.

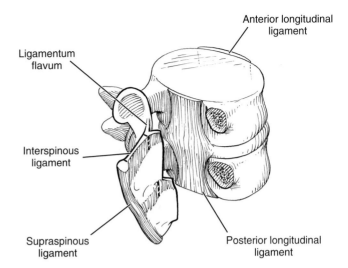

Figure 19–2 Ligaments of spinal column. Supraspinous ligament is a thin ligament that connects the spinous processes. Interspinous ligaments also connect spinous processes. This ligament is prone to degeneration and cavitation with aging. Cavitation can lead to false-positive loss of resistance. Ligamentum flavum is the more dense ligament. Needle entrance into this ligament can be noticed by a "gritty" feeling.

important to the anesthesiologist: the intrathecal space, the subdural space, and the epidural space. The epidural space (containing epidural veins, fat, and exiting vertebral nerve roots) surrounding the spinal dura is separated from the subarachnoid space (containing spinal cord and cerebrospinal fluid [CSF]) by the spinal meninges (dura, arachnoid, and pia mater) (Fig. 19–3).

A potential space bounded by the arachnoid and dura mater is called the subdural space. Needles, catheters, and local anesthetic intended for the subarachnoid or epidural spaces sometimes end up in this space. In the newborn, the spinal cord ends at the level of the third lumbar vertebra, and in the adult, at the level of the first lumbar vertebra (Fig. 19–4). The thecal sac usually has its caudal terminus at the level of the second sacral vertebra. To avoid possible needle trauma to the spinal cord, spinal anesthesia is usually initiated at the second, third, fourth, or fifth lumbar interspace.

Occasionally, the intrathecal space extends for a variable distance along the spinal nerve roots outside the spinal canal. These extensions are called meningoceles

Figure 19–3 Contents of dural sac at level of L-4. The cauda equina are contained within a dural sac filled with cerebrospinal fluid.

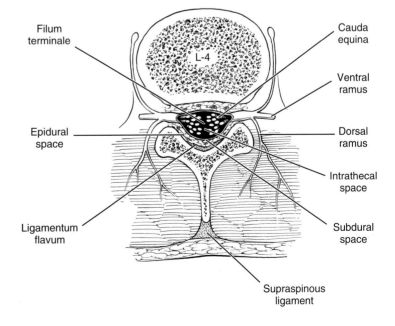

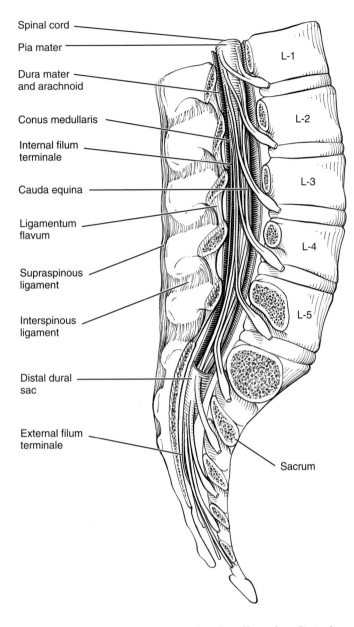

Spinal cord

Pia mater

Dura mater
and arachnoid

Conus medullaris

Internal filum
terminale

Cauda equina

Ligamentum
flavum

Supraspinous
ligament

Interspinous
ligament

Distal dural
sac

External filum
terminale

Sacrum

L-1

L-2

L-3

L-4

L-5

Figure 19–4 Spinal cord anatomy. Note termination of spinal cord (conus medullaris) at L1-2 and termination of dural sac at S-2.

or dilated nerve root sleeves (dural cuffs). The clinical importance of these anatomic variations is that occasionally a needle intended for a paravertebral nerve root block or a lumbar sympathetic block may enter the intrathecal space outside the spinal canal, resulting in an unintended spinal block or in a PDPH.[14]

Spinal Ligaments

Logically, the spinal (or epidural) needle must pass through several structures in order to reach the spinal canal. These are, in order: skin, subcutaneous fat, supraspinous ligament, interspinous ligament, and ligamentum flavum. There are several anatomic and pathologic variations that can complicate this otherwise straightforward needle path. In older patients, there is often a degeneration of the interspinous ligament, resulting in a cavity. This can cause the anesthesiologist to encounter a false loss of resistance superficial to the epidural space during epidural needle insertion.

Additionally, in older patients and in those with advanced osteoarthritis and rheumatoid arthritis, the interspaces between vertebrae may be quite calcified and, thus, narrowed. This can make insertion of a needle more difficult. A paramedian approach may be the only way a needle can be successfully inserted. In some disease states, such as ankylosing spondylitis, calcification of the interspaces and ligamenta flava can be so advanced as to make spinal and epidural needle insertion impractical. If a radiograph of the spine is available, it can provide useful information before neuraxial block is attempted.

Study of a normal human skeleton is instructive for the practitioner of neuraxial block. The spinous processes of the cervical and lumbar vertebrae are perpendicular to the plane of the back. Therefore, to pass between the spinous processes without contacting bone, a needle in these regions should be inserted parallel to the lumbar spinous processes. In the lumbar region, the normal lumbar lordosis, with its apex at the fourth lumbar interspace, can make passage of a needle between spinous processes difficult. For this reason, it is useful for an assistant to position the patient with the back flexed, to minimize the lumbar lordosis. If assuming this position is not possible for the patient, further study of the skeleton reveals that a paramedian approach, with the needle inserted 15° to 20° from the parasagittal plane, provides a much larger target than the midline approach. The skeleton also reveals that the spinous processes of the 4th to 12th thoracic vertebrae are angulated and in some places overlapping. This explains why a midline approach at these segments is difficult. A paramedian approach is much easier at these interspaces. One final observation from the skeleton: not all interspaces are created equal! The largest interspace is the fifth lumbar interspace; the second largest is the seventh cervical interspace. These anatomic trivia can often be put to good use when interspaces are narrowed as a result of arthritic changes.

Anatomy of the Epidural Space

The anatomy of the spinal canal and associated structures is extensively covered in Chapters 3 and 4 and briefly in the first section of this chapter, so it is only highlighted here.

Contents of the Epidural Space

A study[15] of the epidural space anatomy, using cryomicrotome sectioning, has revealed several interesting observations that differ from previous reports using methods more prone to introduction of artifact. The epidural space contents are mainly fat and also veins and nerves. The contents are circumferentially and metamerically segmented compartments rather than a uniform layer, as usually portrayed in textbooks.[16] In many areas, dura is directly in contact with the spinal canal, obliterating the epidural space at these levels. However, these areas of potential space can be distended by injection of local anesthetic or contrast material and do allow passage of catheters.

Ligamenta Flava

The ligamenta flava are paired in nature, arising embryonically from two separate structures. They are high, arched, and fused to a variable degree in the midline. Occasionally, they are not fused at all, resulting in a midsagittal gap. Because the ligamentum flava are dense and usually adherent to the interspinous ligament, an increase in resistance to injection is felt as the epidural needle is advanced through the interspinous ligament into the ligamentum flavum. A loss of resistance after increasing resistance to injection is a good indication of entrance into the epidural space. In the case of a midsagittal gap between unfused ligamenta flava, this may lead to an unintended rapid advancement of the needle and subsequent dural puncture.

The posterior epidural space is filled mainly with a large fat pedicle and some veins. The anterior epidural space is filled mainly with a venous channel and has minimal fat. This compartment vanishes at each disk. The contents of the epidural space depend on the exact longitudinal site of the axial section (Fig. 19–5). Below the L4-5 disk, the anterior epidural space becomes quite capacious. This large space may be, in part, responsible for clinical difficulty in blocking the fifth lumbar and first sacral nerve roots.[17] A membranous lateral extension of the posterior longitudinal ligament was

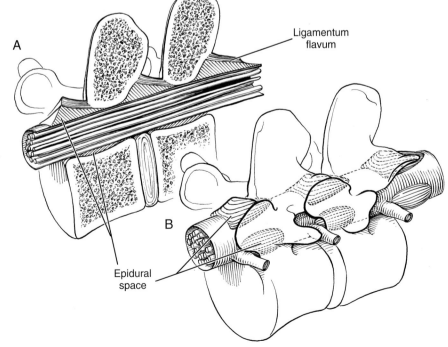

Figure 19–5 *A,* Sagittal section of epidural space demonstrates that the contents of the epidural space depend on level of section. *B,* Three-dimensional drawing of the epidural space shows the discontinuity of the epidural contents. However, this potential space can be dilated by injection of fluid into the epidural space.

Ligamentum flavum

Epidural space

observed to separate the anterior epidural space from the remainder of the space. This and the midline fat pedicle in the posterior epidural space were the only observed potential barriers to spread of epidural solutions.

The lateral epidural space contains spinal nerve roots and radicular arteries. Hogan[15] was unable to find any evidence of fibrous septa enclosing the lateral epidural space. This is consistent with many observations[18, 19] made of contrast material spreading unimpeded out the intervertebral neural foramina into the paravertebral space. There is some evidence these neural foramina may become relatively closed with age. For example, it is known that compliance of the epidural space decreases with advancing age. Perhaps this explains why there is increased spread of local anesthetics in elderly compared with young patients.[20]

Bony Anatomy

As recalled previously, osseous anatomy of the spinal column is important for deciding the angle of needle insertion in spinal and epidural anesthesia. To recapitulate: the spinous processes of the cervical and lumbar vertebrae are perpendicular to the plane of the back (Fig. 19–6). Thoracic spinous processes between T-4 and T-9 are quite angulated, even overlapping in places. This means that a midline approach in the mid to lower thoracic spine is difficult, and the paramedian approach is best at these levels (Fig. 19–7).

Spinal Cord Blood Supply

The spinal cord is supplied with arterial blood from the aorta by segmental arteries associated with the spinal nerve roots via the intervertebral foramina. These segmental arteries supply a single anterior and two posterior spinal arteries running longitudinally with the spinal cord. Although there are small spinal feeder arteries at each vertebral level, the major feeder is the artery radicularis magnus (artery of Adamkiewicz). This usually enters unilaterally (75% on left) via a single foramen between T-8 and L-3.[21] Because there is only one anterior spinal artery, the area of the cord supplied by this artery is thought to be most vulnerable to vascular interruption (Fig. 19–8). The anterior portion of the spinal cord provides innervation mainly to skeletal muscles plus preganglionic sympathetic innervation. The posterior spinal cord provides somatosensory, vibratory, and position sensation. The anterior spinal artery syndrome consists of skeletal muscle weakness, with intact vibratory, position, and somatosensory innervation. Direct needle trauma to a feeder artery, particularly the artery radicularis magnus, could theoretically explain cases of anterior spinal artery syndrome after epidural or spinal anesthesia.

Cerebrospinal Fluid and Baricity

CSF, an ultrafiltrate of plasma, is formed by the choroid plexuses of the lateral, third, and fourth ventricles.[2] It is absorbed by the arachnoid villi in the cranium, normally at a rate equal to the rate of production. This is about 0.35 mL/min or 500 mL/d. Total volume of CSF is 120 to 150 mL, distributed about equally between cranial and spinal CSF. Normal spinal CSF pressure in the lumbar region with the patient horizontal is 60 to 80 mm H$_2$O. Normal CSF specific gravity (density in g/mL per density of water) is 1.0006 $\pm$ 0.0003 at 37° C.

A solution of local anesthetic is considered to be hyperbaric if its baricity (specific gravity of local anesthetic/specific gravity of CSF) is greater than 1.0, iso-

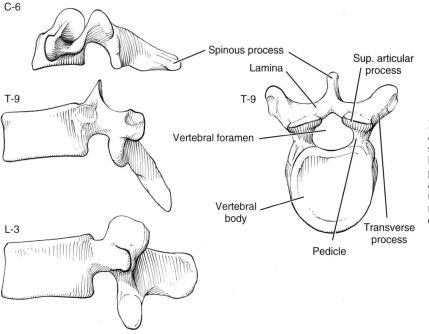

Figure 19–6 Anatomy of cervical, thoracic, and lumbar vertebrae with emphasis on spinous processes. Note that cervical and lumbar spinous processes are perpendicular to plane of back. Thoracic spinous processes are angulated. In the midthoracic region (T-4 through T-9) the spinous processes overlap, necessitating a paramedian approach to the epidural space in this region.

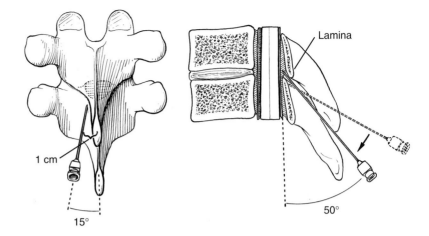

Figure 19–7 Paramedian approach to the midthoracic epidural space. Needle is inserted 1 cm lateral to spinous process and advanced until lamina is contacted, usually 2 to 3 cm deep to skin. Then needle is redirected cephalad and medial toward the interspace.

baric if it is approximately 1.0, and hypobaric if it is less than 1.0. Because of the normal range in specific gravity of CSF, local anesthetic solutions must have specific gravities less than 0.9990 and more than 1.0010 to be predictably hypobaric or hyperbaric, respectively. In the clinical situation, this is done by dissolving the local anesthetic in a dextrose solution (usually 7.5% or 10%) to make a hyperbaric solution or in sterile distilled H_2O to make a hypobaric solution. Commercially available solutions of 0.5% bupivacaine marketed for epidural anesthesia are slightly hypobaric (specific gravity at 37° C = 0.9990) and have characteristics somewhat different from those of isobaric tetracaine: the distribution tends to be more cephalad if the patient sits for any time after injection[22, 23] (Table 19–1).

Factors Affecting Spread of Spinal Anesthesia

Although many other factors have been considered to affect the spread of spinal anesthesia,[24] only those factors considered to be clinically important[25, 26]—baricity and position of the patient, dose (mg) of drug, site of injection, and age of the patient—are discussed here. The practitioner of spinal anesthesia needs to know: "What is the minimum block I can expect?" in order to guarantee there will be adequate spread of anesthesia to perform a given operation. Additionally, the anesthesiologist needs to know: "What is the maximum extent of block I must be prepared to deal with?" to avoid being caught unaware. These questions must be answered before choosing the drug, baricity, and dose.

Because of the various curves in the vertebral column and the effect of gravity, the interplay between baricity and patient position is the single most important determinant of spread of spinal anesthesia. Clinically, this fact can be used to increase the predictability of the spread of local anesthetic in the CSF. For example, when a hyperbaric solution is injected into the CSF in the lumbar region (usually at the third lumbar interspace) and the patient is turned supine, because of the curves in the vertebral column, the hyperbaric solution moves cephalad and caudad along

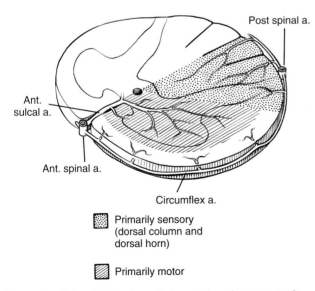

Figure 19–8 Arterial blood supply to spinal cord. Note a single anterior spinal artery supplies blood to anterior portion of cord. The anterior spinal nerve roots (motor fibers) originate here. Two posterior spinal arteries supply blood to the dorsal portions of the spinal cord, where afferent fibers (somatosensory, nociceptive, proprioceptive, and vibratory fibers) enter the cord and synapse.

Table 19–1 Physical Characteristics of Local Anesthetic Solutions at 37° C (Mean)

SOLUTION	DENSITY	SPECIFIC GRAVITY	BARICITY
Water	0.9934	1.0000	0.9931
Cerebrospinal fluid	1.0003	1.0069	1.0000
Tetracaine			
1.0% in water	1.0003	1.0007	1.0000
0.5% in 50% cerebrospinal fluid	0.9998	1.0064	0.9995
0.5% in 5% dextrose	1.0136	1.0203	1.0133
Dibucaine			
0.066% in 0.5% saline	0.9970	1.0036	0.9976
Bupivacaine			
0.5% in water	0.9993	1.0059	0.9990
0.5% in 8% dextrose	1.0210	1.0278	1.0207
Procaine			
2.5% in water	0.9983	1.0052	0.9983
Lidocaine			
2% in water	1.0003	1.0066	1.0003
5% in 7.5% dextrose	1.0265	1.0333	1.0265

Data from Greene NM: Distribution of local anesthetic solutions within the subarachnoid space. Anesth Analg 1985; 64: 715–730.

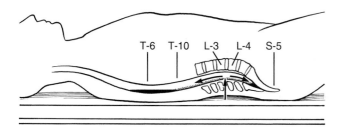

Figure 19–9 Distribution of hyperbaric local anesthetic solution in the intrathecal space after injection at L3-4 (at the apex of the lumbar lordosis) in a patient turned immediately supine. Note higher concentrations in midthoracic and sacral regions as the local anesthetic solution runs "down hill."

the lumbar lordotic curve, spreading to sacral and thoracic regions of the intrathecal space (Fig. 19–9). If the patient is kept sitting for 5 to 10 min after injection of a small dose (e.g., 25 mg lidocaine or 5 mg tetracaine) of a hyperbaric solution, anesthesia confined to the sacral dermatomes can be achieved (saddle block). If a hypobaric solution is injected and the patient is placed prone in the jackknife position (with the buttocks uppermost), local anesthetic will rise in the CSF to the most superior region, in this case providing anesthesia to the sacral dermatomes. Hypobaric solutions can also be effectively used to anesthetize the superior leg of a

patient placed in the lateral decubitus position for total hip arthroplasty, for example. Isobaric solutions should theoretically be unaffected by gravity or patient position. Spread of isobaric and hypobaric solutions is not as predictable as that of hyperbaric solutions.

In practical terms, this means that anesthesia of lumbar but not thoracic dermatomes is reliably achieved after lumbar injection of a hypobaric or isobaric solution (Fig. 19–10).[25] Therefore, to provide reliable anesthesia for intra-abdominal surgery, one must use a hyperbaric solution.

Other important factors influencing the spread of spinal anesthesia are dose (mass = concentration × volume) of drug (for hyperbaric but not for isobaric solutions of tetracaine[25, 26] and for hypobaric solutions of bupivacaine[27]), site of injection (high versus low lumbar interspace),[28] and age of patient (greater spread of anesthesia with advancing age),[22, 29, 30] although the last has not been a universal finding.[31] In fact, although statistically greater spread has been seen in older patients, only a few dermatomes' difference is seen, and this may not be clinically significant. For hyperbaric solutions, increasing dose of drug slightly increases spread of anesthesia, increases duration of block, produces a more complete neural block (better motor block), and thus increases the predictability of spinal anesthesia. Thus, for example, use of 15 mg rather

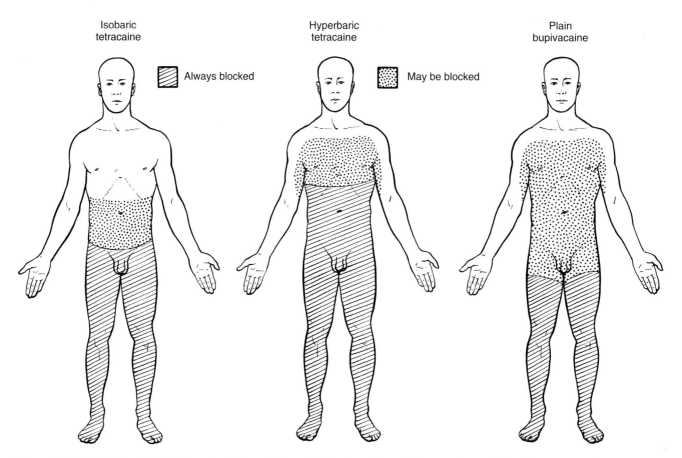

Figure 19–10 Variability of distribution of spinal anesthesia with isobaric and hyperbaric tetracaine, and plain bupivacaine after lumbar intrathecal injection in patients turned immediately supine. Plain bupivacaine is slightly hypobaric. Because of variability with isobaric and hypobaric solutions, they do not reliably provide anesthesia of lower thoracic dermatomes. (Modified from Wildsmith JAW, Rocco AG: Current concepts in spinal anesthesia. Reg Anesth 1985; 10: 119–124.)

than 10 mg hyperbaric bupivacaine produces a more predictable block of the lower thoracic dermatomes and a slightly more extensive cephalad spread.

Factors not believed to significantly affect spread of local anesthetics in the CSF are sex, height, weight,[25] volume of injected solution (assuming constant mass of drug), needle direction, and barbotage.[26] Morbid obesity and third trimester pregnancy result in a slightly higher level of anesthesia compared with controls given the same dose of drug; however, this difference may not be as clinically important in determining spread of local anesthetics as dose and baricity. In the normal situation, CSF volume does not seem to play a role, although prior removal of CSF does produce a higher level of anesthesia.[32]

Duration of Action

Discussion of duration of action is somewhat complicated by definitions. Spinal anesthesia wears off starting at the uppermost segment blocked. Therefore, we commonly speak of time to two-segment regression or time to four-segment regression to measure duration of action during epidural and spinal anesthesia (Fig. 19–11). Of course, there may be anesthesia at lumbar dermatomes a considerable time after anesthesia has dissipated in upper thoracic dermatomes, and this may have significant clinical consequence for the patient (e.g., inability to ambulate). Obviously, clinically meaningful duration of action depends on the dermatome involved in surgery.

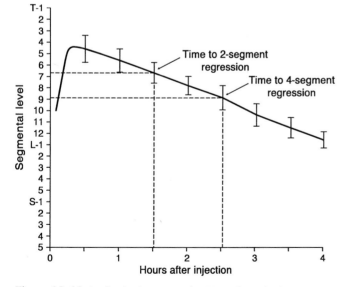

Figure 19–11 Analgesia-time curve for 20 mg hyperbaric bupivacaine after lumbar intrathecal injection; mean dermatome ± SD for $n = 10$. Note that peak block height is reached within 20 min. Regression of block begins almost immediately. Duration of surgical anesthesia depends on location of operation. The patient will be able to ambulate after regression of anesthesia below the lumbar dermatomes. Despite four-segment regression of block after 4 h, the patient would not be ambulatory at this time. (Data from Covino BG: New techniques in regional anesthesia [review course lecture]. Instructional Anesthesia Research Society Annual Meeting, San Antonio, Texas, March 8 to 12, 1990.)

The major factor affecting duration of action is the drug injected. More highly protein-bound drugs—e.g., tetracaine, dibucaine, and bupivacaine—have a longer duration of action than less highly protein-bound drugs such as lidocaine, mepivacaine, or procaine. Effects of vasoconstrictors are discussed separately below. An increase in dose of a given drug increases duration of action.[33] In general, isobaric solutions produce a greater duration of action in those dermatomes blocked than the same dose of a hyperbaric solution. Presumably, this is because the isobaric drug spreads less from the site of injection, resulting in a higher concentration of local anesthetic per spinal segment. Duration is also affected by level of block produced. If x mg of a drug produces anesthesia to a thoracic level, there will be a shorter duration of anesthesia at that dermatome than if the same dose of the same drug had produced anesthesia to a lumbar level. Presumably, a greater spread produces a lower concentration of drug per spinal segment.[25]

Choice of Drug

One important difference among available drugs for spinal anesthesia is the degree of protein binding of drug, which determines, in part, the duration of action (Table 19–2).[34] Dibucaine, tetracaine, and bupivacaine are the most highly protein bound of the drugs commonly used for spinal anesthesia. They also produce the longest duration of action. Lidocaine and mepivacaine are moderately protein bound and produce a shorter duration of action. Procaine is least protein bound and thus produces the shortest duration of action. Another important difference among drugs is the degree to which addition of a vasoconstrictor increases duration of action. This effect is greatest for tetracaine. Addition of 200 μg of epinephrine or 2 to 5 mg phenylephrine increases the time to two-segment regression of tetracaine spinal anesthesia 30% to 70%.[35, 36] A double-blind study has shown that epinephrine (0.2 mg or 0.3 mg) or phenylephrine (1 mg or 2 mg) prolongs the duration of spinal anesthesia with tetracaine equally.[37] These investigators did not include an often used higher dose of phenylephrine (5 mg) in their study. Addition of epinephrine to bupivacaine and lidocaine has no effect on time to two-segment regression but does produce a measurable increase in duration of anesthesia at lumbar dermatomes.[38, 39] Therefore, addition of epinephrine to these last two drugs may be useful if surgery is contemplated on the lower extremities or the perineum.

Bupivacaine and tetracaine are the two most widely used local anesthetics for spinal anesthesia in North America. They are similar in anesthetic potency. One double-blind comparison[40] showed tetracaine produced a significantly longer duration of motor block than bupivacaine. Other than a difference in the efficacy of adding vasoconstrictors to increase duration of anesthesia, differences between these two drugs are small.

A new local anesthetic, ropivacaine, which has a chemical structure homologous to mepivacaine and

Table 19–2 Local Anesthetics for Spinal Anesthesia

LOCAL ANESTHETIC	CONCENTRATION, %	USUAL DURATION, h	MAXIMUM DOSE, mg
Procaine	10.0	0.5–1.0	200
Lidocaine	5.0 (7.5% dextrose)	1.0–1.5	100
Mepivacaine	4.0 (7.5% dextrose)	1.0–1.5	100
Dibucaine	0.25–0.5 (dextrose) 0.667 mg/mL (hypobaric)	2.0–4.0	10
Tetracaine	1.0	2.0–4.0	20
Bupivacaine	0.75 (8.5% dextrose) 0.75% and 0.50% plain	2.0–4.0	20

Data from Covino BG: Clinical pharmacology of local anesthetic agents. In Cousins MJ, Bridenbaugh PO (eds): Neural Blockade in Clinical Anesthesia and Management of Pain, 2nd ed, pp 111–144. Philadelphia, JB Lippincott, 1988.

bupivacaine, will soon be marketed for epidural and peripheral nerve anesthesia in the United States and in Europe. Although the manufacturer (Astra Pharmaceuticals) does not currently intend to market this drug for spinal anesthesia, it has been used for this purpose. A study[41] of 3 mL isobaric ropivacaine (0.5% and 0.75%) for spinal anesthesia showed that sensory anesthesia to the T-10 dermatomes was achieved within 10 min of injection with the 0.75% solution. Fifty percent of the 0.5% group did not achieve analgesia to that level. Motor block of the lower extremities lasted for about 2.5 and 3.0 h with the 0.5% and 0.75% solutions, respectively. Sensory block at the T-10 dermatome (in those patients in whom it was achieved) lasted about 2 h. It appears from this study that 3 mL ropivacaine (0.75%, 22.5 mg) has similar characteristics to 15 mg plain bupivacaine.

Drugs for spinal anesthesia come in various forms. In the United States, tetracaine is marketed as niphanoid crystals (20 mg/ampule), which can be diluted with CSF, sterile water, or 10% dextrose to produce isobaric, hypobaric, or hyperbaric solutions, respectively. Tetracaine is also marketed in a 1% solution in water. In the United States, but not in Europe, lidocaine is marketed in a 5% solution in dextrose. In Germany, a 4% solution of mepivacaine in dextrose is available. Bupivacaine is available in a 0.75% solution in dextrose in the United States and in a 0.5% heavy solution in the United Kingdom. Alternatively, as mentioned above, 0.5% and 0.75% bupivacaine for epidural anesthesia can be used for spinal anesthesia. These last two solutions are slightly hypobaric at 37° C.

Post–dural Puncture Headache

In the opinion of many anesthesiologists, the greatest drawback of spinal anesthesia is the risk of PDPH. Because PDPH is believed to be caused by leakage of CSF through a dural hole made by the spinal needle, decreasing the size of the hole would be a logical way to decrease the incidence of PDPH. In fact, this has been the finding of many studies. After accidental dural puncture with a 17-G Tuohy epidural needle, incidence of PDPH is more than 80%. With 29- to 30-G needles, the reported incidence of PDPH has been as low as 1%.[42, 43] One problem with the use of such fine needles

is that they are easily bent during insertion and penetration of the skin and ligaments, and the success rate may be lower, particularly in inexperienced hands. Therefore, an introducer, such as the Pitkin introducer, is recommended when using needles smaller than 22 G (Fig. 19–12). In addition to needle size, other independent factors contributing to an increased incidence of PDPH are female sex, pregnancy, multiple dural punctures, direction of needle bevel insertion, design of needle, and younger age of the patient.

In older patients, increasing calcification of ligaments and osteoarthritic changes make insertion of such small needles difficult. Fortunately, the decreasing incidence of PDPH with increasing age makes use of larger-gauge needles in older patients feasible. For example, the incidence of PDPH may be as high as 10% to 20% in patients younger than age 50 years, when a 22-G needle is used, but it is approximately 5% in patients older than age 50 years.[44] PDPH is rarely seen in patients older than age 65 years. Because of a better feel for anatomic structures when a larger-gauge needle is used during insertion, the author recommends the use of a 22-G spinal needle in the elderly patient or in the patient in whom significant arthritic changes of the spine are known or suspected.

Design of Needles Available

In an attempt to decrease the leakage of CSF through the dural puncture, various designs of spinal needles

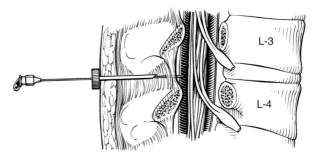

Figure 19–12 Use of the Pitkin introducer for insertion of a spinal needle. An introducer is recommended for spinal needles size 22 G and smaller to keep these relatively flexible needles from being deflected by ligaments along their path to the dura.

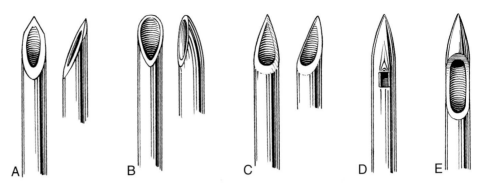

Figure 19–13 Designs of various spinal needle tips. *A,* Standard cutting or Quincke needle. *B,* Directional Tuohy needle, first designed for continuous spinal anesthesia. Pencil-point needles: *C,* Greene; *D,* Whitacre; *E,* Sprotte.

have been developed (Fig. 19–13). Common to all designs is a tight-fitting removable stylet to prevent coring of epidermal tissue, possibly resulting in production of an epidermoid tumor in the spinal canal. The standard spinal needle with a medium length cutting bevel is the Quincke point needle. Greene developed a pencil-point needle designed to separate, rather than cut, the dural fibers.[45, 46] This needle has a hole located just proximal to the needle tip. Further modifications of this principle resulted in development of the Whitacre[47] and Sprotte[48] needles. The Whitacre needle has a smaller hole than the Greene needle. The Sprotte needle is a modification of the Whitacre needle, with a more tapered tip and a larger side hole. The incidence of PDPH when 24-G Sprotte needles were used in an obstetric population has been reported to be as low as 1.5%, compared with 9% with the 25-G Quincke and 8% with the 26-G Quincke needles.[49] However, another study suggested that dural puncture is more difficult with the Sprotte needle than with the sharper Quincke needle and that when the Quincke needle bevel is inserted parallel to the dural fibers (see below), there is no significant difference in incidence of PDPH among needles.[50]

A large study comparing failure rate and incidence of PDPH between 27-G Whitacre and Quincke needles showed no difference. Failure rate was about 5%, and incidence of PDPH was less than 2% in both groups.[51] At present, it is not clear if there is a significant advantage in pencil-point over cutting needles if only ultra-small-gauge needles (27 G or smaller) are considered. It does seem clear that at larger needle sizes, the pencil-point design decreases PDPH incidence compared with cutting needle tip design.

Preparation and Positioning of the Patient

Before a spinal or epidural anesthetic is begun, the patient should be prepared as for general anesthesia, because one must always be ready to manage acute changes in blood pressure, heart rate, or oxygenation. This requires adequate intravenous access and proper patient monitoring. The minimum monitoring necessary includes an electrocardiogram, blood pressure cuff or arterial catheter, and pulse oximeter. Skin temperature monitoring should be available, because patients can become hypothermic during spinal and epidural

block, particularly during longer operations. The anesthetic machine, mask, oxygen source, and suction should be working. At the minimum, the following drugs should be at hand: thiopental, atropine, ephedrine, and succinylcholine. A tracheal tube, laryngoscope, and oropharyngeal airway should also be at hand.

In most instances, the patient is positioned for spinal anesthesia in the lateral decubitus position (Fig. 19–14). If one uses a hypobaric solution for total hip replacement, the patient should be positioned as for surgery, with the operative side up. After light sedation (e.g., 3 mg midazolam for a young, healthy patient), the patient is instructed to assume the "Halloween cat position" with back arched, legs and knees flexed, and chin on chest. This position decreases the lumbar lordosis and increases the target area between spinous processes. Spinous processes are then palpated, and an interspace is chosen. The commonly used intercristal line connecting the iliac crests usually crosses the body of L-4. However, in obese patients, generous adipose tissue overlying the iliac crests can cause one to misjudge the presumed intercristal line, resulting in a lumbar puncture several segments higher than planned. This could lead to unintended subarachnoid puncture in the area of the conus medullaris at L-1.

The author favors placing the patient in the lateral decubitus position for spinal and epidural blocks, because it is usually easier for the patient to assume this position with monitors attached, particularly if she is

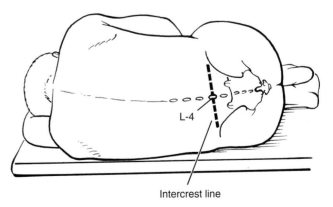

Figure 19–14 Patient in lateral decubitus position for neuraxial block. Intercrest line identifies level of third lumbar interspace or fourth lumbar vertebra.

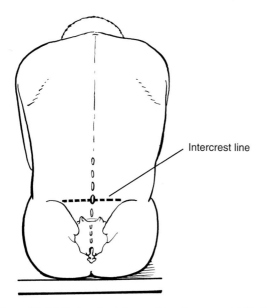

Figure 19–15 Patient in sitting position for neuraxial block.

pregnant. Furthermore, if there is a sudden change in the vital signs (e.g., vasovagal fainting), it is easier to turn the patient supine and manage the problem if the patient is in the lateral decubitus position rather than sitting. However, there are several circumstances when sitting or the prone position is desired. If the patient is morbidly obese and it is difficult to identify midline in the lateral decubitus position, the sitting position is preferred. Additionally, if the CSF pressure is low or CSF cannot be found with the patient in the lateral decubitus position, it may be helpful to have the patient sit, increasing the CSF pressure at the puncture site (Fig. 19–15). If a hyperbaric saddle block is intended for perineal surgery, the patient must be kept sitting for at least 5 min after injection of local anesthetic. If a hypobaric technique for perianal surgery is planned, the prone position can be used. The patient is positioned as for surgery, with pillows raising the buttocks and flexing the lumbar spine slightly (Fig. 19–16). Lumbar puncture can then be accomplished, using a syringe to aspirate for CSF.

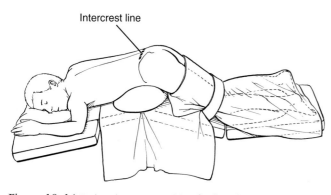

Figure 19–16 Patient in prone position for hypobaric spinal for perianal surgery.

Techniques of Needle Insertion

Midline Approach

Whichever position is chosen, the author favors the following technique for lumbar puncture (Fig. 19–17). First, the midline is identified by following several spinous processes in line. The desired interspace is identified, usually by counting up from the sacrum, and perhaps marked with a skin marker. The skin is prepared with an antiseptic solution, and sterile draping is performed. The nondominant hand is used to place the index and middle fingers to straddle the spinous process, identifying the interspace. These fingers are left in place during local infiltration. Local anesthesia is produced ideally by using a 1.5-in, 25- or 27-G needle. This allows one to raise a skin wheal and infiltrate to the interspinous ligament without changing needles. From the personal experience of the author, while on the receiving end of an epidural needle, generous infiltration of skin and interspinous ligament with 3 to 5 mL of local anesthetic makes lumbar puncture more tolerable. The needle is then grasped with the dominant hand (the fingers of the other hand are still straddling the spinous process) and inserted in the middle of the interspace, advancing the needle just off the spinous process identified by the fingers of the opposite hand into the interspinous ligament.

Judging how deep to insert the needle requires some experience. In a nonobese 75-kg male, the distance from skin to epidural space is approximately 5 cm, with the dura being 3 to 5 mm deeper. In a smaller

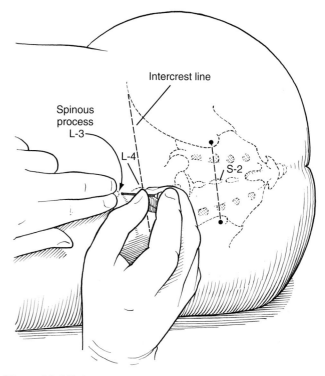

Figure 19–17 Placement of introducer for spinal anesthesia. Fingers of nondominant hand straddle spinous process of vertebra cephalad to interspace to guide needle into interspinous ligament. Needle is inserted perpendicular to long axis of back.

patient, the distance will be less. In a morbidly obese patient, the distance could be 8 to 9 cm (the entire length of the needle). At this point the stylet is removed, and the needle is advanced slowly until CSF is seen in the needle hub (Fig. 19–18). If one is using a spinal needle smaller than 22 G, it is helpful to first insert an introducer (e.g., a Pitkin or similar introducer) to its hub, and then pass the spinal needle through the introducer (Fig. 19–12). One must be careful in small or thin patients, because the introducer may be long enough to puncture the dura.

If CSF is not encountered after reaching a depth of 8 cm, midline position of the needle should be confirmed. The most common cause of failure to obtain CSF is failure to stay in the midline. If the needle is ascertained to be in the midline, but no CSF is forthcoming, the next maneuver is to remove the needle and to replace the stylet, confirming patency of the needle. At the next insertion, after reaching the interspinous ligament and removing the stylet, a 3-mL syringe can be used to aspirate as the needle is advanced (Fig. 19–19). This technique of loss of resistance to negative pressure has been used to increase the success rate of spinal anesthesia when fine-gauge needles are used.[52] If bone is encountered before CSF, despite a midline needle position, the midline approach is abandoned in favor of a paramedian approach.

Once CSF is aspirated, needle advancement is halted. The needle hub is gently rotated through all four quadrants to ensure the tip of the needle is well within the subarachnoid space. If CSF continues to be seen at the hub, local anesthetic is slowly injected, aspirating CSF once or twice to ensure continued subarachnoid position of the needle tip. The patient is then placed in position for operation. The author does not find it generally necessary to place the patient in the Trendelenburg position to obtain anesthesia of the lower abdomen if an adequate dose of hyperbaric drug is injected (e.g., 15 to 20 mg of bupivacaine or tetracaine or 100 mg of lidocaine).

The direction of needle bevel and angle of insertion are important. To decrease the incidence of PDPH, it is important to insert the needle so that the bevel is parallel to longitudinal dural fibers, so that the fibers

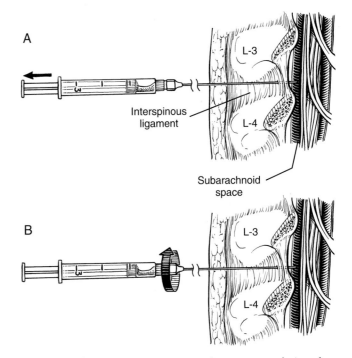

Figure 19–19 Loss of resistance to negative pressure technique for detecting needle entry into subarachnoid space. This is particularly useful for small-gauge needles (24 G or smaller). *A,* Once cerebrospinal fluid (CSF) is aspirated, needle bevel is rotated through 360° *(B)* while CSF is aspirated to ascertain subarachnoid position of needle bevel.

are separated, not cut. This was first suggested by Greene[45] in 1926, confirmed experimentally by Franksson and Gordh[53] in 1946, and demonstrated clinically by Mihic[54] in 1985. Inserting the needle at an acute angle to the dura by using the paramedian approach has also been shown to decrease the incidence of PDPH. Hatfalvi[55] reported absence of PDPH in more than 600 cases of spinal anesthesia by using a 20-G needle with this method. Using an in vitro model, Ready and colleagues[56] showed a small leak of fluid when the dura was punctured with an angle of 30°. The postulated explanation is that the holes in the dura and arachnoid made by the spinal needle do not overlap when puncture is made at an acute angle.[44] These holes could be effectively sealed by movement of the loose inner arachnoid with respect to the outer, stiffer dural layer as the patient is moved from the flexed position after lumbar puncture. The paramedian approach may thus have an advantage over the midline approach of decreasing the incidence of PDPH.

Paramedian Technique

Generally, the midline approach to needle insertion is easiest for neophytes, because one only has to ensure the needle is in midline, in the middle of the interspace, and roughly parallel to the lumbar spinous processes. If one encounters bone with the midline technique, usually it is because the needle is either too cephalad or too caudad in the interspace, causing the needle to strike lamina. Because the lumbar spinous processes are perpendicular to the long axis of the back, the

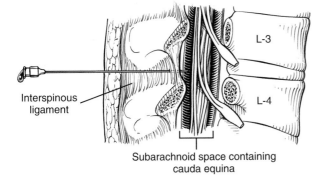

Figure 19–18 Needle in intrathecal space with return of cerebrospinal fluid at needle hub. Note needle direction is perpendicular to the long axis of back. Injection of local anesthetic is done at level of the cauda equina.

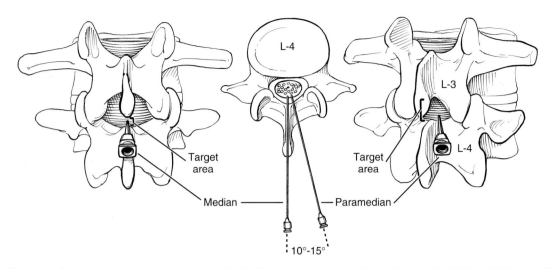

Figure 19–20 Paramedian approach for lumbar neuraxial block. The target area when the needle is angled 10° to 15° from midline is larger than the target area for the midline approach. This is particularly useful in elderly patients who may have osteoarthritic changes narrowing the interspace or degenerative interspinous ligaments, which could produce a false-positive loss of resistance to injection.

needle should also be directed perpendicular to this plane of the back when the midline approach is used. If the patient is unable to arch the back to separate spinous processes or if arthritic changes of the spine are known or suspected, a midline approach may be impossible as a result of bone in the way of the needle. In these circumstances, a paramedian approach is indicated.

There are some clear advantages to the paramedian technique. First, the target area of potential needle entry into the interspace is enlarged. This is particularly important in a patient whose interspaces are narrowed secondary to osteophytes. It is also important if a patient cannot flex the back to separate spinous processes. A paramedian approach again provides the largest target area for needle insertion. Second, the paramedian approach avoids the interspinous ligament, which degenerates with age, particularly in the lumbar region, and may contain interligamentous cysts, which can lead to false-positive loss of resistance. Third, in the midthoracic region, epidural puncture with the midline approach is difficult or impossible because of overlapping spinous processes. The paramedian approach is the only reliable method for puncture in this region. Because of the ability to insert a needle into the spinal canal in situations in which the midline approach has failed, some experienced practitioners of regional anesthesia have adopted the paramedian approach for all spinal or epidural needle insertions.

There are several variations of the paramedian approach. The one favored by the author is detailed here (Fig. 19–20). The spinous process at the caudad side of the interspace is straddled by using the two-finger technique. A skin wheal is raised about one finger-breadth lateral to the spinous process at the caudad side of the interspace. Deeper infiltration is performed, as for the midline approach, by using a 1.5-in (3-cm) needle. The needle is then inserted through the skin, directed at about a 10° to 15° angle toward midline and slightly cephalad. This approach affords a larger

target than the midline approach, and it is sometimes the only way to get into a calcified interspace. In this situation, a 22-G spinal needle is recommended, because smaller needles tend to bend too much and afford less feel if it is necessary to "walk off" bone to find the interspace because of calcification.

Another variation of the paramedian approach is the Taylor approach (Fig. 19–21). This technique takes advantage of the anatomic fact that the fifth lumbar interspace is the largest in the body. A skin wheal is raised 1 cm medial to and 1 cm caudad to the ipsilateral posterior superior iliac spine. The spinous process of L-5 can be straddled with two fingers of the nondominant hand to provide a better idea of the target interspace. The needle is directed medially and cranially toward the midline. If bone is contacted (usually the

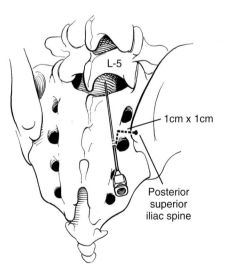

Figure 19–21 Taylor approach for neuraxial block. The L5-S1 interspace is the largest in the body. This approach is particularly useful in cases in which the interspace has been narrowed by pathologic bone encroachment on the interspaces, such as osteoarthritis or rheumatoid arthritis.

sacrum), the needle is walked off cephalad into the interspace. In this scenario, a 22-G spinal needle is recommended.

Testing of the Block

Five minutes are allowed to elapse before the anesthesia is tested. By this time, motor and sensory block should be apparent regardless of the local anesthetic used. Motor block can be tested by asking the patient to raise the leg off the table with a straight knee. Inability to raise the leg (assuming the patient was able to do this before anesthesia) is a good indicator of motor block in the lumbar dermatomes. Anesthesia should be tested at the operative site with a dull needle. Level of analgesia cephalad can be tested by establishing a sharp sensation (again with a dull needle) at an unblocked area, e.g., the shoulder (C-4 dermatome), confirming anesthesia at the operative site, and moving cephalad up the trunk until the sensation is again as sharp as tested at the shoulder. The dermatome just caudad to this point is the highest level of analgesia. Although the highest level of block is usually established by 20 min after spinal injection, in unusual circumstances, it may continue to rise as long as 30 min after injection. The significance of this is that when the level of analgesia is above T-5, there is a 3.8-fold greater risk of hypotension and a 1.8-fold greater risk of bradycardia.[57] It is better to ask the patient to respond only when something is felt (when testing for anesthesia) or something sharp is felt (testing for analgesia) than to ask more general questions (e.g., "What do you feel?"). It is important to be confident that the anesthetic will work so that the patient is not made to believe there may be some question of this. If there are no objective signs of adequate block 5 min after injection, you must either repeat the block or induce general anesthesia.

Continuous Spinal Anesthesia

Continuous spinal anesthesia (CSA) was repopularized in the 1980s with the development of microcatheters (29 to 32 G).[58] The advantage of this technique is that a relatively short-acting local anesthetic, e.g., procaine or lidocaine, could be used, even if the duration of surgery is in doubt, allowing for dissipation of anesthesia 1 to 2 h after the last injection of local anesthetic. Theoretically, small doses of local anesthetic could be titrated to produce only the spread of spinal anesthesia needed, limiting cardiovascular side effects. Additionally, intrathecal opioids for postoperative or cancer pain management could be given. Intrathecal baclofen infusion for control of spasticity in paraplegic patients was also possible with this technique. Interestingly, baclofen is the only drug the Food and Drug Administration has approved for continuous intrathecal infusion.[59]

CSA is not a new technique. It was first used by Dean[60] in 1907. Lemmon[61] used a malleable needle to be left in place in the intrathecal space during operation. Access to the needle during operation was ensured by use of a split mattress. Tuohy[8] passed a 15-G urethral catheter 4 to 5 cm into the subarachnoid space, and he also designed the Tuohy point needle, which carries his name, to facilitate directional control of the spinal catheter.

Problems encountered with microcatheters for CSA centered around technical difficulties in passing a tiny catheter through a small needle.[62] Difficulty inserting the catheter, coiling of the catheter, catheter breakage, and failure to aspirate CSF were all problems encountered, particularly by people inexperienced in the technique. Instances of patchy anesthesia, probably owing to maldistribution of local anesthetic in the subarachnoid space, sometimes tempted anesthesiologists to inject large doses of local anesthetic in an attempt to overcome this problem.

Since 1991, at least 14 cases of cauda equina syndrome after CSA have been reported to the Food and Drug Administration.[63, 64] As a result of these cases, the Food and Drug Administration and the Canadian regulatory authorities withdrew microcatheters from the North American markets. As of this writing, microcatheters are still available in Germany. Research attempting to explain the mechanism of presumed local anesthetic neurotoxicity has suggested that injection of local anesthetic through an intrathecal catheter can lead to pooling of local anesthetic near the roots of the cauda equina, particularly if the catheter is directed sacrally and dextrose-containing solutions are injected.[65] This situation is worse with a single-hole catheter than a multiorifice catheter.[66] Further research in animal models has demonstrated the neurotoxic potential of 5% hyperbaric lidocaine.[67]

After a conference on CSA sponsored by the American Society of Regional Anesthesia,[68] the following guidelines concerning clinical use of CSA were suggested:

1. Examine the lower extremity sensory, motor, and reflex functions before the anesthetic is begun to identify and document preexisting neurologic deficits.

2. Attempt to advance the catheter cephalad when using a Tuohy needle, and do not advance the catheter more than 2 to 3 cm beyond the needle tip.

3. Do not introduce the catheter if severe or persistent paresthesia, involuntary motor activity, or excessive bleeding occurs during needle placement.

4. Limit the initial and subsequent dose and concentration to those that would be used for a single injection. Plain 2% lidocaine may be a better choice than hyperbaric 5% lidocaine, because neurotoxicity has been associated with the latter.

5. Develop criteria for reinjection, e.g., return of motor function or regression of sensory block.

6. Assess initial extent of anesthesia carefully. If inadequate spread occurs, this may be an indication of sacral pooling. It may be best to abandon the technique if this occurs.

7. Use optimal patient position for catheter removal to avoid possible breakage of the catheter.

8. It is inadvisable to use CSA in a patient with already established general, epidural, or spinal anesthesia, because catheter-related paresthesia cannot be assessed.

In addition to this consensus statement, some participants at the conference suggested using only multiport catheters for CSA for better mixing of local anesthetic solutions with CSF.

Combined Spinal and Epidural Anesthesia

Interest has been increasing on both sides of the Atlantic in combining the fast onset of action of intrathecal injection with the flexibility of continuous epidural anesthesia.[69] This technique has been termed "combined spinal-epidural anesthesia" and has been advocated for cesarean section,[70] labor analgesia,[71] and outpatient orthopedic surgery.[72] The technique usually involves placing a 17-G, 3- or 3.5-in Tuohy needle into the epidural space by using a loss of resistance technique, advancing a long (4 11/16 in) 27-G spinal needle by using the Tuohy needle as a guide to the intrathecal space. Then a local anesthetic (for surgery) or 10 μg sufentanil (for labor analgesia) is injected intrathecally, followed by removal of the spinal needle and insertion of an epidural catheter. When used to provide labor analgesia, this technique is claimed to provide fast onset of excellent analgesia lasting about 80 minutes, while allowing the patients to ambulate, at least until epidural local anesthetics are required. In ambulatory patients, knee arthroscopic surgery has been performed by using a small dose (40 mg) of lidocaine given intrathecally and top-up doses of epidural lidocaine only if necessary to extend duration of anesthesia. Compared with results in patients receiving epidural anesthesia with lidocaine, incidence of hypotension was lower and time to ambulation and recovery much shorter.

This appears to be a promising technique for certain indications. In the United States, several manufacturers (e.g., Becton Dickinson and NeuroDelivery) are marketing combination sets of epidural and spinal needles. In Germany, another manufacturer (B. Braun) has marketed a Tuohy needle with a guide for the spinal needle. One problem noted to date is that when a 3.5-in Tuohy needle is used, the spinal needle will sometimes "tent" the dura, particularly when a Whitacre needle is used, making dural puncture difficult. This is less often a problem when a 3-in Tuohy epidural needle is used, because the distance that the spinal needle extends past the tip of the Tuohy needle is increased. Alternatively, a Quincke spinal can be used, which will cut the dural fibers, making dural puncture easier (Kopacz D, Urmey W: Personal communications). When 27-G spinal needles are used, the incidence of PDPH is similar with cutting and pencil-point needles (less than 2%). Once these minor technical problems are worked out, this is likely to become a

popular technique in ambulatory surgery as well as obstetric units.

Intraoperative and Postoperative Management of Spinal Anesthesia

An important issue in the management of spinal (or epidural) anesthesia is to make sure that there is adequate anesthesia before the start of the operation and that a drug with adequate duration of action is chosen (unless one has chosen a continuous catheter technique). One should have objective evidence of an adequate block (i.e., onset of motor block and anesthesia at the operative site) within 5 min of spinal injection. If this is not the case, the block must be repeated or another anesthetic technique instituted. It is not fair to the patient or to your surgical colleagues and will certainly not enhance your reputation as a clinician if this point is not adhered to rigidly.

The next most important issues, once anesthesia is present, are airway maintenance and cardiovascular stability. The cephalad level of analgesia should be monitored with a safety pin for 15 to 20 min after the initial block (Fig. 19–22). If the cephalad level rises above the C-7 dermatome (middle of the hand), one must assume that a total spinal block (unusually high cephalad spread of intrathecal local anesthetic) may occur. One must be prepared to manage the airway (usually this means to intubate the trachea) and give vasopressors to support blood pressure and heart rate.

Assuming that no unusually high spread of anesthesia occurs, one must still be vigilant for sudden bradycardia or hypotension or both. Carpenter and colleagues[57] have shown that there is a greater risk of hypotension and bradycardia when the level of analgesia is higher than T-5. Additional risk factors for bradycardia identified by Carpenter et al are preexisting sinus bradycardia, β-blocker therapy, and American Society of Anesthesiologists physical status 3. This side effect may be responsible for some of the cases of unexpected cardiac arrest reported by Caplan et al[73] in the American Society of Anesthesiologists Closed Claims Study, rather than oversedation as originally suggested by the authors. If bradycardia occurs, it must be rapidly treated. This can be done with atropine given intravenously. However, the author prefers epinephrine, particularly in the situation of bradycardia with a cephalad level of analgesia above the T-5 dermatome, because cardiac accelerator fibers may be impaired. Epinephrine can be given as bolus injections of 10 μg or, better, as an infusion of 1 to 4 μg/min. A solution of 4 μg/mL can be made up easily by injecting 1 mg epinephrine into 250 mL 0.9% NaCl. An infusion (via an infusion pump) of 15 mL/h is equivalent to 1 μg/min. Hypotension unrelated to bradycardia can be treated by intravenous 5-mg bolus injections of ephedrine. An intravenous infusion of ephedrine (50 mg in 250 mL 0.9% NaCl) can also be started at 15 to 45 mL/h if repeated intravenous boluses are necessary. If one expects hypotension because of a high block or if it is unexpectedly

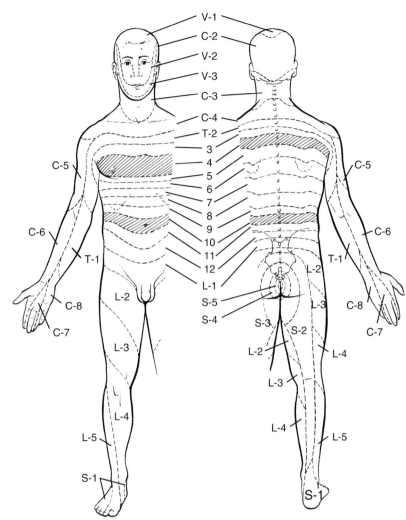

Figure 19–22 Dermatome chart. When testing the upper limit of block on the chest, note that the T-2 dermatome borders on the C-4 dermatome. Dermatomes C-5 through T-1 (brachial plexus) are in the arm.

encountered, insertion of an arterial catheter may ease patient management.

Padding and Sedation

If the patient is comfortable on the operating table, less sedation will be required. The author begins by padding the patient's shoulders, head, and arms well with several pillows. If the patient will be in the lateral decubitus position (e.g., for total hip arthroplasty), the author uses an axillary roll to take some pressure off the shoulder, in addition to pillows under the arms, shoulder, and head. After attaching an oxygen cannula, preferably one capable of attachment to a CO_2 waveform monitor, the author gives a small dose of midazolam intravenously (1 to 4 mg, depending on age and general physical status of the patient). If more sedation is necessary, the author prefers to use an intravenous infusion of propofol. Titrating to clinical effect, the author commonly uses 25 to 75 μg/kg body weight per min to produce a state of light sedation, with acceptable oxygen saturation (by pulse oximetry).

Airway Considerations

If the patient requires deep sedation, bordering on general anesthesia, one must be vigilant about the airway. This can be done by insertion of a nasopharyngeal airway or by an oral tracheal tube for a combined general-regional anesthetic technique. This is particularly useful for procedures that last more than 2 to 3 h.

An exciting development in the United Kingdom has the potential to revolutionize regional anesthesia. The laryngeal mask airway, developed by Dr. Archie Brain, is ideal for combined general-regional anesthesia. The laryngeal mask airway is currently used for approximately 50% of all anesthetics in the United Kingdom.[74] Because the laryngeal mask airway can be tolerated at relatively light planes of anesthesia, it can allow the patient to spontaneously breathe nitrous oxide and oxygen with a low concentration of a volatile anesthetic or an intravenous infusion of propofol. The airway is then much easier to maintain in a heavily sedated patient than with a nasopharyngeal airway or with a face mask. Additionally, capnography with the laryngeal mask airway gives a more reliable indication of the end-tidal CO_2 than when either a nasal cannula or a face mask is used. Because of these advantages, the laryngeal mask airway is useful for patients undergoing longer procedures or for those in a lateral decubitus position, in which airway management of the heavily sedated patient is problematic. For patients unwilling to be awake for their operation, yet otherwise good candidates for regional anesthesia, the laryngeal mask airway will make a significant difference once North American anesthesiologists become familiar with its use.

Postoperative Management

Once the operation is completed and the patient is transported to the recovery room, the patient is monitored until recovery from the effect of sedatives and the motor block is beginning to resolve. Once the motor block starts to regress, in the experience of the author, the hemodynamic effects of spinal and epidural anesthesia also dissipate. However, one must be sure that blood lost has been adequately replaced with crystalloid or colloid. This point is important particularly with patients after total knee arthroplasty. Because a tourniquet is inflated for most of if not the entire surgical procedure, there is little blood loss in the operating theater. In the recovery room, a patient can lose more than 500 mL of blood in the first hours after operation (double this volume if a bilateral procedure is performed). To make the situation worse, because some surgeons wrap the knee in a plaster cast, and some do not insert a drain, this blood loss may not be obvious to the recovery room personnel. In the face of a persistent high spinal or epidural block, this is a recipe for hypotension and bradycardia. The author therefore suggests checking the drains, dressings, and urinary output as well as vital signs before dismissing the patient to the wards.

If the sensory and motor blocks are prolonged more than the usual time for the local anesthetic used, the patient must be closely observed. If an epidural hematoma occurs, this needs to be quickly diagnosed (by magnetic resonance imaging or computed tomographic scan) and evacuated within 6 h to give the patient a reasonable chance of full neurologic recovery. Therefore, if the patient is at risk for this complication (receiving anticoagulants or has inadequate platelet function), orders should be written to follow the neurologic status of the patient and to contact the physician if recovery is unusually delayed.

Once the motor and sensory blocks have fully dissipated and once the patient's surgical condition permits, the patient should be allowed to ambulate, with assistance the first time. There is no evidence that keeping a patient supine prevents development of a PDPH.

Epidural Anesthesia

Identification of the Epidural Space

Over the years, there have been quite a number of techniques used to identify needle entry into the epidural space.[75] For the purposes of this chapter, the discussion is of the two simplest and most widely used techniques: loss of resistance and hanging drop. The hanging drop of Gutiérrez technique[76] relies on the presence of apparent negative pressure in the epidural space.[77] A drop of saline or local anesthetic solution is placed in the hub of the epidural needle, once the tip of the needle is located in the interspinous ligament (Fig. 19–23). The needle is then carefully advanced through the ligamentum flavum until the drop of fluid is drawn into the needle by the negative pressure in the epidural space. The negative pressure in the thoracic epidural space is thought to be related to transmitted negative pleural pressure.[77] Optimal conditions for the hanging drop test are found in the thoracic region, with the patient sitting. Most investigators attribute the existence of negative pressure in the lumbar epidural space to tenting of the dura by the epidural needle.[75] In the lumbar epidural space, pressure is not reliably below atmospheric pressure, particularly if the patient is sitting, if intra-abdominal pressure is increased, or if uterine contractions are in progress. Bromage[75] recommended this test not be used in the lumbar region. One must be careful deciding when to use this technique, particularly when the technique is performed at a level where spinal cord is underlying the dura.

The loss of resistance technique is commonly used with either saline or air. The syringe used for the loss of resistance test can be either glass or plastic. Glass syringes should be lubricated with saline or local anesthetic solution to prevent a sticky plunger and unintentional dural puncture. The author prefers to use a 20-mL plastic syringe and loss of resistance to air; he has used these for more than 2000 cases of epidural anesthesia during the past 4 years, with a dural puncture rate of less than 1 in 300. Loss of resistance to air is simple, does not introduce fluid into the epidural space (which can be confused with CSF), and has been used for many years with relatively few problems. Because air is compressible, intermittent pressure of the plunger of the syringe (versus constant pressure when a saline-filled syringe is used) is used to detect a loss of resistance to injection, once the needle has passed through the ligamentum flavum. Problems with the loss of resistance to air technique include possible subarachnoid or subdural injection of air resulting in headache,[78] venous air embolism,[79] and introduction of air bubbles into the epidural space. These air bubbles have been shown to persist for more than 24 h[80] and to expand when nitrous oxide is inhaled.[81] Large epidural air bubbles have been implicated in inadequate analgesia under certain conditions.[82] Because of these potential problems, the author recommends limiting injection of air to 3 mL or less and avoiding air injection altogether (in favor of saline) if nitrous oxide will be used as part of the anesthetic.

Loss of resistance to saline is another commonly used technique. This technique introduces a fluid into the epidural space, which can be confused with CSF and can dilute local anesthetics. However, it has not been associated with any of the above-mentioned complica-

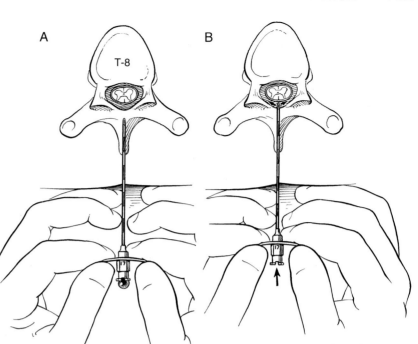

Figure 19–23 *A* and *B,* The hanging drop of Gutiérrez technique for identifying needle entry into epidural space. Presence of negative pressure is reliable only in the thoracic epidural space.

tions of epidural air injection and is the preferred technique of the editor.

A false loss of resistance to either air or saline can occur, leading to failure of epidural anesthesia. This is usually due to deviation of the needle from midline. A loss of resistance can be found with the needle tip lateral to the midline in the paravertebral[83] or prevertebral space. Injection of local anesthetic in either of these spaces results in an inadequate anesthesia for operation. In older patients, degeneration of the interspinous ligaments can result in ligamentous cysts, which can result in a loss of resistance more superficial than expected.[84] These cysts are quite common (85% incidence) in patients older than age 60 years and usually have no associated radiographic findings, so they cannot be anticipated.[85] They can be capacious enough to accept several milliliters of local anesthetic and to allow easy passage of the epidural catheter. For these reasons, some experienced practitioners of regional anesthesia prefer to use the paramedian approach routinely in older patients.

Suggestions for avoiding common pitfalls in identifying the epidural space are (1) make sure the needle tip is in the midline when it enters the epidural space, (2) become familiar with the expected depth of entrance into the epidural space for a given-size patient, and (3) feel for entrance of the needle into the ligamentum flavum. If there is an abnormal loss of resistance or if the ligamentum flavum is not felt before a loss of resistance, the needle should be withdrawn, the landmarks rechecked, and the needle reinserted. In adults, the distance from epidural space to skin is usually 4 to 6 cm[75] (Fig. 19–24). Obesity increases this distance, up to 9 cm in a morbidly obese patient. Distances greater than this are rare. In a thin patient (and in children), distances less than 4 cm can be encountered. Once one has become comfortable in pre-

dicting the distance from skin to epidural space, one will easily recognize a false loss of resistance if it occurs much more superficial or much deeper than is reasonable for a particular patient. In addition to recognizing these pitfalls of the loss of resistance technique, practice is important to develop the feel of the ligaments. This can come only with the experience of several hundred epidural anesthetic procedures.

Choice of Needles and Catheters

Epidural anesthesia is usually performed as a continuous catheter technique. For this reason, thin-walled needles (17 to 20 G) are favored. The incidence of PDPH in young patients after unintentional dural puncture with a needle of this size is quite high (70%

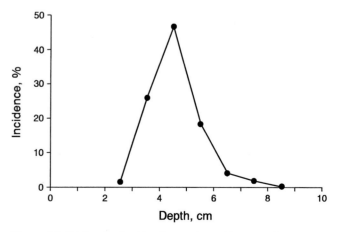

Figure 19–24 Depth of epidural space from skin. (Data from Gutiérrez A: Anestesia Extradural. Rev Cir Buenos Aires 1939; 18: 349; 409.)

to 80%).[86] To decrease the incidence of PDPH if the dura is punctured, some practitioners of epidural anesthesia advocate use of a 22-G spinal needle for single-shot epidural injection, i.e., epidural steroid injections. For continuous epidural anesthesia, the smallest needle and catheter set available in the United States is a 20-G needle and a 24-G catheter. The most common Tuohy needle sizes available are 18 G (20-G catheter) and 17 G (18-G catheter). The 18-G catheter is a bit easier to insert than the 20 G because it is stiffer.

Although many epidural needle designs are available, the two most widely used are the Tuohy, which has a directional tip, and the Crawford needle, which has a 45° bevel. The Weiss needle adds wings to the Tuohy needle, to assist in needle insertion. This is particularly helpful for cervical epidural puncture or any time the hanging drop test is used. Some clinicians believe the Tuohy needle, because of its directional tip, is less likely to accidentally puncture the dura than is a Crawford needle. However, data to support this assertion are lacking. It should also be mentioned that the design of the Tuohy needle does not guarantee the direction a catheter will take in the epidural space. Indeed, an epidural catheter can be deflected by nerve roots or other structures, change directions, or coil independently of the type and direction of needle used for insertion.

Epidural catheters come in two basic designs: open tip, single orifice; and bullet tip, multiorifice catheters. Catheters marketed in the United States range in size from 18 to 24 G. The multiorifice (usually three orifices) catheter was designed to provide a more even distribution of epidural local anesthetic in case of blockage or obstruction of one of the orifices. Some detractors of this type of catheter point out that different orifices may be in different anatomic spaces at the same time. For example, a subdural or subarachnoid catheterization may have occurred, leaving the distal orifice in the subarachnoid or subdural space and the two proximal orifices in the epidural space. Similarly, the distal orifice may be in an epidural vein and the proximal two orifices in the epidural space. To the author's knowledge, there are no good studies comparing the efficacy or complication rates of these two catheter types.

In addition to differences in orifices, catheters may have a stylet, have no stylet, or be constructed around a coil of wire (Racz Catheter, Arrow International, Inc) similar to an armored tracheal tube. Catheters constructed from polyamide (Burron Medical, Inc) are fairly stiff, making insertion without a stylet easier. More pliable material used for construction of catheters requires use of a stylet (e.g., some catheters manufactured by Abbott, Inc). Stiffer catheters theoretically would be more likely to puncture a blood vessel or the dura. One manufacturer (Arrow) has marketed a catheter with a flexible tip to minimize these complications. Catheters that are pliable enough to require a stylet for insertion may be more prone to kinking or obstruction or more difficult to insert than a stiffer catheter. No data comparing the efficacy of various catheter designs are available at present.

Administering the Anesthetic

The principles of intravenous sedation and patient positioning are the same as for spinal anesthesia. Generally, the patient is placed in the lateral decubitus position for the block, unless it is necessary for the patient to sit so that the anesthesiologist can identify midline in a morbidly obese or scoliotic patient. The patient is placed with the operative side down. Although studies of position have not shown a clinically significant effect of position on spread of epidural anesthesia, the dependent side usually becomes anesthetized a few minutes earlier and the block can be one to two dermatomes higher on the dependent side. This may be useful when trying to increase operating room efficiency. An intravenous catheter is started, and monitors are placed consisting of, at the minimum, a blood pressure cuff, an electrocardiograph, or a pulse oximeter, and, if indicated for surgery, an arterial catheter. Intravenous sedation is usually achieved by injecting 1 to 4 mg of midazolam, as appropriate to the patient's age and physical condition. More can be given if necessary.

If the anesthesiologist is well trained in thoracic and cervical epidural anesthesia, puncture at any level of the vertebral column is reasonable. However, less experienced residents and occasional epidural anesthetists should be restricted to puncture below the termination of the spinal cord. In the former case, the puncture site is chosen by finding the dermatome in the center of the intended surgical incision. A midline or paramedian approach is chosen on the basis of the location of epidural puncture, the age, and the degree of expected arthritic changes of the spine. Antiseptic preparation, sterile draping, and local anesthetic infiltration are performed, as for spinal anesthesia. Specifically, a spinous process is identified with the index and middle fingers of the nondominant hand and straddled by these two fingers to identify the interspace. A skin wheal is raised in the middle of the interspace (for the midline approach) or 1 cm lateral and slightly caudad to the middle of the interspace (for the paramedian approach) with a 27-G, 3-cm needle to infiltrate local anesthetic into the interspinous ligament. The epidural needle is grasped in the dominant hand and inserted about 3 to 4 cm (adult patient) into the interspinous ligament, depending on expected distance from skin to epidural space. Then the stylet is removed, and a syringe containing either air or saline is attached. The needle is grasped between the bent fingers and thumb of the nondominant hand. Forward motion of the needle is controlled by extending the wrist (Fig. 19–25). As the needle is advanced, the thumb of the dominant hand exerts intermittent pressure on the plunger of the syringe (using air) or constant pressure (using saline).

It is important that the needle penetrate the ligamentum flavum near the midline to avoid misidentification of the epidural space. Needle entry into the ligamentum flavum is characterized by a gritty feeling, because this ligament is denser than the interspinous ligament. Within 3 to 5 mm after entry of the needle tip into the ligamentum flavum, a loss of resistance

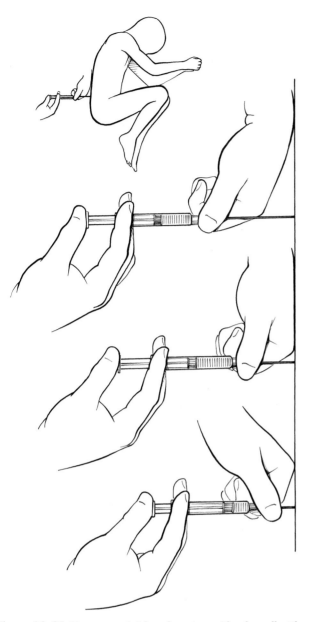

Figure 19–25 "Bromage grip" for advancing epidural needle. The needle is firmly gripped between the thumb and index finger of the nondominant hand. The dorsum of the wrist is placed against the patient's back, and the needle is advanced by extension of the wrist. The dominant hand provides intermittent (for loss of resistance to air) or constant (for loss of resistance to saline) pressure on the plunger of the syringe.

has occurred with a 17-G Tuohy needle, it will be evident, except in the rarest circumstances.

After 60 s, if there has been no change in heart rate and no CSF observed, several approaches to delivering the therapeutic dose of local anesthetic are available. Some inject the entire epidural dose incrementally, 5 mL at a time, via the needle and then thread the epidural catheter for subsequent injections. Others inject one half of the intended local anesthetic dose (containing epinephrine) via the needle, again incrementally, with no more than 5 mL at a time, and then thread the catheter into the epidural space. At this point, an additional 3-mL test dose of local anesthetic containing epinephrine is given, and if the reaction to this test dose is negative, the remainder of the therapeutic dose of local anesthetic is injected. Still others insert the epidural catheter after the initial 3-mL test dose and deliver the therapeutic dose via the epidural catheter incrementally, in 5-mL aliquots.

By limiting the local anesthetic injection via the needle or catheter to incremental aliquots, usually an intravascular injection can be detected before sufficient drug has been injected to cause a seizure.

If clear liquid is aspirated, one must determine if this is local anesthetic or CSF. This can easily be determined by one of three tests. (1) A drop or two of the fluid can be dropped on to the forearm. If it is cold (room temperature), the fluid is likely local anesthetic. If it is warm, it is likely CSF. (2) Mix a drop or two of the fluid with an equal volume of thiopental. If there is an immediate precipitate, the fluid is local anesthetic. (3) Place a drop of the aspirated fluid on a glucose test paper. If the test paper is positive for glucose, the fluid is CSF. If the catheter is intrathecal, the catheter can still be used, provided doses are adjusted accordingly and guidelines for continuous spinal anesthesia are followed. Be sure to label this catheter as intrathecal so that it is not mistaken for an epidural catheter.

As with spinal anesthesia, close attention to the airway, oxygenation, heart rate, and blood pressure is crucial. If a total spinal block occurs, because of injection of an epidural dose into the intrathecal space, it will occur within 15 min of local anesthetic injection. A subdural block will make its appearance within 30 min and may be detected when the block is much more extensive than expected or markedly asymmetric.

Technical Problems With Needle and Catheter Insertion

Problems with needle insertion in general relate to inability to find the midline, owing to obesity, or inability to enter the interspace as a result of significant calcification of ligaments or intervertebral space. These problems are addressed above in the section on spinal anesthesia. In the case of suspected or proved abnormal calcification (elderly patients, osteoarthritis, rheumatoid arthritis), it is usually easier to walk the needle off bone into the interspace when using a 17- or 18-G epidural needle versus a 22-G spinal needle, because the large-gauge needle will bend less and provide a

will be felt. A tight grip on the needle is important to control the forward motion of the needle as it pierces the ligamentum flavum and to avoid dural puncture. It is important at this juncture to avoid injecting more air or saline into the epidural space than is necessary to detect a loss of resistance.

Once loss of resistance has been detected, the syringe is used to aspirate for blood or CSF. If neither is obtained, a test dose of 3 mL of local anesthetic containing epinephrine 1:200,000 is injected while monitoring the heart rate. The syringe is disconnected from the needle to look for egress of CSF. If a dural puncture better feel. Additionally, when calcification has narrowed the interspace, a paramedian approach from the outset would be recommended because of the larger target provided.

Other technical problems include dural puncture with the needle, aspiration of blood or CSF via the catheter, shearing of the catheter, and accidental subdural catheterization. If dural puncture with the needle occurs during placement of an epidural agent for labor analgesia, the author's approach is to replace the needle (and catheter) at another interspace. After delivery of the infant, the catheter can be used to give a prophylactic epidural autologous blood patch, because the incidence of PDPH in this situation is 70% to 80% (see discussion of complications). If accidental dural puncture occurs during the placement of a lumbar epidural needle for surgical anesthesia, it is the author's usual practice to pass the epidural catheter 3 cm into the intrathecal space and to inject 2 to 3 mL of the intended epidural local anesthetic. This gives adequate, reliable anesthesia for surgery on the lumbar and sacral dermatomes. Anesthesia of lower thoracic dermatomes by using plain local anesthetic solutions (slightly hypobaric) is not reliable. A hyperbaric local anesthetic solution would have to be used to reliably obtain anesthesia of thoracic dermatomes. At any rate, conversion of an intended epidural to continuous spinal anesthesia will not make the risk of PDPH worse. However, the guidelines for CSA should be followed.

If CSF is aspirated via the epidural catheter, the technique is converted to a CSA technique, unless there is some compelling reason not to do so, such as necessity for continuous postoperative epidural analgesia and unfamiliarity of postoperative nurses with intrathecal catheters. A single dose of intrathecal morphine before removing the intrathecal catheter may be the ideal way to solve this problem. However, if an intrathecal catheter is left in place, it must be clearly labeled as such and all personnel informed, to prevent accidental intrathecal injection of an epidural dose of drug. If for some reason it is decided that an epidural catheter is indicated, the intrathecal catheter should be removed, together with the needle (if it is still in place) to avoid shearing of the catheter. The needle and catheter should be reinserted at another interspace.

Aspiration of frank blood via the epidural catheter means the catheter has entered an epidural vein. However, aspiration of slightly blood-tinged local anesthetic does not necessarily mean venous cannulation. Because most of the epidural veins are located in the anterior epidural space, it may be possible to reinsert the needle at the same interspace, at a slightly different angle. The next catheter insertion would then be at a different location in the epidural space. If this again leads to aspiration of blood, a new interspace should be chosen.

Occasionally, despite a normal loss of resistance to injection, a catheter cannot be advanced into the epidural space. This is probably due to impingement of the catheter on some portion of the high arched ligamentum flavum. This problem calls for the catheter and needle to be withdrawn together and the needle

reinserted at the same interspace, with a slightly different angle. If the patient complains of a sudden, severe paresthesia (a radiating electrical or a burning sensation), one must assume the epidural catheter is abutting a nerve root. Because of the unpleasantness of this sensation and the potential danger of damaging the radicular artery, the epidural needle and catheter should be removed and replaced at the same interspace, again with a slightly different angle of approach. If the same problem results, another interspace is chosen.

If an epidural catheter has been inserted, it should be tested immediately by injection of a 3-mL test dose of an epinephrine-containing (15 µg) local anesthetic solution after a negative aspiration test to minimize the possibility of intravascular position of the catheter. However, it should be recognized that a negative test result gives no information as to where the catheter tip is located; it merely tells you where the catheter tip is not. Some suggest that the 3-mL test dose of local anesthetic and epinephrine will eliminate subarachnoid position of the catheter; however, often sufficient time is not allowed to pass after the test dose injection to reliably confirm whether a subarachnoid block is or is not developing.

There are only two ways to ensure a catheter is located in the epidural space: injection of a radiopaque dye and radiography (epidurogram) or injection of sufficient mass of a local anesthetic to produce a bilateral motor and sensory block. Although the former technique is usually performed after placement of permanent epidural catheters for cancer pain therapy, it is not practical for the usual operating room anesthetic. The anesthesiologist should inject 10 to 15 mL of 2% lidocaine or 0.5% to 0.75% bupivacaine after the possibility of intravascular placement of the catheter is eliminated. If a bilateral sensory and motor block is not apparent within 10 to 15 min, the catheter tip is not in the epidural space. The catheter should be removed and either replaced or an alternative anesthetic technique should be instituted.

Occasionally, a catheter will become kinked during insertion. It will be impossible to inject solution through the catheter. In this situation, the only recourse is to remove the catheter and to start again. If this situation is recognized immediately after catheter insertion, it should be no problem to rectify. However, if it occurs after the patient has been positioned and prepared for surgery, the only alternative may be to induce general anesthesia. It is to avoid this scenario that some anesthesiologists prefer to inject the therapeutic dose of local anesthetic via the Tuohy needle before catheter insertion. In this way, even if the catheter were to become kinked or dislodged, adequate anesthesia for the operation would be ensured if a local anesthetic of adequate duration was chosen.

Subdural catheterization is a clinically rare problem, which is detected only because of the unusual nature of the block that develops after local anesthetic injection.[87, 88] Typically, a subdural block is much more extensive than expected, with analgesia sometimes reaching cervical dermatomes after injection of 6 to 8 mL of local anesthetic. Analgesia may be markedly asymmetric. Onset of block is more like an epidural than a spinal block. Usually, blood pressure and heart rate are well maintained without pharmacologic intervention, in contrast to total spinal anesthesia. The diagnosis of subdural catheterization is usually only presumptive, but it can be confirmed by the injection of a small volume (3-5 mL) of a water-soluble, nonionic contrast material and a computed tomographic scan. Plain radiographs may not be sufficient to definitely state whether the contrast material is intrathecal or subdural. Management of this problem is to remove the catheter. If an epidural catheter is necessary for the patient, reinsertion should be performed at another interspace, because the dura has been punctured at this level.

If one shears a catheter tip in the epidural space, it should be left in place.[89] Catheter tips in the epidural space are eventually walled off by fibrosis and do not pose a problem of further migration. The risks of surgical exploration are likely higher than the risks of leaving a small piece of plastic in the epidural space. In the intrathecal space, in contrast, fibrosis of catheters does not occur, leaving migration of a sheared-off catheter tip a possibility. Surgical exploration should be discussed with a neurosurgeon in the event of intrathecal shearing.

Pharmacology

The pharmacology of local anesthetics is extensively covered in Chapters 8 and 12. This section deals only with issues specific to the use of these local anesthetics for epidural anesthesia. In the United States, the following local anesthetics are available: 2% and 3% 2-chloroprocaine HCl; 1.5% and 2.0% lidocaine HCl; 1.5% and 2% mepivacaine HCl; 0.25%, 0.5%, and 0.75% bupivacaine HCl; and 1.0% and 1.5% etidocaine HCl. In Canada 1.75% lidocaine HCO_2 and in Germany 0.5% bupivacaine HCO_2 also are available. Generally, the more concentrated solutions are better

for surgical indications, particularly for the initial dose, because the resultant anesthesia has shorter latency, is more profound, and has longer duration than equal volumes of more dilute solutions. Once the block has developed, a lower concentration of local anesthetic can be used to maintain anesthesia. The less concentrated solutions are also useful for lithotripsy and labor analgesia, when a profound motor and sensory block is neither necessary nor desired. The local anesthetics with longest duration of action—bupivacaine, etidocaine, and perhaps mepivacaine with epinephrine—are not recommended for outpatient epidural anesthesia because 6 to 12 h are required for the patients to be ambulatory after local anesthetic injection.

Duration of Anesthesia

Because epidural anesthesia has its initial action at the intradural spinal roots, its onset and offset of action follow a dermatomal pattern.[90] When comparing local anesthetics used in the epidural space, it is useful to understand four variables (Fig. 19–26). The first is latency to initial onset. This is the time from injection of the drug until there is a demonstrable clinical effect. The second is time to maximum spread of anesthesia. The third is time to two-segment regression of analgesia. The final variable is time to complete resolution of the block. The first two variables are measures of how fast one can expect to detect a block. The second two are measures of duration of action. Duration of action at a particular surgical site depends not only on which local anesthetic is used but also on how extensive the initial block is and where the surgical site is located.

For example, a patient is undergoing inguinal herniorrhaphy under lumbar epidural anesthesia (injected at L3-4). After a single injection of 25 mL 2% lidocaine (with epinephrine), a maximum spread to the T-2 dermatome is obtained. The mean time to two-segment regression will be approximately 97 min. However, duration of action at the surgical site (T-12 dermatome) will be longer than this. Anesthesia will persist longer

Figure 19–26 Analgesia-time plot of epidural analgesia. Note time to initial onset (latency), time to maximum spread, time to two-segment regression, and time to complete resolution of analgesia. For an unconscious patient, the optimum time to reinjection to avoid regression of anesthesia is calculated as mean time to two-segment regression minus 1.5 times the standard deviation. (Data from Bromage PR: Epidural Analgesia, p 239. Philadelphia, WB Saunders Co, 1978.)

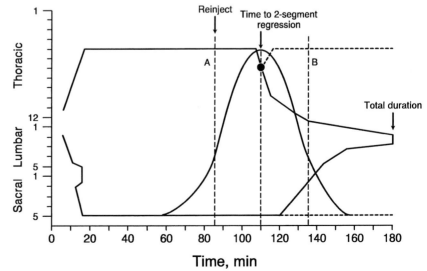

still at the L-3 dermatome, where the initial injection was made. Thus, this patient will not be able to ambulate (nor be ready for dismissal) until perhaps 3 to 4 h have passed after the initial injection.[91] If instead of lidocaine, 25 mL of 0.75% bupivacaine had been given, the patient would have been ambulatory in 8 to 12 h. Planning just the right dose of the right local anesthetic for the right patient for the right operation requires considering many factors in addition to the time to two-segment regression. Unfortunately, it is not possible to look up all these variables, although time to two-segment regression is well documented for most local anesthetics. Latency and time to two-segment regression of several epidural local anesthetics are given in Table 19–3.

Addition of Epinephrine

Addition of a vasoconstrictor, usually epinephrine 5 μg/mL, significantly increases the duration of action, as measured by time to two-segment regression, only for 2-chloroprocaine and lidocaine. However, even with bupivacaine and etidocaine, there are other reasons for adding epinephrine. First, because relatively large volumes of local anesthetic are injected, an accidental intravenous injection can be fatal. It is useful not only to give a test dose of 3 mL of local anesthetic (with epinephrine 1:200,000, containing 15 μg of epinephrine) but also to use every dose as a test dose. If a sudden tachycardia occurs after local anesthetic injection, an intravascular catheter must be suspected. Second, epinephrine decreases peak plasma local anesthetic concentrations by 20% to 50%.[92, 93] Third, epinephrine increases the quality of motor block.[94] Therefore, the author adds epinephrine to all local anesthetics unless there is a good reason not to do so.

Relative contraindications to use of epinephrine, in the view of the author, are (1) uncontrolled hypertension, (2) known cerebrovascular aneurysm, (3) severe preeclampsia, (4) untreated thyrotoxicosis, (5) monoamine oxidase inhibitor therapy, and (6) history of malignant hyperthermia. However, even in these cases, the author would use a 3-mL test dose containing epinephrine, as recommended by Moore and Batra.[95] Some authors consider all intrauterine pregnancies to be contraindications for use of epinephrine, because of transient decreased placental blood flow observed in sheep receiving an intravascular epinephrine bolus.[96] However, in the last study, uterine blood flow returned to normal after 3 min, and there were no changes in fetal blood gases. To date, there have been no reports of adverse fetal outcomes after intravenous bolus injection of 15 μg epinephrine. In the view of the author, the risk of an accidental intravascular bolus of local anesthetic outweighs the risk of a transient decrease in placental flow. If the mother were to have a seizure or to experience cardiac arrest, placental flow might even be more compromised.

Choice of Local Anesthetics

Chloroprocaine is an aminoester local anesthetic with a plasma half-life of approximately 22 s. This property reportedly makes this drug the least toxic local anesthetic available, from the point of view of accidental intravascular injection. Because of its short latency and short duration, it seems to be the perfect local anesthetic for outpatient surgical treatment. However, accidental intrathecal injection of large doses of chloroprocaine has caused neurotoxicity.[97–99] Subsequent laboratory investigations linked neurotoxicity to low pH and high concentrations of sodium bisulfite used as a preservative in a commercial preparation of chloroprocaine.[100, 101] Since reformulation and replacement of sodium bisulfite with disodium ethylenediaminetetraacetic acid (EDTA) in 1987, there have been several reports of post–epidural anesthesia back pain. The author's research group has shown that use of doses of this formulation greater than 25 mL can produce an unacceptably high incidence of post–epidural anesthesia back pain.[102] A mechanism has not yet been established for this back pain, but evidence to date suggests that it is related to the disodium EDTA, with increasing dose of this drug resulting in both increased incidence and severity of back pain. The author and his colleagues recommend that if a 2-chloroprocaine solution containing EDTA is used, the total dose be limited to 25 mL and the epidural catheter be left in place until after the anesthesia fully resolves. This way,

Table 19–3 Latency and Regression Times for Lumbar Epidural Anesthesia*

LOCAL ANESTHETIC	INITIAL LATENCY	TIME TO MAXIMUM SPREAD	TIME TO TWO-SEGMENT REGRESSION (PLAIN)	TWO-SEGMENT REGRESSION WITH EPINEPHRINE (1:200,000)
3% 2-chloroprocaine	4.9	12.3	45	57 ± 7
2% lidocaine	5.0 ± 1.1	16.2 ± 2.6	46 ± 5	97.5 ± 19
2% mepivacaine	6.2	17.5	—	117
0.5% bupivacaine	5.8	18.2	165	196 ± 31
0.75% bupivacaine	5.0	16.8	164 ± 46	201 ± 40
1% ropivacaine (plain)	6.0	24.5	177.5	—
1% etidocaine	3.6	10.9	128 ± 43	170 ± 57

*Time in min; means ± SD. All solutions with epinephrine 1:200,000, unless noted.
Data from Bromage PR: Epidural Analgesia. Philadelphia, WB Saunders Co, 1978.

epidural fentanyl analgesia can be given if severe back pain occurs.

Etidocaine is a potent local anesthetic with a long duration of action but with a latency similar to that of lidocaine. Etidocaine never achieved wide popularity, probably because of its profound motor blocking properties, which occasionally outlast analgesia.[103, 104] It was associated with cardiac toxicity after accidental intravenous injection, as was bupivacaine.

In an attempt to decrease the latency of local anesthetic drugs, it was discovered that the bicarbonate salts of lidocaine and prilocaine have a much faster onset of action than their hydrochloride salts.[105, 106] This seemed to work well for lidocaine and prilocaine[105, 106] but less well for bupivacaine.[107] Unfortunately, none of these three compounds are likely to be marketed in the United States.

In the United States and Canada, the use of 0.75% bupivacaine for cesarean section anesthesia is not approved by federal regulatory agencies. The reason for this is several well-publicized cases of cardiac arrest after accidental intravascular injection of this local anesthetic.[108, 109] Rapid intravenous bolus doses of bupivacaine and etidocaine can lead to ventricular fibrillation, from which it is difficult to resuscitate laboratory animals.[110, 111] Because the risk of a cardiac arrhythmia after intravascular injection depends on dose and rapidity of intravascular injection, it is possible that 0.5% bupivacaine could also result in cardiac arrest if given accidentally into a vein.

In an attempt to decrease the cardiotoxicity of local anesthetics, a new agent, structurally related to mepivacaine and bupivacaine, has been developed. Ropivacaine is less cardiotoxic and arrhythmogenic than bupivacaine in dogs.[112] This is probably because ropivacaine is manufactured as the *S*-stereoisomer, which is much less arrhythmogenic than the *R*-stereoisomer. Bupivacaine and other local anesthetics as well are manufactured as racemic mixtures of *R*- and *S*-isomers. Clinical trials of ropivacaine for epidural anesthesia have shown this drug to be somewhat less potent than bupivacaine (1.0% ropivacaine is similar in potency to 0.75% bupivacaine) but similar in onset and duration of action.[113–115]

Factors Affecting Spread of Epidural Anesthesia

This discussion is limited to factors that have been shown to have a clinically significant effect: dose (volume × concentration), site of injection, and age.[116] Other factors, which probably have only minor and not clinically significant effects, are position of the patient[117, 118] and morbid obesity.[119] Epidural dose requirements are generally accepted to be lower in pregnant than in nonpregnant patients,[120, 121] although this has been disputed.[122] Factors that probably have no significant independent effects include height, weight, speed of injection, direction of needle, arteriosclerosis, and mode of injection (fractionated versus bolus injection).[116]

Dose is the most important factor.[123] The higher the volume of a given local anesthetic, the greater the spread. Mass of the drug appears to be more important than either concentration or volume: 20 mL 2% lidocaine (400 mg) would be expected to produce the same extent of block as 8 mL 5% lidocaine (400 mg). Bromage[123] calculated linear segmental dose requirements (mg/dermatome), which depend only on patient age and site of injection (thoracic, lumbar, caudal). However, other investigators have called this linearity into question.[124–126] For example, doubling the volume from 10 to 20 mL of either 0.75% bupivacaine or 1.5% lidocaine resulted in a spread of three to four more spinal segments, not twice as many, as would have been predicted if the dose-response relationship were perfectly linear. The probable explanation for this is that significant leakage of local anesthetics from the neural foramina limits the cephalad spread of block (a plateau effect), at least in young adults. The epidural space has been shown to behave as a Starling resistor during injection into the lumbar epidural space, as a constant pressure is maintained, despite increasing volume of injectant.[127] This suggests increasing leakage of fluid from the epidural space with increasing injected volume. It appears that the practical limit of spread of analgesia with lumbar epidural injection in young individuals, exclusive of intrathecal and subdural injections, is between the C-8 and C-6 dermatomes, even after injection of 60 mL of 3% 2-chloroprocaine.[128]

Although mass of drug injected is more important than volume or concentration, given equal mass of drug, injection of a larger volume may give a better block than a smaller volume of more concentrated solution. This may be because of better filling of the anterior and posterior epidural space with higher volumes.[19] Early practitioners of epidural anesthesia commonly used 60 to 100 mL of 1% to 1.5% procaine or 20 to 50 mL of more potent local anesthetics such as 0.15% to 0.2% tetracaine or dibucaine. These large volumes of dilute local anesthetic solutions would generally produce blocks extending approximately to the T-4 dermatome.[123]

Site of epidural injection is also important to the spread of block. The overall size of the segmental epidural space increases as one descends from the cervical to thoracic to lumbar epidural space, because of the volume taken up by the spinal cord. Not surprisingly, most investigators have found greater spread when anesthetic is injected into the epidural space above the termination of the spinal cord than below this level.[116, 117]

The closer to the site of operation that a local anesthetic is injected into the epidural space, the higher the local anesthetic concentration at the site of stimulation, the sooner the onset of block, and the greater the density of block.[129] A study[128] demonstrated the existence of a differential block during lumbar epidural anesthesia, similar to that seen with spinal anesthesia. Close to the injection site, there is a zone of intense anesthesia. As one moves cephalad up the trunk, the anesthesia becomes less intense until one encounters a zone of analgesia. Further cephalad, analgesia disappears. Because the site of injection is important to the extent of block, common practice is to choose for the site of epidural injection the spinal level of the dermatome in the middle of the proposed surgical incision. This provides the most intense anesthesia and motor block at the site of operation. Injection at or near the site of operation also allows one to use the lowest possible dose of local anesthetic.

Advancing age also increases the spread of epidural anesthesia. For some time, this relationship was assumed to be linear,[130] but more recent work has shown that this is not so.[125, 126] There are two possible anatomic reasons for increased spread with advancing age. The first is that with aging there is a decrease in the number of myelinated nerve fibers in the nerve roots as well as general deterioration in the mucopolysaccharides of the ground substance, allowing more local anesthetic penetration of nerve sheaths.[131] The second is that age and increasing calcification of neural foramina and density of areolar tissue surrounding the neural foramina decrease the egress of local anesthetic from the epidural space, increasing the longitudinal spread in the epidural space.[132] Park et al[125] showed the effect of age is probably not clinically significant until ages older than 40 years. Thereafter, an increase of two to three dermatomes was noted with injectant volumes of 10, 15, and 20 mL of 1.5% lidocaine. However, these are mean changes. Certainly, specific individuals may exhibit a much more dramatic effect of increased spread. For this reason, with patients older than age 70 years, the author recommends an initial dose (including test dose) of 15 mL or less, until the maximum spread of anesthesia is evident.

Testing of the Block

After injection of local anesthetic, the next step is to test for the appearance of an adequate block. Testing should start about 5 min after completion of local anesthetic injection. Patients are asked if their legs feel noticeably warmer. They are then asked to perform a straight leg raise to test for onset of a motor block. Testing for a level of cold sensation is performed with an alcohol wipe. The cold sensation on an unblocked dermatome (e.g., shoulder) is compared with a dermatome that you expect to be blocked (e.g., the knee). Once the block has set up, you will find that there are several zones of differential block. Close to the site of injection is the most intense zone of complete anesthesia. Further cephalad up the trunk above the level of anesthesia, you will find a zone of insensitivity to cold. Above this level is a zone of analgesia to pinprick.[128] If an adequate dose of local anesthetic is administered, within 10 min of injection some detectable block should be apparent. If it is not, there is no point in waiting longer. An alternative plan should be immediately put into action: either repeat the block or induce general anesthesia.

Sedation

After the block has been determined to be setting up, the patient can be positioned for operation. As with spinal anesthesia, attention to padding the patient as well as possible, including the use of pillows, decreases the amount of sedation necessary. Sedation can be accomplished with small doses of midazolam or a propofol infusion of 25 to 75 μg/kg body weight per min. For procedures longer than 2 h, or for upper abdominal or thoracic surgery, combined epidural and light general anesthesia may be indicated. The airway can be managed with either tracheal intubation or laryngeal mask airway when muscle relaxation and ventilation are not necessary.

Special Monitoring

In the setting in which the patient has a partial sympathetic block when general anesthesia is induced, there is almost always a marked decline in blood pressure after induction of general anesthesia. In the view of the author, this eventuality is an indication for arterial catheter placement before induction of general anesthesia. Particularly for extensive intra-abdominal or intrathoracic procedures with the possibility of large fluid shifts, an arterial catheter makes management of combined epidural and general anesthesia easier, as may a central venous catheter. At a minimum, a urinary catheter should be placed to help judge fluid therapy. If epidural opioids are used for postoperative pain relief, a catheter will be needed to prevent urinary retention.

Hemodynamic Management

Management of blood pressure and heart rate is as for spinal anesthesia. The major difference is that hypotension and bradycardia tend to occur earlier after spinal injection of local anesthetic than with epidural injection. If a central venous or pulmonary catheter is in place, filling pressure should be kept close to the preoperative values during the procedure. For less extensive surgeries, the urinary catheter can be used to guide fluid replacement, maintaining at least 0.5 mL/kg body weight per h urine output.

If patients become hypovolemic during combined epidural and general anesthesia, they will become hypotensive and possibly bradycardiac. Therefore, careful attention to fluid replacement is important. Bradycardia during hypotension must be immediately treated. This is best done with intravenous infusion of epinephrine (1 to 4 μg/min) or ephedrine (5- to 10-mg bolus). Atropine given intravenously is often effective despite a presumed block of cardioaccelerator fibers.

Once intravascular volume has been optimized with volume replacement, an infusion of an adrenergic agonist such as ephedrine, epinephrine, norepinephrine, or phenylephrine can be used to support blood pressure if necessary. Mild hypotension is well tolerated, as long as heart rate (and thus cardiac output) is well maintained.[133, 134]

"Top-Up" Dosing

If the patient is heavily sedated or receiving general anesthesia, it is not possible to detect time to two-segment regression of the block. Therefore, one uses a table (see Table 19–3) to determine when to redose local anesthetic. As a general rule, one half to two thirds of the initial dose of drug is reinjected before the time to two-segment block is reached. Bromage[135] suggested reinjecting at a time equal to 1.5 standard deviations before the mean time to two-segment regression. For example, with 2% lidocaine (with epinephrine 1:200,000), initial dose 20 mL, a top-up dose of 10 to 12 mL is given approximately 70 min after the initial dose. This timing is necessary to prevent dissipation of the block or the appearance of tachyphylaxis. One note of caution: The author recommends that a top-up dose not be given shortly before the end of the operation. If hypotension appears, it is preferable for this to happen in the operating theater, not in the recovery room or during transport to the intensive care unit. Therefore, some thought must be given to the timing of top-up doses.

Combined Epidural and "Light" General Anesthesia

Because the epidural block provides anesthesia and muscle relaxation for operation, inhalational or intravenous anesthetics are necessary only to provide amnesia. This can be accomplished in many ways. The author's usual approach is to use nitrous oxide 50% to 70% in oxygen (sometimes with 0.2% to 0.3% isoflurane) via a laryngeal mask airway and with spontaneous ventilation. For intrathoracic and upper abdominal operations, the trachea is intubated, muscle relaxants are given, and the lungs are ventilated. This light general anesthesia provides adequate amnesia, particularly if midazolam had been used to provide sedation for epidural catheter insertion.

At the end of the surgical procedure, the inhalational or intravenous anesthetics are discontinued and the trachea is extubated when indicated by the clinical situation. The patient should be awake, if excessive amounts of inhalational or intravenous anesthesia have not been given, and should be pain-free. This combination, after a long procedure, is particularly reassuring to our surgical colleagues, nursing staff, and patients. Once the patient is in the recovery room or intensive care unit, vital signs should be immediately assessed and corrective action, as indicated, taken immediately. It is possible that hypotension has developed during transport from the operating room. Once vital signs are stable, the catheter can be attached to a continuous infusion source for postoperative analgesia.

Specific Recommendations for Various Approaches to Epidural Anesthesia

Lumbar Epidural Anesthesia

Indications. Operation on lumbar, sacral, or lower thoracic dermatomes, e.g., cesarean section, herniorrhaphy, postoperative analgesia, labor analgesia, treatment of various chronic pain states.

Optimal Patient Position. Lateral decubitus, with operative side dependent; alternative: sitting.

Optimal Site of Needle Insertion. For lower abdominal surgical procedures, second or third lumbar interspace; for operations on lumbar dermatomes, third or fourth lumbar interspace; for operations on sacral dermatomes (e.g., ankle surgery), fifth lumbar interspace.

Optimal Approach to Interspace. Either midline or paramedian, depending on age of patient and calcification of interspace and ligaments.

Initial Local Anesthetic Dose. 15 to 20 mL, depending on age and physical status of patient. Spread of local anesthetic is approximately 1.25 mL/segment in young adult.[136]

Special Precautions. Hanging drop test may be unreliable, particularly if intra-abdominal pressure increased. Anesthesia of L-5 and S-1 nerve roots has prolonged latency and higher failure rate than other roots. To ensure anesthesia of these dermatomes, epidural needle should be placed at L5-S1 and the initial dose of local anesthetic given via the needle. It may be necessary to give a top-up dose via the catheter to achieve adequate analgesia.

Thoracic Epidural Anesthesia

Indications. Operation on the abdomen, thorax; postoperative analgesia; analgesia for fractured ribs; treatment of various chronic pain states.

Optimal Patient Position. Lateral decubitus, with operative side dependent; alternative: sitting.

Optimal Site of Needle Insertion. As close to the center of surgical stimulus as practical, e.g., T4-5 for thoracotomy, T9-10 for gastrectomy.

Optimal Approach to Interspace—Paramedian. Note angulated spinous processes between circa T-4 and T-9. Midthoracic spinous processes overlap, making the midline approach difficult, if not impossible. The technique favored by the author for midthoracic epidural puncture is as follows: The patient is placed either in the lateral decubitus position (preferred) or in the sitting position (for obese patients). The skin is prepared and draped in sterile fashion. A skin wheal is raised with local anesthetic 0.5 to 1.0 cm lateral to the spinous process chosen. Additional infiltration is performed with a 1.5-in finder needle by advancing the needle perpendicular to the long axis of the back until the lamina is encountered. The needle is withdrawn to skin and reinserted, directed medial and cephalad, until contact with the lamina is lost. A Tuohy needle is exchanged for the finder needle, and the process is repeated. Once contact with the lamina is lost, a syringe is placed on the Tuohy needle and resistance to injection is sought.

Initial Local Anesthetic Dose. 7 to 10 mL. Spread of local anesthetic is approximately 0.7 to 1.0 mL/ segment in a young adult.[136] Spread is greater than in the lumbar epidural space because of a decreased potential volume of the space as a result of the volume of the dural sac and spinal cord.

Comment. Thoracic and cervical epidural puncture should be learned under the close supervision of an expert, because of the potential consequences of damage to the underlying spinal cord. Epidural puncture in the midthoracic region is more difficult than in the lower thoracic region owing to the increased angulation of the spinous processes. Refreshing one's memory of the osseous anatomy by examining a skeleton immediately before epidural puncture is highly recommended. Because of overlapping spinous processes, if one inserts a needle 1 cm lateral to a midthoracic spinous process, as it is inserted perpendicular to the long axis of the back, it will sooner or later strike the lamina of the vertebral body immediately caudal to the vertebra belonging to the spinous process. The angle that an epidural needle must take to reach the interspace (medial and cephalad) can be much better appreciated by reference to a skeleton than to a textbook.

As in the lumbar region, depth of the epidural space from skin depends on body size. Because the paramedian approach is used, the epidural needle bypasses the interspinous ligament and encounters the ligamentum flavum. The first good resistance to injection is felt once the needle tip is at this point. Before this, resistance to injection is poor.

Special Precautions. Spinal cord underlies thoracic epidural space; spread of local anesthetic is greater than in lumbar space as a result of relatively smaller space. Hypotension is possible, particularly with a top-up dose if local anesthetic spreads to lumbar segments. Care must be taken to avoid hypovolemia, particularly if a combined epidural and light general anesthetic is used.

Attention must be paid to central venous or pulmonary artery pressures.

Cervical Epidural Anesthesia

Indications. Operations on breast, shoulders, upper extremities, and neck; treatment of various chronic pain states.

Optimal Patient Position. Sitting; alternative: lateral decubitus.

Optimal Site of Needle Insertion. C7-T1 (second largest interspinous interspace in vertebral column).

Optimal Approach to Epidural Space. Midline.

Initial Local Anesthetic Dose. 10 mL. Spread of local anesthetic is approximately 0.7 to 1.0 mL/segment in a young adult.

Comment. Spinal cord underlies the cervical epidural space. Anesthesia of cervical dermatomes causes patients to lose motor control of upper extremities, so patients should be forewarned. The diaphragm is apparently unaffected by these doses of epidural local anesthetics. The C7-T1 interspace is fairly large, so this seems to be the best choice for cervical epidural puncture. The spinous processes of C-7 and T-1 are the most prominent in the neck. When one palpates these spinous processes, they are most prominent when the neck is flexed; when the neck is extended, the C-7 spinous process disappears. The cervical spinous processes are perpendicular to the long axis of the spine; thus the epidural needle should also be directed perpendicular to the long axis of the back. The depth of the epidural space is similar to that in the lumbar space, i.e., 4 to 6 cm from the skin. The feeling as the needle enters the ligamentum flavum is similar to that in the lumbar region. Although the hanging drop technique is often advocated for cervical epidural puncture, the author prefers the loss of resistance technique, on the premise that one should use the technique with which one is most familiar.

Caudal Epidural Anesthesia

Indications. Operations on sacral dermatomes— e.g., hemorrhoidectomy or anal fissurectomy; postop-

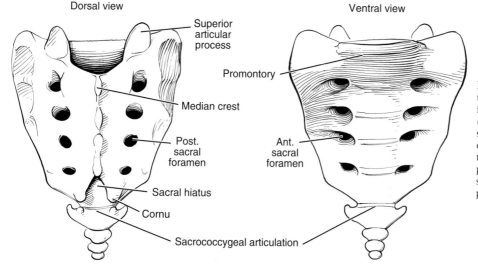

Figure 19–27 The bony anatomy of the sacrum. Note dorsal sacral foramina, large ventral foramina (which allow easy escape of injected solution), sacral hiatus, and articulation of sacrum with coccyx. In thin patients, the midline can be identified by palpating the median crest (vestigial spinous processes). Ant., anterior; Post., posterior.

Dorsal view

Superior articular process

Median crest

Post. sacral foramen

Sacral hiatus

Cornu

Sacrococcygeal articulation

Ventral view

Promontory

Ant. sacral foramen

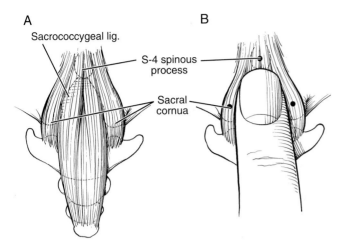

Figure 19–28 *A* and *B,* The anatomy of the sacral hiatus. Note sacral cornua lateral to hiatus. These are vestiges of the S-5 lamina that failed to fuse. Sacrococcygeal ligament covers the sacral hiatus.

erative analgesia (particularly for pediatric urologic and lower extremity orthopedic surgery); labor and delivery; and treatment of various chronic pain states. An epidural catheter can be advanced through the sacral hiatus to lie at the lumbosacral juncture. With the catheter tip in this position, the block produces results like a lumbar epidural block, and surgery on lumbar and low thoracic dermatomes can be performed. This technique might be used in the case of a patient who has had fusion of the lumbar spine, where the sacral hiatus is the only opening to the epidural space easily available.

Optimal Patient Position. Prone (adults), with a pillow under the sacrum; alternative: lateral decubitus (preferred in children).

Initial Local Anesthetic Dose. 20 to 30 mL (adults), 0.5 mL/kg body weight (children). Spread of local anesthetic is approximately 2.5 to 3.0 mL/segment in a young adult[136] or 0.1 mL/segment per year of age (using 1% lidocaine or 0.25% bupivacaine) in a prepubescent child.[137, 138] Maximum doses recommended are 10 mg/kg body weight lidocaine or mepivacaine and 2.5 mg/kg body weight bupivacaine.[139]

The anatomy and spread of local anesthetic within the caudal epidural space are sufficiently different from other approaches to the epidural space to warrant separate discussion.

Anatomy

The sacrum is formed by fusion and flattening of five sacral vertebrae to form a triangular bone, dorsally convex, that articulates cephalad with the fifth lumbar vertebra and caudally with the coccyx (Fig. 19–27). In the sacrum, the epidural space ends at the sacrococcygeal ligament, which covers the sacral hiatus (Fig. 19–28). The sacral hiatus is the failure of the laminae of the fifth and usually fourth sacral vertebrae to fuse. This inverted U-shaped opening into the sacral canal is flanked by the prominent sacral cornua—the remnants

of the S-5 inferior articular processes. The extent of this "spina bifida" varies in adults (Fig. 19–29). Anatomic variants have been reported, several of which can pose problems for the anesthesiologist. Among these are extensive bifida, including the third sacral lamina, or even complete bifida of the entire sacrum; abnormalities of the sacral cornua; false or decoy hiatus; and absence of a hiatus. There is a reported 7.7% incidence of the last variant,[140] which would make caudal epidural block theoretically impossible in those patients.

The sacrum is pierced anteriorly by four neural foramina, through which pass rather large anterior primary rami, and posteriorly by posterior sacral foramina, from which pass smaller posterior primary rami. In contrast with the posterior foramina, the large anterior neural foramina provide a ready route of escape from the sacral epidural space for local anesthetic solution. Within the sacral canal is a plexus of epidural veins. The dural sac usually terminates at the level of S-2 in adults (S-3 in newborns). A line connecting the posterior superior iliac spines approximates the S-2 level.

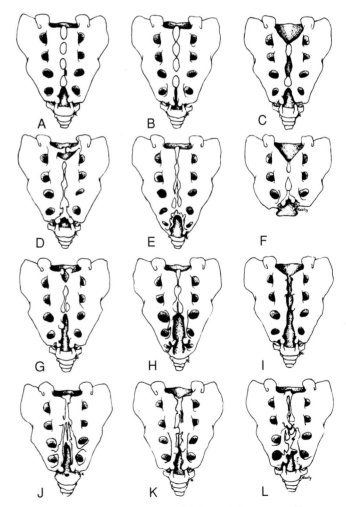

Figure 19–29 Normal anatomic variations of the sacrum. (From Willis RJ: Caudal epidural blockade. In Cousins MJ, Bridenbaugh PO [eds]: Neural Blockade in Clinical Anesthesia and Management of Pain, 2nd ed, pp 361–383. Philadelphia, JB Lippincott, 1988.)

Clinical Applications

Although the current resurgence in popularity of epidural anesthesia owes much to the former practice of continuous caudal epidural anesthesia for labor analgesia, caudal anesthesia is seldom used for this indication today. In the United States, caudal anesthesia is used largely for postoperative analgesia or combined epidural and light general anesthesia in children. The reasons for this are anatomic. Because the spinal cord ends in the lumbar region and the dural sac ends at S-2, the potential complications of neural trauma or intrathecal injection are decreased with the caudal approach vis-à-vis the lumbar approach to the epidural space.[141] In preadolescent children, the approach to the sacral coccygeal membrane is straightforward. Studies by Schulte-Steinberg and Rahlfs[137, 138] have demonstrated a high degree of predictability in spread of caudal anesthesia in children up to age 12 years. During adolescence, there is marked growth of the sacrum and alteration of its shape. These changes lead to much less predictable spread of caudal anesthesia in the adult compared with the child (Fig. 19–30). These advantages have helped popularize this technique among pediatric anesthesiologists in recent years.[142]

Technique of Caudal Block

If the patient is a preadolescent child, general anesthesia is usually induced before the block is placed. There are several formulae to calculate dose.[137, 143] For children, the author uses 0.5 mL/kg body weight of either 0.25% or 0.5% bupivacaine, containing epinephrine 1:200,000, depending on what duration of analgesia is desired and how much postoperative motor block is acceptable. This dose should provide a level of analgesia to the umbilicus if the 0.5% solution of bupivacaine is used. If lidocaine or mepivacaine is used for a block of shorter duration, the author uses 7 mg/kg body weight of an epinephrine-containing solution. The practical limit of reliably attainable anesthesia with caudal anesthesia is roughly the umbilicus. This technique is not recommended for operations above that level, because of high doses of local anesthetic required and consequently potentially toxic plasma concentrations of local anesthetic.

To begin the pediatric caudal block, monitors are applied, anesthesia is induced, the airway is secured (either with a tracheal tube or by a colleague holding a mask), intravenous access is attained, and the patient is turned to the lateral decubitus or the prone position (Fig. 19–31). The osseous landmarks (sacral cornua and sacral hiatus) are palpated and identified. It is best to be sure of the landmarks at this step. A quick look at a textbook of the anatomy or at a skeleton is helpful immediately before performing this block. Skin is cleansed with antiseptic, and a no-touch technique is used. Using the nondominant hand to palpate the sacral cornua, the dominant hand guides a 22-G needle attached to a 5- or 10-mL syringe of local anesthetic into the hiatus at about 60° to the skin. Once the needle is felt to pass through the sacrococcygeal ligament, the angle is decreased to about 30° to the skin and advanced a further 1 cm or so into the sacral canal (Fig. 19–31). If bone is unexpectedly encountered or if there is any resistance to injection, the needle is removed, landmarks are reassessed, and the needle is reinserted. After a negative aspiration test for blood and CSF, a test dose of 1 to 2 mL of local anesthetic is injected. There should be little resistance to injection (similar to injecting local anesthetic into the lumbar epidural space). If the test dose is negative, the remainder of the dose is given (fractionated), with repeated aspiration tests. Any swelling of the skin under the injection needle or resistance to injection indicates the local anesthetic is not being injected into the sacral canal. If all signs indicate correct injection into the epidural space, the patient can be positioned for operation.

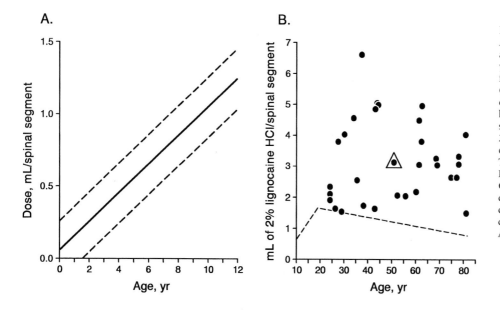

Figure 19–30 Epidural anesthesia. *A,* Linear relationship between age and anesthetic dose in children younger than age 12 years. (Data from Schulte-Steinberg O, Rahlfs VW: Caudal anesthesia in children and the distribution of 0.25 per cent bupivacaine solution. A statistical study [German]. Anaesthesist 1972; 21:96.) *B,* Scattergram of age versus dose requirements/segment in adults. There is no predictable relationship. Lignocaine = lidocaine. (From Cousins MJ, Bromage PR: A comparison of the hydrochloride and carbonated salts of lignocaine for caudal analgesia in out-patients. Br J Anaesth 1971; 43: 1149–1154.)

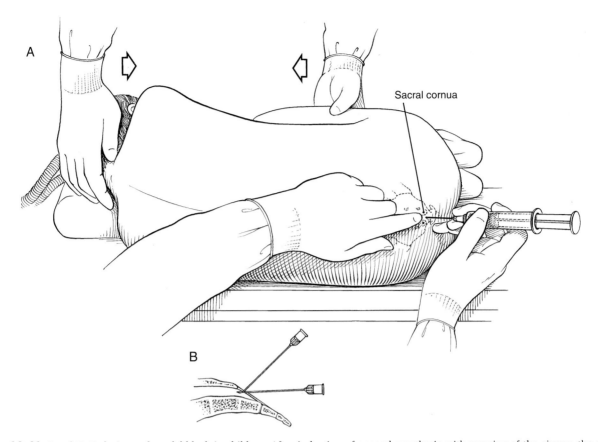

Figure 19–31 *A* and *B*, Technique of caudal block in children. After induction of general anesthesia with securing of the airway, the child is placed in left lateral decubitus position (for a right-handed anesthesiologist). Povidone-iodine is used to prepare the skin, and a no-touch technique is used to insert a 22-G needle attached to a syringe filled with local anesthetic. After popping through the sacrococcygeal ligament, the angle of the needle is lowered, and the needle is advanced 0.5 to 1.0 cm further in the sacral canal. If the aspiration test is negative for blood and cerebrospinal fluid, the local anesthetic is injected 1 to 2 mL at a time, with frequent repeated aspiration. There should be no resistance to injection.

Continuous Caudal Anesthesia

A continuous caudal technique can also be performed in children. In small children, a 20-G intravenous cannula can be placed, using a 3-mL syringe to detect a loss of resistance to injection and threading off the plastic cannula into the sacral canal. Cannulae smaller than 20 G tend to kink and have not been satisfactory. It is possible to puncture the dural sac if the cannula is threaded more cephalad than S-3 in newborns. In larger children (e.g., greater than 15 kg), a 20-G epidural catheter can be inserted via an 18-G Tuohy needle.

Adult patients should be placed in the prone position, with a pillow under the sacrum. This position maximizes the bony landmarks, which can otherwise be obscured by fatty buttocks with the patient in the lateral decubitus position. Sterile gloves, antiseptic preparation, and sterile draping are used, as with other approaches to the epidural space. The sacral cornua and sacral hiatus are identified. Again, extra time is taken to carefully identify landmarks. After a skin wheal is raised with local anesthetic, a 22-G, 1.5-in needle is used to pop through the sacrococcygeal ligament, feeling a loss of resistance to injection. A 17- or 18-G Tuohy needle can be used to achieve a loss of

resistance if a catheter technique is planned. After a negative aspiration test for blood and CSF, a 3-mL test dose of epinephrine-containing local anesthetic is given via the needle. The main dose of local anesthetic should not be injected if there is any resistance to injection of the test dose. If the result with the test dose is negative, the remainder of the local anesthetic solution can be given (fractionated), again with frequent aspiration tests. An epidural catheter can be inserted and should be aspirated again and a test dose given before assuming the catheter is in the epidural space.

It is crucial to demonstrate analgesia of the operative site (within 10 min of injection) before allowing preparation and draping. There is a high failure rate for this technique with adult patients, particularly in inexperienced hands. Because it would be difficult to induce general anesthesia with the patient in the prone position, inadequate caudal blocks must be discovered before preparation and draping while there still is time to either repeat the block or induce general anesthesia.

Complications of Caudal Anesthesia

Potential complications are similar to those with lumbar epidural anesthesia. There is a sacral epidural

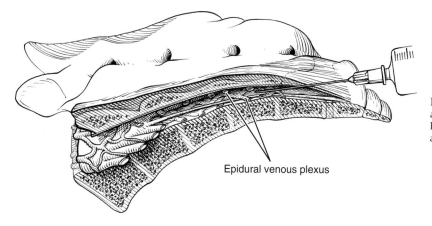

Figure 19–32 Caudal epidural venous plexus. An accidental intravascular or intrathecal injection of local anesthetic must be considered during caudal anesthesia.

Epidural venous plexus

venous plexus, which can be unintentionally cannulated (Fig. 19–32). Injection into the sacrum, with resultant rapid intravenous uptake of local anesthetics, is possible. In a pregnant patient, with the fetal head into the perineum, injection into the fetal head, with disastrous consequences, has been reported.[144] Dural puncture, and resultant high spinal block, is a possibility if the dural sac terminates more caudad than usual or if the sacral hiatus extends more cephalad than expected.[145] Finally, in the adult patient, failure rates for this technique are reported to be high (5% to 10%) for reasons of anatomic variability.[146] The needle can be unintentionally inserted into several decoys, such as a decoy hiatus or into a dorsal sacral foramen (Fig. 19–33). For these anatomic reasons, lumbar epidural anesthesia is often preferred over caudal anesthesia in the adult patient.

Complications of Neuraxial Block

Dural Puncture and Post–dural Puncture Headache

If during the course of an epidural needle insertion, an accidental dural puncture occurs, it is the author's practice to convert the technique to a continuous spinal technique whenever possible. Two to three milliliters

of the same local anesthetic originally planned for the epidural, i.e., either 2% lidocaine or 0.5% to 0.75% bupivacaine, can be injected via the catheter. If an epidural catheter is clearly indicated, it is best to choose a different interspace. An epidural catheter inserted at a different interspace can also be used to give a prophylactic autologous blood patch.[147] Although this is controversial, present evidence suggests the rate of PDPH after prophylactic blood patch is in the range of 10% to 21%. Patients in whom this treatment fails usually respond to a second blood patch. Other described treatments for PDPH include intravenous caffeine injection, epidural saline infusions, and epidural dextran injection. These methods are effective, but their effects are usually transient. To date, autologous epidural blood patch remains the best treatment of severe PDPH.

If a patient complains of headache after spinal or epidural anesthesia, it is important to establish the postural nature of this headache, because there are other types of headache, requiring different treatments, which can be confused with PDPH. These include paranasal sinusitis, cortical vein thrombosis, and subdural hematoma.[148] If a PDPH does not respond to 2 days of bed rest and orally administered analgesics, or in the case of a new mother, immediately after headache develops, the author administers an autologous epidural blood patch, using 10 to 15 mL of blood. Contra-

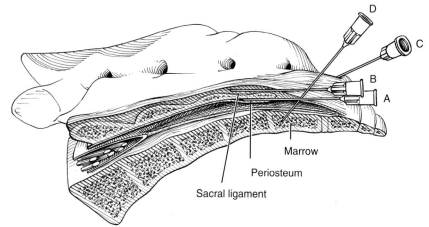

Figure 19–33 Potential needle malposition during caudal epidural injection. Needle may enter A, periosteum; B, subcutaneous tissues; C, a decoy hiatus; D, bone of the sacrum.

Marrow

Periosteum

Sacral ligament

indications to an autologous blood patch are the same as for epidural anesthesia. Epidural abscess has been known to occur after autologous blood patch in a bacteremic patient. AIDS (acquired immunodeficiency syndrome) is not a contraindication to epidural blood patch.[149]

Hypotension and Bradycardia

Bradycardia during high epidural or spinal anesthesia can rapidly deteriorate if not treated immediately. There have been several reports of cardiac arrest with poor neurologic outcomes.[74] In some cases, cardiac arrests have been attributed to intravenously given sedatives and hypoventilation, when in fact hypotension and bradycardia may have been the central problem. For reasons not currently well understood, some individuals are prone to vasovagal episodes during epidural anesthesia, perhaps related to pooling of blood in the splanchnic circulation.[150] Arndt et al[150] reported vasovagal syncope in healthy young male volunteers with levels of analgesia at T-5 or below, suggesting that impairment of cardioaccelerator fibers is not the cause. Often this is seen in young athletic men, suggesting that high vagal tone may be responsible. Carpenter and coworkers[57] found several factors associated with bradycardia during spinal anesthesia. These included preexisting bradycardia, β-adrenergic receptor blocker therapy, and a block at or above the T-5 dermatome.

Treatment of bradycardia during spinal or epidural anesthesia should be directed at restoring cardiac output as rapidly as possible. Depending on the urgency, the first drug given should be either atropine (0.4 to 0.6 mg) or epinephrine (10 μg) to speed the heart rate. These drugs can be repeated as necessary. Next, ventilation and oxygenation should be assessed. If cardiac or respiratory arrest is imminent, call for help immediately. It may be necessary to intubate, ventilate, and give external cardiac massage to circulate the epinephrine. Extra hands will be needed. Patients who have experienced bradycardiac arrest during epidural and spinal anesthesia have been successfully resuscitated without neurologic sequelae, if they have been treated immediately.[151]

Permanent Neurologic Sequelae

A large study performed in the 1950s by Vandam and Dripps[152] suggested that the incidence of permanent neurologic sequelae after spinal anesthesia was less than 1/10,000. Nonetheless, there are reported cases of this complication after neuraxial block. Already mentioned are unexpected cardiac arrest,[74] neurotoxicity after continuous spinal anesthesia,[98] and accidental intrathecal injection of 2-chloroprocaine.[64] Additionally, cases of paralysis due to suspected anterior spinal artery syndrome[21]; epidural, subdural, or subarachnoid hematoma[153]; and epidural abscess[154] have been reported. Of these complications resulting in permanent

neurologic deficits, all are quite rare, and only the last two are treatable.

Spinal Hematoma

Hematoma in the epidural, subdural, and intrathecal spaces is a rare complication of neuraxial block. In the combined series by Vandam and Dripps,[152] Moore and Bridenbaugh,[155] Phillips et al,[156] and Sadove and associates[157] totaling more than 50,000 administrations of spinal anesthetics, not one case of spinal hematoma was reported. Owens and colleagues,[153] in a review of the English language medical literature, compiled reports of 33 cases of spinal hematoma after lumbar puncture for diagnostic puncture (27 cases) and anesthesia (6 cases). Thirteen of these patients had received anticoagulants; nine had thrombocytopenia; one was treated with ticlopidine, an antiplatelet drug[158]; and one received aspirin post–lumbar puncture.[159] Two others had hepatic abnormalities. Thus, 26 of 33 cases (79%) occurred in patients with evidence of hemostatic abnormality. Although there is one reported series of patients undergoing epidural anesthesia during partial anticoagulation,[160] this practice seems inadvisable in light of the findings of Owens et al.[153]

Except for one case report,[158] there is no evidence to suggest that a patient taking nonsteroidal anti-inflammatory drugs is at risk for this complication. A large study at the Mayo Clinic by Horlocker et al[161] showed that patients taking nonsteroidal anti-inflammatory drugs probably are not at any higher risk for major bleeding problems when undergoing epidural or spinal anesthesia. Furthermore, it is probably safe to use heparin in a patient in whom a spinal or epidural catheter has been inserted, provided that the insertion was not traumatic and that the catheter is not removed until after the coagulation status of the patient has returned to normal.[162]

The author's practice in patients without a dominating indication for regional block is to avoid epidural or spinal anesthesia in the following situations:

1. Partial thromboplastin time is longer than control
2. Prothrombin time is 2 s longer than control
3. Bleeding time is grossly abnormal on two occasions (longer than 15 min)
4. Patient has a known coagulopathy, unless the coagulopathy is von Willebrand's disease and the patient is known to have normal coagulation and bleeding studies at the time of anesthesia
5. Platelet count less than 80 cells × 10⁹/L
6. If a coagulopathy may develop in the course of treatment (e.g., HELLP [hemolysis, elevated liver enzymes, low platelets] syndrome or severe hepatic dysfunction)

If heparin has been administered during operation, the author makes sure the activated clotting time or partial thromboplastin time is normal before removal of an epidural or spinal catheter.

Signs and symptoms of epidural hematoma are severe back pain and motor or sensory block (or both) of the lower extremities persisting after the epidural or spinal anesthesia should have dissipated or recurring after dissipation of the block. If an epidural hematoma or abscess is thought to have developed, the patient should have immediate computed tomography or magnetic resonance imaging of the appropriate area of the spine. Evidence indicates that of the two, magnetic resonance imaging is a better diagnostic test, because of higher sensitivity to soft tissue densities in the spinal canal.[163] A neurosurgeon or orthopedic spine surgeon should be consulted at once if there is any question of an epidural hematoma or abscess. If evacuation of the hematoma is performed within 6 h, there is a chance of full neurologic recovery. Delayed evacuation will have poorer results.[154]

Epidural Abscess

This rare complication can result in permanent neurologic deficits. Epidural abscess has been reported to occur spontaneously in patients with sepsis, after epidural anesthesia,[154] and with indwelling epidural catheters for chronic pain relief (15 of 350 cancer patients reported by Du Pen et al[164]). Signs and symptoms of epidural abscess may be similar to those of epidural hematoma, except that these patients are febrile. Other symptoms are slowly developing severe back pain and motor and sensory block of the lower extremities. Diagnosis of epidural abscess is best made by magnetic resonance imaging (Fig. 19–34), although computed tomography would be necessary if the patient had an implanted metal port. Treatment of epidural abscess is immediate surgical evacuation, culture, drainage, and intravenous administration of antibiotics appropriate to the organism. Du Pen et al[164] reported successful treatment of epidural abscess and deep catheter tract infections in cancer patients with indwelling epidural catheters by removal of the catheter, culture, intravenous administration of antibiotics, and repeated magnetic resonance images to follow the abscess. None of their patients required laminectomy for decompression of the epidural space. However, if neurologic signs develop, it is the author's opinion that a surgeon capable of decompressive surgery should be consulted.

Infection of Epidural Catheter Insertion Sites

A local infection can develop around the insertion site of an epidural catheter if it is left in place long enough. Because of the potential for this problem, most catheters that are to be left in place longer than 5 to 7 days should be tunneled, and of course strict sterile technique must be adhered to during placement, just as for indwelling central venous catheters. Tunneling a catheter will not prevent the occurrence of an infection, but it will increase the distance from catheter entry site to epidural space. An intravenous dose of a first-generation cephalosporin antibiotic before insertion is routinely given by the author. Daily inspection of the catheter site for signs of infection is highly recommended. Even with these precautions, skin infections do occur. They are almost always limited to the skin or catheter tract, but rarely they can extend into the epidural space.[164] Du Pen and colleagues[164] successfully managed many cancer patients with superficial catheter infections by thorough daily cleaning with povidone-iodine and antibiotics given topically or orally. The tunneled epidural catheters were left in place. In the case of patients with epidural catheters for acute postoperative analgesia, treatment of these infections should include removal of the catheter, culture of the organism, antibiotics given intravenously, and local incision and drainage (if indicated).

Back Pain

Post–epidural anesthesia back pain has become an area of interest, as a result of its suspected link to disodium EDTA used as an antioxidant for a commercial preparation of 2-chloroprocaine.[102] However, there are other possible causes of post–epidural or post–spinal anesthesia back pain. Two studies showed there is a surprisingly high incidence of needle-related post–epidural[102] or post–spinal anesthesia back pain,[165] which can last more than 24 hours after anesthesia. Usually this is a minor annoyance for the patient, which is confined to the site of needle insertion and disappears without treatment. However, if a patient does not expect any backache, its presence may be alarming. For this reason, the author makes it a practice to warn patients they may experience transient, but inconsequential, backache related to needle insertion.

Another possible cause of postanesthesia back pain is the unphysiologic condition of lying anesthetized on an operating room table or recovery room bed for several hours.[166] This can result in transient musculoskeletal changes and backache unrelated to epidural

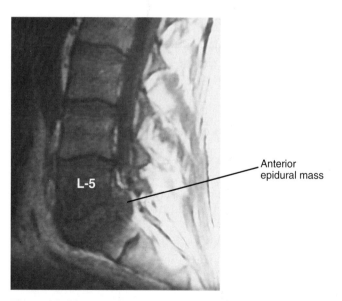

L-5

Anterior epidural mass

Figure 19–34 A magnetic resonance imaging scan of lumbar epidural abscess.

block. For example, it has been shown that women undergoing childbirth have a relatively high incidence of postdelivery backache, independent of whether they received any anesthesia.[148]

Diagnosis of minor, needle-related pain can usually be made over the telephone, because this pain is always localized to the site of needle insertion. Chloroprocaine-related back pain develops as the anesthesia dissipates or shortly thereafter.[102] It will be localized to the lumbar region but in the deep back muscles. It has a burning, aching quality. Muscle spasm is usually not evident. This pain may be severe enough to require epidural fentanyl (100 to 150 µg). Orally administered nonsteroidal anti-inflammatory medications or opioids should be given to the patients with instructions to take them as needed and to call for a follow-up appointment in 24 h. Usually, by that time the pain has subsided to the level of a minor nuisance. Recurrence of previous, chronic back pain, sometimes with a radicular component, can also occur. However, other, more serious causes of back pain, such as epidural hematoma and abscess, must be eliminated. If there is any question as to the diagnosis, it is obligatory that the patient be seen and examined by an anesthesiologist familiar with the complications of epidural and spinal anesthesia. This can often best be done by having the patient seen in the Anesthesia Pain Clinic.

References

1. Bier A: Versuche über Cocainisirung des Rückenmarkes. Dtsch Z Chir 1899; 51: 361–369.
2. Bridenbaugh PO, Greene NM: Spinal (subarachnoid) neural blockade. In Cousins MJ, Bridenbaugh PO (eds): Neural Blockade in Clinical Anesthesia and Management of Pain, 2nd ed, pp 213–251. Philadelphia, JB Lippincott, 1988.
3. Bromage PR: Epidural Analgesia, pp 1–7. Philadelphia, WB Saunders Co, 1978.
4. Dogliotti AM: Anesthesia. Chicago, SB Dubour, 1939. [English translation by CS Scuderi].
5. Gutiérrez A: Anestesia Extradural. Rev Cir Buenos Aires 1939; 18: 349; 409.
6. Düttmann G: Die peridurale, segmentäre Anästhesie. Zentralbl Chir 1941; 68: 530–535.
7. Goepel H: Erfahrungsbericht über die Periduralanästhesie. Die Pontocain-Periston-Plombe zur segmentären Anästhesie. Zentralbl Chir 1947; 72: 467–473.
8. Tuohy EB: The use of continuous spinal anesthesia: utilizing the ureteral catheter technic. JAMA 1945; 128: 262–263.
9. Kehlet H: Surgical stress: the role of pain and analgesia. Br J Anaesth 1989; 63: 189–195.
10. Modig J, Borg T, Bagge L, et al: Role of extradural and of general anaesthesia in fibrinolysis and coagulation after total hip replacement. Br J Anaesth 1983; 55: 625–629.
11. Modig J, Borg T, Karlstrom G, et al: Thromboembolism after total hip replacement: role of epidural and general anesthesia. Anesth Analg 1983; 62: 174–180.
12. Tuman KJ, McCarthy RJ, March RJ, et al: Effects of epidural anesthesia and analgesia on coagulation and outcome after major vascular surgery. Anesth Analg 1991; 73: 696–704.
13. Ready LB, Loper KA, Nessly M, et al: Postoperative epidural morphine is safe on surgical wards. Anesthesiology 1991; 75: 452–456.
14. Artuso JD, Stevens RA, Lineberry PJ: Post dural puncture headache after lumbar sympathetic block: a report of two cases. Reg Anesth 1991; 16: 288–291.
15. Hogan QH: Lumbar epidural anatomy: a new look by cryomicrotome section. Anesthesiology 1991; 75: 767–775.
16. Covino B, Scott DB: Handbook of Epidural Anaesthesia and Analgesia, pp 16–26. Orlando, Grune & Stratton, 1985.
17. Galindo A, Hernandez J, Benavides O, et al: Quality of spinal extradural anaesthesia: the influence of spinal nerve root diameter. Br J Anaesth 1975; 47: 41–47.
18. Savolaine ER, Pandya JB, Greenblatt SH, et al: Anatomy of the human lumbar epidural space: new insights using CT-epidurography. Anesthesiology 1988; 68: 217–220.
19. Burn JM, Guyer PB, Langdon L: The spread of solutions injected into the epidural space. A study using epidurograms in patients with the lumbosciatic syndrome. Br J Anaesth 1973; 45: 338–345.
20. Bromage PR: Epidural Analgesia, pp 171–175. Philadelphia, WB Saunders Co, 1992.
21. Cousins MJ, Bromage PR: Epidural neural blockade. In Cousins MJ, Bridenbaugh PO (eds): Neural Blockade in Clinical Anesthesia and Management of Pain, 2nd ed, pp 253–360. Philadelphia, JB Lippincott, 1988.
22. Wildsmith JSW, McClure JH, Brown DT: Plain bupivacaine 0.5%: a preliminary evaluation as a spinal anaesthetic agent (comment). Ann R Coll Surg Engl 1983; 65: 277–278.
23. Veering BT, Burm AG, Spierdijk J: Spinal anaesthesia with hyperbaric bupivacaine. Effects of age on neural blockade and pharmacokinetics. Br J Anaesth 1988; 60: 187–194.
24. Greene NM: Uptake and elimination of local anesthetics during spinal anesthesia. Anesth Analg 1983; 62: 1013–1024.
25. Wildsmith JAW: Current concepts in spinal anesthesia. Reg Anesth 1985; 10: 119–124.
26. Stienstra R, Greene NM: Factors affecting the subarachnoid spread of local anesthetic solutions. Reg Anesth 1991; 16: 1–6.
27. Sheskey MC, Rocco AG, Bizzarri-Schmid M, et al: A dose-response study of bupivacaine for spinal anesthesia. Anesth Analg 1983; 62: 931–935.
28. Tuominen M, Taivainen T, Rosenberg PH: Spread of spinal anaesthesia with plain 0.5% bupivacaine: influence of the vertebral interspace used for injection. Br J Anaesth 1989; 62: 358–361.
29. Cameron AE, Arnold RW, Ghorisa MW, et al: Spinal analgesia using bupivacaine 0.5% plain. Variation in the extent of the block with patient age. Anaesthesia 1981; 36: 318–322.
30. Pitkanen M, Haapaniemi L, Tuominen M, et al: Influence of age on spinal anaesthesia with isobaric 0.5% bupivacaine. Br J Anaesth 1984; 56: 279–284.
31. Veering BT, Burm AG, van Kleef JW, et al: Spinal anesthesia with glucose-free bupivacaine: effects of age on neural blockade and pharmacokinetics. Anesth Analg 1987; 66: 965–970.
32. Foelschow J, Batra M, Mulroy M: Previous withdrawal of spinal fluid produces higher hypobaric spinal anesthesia. Reg Anesth 1982; 7: 79.
33. Brown DT, Wildsmith JA, Covino BG, et al: Effect of baricity on spinal anaesthesia with amethocaine. Br J Anaesth 1980; 52: 589–596.
34. Covino BG: Clinical pharmacology of local anesthetic agents. In Cousins MJ, Bridenbaugh PO (eds): Neural Blockade in Clinical Anesthesia and Management of Pain, 2nd ed, pp 111–144. Philadelphia, JB Lippincott, 1988.
35. Armstrong IR, Littlewood DG, Chambers WA: Spinal anesthesia with tetracaine—effect of added vasoconstrictors. Anesth Analg 1983; 62: 793–795.
36. Meagher RP, Moore DC, DeVries JC: Phenylephrine: the most effective potentiator of tetracaine spinal anesthesia. Anesth Analg 1966; 45: 134–139.
37. Concepcion M, Maddi R, Francis D, et al: Vasoconstrictors in spinal anesthesia with tetracaine—a comparison of epinephrine and phenylephrine. Anesth Analg 1984; 63: 134–138.
38. Chambers WA, Littlewood DG, Scott DB: Spinal anesthesia with hyperbaric bupivacaine: effect of added vasoconstrictors. Anesth Analg 1982; 61: 49–52.
39. Chambers WA, Littlewood DG, Logan MR, et al: Effect of added epinephrine on spinal anesthesia with lidocaine. Anesth Analg 1981; 60: 417–420.
40. Rocco AG, Mallampati SR, Boon J, et al: Double blind evaluation of intrathecal bupivacaine and tetracaine. Reg Anesth 1984; 9: 183–187.
41. van Kleef JW, Veering BT: Spinal anesthesia with ropivacaine.

A double blind study on efficacy and safety of 0.5% and 0.75% solutions in patients undergoing minor lower limb surgery. (Abstract.) Reg Anesth 1993; 18(2S): 60.

42. Flaatten H, Rodt SÅ, Vamnes J, et al: Post dural puncture headache using 26- or 29-gauge needles in young patients. (Abstract.) Reg Anaesth 1988; 11: 109.

43. Kho HG: Spinal anesthesia without postspinal headache: a new technique. (Abstract.) Reg Anaesth 1988; 11: 119.

44. Gielen M: Post dural puncture headache (PDPH): a review. Reg Anesth 1989; 14: 101–106.

45. Greene HM: Lumbar puncture and prevention of postpuncture headache. JAMA 1926; 86: 391–392.

46. Greene HM: A technique to reduce the incidence of headache following lumbar puncture in ambulatory patients with a plea for more frequent examinations of the cerebrospinal fluid. Northwest Med 1943; 22: 240–245.

47. Hart JR, Whitacre RJ: Pencil-point needle in prevention of postspinal headache. JAMA 1951; 147: 657–658.

48. Sprotte G, Schedel R, Pajunk H, et al: An "atraumatic" universal needle for single-shot regional anesthesia: clinical results and a 6 year trial in over 30,000 regional anesthesias [German]. Reg Anaesth 1987; 10: 104–108.

49. Ross BK, Chadwick HS, Mancuso JJ, et al: Sprotte needle for obstetric anesthesia: decreased incidence of post dural puncture headache. Reg Anesth 1992; 17: 29–33.

50. Tarkkila PJ, Heine H, Tervo RR: Comparison of Sprotte and Quincke needles with respect to post dural puncture headache and backache. Reg Anesth 1992; 17: 283–287.

51. Lynch J, Kasper S-M, Strick K, et al: The use of Quincke and Whitacre 27-gauge needles in orthopedic patients: incidence of failed spinal anesthesia and postdural puncture headache. Anesth Analg 1994; 79: 124–128.

52. Bromage PR, Van Zundert A, Van Steenberge A, et al: A loss of resistance to negative pressure technique for subarachnoid puncture with narrow gauge needles. Reg Anesth 1993; 18: 155–161.

53. Franksson C, Gordh T: Headache after spinal anesthesia and technique for lessening its frequency. Acta Chir Scand 1946; 94: 443–454.

54. Mihic DN: Postspinal headache and relationship of needle bevel to longitudinal dural fibers. Reg Anesth 1985; 10: 76–81.

55. Hatfalvi BI: The dynamics of post-spinal headache. Headache 1977; 17: 64–66.

56. Ready LB, Woodland RV, Haschke RH: Spinal needle angle affects rate of fluid leak across human dura. (Abstract.) Anesthesiology 1985; 63: A241.

57. Carpenter RL, Caplan RA, Brown DL, et al: Incidence and risk factors for side effects of spinal anesthesia. Anesthesiology 1992; 76: 906–916.

58. Hurley RJ, Lambert DH: Continuous spinal anesthesia with a microcatheter technique: preliminary experience. Anesth Analg 1990; 70: 97–102.

59. Abram SE: Continuous spinal anesthesia for cancer and chronic pain. Reg Anesth 1993; 18(6S): 406–413.

60. Sykes WS: Essays on the First Hundred Years of Anaesthesia, vol 1, plate XI. Edinburgh, E & S Livingstone, 1960.

61. Lemmon WT: A method for continuous spinal anesthesia: a preliminary report. Ann Surg 1940; 111: 141–144.

62. Covino BG: New techniques in regional anesthesia (review course lecture). International Anesthesia Research Society Annual Meeting, San Antonio, Texas, March 8–12, 1991.

63. FDA Safety Alert: Cauda equina syndrome associated with the use of small-bore catheters in continuous spinal anesthesia, May 29, 1992.

64. Rigler ML, Drasner K, Krejcie TC, et al: Cauda equina syndrome after continuous spinal anesthesia. Anesth Analg 1991; 72: 275–281.

65. Lambert DH, Hurley RJ: Cauda equina syndrome and continuous spinal anesthesia. Anesth Analg 1991; 72: 817–819.

66. Rigler ML, Drasner K: Distribution of catheter-injected local anesthetic in a model of the subarachnoid space. Anesthesiology 1991; 75: 684–692.

67. Lambert DH, Lambert LA, Strichartz GR: Potential neurotoxicity of lidocaine solutions used for spinal anesthesia. (Abstract.) Anesthesiology 1992; 77 (suppl): A898.

68. Continuous Spinal Anesthesia, ASRA Symposium, Milwaukee, August 14–15, 1993. Reg Anesth 1993; 18(6S): 387–484.

69. Carrie LES: Extradural, spinal or combined block for obstetric surgical anaesthesia. Br J Anaesth 1990; 65: 225–233.

70. Rawal N, Schollin J, Wesstrom G: Epidural versus combined spinal epidural block for cesarean section. Acta Anaesthesiol Scand 1988; 32: 61–66.

71. Camann WR, Denney RA, Holby ED, et al: A comparison of intrathecal, epidural, and intravenous sufentanil for labor analgesia. Anesthesiology 1992; 77: 884–887.

72. Urmey WF, Stanton J, Sharrock NE: Initial experience with combined spinal-epidural technique using a 27 gauge Whitacre spinal needle for ambulatory knee arthroscopy. (Abstract.) Reg Anesth 1993; 18(2S): 1.

73. Caplan RA, Ward RJ, Posner K, et al: Unexpected cardiac arrest during spinal anesthesia: a closed claims analysis of predisposing factors. Anesthesiology 1988; 68: 5–11.

74. Pennant JH, White PF: The laryngeal mask airway. Its uses in anesthesiology. Anesthesiology 1993; 79: 144–163.

75. Bromage PR: Epidural Analgesia, pp 176–214. Philadelphia, WB Saunders Co, 1978.

76. Gutiérrez A: Valor de la aspiración líquida en el espacio peridural en la anestesia peridural. Rev Cir Buenos Aires 1933; 12: 225–227.

77. Bromage PR: Epidural Analgesia, pp 160–175. Philadelphia, WB Saunders Co, 1978.

78. Hogan QH, Haddox JD: Headache from intracranial air after a lumbar epidural injection: subarachnoid or subdural? Reg Anesth 1992; 17: 303–305.

79. Naulty JS, Ostheimer GW, Datta S, et al: Incidence of venous air embolism during epidural catheter insertion. Anesthesiology 1982; 57: 410–412.

80. Stevens RA, Mikat-Stevens M, Van Clief M, et al: Deliberate epidural air injection in dogs: a radiographic study. Reg Anesth 1989; 14: 180–182.

81. Stevens R, Petty R, Teague P, et al: Does nitrous oxide expand epidural air bubbles? (Abstract.) Anesthesiology 1993; 79(suppl): A883.

82. Dalens B, Bazin JE, Haberer JP: Epidural bubbles as a cause of incomplete analgesia during epidural anesthesia. Anesth Analg 1987; 66: 679–683.

83. Santos DJ, Bridenbaugh PO, Heins S, et al: Unilateral epidural analgesia for labor. (Abstract.) Reg Anesth 1985; 10: S41–S42.

84. Sharrock NE: Recordings of, and an anatomical explanation for, false positive loss of resistance during lumbar extradural analgesia. Br J Anaesth 1979; 51: 253–258.

85. Rissanen PM: The surgical anatomy and pathology of the supraspinous and interspinous ligaments of the lumbar spine with special reference to ligament ruptures. Acta Orthop Scand Suppl 1960; 46: 1–100.

86. Crawford JS: The prevention of headache consequent upon dural puncture. Br J Anaesth 1972; 44: 598–600.

87. Stevens RA, Stanton-Hicks MD: Subdural injection of local anesthetic: a complication of epidural anesthesia. Anesthesiology 1985; 63: 323–326.

88. Lubenow T, Keh-Wong E, Kristof K, et al: Inadvertent subdural injection: a complication of an epidural block. Anesth Analg 1988; 67: 175–179.

89. Bromage PR: Epidural Analgesia, pp 665–666. Philadelphia, WB Saunders Co, 1978.

90. Bromage PR: Mechanism of action of extradural analgesia. Br J Anaesth 1975; 47 (Suppl): 199–211.

91. Kopacz DJ, Mulroy MF: Chloroprocaine and lidocaine decrease hospital stay and admission rate after outpatient epidural anesthesia. Reg Anesth 1990; 15: 19–25.

92. Mather LE, Tucker GT, Murphy TM, et al: The effects of adding adrenaline to etidocaine and lignocaine in extradural anaesthesia II: Pharmacokinetics. Br J Anaesth 1976; 48: 989–994.

93. Bromage PR: Epidural Analgesia, pp 85–86. Philadelphia, WB Saunders Co, 1978.

94. Bromage PR, Burfoot MF, Crowell DE, et al: Quality of epidural blockade. I: Influence of physical factors. Br J Anaesth 1964; 36: 342–352.

95. Moore DC, Batra MS: The components of an effective test dose prior to epidural block. Anesthesiology 1981; 55: 693–696.

96. Hood DD, Dewan DM, James FM III: Maternal and fetal effects of epinephrine in gravid ewes. Anesthesiology 1986; 64: 610–613.

97. Ravindran RS, Bond VK, Tasch MD, et al: Prolonged neural blockade following regional analgesia with 2-chloroprocaine. Anesth Analg 1980; 59: 447–451.

98. Reisner LS, Hochman BN, Plumer MH: Persistent neurologic deficit and adhesive arachnoiditis following intrathecal 2-chloroprocaine injection. Anesth Analg 1980; 59: 452–454.

99. Moore DC, Spierdijk J, vanKleef JD, et al: Chloroprocaine neurotoxicity: four additional cases. Anesth Analg 1982; 61: 155–159.

100. Gissen AJ, Datta S, Lambert DH: The chloroprocaine controversy. I. Hypothesis to explain the neural complications of chloroprocaine epidurals. Reg Anesth 1984; 9: 124–134.

101. Gissen AJ, Datta S, Lambert DH: The chloroprocaine controversy. II. Is chloroprocaine neurotoxic? Reg Anesth 1984; 9: 135–145.

102. Stevens RA, Urmey WF, Urquhart BL, et al: Back pain after epidural anesthesia with chloroprocaine. Anesthesiology 1993; 78: 492–497.

103. Bridenbaugh PO, Tucker GT, Moore DC, et al: Etidocaine: clinical evaluation for intercostal nerve block and lumbar epidural block. Anesth Analg 1973; 52: 407–413.

104. Bromage PR, O'Beirn P, Dunford LA: Etidocaine: a clinical evaluation for regional analgesia in surgery. Can Anaesth Soc J 1974; 21: 523–534.

105. Bromage PR: A comparison of the hydrochloride and carbon dioxide salts of lidocaine and prilocaine in epidural analgesia. Acta Anaesth Scand Suppl 1965; 16: 55–69.

106. Cousins MJ, Bromage PR: A comparison of the hydrochloride and carbonated salts of lidocaine for caudal analgesia in outpatients. Br J Anaesth 1971; 43: 1149–1155.

107. Schulte-Steinberg O: Spread of local anesthetic solutions in caudal blocks in children. (Abstract.) Excerpta Medica Int Congr Series 1976; 387: 132.

108. Albright GA: Cardiac arrest following regional anesthesia with etidocaine or bupivacaine. (Editorial.) Anesthesiology 1979; 51: 285–287.

109. Prentiss JE: Cardiac arrest following caudal anesthesia. Anesthesiology 1979; 50: 51–53.

110. de Jong RH, Ronfeld RA, DeRosa RA: Cardiovascular effects of convulsant and supraconvulsant doses of amide local anesthetics. Anesth Analg 1982; 61: 3–9.

111. Kotelko DM, Shnider SM, Dailey PA, et al: Bupivacaine-induced cardiac arrhythmias in sheep. Anesthesiology 1984; 60: 10–18.

112. Feldman HS, Arthur GR, Covino BG: Comparative systemic toxicity of convulsant and supraconvulsant doses of intravenous ropivacaine, bupivacaine, and lidocaine in the conscious dog. Anesth Analg 1989; 69: 794–801.

113. Brockway MS, Bannister J, McClure JH, et al: Comparison of extradural ropivacaine and bupivacaine. Br J Anaesth 1991; 66: 31–37.

114. Wood MB, Rubin AP: A comparison of epidural 1% ropivacaine and 0.75% bupivacaine for lower abdominal gynecologic surgery. Anesth Analg 1993; 76: 1274–1278.

115. Niesel HC, Eilingsfeld T, Hornung M, et al: Ropivacain 1% versus Bupivacain 0.75% ohne Vasokonstriktor. Vergleichende Untersuchung zur Epiduralanasthesie bei orthopadischen Eingriffen. Anaesthesist 1993; 42: 605–611.

116. Park WY: Factors influencing distribution of local anesthetics in the epidural space. Reg Anesth 1988; 13: 49–57.

117. Grundy EM, Rao LN, Winnie AP: Epidural anesthesia and the lateral position. Anesth Analg 1978; 57: 95–97.

118. Park WY, Hagins FM, Massengale MD, et al: The sitting position and anesthetic spread in the epidural space. Anesth Analg 1984; 63: 863–864.

119. Hodgkinson R, Husain FJ: Obesity, gravity, and spread of epidural anesthesia. Anesth Analg 1981; 60: 421–424.

120. Bromage PR: Epidural Analgesia, pp 141–142. Philadelphia, WB Saunders Co, 1978.

121. Fagraeus L, Urban BJ, Bromage PR: Spread of epidural analgesia in early pregnancy. Anesthesiology 1983; 58: 184–187.

122. Grundy EM, Zamora AM, Winnie AP: Comparison of spread of epidural anesthesia in pregnant and nonpregnant women. Anesth Analg 1978; 57: 544–546.

123. Bromage PR: Epidural Analgesia, pp 142–147. Philadelphia, WB Saunders Co, 1978.

124. Grundy EM, Ramamurthy S, Patel KP, et al: Extradural analgesia revisited. A statistical study. Br J Anaesth 1978; 50: 805–809.

125. Park WY, Hagins FM, Rivat EL, et al: Age and epidural dose response in adult men. Anesthesiology 1982; 56: 318–320.

126. Sharrock NE: Epidural anesthetic dose responses in patients 20 to 80 years old. Anesthesiology 1978; 49: 425–428.

127. Rocco AG, Scott DA, Boas RA, et al: The epidural space behaves as a Starling resistor and inflow resistance is elevated in a diseased epidural space. (Abstract.) Reg Anesth 1990; 15: S39.

128. Stevens RA, Bray JG, Artuso JD, et al: Differential epidural block. Reg Anesth 1992; 17: 22–25.

129. Foldes FF, Colavincenzo JW, Birch JH: Epidural anesthesia: a reappraisal. Curr Res Anesth Analg 1956; 35: 33–47.

130. Bromage PR: Ageing and epidural dose requirements: segmental spread and predictability of epidural analgesia in youth and extreme age. Br J Anaesth 1969; 41: 1016–1022.

131. Bromage PR: Exaggerated spread of epidural analgesia in arteriosclerotic patients: dosage in relation to biological and chronological ageing. Br Med J 1962; 2: 1634–1638.

132. Bromage PR: Epidural Analgesia, pp 31–32. Philadelphia, WB Saunders Co, 1978.

133. Sharrock NE, Mineo R, Urquhart B: Hemodynamic response to low-dose epinephrine infusion during hypotensive epidural anesthesia for total hip replacement. Reg Anesth 1990; 15: 295–299.

134. Sharrock NE, Mineo R, Urquhart B: Haemodynamic effects and outcome analysis of hypotensive extradural anaesthesia in controlled hypertensive patients undergoing total hip arthroplasty. Br J Anaesth 1991; 67: 17–25.

135. Bromage PR: Epidural Analgesia, pp 100–105. Philadelphia, WB Saunders Co, 1978.

136. Bromage PR: Epidural Analgesia, pp 131–135. Philadelphia, WB Saunders Co, 1978.

137. Schulte-Steinberg O, Rahlfs VW: Caudal anaesthesia in children and spread of 1 per cent lignocaine. A statistical study. Br J Anaesth 1970; 42: 1093–1099.

138. Schulte-Steinberg O, Rahlfs VW: Caudal anaesthesia in children and the distribution of 0.25 per cent bupivacaine solution. A statistical study [German]. Anaesthesist 1972; 21: 94–100.

139. Bromage PR: Epidural Analgesia, pp 272–273. Philadelphia, WB Saunders Co, 1978.

140. Thompson JE: An anatomical and experimental study of sacral anaesthesia. Ann Surg 1917; 66: 718–727.

141. Broadman LM, Hannallah RS, Norden JM, et al: "Kiddie caudals": experience with 1154 consecutive cases without complications. (Abstract.) Anesth Analg 1987; 66: S18.

142. Dalens B: Regional anesthesia in children. Anesth Analg 1989; 68: 654–672.

143. Takasaki M, Dohi S, Kawabata Y, et al: Dosage of lidocaine for caudal anesthesia in infants and children. Anesthesiology 1977; 47: 527–529.

144. Sinclair JC, Fox HA, Lentz JF, et al: Intoxication of the fetus by a local anesthetic: a newly recognized complication of maternal caudal anesthesia. N Engl J Med 1965; 273: 1173–1177.

145. Trotter M: Variations of the sacral canal: their significance in the administration of caudal analgesia. Curr Res Anesth Analg 1947; 26: 192–202.

146. Bromage PR: Epidural Analgesia, pp 258–282. Philadelphia, WB Saunders Co, 1978.

147. Cheek TG, Banner R, Sauter J, et al: Prophylactic extradural blood patch is effective. A preliminary communication. Br J Anaesth 1988; 61: 340–342.

148. Bromage PR: Neurologic complications of regional anesthesia for obstetrics. In Shnider SM, Levinson G (eds): Anesthesia for Obstetrics, 3rd ed, pp 433–453. Baltimore, Williams & Wilkins, 1993.

149. Tom DJ, Gulevich SJ, Shapiro HM, et al: Epidural blood patch in the HIV-positive patient. Review of clinical experience. San Diego HIV Neurobehavioral Research Center. Anesthesiology 1992; 76: 943–947.

150. Arndt JO, Hock A, Stanton-Hicks M, et al: Peridural anesthesia and the distribution of blood in supine humans. Anesthesiology 1985; 63: 616–623.

151. Chester WL: Spinal anesthesia, complete heart block, and the precordial chest thump: an unusual complication and a unique resuscitation. Anesthesiology 1988; 69: 600–602.

152. Vandam LD, Dripps RD: Long-term follow-up of patients who received 10,098 spinal anesthetics. IV. Neurological disease incident to traumatic lumbar puncture during spinal anesthesia. JAMA 1960; 172: 1483–1487.

153. Owens EL, Kasten GW, Hessel EA II: Spinal subarachnoid hematoma after lumbar puncture and heparinization: a case report, review of the literature, and discussion of anesthetic implications. Anesth Analg 1986; 65: 1201–1207.

154. Bromage PR: Epidural Analgesia, pp 682–690. Philadelphia, WB Saunders Co, 1978.

155. Moore DC, Bridenbaugh LD: Spinal (subarachnoid) block: a review of 11,574 cases. JAMA 1966; 195: 907–912.

156. Phillips OC, Ebner H, Nelson AT, et al: Neurologic complications following spinal anesthesia with lidocaine: a prospective review of 10,440 cases. Anesthesiology 1969; 30: 284–289.

157. Sadove MS, Levin MJ, Rant-Sejdinaj I: Neurological complications of spinal anaesthesia. Can Anaesth Soc J 1961; 8: 405–416.

158. Mayumi T, Dohi S: Spinal subarachnoid hematoma after lumbar puncture in a patient receiving antiplatelet therapy. Anesth Analg 1983; 62: 777–779.

159. Greensite FS, Katz J: Spinal subdural hematoma associated with attempted epidural anesthesia and subsequent continuous spinal anesthesia. Anesth Analg 1980; 59: 72–73.

160. Odoom JA, Sih IL: Epidural analgesia and anticoagulant therapy. Experience with one thousand cases of continuous epidurals. Anaesthesia 1983; 38: 254–259.

161. Horlocker TT, Wedel DJ, Offord KP: Does preoperative antiplatelet therapy increase the risk of hemorrhagic complications associated with regional anesthesia? Anesth Analg 1990; 70: 631–634.

162. Rao TL, El-Etr AA: Anticoagulation following placement of epidural and subarachnoid catheters: an evaluation of neurologic sequelae. Anesthesiology 1981; 55: 618–620.

163. Mamourian AC, Dickman CA, Drayer BP, et al: Spinal epidural abscess: three cases following spinal epidural injection demonstrated with magnetic resonance imaging. Anesthesiology 1993; 78: 204–207.

164. Du Pen SL, Peterson DG, Williams A, et al: Infection during chronic epidural catheterization: diagnosis and treatment. Anesthesiology 1990; 73: 905–909.

165. Jorgensen NH, Lineberry PJ: Hyperbaric bupivacaine spinal anesthesia is associated with less back pain postoperatively than hyperbaric lidocaine spinal anesthesia. (Abstract.) Reg Anesth 1992; 17: S51.

166. Healy TE, Wilkins RG: Patient posture and the anaesthetist. Ann R Coll Surg Engl 1984; 66: 56–58.

CHAPTER 20
Sympathetic Nerve Blocks

Tim J. Lamer, M.D.

Anatomy of the Sympathetic Nervous System

The sympathetic neurons have their cell bodies in the intermediolateral column of the thoracic and upper lumbar spinal cord. The axons leave the cord through the ventral roots and reach the sympathetic trunks (or chains) through the white rami communicantes (Figs. 20–1 and 20–2). On reaching the sympathetic trunk, preganglionic sympathetic fibers may take one of three courses (Figs. 20–1 and 20–3): synapse with postganglionic sympathetic neurons in the homologous paravertebral sympathetic ganglion; continue up or down the sympathetic trunk a variable distance to synapse with postganglionic sympathetic neurons in a distant paravertebral ganglion; or pass through the sympathetic trunk to synapse with postganglionic sympathetic neurons in a remote prevertebral ganglion (e.g., celiac ganglion). Postganglionic sympathetic fibers pass from the paravertebral sympathetic trunks through gray rami communicantes or from the prevertebral plexuses to their final destination. Major targets of sympathetic efferent fibers include blood vessels, visceral smooth muscles, and visceral secretory organs (Table 20–1 and see Fig. 20–3).[1]

The paravertebral sympathetic trunks are a series of ganglia and connecting cords along the anterolateral vertebral column (see Fig. 20–2). Although the preganglionic sympathetic cell bodies are confined to the thoracolumbar cord, the sympathetic trunk is located along the entire length of the vertebral column, from the foramen magnum to the distal sacrum. At the caudal end, the right and left trunks fuse together to form a small but recognizable ganglion, the ganglion impar (see Fig. 20–2). A technique to block the ganglion impar has been described but is of dubious value because few if any pain fibers pass through this structure.[2] The regional anatomy of the sympathetic trunks is considered in more detail in subsequent sections.

Preverterbral Sympathetic Nerves and Plexuses

Thoracic Splanchnic Nerves

Several sympathetic fibers originating from approximately T-5 to T-12 coalesce anterior to the lower thoracic vertebral bodies into one to three recognizable splanchnic nerves (see Fig. 20–2). When all three nerves are present, they are named the greater, lesser, and least splanchnic nerves. These splanchnic nerves consist of preganglionic sympathetic fibers that relay sympathetic efferent input to the abdominal viscera by forming synapses with postganglionic sympathetic neurons in the aortic plexuses. Additionally, the tho-

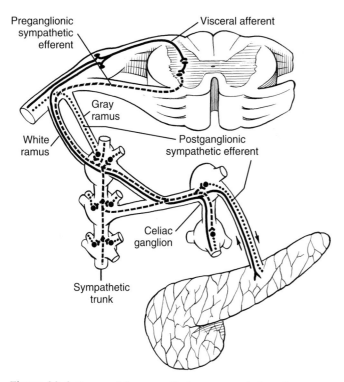

Figure 20–1 Course of the sympathetic nerves and visceral afferent (pain) fibers.

racic splanchnic nerves relay afferent impulses from the abdominal viscera. The thoracic splanchnic nerves lie along the thoracic vertebral column and enter the abdomen through the crus of the diaphragm or, more commonly, through a small defect in the diaphragm just lateral to the crus. The fibers then become enmeshed in and part of the celiac plexus.

Lumbar Splanchnic Nerves

Several sympathetic fibers from the upper lumbar sympathetic ganglia coalesce into lumbar splanchnic nerves, consisting of sympathetic efferent fibers to the lower abdominal and pelvic viscera (see Fig. 20–2). Lower abdominal and pelvic viscera may receive sympathetic efferent input from thoracic and lumbar splanchnics. As a result of this dual sympathetic input, interruption of thoracic splanchnic nerves does not completely abolish sympathetic efferent input to the lower abdominal and pelvic viscera.

Table 20–1 Effect of Sympathetic Block on Effector Organ Function

ORGAN	RESPONSE TO SYMPATHETIC BLOCK
Pupil	Constriction
Sweat glands	Decreased secretion
Salivary glands	Decreased secretion
Cutaneous blood vessels	Vasodilation
Heart	Decreased rate
	Decreased contractility
Intestines	Increased peristalsis

Aortic Plexuses

The thoracic splanchnic nerves pierce through the diaphragm and, on entering the abdomen, diverge into a network of fibers along the anterior surface of the aorta. Similarly, there is a contribution of sympathetic efferent fibers to this plexus from the lumbar splanchnic nerves. This network or plexus extends from the diaphragm caudad into the pelvis (see Fig. 20–2). This aortic plexus has several named structures, most notably the celiac, superior mesenteric, inferior mesenteric, and superior hypogastric plexuses. These plexuses contain preganglionic sympathetic efferent fibers from approximately T-5 to L-2, postganglionic sympathetic efferent fibers to the abdominal viscera, parasympathetic efferent fibers from the vagus nerves, and visceral afferent (sensory) fibers. Distinct ganglia exist within these plexuses, formed by synaptic connections between preganglionic and postganglionic sympathetic efferents.

Visceral Afferent Fibers and Visceral Pain

Visceral afferent fibers, including nociceptive (pain) afferents, course from the abdominal and thoracic viscera to the spinal cord along the path of the visceral sympathetic efferent fibers (see Fig. 20–1).[3] It is this anatomic convenience that allows us to block visceral nociceptive (pain) fibers when we block the celiac plexus and other visceral sympathetic plexuses and nerves. In addition to nociceptive transmission, these afferent fibers convey other sensory information, including hunger, nausea, and stretch (e.g., airway smooth muscle, baroreceptors).

In general, visceral afferent fibers from the abdomen course through the aortic plexuses, then through the thoracic splanchnics, and then through the thoracic and upper lumbar paravertebral sympathetic trunks on their way to the dorsal horn of the spinal cord. Some fibers from pelvic and lower abdominal viscera also course through the lumbar splanchnic nerves.[4]

Although anatomists disagree about their significance, there are visceral afferent fibers from the pelvic viscera coursing through the pelvic splanchnic nerves.[2, 4] The pelvic splanchnic nerves originate from S-1 through S-4 and consist primarily of parasympathetic efferent fibers to the pelvic viscera. The pelvic splanchnic nerves do not contain sympathetic fibers. Lower abdominal and pelvic structures may send visceral nociceptive afferents back to the spinal cord through the lumbar splanchnics, the pelvic splanchnics, and the thoracic splanchnics through the aortic plexuses.[2, 4] The existence of these multiple pathways makes it difficult to effectively block pain originating from lower abdominal and pelvic structures, unlike the upper abdominal visceral afferents, which course almost exclusively through the celiac plexus and thoracic splanchnic nerves.

Cranial Sympathetic System

The sympathetic efferents to the head and face originate from T-1 to T-4 and course through the cervical sympathetic trunk and the jugular foramen and then

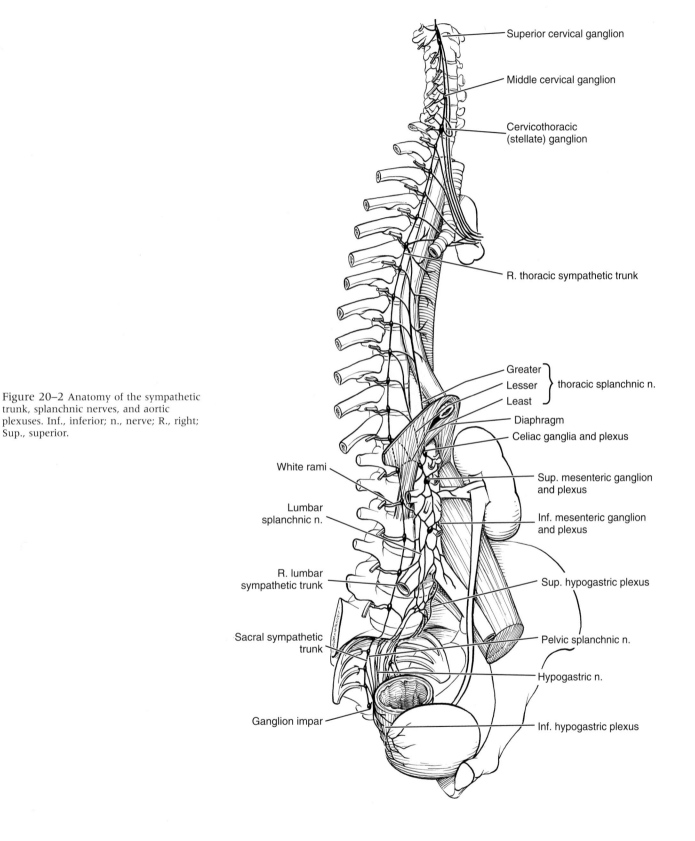

Figure 20–2 Anatomy of the sympathetic trunk, splanchnic nerves, and aortic plexuses. Inf., inferior; n., nerve; R., right; Sup., superior.

Superior cervical ganglion

Middle cervical ganglion

Cervicothoracic (stellate) ganglion

R. thoracic sympathetic trunk

Greater
Lesser } thoracic splanchnic n.
Least

Diaphragm

Celiac ganglia and plexus

Sup. mesenteric ganglion and plexus

Inf. mesenteric ganglion and plexus

Sup. hypogastric plexus

Pelvic splanchnic n.

Hypogastric n.

Inf. hypogastric plexus

White rami

Lumbar splanchnic n.

R. lumbar sympathetic trunk

Sacral sympathetic trunk

Ganglion impar

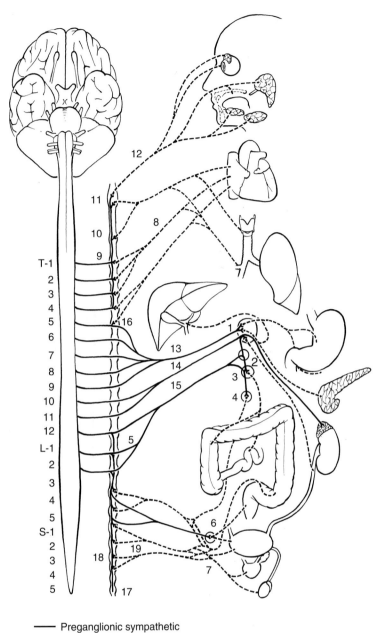

Figure 20–3 Course of preganglionic and postganglionic sympathetic fibers to effector organs. 1, Celiac ganglia and plexus; 2, aorticorenal ganglia and plexus; 3, superior mesenteric ganglion and plexus; 4, inferior mesenteric ganglion and plexus; 5, lumbar sympathetic trunk; 6, superior hypogastric ganglion and plexus; 7, inferior hypogastric plexus; 8, cardiac nerves; 9, cervicothoracic (stellate) ganglion; 10, middle cervical ganglion; 11, superior cervical ganglion; 12, carotid nerve; 13, greater thoracic splanchnic nerve; 14, lesser thoracic splanchnic nerve; 15, least thoracic splanchnic nerve; 16, thoracic sympathetic trunk; 17, ganglion impar; 18, sacral sympathetic trunk; 19, pelvic splanchnic nerves.

—— Preganglionic sympathetic
----- Postganglionic sympathetic

distribute along the sensory nerves of the head and neck and internal and external carotid arteries and their branches. Sympathetic efferents project to the intrinsic eye muscles, sweat glands, salivary glands, mucous membranes of the nose and pharynx, and cutaneous blood vessels.[4, 5] Some afferent sensory nerves from intracranial structures (e.g., meninges, blood vessels) pass along the course of these sympathetic efferent fibers. Sympathetic efferents and possibly some intracranial afferent fibers course through the ciliary, otic, and pterygopalatine ganglia.

Physiology of Sympathetic Block

Vascular Effects

Sympathetic stimulation usually results in arterial and venous constriction, and sympathetic block gener-

ally results in arterial and venous dilation. The net clinical effect of sympathetic block is an increase in blood flow to the affected body region. Extensive sympathetic block, such as occurs after celiac plexus or bilateral lumbar sympathetic block, results in extensive venodilation and sequestration of large volumes of blood in the affected vascular beds. This accumulation of blood within dilated vascular beds can be sufficient to lower venous return to the heart, leading to decreased cardiac output, decreased blood pressure, or both.

Block of sympathetic fibers to the limbs leads to a significant increase in blood flow in the extremity, with the distal limb blood flow increasing proportionately more than the proximal limb blood flow. Skin blood flow, measured by laser Doppler flowometry and transcutaneous oxygen tension, increases to a greater degree than does muscle blood flow. Extremity blood flow is profoundly affected by muscle activity, the temperature of the environment, the presence of vascular disease, and the existence of collateral blood flow and arteriovenous shunts. In patients with severe peripheral vascular disease, a paradoxical reduction in blood flow to ischemic areas may develop after sympathetic block.[6] Presumably, severely ischemic areas are already maximally vasodilated in their preblock state and will not vasodilate in response to sympathetic block. Nearby nonischemic tissue may vasodilate and blood may be diverted away from the ischemic tissue. This vascular steal phenomenon is well described in the literature, but it is not clear how often it occurs. Extensive experience with sympathetic block in patients with vascular disease suggests that this steal phenomenon is not a common occurrence.

Fujita[7] studied the effect of celiac plexus block on splanchnic circulation and found venous dilation was much more prominent than arterial dilation. The net effect was venous pooling of blood in the splanchnic bed, with a significant decrease in arterial blood pressure and cardiac output. This effect on the systemic circulation overshadowed the minimal increase in splanchnic arterial blood flow, and the net effect was a decrease in splanchnic blood flow owing to decreased cardiac output.

Cardiac Effects

Sympathetic stimulation of the heart results in positive inotropic and positive chronotropic effects. Extensive (bilateral) sympathetic block of the heart leads to decreased contractility, decreased heart rate, and a significant decrease in myocardial oxygen demand. Unilateral sympathetic block of the heart does not affect myocardial contractility.

Unilateral sympathetic block of the heart has a variable effect on the heart rate and rhythm. In a study[8] performed in normal volunteers, right stellate ganglion block resulted in a diminished heart rate and a prolonged QT interval, but a left stellate ganglion block had no effect on the rate or rhythm. This observation is consistent with the identification of asymmetric sympathetic activity to the heart in patients with prolonged QT syndromes (e.g., torsade de pointes) in which dominant left-sided sympathetic input seems to facilitate the development of the prolonged QT interval. Left stellate ganglion block in this group of patients provides benefit by shortening the QT interval and decreasing the propensity for arrhythmias to develop.[9, 10]

Effects on Visceral Smooth Muscle

Postganglionic sympathetic fibers innervate the myenteric and submucosal plexuses of the intestinal tract. Strong sympathetic stimulation inhibits gastrointestinal motility and secretory activity. Clinically, increased sympathetic activity, such as occurs as part of the stress response after trauma or surgery, can lead to gastric

stasis and intestinal ileus. Sympathetic block results in a transient increase in gastric emptying and intestinal motility. There is no effect on esophageal motility, gallbladder activity, and sphincter of Oddi tone.[1]

Bladder control, ejaculation, and erection are controlled mainly by parasympathetic activity, but the bladder neck, trigone, and seminal vesicles are controlled by sympathetic efferents. Bilateral sympathetic block of these structures can impair seminal emission and bladder neck closure, resulting in retrograde ejaculation and impotence.

Methods to Measure Sympathetic Block

To perform sympathetic blocks, a thorough understanding of anatomy is essential. Anesthesiologists rely heavily on cutaneous topographic landmarks and their relationship to underlying structures. These landmarks can be supplemented with radiologic imaging techniques, and correct needle placement and spread of injectant can be verified by using radiopaque contrast materials. However, none of these methods guarantees a successful block, nor does the mere demonstration of a properly placed needle or an appropriate contrast pattern indicate a successful block. Confirmation of a physiologic block can be accomplished by various techniques (Table 20–2).

Pain Relief

In most cases, a sympathetic block is performed to relieve some painful condition, and some clinicians could argue that the ultimate confirmatory test is whether the patient's pain is relieved by the block. Although pain relief is a crucial indicator, sole reliance on this indicator may lead to erroneous conclusions regarding the nature of the patient's pain problem and can lead to erroneous follow-up treatment.

The interpretation of the pain relief experienced by a patient after a sympathetic block may be influenced by the effect of systemic local anesthetic absorption on the painful condition, coincidental block of other structures that may affect the patient's pain, and the placebo effect.

Most sympathetic blocks are performed with dosages of local anesthetics that lead to significant systemic

Table 20–2 Methods to Confirm Sympathetic Block

Pain relief
Functional improvement
Sweat tests
Laser Doppler flowometry
Ultrasonography
Cutaneous temperature
Transcutaneous oximetry
Thermography
Limb plethysmography
Quantitative sudomotor axon reflex test (QSART)
Skin conductance

vascular uptake of the anesthetic. Several studies[11, 12] have demonstrated that systemic local anesthetics may result in significant pain relief in various neuropathic pain states. It is often useful to assess a patient's response to systemic lidocaine with an intravenous injection of lidocaine before embarking on a course of invasive sympathetic blocks.

In most areas of the body, the somatic nerves are not far from the sympathetic trunk. Because sympathetic nerves accompany somatic nerves to the periphery, a somatic nerve block usually is accompanied by signs of sympathetic block. Unintentional and unrecognized block of the brachial plexus during a stellate ganglion block or block of the lumbar plexus during a lumbar sympathetic block is accompanied by some or all the usual signs of a successful sympathetic block. However, it may not be possible to determine whether pain relief in this situation results from the somatic block or the sympathetic block. It is essential to assess the presence of sensory or motor block, or both, after a sympathetic block to make an accurate assessment of the block. It would be unfortunate to subject a patient to an unnecessary neurolytic sympathetic block on the basis of pain relief from an unrecognized somatic nerve or plexus block.

Patients with chronic painful conditions hope and anticipate that the physician will be able to relieve their pain. This setting is conducive to a placebo response. Unfortunately, there is no reliable way to identify this response. Some clinicians routinely include a sham injection as part of their therapeutic intervention when performing a series of blocks. There are advantages and disadvantages to this approach; however, it is essential to obtain informed consent from the patient before embarking on a series of injections that includes a sham injection. Haddox and Kettler[13] demonstrated that saline is a reasonable vehicle for a sham injection, because saline stellate ganglion injection does not result in a sympathetic block.

Functional Improvement

When starting a series of sympathetic blocks, it is useful to look for functional improvement in addition to pain relief. Increased range of motion after a sympathetic block in patients with reflex sympathetic dystrophy, increased walking tolerance in patients with claudication, decreased consumption of potent analgesics, and improved gastrointestinal function after celiac plexus block are just a few examples of clinical indicators.

Clinical Tests of Sympathetic Function

Several tests are available to help document objective evidence of successful sympathetic block. Cutaneous temperature monitoring is a useful and readily available test. Sweat testing, skin conductance, thermography, limb blood flow, and quantitative sudomotor axon reflex testing require specialized equipment.

Cutaneous temperature measurement is an indirect measure of sympathetic function and is the method most commonly used to assess the response to sympathetic block. The necessary equipment is relatively inexpensive and does not require special training for use and interpretation. Conversely, thermography requires expensive equipment and specially trained personnel, and there is no evidence that thermography is of any more benefit than cutaneous temperature monitoring.[14] Skin temperature should be monitored bilaterally, taking care to avoid placing the patient near air-conditioning or heating vents. Temperature sensors or thermometers should be placed on the palmar surface of the hands or the plantar surface of the feet. Additional measurements should be taken along the axis of the extremities. In general, an increase of 2° C or more indicates a successful block. Patients with severe peripheral vascular disease and patients with a high preblock skin temperature (34° C or more) may not have a significant temperature increase after a block.

Sweat gland secretion is under sympathetic efferent control. Sympathetic denervation from a sympathetic block can be measured by applying a moisture-sensitive indicator.[15] I use a powdered starch alizarin indicator, which is dusted on the patient's limb and changes from yellow to purple when exposed to moisture. Lack of sweating is indicated by failure of the indicator to turn purple when the patient is exposed to a warm temperature and humidity-controlled environment and is strong confirmatory evidence of a sympathetic block.

Various techniques are available to measure blood flow in a limb. They are most valuable in assessing the response to sympathetic block in patients with severe peripheral vascular disease. Skin blood flow can be measured by laser Doppler flowometry or indirectly by transcutaneous oximetry.[16] Muscle blood flow is most often determined indirectly by venous occlusion plethysmography.[17] Limb blood flow can be measured intraoperatively by placing an electromagnetic flowmeter directly on surgically exposed blood vessels or percutaneously by using an ultrasound probe. These techniques require special equipment and training to operate and interpret.

Changes in skin conductance in response to a sensory stimulus such as a skin pinch or exposure to cold can be used to assess sympathetic function. In the cold pressor test, failure of the skin conductance to change in response to a cold stimulus is strong confirmatory evidence of sympathetic block, but a successful sympathetic block does not always abolish the response.[18]

The quantitative sudomotor axon reflex test is another measure of sweat output as a test of sympathetic function. A sympathetic block diminishes or abolishes the sweat output after methacholine iontophoresis (Catherine Willner, M.D.: personal communication). This technique is used in a few centers with sophisticated autonomic testing capabilities.

Cervical Sympathetic Block

Anatomy

Sympathetic efferent fibers to the head, neck, and upper extremities originate in the upper thoracic spinal cord from T-1 to approximately T-6. These sympathetic efferent fibers enter the thoracic sympathetic trunks and course cephalad to the cervical sympathetic trunks and ganglia. In the 1920s, Kuntz[19] described sympathetic fibers to the upper extremities that bypass the cervical sympathetic trunk. Their significance remains uncertain, but it is clear that these fibers are not blocked by the usual cervical sympathetic (stellate ganglion) block.

The cervical sympathetic trunk extends from the base of the skull to the first thoracic vertebra, lying on the ventral surface of the longus colli and longus capitis muscles (Fig. 20–4). There are one to four identifiable cervical ganglia. The inferior cervical ganglion often is fused with the first thoracic ganglion to form the cervicothoracic or stellate ganglion. The middle cervical ganglion is usually identified overlying the C-6 transverse process. The superior cervical ganglion is identified overlying the upper two to three cervical vertebral transverse processes.

Cervical sympathetic block is usually performed at approximately C-6. The block is technically easier and safer at this level than at the cervicothoracic or stellate ganglion. At the level of C-6, the sympathetic trunk is bounded posteriorly by the longus colli muscle and prevertebral fascia overlying the C-6 transverse process, anteromedially by the laryngopharyngeal structures, and anterolaterally by the scalene muscles, the carotid sheath (i.e., carotid artery, internal jugular vein, and vagus nerve), and the sternocleidomastoid muscle (Figs. 20–4 through 20–7). The vertebral artery and cervical nerve roots lie just deep to the anterior tubercle of the transverse process and are easily accessible to a needle that has passed a bit too deep (see Fig. 20–4). Other structures in the vicinity include the recurrent laryngeal nerve, the phrenic nerve, and the thyroid gland and vessels.

Indications and Efficacy

Sympathectomy was first used to treat epilepsy in the late 1800s and spastic paraplegia in the early 1900s.[5] Since then, cervical sympathetic block has been used to treat a seemingly endless list of conditions, ranging from chronic tinnitus to quinine poisoning (Table 20–3). As our understanding of disease pathophysiology has advanced, the indications for sympathetic block have been reduced to the treatment of reflex sympathetic dystrophy and causalgia, hyperhidrosis of the extremities, peripheral vascular disease with painful ischemic neuropathy or poor tissue perfusion, and possibly herpetic neuralgia.[20–27] The use of sympathetic blocks for all of these conditions is based on anecdotal series and case reports, rather than controlled clinical trials. Even the time-honored series of sympathetic blocks for reflex sympathetic dystrophy is based on a large body of case reports and anecdotes, and it is possible that the role of sympathetic blocks will diminish as our understanding of reflex sympathetic dystrophy and other painful neuropathic conditions advances.[28]

Because a large body of evidence lends support to the role of sympathetic block for certain conditions and because they are, for the most part, debilitating conditions, sympathetic blocks will continue to play a significant role in their treatment until further study identifies alternative treatment modalities. Studies with systemic sympatholytic drugs for reflex sympathetic dystrophy, systemic lidocaine or lidocaine-like drugs for neuropathic pain, and N-methyl-D-aspartate acid receptor antagonists for neuropathic pain are examples of promising therapy.[11, 29, 30]

There are many published recipes and algorithms for the use of cervical sympathetic block for reflex sympathetic dystrophy and other neuropathic painful

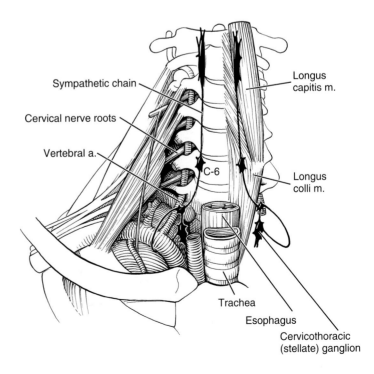

Figure 20–4 Regional anatomy of the cervical sympathetic trunk. Notice the proximity of the sympathetic trunk to the vertebral artery (a.) and the cervical nerve roots. m., muscle.

Sympathetic chain

Cervical nerve roots

Vertebral a.

Longus capitis m.

C-6

Longus colli m.

Trachea

Esophagus

Cervicothoracic (stellate) ganglion

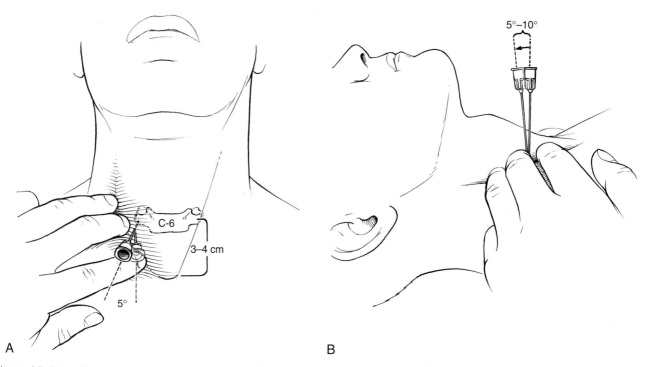

Figure 20–5 Needle placement for cervical sympathetic block at C-6. *A,* If the transverse process is not encountered on the first pass, the needle is withdrawn to the subcutaneous tissue and advanced 5° to 10° more medially. *B,* If the transverse process is not encountered on this pass, the needle is withdrawn and advanced 5° to 10° caudally.

conditions. Many experienced clinicians have developed their own successful approaches, and it is necessary to interview only a handful of pain management specialists to see that there are various algorithms or approaches.

My usual approach is based on the current literature and clinical experience. In a blinded fashion, the patient receives an intravenous infusion of lidocaine (1 to 2 mg/kg over 5 min). If the patient achieves significant pain relief, I perform a series of intravenous

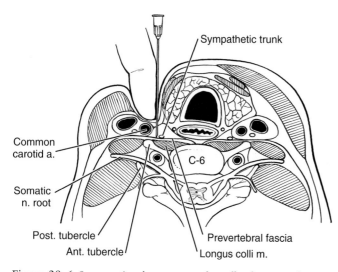

Figure 20–6 Cross-sectional anatomy and needle placement for cervical sympathetic block at C-6. Notice the gentle retraction of the carotid artery (a.) and sheath by the fingertips of the nondominant hand. Ant., anterior; m., muscle; Post., posterior.

injections of lidocaine, or if there are no contraindications, I treat the patient with mexiletine given orally.[31, 32] If the patient does not obtain relief from the lidocaine, I perform a blinded intravenous infusion of phentolamine (0.4 mg/kg over 20 to 30 min). If the patient achieves pain relief, I perform a series of intravenously administered phentolamine blocks or treat the patient with an adrenergic blocking agent given orally.[29, 33] The rationale for the diagnostic and therapeutic use of lidocaine and phentolamine in patients with reflex sympathetic dystrophy is based on relatively recent investigations. The role of these and other agents for reflex sympathetic dystrophy and other neuropathic pain states may change as our understanding of these conditions advances.

If the patient does not respond to lidocaine or phentolamine, I perform a diagnostic cervical sympathetic ganglion block. If the patient achieves pain relief from

Table 20–3 Conditions Reported to Respond to Sympathetic Block

Reflex sympathetic dystrophy
Raynaud's disease
Chronic tinnitus (stellate block)
Visceral thoracic pain
Herpetic neuralgia
Phantom limb pain
Causalgia
Peripheral vascular disease
Quinine poisoning (stellate block)
Hyperhidrosis
Post–cardiac surgery pain syndrome
Frostbite injury

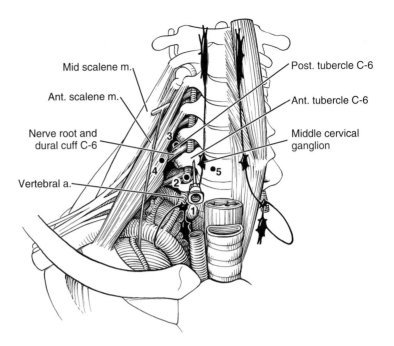

Figure 20–7 1, Correct needle placement for cervical sympathetic block; 2, incorrect placement in the vertebral artery (a.); 3, incorrect placement near a cervical nerve root; 4, incorrect placement laterally in the scalene muscle (m.); 5, incorrect placement too far medial. Ant., anterior; Mid, middle; Post., posterior.

the diagnostic block, I perform a series of blocks in conjunction with a physical therapy program. To perform a series, it is necessary to determine how long the diagnostic block produces pain relief. If the duration of the block is less than 24 h, blocks are performed daily, and if greater than 24 h, an every-other-day schedule is reasonable. I continue the series as long as the patient shows improvement in function and pain relief (usually three to seven blocks). When the patient can tolerate appropriate physical therapy without the blocks, I stop the series. If after three to seven blocks, the patient achieves temporary relief only for the duration of the anesthetic, followed by regression to baseline as the anesthetic wears off, I consider neurolytic or surgical sympathectomy or a trial of spinal cord stimulation. Neurolytic and surgical cervical sympathectomy are not recommended because of a high frequency of side effects and complications. The ablative procedures of choice are upper thoracic neurolytic sympathetic block or endoscopic thoracic sympathectomy.[34, 35]

There are physicians who reverse my approach to sympatholysis and use cervical sympathetic ganglion block before attempts with intravenous injection of lidocaine or phentolamine.

Technique

The most commonly used anterior paratracheal approach to the cervical sympathetic trunk is described in this section. The block is most commonly performed at the C-6 level, rather than at the stellate ganglion. Although it is a misnomer, the block at C-6 is commonly referred to as a stellate ganglion block. A block more caudally at C-7 carries a greater risk of intravascular injection and pneumothorax, and caudal spread of the injectant toward the stellate ganglion is no

greater with injection at C-7 than it is at C-6. The procedure is performed as follows:

1. The patient is placed in the supine position with the head extended and the lower jaw relaxed. If the patient has a short neck, it helps to place a small pillow or rolled-up towel under the shoulders to facilitate neck extension.

2. Surface landmarks are identified. The nondominant hand is used to identify the anterior surface of the C-6 transverse process (i.e., Chassaignac tubercle) by gentle palpation with the index and middle finger in the groove between the trachea and the sternocleidomastoid muscle at the level of the cricoid cartilage. If the cricoid cartilage is difficult to identify, the C-6 transverse process can be readily identified 3 to 4 cm cephalad to the sternal notch (see Fig. 20–5A).

3. The puncture area is prepared with alcohol or a povidone-iodine solution.

4. Skin and subcutaneous local anesthesia is optional but may be beneficial in patients in whom the procedure is anticipated to be difficult because of the anatomy or when a less experienced physician is performing the block.

5. The index, middle, and ring fingers of the nondominant hand of the physician are placed in the groove between the trachea and the sternocleidomastoid muscle of the patient. The previously marked spot overlying the C-6 transverse process should be between the index and middle fingers. The sternocleidomastoid muscle is gently retracted laterally. The carotid pulse should be felt on the palmar surface of the fingertips and provides reassurance that the artery is not in the path of the needle (see Figs. 20–5 and 20–6).

6. With the anesthesiologist's dominant hand, a 4-cm, 23- to 25-G needle attached to a prefilled syringe is carefully advanced directly perpendicular to the anticipated location of the C-6 transverse process between

the index and middle fingers of the physician's non-dominant hand. The C-6 transverse process should be contacted at a depth of 2.5 to 3 cm, except in patients with obese or muscular necks.

7. When the C-6 transverse process is contacted with the needle, the physician's nondominant hand is removed from the patient's neck and is used to stabilize the needle. The needle is grasped at the hub, using the thumb and index finger while the ulnar or hypothenar aspect of the hand gently rests on the patient's neck. This ensures needle stability if the patient coughs or swallows.

8. The nondominant hand withdraws the needle 3 mm to avoid injection within the longus colli muscle (see Fig. 20–6).

9. The dominant hand gently aspirates for blood and cerebrospinal fluid. After negative aspiration, a 0.5-mL test dose of local anesthetic is injected. After waiting 30 s, the injection can be completed by injecting 10 mL of local anesthetic over 30 s. Faster injection overdistends the soft tissues in the neck and results in the patient experiencing pain in the back of the neck or interscapular region. A 0.25% concentration of bupivacaine is a suitable agent for most blocks.

10. The anesthesiologist monitors for evidence of a successful sympathetic block. Block of the sympathetic supply to the head is indicated by Horner's syndrome: ptosis, miosis, enophthalmos, and anhidrosis of the ipsilateral eye and side of the face. Successful block of the sympathetic supply to the upper extremity is indicated by increased temperature ($\geq 2°$ C increase) and decreased sweating. Occasionally, it is necessary to conduct specialized testing. A successful cervical sympathetic block should result in Horner's syndrome, but the Horner's syndrome indicates a sympathetic block to the head and does not necessarily indicate a successful sympathetic block of the upper extremity.

Troubleshooting

Failure to Contact the Transverse Process

Failure to contact the transverse process indicates that the needle trajectory is too lateral, too cephalad, or too caudad. The needle is withdrawn to the subcutaneous tissue and redirected 5° to 10° medially and then advanced again (see Fig. 20–5A). If bone is not contacted, the needle is withdrawn again, redirected 5° to 10° caudally, and advanced again (see Fig. 20–5B). If bone is not contacted on this attempt, it is best to remove the needle, reassess the landmarks, and start over.

Paresthesia of the Arm or Shoulder

Arm or shoulder paresthesia indicates that the needle has contacted the brachial plexus or a nerve root and that the advancing needle is too deep, too far lateral, or too cephalad (see Fig. 20–7). The needle is withdrawn, and the procedure is begun again.

Blood or Fluid in the Syringe

If blood or clear fluid (i.e., cerebrospinal fluid) appears in the hub of the needle or the syringe, the needle has gone too deep. The anesthesiologist must withdraw, redirect, and again advance the needle.

Signs of a Successful Sympathetic Block Are Absent Despite a Technically Successful Block

The signs of a successful sympathetic block may not be apparent for any of three reasons. First, the needle makes proper contact with the anterior tubercle of the C-6 transverse process but is not withdrawn sufficiently, resulting in an intramuscular injection into the longus colli muscle. Second, the posterior tubercle of the transverse process is contacted and incorrectly assumed to be the anterior tubercle. This leads to injection in the area of the cervical nerve roots and often results in a paravertebral nerve root or brachial plexus block. Third, the needle is withdrawn too far, and the injection is too superficial.

Evidence of Adequate Sympathetic Block to the Head but Inadequate Sympathetic Block to the Extremity

There are three possible explanations for evidence of adequate sympathetic block to the head (Horner's syndrome) but inadequate sympathetic block to the extremity. First, the vasculature of the upper extremity is severely diseased and is incapable of vasodilation in response to sympathectomy. In this case, evidence of a successful sympathetic block can be obtained with one of the sweat testing methods. Second, the attempt may have resulted in a failure to block the nerves of Kuntz. Third, the injectant may not have spread caudally to anesthetize the stellate (cervicothoracic) ganglion. This is the most likely explanation.

Investigations indicate that failure of the injectant to spread caudally occurs commonly as a result of an anatomic barrier. Guntamukkala and Hardy[36] injected methylene blue around the cervical sympathetic trunk at C-6 in cadavers and demonstrated that as the dye spread caudally, it tracked anteriorly into the prevertebral space and posterior mediastinum, rather than into the region of the cervicothoracic and upper thoracic sympathetic trunk. Hogan and colleagues[37] used magnetic resonance imaging to determine the spread of saline injected at C-6 and C-7 in humans. As the solution tracked caudally beyond C-7, it failed to spread to the stellate ganglion, instead tracking anterior to the ganglion along the prevertebral fascia of the neck and chest. Other studies[38–40] have demonstrated that cervical sympathetic blocks frequently fail to produce evidence of complete sympathetic block to the upper extremity. In cases in which complete sympathetic denervation is necessary and cannot be achieved by using an anterior paratracheal approach, it may be preferable to use a posterior approach to the upper thoracic sympathetic trunk.

Prolonged Cervical Sympathetic Block

When a series of sympathetic blocks results in temporary relief of symptoms and a long-term sympathectomy is desired, there are three options available: catheter techniques for continuous infusion, neurolytic sympathectomy, or surgical sympathectomy.

Various convenient cervical sympathetic or stellate ganglion catheter kits are available from several manufacturers. The technique involves placing a needle in the area of the cervical sympathetic trunk and then passing a catheter through the needle.[41, 42] The needle is removed, the catheter is secured, and the position is confirmed with 1 to 2 mL of radiopaque contrast material, followed by injection of 10 mL of local anesthetic to confirm a satisfactory sympathetic block. An infusion pump for ambulatory use can be attached to the catheter for continuous local anesthetic infusion, or the catheter can be injected daily.

Surgical and neurolytic sympathetic blocks of the cervical sympathetic trunk are attended by a significant risk of side effects and complications and are best avoided in most circumstances. Surgical or neurolytic sympathetic blocks for the upper extremity are best accomplished by an upper thoracic sympathectomy.

Complications and Side Effects

Side effects to be expected as an extension of the physiologic response to cervical sympathetic block include nasal stuffiness, hemicranial (migraine-like) headache, conjunctival injection, ptosis, erythema, and warmth of the face and arm.

Side effects from local anesthetic spread to other tissues and nerves in the area include phrenic nerve block; unilateral vocal cord paralysis from recurrent laryngeal nerve block, which manifests clinically as hoarseness; and brachial plexus or cervical nerve root anesthesia. Bilateral cervical sympathetic blocks are not recommended because of possible bilateral recurrent laryngeal or phrenic nerve blocks.

Complications include intravascular injection (usually into the vertebral artery) leading to seizure or cardiovascular collapse, intrathecal or epidural injection if the needle penetrates a dural cuff accompanying a cervical nerve root, pneumothorax, and trauma to the thoracic duct, thyroid gland, trachea, esophagus, and cervical nerve roots.

Summary

The cervical sympathetic trunk is most commonly blocked at C-6 because of the accessible location and lower likelihood of complications at this site. The injectant spreads caudally toward the stellate ganglion but does not reliably anesthetize the stellate ganglion and the nerves of Kuntz. If complete interruption of the sympathetic efferent supply to the arm is necessary, the block should be performed in the upper thoracic area.

Thoracic Sympathetic Block

Anatomy and Physiology

The right and left thoracic sympathetic trunks consist of a series of 10 to 12 ganglia and the connecting interganglionic cords. The thoracic trunks course along the thoracic vertebral column, lying posterior to the pleura and in front of the neck of the first rib (Fig. 20–8). The thoracic trunk sends sympathetic efferents to the head, neck, upper extremities, and thoracic and abdominal viscera and blood vessels. Visceral afferent sensory fibers from the abdomen and thorax lie along the course of the thoracic sympathetic trunks on their way to the spinal cord.

Yarzebski and Wilkinson[43] studied the location of the T-2 and T-3 sympathetic ganglia and found them along the dorsolateral surface of the vertebral body, just rostral to the midpoint of the vertebral bodies and between the heads of the ribs. A sympathetic block at T-2 or T-3 blocks sympathetic efferent output to the head, neck, and upper extremity, including fibers that often are missed when performing an anterior paratracheal cervical sympathetic block.[44] Because oculopupillary efferents originate primarily from T-1, interruption of the trunk at T-2 or T-3 often does not produce Horner's syndrome.[5]

Indications

The upper (T-2 or T-3) thoracic sympathetic block is used for the same conditions outlined in the section on cervical sympathetic blocks.[45–47] Because the anterior paratracheal approach is less cumbersome, easier to perform, and less invasive and because most patients seem to respond adequately to this approach, most patients can be managed with a cervical sympathetic block. The upper thoracic sympathetic block should be considered for a patient who does not respond to cervical sympathetic blocks but for whose condition the physician strongly suspects there is a sympathetic component.

There are few specific indications in the literature for middle and lower thoracic sympathetic block. In theory, visceral pain from the heart, esophagus, and other thoracic structures should be amenable to treatment with thoracic sympathetic blocks; however, such treatment would require multiple needles placed bilaterally to provide complete visceral afferent interruption. The risk of bilateral pneumothoraces would be considerable and perhaps prohibitive.

Technique

To minimize the risk of pneumothorax, this block should be performed with radiologic imaging. Fluoroscopy and computed tomography have been used successfully, although pneumothorax would seem to be less likely with computed tomographic guidance, because the lung can be visualized and the needle

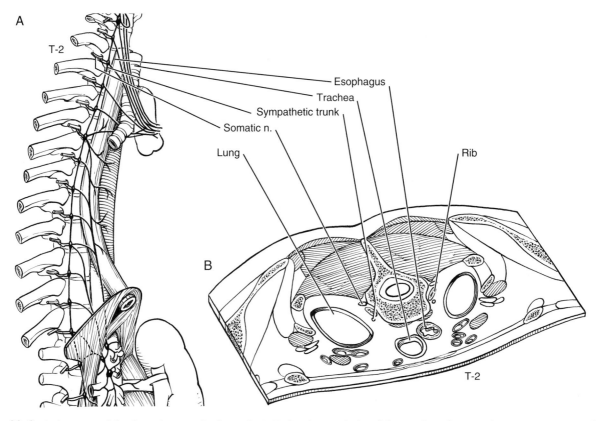

Figure 20–8 *A,* Anatomy of the thoracic sympathetic trunk. *B,* Notice the proximity of the trunk to the somatic nerve (n.) roots and the lung.

trajectory planned to avoid the lung. The technique is performed as follows:

1. The patient is placed prone.
2. Surface landmarks for needle placement at T2-3 are delineated with fluoroscopy or computed tomographic guidance. The correct needle entry site and approximate needle angle can be determined from a preblock computed tomography spot film. In most patients, the needle entry site is 4 to 5 cm from the midline, located such that the needle can pass between the transverse processes of the second and third thoracic vertebrae.
3. The skin is prepared with alcohol or povidone-iodine, and the skin and subcutaneous tissues are anesthetized with 1% lidocaine by using a 30-G needle.
4. A 22-G, 6- to 8-cm needle is advanced by using radiologic guidance to contact the edge of the T-2 lamina. The needle is withdrawn to the subcutaneous tissues and then readvanced in a slightly more lateral and caudal direction to slip past the lamina. The needle is advanced approximately 2 cm deep to the lamina to contact the dorsolateral aspect of the vertebral body (Figs. 20–9 and 20–10). After the body is contacted, the needle is withdrawn 3 to 4 mm.

If careful aspiration for blood, cerebrospinal fluid, and air is negative, 0.5 to 1.0 mL of contrast agent is injected to ensure spread along the anticipated path of the sympathetic trunk. Then, 2 to 3 mL of 0.5% bupivacaine are injected. For neurolytic blocks, 1 to 2 mL of a 6% to 10% phenol solution mixed with a radiopaque dye are injected. During a neurolytic injection, the patient must be observed for paresthesia to the arm, indicating spread of the injectant to the T-1 somatic nerve root. As an alternative to neurolytic block, the procedure can be performed with a radiofrequency probe, with a lower risk of somatic nerve neuralgia.[46, 47]

Complications and Side Effects

Side effects are an extension of the physiologic effects of the upper thoracic sympathetic block. By using a small volume of injectant (1 to 2 mL), it is usually possible to block the sympathetic output to the arm without producing Horner's syndrome, which is desirable when performing a neurolytic block. It is unknown if this approach spares some of the sympathetics to the arm.

Several serious complications are possible when this technique is used. Pneumothorax is a possibility. The needle may enter an intervertebral foramen, resulting in epidural or intrathecal injection. Somatic nerve block occurs, commonly as a result of the proximity in the thoracic area of the sympathetic trunk to the somatic nerves. This is a minor concern when a local anesthetic is injected, but spread of a neurolytic agent to the T-1 somatic nerve root can have serious conse-

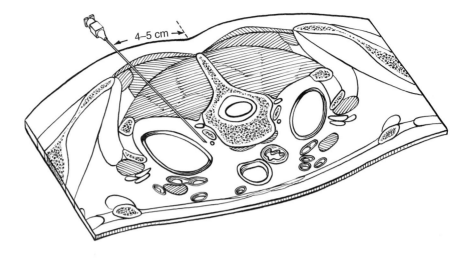

Figure 20–9 Correct needle position for thoracic sympathetic block.

quences because of the significant sensory and motor supply to the arm and hand by the T-1 nerve root.

Lumbar Sympathetic Block

Anatomy

The paired lumbar sympathetic trunks course along the anterior vertebral bodies at the inferomedial margin of the psoas muscle (Fig. 20–11). The lumbar trunk sends sympathetic efferents to the lower extremities and the lower abdominal and pelvic viscera. Visceral afferent fibers from lower abdominal and pelvic viscera reach the lumbar sympathetic trunk and, ultimately, the spinal cord through lumbar splanchnic nerves. The lumbar ganglia vary in number and appearance and do not necessarily correspond to the number of lumbar vertebrae.[48, 49] The postganglionic sympathetic fibers to the lower extremity originate in the ipsilateral lumbar ganglia, and interruption of the trunk and ganglia in the upper lumbar area effectively blocks the sympathetic efferents to the lower extremity. Some researchers have mentioned the existence of sympathetic fibers

that cross the midline to the contralateral lumbar trunk, but some anatomists have failed to demonstrate their existence.[2, 49] The significance of such fibers is uncertain. They have been posited by some as an explanation (or excuse) when a sympathetic block fails to produce symptomatic improvement despite a seemingly technically successful block.

The lumbar sympathetic trunks, unlike the thoracic trunks, are well separated from the somatic nerve roots by the psoas muscle and fascia, making it less likely that injection of an anesthetic or neurolytic agent through a correctly placed needle will spread to somatic nerves (see Fig. 20–11). The lumbar nerve roots and lumbar plexus course through the psoas muscle, and a needle placed improperly within the substance of the psoas muscle can result in anesthesia of the lumbar somatic nerves. Fibrous sheaths overlying the rami communicantes between the somatic and sympathetic nerves have been described, through which an injectant can spread from the area of the sympathetic trunk to a somatic nerve root.[50]

Other important structures in the area of the sympathetic trunks include the kidneys, aorta, vena cava, lumbar vessels, and lymphatic duct (see Fig. 20–11).

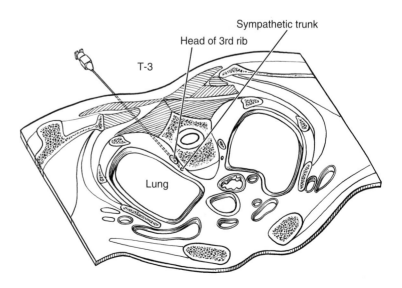

Figure 20–10 Percutaneous computed tomography–guided thoracic sympathetic block at T-3.

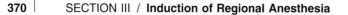

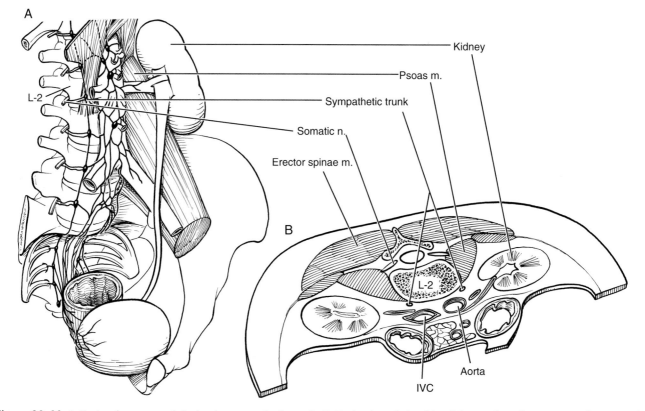

Figure 20–11 *A*, Regional anatomy of the lumbar sympathetic trunk. *B*, Notice the relationship of the trunk to the psoas muscle (m.) and fascia. IVC, inferior vena cava; n., nerve.

The kidneys are situated quite laterally and are in little danger of being punctured during lumbar sympathetic block.[51]

Indications and Efficacy

As with cervical sympathetic blocks, lumbar sympathetic blocks have been used in the past to treat various unrelated conditions (see Table 20–3). Current indications for lumbar sympathetic block include reflex sympathetic dystrophy, causalgia, peripheral vascular disease with painful ischemic neuropathy or poor tissue perfusion (or both), and perhaps some visceral pain syndromes.[20, 52–55] As with cervical sympathetic blocks, the use of lumbar sympathetic blocks for these conditions is based on anecdotal series and case reports rather than controlled clinical trials.

Leriche and Fontaine[56] first described the use of sympathectomy for reflex sympathetic dystrophy and causalgia in the 1930s. The role of sympathetic blocks for the diagnosis and treatment of reflex sympathetic dystrophy and causalgia is based on a large body of case reports and extensive clinical experience. My approach to lower extremity reflex sympathetic dystrophy is similar to that described for upper extremity reflex sympathetic dystrophy. I perform intravenously administered lidocaine and phentolamine tests, as described previously. If the patient does not respond to the lidocaine and phentolamine infusions, I perform a diagnostic lumbar sympathetic block. If the patient

achieves satisfactory pain relief, I proceed with a series of lumbar sympathetic blocks in conjunction with a good physical therapy program. I continue the series in a fashion similar to that described for upper extremity blocks. If the patient achieves excellent symptomatic relief from the blocks but the relief is short lived, three options are available: neurolytic lumbar sympathetic block, surgical sympathectomy, or use of implantable devices (spinal cord stimulation or spinal infusion systems). An in-depth discussion of the pros and cons of each technique is beyond the scope of this chapter. Some physicians reverse the order of lumbar sympathetic block and diagnostic infusion tests, similar to their use in upper extremity pain states.

Lower extremity occlusive vascular disease is a common medical problem. Definitive management usually consists of surgical bypass of one or more obstructed segments, unless the disease process is too diffuse to permit a bypass or the patient's underlying medical condition makes surgical treatment too risky. Patients who are not candidates for operation may be candidates for sympathetic blocks or surgical sympathectomy for intractable pain due to an ischemic neuropathy, intractable pain due to tissue ischemia, and poor tissue perfusion.

Sympathetic blocks and sympathectomy have been used to treat lower extremity occlusive vascular disease since the 1940s.[57] A large body of literature consisting mainly of a series of case reports fails to clearly define the role of sympathetic blocks for lower extremity vascular disease, but several series demonstrated improvement in blood flow and pain relief (Table 20–4). However, a controlled clinical trial of phenol sympathectomy for the treatment of intermittent claudication failed to demonstrate objective or subjective improvement.[62]

A sensible approach can be constructed based on the current literature. Patients who have failed medical therapy, who are not candidates for reconstructive or bypass surgery, and who have ischemic pain or evidence of poor tissue perfusion are candidates for sympathetic blocks. Symptoms of rest pain, a cold limb, and cyanosis are more likely to respond to blocks than are symptoms of claudication and skin or muscle necrosis. In most cases, it is wise to perform a diagnostic block with a local anesthetic to assess the degree of pain relief and objective improvement in tissue perfusion. A successful local anesthetic block can be followed by a neurolytic block.

The use of lumbar sympathetic blocks for visceral pain syndromes is based on the knowledge that some visceral afferent fibers from some of the abdominal and pelvic viscera pass through the lumbar sympathetic trunk. There are many anecdotal reports of pain relief after lumbar sympathetic blocks for patients with a wide variety of conditions. Although I have seen a few patients with chronic renal colic improve after lumbar sympathetic blocks, most patients with visceral abdominal pain do not achieve significant improvement after lumbar sympathetic block, because most of the visceral afferents pass through the aortic plexuses and thoracic splanchnic nerves.

Techniques

The various techniques described in the literature can be categorized as needle entry greater than or less than 6 cm from the midline; block with or without radiologic imaging; single- or multiple-needle techniques; catheter techniques; and neurolytic blocks.

Needle Entry Site

Lumbar sympathetic block techniques in which the site of needle entry is less than 6 cm from the midline have been described in detail elsewhere. I do not recommend this method, because it frequently leads to a somatic nerve block. As demonstrated in Figure 20–12A, if a needle entry site 5 cm from the midline is used, the needle has difficulty clearing the vertebral body to achieve the necessary final position near the sympathetic trunk along the anterior vertebral column. Instead, the needle often slides tangentially along the lateral vertebral body, with the needle tip resting within the psoas muscle. This is especially true in patients with vertebral osteophytes, which tend to direct the needle even further laterally. Block of the psoas muscle and the lumbar plexus as it runs through the muscle usually leads to a significant temperature increase in the lower extremity because of block of the sympathetic fibers accompanying the somatic nerves. However, if the patient's pain improves, it is not clear if the sympathetic or the somatic block is responsible for the improvement.

A more reliable technique is to use a needle entry point 7 to 8 cm from the midline:

1. The patient is placed prone, with a pillow under the pelvis and lower abdomen to straighten the lumbar lordosis.

2. Surface landmarks are identified. A single-needle technique should be performed at L-2. If two- or three-needle techniques are chosen, they should be performed at L-2, L-3, and L-4. The spinous process of L-4 is identified by palpating the spinous process that is intersected by a line drawn between the right and left iliac crests (Fig. 20–13).

3. The needle entry site is marked 7 to 8 cm lateral to the midpoint of the spinous processes (see Fig. 20–13). Eight centimeters generally works better for muscular or obese patients and patients with extensive degenerative disk disease.

4. The skin, subcutaneous tissues, and muscle are anesthetized with a local anesthetic (1% lidocaine). A 5-cm, 25-G needle is advanced at a 45° angle toward the midline in the cross-sectional plane, and 2 to 3 mL of anesthetic are injected along the anticipated track of the block needle. Large volumes of anesthetic should be avoided to prevent anesthetizing somatic nerves during deep infiltration.

5. A 20- or 22-G, 12.5- to 15-cm needle is used to perform the block. The needle should be graduated or it should have a movable collar to use as a depth marker. The needle is advanced carefully at a 45° angle until the vertebral body is contacted. Because the peri-

Table 20–4 Sympathetic Blocks and Sympathectomy for Peripheral Vascular Disease

INVESTIGATION	PATIENTS, NO.	PROCEDURE*	SATISFACTORY RESPONSE, %	NO RESPONSE, %
Hughes-Davies and Redman[58]	97	1	69	31
Strand[57]	167	3	56	44
Cousins et al[54]	368	1, 2	80	20
Haimovici et al[59]	171	3	55	45
Froysaker[60]	32	3	5.5	94.5
Myers and Irvine[61]	26	3	69	31
Vulpio et al[52]	20	4	68	32
Rosen et al[53]	37	1	38	62
Fyfe and Quin[62]	25	1	25	75

*1, phenol sympathetic block; 2, alcohol sympathetic block; 3, surgical sympathectomy; 4, series of local anesthetic sympathetic blocks.

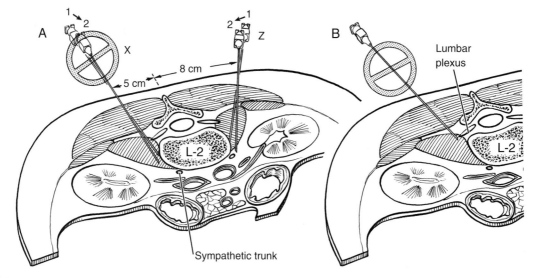

Figure 20–12 Cross-sectional anatomy at L-2 demonstrates correct and incorrect needle placement for lumbar sympathetic block. *A,* Needle x enters the skin too close to the midline (5 cm) and cannot get past the lateral vertebral body to reach the sympathetic trunk. The final needle position is too lateral and within the psoas muscle. Needle z enters the skin 8 cm from the midline, a more favorable approach to slide past the vertebral body and achieve satisfactory position in the area of the sympathetic trunk. *B,* Needle placement too superficial, within the psoas muscle and near the lumbar plexus.

osteum and the intervertebral disk are quite sensitive, 0.5 mL of anesthetic is deposited at this point. In an average-sized patient, the vertebral body is contacted at a depth of 7 to 8 cm, and more superficial bone contact represents the transverse process.

6. The final needle position is 2 to 3 cm beyond the depth at which the vertebral body is contacted. The needle is withdrawn to the subcutaneous tissue but not so much that the needle exits the skin. The angle of the needle is raised 5° to 10°, and it is readvanced. If the vertebral body is contacted again, the needle is withdrawn, raised another 5° to 10°, and readvanced

until it slips past the body to the predetermined depth. The physician should feel the needle pop as it advances through the anterior psoas fascia to rest in the area of the lumbar sympathetic trunk (see Fig. 20–12*A*).

7. If a single-needle technique is used, after careful aspiration for blood and cerebrospinal fluid, 10 to 15 mL of local anesthetic (bupivacaine) are injected in incremental doses. It is advisable to use a solution containing a 1:200,000 concentration of epinephrine to help monitor for intravascular injection. If multiple needles are used, 3 to 5 mL of anesthetic are injected through each needle.

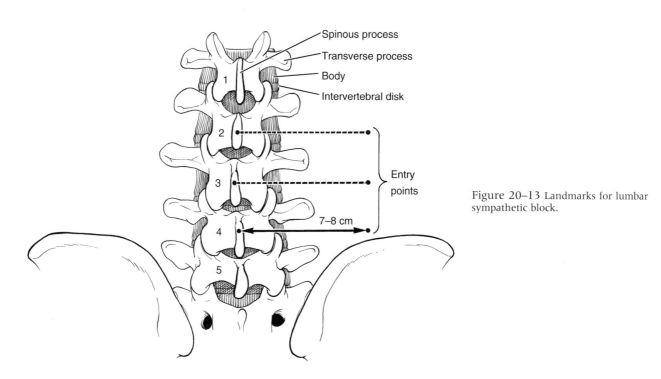

Figure 20–13 Landmarks for lumbar sympathetic block.

Radiologic Imaging

The use of radiologic imaging to perform lumbar sympathetic block, although helpful, is not always necessary. In general, a series of local anesthetic sympathetic blocks to treat reflex sympathetic dystrophy can be performed without radiographic guidance by using percutaneous landmarks, if documentation of sympathetic block is provided. Radiographic guidance is indicated for a neurolytic lumbar sympathetic block; if the patient's anatomy precludes the use of surface landmarks (e.g., obesity, spinal deformities); failure to achieve evidence of sympathetic block without the use of radiographic guidance; and for a prognostic local anesthetic block before a neurolytic or surgical sympathectomy.

The most common imaging techniques are fluoroscopy and computed tomography.[63, 64] In most cases, the considerable expense of computed tomography and the inconvenience of scheduling the procedure with radiology is not worth the negligible benefit of computed tomography over fluoroscopy. Because the lumbar trunk is too small to be visualized on computed tomography, there is little reason to use computed tomographic guidance. On the other hand, C-arm fluoroscopy can be extremely helpful to visualize and avoid intervertebral disks and transverse processes, to visualize and avoid large vertebral osteophytes, to obtain final needle placement with fewer needle passes and less discomfort to the patient, to confirm needle placement to be in correct relationship to the vertebral body, and to avoid psoas muscle injection (requires the use of a small amount of radiopaque dye).

The technique is similar to that previously described. The fluoroscope can be used to confirm landmarks and to map out a needle path that avoids the intervertebral disk and transverse processes. Posteroanterior and lateral fluoroscopy can be used to guide the needle and confirm final placement to be in the anticipated location of the sympathetic trunk. Injection of 0.5 to 1.0 mL of radiopaque dye, such as diatrizoate meglumine or a similar agent, produces a linear pattern along the course of the sympathetic trunk (Fig. 20–14). It is essential to inquire about intravenous iodine allergy before injecting iodinated contrast agents. If the needle is too superficial or too lateral and located within the psoas muscle, the dye reveals a psoas muscle cast and the needle can be advanced until the pop of the psoas fascia is identified.

Single Versus Multiple Needles

The technique of lumbar sympathetic block is classically described as requiring three needles, one each at L-2, L-3, and L-4. Subsequent studies by Hatangdi and Boas[65] and others[66] using radiographic confirmation and clinical results have demonstrated equally satisfactory results with a single-needle technique, provided the needle is in the correct location. A single-needle technique is preferred by the patient. For a local anesthetic block, a single-needle technique with 10 to 15 mL of local anesthetic is the preferred technique. Large volumes of injectant through a single needle may result

in a small amount of injectant tracking along the medial surface of psoas muscle, between the psoas and the vertebral body, to reach the somatic nerve root.[50] For this reason, it may be advisable to use a two- or three-needle technique with lower injectant volumes per needle (3 mL) for neurolytic lumbar sympathetic blocks.

Catheter Techniques

In situations in which a series of sympathetic blocks is being considered, placement of a catheter in the area of the sympathetic trunk is an alternative to repeated percutaneous blocks.[67] From the patient's perspective, daily injection or continuous infusion through a catheter is preferable to serial percutaneous blocks. An 18- to 20-G needle is placed in the area of the sympathetic trunk using radiographic guidance. A catheter is threaded through the needle, 3 to 4 cm beyond the needle tip. Proper location is confirmed with contrast dye and an appropriate confirmation of sympathetic block (e.g., temperature increase) after injection of local anesthetic. The needle is carefully removed, and the catheter is secured and dressed. The usual monitoring, aspiration, and injection precautions should be used with subsequent injections, because the catheter can migrate.

Neurolytic Block

Neurolytic block can be considered after a successful diagnostic block in patients with lower extremity vascular disease or in patients with reflex sympathetic dystrophy who achieve temporary relief from a series of local anesthetic blocks. A two- or three-needle technique is recommended and the use of fluoroscopy or computed tomography guidance is mandatory. After appropriate needle placement is confirmed, 2 to 3 mL of absolute alcohol or 10% phenol are injected through each needle. The needles are flushed with 0.5 mL of local anesthetic or air and removed. The use of a radiofrequency generator and probe to produce a lesion of the sympathetic trunk has been described.[68] The equipment is expensive, the probes have a much greater diameter than a 20- to 22-G block needle, and there is no demonstrated advantage over neurolytic block.

Troubleshooting

Failure to Achieve Evidence of a Sympathetic Block

Evidence of a sympathetic block should be apparent within 20 to 30 min of injecting the anesthetic. Failure to obtain an increase in temperature or other confirmatory sign is almost always the result of needle placement too lateral or superficial or both.

Sympathetic Block Accompanied by Sensory or Motor Block of the Extremity

Signs of a successful sympathetic block may be accompanied by a sensory or motor block of the extrem-

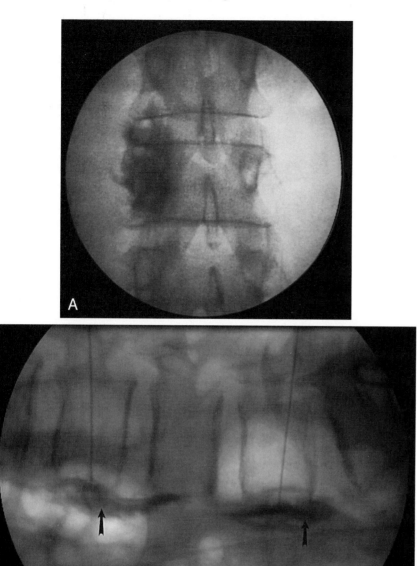

Figure 20–14 *A*, Posteroanterior view of contrast pattern from lumbar sympathetic block at L-2. *B*, Lateral view of contrast pattern (arrows) from lumbar sympathetic block at L-2 and L-4. Each injection was performed with 1 mL of diatrizoate meglumine.

ity. This can result from overzealous local anesthetic infiltration before the block or from needle placement that is too superficial, as within the psoas muscle.

Pain During the Procedure

Careful local infiltration before placing the block needles minimizes the patient's discomfort. There are two portions of the block that can be quite uncomfortable. First, needle contact with the periosteum of the vertebral body may produce pain. Patients often report back pain with radiation to the hip area. Gentle needle placement and judicious use of sedation can minimize this discomfort. Injection of 0.5 mL of anesthetic (after aspiration) on initial bone contact prevents further discomfort if the vertebral body is contacted on subsequent passes. Second, a paresthesia may occur during needle placement. The paresthesia usually is transient, but if it persists, the needle should be withdrawn and replaced 0.5 cm more cephalad or caudad to avoid the somatic nerve.

Pain During Injection

Injection through a needle that is in the correct location should be painless. Pain with injection indicates incorrect needle placement, usually within an intervertebral disk or the psoas muscle.

Resistance to Injection

Injection through a correctly placed needle should require little effort. Injection of 1 mL of air can help as a test. If the air is not easily injected, similar to a correctly placed epidural needle, the needle is incorrectly located, probably in a disk or muscle. Most of these problems can be avoided or minimized by using fluoroscopy to assist with needle placement.

Complications and Side Effects

Several complications may occur after local anesthetic sympathetic block.

Intravascular injection of local anesthetic into the aorta (left-sided block), vena cava (right-sided block), or lumbar vessels can be minimized by careful aspiration, use of an appropriate test dose, and use of fluoroscopy.

During a lumbar sympathetic block, unrecognized needle placement near the intervertebral foramen, followed by injection of local anesthetic, can lead to epidural or spinal anesthesia. Careful attention to needle depth, use of fluoroscopy, or both methods can prevent this complication.

Complications after neurolytic block are related to injection of the neurolytic agent near a somatic nerve (i.e., within the psoas muscle) or from spread of the neurolytic solution from a correctly placed needle to a somatic nerve. The use of fluoroscopy, small volumes of injectant, and observation of the spread of the injectant to which a radiopaque dye has been added can minimize but not prevent these complications.

Even the most carefully performed block can result in small amounts of the injectant tracking along tissue planes to contact a somatic nerve. The genitofemoral nerve or L-2 nerve roots are most often affected. Such tracking of small amounts of agent is more likely to lead to sensory loss than motor deficit, and the loss usually resolves with time. This postneurolysis neuralgia occurs with a reported frequency of 5% to 15% and usually presents as burning, dysesthesia, and allodynia in the groin or anterior thigh.[54, 69]

Celiac Plexus and Splanchnic Nerve Block

Anatomy and Physiology

The terms "celiac plexus block" and "splanchnic nerve block" often are used synonymously, but the celiac plexus and splanchnic nerves are anatomically and regionally distinct structures (Fig. 20–15*B*). Most of the sympathetic efferent fibers to the abdominal viscera originate in the thoracic spinal cord and reach the abdominal viscera through the thoracic splanchnic nerves and celiac plexus. The thoracic splanchnic nerves lie cephalad to the diaphragm, anterior to the lower thoracic vertebral bodies (see Fig. 20–15). The celiac plexus lies just caudad to the diaphragm, at the level of the first (and occasionally the second) lumbar vertebra.[70, 71] It encases the anterolateral surface of the aorta and the origin of the celiac artery. The plexus continues inferiorly as the superior mesenteric plexus and then as the inferior mesenteric plexus. The celiac plexus and splanchnic nerves are near the diaphragm, lungs, vena cava, aorta, kidneys, pancreas, and liver.

Successful block of the splanchnic nerves or celiac plexus leads to vasodilation of the splanchnic vascular bed and significant pooling or accumulation of blood within the dilated splanchnic veins. Celiac plexus block results in block of sympathetic and parasympathetic fibers to the abdominal viscera, and the net effect on gastrointestinal motility varies. Although few objective data are available, patients often exhibit signs of increased bowel motility, as evidenced by diarrhea and increased passage of flatus.

Indications and Efficacy

Celiac plexus and splanchnic nerve block are performed most often for pain from an intra-abdominal malignancy. Many series[72–78] reported neurolytic celiac or splanchnic blocks successfully relieved pain in 70% to 90% of patients with pancreatic and other upper gastrointestinal tract malignancies. Sharfman and Walsh[79] reviewed the literature regarding the efficacy of celiac plexus blocks, found methodologic flaws in many of the reports, and concluded that there are insufficient data to judge the efficacy and long-term morbidity of neurolytic celiac plexus block.

Ischia and colleagues[78] reported a prospective study of 61 patients with pancreatic cancer pain treated with celiac plexus block who were followed until death. Complete pain relief occurred in only 24% of patients. However, celiac plexus block in conjunction with adjuvant techniques resulted in satisfactory pain relief in 80% to 90% of patients. Lillemoe and coworkers[80] showed that the intraoperative use of alcohol celiac plexus blocks in patients with preoperative pancreatic cancer pain (undergoing exploratory laparotomy) significantly prolonged life compared with saline celiac blocks.

Pancreatic cancer can invade the body wall, which is not innervated by nerves passing through the celiac plexus. Some visceral afferent fibers from other abdominal structures may bypass the celiac plexus. For these and perhaps other reasons, celiac plexus block may not always result in satisfactory or complete relief of pain. A celiac plexus block for pain from upper abdominal malignancy is likely to be most beneficial when the pain is primarily visceral in origin and when used in conjunction with other pain-management modalities.

The role of celiac plexus and splanchnic nerve blocks for abdominal pain from noncancerous conditions such as chronic pancreatitis and postsurgical visceral pain syndromes is controversial. Few data are available other than small series or case reports.[81–83] Until additional data are available, it seems reasonable to consider a series of splanchnic or celiac blocks in patients with intractable abdominal pain from nonmalignant causes that is unresponsive to more conservative modalities, such as medications and physiotherapy. Some practitioners advocate the addition of a corticosteroid suspension, such as methylprednisolone or triamcinolone. The role of neurolytic blocks in this patient population is even more controversial, and the potential risks and complications should be considered in light of the patient having a nonterminal illness.[83] As a result of neural regrowth, most neurolytic blocks provide only temporary relief. I consider neurolytic splanchnic or celiac blocks in patients who have not responded to more conservative therapy, who are debilitated by their pain, and who consistently obtain temporary relief from a local anesthetic or local anesthetic plus corticosteroid block.

The terms "visceral or abdominal reflex sympathetic dystrophy" and "sympathetically mediated pain of the abdomen" have crept into the pain and regional anesthesia literature. These phrases should be avoided be-

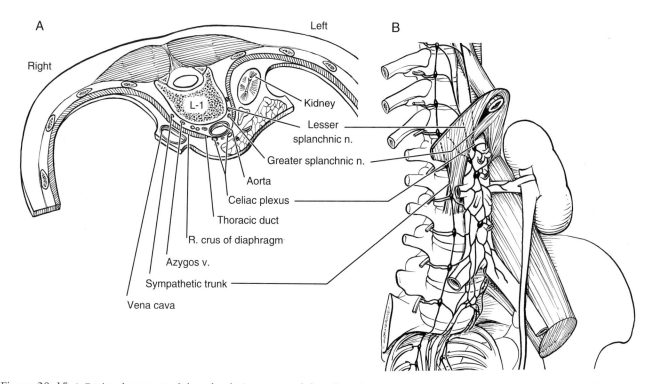

Figure 20–15 *A*, Regional anatomy of the splanchnic nerves and the celiac plexus. v., vein. *B*, Notice the relationship of the celiac plexus and splanchnic nerves (n.) to the diaphragm.

cause there is no evidence that such entities exist. A celiac plexus block interrupts the sympathetic efferent fibers and the visceral nociceptive afferent fibers, preventing inferences regarding pain mechanisms from the results of a celiac plexus block.

Techniques

Of the many techniques that have been described, the splanchnic nerve or retrocrural celiac plexus block and the transcrural celiac plexus block are the most frequently used approaches. Other techniques include the transaortic approach, anterior approach, paramedian approach at T-12, and a transdiskal approach. Other variations include the use of fluoroscopy, computed tomographic guidance, catheter techniques, and neurolytic blocks.

The term "retrocrural celiac plexus block" is a misnomer, because the celiac plexus proper is not blocked. "Splanchnic nerve block" is better, because the goal is to direct the needles and injectant cephalad to (or posterior to) the diaphragm (i.e., retrocrural) and anterior to the T-12 or L-1 vertebral bodies (Fig. 20–16) to

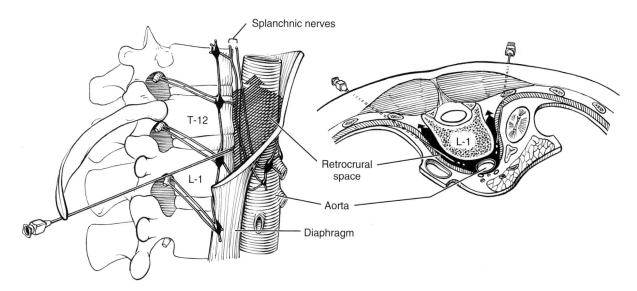

Figure 20–16 Splanchnic (retrocrural) nerve block. The needles are positioned posterior to the diaphragm.

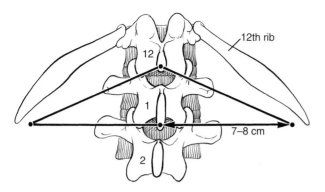

Figure 20–17 Landmarks for celiac plexus and splanchnic nerve blocks. See text for explanation.

block the splanchnic nerves just before they pierce the diaphragm to enter the abdomen. The technique is performed as follows:

1. The patient is placed prone, with one to two pillows under the hips and abdomen to flatten the lumbar lordosis.

2. The spinous processes of T-12 to L-4 are identified by palpation or with fluoroscopic guidance and marked.

3. The inferior margins of the 12th rib are identified. The needle entry site is determined by marking a point immediately caudal to each of the 12th ribs and 7 to 8 cm from the midline (Fig. 20–17). Be careful to identify the 12th rib; identifying the 11th rib instead of the 12th rib significantly increases the risk of pneumothorax.

4. To help guide the needle trajectory, draw a straight line to connect the needle entry points to the caudal edge of the T-12 spinous process.

5. After sterile preparation and draping, infiltrate the skin, subcutaneous, and muscle layers with lidocaine along the anticipated course of the block needles. Use a 25-G, 5- to 6-cm needle to inject 4 to 5 mL per side.

6. The block is performed with 15-cm, 20- to 22-G needles. The use of a calibrated needle or an adjustable needle collar as a depth marker is helpful. Place the left-sided needle first because the aorta is a helpful landmark to assist with correct placement.

7. Using the previously drawn line between the needle entry site and the interspace between T-12 and L-1 to guide the needle direction, the needle is advanced at a 45° angle from the horizontal plane toward the interspace. If radiography is used, aim for the cephalad aspect of the L-1 or caudal aspect of the T-12 vertebral bodies. Observe the distance that the vertebral body is contacted.

8. Withdraw the needle, although not through the skin. Increase the angle of the needle 5° to 10° to slide past the vertebral body. In approaching the anticipated depth, advance the needle carefully (Figs. 20–18 and 20–19). Stop the advancing needle at the first sign of increased tissue resistance, because this probably represents the aorta. By applying gentle pressure on the needle, the aortic pulsations transmitted through the needle can be felt. The fluoroscopic view shows the needle tip pulsating.

9. Repeat the procedure on the right side. The aorta is not present on the right, and the needle is advanced approximately 1 cm deeper on the right.

10. If fluoroscopy is used, injection of 3 to 4 mL of radiopaque dye (diatrizoate meglumine) reveals a dye pattern spreading cephalad to the diaphragm and anterior to the vertebral column in the area of the splanchnic nerves (Fig. 20–20). After careful aspiration, 10 to 15 mL of local anesthetic with 1:200,000 epinephrine are slowly injected through each needle after a 3-mL test dose is negative for intravascular or neuraxial injection.

11. The patient should be well hydrated and observed for a sufficient time after the block to ensure that postural hypotension is not a problem.

The transcrural celiac plexus block is truly a celiac plexus block.[84] The technique and landmarks are similar to those of the splanchnic nerve block, although some modifications are needed:

1. Needle entry sites are the same.

2. The needles are projected toward the L-1 body.

3. The needles must be advanced in a transcrural approach through the diaphragm (see Fig. 20–18). This is difficult to accomplish on the left side unless the

Figure 20–18 Cross-sectional representation of splanchnic nerve and celiac plexus block. Notice the position of the splanchnic needle posterior to the diaphragm and the celiac needle anterior (transcrural) to the diaphragm. (1) The initial needle approach contacts the L-1 vertebral body; (2) the needle is withdrawn to the subcutaneous tissue, the angle is increased 10° and advanced.

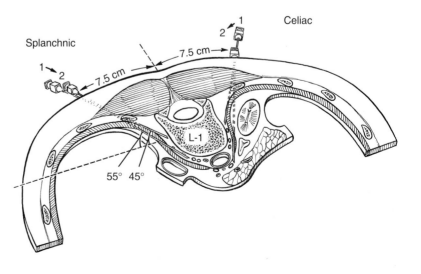

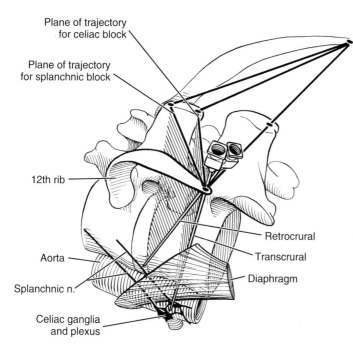

Plane of trajectory for celiac block

Plane of trajectory for splanchnic block

12th rib

Aorta

Splanchnic n.

Celiac ganglia and plexus

Retrocrural

Transcrural

Diaphragm

Figure 20–19 Three-dimensional view of celiac plexus and splanchnic nerve block needle placement. n., nerve.

block is performed with computed tomographic guidance (Fig. 20–21) or unless the transaortic technique is used, because the aorta blocks the path of the advancing needle.[84]

4. The right-sided needle usually can be advanced through the diaphragm without encountering vascular structures. The position can be confirmed with fluoroscopy and a small amount of contrast medium.

5. Injection is performed.

The transaortic method was described by Ischia and

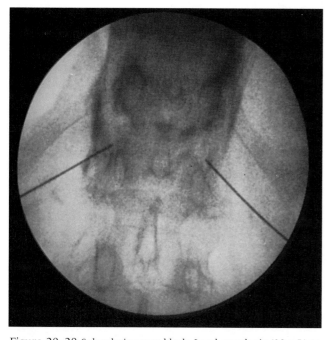

Figure 20–20 Splanchnic nerve block. Local anesthetic (10 mL) to which contrast material was added was injected through each needle. Cephalad spread (above the diaphragm) is evident.

associates[85] and is a variation of the transcrural celiac plexus block. A left-sided needle is advanced under computed tomographic or fluoroscopic guidance by using landmarks. Instead of stopping the needle posterior to the aorta, the needle is advanced carefully through the aorta until it is just anterior to the aorta. The position is confirmed with fluoroscopy or computed tomography, and 20 mL of anesthetic are injected incrementally after negative response to aspiration and to a test dose. A study by Ischia and coworkers[78] comparing the efficacy of the transcrural and the retrocrural techniques for pancreatic cancer pain showed no significant difference between the two techniques.

Montero Matamala and colleagues[86] reported a computed tomography–guided anterior approach to the celiac plexus. The patient is placed supine, and after sterile preparation and local anesthesia, a 22-G, 15-cm needle is advanced with computed tomographic guidance through a subxiphoid approach to the area of the celiac plexus. The needle position and spread of injectant are confirmed with computed tomography. Ten milliliters of local anesthetic (or neurolytic agent) are injected in incremental doses.

The T-12 paramedian and transdiskal approaches have been described briefly in the literature. They have no readily identifiable advantages over the techniques described here.[87]

The use of fluoroscopy may facilitate the performance of a splanchnic or celiac plexus block. Fluoroscopy can be used to confirm surface landmarks, facilitate needle advancement, identify aortic pulsations, and confirm the spread of radiopaque dye. It can be used to help avoid complications such as injection that is too superficial (somatic nerve block), injection in the epidural or subarachnoid space, and pneumothorax. Computed tomographic guidance is useful when unusual patient anatomy makes traditional approaches

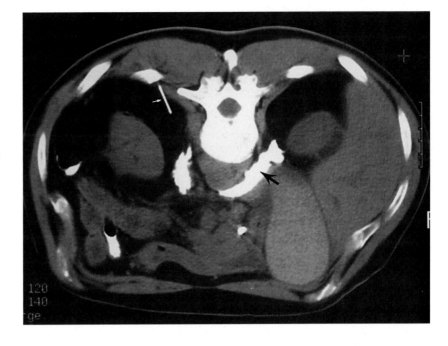

Figure 20–21 Computed tomography–guided transcrural celiac plexus block. Contrast material (large arrow) can be seen from injection on the right side. A portion of the left-sided needle is visible (small arrow) and has not been used for injection.

difficult and is essential when an anterior approach is used.[84, 88, 89] Although the celiac plexus itself cannot be visualized on a computed tomographic scan, the needles can be guided to the approximate location of the celiac plexus by locating the origin of the celiac artery from the aorta.

Clinical Approach to the Patient With Cancer Pain

Nerve blocks can provide relief for the patient with intractable pain from upper abdominal malignancy. If the patient is able to lie prone, I perform a diagnostic splanchnic nerve block using 0.5% bupivacaine with 1:200,000 epinephrine. If the patient experiences significant pain relief for the duration of the anesthetic, I perform a neurolytic splanchnic block with a 100% alcohol solution. I use fluoroscopy to assist needle placement. After satisfactory needle placement, I inject 10 to 15 mL of 0.25% bupivacaine with epinephrine through each needle. I wait 10 min and verify pain relief and normal lower extremity neurologic function. I then inject 8 to 10 mL of absolute alcohol through each needle, flush the needles with anesthetic or air, and remove the needles.

If the patient does not achieve pain relief despite a technically satisfactory block and the pain pattern appears amenable to block therapy, I consider a repeat diagnostic block with a transcrural celiac plexus block. If successful, I follow up with a transcrural neurolytic block.

If the patient is unable to lie prone or if a posterior approach is limited by anatomic factors, I use a computed tomography–guided anterior approach (Fig. 20–22). Occasionally, patients with previous radiation or surgical therapy or patients with extensive retroperitoneal metastatic disease do not achieve satisfactory relief from a posterior approach because of impairment of anesthetic spread through the diseased tissue. The anterior approach is a useful alternative for this group of patients.

Clinical Approach to the Patient With Benign Pain

The most common visceral chronic pain syndromes are pain in the setting of chronic pancreatitis and pain in the setting of the multiply operated abdomen. Pain that persists in the absence of identifiable organ abnormality and that is refractory to more conservative management techniques occasionally responds to splanchnic or celiac plexus block. My initial approach is to perform a splanchnic block and inject a solution of 0.25% bupivacaine with 40 to 60 mg of triamcinolone or methylprednisolone. If the patient achieves long-term relief (3 to 6 mo), the procedure can be repeated on a periodic basis. If the patient does not achieve relief, I avoid further blocks. If the patient achieves relief for the duration of the local anesthetic, a series of blocks every other day or a series of injections through celiac plexus catheters (placed like lumbar sympathetic catheters) can be performed.[90] If this results in short-term relief, a neurolytic block can be considered, taking into account the potential complications and the likelihood of neural regrowth and recurrent pain.

Complications and Side Effects

The side effects are usually transient. They are an extension of the physiologic effects of the block and include diarrhea and postural hypotension. The postural hypotension can be minimized with sufficient intravenous hydration.

There are many possible complications:

1. Local anesthetic toxicity.
2. Spinal or epidural injection can be a transient

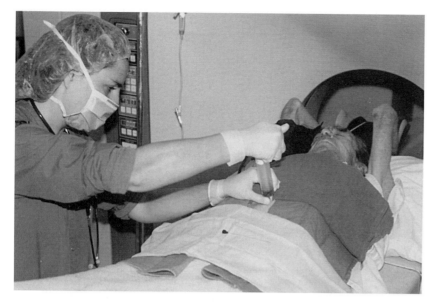

Figure 20–22 Computed tomography–guided anterior approach to the celiac plexus.

problem when a local anesthetic is injected and catastrophic if a neurolytic agent is injected.

3. Pneumothorax may result from a needle placed too far cephalad.

4. Puncture of the aorta or vena cava rarely leads to serious bleeding sequelae, and even the transaortic technique appears to be a safe technique in the absence of a coagulopathy.

5. Visceral organ puncture, including bowel, pancreas, and kidney, can occur but only rarely leads to serious organ dysfunction or damage.[51] Complications from visceral puncture have not been reported from the anterior approach.

6. Injury to the thoracic duct has been reported.

7. Placement of needles and injection of anesthetic and neurolytic agents near the aorta can cause an anterior spinal artery syndrome, presumably the result of trauma to or vasospasm of the artery of Adamkiewicz.[91, 92] Paralysis appears to be a rare complication.

8. Somatic nerve block or neuralgia can occur as described for lumbar sympathetic block. Local anesthetic or a neurolytic agent can spread to the lumbar somatic nerves (especially L-1) if the needles are unintentionally placed in the psoas muscle (Fig. 20–23). On occasion, some of the injectant can spread to the thoracic somatic nerves during a splanchnic nerve block.

9. An acetaldehyde syndrome has been reported after alcohol block of the celiac plexus in patients with aldehyde dehydrogenase I deficiency.[93] This manifests clinically as facial flushing, palpitations, and diaphoresis. Among the Japanese, the frequency of aldehyde dehydrogenase I deficiency may be as high as 38%.

Superior Hypogastric Plexus Block

Anatomy and Physiology

The superior hypogastric plexus is a continuation of the aortic plexus and is located anterior to the L-5 vertebral body and upper sacrum in the area of the bifurcation of the iliac vessels (Fig. 20–24). Visceral afferent fibers pass through the superior hypogastric plexus.[94] Important structures in the vicinity of the plexus include the psoas muscle, the lumbar somatic nerves, and the iliac vessels.

Indications and Efficacy

Superior hypogastric plexus block was initially reported to be an effective treatment for intractable pain from neoplastic involvement or radiation injury of the pelvic organs, including the cervix, prostate, and testicles.[95] Subsequent series[96, 97] reported the successful

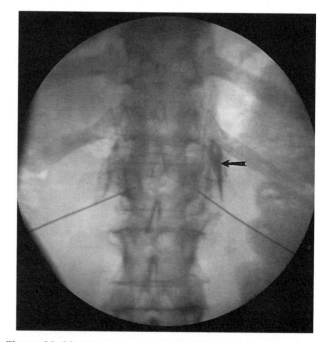

Figure 20–23 Splanchnic nerve block. The needle on the right side of the photograph is too superficial, and a 1-mL injection of contrast material can be seen outlining the psoas muscle (arrow).

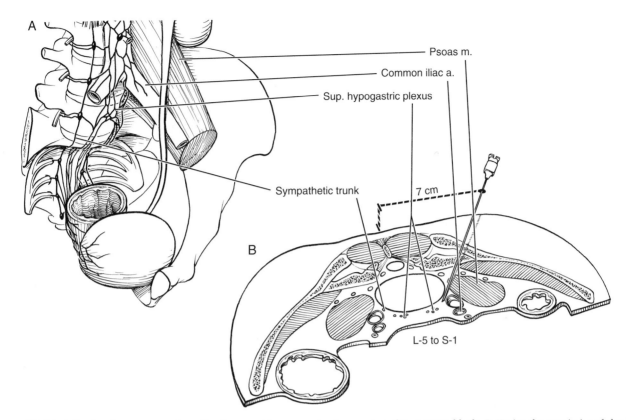

Figure 20–24 *A*, Regional anatomy and needle placement for a superior hypogastric plexus (SHP) block. *B*, Notice the proximity of the SHP to the iliac vessels. a., artery; m., muscle; Sup., superior.

treatment of neoplastic and nonneoplastic pelvic pain syndromes involving the ovaries, bladder, distal colon, and rectum. Reported success was high in these series, despite the fact that visceral nociceptive afferent fibers from most of these structures do not pass through the hypogastric plexus or they send a significant population of visceral afferents through additional pathways such as lumbar and pelvic splanchnic nerves.[94]

My experience with hypogastric plexus block has been less encouraging than these reports. I have had a few responses in patients with pain from endometrial cancer, one patient with dysmenorrhea, and a few patients with low back and pelvic pain secondary to extensive retroperitoneal tumor involvement. Further studies are needed to define the role of hypogastric plexus block for pelvic pain syndromes.

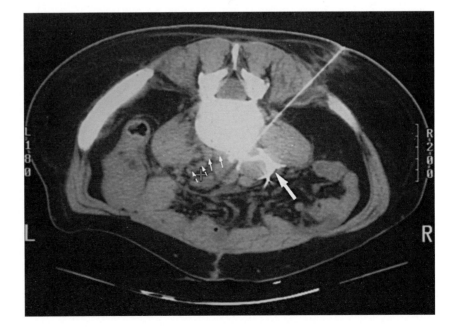

Figure 20–25 Computed tomography (CT)–guided superior hypogastric plexus block. Notice the extensive prevertebral lymphadenopathy (small arrows). CT-aided needle placement was used to avoid vascular structures and lymph nodes in the region. Contrast material was injected (large arrow) through the needle on the right side. The procedure was repeated on the left side.

Because the rate of complications seems to be low, it seems reasonable to offer a diagnostic block to patients with intractable visceral pelvic pain as a result of cancer and to follow a successful diagnostic block with a neurolytic block. In my opinion, superior hypogastric plexus block has a limited or no role in the treatment of chronic benign pelvic pain.

Technique

The technique was originally described by Plancarte and colleagues[95] and subsequently modified by others. It is best performed with fluoroscopy. Computed tomographic guidance is helpful when extensive neoplastic disease in the area of the plexus is expected to impede diffusion of the injectant (Fig. 20–25).

1. The patient is placed prone, as for celiac and sympathetic blocks.
2. Identify the L-4, L-5, and S-1 spinous processes.
3. The needle entry sites are lateral to the L-4 spinous process, 7 cm from the midline (Fig. 20–26).
4. Use a marking pen to draw a straight line to connect the needle entry points to the interspace between L-5 and S-1, because these lines help guide the needle trajectory.
5. Perform sterile preparation and draping.
6. Infiltrate the skin, subcutaneous, and muscle layers in the anticipated path of the block needle with 4 to 5 mL of lidocaine and a 25-G, 5- to 6-cm needle.
7. The 12- to 15-cm, 22- or 20-G needles are advanced during fluoroscopic guidance to contact the inferior portion of the L-5 vertebral body.
8. The needles are withdrawn, the angles of the needles are increased 5° to 10°, and then the needles are readvanced approximately 2 to 3 cm beyond the

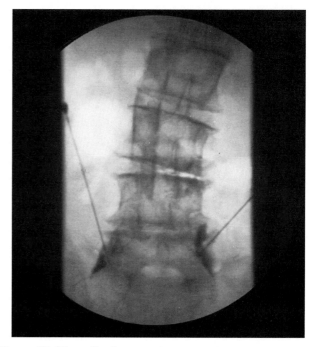

Figure 20–27 Needle placement for superior hypogastric plexus block. Contrast material (1 mL) was injected through each needle.

point of initial bone contact to slip past the L-5 vertebral body.
9. Posteroanterior and lateral fluoroscopy can be used to confirm needle placement. Injection of a small amount of contrast dye helps to confirm spread of the injectant in the appropriate area (Fig. 20–27).
10. After negative results of aspiration and an appropriate test dose, 10 mL of 0.25% to 0.5% bupivacaine with 1:200,000 epinephrine are injected in divided doses through each needle. For a neurolytic block, this procedure can be followed 10 min later by injection of 7 mL of absolute alcohol or 6% to 10% phenol. The needles are flushed to clear the injectant and then removed.

Complications and Side Effects

Superior hypogastric plexus block can have several side effects and complications:

1. Local anesthetic toxicity.
2. Puncture of the iliac vessels usually occurs without sequelae, unless the patient has a coagulopathy.
3. Somatic nerve block is a nuisance with a local anesthetic block and a catastrophe with a neurolytic block.
4. Visceral organ puncture is possible.
5. Bowel and bladder dysfunction seem to be a theoretical concern but have not been reported.
6. Ejaculatory and sexual dysfunction seem to be likely complications of bilateral neurolytic block but have not been reported.[98]

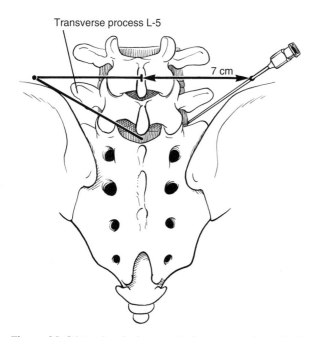

Figure 20–26 Landmarks for superior hypogastric plexus block.

References

1. Guyton AC: Textbook of Medical Physiology, 7th ed, pp 686–698. Philadelphia, WB Saunders Co, 1986.
2. Goss CM: The visceral nervous system. In Gray H (ed): Anatomy of the Human Body, 29th ed, pp 1004–1036. Philadelphia, Lea & Febiger, 1973.
3. Cervero F: Visceral pain. In Dubner R, Gebhart GF, Bond MR (eds): Proceedings of the Vth World Congress on Pain, pp 216–226. Amsterdam, Elsevier Science–Biomedical Division, 1988.
4. Hollinshead WH, Rosse C: Textbook of Anatomy, 4th ed, pp 577–734. Philadelphia, Harper & Row, 1985.
5. Collins SL: The cervical sympathetic nerves in surgery of the neck. Otolaryngol Head Neck Surg 1991; 105: 544–555.
6. Uhrenholdt A, Dam WH, Larsen OA, et al: Paradoxical effect on peripheral blood flow after sympathetic blockades in patients with gangrene due to arteriosclerosis obliterans. Vasc Surg 1971; 5: 154–163.
7. Fujita Y: Splanchnic circulation following coeliac plexus block. Acta Anaesthesiol Scand 1988; 32: 323–327.
8. Kashima T, Tanaka H, Minagoe S, et al: Electrocardiographic changes induced by the stellate ganglion block in normal subjects. J Electrocardiol 1981; 14: 169–174.
9. Crampton R: Preeminence of the left stellate ganglion in the long Q-T syndrome. Circulation 1979; 59: 769–778.
10. Mesa A, Kaplan RF: Dysrhythmias controlled with stellate ganglion block in a child with diabetes and a variant of long QT syndrome. Reg Anesth 1993; 18: 60–62.
11. Marchettini P, Lacerenza M, Marangoni C, et al: Lidocaine test in neuralgia. Pain 1992; 48: 377–382.
12. Devor M, Wall PD, Catalan N: Systemic lidocaine silences ectopic neuroma and DRG discharge without blocking nerve conduction. Pain 1992; 48: 261–268.
13. Haddox JD, Kettler RE: Stellate ganglion block: normal saline as placebo. Anesthesiology 1987; 67: 832–834.
14. LeRoy PL, Filasky R: Thermography. In Bonica JJ (ed): The Management of Pain, 2nd ed, vol I, pp 610–621. Philadelphia, Lea & Febiger, 1990.
15. Low PA: Non-invasive evaluation of autonomic function. Neurol Chronicle 1992; 2: 1–8.
16. Lantsberg L, Goldman M: Lower limb sympathectomy assessed by laser Doppler blood flow and transcutaneous oxygen measurements. J Med Eng Technol 1990; 14: 182–183.
17. Joyner MJ, Nauss LA, Warner MA, et al: Sympathetic modulation of blood flow and O_2 uptake in rhythmically contracting human forearm muscles. Am J Physiol 1992; 263: H1078–H1083.
18. Walsh JA, Glynn CJ, Cousins MJ, et al: Blood flow, sympathetic activity and pain relief following lumbar sympathetic blockade or surgical sympathectomy. Anaesth Intensive Care 1984; 13: 18–24.
19. Kuntz A: Distribution of the sympathetic rami to the brachial plexus: its relation to sympathectomy affecting the upper extremity. Arch Surg 1927; 15: 871–877.
20. Wang JK, Johnson KA, Ilstrup DM: Sympathetic blocks for reflex sympathetic dystrophy. Pain 1985; 23: 13–17.
21. Payne R: Neuropathic pain syndromes, with special reference to causalgia and reflex sympathetic dystrophy. Clin J Pain 1986; 2: 59–73.
22. Olson ER, Ivy HB: Stellate block for trigeminal zoster. J Clin Neuroophthalmol 1981; 1: 53–55.
23. Lipton JR, Harding SP, Wells JCD: The effect of early stellate ganglion block on postherpetic neuralgia in herpes zoster ophthalmicus. Pain Clin 1987; 1: 247–251.
24. Milligan NS, Nash TP: Treatment of post-herpetic neuralgia. A review of 77 consecutive cases. Pain 1985; 23: 381–386.
25. Shih CJ, Wu JJ, Lin MT: Autonomic dysfunction in palmar hyperhidrosis. J Auton Nerv Syst 1983; 8: 33–43.
26. Tenicela R, Lovasik D, Eaglstein W: Treatment of herpes zoster with sympathetic blocks. Clin J Pain 1985; 1: 63–67.
27. Lilley J-P, Su WPD, Wang JK: Sensory and sympathetic nerve blocks for postherpetic neuralgia. Reg Anesth 1986; 11: 165–167.
28. Ochoa JL: Reflex sympathetic dystrophy: a disease of medical understanding. Clin J Pain 1992; 8: 363–366.
29. Campbell JN, Meyer RA, Raja SN: Is nociceptor activation by alpha-1 adrenoreceptors the culprit in sympathetically maintained pain? Am Pain Soc J 1992; 1: 3–11.
30. Woolf CJ, Thompson SW: The induction and maintenance of central sensitization is dependent on N-methyl-D-aspartic acid receptor activation; implications for the treatment of post-injury pain hypersensitivity states. Pain 1991; 44: 293–299.
31. Chabal C, Jacobson L, Mariano A, et al: The use of oral mexiletine for the treatment of pain after peripheral nerve injury. Anesthesiology 1992; 76: 513–517.
32. Tanelian DL, Brose WG: Neuropathic pain can be relieved by drugs that are use-dependent sodium channel blockers: lidocaine, carbamazepine, and mexiletine. Anesthesiology 1991; 74: 949–951.
33. Arner S: Intravenous phentolamine test: diagnostic and prognostic use in reflex sympathetic dystrophy. Pain 1991; 46: 17–22.
34. Drott C, Gothberg G, Claes G: Endoscopic procedures of the upper-thoracic sympathetic chain. A review. Arch Surg 1993; 128: 237–241.
35. Robertson DP, Simpson RK, Rose JE, et al: Video-assisted endoscopic thoracic ganglionectomy. J Neurosurg 1993; 79: 238–240.
36. Guntamukkala M, Hardy PA: Spread of injectate after stellate ganglion block in man: an anatomical study. Br J Anaesth 1991; 66: 643–644.
37. Hogan QH, Erickson SJ, Haddox JD, et al: The spread of solutions during stellate ganglion block. Reg Anesth 1992; 17: 78–83.
38. Hogan QH, Taylor ML, Goldstein M, et al: Success rates in producing sympathetic blockade by paratracheal injection. Clin J Pain 1994; 10: 139–145.
39. Malmqvist EL, Bengtsson M, Sorensen J: Efficacy of stellate ganglion block: a clinical study with bupivacaine. Reg Anesth 1992; 17: 340–347.
40. Hardy PA, Wells JC: Extent of sympathetic blockade after stellate ganglion block with bupivacaine. Pain 1989; 36: 193–196.
41. Linson MA, Leffert R, Todd DP: The treatment of upper extremity reflex sympathetic dystrophy with prolonged continuous stellate ganglion blockade. J Hand Surg [Am] 1983; 8: 153–159.
42. Hoepp HW, Eggeling T, Hombach V: Pharmacologic blockade of the left stellate ganglion using a drug-reservoir-pump system. Chest 1990; 97: 250–251.
43. Yarzebski JL, Wilkinson HA: T2 and T3 sympathetic ganglia in the adult human: a cadaver and clinical-radiographic study and its clinical application. Neurosurgery 1987; 21: 339–342.
44. Hogan Q, Erickson S: Success rates of sympathetic blockade: CT guided T1 injection vs C6 paratracheal injection. Reg Anesth 1993; 18: S23.
45. Dondelinger RF, Kurdziel JC: Percutaneous phenol block of the upper thoracic sympathetic chain with computed tomography guidance. A new technique. Acta Radiol 1987; 28: 511–515.
46. Wilkinson HA: Percutaneous radiofrequency upper thoracic sympathectomy: a new technique. Neurosurgery 1984; 15: 811–814.
47. Chuang K-S, Liou N-H, Liu J-C: New stereotactic technique for percutaneous thermocoagulation upper thoracic ganglionectomy in cases of palmar hyperhidrosis. Neurosurgery 1988; 22: 600–604.
48. Simeone FA: The anatomy of the lumbar sympathetic trunks in man (with special reference to the question of regeneration after sympathectomy). J Cardiovasc Surg (Torino) 1979; 20: 283–288.
49. Cowley RA, Yeager GH: Anatomic observations on the lumbar sympathetic nervous system. Surgery 1949; 25: 880–890.
50. Löfström JB, Cousins MJ: Sympathetic neural blockade of upper and lower extremity in Cousins MJ, Bridenbaugh PO (eds): Neural Blockade in Clinical Anesthesia and Management of Pain, 2nd ed, pp 461–500. Philadelphia, JB Lippincott, 1988.
51. Cherry DA, Rao DM: Lumbar sympathetic and coeliac plexus blocks. An anatomical study in cadavers. Br J Anaesth 1982; 54: 1037–1039.
52. Vulpio C, Borzone A, Iannace C, et al: Lumbar chemical sympathectomy in end stage of arterial disease: early and late results. Angiology 1989; 40: 948–952.
53. Rosen RJ, Miller DL, Imparato AM, et al: Percutaneous phenol sympathectomy in advanced vascular disease. AJR Am J Roentgenol 1983; 141: 597–600.
54. Cousins MJ, Reeve TS, Glynn CJ, et al: Neurolytic lumbar sympathetic blockade: duration of denervation and relief of rest pain. Anaesth Intensive Care 1979; 7: 121–135.

55. Skeehan TM, Cory PC Jr: Neurolytic lumbar sympathetic block in the treatment of Raynaud's phenomenon. Anesthesiology 1986; 64: 119–120.

56. Leriche R, Fontaine R: L'anesthésie isolée du ganglion étoilé: sa technique, ses indications, ses resultats. Presse Med 1934; 42: 849–850.

57. Strand L: Lumbar sympathectomy in the treatment of peripheral obliterative arterial disease. An analysis of 167 patients. Acta Chir Scand 1969; 135: 597–600.

58. Hughes-Davies DI, Redman LR: Chemical lumbar sympathectomy. Anaesthesia 1976; 31: 1068–1075.

59. Haimovici H, Steinman C, Karson IH: Evaluation of lumbar sympathectomy: advanced occlusive arterial disease. Arch Surg 1964; 89: 1089–1095.

60. Froysaker T: Lumbar sympathectomy in impending gangrene and foot ulcer. Scand J Clin Lab Invest Suppl 1973; 128: 71–72.

61. Myers KA, Irvine WT: An objective study of lumbar sympathectomy. II. Skin ischaemia. Br Med J 1966; 1: 943–947.

62. Fyfe T, Quin RO: Phenol sympathectomy in the treatment of intermittent claudication: a controlled clinical trial. Br J Surg 1975; 62: 68–71.

63. Eaton AC, Wright M, Callum KG: The use of the image intensifier in phenol lumbar sympathetic block. Radiography 1980; 46: 298–300.

64. Zagzag D, Fields S, Romanoff H, et al: Percutaneous chemical lumbar sympathectomy with alcohol with computed tomography control. Int Angiol 1986; 5: 83–86.

65. Hatangdi VS, Boas RA: Lumbar sympathectomy: a single needle technique. Br J Anaesth 1985; 57: 285–289.

66. Umeda S, Arai T, Hatano Y, et al: Cadaver anatomic analysis of the best site for chemical lumbar sympathectomy. Anesth Analg 1987; 66: 643–646.

67. Strumpf M, Zenz M, Donner B, et al: Continuous block of the lumbar sympathetic trunk via catheter. Pain Digest 1994; 1: 21–28.

68. Haynsworth RF Jr, Noe CE: Percutaneous lumbar sympathectomy: a comparison of radiofrequency denervation versus phenol neurolysis. Anesthesiology 1991; 74: 459–463.

69. Buche M, Randour P, Mayne A, et al: Neuralgia following lumbar sympathectomy. Ann Vasc Surg 1988; 2: 279–281.

70. Ward EM, Rorie DK, Nauss LA, et al: The celiac ganglia in man: normal anatomic variations. Anesth Analg 1979; 58: 461–465.

71. Paz Z, Rosen A: The human celiac ganglion and its splanchnic nerves. Acta Anat (Basel) 1989; 136: 129–133.

72. Thompson GE, Moore DC, Bridenbaugh LD, et al: Abdominal pain and alcohol celiac plexus nerve block. Anesth Analg 1977; 56: 1–5.

73. Gorbitz C, Leavens ME: Alcohol block of the celiac plexus for control of upper abdominal pain caused by cancer and pancreatitis. Technical note. J Neurosurg 1971; 34: 575–579.

74. Hegedus V: Relief of pancreatic pain by radiography-guided block. AJR Am J Roentgenol 1979; 133: 1101–1103.

75. Brown DL, Bulley CK, Quiel EL: Neurolytic celiac plexus block for pancreatic cancer pain. Anesth Analg 1987; 66: 869–873.

76. Brown DL: A retrospective analysis of neurolytic celiac plexus block for nonpancreatic intra-abdominal cancer pain. Reg Anesth 1989; 14: 63–65.

77. Lebovits AH, Lefkowitz M: Pain management of pancreatic carcinoma: a review. Pain 1989; 36: 1–11.

78. Ischia S, Ischia A, Polati E, et al: Three posterior percutaneous celiac plexus block techniques. A prospective, randomized study in 61 patients with pancreatic cancer pain. Anesthesiology 1992; 76: 534–540.

79. Sharfman WH, Walsh TD: Has the analgesic efficacy of neurolytic celiac plexus block been demonstrated in pancreatic cancer pain? Pain 1990; 41: 267–271.

80. Lillemoe KD, Cameron JL, Kaufman HS, et al: Chemical splanchnicectomy in patients with unresectable pancreatic cancer: a prospective randomized trial. Ann Surg 1993; 217: 447–455.

81. Dale WA: Splanchnic block in the treatment of acute pancreatitis. Surgery 1952; 32: 605–614.

82. Bell SN, Cole R, Roberts-Thomson IC: Coeliac plexus block for control of pain in chronic pancreatitis. Br Med J 1980; 281: 1604.

83. Hastings RH, McKay WR: Treatment of benign chronic abdominal pain with neurolytic celiac plexus block. Anesthesiology 1991; 75: 156–158.

84. Singler RC: An improved technique for alcohol neurolysis of the celiac plexus. Anesthesiology 1982; 56: 137–141.

85. Ischia S, Luzzana A, Ischia A, et al: A new approach to the neurolytic block of the coeliac plexus: the transaortic technique. Pain 1983; 16: 333–341.

86. Montero Matamala A, Vidal Lopez F, Inaraja Martinez L: The percutaneous anterior approach to the celiac plexus using CT guidance. Pain 1988; 34: 285–288.

87. Ina H, Kobayashi M, Narita M, et al: A new approach to neurolytic block of the celiac plexus: transintervertebral disc technique. (Abstract.) Anesthesiology 1991; 75: A718.

88. Buy J-N, Moss AA, Singler RC: CT guided celiac plexus and splanchnic nerve neurolysis. J Comput Assist Tomogr 1982; 6: 315–319.

89. Filshie J, Golding S, Robbie DS, et al: Unilateral computerised tomography guided coeliac plexus block: a technique for pain relief. Anaesthesia 1983; 38: 498–503.

90. Humbles FF, Mahaffey JE: Teflon epidural catheter placement for intermittent celiac plexus blockade and celiac plexus neurolytic blockade. Reg Anesth 1990; 15: 103–105.

91. Lo JN, Buckley JJ: Spinal cord ischemia: a complication of celiac plexus block. Reg Anesth 1982; 7: 66–68.

92. Cherry DA, Lamberty J: Paraplegia following coeliac plexus block. Anaesth Intensive Care 1984; 12: 59–61.

93. Noda J, Umeda S, Mori K, et al: Acetaldehyde syndrome after celiac plexus alcohol block. Anesth Analg 1986; 65: 1300–1302.

94. Hollinshead WH, Rosse C: Textbook of Anatomy, 4th ed, pp 735–814. Philadelphia, Harper & Row, 1985.

95. Plancarte R, Amescua C, Patt RB, et al: Superior hypogastric plexus block for pelvic cancer pain. Anesthesiology 1990; 73: 236–239.

96. de Leon-Casasola OA, Kent E, Lema MJ: Neurolytic superior hypogastric plexus block for chronic pelvic pain associated with cancer. Pain 1993; 54: 145–151.

97. Waldman SD, Wilson WL, Kreps RD: Superior hypogastric plexus block using a single needle and computed tomography guidance: description of a modified technique. Reg Anesth 1991; 16: 286–287.

98. Johnson RM, McGuire EJ: Urogenital complications of anterior approaches to the lumbar spine. Clin Orthop 1981; 154: 114–118.

CHAPTER 21

Intravenous Regional Anesthesia

Per H. Rosenberg, M.D., Ph.D.

History

In 1908, August Bier (professor of surgery in Berlin) described[1] the principles of the technique that today is called intravenous regional anesthesia (IVRA) and sometimes Bier's block. A surgical cutdown during infiltration local anesthesia was performed to locate a superficial vein of the limb between two tourniquets. After injection of procaine (0.25% or 0.5%) into a vein, Bier noted an initial rapidly developing analgesia in the region between the tourniquets, which allowed the start of surgery. A slower developing analgesia was noted distal to the more distally positioned tourniquet.

The original version of the modern pneumatic tourniquet, an adaptation of the sphygmomanometer, was introduced by Harvey Cushing in 1904. His design was supplied by a bicycle pump, which later was improved by including a manometer and a connection to compressed air pipelines.

Equipment

Tourniquets

A pneumatic tourniquet for application on the extremity is an essential component of IVRA. Tourniquets similar to those used in orthopedic surgery for bloodless operations may be used (e.g., 5, 7, or 9 cm wide for adults). Pneumatic tourniquets are available in several widths with Velcro strap fasteners. Usually, a double-tourniquet technique should be used, but there may not be space on the upper arm for two separate tourniquet cuffs. Specially designed IVRA double-cuff tourniquets, i.e., two cuffs attached to each other, are commercially available. These are quite practical, particularly for use in IVRA of the upper extremity.

The incidence of the so-called tourniquet paralysis was significantly decreased (to almost nil) when the use of the Martin (von Esmarch) bandage tourniquet was abandoned and instead pneumatic tourniquets with pressure gauges were introduced.[2, 3] Unfortunately, the gauges used in most commercially available pneumatic tourniquets are subject to inaccuracy and each tourniquet manometer must undergo routine and regular calibration (record keeping). This is easily done with a commercial test gauge or a standard manually operated blood pressure manometer.

It is important to apply a soft and smooth padding (e.g., cast padding) between the skin and the rough tourniquets. This protects the skin from possible injuries by the hard surface of the inflated tourniquet cuffs. The pad will not decrease the pressure effect on the underlying tissue mass. Care should be taken to prevent flow of scrubbing disinfectant under the cuffs because the ischemic skin may be easily damaged.

The best way of preventing nerve injuries due to tourniquets is to minimize as much as possible the destructive effect of the cuff pressure, especially the shear stress under the cuff edges. The pressure in the cuff should be kept as low as possible, and the pressure applied should always be related to the patient's arterial blood pressure at the time of operation. It is recommended that the pressure in the cuff used for the upper extremity not be more than 50 to 100 mm Hg above the systolic pressure, usually 250 to 300 mm Hg in adults.[4, 5] For the lower limb (thigh), twice the systolic pressure, usually 350 to 400 mm Hg, is used.[6, 7] The use of sufficiently wide cuffs enables lower-range pressures to be used, decreasing the risk of tissue injury under the cuff edges.

After inflation of the tourniquet, there is a rapid change in cell metabolism, fibrinolytic activity, and electrolyte balance in the ischemic extremity.[8–12] There is rapid decrease in tissue Po_2, which reaches low values after only 20 to 25 min, accompanied by a corresponding increase in P_{CO_2} and a decrease in pH. During the period of ischemia, the metabolism of muscle cells switches from aerobic to anaerobic. The glycogen level in the tissue decreases gradually during the ischemia at the same time as there is an increased lactate level in the muscle. After deflation of the tourniquet cuff and the restitution of blood flow, the values of P_{O_2} and P_{CO_2} revert to normal within 10 min after 1 h of ischemia and within 15 to 20 min after 3 h of ischemia.[13]

Reversible histologic and ultrastructural changes as well as disturbance in neuromuscular transmission have been observed after only 1.5 to 2 h of ischemia.[8, 14]

There is no absolute rule as to how long a tourniquet may safely remain inflated on the extremity. In practice, 1.5 h (sometimes up to 2 h) is considered the limit. In an awake patient, e.g., in IVRA, tourniquet pain usually limits the time to 1 h.

Martin (von Esmarch) Bandage

Although von Esmarch introduced the principle of limb exsanguination by a rubber-containing bandage in 1873, the rubber bandage still used clinically today for exsanguination is the design of the surgeon Henry A. Martin in 1877.

Like von Esmarch, Martin also did not use his bandage as an actual tourniquet but rather as a method of applying diffuse pressure to an entire lower extremity for the treatment of stasis ulcers and to prevent recurrence of effusion after aspiration of the knee or elbow joint.

Today, the Martin bandage, usually 10 to 12 cm wide, is used for emptying the extremity of blood. The bandage is wound from the periphery toward the tourniquet cuff as tightly as possible, creating an intratissue pressure that markedly exceeds the arterial pressure along the whole extremity. When the final turns of the bandage have been applied over the more distal of the two tourniquet cuffs, the cuff is inflated to the proper pressure. For the exsanguination of the lower limb, tight and slightly elastic rubber rings of different sizes may be used to roll on the extremity and compress the underlying arteries.

Both the upper and the lower extremities may be partly (sufficiently) exsanguinated just by elevating the limb for 2 to 3 min. The inflow of arterial blood may be restricted by manually compressing the main artery (axillary artery and femoral artery, respectively). Adequate artery compression can be monitored by attaching a pulse oximeter probe on a finger or a toe.

Pressure Gauge

Tourniquet paralysis was more frequent when the Martin bandage itself was routinely used as a tourniquet,[15, 16] and it is well documented that these rubber bandages can easily generate pressures far in excess of those considered safe. The incidence of this complication has been significantly decreased, but not completely eliminated, with the use of pneumatic tourniquets.[2, 16] The gauges currently in use in most commercially available pneumatic tourniquets are subject to significant inaccuracies[16]; therefore, regular and routine calibration must be performed before use. Although the relative roles of ischemia and pressure have been debated, it appears that direct pressure beneath the cuff is the major causative factor in the production of posttourniquet paralysis.[17] By the use of double-cuff tourniquets or two tourniquet cuffs and alternating inflation-deflation at 30- to 45-min intervals, continuous compression of localized segments of nerves and vessels is prevented.

Drugs for IVRA

Local Anesthetics

All available local anesthetics have been used for IVRA (Table 21–1). Because of the administration of a substantial dose of the local anesthetic directly intravenously, toxicologic aspects have determined, to a great extent, the choices of clinically suitable local anesthetics for IVRA. Thus, 0.5% lidocaine and 0.5% prilocaine are the most common local anesthetics for IVRA at present. Prilocaine, which is slightly less toxic to the central nervous system and the heart, is not available in the United States. Obviously, epinephrine (adrenaline) is not added to the solutions, which should be preservative-free.

For IVRA of the whole lower extremity, a local anesthetic volume of approximately 100 mL is needed in an adult. Therefore, in the case of lidocaine, a more dilute solution, 0.2% to 0.25%, should be used to meet the recommendations regarding maximum doses. With prilocaine, the solution may still be undiluted (0.5%) because the maximum recommended dose in adults is 600 mg. After the use of prilocaine for IVRA, there is a moderate increase in blood methemoglobin levels[27, 28] but not to a level that is accompanied by cyanosis and hypoxemia (Fig. 21–1).

Table 21–1 Local Anesthetics Used in Intravenous Regional Anesthesia (IVRA)

ANESTHETIC	CONCENTRATION (%)	REFERENCE
Esters		
2-Chloroprocaine	0.5–1	Dickler et al, 1965[18]
Cocaine	0.5	Hitzrot, 1909[19]
Procaine	0.25–0.5	Bier, 1908[1]
Tetracaine	0.5	Durrani et al, 1982[20]
Amides		
Articaine	0.5	Simon et al, 1995[21]
Bupivacaine	0.2–0.5	Ware, 1975[22]
Etidocaine	0.25	Evans et al, 1974[23]
Lidocaine	0.15–1	Holmes, 1963[24]
Mepivacaine	0.5	Cox, 1964[25]
Prilocaine	0.25–2	Hooper, 1964[26]

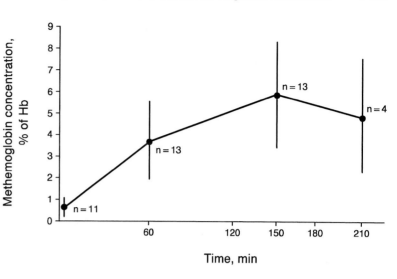

Figure 21–1 Mean methemoglobin concentrations (percentage of hemoglobin [Hb] ± standard deviation) after intravenous regional anesthesia (6 mg/kg prilocaine) of the whole lower extremity of patients. Hypoxemia usually does not develop at methemoglobin levels below 10% to 15%. (From Valli HK, Rosenberg PH, Hekali R: Comparison of lidocaine and prilocaine for intravenous regional anesthesia of the whole lower extremity. Reg Anesth 1987; 12: 128–134.)

More concentrated prilocaine solutions (0.75% to 2%) have been used for IVRA of the upper and lower extremities.[29, 30] The onset time is decreased, but otherwise the block characteristics are quite similar to those of IVRA with 0.5% prilocaine. The occurrence of mild symptoms of central nervous system toxicity may be more frequent in patients who have received the more concentrated solutions if the dose is not decreased.

Mepivacaine 0.5% produces an equivalent IVRA block to that of lidocaine or prilocaine,[31, 32] but it does not offer any clinical advantage, and it is more toxic than prilocaine.[33]

Bupivacaine at concentrations from 0.2% to 0.5% was popular for IVRA in the early 1980s.[34, 35] However, as a result of severe toxic reactions[36] and deaths[37] associated with bupivacaine-IVRA, bupivacaine is no longer recommended for use in IVRA.

Etidocaine 0.25% has been found to produce an IVRA block similar in anesthetic quality to that produced by 0.5% lidocaine, but after the release of the tourniquet the motor block caused by etidocaine persists for about 2 h.[38]

Articaine (4-methyl-3-[2-propylaminopropionamido]-thiophene-2-carboxylic acid hydrochloride), an amide-type local anesthetic with a sulfur atom included in the aromatic part of the molecule, appears to be a suitable drug for IVRA.[21] As a 0.5% solution, it has a faster onset and anesthetic characteristics similar to 0.5% lidocaine and prilocaine.

Ester-type local anesthetics have also been used for IVRA. In fact, procaine was the first one used, as described by Bier,[1] followed by cocaine.[25] Tetracaine has been studied[20] but not widely used in IVRA. On the other hand, 2-chloroprocaine has been more commonly used, but the solution that contained both preservative and antioxidant was abandoned already in the late 1960s because of the occurrence of thrombophlebitis in the veins exposed to 2-chloroprocaine.[18, 39] A new additive-free 0.5% 2-chloroprocaine solution seems to be better tolerated, but still, postinflation irritation of the exposed veins occurs.[40, 41] Because of the rapid breakdown of ester-type local anesthetics in the blood by serum pseudocholinesterase,[42] the systemic toxicity of 2-chloroprocaine should be lower than that of prilocaine.[43]

Drugs Combined with Local Anesthetics

The addition of fentanyl[44, 45] or morphine[46] to local anesthetic solutions does not improve the quality of surgical anesthesia or analgesia. After the release of the tourniquet, the released opioid delays the need for the first postoperative analgesic,[45] and some patients experience nausea and vomiting. When 0.2 mg of fentanyl has been mixed with 0.5% prilocaine for upper extremity IVRA, the plasma concentrations of prilocaine after tourniquet release have been significantly higher than when prilocaine alone has been given.[45] This may be due to a vasodilatory action of fentanyl on the exposed limb and a pharmacokinetic interaction after release into the circulation. Opioids alone (small doses) do not seem to have any analgesic action when injected intravenously to an isolated arm.[44, 47]

Pancuronium (0.5 mg) has been added to 0.25% lidocaine for IVRA of the arm.[48] There was no influence on the sensory block, but the motor block developed faster and lasted longer after the tourniquet release when pancuronium had been given. Dilute d-tubocurarine (3 mg in 40 mL saline), injected instead of lidocaine, produced a marked muscle relaxation without influence on analgesia.[49] Although interesting, these findings have little clinical relevance because normally there is profound motor block during local anesthetic IVRA.

Other Drugs Used in IVRA or Given by IVRA Technique

Ketamine, 0.2% to 0.5%, has been used for IVRA of the arm in patients and volunteers.[50, 51] With the more concentrated solutions, sensory analgesia is good but loss of consciousness[50] and psychotomimetic side effects[51] occur after the release of the tourniquet in some of the subjects.

Most of the other drugs administered by the IVR technique have been intended for the treatment of chronic pain syndromes (mostly, reflex sympathetic dystrophy) of the extremities. This group includes guanethidine, bretylium, reserpine, droperidol, phentolamine, calcium channel blockers, clonidine, methylprednisolone, ketanserin, and ketorolac. The true value of these drugs is hard to assess because of the difficulty in arranging masked and controlled study conditions. Among those that have undergone controlled evaluations, bretylium,[52] ketanserin (a serotonin antagonist),[53] and ketorolac[54] appear to be beneficial in the treatment of reflex sympathetic dystrophy with the IVR technique.

Clinical Pharmacology and Toxicity of Local Anesthetics in IVRA

Peak plasma concentrations of local anesthetics are significantly greater after a rapid intravenous infusion than after tourniquet cuff deflation in upper extremity IVRA, with the same dose.[55] Prolongation of the tourniquet inflation time (tourniquet time) decreases peak arterial plasma concentrations after cuff deflation (Fig. 21–2). Possible secondary plasma concentration peaks[56, 57] may result from exercise (motor testing, movements) of the limb in the immediate recovery and blood-sampling period. By using larger volumes of more dilute solutions (same dose), plasma concentrations of the local anesthetic are slightly lower[55] or remain virtually unchanged.[58]

The amount of local anesthetic that is immediately washed away into the circulation on release of the tourniquet cuff depends on the tourniquet time. After 10 min with a tourniquet on (1% lidocaine), about 30% of the dose is released immediately in the first flush, and after 30 min, still about 45% of the dose remains in the arm.[55] When the tourniquet is on 45 min, the release is much slower, and the release of a 30% fraction of the total dose takes almost 4 min. It has been estimated that about 55% of the dose remains in the arm after 30 min.[55]

Drugs released from the blocked extremity must first pass through the lungs (Fig. 21–3) before entering the systemic arterial circulation. The lungs, therefore, are in a strategic position for clearing the blood of drug, thereby protecting the central nervous system and heart from a high concentration (bolus-type effect) of the drug. It has been shown that lung uptake of prilocaine in humans is greater than that of lidocaine, which contributes to its greater safety margin systemically and in IVRA.[59] The extravascular pH of the lung tissue is low relative to plasma pH, and this enhances ion trapping of local anesthetics.[60]

Certain practical aspects can be derived from known pharmacokinetic facts. For instance, if IVRA of an extremity needs to be reestablished following tourniquet cuff release, this may be possible 10 to 30 min after the release, and the dose of local anesthetic should be about half the dose given for the original block.[55]

In order to avoid toxic reactions, the tourniquet should be kept inflated for a minimum of 20 min, even when the operation would have been completed earlier. If, on the other hand, the cuff must be released earlier (e.g., increasing venous congestion, sharp pain under the cuff), this should be done in cycles with a reinflation interval less than 30 s. The cuff is deflated and inflated in cycles until there is certainty that toxic symptoms have not developed (usually in 2 to 3 min). In order to avoid venous congestion during the cycling, it has been recommended that the deflation phase of the cycling be shortened to just 10 s.[61]

Mild central nervous system toxicity sometimes occurs after the deflation of the cuff, even with the use of prilocaine.[28, 41, 45] These symptoms range from numbness of the tongue to tinnitus and visual disturbances.[28] Convulsions and loss of consciousness associated with IVRA are rare when prilocaine or lidocaine is used. However, severe local anesthetic intoxications have been reported when bupivacaine has been used for IVRA, owing to either leakage under the tourniquet cuff (Fig. 21–4)[36] or rapid release into the circulation because of faulty equipment.[37]

Signs (electrocardiogram and arterial blood pressure) of mild cardiovascular toxicity sometimes occur after

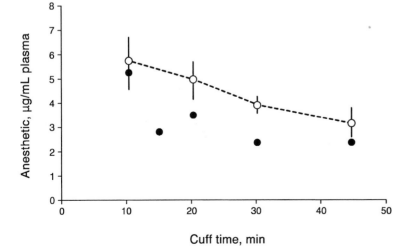

Figure 21–2 Relationship between tourniquet inflation time during intravenous regional anesthesia and arterial concentrations (μg/mL) of lidocaine in plasma at 1 min after cuff release. Open circles, mean data, 1% solution; closed circles, individual data, 0.5% solution. The difference between the two groups (solutions) is statistically significant, $P < .05$. (From Tucker GT, Boas RA: Pharmacokinetic aspects of intravenous regional anesthesia. Anesthesiology 1971; 34: 538–549.)

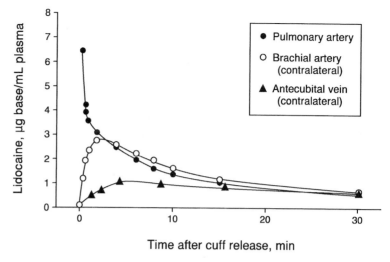

Figure 21–3 Plasma concentrations of lidocaine in a subject following tourniquet cuff release after intravenous regional anesthesia with 3 mg/kg lidocaine (tourniquet time was 45 min). Note the indications of the uptake of lidocaine in the lung, as evidenced by the differences between pulmonary arterial and peripheral arterial concentrations. (From Tucker GT, Boas RA: Pharmacokinetic aspects of intravenous regional anesthesia. Anesthesiology 1971; 34: 538–549.)

the release of the tourniquet cuff.[62, 63] This seems to occur more often after 0.5% 2-chloroprocaine than after 0.5% prilocaine.[40, 64] Severe cardiovascular toxicity of local anesthetics in IVRA has occurred only as a result of technical defects, perhaps in addition to inability to recognize early symptoms of toxicity.

The majority of patients with a history of allergy to local anesthetic drugs are not allergic,[65] and true allergy, particularly to amide-type local anesthetics, is rare. However, there are a few case reports of adverse reactions to prilocaine in association with IVRA of the upper extremity[66] as well as skin reaction and venous irritation after tourniquet release with the use of either prilocaine or 2-chloroprocaine.[41] It has been suggested that some of the skin reactions after the use of prilocaine could be due to the antimicrobial preservative methylparaben, which is known to cause hypersensitivity-type skin reactions.[65, 67] In order to avoid this possibility, preservative-free local anesthetic solutions should be used in IVRA.

Mechanisms of Action of IVRA

Although the large superficial veins contain valves, they can be filled retrogradely, even by a relatively slow peripheral injection of local anesthetic. Smaller veins are valveless, and they communicate with a rich network to the venules of the nerve trunks, probably more to the core than to the periphery.[68]

The nerve trunks of the extremity consist of several fascicles united by a connective tissue layer called *epineurium*. Blood vessels supplying the nerve are contained in the epineurium. The *endoneurium* forms an envelope around each individual nerve fiber and contains capillary plexuses that extend interneurally as *vasa nervorum*. The capillaries drain directly into small veins. Nerve fibers at the center of the fascicle are more distant from the lipoprotein-rich epineurium, and they are not encumbered by any great diffusion barrier between the vessels and the nerve axon. Therefore, local anesthetic diffusion from the nerve core to the periph-

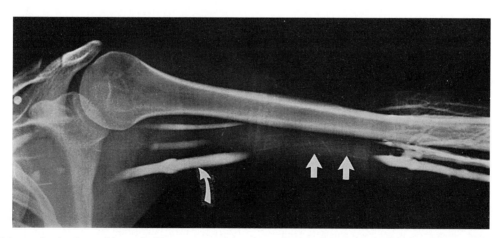

Figure 21–4 Phlebography (performed instead of intravenous regional anesthesia) of the arm of a female volunteer. The tourniquet cuff pressure was 250 mm Hg, and 50 mL of contrast medium was injected at a rate of 1 mL/s. Note the filling of axillary veins with contrast medium already in the first (15 s) roentgenogram (curved arrow). The straight arrows indicate narrow contrast medium streaks under the inflated cuff. (From Rosenberg PH, Kalso EA, Tuominen MK, et al: Acute bupivacaine toxicity as a result of venous leakage under the tourniquet cuff during a Bier block. Anesthesiology 1983; 58: 95–98.)

ery may account for an often-noted centripetal progression of the anesthesia in IVRA.

Some areas are not supplied by nerve fibers emanating from assembled nerve trunks near regions rich in vascularity. Such nerves as the intercostobrachial nerves are not near a tight vessel network and, therefore, are not rapidly anesthetized in IVRA unless they are specifically blocked. Nerve endings in the skin may be reached by local anesthetic solution through a multitude of valveless venules.

Surgical anesthesia in IVRA is produced by multiple and complementary mechanisms (Table 21–2). The initial observable effect is block of the skin along the veins filled with local anesthetic, i.e., block of nerve endings and small nerves (peripheral action). Some radiographic studies[69] have shown that the development of analgesia follows the distribution of the injected mixture of local anesthetic and contrast medium. Others have found accumulation of injected contrast medium[68, 70] or radioactive lidocaine[71] in the vicinity of major nerve trunks near the elbow in IVRA of the arm. When distal flow of a solution of local anesthetic and contrast medium is prevented by a tourniquet, anesthesia develops to the most distal parts of the arm.[68] This phenomenon, in fact, was shown already in 1908 by August Bier.[1]

The uptake of lidocaine into nerve trunks occurs rapidly (2 to 4 min), as shown by positron emission tomography, after the injection of [^{11}C]lidocaine for IVRA.[71] After tourniquet release, positron emission in the nerves decreases rapidly. More lipid-soluble and strongly protein-bound local anesthetics, such as bupivacaine and etidocaine, stay in the nerve trunks longer, which in IVRA has been associated with prolonged analgesia after deflation of the tourniquet cuff.[34, 38]

The ischemic component of IVRA is usually regarded as a major determinant in the nerve-blocking mechanisms.[72] In fact, complete pinprick analgesia of the skin of the arm, as well as motor block of the hand, can be achieved in 20 to 25 min when saline, or nothing at all, is administered as in IVRA.[72, 73]

Clinical Aspects of IVRA

IVRA of the Arm

Indications for IVRA of the arm (upper extremity) are surgical treatment of the hand, forearm, or elbow, which will last, usually, less than an hour. Typical surgical diagnoses are carpal tunnel syndrome, ganglion of

Table 21–2 Mechanisms of Action of Intravenous Regional Anesthesia (IVRA)

Block of peripheral small nerve endings and nerves (initial effect)
Block of nerve trunks at a proximal site (e.g., cubital area in IVRA of the arm)
Ischemia (blocks nerve conduction and motor end plate function)
Compression on nerve trunks (slow component)

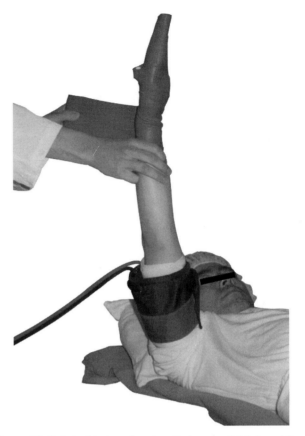

Figure 21–5 A double tourniquet applied over soft fabric padding. A Martin (von Esmarch) bandage is tightly wound from the periphery to the distal cuff for exsanguination.

the carpal or hand region, tendon ruptures, and Colles fracture.

Usually no premedication is needed in adult cooperative patients, but in anticipation of a prolonged operation, premedication with diazepam, 0.1 to 0.2 mg/kg, given orally may be warranted. The administration of opioid premedication, in addition, may prevent or ease tourniquet-induced pain.[74]

A plastic venous cannula (20 to 22 G) is placed as far peripherally as possible (dorsum of the hand) on the arm to be blocked. Another cannula is placed in a suitable vein of the other arm.

The brachium of the arm to be blocked is wrapped by two or three layers of thin cast padding (or other suitable nonirritant fabric). A double tourniquet or two separate tourniquets (usually each 7 cm wide) are fitted around the padding so that no wrinkles are formed and so that the tourniquet cuff edges are not in contact with the skin (Fig. 21–5). The tourniquet cuff straps are fastened, and the security cords are thoroughly tied around both cuffs (over the straps).

Exsanguination of the arm is accomplished by elevating the arm for 1 to 2 min and then wrapping a Martin (von Esmarch) rubber bandage (Fig. 21–5) around the arm, from the fingertips all the way to and partly over the more distal of the tourniquet cuffs. The wrapping should be tight, but not enough to hurt, in order to occlude arterial flow past the bandaged level. First, the distal cuff is inflated to a pressure approximately 100 mm Hg higher than the patient's systolic blood pressure, normally to 250 to 300 mm Hg. Then, when the cuff has been inflated, as verified both by the reading on the manometer gauge and by palpating the cuff, the proximal cuff is inflated to the same pressure. Again, the pressure and filling are verified and then the distal cuff is deflated. The Martin bandage is removed, and the injection of the local anesthetic solution can start. It is advisable to observe the superficial veins for 1 to 2 min before injection. If the veins start to fill, indicating arterial inflow under the cuff, the exsanguination procedure should be repeated, and the tourniquet inflation pressure may be raised by 50 mm Hg. If there is still arterial inflow that distends the veins, the IVRA technique should be abandoned and another anesthesia technique should be chosen (e.g., axillary brachial plexus block, local infiltration anesthesia, or general anesthesia).

In certain conditions, e.g., Colles fracture, a Martin bandage cannot be wrapped tightly. Often sufficient exsanguination can be achieved by elevating the arm for 2 to 3 min while compressing the axillary artery enough to occlude arterial inflow. This can be monitored by palpating the radial artery or by pulse oximetry from a finger.

In adults, 3 mg/kg of 0.5% lidocaine or 0.5% prilocaine (preservative-, antioxidant-, and epinephrine-free) is injected at a rate of approximately 20 mL/min. Faster rates of injection may result in an increase in venous pressure approaching that of the tourniquet pressure.[75, 76] At present, there are no reasons to use any of the other amide- or ester-type local anesthetics for IVRA.

The onset of analgesia of the skin normally occurs in 2 to 4 min, but surgical anesthesia after the administration of 0.5% lidocaine or prilocaine may not develop until after 15 to 20 min. With the use of more concentrated solutions of these local anesthetics (e.g., 0.75% or 1% prilocaine), the onset of pinprick analgesia and surgical anesthesia occurs faster. Usually, there is no need to supplement the block with local anesthetic infiltration because ischemia is also a powerful supplement.[72] Therefore, if time allows, waiting for just a few more minutes guarantees complete anesthesia of the extremity.

Tourniquet-induced pain, which may occur in spite of alternating pressurization of the cuffs, may be treated with small doses of fentanyl or alfentanil given intravenously.

Modifications of IVRA of the Arm

"Second-Wrap" Technique

Oozing at the site of operation is an infrequent but irritating problem that may occur in spite of a meticulous technique. A second wrap with a sterile Martin bandage has been shown to dry up the operative field.[77] A second wrap, performed 15 to 20 min after the local anesthetic injection, has no influence on the sensory and the motor block, but tolerance of the tourniquet seems to be improved.[78] When carefully performed, with lidocaine or prilocaine, the amount of local anesthetic removed from the arm to the circulation usually causes no toxic symptoms.

Preischemia IVRA Technique

Preinjection ischemia resulted in a significant reduction in the amount of local anesthetic needed for satisfactory anesthesia.[39, 79] With 20 to 30 min of preischemia, the lidocaine dose may be halved. However, this modification of IVRA has not gained popularity because of the substantial discomfort the patients may experience from the tourniquet and ischemia and because of the inevitable loss of active surgical time.

Additional Tourniquets

The peripherally injected local anesthetic solution may be forced to stay as peripherally as possible by applying a tight temporary tourniquet (e.g., Penrose drain) around the forearm for the duration of the injection and 5 to 10 min after it. Nerve endings in the more distal parts of the arm may become rapidly blocked, and operation on the hand can begin a few minutes earlier than usual.[80]

IVRA of the Lower Extremity

Indications for IVRA of the leg (lower extremity) include orthopedic surgery of short duration on the foot, removal of fixation plates and screws from the bones below the knee, and foreign body removal from the foot.

There are two significant differences between IVRA of the arm and IVRA of the leg. First, the local anesthetic volume (and dose) in IVRA of the whole lower extremity has to be approximately double that used for the arm. This obviously may increase the risk of local anesthetic intoxication due to leakage under the inflated cuff and to release of a large bolus dose of local anesthetic when the cuff is deflated. Second, in order to occlude the arterial inflow at the thigh level (femoral artery), the tourniquet pressure must be higher than in the arm (usually 350 to 400 mm Hg), which increases the occurrence and the intensity of tourniquet pain.[28]

Two separate 9-cm-wide tourniquet cuffs (adult patient) are applied, and care must be taken that the pneumatic parts of the tourniquets surround the thigh by more than 1.5 turns. Otherwise, the technique is similar to that described for IVRA of the arm. The preferred local anesthetic is prilocaine: dose, 6 mg/kg; injected volume, 90 to 100 mL.

In short-lasting surgery of the foot or ankle, the distal tourniquet cuff may be applied on the calf, clearly below the head of the fibula (away from the peroneal nerve), and the proximal cuff on the thigh (Fig. 21–6). The local anesthetic solution is injected with the distal tourniquet cuff inflated; therefore, the volume and the dose can be the same as for the arm of an adult,

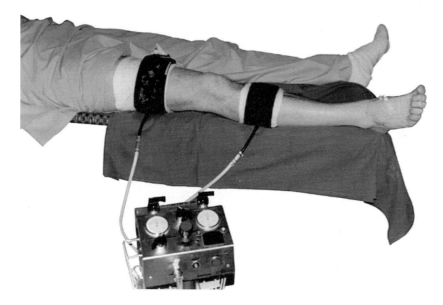

Figure 21–6 Intravenous regional anesthesia below the knee. The distal cuff is placed around the calf and kept inflated during the short surgical procedure, while the proximal cuff around the thigh is inflated only in an emergency, i.e., if the distal cuff fails.

i.e., 35 to 45 mL of 0.5% lidocaine or prilocaine. The proximal tourniquet is usually not inflated at all, but it is kept prepared as security in case the distal cuff fails.

Tourniquet Release

Severe local anesthetic intoxication after the release of the tourniquet cuff is rare when lidocaine or prilocaine (or 2-chloroprocaine) is used for IVRA. It has been generally accepted, in part from pharmacokinetic data,[55] that the tourniquet should never be released less than 20 min after the injection of the local anesthetic. If the patient is otherwise healthy, the amount of local anesthetic suddenly released into the circulation after such a latency does not seem to be deleterious to the heart. Occasional mild central nervous system symptoms (dizziness, tinnitus, lightheadedness) may occur. Such symptoms may be observed even when the subject has been heavily premedicated.[81] The tourniquet may be released in one step, but if the patient has some disease that may predispose the patient to severe toxic reactions (e.g., atrial fibrillation, hepatic dysfunction), a cycling deflation-inflation-deflation system is recommended. The reinflation interval should be less than 30 s. After final tourniquet release, the cuffs should be immediately removed in order to allow free circulation in the skin.

Monitoring of the Patient During IVRA

The patient should be monitored exactly as any other surgical patient who is receiving regional anesthesia. Therefore, electrocardiogram, noninvasive arterial blood pressure, and pulse oximetry are routine monitoring of such patients.

Special attention is paid to identifying possible signs or symptoms of local anesthetic intoxication during injection, during switch of pressurization of cuffs, and during the tourniquet release.

All equipment and drugs necessary for cardiopulmonary resuscitation should be immediately available. Thiopental (prepared) or propofol[82] must be at hand in case of severe central nervous system intoxication, including grand mal convulsions.

Contraindications to the Use of IVRA

In addition to a patient's refusal, contraindications are moderate or severe hypertensive disease, athletic build (strong muscles) of the patient, skeletal muscle disorders, and hypersensitivity to ester- or amide-type local anesthetics.

IVRA in Pediatric Patients

The IVRA technique is also applicable in children from age 3 years[83, 84] for operations of short duration. Indications include repositioning of painful fractures of the elbow, forearm, or hand as well as minor operations on the hand or foot. Technique-related pain may be avoided by omitting the use of the Martin (von Esmarch) bandage for exsanguination (elevation only), using eutectic lidocaine-prilocaine cream topically at the sites of venous cannulations, and restricting the use of IVRA to operations shorter than 20 min. In small children a single tourniquet is used, but in older ones (bigger) a double tourniquet or two cuffs should be applied as in adults. The sizes of the cuffs have to be selected according to size of the extremity. In the upper extremity, the tourniquet pressure should be 50 to 75 mm Hg above the patient's systolic blood pressure, whereas in the lower extremity, the pressure in a thigh tourniquet cuff should be 250 to 300 mm Hg (applicable only in older children).

The local anesthetics are either lidocaine or prilocaine 0.5%, and the volume (dose) for IVRA of the upper extremity may vary from 10 to 15 mL in a 3- to 4-year-old child to 25 to 30 mL in an 11- to 12-year-old.[83] For the lower extremity, the doses are approximately double (whole extremity), with prilocaine being the drug of choice.

References

1. Bier A: Ueber einen neuen Weg Localanästhesie an den Gliedmassen zu erzeugen. Arch Klin Chir 1908; 86: 1007–1016.
2. Bolton CF, McFarlane RM: Human pneumatic tourniquet paralysis. Neurology 1978; 28: 787–793.
3. Larsen UT, Hommelgaard P: Pneumatic tourniquet paralysis following intravenous regional analgesia. Anaesthesia 1987; 42: 526–528.
4. Flatt AE: Tourniquet time in hand surgery. Arch Surg 1972; 104: 190–192.
5. Klenerman L: Tourniquet time—how long? Hand 1980; 12: 231–234.
6. Klenerman L, Hulands GH: Tourniquet pressures for the lower limb (abstract). J Bone Joint Surg [Br] 1979; 61: 124.
7. Klenerman L: Tourniquet paralysis (editorial). J Bone Joint Surg [Br] 1983; 65: 374–375.
8. Solonen KA, Hjelt L: Morphological changes in striated muscle during ischaemia. A clinical and histological study in man. Acta Orthop Scand 1968; 39: 13–19.
9. Haljamäe H, Enger E: Human skeletal muscle energy metabolism during and after complete tourniquet ischemia. Ann Surg 1975; 182: 9–14.
10. Klenerman L, Chakrabarti R, Mackie I, et al: Changes in haemostatic system after application of a tourniquet. Lancet 1977; 1: 970–972.
11. Santavirta S, Höckerstedt K, Niinikoski J: Effect of pneumatic tourniquet on muscle oxygen tension. Acta Orthop Scand 1978; 49: 415–419.
12. Newman RJ: Metabolic effects of tourniquet ischaemia studied by nuclear magnetic resonance spectroscopy. J Bone Joint Surg [Br] 1984; 66: 434–440.
13. Haljamäe H, Hagberg H, Jennische E: Cellular effects of complete tourniquet ischemia. In Lewis DH (ed): Induced Skeletal Muscle Ischemia, p 33. Basel, Karger, 1982.
14. Patterson S, Klenerman L: The effect of pneumatic tourniquets on the ultrastructure of skeletal muscle. J Bone Joint Surg [Br] 1979; 61: 178–183.
15. Eckhoff NL: Tourniquet paralysis: plea for extended use of pneumatic tourniquet. Lancet 1931; 2: 243–245.
16. Green DP (ed): Operative Hand Surgery, pp 5–7. New York, Churchill Livingstone, 1982.
17. Lundborg G: Nerve Injury and Repair, pp 64–101. Edinburgh, Churchill Livingstone, 1988.
18. Dickler DJ, Friedman PL, Susman IC: Intravenous regional anesthesia with chloroprocaine (abstract). Anesthesiology 1965; 26: 244–245.
19. Hitzrot JM: Intravenous local anaesthesia. Ann Surg 1909; 1: 782–785.
20. Durrani Z, Russell J, Zsigmond EK, et al: Tetracaine for intravenous regional anesthesia. Reg Anesth 1982; 7: 81–82.
21. Simon MAM, Gielen MJM, Alberink N, et al: Intravenous regional anaesthesia with articaine 0.5% lidocaine 0.5% or prilocaine 0.5%. A double-blind clinical study. Reg Anesth (in press).
22. Ware RJ: Intravenous regional analgesia using bupivacaine. Anaesthesia 1975; 30: 817–822.
23. Evans CJ, Dewar JA, Boyes RN, et al: Residual nerve block following intravenous regional anaesthesia. Br J Anaesth 1974; 46: 668–670.
24. Holmes C McK: Intravenous regional analgesia: a useful method of producing analgesia of the limbs. Lancet 1963; 1: 245–247.
25. Cox JMR: Intravenous regional anaesthesia. Can Anaesth Soc J 1964; 11: 503–508.
26. Hooper RL: Intravenous regional anaesthesia: a report on a new local anaesthetic agent. Can Anaesth Soc J 1964; 11: 247–251.
27. Harris WH, Cole DW, Mital M, et al: Methemoglobin formation and oxygen transport following intravenous regional anesthesia using prilocaine. Anesthesiology 1968; 29: 65–69.
28. Valli HK, Rosenberg PH, Hekali R: Comparison of lidocaine and prilocaine for intravenous regional anesthesia of the whole lower extremity. Reg Anesth 1987; 12: 128–134.
29. Tryba M, Zenz M, Hausmann E: Controlled study on intravenous regional anesthesia using high and low concentration prilocaine. [German] Reg Anaesth 1983; 6: 27–29.
30. Prien T, Goeters C: Intravenose Regionalanesthesie an Arm und Fuss mit 0,5-, 0,75- und 1,0prozentigem Prilocain. [German] [Intravenous regional anesthesia of the arm and foot using 0.5, 0.75 and 1.0 percent prilocaine.] Anasth Intensivther Notf Med 1990; 25: 59–63.
31. Solonen KA, Tarkkanen L: Intravenous anaesthesia in surgery of the hand. Arch Orthop Unfallchir 1966; 60: 115–121.
32. Thorn-Alquist AM: Intravenous regional anaesthesia. Acta Anaesthesiol Scand Suppl 1971; 40: 1–35.
33. Englesson S: The influence of acid-base changes on central nervous system toxicity of local anaesthetic agents. I. An experimental study in cats. Acta Anaesthesiol Scand 1974; 18: 79–87.
34. Magora F, Stern L, Zylber-Katz E, et al: Prolonged effect of bupivacaine hydrochloride after cuff release in i.v. regional anaesthesia. Br J Anaesth 1980; 52: 1131–1136.
35. Gooding JM, Tavakoli MM, Fitzpatrick WO, et al: Bupivacaine: preferred agent for intravenous regional anesthesia? South Med J 1981; 74: 1282–1283.
36. Rosenberg PH, Kalso EA, Tuominen MK, et al: Acute bupivacaine toxicity as a result of venous leakage under the tourniquet cuff during a Bier block. Anesthesiology 1983; 58: 95–98.
37. Heath ML: Deaths after intravenous regional anaesthesia (editorial). Br Med J 1982; 285: 913–914.
38. Finucane BT, McClain DA, Smith SR: A double-blind comparison of etidocaine and lidocaine for IV regional anesthesia. Reg Anesth 1980; 5 no. 4: 17–18.
39. Harris WH: Choice of anesthetic agents for intravenous regional anesthesia. Acta Anaesthesiol Scand Suppl 1969; 36: 47–52.
40. Pitkänen MT, Suzuki N, Rosenberg PH: Intravenous regional anaesthesia with 0.5% prilocaine or 0.5% chloroprocaine. A double-blind comparison in volunteers. Anaesthesia 1992; 47: 618–619.
41. Pitkänen M, Kyttä J, Rosenberg PH: Comparison of 2-chloroprocaine and prilocaine for intravenous regional anaesthesia of the arm: a clinical study. Anaesthesia 1993; 48: 1091–1093.
42. Aven M, Foldes FF: The chemical kinetics of procaine and chloroprocaine hydrolysis. Science 1951; 114: 206–208.
43. Rosenberg PH, Zou J, Heavner JE: Comparison of acute central nervous system and cardiovascular toxicity of 2-chloroprocaine and prilocaine in the rat. Acta Anaesthesiol Scand 1993; 37: 751–755.
44. Arthur JM, Heavner JE, Mian T, et al: Fentanyl and lidocaine versus lidocaine for Bier block. Reg Anesth 1992; 17: 223–227.
45. Pitkänen MT, Rosenberg PH, Pere PJ, et al: Fentanyl-prilocaine mixture for intravenous regional anaesthesia in patients undergoing surgery. Anaesthesia 1992; 47: 395–398.
46. Gupta A, Björnsson A, Sjöberg F, et al: Lack of peripheral analgesic effect of low-dose morphine during intravenous regional anesthesia. Reg Anesth 1993; 18: 250–253.
47. Arendt-Nielsen L, Oberg B, Bjerring P: Laser-induced pain for quantitative comparison of intravenous regional anesthesia using saline, morphine, lidocaine, or prilocaine. Reg Anesth 1990; 15: 186–193.
48. Prippenow G, Fruhstorfer H, Seidlitz P, et al: Addition of muscle relaxants to intravenous regional anaesthesia. Reg Anaesth 1985; 8: 15–20.
49. Atkinson DI, Modell J, Moya F: Intravenous regional anesthesia. Anesth Analg 1965; 44: 313–317.
50. Amiot JF, Bouju P, Palacci JH, et al: Intravenous regional anaesthesia with ketamine. Anaesthesia 1985; 40: 899–901.
51. Durrani Z, Winnie AP, Zsigmond EK, et al: Ketamine for intravenous regional anesthesia. Anesth Analg 1989; 68: 328–332.
52. Hord AH, Rooks MD, Stephens BO, et al: Intravenous regional bretylium and lidocaine for treatment of reflex sympathetic dystrophy: a randomized, double-blind study. Anesth Analg 1992; 74: 818–821.
53. Hanna MH, Peat SJ: Ketanserin in reflex sympathetic dystrophy. A double-blind placebo controlled cross-over trial. Pain 1989; 38: 145–150.
54. Vanos DN, Ramamurthy S, Hoffman J: Intravenous regional

block using ketorolac: preliminary results in the treatment of reflex sympathetic dystrophy. Anesth Analg 1992; 74: 139–141.

55. Tucker GT, Boas RA: Pharmacokinetic aspects of intravenous regional anesthesia. Anesthesiology 1971; 34: 538–549.

56. Cotev S, Robin GC: Experimental studies on intravenous regional anaesthesia using radioactive lignocaine. Br J Anaesth 1966; 38: 936–940.

57. Thorn-Alquist AM: Blood concentrations of local anaesthetics after intravenous regional anaesthesia. Acta Anaesthesiol Scand 1969; 13: 229–240.

58. Valli H, Rosenberg PH: Intravenous regional anaesthesia below the knee. A cross-over study with prilocaine in volunteers. Anaesthesia 1986; 41: 1196–1201.

59. Arthur GR: Distribution and elimination of local anaesthetic agents: the role of lung, liver and kidney. PhD Thesis, University of Edinburgh, Scotland, 1981.

60. Post C, Eriksdotter-Behm K: Dependence of lung uptake of lidocaine in vivo on blood pH. Acta Pharmacol Toxicol (Copenh) 1982; 51: 136–140.

61. Sukhani R, Garcia CJ, Munhall RJ, et al: Lidocaine disposition following intravenous regional anesthesia with different tourniquet deflation technics. Anesth Analg 1989; 68: 633–637.

62. Kerr JH: Intravenous regional analgesia. A clinical comparison of lignocaine and prilocaine. Anaesthesia 1967; 22: 562–567.

63. Ware RJ: Intravenous regional analgesia using bupivacaine. A double blind comparison with lignocaine. Anaesthesia 1979; 34: 231–235.

64. Gerber H, Koller R, Hodel D: Intravenous regional anesthesia (IVRA) with chloroprocaine in the lower extremity. Reg Anesth 1991; 16: S1.

65. Sindel LJ, deShazo RD: Accidents resulting from local anesthetics. True or false allergy? Clin Rev Allergy 1991; 9: 379–395.

66. Ruiz K, Stevens JD, Train JJ, et al: Anaphylactoid reactions to prilocaine. Anaesthesia 1987; 42: 1078–1080.

67. Adriani J: Drug allergy: local anesthetics. Anesth Rev 1984; 11: 14–21.

68. Raj PP, Garcia CE, Burleson JW, et al: The site of action of intravenous regional anesthesia. Anesth Analg 1972; 51: 776–786.

69. Fleming SA, Veiga-Pires JA, McCutcheon RM, et al: A demonstration of the site of action of intravenous lignocaine. Can Anaesth Soc J 1966; 13: 21–27.

70. Sorbie C, Chacha P: Regional anaesthesia by the intravenous route. Br Med J 1965; 1: 957–960.

71. Hallén J, Rawal N, Hartvig P, et al: Pharmacokinetic and pharmacodynamic studies of ^{11}C-lidocaine following intravenous regional anesthesia (IVRA) using positron emission tomography (abstract). Acta Anaesthesiol Scand 1991; 35 suppl 96: 214.

72. Rosenberg PH, Heavner JE: Multiple and complementary mechanisms produce analgesia during intravenous regional anesthesia (letter to the editor). Anesthesiology 1985; 62: 840–842.

73. Heavner JE, Leinonen L, Haasio J, et al: Interaction of lidocaine and hypothermia in Bier blocks in volunteers. Anesth Analg 1989; 69: 53–59.

74. Korttila K, Tarkkanen L, Aittomaki J, et al: The influence of intramuscularly administered pethidine on the amnesic effects of intravenous diazepam during intravenous regional anaesthesia. Acta Anaesthesiol Scand 1981; 25: 323–327.

75. Lawes EG, Johnson T, Pritchard P, et al: Venous pressures during simulated Bier's block. Anaesthesia 1984; 39: 147–149.

76. Haasio J, Hiippala S, Rosenberg PH: Intravenous regional anaesthesia of the arm. Effect of the technique of exsanguination on the quality of anaesthesia and prilocaine plasma concentrations. Anaesthesia 1989; 44: 19–21.

77. Haas LM, Lendeen FH: Improved intravenous regional anesthesia for surgery of the hand, wrist, and forearm. The second wrap technique. J Hand Surg [Am] 1978; 3: 194–195.

78. Rawal N, Hallén J, Amilon A, et al: Improvement in i.v. regional anaesthesia by re-exsanguination before surgery. Br J Anaesth 1993; 70: 280–285.

79. Bell HM, Slater EM, Harris WH: Regional anesthesia with intravenous lidocaine. JAMA 1963; 186: 544–549.

80. Eastwood D, Griffiths S, Jack J, et al: Bier's block—an improved technique. Injury 1986; 17: 187–188.

81. Haasio J, Hekali R, Rosenberg PH: Influence of premedication on lignocaine-induced acute toxicity and plasma concentrations of lignocaine. Br J Anaesth 1988; 61: 131–134.

82. Heavner JE, Arthur J, Zou J, et al: Comparison of propofol with thiopentone for treatment of bupivacaine-induced seizures in rats. Br J Anaesth 1993; 71: 715–719.

83. FitzGerald B: Intravenous regional anaesthesia in children. Br J Anaesth 1976; 48: 485–486.

84. Rudzinski JP, Ampel LL: Pediatric application of intravenous regional anesthesia. Reg Anesth 1983; 8: 69–72.

IV

Concurrent Medical Problems, Side Effects, and Complications With Regional Anesthesia

CHAPTER 22

Physiologic Effects of Regional Block

David C. Mackey, M.D.

The earliest reports on local and regional anesthesia by Koller, Corning, Bier, and others noted that local anesthetic block was a technique distinctly different from the ether, chloroform, and nitrous oxide general anesthetics of the time.[1-5] These early impressions were soon followed by investigations into the anatomic and physiologic elements of regional anesthesia and into the mechanisms that produced the benefits and liabilities seen clinically.[6-9] Regional anesthesia may cause or influence various physiologic perturbations, depending on the patient's surgical pathology, operation, and comorbidity and on the type and extent of block used. For optimal use of local and regional anesthetics, the anesthesiologist must have a firm grasp of normal physiology and pathophysiologic processes and must understand how local and regional anesthesia may affect and be affected by normal physiology and disease states. This chapter reviews several physiologic implications of regional anesthesia.

Central and Peripheral Nervous System Effects of Regional Anesthesia

The clinical consequences of regional anesthetic and analgesic techniques on the central and peripheral nervous system depend on the local anesthetics, opioids, and α_2-adrenergic agonists used in neuraxial techniques and on the systemic levels of local anesthetics resulting from the peripheral regional block and, in the case of mexiletine, a structural analogue of lidocaine used in the treatment of neuropathic pain syndromes, from oral administration.[10, 11] Additional considerations in performing a regional block are the effects of deafferentation on the central nervous system and the effects of adjunct sedative-hypnotic and opioid medications.

Spinal Cord Function and Spinal and Epidural Anesthesia

The primary site of action of local anesthetics used in neuraxial block is on the nerve roots, although drugs such as opioids, α-adrenergic agonists, and local anesthetics do act on the spinal cord itself.[12, 13] Drugs injected into the subarachnoid space can act directly on the nerve roots and spinal cord, but drugs administered into the epidural space must first diffuse through the spinal meninges or reach the spinal cord through the spinal radicular arteries.[14-16] Although local anesthetics can penetrate and affect the spinal cord, neuraxial blocks do not result in a chemical transection of the cord.[17-19] The fact that the spinal cord is still functional is graphically illustrated by the practice of early regional anesthesiologists, who administered regional spinal anesthesia alone for a wide range of neurosurgical, ophthalmologic, and otolaryngologic procedures, without the need for ventilatory support (Fig. 22–1).[20-22]

Spinal Cord Blood Flow and Spinal and Epidural Anesthesia

Investigators using plain lidocaine and tetracaine in laboratory animals to examine the effect of spinal anesthesia on spinal cord blood flow have found an increase[23, 24] or no change.[25-27] The increase in spinal cord blood flow observed by Kozody and colleagues[23, 24] was not found when they added 200 μg of epinephrine to the lidocaine or tetracaine. Other studies[25, 27] using animal models found no change in spinal cord blood flow when epinephrine was added to subarachnoid

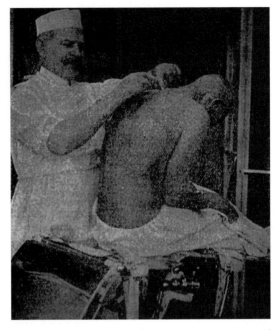

Figure 22–1 Professor T. Jonnesco is administering an intrathecal injection in the interspace between T-1 and T-2. Head and neck surgery was completed with spinal anesthesia alone. (From Jonnesco T: Remarks on general spinal analgesia. Br Med J 1909; 2: 1396–1401.)

administration of lidocaine or tetracaine. Kozody and coworkers[28] also found no change in spinal cord blood flow after intrathecal administration of 200 μg of epinephrine or 5 mg of phenylephrine alone. Kozody and colleagues[29] also showed that lumbosacral spinal cord blood flow was decreased by subarachnoid administration of bupivacaine in dogs, although the clinical importance of this observation seems minimal. Animal studies[25, 27] of spinal anesthesia have found maintenance of spinal cord blood flow in the setting of moderate decreases in mean arterial blood pressure.

In the normal clinical setting it is unlikely that spinal anesthesia with or without use of a vasoconstrictor has any adverse effect on spinal cord blood flow by means of a direct effect or a loss of autoregulation. Similarly, there is little reason to believe that epidural anesthesia under normal clinical conditions has any adverse effect on spinal cord blood flow, although data supporting this assumption are lacking.

Regional Anesthesia and the Brain

Regional anesthesia potentially affects brain function by several mechanisms, including alteration in cerebral blood flow, block of sensory afferents, and direct effects of systemic blood levels of local anesthetics. Alteration of cerebral blood flow may result from changes in cerebrovascular resistance or mean arterial pressure, both potentially mediated by sympathectomy. The current belief[30] that sympathetic supply to intracranial vessels has little role in regulation of cerebral blood flow and the finding that unilateral[31] or bilateral[32] stellate ganglion block has no significant effect on cerebral blood flow suggest that sympathectomy itself probably has no significant effect on cerebral blood flow. Cerebral blood flow may also be disturbed by the effect of decreased mean arterial blood pressure on cerebral perfusion pressure.

Investigators[33, 34] using spinal anesthesia have found that normotensive subjects are able to maintain cerebral blood flow unchanged despite a moderate decrease in mean arterial pressure, but hypertensive subjects are vulnerable to significant decreases in cerebral blood flow in this setting, presumably due to altered cerebral blood flow autoregulation. This is much like the situation for general anesthesia. There is no evidence that cerebral blood flow is more or less vulnerable to mean systemic blood pressures above or below the autoregulatory thresholds with general anesthesia or neuraxial blocks.

The number of sensory impulses reaching the brainstem reticular excitatory area is a primary determinant of its level of activity, and the activity of this brainstem structure is principally responsible for the overall level of brain arousal. Afferent nociceptive traffic is a particularly potent stimulus of reticular excitatory area activity and of overall brain activity. Sectioning all afferent nerves up to and including the fifth cranial nerve results in a greatly decreased level of overall brain activity that approaches a state of coma.[35] Deafferentation is a possible explanation of the clinical observation that patients frequently become somnolent during spinal anesthesia with high levels of sensory block.[9, 36, 37] Deafferentation has also been described as the cause of phantom limb phenomena appearing during spinal anesthesia, presumably due to decreased spinal cord and brain inhibition secondary to block of somatic input.[38]

Systemic absorption of local anesthetics used in regional anesthetic techniques, particularly intercostal, caudal, and epidural blocks, may be sufficient to affect the central nervous system.[39, 40] The degree to which the central nervous system is affected is directly related to the potency of the local anesthetic agent and to the systemic blood level. Early manifestations may include sedation, slurred speech, or signs of central nervous system excitation, including restlessness and tremulousness, which may be accompanied by increased sympathetic tone, heart rate, and blood pressure. The patient may report blurred vision, lightheadedness, circumoral numbness or tingling, metallic taste, or tinnitus, but these symptoms may be obscured by premedication. Signs of toxic central nervous system reactions accompanying higher systemic blood levels of local anesthetic include obtundation, seizure activity, and central nervous system–mediated cardiac arrhythmias and cardiovascular collapse.[41–43]

Investigators[44] have shown that lidocaine depresses the activity of excitatory and inhibitory neurons, with block of inhibitory neuron function occurring at lower concentrations than that of excitatory neuron activity. This may explain the clinical observation that toxic systemic levels of lidocaine may cause tremulousness or seizures, with even higher levels producing a state of general anesthesia.

The Central Nervous System and Therapeutic Effects of Systemic Local Anesthetic Administration

Clinically significant systemic levels of local anesthetic are normally addressed in terms of toxicity. However, a growing body of literature[10] suggests that systemic administration of local anesthetic agents may have a therapeutic effect on the central nervous system in certain clinical situations. Systemic levels of local anesthetic agent may affect the brain and the spinal cord.[45–47] Intravenous administration of lidocaine has been used to alter the sympathetic response to operation[48]; suppress the cough response to tracheal intubation[49]; decrease the incidence of vomiting in children after strabismus surgery[50]; and treat postoperative pain,[51] pain after stroke,[52] vascular headache,[53] and diabetic neuropathy.[54] Some of these therapeutic systemic local anesthetic effects may be mediated through direct action on peripheral nerve fibers as well.

Thermoregulation and Neuraxial Anesthesia

Thermoregulation in homeotherms depends on central nervous system integration of afferent temperature information that is received from deep thoracic and abdominal structures, skin, muscle, brain, and spinal cord. This centrally processed information is compared with thresholds for autonomic thermoregulatory mechanisms, such as vasodilation, sweating, vasoconstriction, shivering, and nonshivering thermogenesis, and if the thresholds for temperature decreasing or temperature increasing mechanisms are exceeded, the central nervous system initiates the appropriate effector organ activity.[55] The narrow range in core temperature between the activation of various thermoregulatory responses, called the interthreshold range, is normally about $0.2°$ C in men and women.[56] The intensity of each thermoregulatory response increases as the difference between its given response threshold and the centrally integrated thermal signal increases; the rate of this increase in thermoregulatory action in response to a given change in thermal signal is the response gain. However, within the interthreshold range, thermoregulatory responses are not triggered, and core temperature varies passively.[55]

General anesthesia and neuraxial anesthesia impair thermoregulation, and the perioperative hypothermia that can result from this process may adversely affect outcome.[57–59] Epidural and spinal anesthesia[60–63] as well as inhaled and intravenous anesthetic agents[64, 65] widen the interthreshold range without altering the response gain or the maximal intensity of thermoregulatory effector organ activity. The mechanism by which epidural and spinal anesthesia affect thermoregulation is probably through block of afferent temperature information; regional anesthesia impairs thermoregulatory control to a lesser extent than does general anesthesia.[63, 66, 67] Epidural and spinal anesthesia also may promote perioperative hypothermia by redistribution of heat within the body, by increasing cutaneous blood flow and environmental heat loss, and by decreasing the effectiveness of shivering thermogenesis by motor block.[61, 68] Clinical studies[69–73] of the comparative risk of general versus regional anesthesia as contributors to perioperative hypothermia have produced conflicting findings, with no consensus about the superiority of either technique.

Regional Anesthesia and Differential Block

Differential block refers to the ability of local anesthetic solutions to block impulse conduction in certain nerve fibers while not affecting conduction in others.[74] The clinical manifestation of this pharmacologic property of local anesthetics was first reported by Greene,[75] who noticed that the levels of anesthesia for temperature discrimination and for pinprick were not the same (Fig. 22–2). A similar observation for epidural block

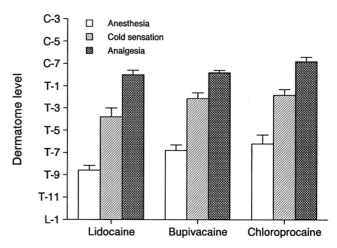

Figure 22–3 The property of differential block in epidural anesthesia does not depend on the local anesthetic used. Extent of epidural block 20 min after injection. Note the lack of significant differences in each level of anesthesia, analgesia, and cold sensation among the three local anesthetics tested. (Redrawn from White JL, Stevens RA, Beardsley D, et al: Differential epidural block: does the choice of local anesthetic matter? Reg Anesth 1994; 19: 335–338.)

was subsequently made by Bromage[76] and confirmed by others.[77, 78] Greene initially ascribed this phenomenon to the increased sensitivity of smaller nerve fibers to local anesthetic block and to the progressive decrease in local anesthetic concentration in the spinal fluid as the distance from the site of injection increases.[79, 80] Fink[81] suggested that the basic mechanism of differential block does not involve fiber size directly but rather the number of consecutive nodes blocked in each individual nerve fiber.[74]

Clinicians often assume that the extent of sympathetic denervation during a neuraxial block may be reasonably approximated by the level of loss of temperature discrimination and that this is usually about two dermatomal levels higher than the level of sensory block. However, Chamberlain and Chamberlain,[82] in a study using skin thermography measurements during tetracaine and lidocaine spinal anesthesia, suggested that the level of sympathetic block may be six or more dermatomal levels higher than that of the sensory block. They suggested that this may explain the occasional observation of hypotension or bradycardia that is more profound than would ordinarily be expected for a relatively low sensory block level. Later investigations[78, 83] indicated that the quality of differential spinal or epidural block did not depend on the specific local anesthetic agent used (Fig. 22–3). There may not be any potential clinical advantage in using one local anesthetic instead of another in attempting to exploit the properties of a differential block.

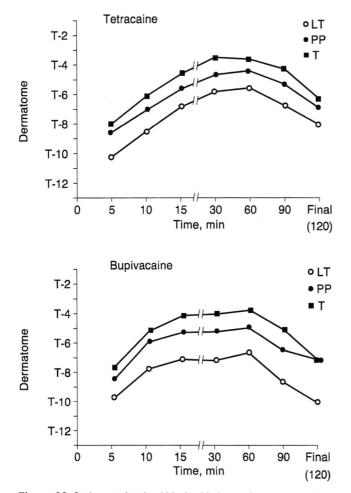

Figure 22–2 Thoracic levels of block of light touch (LT), pinprick (PP), and temperature (T) discrimination as a function of time during tetracaine and bupivacaine spinal anesthesia. The widths of the zones of differential block within either anesthetic show no statistically significant change during onset, maintenance, or regression. (Redrawn from Brull SJ, Greene NM: Time-courses of zones of differential sensory blockade during spinal anesthesia with hyperbaric tetracaine or bupivacaine. Anesth Analg 1989; 69: 342–347.)

Pulmonary Effects of Regional Anesthesia

Pulmonary complications such as atelectasis and pneumonia are major factors contributing to perioperative morbidity in patients undergoing major surgery. Regional anesthesia has long been recognized for its potential to moderate cardiopulmonary morbidity, even though the existence of this property has not always been supported by scientific data. For anesthesiologists to understand the appropriate role of regional anesthesia and analgesia in their practices, they must first understand the effects of various regional anesthetic techniques on normal pulmonary mechanics. Many patients are not normal because of preexisting cardiopulmonary disease, and major operative procedures often induce profound derangements in baseline pulmonary function, whether it was initially normal or not. Medications routinely administered in the perioperative period also affect cardiopulmonary performance. All of these factors, in addition to the anesthesiologist's competence with various regional anesthetic procedures, affect decisions to use various regional anesthetic and analgesic techniques.

Ventilatory Mechanics and Major Surgery

General anesthesia and major surgery are often associated with impaired pulmonary function. Atelectasis, shunt, and ventilation-perfusion mismatch, augmented by the influences of residual anesthesia, immobilization, pain, and administration of analgesic and sedative drugs, may adversely affect perioperative oxygenation and ventilation (Fig. 22–4).[84-87] Functional residual capacity and residual volume are decreased after abdominal operation, at least partially as a result of incisional pain and diaphragmatic dysfunction.[88-91] Some reports[92-94] suggest that regional anesthesia and postoperative analgesia may attenuate some of these deleterious perturbations in perioperative pulmonary function.

Regional Block and Normal Ventilatory Mechanics

Neither spinal nor epidural anesthesia alters resting ventilation significantly in healthy persons who have not been premedicated, although ventilatory reserve may be decreased by decrements in peak negative and positive airway pressures, inspiratory capacity, expiratory reserve volume, and vital capacity.[95-98] Normal, unmedicated persons receiving high-thoracic dermatome neuraxial blocks are able to maintain normal arterial blood gas tensions, and the hypercapnic ventilatory response is unchanged or increased.[98-102] However, motor block of the abdominal and intercostal musculature does interfere with the ability to cough and has the potential to impair the ability to clear pulmonary secretions and perhaps may increase the risk of atelectasis in the perioperative setting.

Moir[96] examined the effect of high epidural (T-2 to T-5 sensory level) anesthesia on pulmonary function in 30 healthy patients without a history of pulmonary disease and found insignificant decreases in resting tidal volume, resting minute volume, and vital capacity and a 5% decrease in peak expiratory flow rate. In the same study, Moir examined 12 patients with chronic bronchopulmonary disease and found no significant change in resting tidal volume or resting minute volume but an 8.5% decrease in vital capacity and a 10% decrease in peak expiratory flow rate. In a study of ventilatory reserve during high spinal (T-2 sensory block level and T-5 motor block level) and high epidural (T-4 sensory block level and T-8 motor block level) anesthesia, Freund and associates[97] found inspiratory capacity was decreased by 8% with spinal anesthesia and by 3% with epidural anesthesia. Expiratory reserve volume was decreased by 48% with spinal anesthesia and by 21% with epidural anesthesia. McCarthy[103] examined the effect of thoracic epidural anesthesia (block extending from T-1 or T-2 to T-12 or L-1, as assessed by loss of temperature discrimination) and found no significant change in closing capacity or functional residual capacity. Similar findings have been reported by other investigators examining the effects of thoracic epidural anesthesia.[104]

In a study of high spinal and epidural anesthesia (sensory block heights of T-4 and T-5, respectively) in preoperative cesarean section patients, Harrop-Griffiths and colleagues[105] found statistically significant decreases in forced vital capacity, forced expiratory volume in 1 s, peak expiratory flow rate, and maximum expiratory pressure after block. The greatest decreases were found in maximum expiratory pressure: 32% in the spinal anesthesia group and 25% in the epidural group. They concluded that the observed changes were unlikely to impair the ability of a normal subject to cough effectively, but they cautioned that significant cough impairment might occur in the setting of higher block level or preexisting pulmonary disease. Similar findings have been reported for intercostal nerve block. In a study of seven healthy males who underwent resting and exercise pulmonary function testing, including determination of hypercapnic ventilatory response, during bilateral T-6 to T-12 intercostal nerve block, Hecker and coworkers[106] found no clinically significant adverse effects at rest or during extremes of exercise.

The results of studies examining the effects of re-

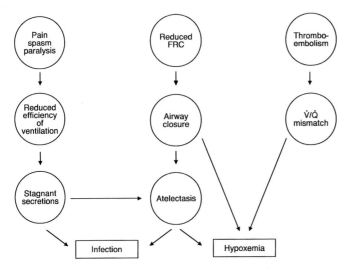

Figure 22–4 Factors contributing to postoperative pulmonary morbidity. FRC, functional residual capacity. (Redrawn from Hedenstierna G: Mechanisms of postoperative pulmonary dysfunction. Acta Chir Scand Suppl 1988; 550: 152–158.)

gional block on pulmonary function in healthy persons must be applied to clinical scenarios with caution, because adequate ventilatory ability may be adversely impacted by factors such as coexisting disease, systemic depressant medication, hypotension and hemorrhage, patient positioning, and type of operation, particularly if an upper abdominal or thoracic incision is involved. The optimal anesthetic for major surgery is given by a knowledgeable and experienced anesthesiologist who has facility with general anesthesia and regional anesthetic techniques and who tailors the anesthetic to the specific patient and specific operation.

Influence of Regional Anesthesia on Perioperative Pulmonary Morbidity

Spinal or epidural anesthesia and analgesia, with or without concurrent light general anesthesia, are often preferred to general anesthesia for decreasing the risk of postoperative pulmonary complications, particularly in patients with preexisting pulmonary impairment. However, reported data[107-113] do not consistently support this bias. This is undoubtedly a reflection of the multifactorial composition of perioperative risk and of the varied facility with which individual institutions and practitioners use different anesthetic and analgesic modalities.

Opioids and Other Systemic Medications and Respiratory Function

Respiratory depression, defined as the failure to respond appropriately to hypoxemia or hypercapnia, is a well-known side effect of all opioids used clinically, whatever their mode of administration.[114] Neuraxial (intrathecal and epidural) administration of opioids shifts the carbon dioxide response curve down and to the right and decreases the response to hypoxemia. The opioids may decrease minute volume by decreasing tidal volume and rate, and breathing patterns may become periodic or irregular.[115, 116]

Although advanced age, residual anesthetic or relaxant drugs, history of respiratory insufficiency, concomitant parenteral administration of opioids or sedatives, lack of history of exposure to opioids, and spinal administration of large opioid doses increase the risk of respiratory depression induced by spinal administration of opioids, there is no evidence[114, 117-120] that spinal administration of opioids poses a greater risk of postoperative respiratory depression than other modalities of opioid administration. Local or regional anesthesia can interact with systemic administration of opioids to induce respiratory depression. Pain is a ventilatory stimulus, and several reports[121-124] described the precipitation of respiratory arrest following analgesic regional blocks in narcotized patients. Inagaki and colleagues[125] reported that analgesia provided by epidural administration of lidocaine anesthesia delayed arousal from isoflurane anesthesia. Lidocaine plasma levels were too low to have provided any sedative effect in this study. There also are reports[126, 127] of decreases in oxygen saturation in patients who have received major regional blocks with sedation, and those researchers recommended concomitant administration of supplemental oxygen.

Systemic Local Anesthetic Levels and Respiratory Function

Because high systemic levels of local anesthetic can cause central nervous system depression, it has been speculated that systemic levels of local anesthetic agent resulting from regional anesthetic procedures may induce or contribute to respiratory depression. Although data from studies examining this potential phenomenon are conflicting, it may be prudent to avoid relatively high systemic local anesthetic levels in patients with severe respiratory impairment.[128-130]

Regional Anesthesia and the Patient With Hyperreactive Airway Disease

Asthma and other clinical processes associated with bronchospasm occur in up to 4% of the general population and are characterized by airway hyperresponsiveness to various stimuli, manifested by inflammatory and neural mechanisms.[131, 132] The muscular walls of the bronchi and bronchioles receive sympathetic, parasympathetic, and nonadrenergic, noncholinergic inhibitory innervation.[133-136] Cholinergic stimulation increases airway smooth muscle tone and promotes pulmonary vasodilation and glandular secretion. β_2-Adrenergic stimulation causes bronchodilation and decreased bronchial secretion and constricts pulmonary blood vessels. The nonadrenergic, noncholinergic inhibitory system promotes bronchodilation, probably mediated by vasoactive intestinal peptide.

It is theoretically possible that a thoracic level of spinal or epidural block promotes bronchoconstriction by blocking direct pulmonary sympathetic innervation (T-2 to T-4) or lowering systemic catecholamine levels through the block of adrenal medullary sympathetic innervation (T-10 to L-1), allowing unopposed cholinergic tone in either case.[137-139] This proposition is supported somewhat by the work of Barnes and associates,[140] who reported a strong correlation between the diurnal variation in plasma epinephrine and plasma cyclic adenosine monophosphate (peak at 4 PM and nadir at 4 AM) and the circadian variation in peak flow (peak at 4 PM and nadir at 4 AM) and proposed this as a cause of nocturnal wheezing in asthmatics. However, bronchospasm during epidural or spinal anesthesia has been reported only occasionally.[138, 139, 141-145]

In a review[141] of 681 anesthetics given to patients with a history of bronchospasm, the overall incidence of intraoperative bronchospasm was 3.9%, with an incidence of 6.4% in those patients administered general tracheal anesthesia and a significantly lower incidence in those patients who received regional anesthesia or general anesthesia without tracheal intubation (1.9% and 1.6%, respectively). Other possible causes of intraoperative bronchospasm include anxiety, airway exposure to cold gases, and anaphylaxis, and these are much more likely to be the etiologic agents of bronchospasm than unopposed vagal tone in the setting of major regional blocks.[146–148]

Although it is theoretically possible that autonomic imbalance associated with regional blocks may promote intraoperative bronchospasm, the potent mechanical stimulus of a tracheal tube is an undeniable reality, and regional anesthesia (or general anesthesia administered by mask) is preferable to general tracheal anesthesia in a patient with a history of airway hyperreactivity. However, this depends on the appropriateness of regional anesthesia to the operation and on possession of the requisite skills for administering a regional block by the attending anesthesiologist.[149, 150]

Cardiovascular Effects of Regional Anesthesia

Circulatory alterations associated with regional anesthesia are well known and were appreciated by the earliest practitioners of these techniques.[5, 6, 8, 151] The therapeutic and adverse cardiovascular effects of regional anesthesia are a sum of the actions of local and systemic levels of local anesthetic agents on cardiac, vascular, neural, and hematologic tissues. Local anesthetic agents used in regional anesthesia may affect hemodynamic perturbations directly and indirectly in various ways, including direct action on the central nervous system or on autonomic nerve fibers, direct effects on the myocardium and vascular smooth muscle, influence on coronary blood flow and cardiac preload and afterload, provocation of cardiovascular reflexes, and modification of hemostatic status. In clinical practice, significant hemodynamic alteration is most likely to occur in the setting of neuraxial blocks reaching the thoracic level, with accompanying widespread sympathectomy and relatively unopposed vagal tone.[152–154]

Most peripheral blocks rarely result in clinically significant circulatory changes, with the exception of unintentional intravascular administration or systemic absorption of toxic amounts of local anesthetic solution. The sites of injection associated with the highest plasma levels of local anesthetic agent are, in descending order of systemic absorption, intercostal, caudal, epidural, brachial plexus, and femoral and sciatic.[39]

Hypotension Induced by the Sympathectomy of Spinal and Epidural Block

Hypotension secondary to peripheral vasodilation from preganglionic sympathetic block commonly occurs in the setting of neuraxial regional anesthesia, and a decrease in arterial blood pressure is often used by the clinician to monitor the onset and duration of sensory analgesia. The strong association between hypotension and spinal anesthesia was recognized by the earliest investigators[6] of regional anesthesia. The anesthesia literature has reflected a 10% to 40% incidence of hypotension during neuraxial blocks. In a well-documented study[153] of 932 patients who received spinal anesthesia, hypotension defined as a systolic blood pressure of less than 90 mm Hg occurred in 33% of cases.

The decrease in blood pressure during spinal and epidural anesthesia is related primarily to the extent of sympathetic block. The lowered blood pressure results from the decrease in systemic arteriolar and venous tone, secondary to sympathectomy, and from the attenuation of cardiac output, secondary to decreased venous return and cardiac sympathetic block, with resultant decreases in heart rate and stroke volume (Fig. 22–5).[152–155] The hypotensive effect of sympathectomy during neuraxial blocks is principally caused by venodilation and decreased cardiac venous return. Systemic vascular resistance decreases only moderately, probably because of the ability of denervated arteriolar smooth muscle to maintain much of its intrinsic tone. A study of high spinal anesthesia found a decrease in systemic vascular resistance of only 19%.[156–159]

The mechanism of sympathectomy-induced heart rate slowing is related to removal of cardiac sympathetic tone, to intrinsic cardiac stretch receptor-induced reflex decrease in sinus rate, and perhaps to unopposed or enhanced vagal outflow.[160–162] The vasodilatory effects of lower levels of sympathetic block may be moderated by a compensatory increase in sympathetic tone and vasoconstriction in unblocked regions, resulting in an essentially unchanged total systemic vascular resistance. However, this compensatory mechanism may be obliterated by higher levels of sympathetic block or by concomitant administration of general anesthesia, in-

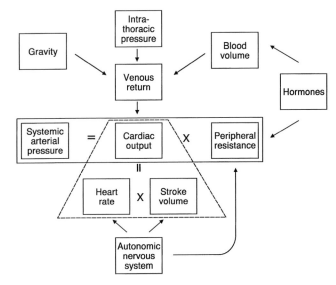

Figure 22–5 Major factors influencing systemic arterial pressure during neuraxial block. (Modified from McCrae AF, Wildsmith JAW: Prevention and treatment of hypotension during central neural block. Br J Anaesth 1993; 70: 672–680.)

creasing the propensity for a decrease in systemic blood pressure in these situations. In addition, the effects of sympathectomy on epidural anesthesia are compounded by the variable effects of systemic levels of local anesthetic and vasoconstrictor agents.[99, 159, 163–168]

The varied observations of hemodynamic changes with epidural and spinal anesthesia as well as the difficulty in reliably anticipating the hemodynamic effects of neuraxial blocks in the clinical setting may be related to the difficulty in predicting the correlation between degree of sympathetic block and the level of sensory analgesia. Studies[82, 169–172] have not provided a consensus of opinion on the correlation of sympathetic and sensory block levels or on the relationship between skin blood flow and skin temperature. For example, clinicians may encounter a degree of hypotension much greater than they would expect with a relatively low level of sensory analgesia, which may reflect a level of sympathetic block disproportionately high relative to the level of sensory block.

Patients who are hypovolemic are at increased risk for severe hypotension during neuraxial blocks.[173, 174] However, studies examining the efficacy of routine prophylactic administration of a fluid bolus to patients who are judged not to be significantly hypovolemic before administration of spinal or epidural anesthesia are without consensus regarding its potential benefit. The recommendation that fluid loading be routinely administered to prevent hypotension during spinal anesthesia may be unwarranted.[154, 175–178] Moderate hypotension in this latter group can be treated by administration of a 300- to 500-mL bolus of balanced salt solution or a mixed α- and β-adrenergic agonist, such as ephedrine, with head-down tilt added to treat more severe hypotension.[179, 180] In addition to a high thoracic level of block and preexisting hypovolemia, a patient older than 40 to 50 years of age presents an increased risk of hypotension during neuraxial blocks.[153, 155, 175]

Additional Vasoactive Effects of Local Anesthetic Agents and Additives

Local anesthetics act directly on vascular smooth muscle and can produce vasoconstriction or vasodilation.[181–183] In a series of reports by Johns and colleagues,[184–186] lidocaine and bupivacaine were shown to exhibit a biphasic effect on vascular smooth muscle, with vasoconstriction present at lower concentrations, comparable to clinical blood levels present with regional anesthetic procedures, and vasodilation present at local anesthetic concentrations much higher than clinical blood levels, such as typical local tissue concentrations accompanying infiltration blocks. Johns[186] suggested that the mechanism of vasoconstriction seen with lower local anesthetic concentrations may be local anesthetic inhibition of endothelium-derived relaxing factor.

Cocaine continues to enjoy limited medical use as a local anesthetic, principally as a topical agent for nasal examination and surgery, because of its potent vasoconstrictor properties. However, undesirable side effects of cocaine administration have been recognized since the earliest days of regional anesthesia. Medical and recreational use of cocaine have been associated with hypertension, tachycardia, cardiac arrhythmias, and seizures.[187, 188] Cocaine is also a potent coronary artery constrictor, and this property, in the setting of concomitant tachycardia and systemic vasoconstriction, is probably the reason why illegal and medical use of cocaine have been associated with myocardial ischemia and infarction.[189–191]

Vasoconstrictor agents are commonly used in local anesthetic solutions to decrease the rate of vascular absorption to prolong the blocks, to lower systemic anesthetic levels, and in the case of epinephrine, to increase the quality of block. The systemic levels of these vasoactive agents resulting from this practice may have physiologic consequences that are beneficial or deleterious. In the setting of epidural block, the β$_1$-adrenergic stimulation provided by epinephrine added to the local anesthetic solution augments cardiac output by increasing heart rate and stroke volume, but the β$_2$-adrenergic–induced vasodilation augments the decrease in systemic vascular resistance resulting from the regional block–induced sympathectomy. The summation of these effects in epidural blocks is a greater decrease in mean arterial blood pressure with an epinephrine-containing local anesthetic solution than with a plain local anesthetic solution.[174, 192–194]

The decrease in systemic vascular resistance resulting from the additive or synergistic effect of combined sympathetic block and epinephrine-induced β$_2$-adrenergic activity has been credited with the increased lower extremity blood flow and lower rates of deep vein thrombosis accompanying hip surgery performed during lumbar epidural anesthesia. Epinephrine contained in local anesthetic solutions used for hip surgery and sympathomimetic agents such as ephedrine administered to maintain blood pressure may also decrease the occurrence of deep vein thrombosis in this setting by increasing fibrinolytic activity, although this assertion has been challenged.[195, 196] In addition, the β$_1$ effects of epinephrine may help offset the myocardial depressant effects of high systemic levels of local anesthetics.[197, 198]

The addition of epinephrine to local anesthetic solutions used for regional anesthetic procedures has been shown to cause a significant decrease in serum potassium concentrations.[199–201] A study[202] of low-dose epinephrine infusion in healthy volunteers documented a significant decrease in serum potassium levels; significant decreases in serum magnesium, calcium, and phosphate levels; and a significant increase in blood glucose concentrations. Electrocardiographic changes, including QT$_c$ prolongation, ST-segment depression, T-wave flattening, and the appearance of a U wave, have occurred in the setting of regional anesthesia with epinephrine-containing local anesthetics and with experimental epinephrine infusion.[199, 200, 202] These minor electrocardiographic changes may be the result of hypokalemia and β-adrenergic stimulation.

The anesthetic risk of cardiac arrhythmias in the setting of chronic hypokalemia is controversial, and the risk in the setting of acute hypokalemia (absolute or an acutely lowered value that is still within the normal range) is similarly undetermined.[203, 204] However, this phenomenon must be part of the differential diagnosis of perioperative arrhythmias and ST-segment and T-wave changes in the setting of local or regional anesthesia administered with an epinephrine-containing local anesthetic solution.

Cardiac Electrophysiology: Direct Effects on Myocardium and on Central Nervous System-Induced Cardiac Arrhythmias

The characteristic membrane excitability possessed by myocardial pacemaker, conduction, and contractile fibers renders them vulnerable to the sodium channel blocking properties of systemic local anesthetic agents.[205] Local anesthetics directly affect cardiac tissue by producing a dose-related decrease in automaticity, conductivity, and contractility.[206–208] This phenomenon is exploited in antiarrhythmia therapy (class I antiarrhythmic agents) but is a disadvantage in local anesthetic toxicity.[209–211] However, the direct effect of local anesthetics on myocardial tissue is probably only a partial explanation of the cardiovascular effects of pathophysiologically significant systemic local anesthetic levels, because laboratory animal investigations have demonstrated central nervous system-induced ventricular arrhythmias, hypertension or hypotension, and bradycardia by intracerebroventricular or intramedullary injection of local anesthetic agents.[212–214]

Sympathetic Autonomic Imbalance and Cardiac Electrophysiology

The degree of lateralization of cardiac sympathetic input is one of several autonomic neural control mechanisms that influence cardiac electrophysiology. Sympathetic imbalance, or the abnormal ratio of sympathetic tone existing between the right and left elements of cardiac sympathetic innervation, is associated with reentrant cardiac arrhythmias and sudden death. It has practical implications for the anesthesiologist contemplating a general anesthetic or a regional anesthetic in which unilateral cardiac sympathectomy is a component of the block.[215–217] Animal and human studies have shown that left sympathetic dominance is arrhythmogenic, with the subsequent clinical implication that a right stellate block may be proarrhythmic and a left stellate block may be antiarrhythmic.[215, 218–220]

Sympathetic imbalance has been implicated as the cause of lethal arrhythmias in several clinical processes, including congenital (Jervell and Lange-Nielsen and Romano-Ward syndromes) and acquired long QT syndromes, sudden infant death syndrome, central nervous system pathology, and psychologic stress.[221–225] In addition to the direct electrophysiologic effects, animal models of sympathetic imbalance have produced alterations in the distribution of myocardial blood flow, with left stellate ganglion stimulation increasing epicar-

dial blood flow relative to endocardial blood flow and left stellectomy improving endocardial perfusion.[226, 227] Sympathetic imbalance may also induce or affect myocardial ischemia-related arrhythmias by affecting the degree of ischemia.

Experimental and clinical observations regarding the influence of sympathetic balance on cardiac electrophysiologic stability are of clinical interest to the anesthesiologist, because interventions that acutely alter sympathetic balance may acutely affect cardiac rhythm. Left stellate block and left cardiac sympathetic denervation have been used for control of potentially life-threatening cardiac arrhythmias.[228–230] Moreover, QT-interval prolongation and sudden cardiac arrest have been reported[231] after right-sided radical neck dissection. However, the clinical data regarding unilateral stellate block are limited and conflicting.

Kashima and coworkers[232] performed unilateral stellate blocks on 19 patients without heart disease and found a significant decrease in heart rate with the right stellate block and no change in atrioventricular conduction times with the right or left stellate block. The investigators also found a significant increase in the average QT_c interval, but they were unable to draw a conclusion from this QT_c change because of its small magnitude (0.40 s ± 0.04 to 0.43 s ± 0.04). Gardner and colleagues[233] performed standard 12-lead electrocardiograms and systemic blood pressure determinations, body surface potential mapping, and radionuclide angiography in 13 patients who were undergoing stellate ganglion blocks for arm pain. Eleven patients received right stellate ganglion blocks, and two received left stellate ganglion blocks. No cardiac rhythm disturbances occurred, and no alterations in body surface potential maps, blood pressure, or resting or exercise cardiac ejection fractions were observed.

In a study of unilateral stellate blocks in six patients with Romano-Ward prolonged QT syndrome, the QT_c lengthened significantly in all four patients with right stellate blocks and shortened significantly in all five patients with left stellate blocks. However, the same study also examined unilateral stellate block in patients with reflex sympathetic dystrophy and found significant QT_c shortening in 10 of 10 patients with right stellate blocks and significant QT_c lengthening in 8 of 9 patients with left stellate blocks.[234] In a study of 27 patients with upper extremity reflex sympathetic dystrophy, a block of either stellate ganglion caused QT_c lengthening.[235]

The conflicting nature of the limited data available, particularly compared with surgical cervicothoracic sympathectomy, may reflect differences in the relative extent of local anesthetic block or the fact that a unilateral stellate block in humans does not result in complete ipsilateral cardiac sympathetic denervation.[230]

Cardiac Electrophysiologic Stability and Sympathetic-Parasympathetic Autonomic Imbalance

Under normal circumstances, sinus arrhythmia is the result of the summation of the influences of vagal and β-adrenergic tone on the cardiac pacemaker and conduction system. Periodic inhibition of vagal tone by afferent barrages from the medullary respiratory center, baroreceptors, and thoracic stretch receptors induces continuous fluctuations of the sinus rhythm around the mean heart rate, a phenomenon known as heart rate variability, which can be influenced by additional factors such as exercise, mental and physical stress, and metabolic alterations.[224, 236, 237]

Analysis of heart rate variability may be performed by statistical analysis of fluctuations in sinus rate (time domain analysis) or by dividing the heart rate signal into various frequency components and quantifying their relative intensity (frequency domain or power spectrum analysis).[238–241] Analysis of heart rate variability is an important method for assessment of sympathetic-parasympathetic autonomic balance. The rhythm is altered in many disorders incorporating autonomic dysfunction, including ischemic cardiovascular disease, hypertension, diabetes, acute intracranial diseases, Guillain-Barré syndrome, multiple sclerosis, chronic alcohol abuse, uremic neuropathy, sudden infant death syndrome, antepartum fetal distress, and industry-related neurotoxicity.[237, 241] Normal aging is also accompanied by decreased heart rate variability.[242]

Autonomic sympathetic-parasympathetic balance is clinically important as a primary determinant of cardiac electrical stability, with increased sympathetic tone promoting arrhythmias by decreasing ventricular refractoriness and fibrillation thresholds and by generating late potentials and with increased vagal tone opposing these proarrhythmic manifestations of increased sympathetic output.[243] In addition to the more commonly used systemic β-adrenergic block, treatment of recurrent ventricular tachycardia with bilateral cervicothoracic sympathetic ganglionectomy has been reported.[244] Clinical assessment of sympathetic-parasympathetic balance provides important prognostic information regarding the risk of sudden cardiac death in patients with ischemic heart disease, and it is used to evaluate other disease processes associated with autonomic dysfunction and increased morbidity and mortality.[223, 245–252] Alteration of sympathovagal interaction by mental stress has also been implicated as a cause of lethal arrhythmias and sudden death.[253–255]

Autonomic dysfunction related to age (older than 39 years), cardiovascular disease, and diabetes, as assessed by heart rate variability studies, has been shown to correlate with increased risk of hypotension during general anesthesia, postoperative ventricular dysfunction, and atrial fibrillation after cardiac surgery.[256–259] The altered autonomic balance occurring with general anesthesia and regional anesthesia can be assessed by heart rate variability studies. Sympathovagal balance in general anesthetic regimens is determined by the relative degree of vagal and β-adrenergic depression produced by different general anesthetic agents.[260–262] Altered autonomic balance indicative of parasympathetic predominance has been demonstrated in total spinal anesthesia and in spinal anesthesia for cesarean section.[263, 264]

In a comparison of lumbar epidural anesthesia (bupivacaine, 0.25 mL/kg) and general anesthesia (morphine, thiopental, nitrous oxide, and isoflurane) for radical retropubic prostatectomy, epidural anesthesia was associated with a shift in cardiac sympathovagal autonomic balance to sympathetic predominance intraoperatively relative to general anesthesia. Postoperatively, general anesthesia was associated with a marked increase in sympathetic tone.[265]

The utility of heart rate variability analysis is a topic of active investigation, and much additional information useful to the clinical and the research anesthesiologist will undoubtedly appear in the scientific literature in the near future.

Coronary Perfusion and Myocardial Ischemia and Regional Block

Perioperative myocardial ischemia is relatively common in patients with coronary artery disease and is associated with adverse outcomes.[266–268] Anesthesiologists who care for patients possessing one or more risk factors for coronary artery disease must consider myocardial ischemia as well as normal cardiac physiology, particularly in relatively stressful operative procedures.

A review of the cardiovascular effects of regional anesthesia must include an examination of the influence of regional block on the occurrence and severity of myocardial ischemia. Spinal[269] and epidural[270] anesthesia have been reported to lessen acute ischemic electrocardiographic ST-segment changes in patients with coronary artery disease. Studies[271, 272] examining the potential myocardial protective effect of thoracic epidural anesthesia in a canine model of coronary occlusion have demonstrated a lessening of ischemic ST-segment elevation and extent of myocardial infarction. Thoracic epidural local anesthetic infusion[270, 273] and the epidural and intrathecal administration of opioids[274–276] have been used to control chest pain associated with myocardial ischemia and infarction. These phenomena may be the basis for reports of the salutary effect of regional anesthesia and analgesia on perioperative cardiovascular complications.[277, 278]

Although local metabolic phenomena play a major role in coronary artery vasoactivity,[279] there are several theoretical means by which neuraxial regional block may exert a protective effect on an ischemic or potentially ischemic myocardium: moderation of the hypercoagulable state, decrease in myocardial workload through the direct effects of sympathectomy and the secondary effects of stress response moderation,[280] and block of sympathetic fibers innervating coronary arteries (Fig. 22–6). Epidural anesthesia and spinal anesthesia induce vasodilation in the region of sympathectomy and compensatory vasoconstriction in the unblocked regions. Sufficiently extensive sympathectomy decreases cardiac preload and afterload, and decreased venous return promotes reflex bradycardia, which are principal determinants of myocardial oxygen demand. Block of the upper thoracic region also blocks cardiac sympathetic innervation, depressing the heart rate and

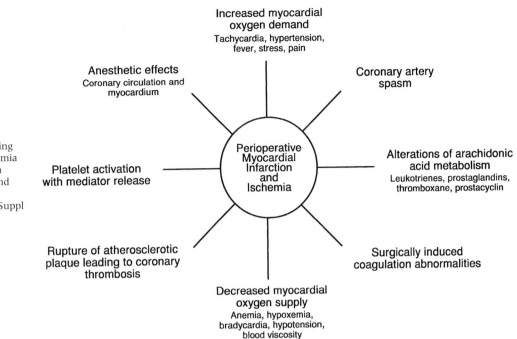

Figure 22–6 Factors influencing perioperative myocardial ischemia and infarction. (Redrawn from London MJ: Silent ischemia and postoperative infarction. J Cardiothorac Anesth 1990; 4[Suppl 1]: 58–67.)

contractility, also affecting myocardial oxygen demand. The increased vagal tone initiated by withdrawal of sympathetic activity may produce marked bradycardia and vasodilation. All of these factors may improve the myocardial supply-demand ratio, unless mean arterial pressure is decreased sufficiently to jeopardize coronary blood flow by means of an extensive local anesthetic-induced sympathectomy or removal of increased vasoconstriction in unblocked regions by increased vagal tone or by addition of general anesthetics.[167]

The beneficial effects of neuraxial block are probably not solely the result of favorable systemic hemodynamic changes on myocardial workload. Many perioperative electrocardiographic ST-segment deviations indicative of ischemia are not associated with significant hemodynamic changes[281–283] but may involve modulation of cardiac autonomic activity. The coronary vascular beds are richly innervated by sympathetic and parasympathetic fibers. Alterations in cardiac autonomic tone have been implicated in the genesis of myocardial ischemia, cardiac pain, and arrhythmias.[284–287]

The presence of reflex arcs promoting a vicious cycle of ischemia-induced cardiac sympathetic activation prompts the idea that regional block of cardiac sympathetic innervation may have a therapeutic effect on patients vulnerable to or experiencing myocardial ischemia. The concept of sympathetic involvement in coronary artery disease is not new; surgical sympathectomy was used as a basis of therapy for angina as early as 1916.[288, 289] Animal studies using epidural blocks of cardiac sympathetic innervation have demonstrated an interruption of the sympathetic feedback cycle that would otherwise worsen ischemia by α-mediated poststenotic coronary vasoconstriction and β-mediated increases in myocardial oxygen demand,[290] a favorable increase in the ratio of endocardial to epicardial blood flow,[291] and an attenuation of ischemia-induced ST-

segment deviation and subendocardial acidosis.[292] Clinical correlation of the potentially beneficial effects of the regional block of cardiac innervation has been provided by Blomberg and colleagues, who, in a series of studies[270, 273, 293–295] using thoracic epidural anesthesia, demonstrated its therapeutic effects on coronary artery disease patients with unstable angina and stress-induced myocardial ischemia.

Animal and human observations implicate sympathetic and vagal afferent involvement in cardiac nociceptive traffic, including the sensation of cardiac pain (Fig. 22–7). They suggest that perturbations involving different regions of the myocardium result in characteristically different autonomic activity. Experimental or pathologic derangements involving the anterior surface of the heart, supplied by the left anterior descending and proximal circumflex coronary arteries, result in sympathetic reflexes, producing tachycardia or hypertension or both. In this situation, upper thoracic and lower cervical sympathectomy provides relief of angina, and vagotomy does not affect afferent nerve traffic. In contrast, experimental or pathologic alterations involving the inferoposterior myocardium, supplied by the right and distal circumflex coronary arteries, result in vagal efferent activity, producing bradycardia or hypotension or both. In this setting, upper thoracic and lower cervical sympathectomy does not usually relieve angina.[286]

Bezold-Jarisch Reflex

The Bezold-Jarisch reflex is a vasodepressor reflex of intracardiac origin that is well known to cardiologists.[296, 297] Activity of inhibitory nonmyelinated C-fiber vagal afferents induced by mechanoreceptors, located primarily in the inferoposterior wall of the left ventri-

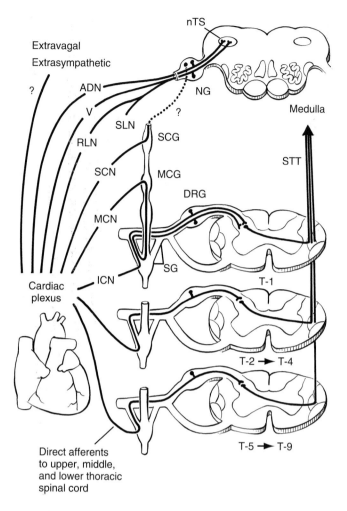

Figure 22–7 Summary of afferent cardiac nociceptor fiber pathways to the central nervous system. Afferent sympathetic fibers from the heart course through the middle cardiac nerve (MCN) to enter the middle cervical sympathetic ganglion (MCG), where they project through the stellate ganglion (SG) to the upper thoracic and lower cervical spinal cord. They may also course from the heart by way of the inferior cardiac nerve (ICN) and stellate ganglion to enter the upper thoracic spinal cord. The upper, middle, and lower thoracic spinal cord (T-2 to T-9) also may receive afferent sympathetic fibers directly from the upper, middle, and lower thoracic sympathetic ganglia. The cell bodies for the afferent sympathetic fibers are located in the dorsal root ganglia (DRG), and information is carried from these ganglia to the thalamus through the spinothalamic tract (STT). The nucleus of the solitary tract (nTS), located in the dorsal medulla, is the primary destination of vagal afferent fibers, with subsequent rostral and caudal relay. Additional vagal fibers course within the recurrent laryngeal nerve (RLN), which subsequently joins the superior laryngeal nerve (SLN), and within the aortic depressor nerve (ADN). The nodose ganglion (NG), which contains the cell bodies of these cardiac vagal afferents, may receive additional vagal afferent fibers through the superior cardiac nerve (SCN) and superior cardiac ganglion (SCG). Extravagal extrasympathetic afferent fibers may lie outside of these conventionally defined sympathetic and vagal pathways. (Reprinted from Meller ST, Gebhart GF: A critical review of the afferent pathways and the potential chemical mediators involved in cardiac pain. Neuroscience 1992; 48: 501–524. With kind permission from Elsevier Science Ltd, The Boulevard, Langford Lane, Kidlington 0X5 1GB, UK.)

cle, normally decreases during orthostatic stress or hemorrhage. This allows a reflex increase in sympathetic tone and protects against hypotension. However, a rapid decrease in central venous return may induce a paradoxical increase in the firing of these inhibitory left ventricular receptors as the ventricle contracts vigorously around its relatively empty chamber. This situation can trigger an abrupt, generalized withdrawal of sympathetic tone concomitant with an increase in vagal outflow and result in reflex bradycardia and hypotension.

The Bezold-Jarisch reflex is a variant of a normally protective physiologic process, and several clinical scenarios in which abrupt onset of severe hypotension and bradycardia or asystole occur have been attributed to paradoxical activation of these left ventricular receptors and initiation of this reflex. The clinical situations include sudden death,[298] vasovagal syncope,[299, 300] exertional syncope in aortic stenosis,[301] administration of nitroglycerin,[302] myocardial ischemia and infarction,[303] coronary arteriography and thrombolysis,[304, 305] pulmonary embolism,[306] hypoxemia,[307] and acute hypovolemia.[308, 309]

Any physiologic reflex with the potential for initiating abrupt, severe hypotension and bradycardia or asystole in the setting of decreased venous return, such as the Bezold-Jarisch reflex, is of practical interest to

anesthesiologists. In a 1988 closed insurance claim analysis, Caplan and associates[310] reported 14 cases of sudden cardiac arrest in healthy patients who had received a spinal anesthetic. The researchers speculated that unappreciated respiratory insufficiency may have been an important factor, but they also observed that these cardiac arrests seemed to evolve quite rapidly in a setting of apparent hemodynamic stability. A subsequent report[311] noted one case of extreme bradycardia and two cases of asystole during spinal anesthesia that were not associated with hypoxemia, obvious respiratory depression, or adverse outcome. The investigators remarked that the abrupt onset of severe bradycardia or asystole, in a setting of relative hemodynamic stability with a gradual downward trend in heart rate, implied the presence of a reflex mechanism as the cause of this phenomenon, and they suggested the Bezold-Jarisch reflex might be responsible (Fig. 22–8).

Review of earlier literature[174, 312–315] reveals that the potential for sudden and unexpected hemodynamic collapse during neuraxial anesthesia, particularly in the situation of relative or absolute hypovolemia, had been considered by previous investigators. The fact that this phenomenon of sudden onset of profound bradycardia is recognized on a regular basis, particularly in centers performing large numbers of spinal anesthesias, and treated without adverse sequelae suggests that it could

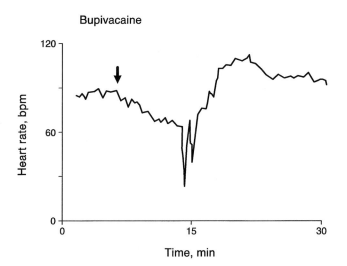

Bupivacaine

Figure 22–8 Trended heart rate during spinal anesthetic in which abrupt onset of severe bradycardia occurred. Notice the gradual slowing of heart rate before the abrupt decline. Atropine (0.2 mg) and ephedrine (20 mg) were administered intravenously, and chest compressions were immediately instituted, producing rapid heart rate recovery. (Redrawn from Mackey DC, Carpenter RL, Thompson GE, et al: Bradycardia and asystole during spinal anesthesia: a report of three cases without morbidity. Anesthesiology 1989; 70: 866–868.)

be classified as a variant of the normal physiologic response to neuraxial block and not as a complication.

Coagulation Function and Regional Block

A hypercoagulable state accompanies major surgery as a result of tissue trauma and activation of the neuroendocrine stress response.[316–318] This perioperative derangement in coagulation status, which would ordinarily be protective in the situation of major trauma, may be maladaptive in the surgical patient and the source of considerable morbidity and mortality. For example, cardiovascular disease is a principal risk factor in major operations and critical illnesses, and elements of a hypercoagulable state have been postulated to be important aspects of unstable angina, myocardial infarction, transient ischemic attacks, and stroke.[279, 319–321]

Regional anesthetic and analgesic techniques incorporating epidural or spinal anesthesia for major surgery have demonstrated decreased perioperative graft occlusion and thromboembolic events compared with general anesthesia.[111, 113, 195, 322–325] The mechanisms by which neuraxial blocks may moderate perioperative hypercoagulability include decreased peripheral vascular stasis that accompanies sympathetic block,[326–329] attenuated trauma-associated procoagulant phenomena such as enhanced platelet aggregation and depressed fibrinolysis and antithrombin III levels,[111, 323, 330] and in the case of epidural anesthesia, direct impairment of platelet activity by systemic levels of local anesthetic.[331–333] Many of these beneficial mechanisms may be related to the moderating impact of neuraxial blocks on the stress response to a major operation and its precipitation of a hypercoagulable state.

Endocrine and Metabolic Effects of Regional Anesthesia

The neuroendocrine stress response is composed of a wide range of neural, endocrine, metabolic, inflammatory, and immune phenomena that accompany tissue trauma during surgery and critical illness.[334, 335] The physiologic mechanisms affected by the neuroendocrine stress response normally are protective in other settings, but the cumulative effect of their perioperative derangements, including tachycardia, hypertension, catabolic metabolic state, hypercoagulability, and immunosuppression, may be particularly deleterious to the critically ill patient. Tissue injury and pain are the principal initiators of the perioperative stress response, with additional contributions from hemorrhage, infection, acidosis, hypoxemia, anxiety, starvation, and hypothermia. Regional blocks may moderate or abolish elements of the stress response to surgery, particularly in operations on the lower abdomen and lower extremities.[336–339]

Regional Anesthesia and Immunocompetence

Neuroendocrine Stress Response and Its Effect on Immune Status

Various humoral and cellular immunologic reactions accompany the stress response in proportion to the degree of acute tissue injury and critical illness, with a cumulative effect of depressed immunocompetency that may last for several weeks.[340–345] The neuroendocrine and immune systems are closely linked by common hormones, neurotransmitters, and receptors that integrate the two systems and facilitate the immunosuppression observed with activation of the neuroendocrine stress response.[346–349] Acute and chronic inflammatory processes traditionally known to involve immunologic mechanisms are influenced by peripheral nervous system activity.[350–352]

The initial inflammatory and immune responses to tissue trauma include activation of the complement, coagulation-fibrinolytic, arachidonic acid, and kinin-kallikrein cascades and release of the cytokines interleukin-1, interleukin-2, interleukin-6, tumor necrosis factor-a (or cachectin), and interferon-γ. B-lymphocyte numbers in the peripheral blood decrease, and immunoglobulin concentrations may decrease secondary to protein extravasation, immunoglobulin consumption, or hemodilution. Cell-mediated immunity, including natural killer cell activity, is also impaired.[353, 354] Natural killer cells are lymphocytes particularly cytotoxic to tumor cells and cells infected with viruses; the lymphocytes possess antibacterial activity as well.[355–357] Animal studies have demonstrated suppression of natural killer cell activity mediated by endogenous opioid peptides and by exogenously administered opioids. These studies have shown enhanced tumor growth by stress-induced endogenous opioid peptides and by morphine administration, although the natural killer cell suppression by morphine appears to be transient and less potent than that of stress-released endogenous opioids.[358-362] Although morphine may transiently increase natural killer cell suppression, it may improve overall resistance to tumor growth if it decreases endogenous opioid released by stress-related mechanisms.[363]

The Immune Response and Anesthetic Agents

In addition to the immunosuppressive effects of the neuroendocrine stress response and exogenous opioids, several anesthetic agents may negatively affect perioperative immunocompetence.[364-369] Anesthetic agents implicated in in vitro or in vivo studies include halothane, isoflurane, thiopental, and ketamine. In animal studies,[370, 371] halothane has been shown to depress natural killer cell activity and enhance the metastatic activity of inoculated tumor cells. In clinical studies comparing regional and general anesthesia in lower abdominal and pelvic operative procedures, in which regional anesthetic block of the stress response is the most complete, regional anesthesia consistently avoided the depression of immune response components seen with the administration of general anesthesia.[372-379]

Regional Anesthesia, Blood Transfusion, and Immunocompetence

Homologous blood transfusion impairs immune function by various mechanisms, including decreased cytokine production, increased suppressor T-cell number or function, decreased monocyte function, and decreased natural killer cell function and helper T-cell number.[380] Although this phenomenon is routinely exploited to increase renal allograft survival, homologous blood transfusion has repeatedly been associated with increased incidence of bacterial and viral infections and with cancer recurrence.[381-383] Any anesthetic method that decreases intraoperative blood loss may decrease the need for homologous blood transfusion, with its attendant transfusion-related immunodepression. Regional anesthesia has been found by some investigators[384-386] to decrease intraoperative blood loss, and the technique may be a useful component of any anesthetic strategy designed to minimize blood loss in operative procedures typically associated with major hemorrhage.

Immunologic Implications of Regional Anesthesia in the Perioperative Environment

Because the anesthesiologist has the ability to moderate the neuroendocrine stress response to operative procedures and to postoperative pain through local and regional blocks, the resultant salutary effects on the typical immune response to surgical trauma and pain may beneficially influence the perioperative outcome. Moreover, regional anesthesia may decrease the possi-

bility of transfusion-related immunosuppression if it lessens the risk of homologous blood transfusion by minimizing intraoperative hemorrhage.

The Gastrointestinal System and Regional Anesthesia

Regional anesthetic procedures that may affect the gastrointestinal system are rarely used outside the perioperative environment. Any review of these effects must include the potential influence of regional anesthesia on perturbations of physiologic gastrointestinal function that are commonly found in the perioperative setting. Regional anesthetic procedures may have a profound influence on visceral pain and other phenomena such as ileus, nutritional status, and infection.

Gastrointestinal Innervation and Regional Block

The gastrointestinal tract receives a dual innervation from the parasympathetic and sympathetic nervous systems through essentially its entire length.[387] Parasympathetic preganglionic fibers from the dorsal motor nucleus of the vagus course principally through the vagus nerves to innervate the upper abdominal viscera and from the middle sacral segments of the spinal cord through pelvic splanchnic nerves to innervate the pelvic viscera. The parasympathetic postganglionic neurons are located in the myenteric and submucosal plexuses. The vagus nerves supply all but the upper portion of the esophagus and the stomach, small intestine, colon to the splenic flexure, pancreas, and liver and biliary tree, and although they are usually thought of as motor nerves, the vagus nerves contain at least 80% afferent fibers.[388, 389] Visceral afferent parasympathetic fibers transmit sensations of satiety, distension, and nausea, but not pain, which is conveyed by sympathetic afferents.[390-393] In general, parasympathetic efferent outflow increases the activity of most gastrointestinal functions, such as tonic contraction, sphincter relaxation, peristalsis, and secretion.

Sympathetic preganglionic neuron cell bodies innervating the gastrointestinal tract are located principally in the fifth thoracic through the second lumbar spinal cord segments. Their fibers extend to the paravertebral sympathetic chain ganglia, where they synapse directly with postganglionic neurons or continue on to leave the paravertebral chain to synapse within one of the prevertebral ganglia (celiac, mesenteric, or hypogastric ganglion). In addition to transmitting pain information through sympathetic afferents, sympathetic efferents inhibit peristalsis and gastric secretion, and they produce sphincter contraction and vasoconstriction.[394] Sympathetic hyperactivity can bring gastrointestinal motility to a standstill, and block of the gastrointestinal sympathetic innervation leads to generalized contraction of the bowel and increased intraluminal pressure due to the unopposed parasympathetic efferent activity.

Table 22–1 Sympathetic Innervation of Gastrointestinal Structures

STRUCTURE	PRINCIPAL AFFERENT PATHWAYS		EFFERENT PATHWAYS		
	Entrance Into Neuraxis	Location of Cell Body in Spinal Cord and Course of Preganglionic Neurons*	Site of Preganglionic-Postganglionic Synapse	Course of Postganglionic Fibers	PRINCIPAL FUNCTIONS
Esophagus Upper Lower	Follow esophageal sympathetic nerves → T-2 to T-7(8)†	T-2 to T-4 → thoracic sympathetic chain T-5 to T-7 → thoracic sympathetic chain	Stellate ganglion and T-2 to T-4 ganglia T(4)-5 to T-7(8) ganglia	Esophageal branches from sympathetic trunk → esophageal plexuses	Decreased motility and contraction of sphincters
Stomach	Follow sympathetic nerves → T-6 to T-9	T-6 to T-9(10); greater splanchnic nerves and celiac plexus	Celiac ganglia	Right and left gastric and gastroepiploic plexuses	Diminution of peristalsis and secretion; contraction of pylorus; vasoconstriction
Gallbladder and bile ducts	Follow sympathetic nerves → T-5 to T-9	T-5 to T-9(10); greater splanchnic nerves and celiac plexus	Celiac ganglia	Hepatic and gastroduodenal plexuses	Diminution of peristalsis
Liver	Follow sympathetic nerves → T-5 to T-9	T-6 to T-9(10); greater splanchnic nerves and celiac plexus	Celiac ganglia	Hepatic plexus	Vasoconstriction
Pancreas	Follow sympathetic nerves → T-6 to T-10	T-6 to T-10; greater splanchnic nerves and celiac plexus	Celiac ganglia	Direct branches from celiac plexus and offshoots from splenic, gastroduodenal, and pancreaticoduodenal plexuses	Vasoconstriction and secretion
Small intestine	Follow sympathetic nerves → T-6 to T-8(10) (duodenum), T-9 to T-11 (jejunum and ileum)	T-6 to T-11; greater and lesser splanchnic nerves to celiac plexus	Celiac and superior mesenteric ganglia	Superior mesenteric plexus → nerves alongside jejunal and ileal arteries	Motility decreased; sphincters relaxed; secretion inhibited
Cecum and appendix	Follow sympathetic nerves → T-10 to T-12	T-10 to T-12; greater and lesser splanchnic nerves → celiac and superior mesenteric plexuses	Celiac and superior mesenteric ganglia	Nerves alongside ileocolic artery	Diminution of peristalsis and secretion
Colon to splenic flexure	Follow sympathetic nerves → T-12 to L-1	T-12(11) to L-1; lesser, least, and lumbar splanchnic nerves	Superior and inferior mesenteric ganglia	Mesenteric plexuses → nerves alongside right, middle, and superior left colic arteries	Diminution of peristalsis and secretion
Colon from splenic flexure to rectum	Follow sympathetic nerves → L-1 to L-2	L-1 to L-2; lumbar and sacral branches of sympathetic trunks; inferior mesenteric and hypogastric plexuses	Ganglia in inferior mesenteric and superior and inferior hypogastric plexuses	Nerves alongside inferior left colic and rectal arteries	Diminution of peristalsis and secretion; contraction of sphincter and internus

*Each preganglionic fiber passes peripherally through the anterior root and white ramus communicans to the sympathetic trunk.
†Segments in parentheses are inconsistent.
From Bonica JJ: Autonomic innervation of the viscera in relation to nerve block. Anesthesiology 1968; 29: 793–813.

The degree to which the gastrointestinal tract is affected by regional block depends on the type and extent of block (Table 22-1 and Fig. 22-9). Block of sympathetic and pelvic parasympathetic fibers commonly occurs in clinical practice, as in cases of spinal and epidural anesthesia, although parasympathetic innervation of the upper gastrointestinal tract usually remains intact in most clinical situations because of the unblocked vagal nerves.

Neuraxial Block and the Risk of Enteric Anastomosis Dehiscence

The clinical scenario of increased gastrointestinal motility due to unopposed vagal activity has caused concern among some clinicians because of reports[395, 396] suggesting the possibility that increased intraluminal pressure from unopposed parasympathetic activity in the setting of neuraxial block may lead to an increased risk of postoperative intestinal anastomotic disruption. However, Schnitzler and colleagues,[397] using a porcine model of colonic anastomosis with intraoperative and postoperative epidural bupivacaine, morphine, or saline infusion, found no anastomotic complications and no significant difference in anastomotic weakness. Two clinical studies,[398, 399] one retrospective and one prospective, comparing colon anastomosis during general or neuraxial block anesthesia revealed no statistically significant difference in the rate of anastomotic dehiscence. The last two studies plus the rarity of the reported event in the setting of common use of neuraxial block for bowel operation support the contention that spinal and epidural anesthesia and analgesia pose no increased risk for anastomotic breakdown in bowel operation.

Because anastomotic wound healing is affected by tissue hypoxia, colonic and small intestinal tissue oxygen tension correlates with blood flow, and spinal and epidural anesthesia increases gastrointestinal blood flow by means of sympatholysis, it could be argued that a neuraxial block actually has the potential to lessen the risk of anastomotic breakdown in bowel surgery.[400–402] The risk of anastomotic disruption may be moderated by any anesthetic technique, including spinal and epidural anesthesia and analgesia, that helps preserve normal peristalsis in the perioperative period and minimizes gaseous distension of the viscus.

Postoperative Adynamic Ileus and Regional Anesthesia

Because postoperative ileus is virtually a universal phenomenon in patients undergoing major intra-abdominal and pelvic surgery, any discussion of the effects of regional anesthesia on the gastrointestinal tract would be incomplete without a discussion of the potential effects of neuraxial block on postoperative gastrointestinal function. Because postoperative ileus is a major determinant of the length of hospital stay and of hospital cost and because it affects the patient's nutritional and immune status, any possible moderating effect that could be provided by epidural or spinal anesthesia is a relevant consideration for clinicians searching for means to improve perioperative outcome.

Postoperative ileus represents a temporary state of gastrointestinal motor dysfunction that occurs after intraperitoneal surgery and after operations remote from the abdominal cavity, such as neurosurgical and orthopedic procedures. Uncomplicated postoperative ileus is principally caused by decreased or absent transit in the stomach (lasting 24–48 h) and the colon (lasting 48–72 h).[403] This common problem adds to overall patient

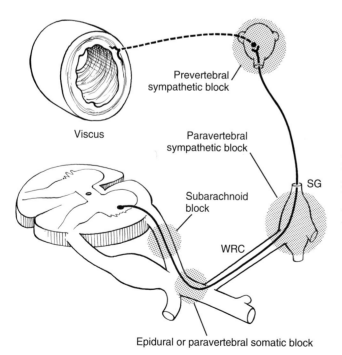

Figure 22–9 Various regional anesthetic techniques that may be used to block preganglionic and postganglionic sympathetic fibers innervating the gastrointestinal tract. SG, sympathetic ganglion; WRC, white ramus communicans. (Modified from Bonica JJ: Autonomic innervation of the viscera in relation to nerve block. Anesthesiology 1968; 29: 793–813.)

discomfort, increases perioperative morbidity, prolongs hospital stay, and increases cost.[404] Ileus is produced by sympathetic fibers innervating the gut that constrain motility by inhibiting the release of acetylcholine and peptidergic transmitters from excitatory fibers within the myenteric plexus and by directly inhibiting smooth muscle cells through activation of the α- and β-receptors on their surfaces. Activation of these sympathetic efferents may occur secondary to generalized surgical stress or through a spinal reflex arc in which afferent fibers project to the prevertebral and sympathetic chain ganglia.[403, 405, 406] Postoperative ileus may be potentiated by gastrointestinal ischemia, by anesthetic agents such as opioids and anticholinergics, and by psychologic influences.[407–412]

Because of its beneficial effects on gastrointestinal blood flow, ability to moderate or abolish perioperative pain and stress, ability to block the afferent and efferent limbs of sympathetically mediated gastrointestinal reflexes, and ability to spare the use of opioids and other systemic anesthetic and analgesic agents, epidural and spinal anesthesia and local anesthetic epidural analgesia are ideal instruments to consider as potential modalities for moderating, if not abolishing, the problem of postoperative ileus.[401, 402, 413–415] This is not a new concept. Although the precise mechanisms of action may not have been entirely appreciated at the time, neuraxial block was proposed for treating ileus by several investigators as early as the 1920s.[416, 417]

In addition to techniques of regional block, Rimbäck and coworkers[418] used systemic lidocaine infusion successfully to moderate postoperative ileus in cholecystectomy patients. They suggested that the beneficial action of systemic local anesthetics in this scenario could be attributed to suppression of inhibitory sympathetic spinal and prevertebral reflexes, attenuation of the neuroendocrine stress response, and the anti-inflammatory effects of amide local anesthetics. Similar results reported by Rimbäck and colleagues[419] using intra-abdominal instillation of bupivacaine in patients undergoing cholecystectomy or gastric surgery support the contention that at least a portion of the salutary effect on postoperative ileus provided by epidural anesthesia and potentially by other anatomically relevant blocks accompanied by significant systemic absorption of local anesthetic, such as splanchnic, hypogastric, or celiac plexus block, may result from the effect of systemic local anesthetic levels.[420]

Several clinical reports have addressed the issue of epidural anesthesia and analgesia and its effect on the recovery of bowel function, with the preponderance of evidence suggesting that, although parenteral and epidural opioid administration delay gastric emptying and prolong intestinal transit time, epidural local anesthetic infusion hastens recovery of postoperative bowel function.[108, 109, 112, 421–430] Reports by England and associates[431] and by Rawal and colleagues[423] suggest that neuraxial administration of opioid alone may have less adverse effect on postoperative bowel function than conventional parenteral opioid administration. Although epidural local anesthetic infusion alone does not contribute to postoperative gastrointestinal stasis and does accelerate recovery from ileus, this modality is not practical in most clinical settings because of the side effects, such as motor block and hypotension, that often accompany epidural local anesthetic infusions of sufficiently high concentration to provide adequate analgesia. The optimal epidural anesthetic and analgesic strategy to promote adequate analgesia and rapid convalescence therefore may be the use of epidural local anesthetic infusion as a means of minimizing the unavoidable patient exposure to epidural or systemic administration of opioids, which is the goal of balanced analgesia.

Regional Anesthesia and Postoperative Gastrointestinal Function: Implications for Nutrition, Immunocompetence, and Perioperative Outcome

Early postoperative nutritional support is important for the maintenance of immunocompetence, attenuation of septic morbidity, and rapid wound healing in the high-risk surgical patient. Enteral feeding is probably the optimal route in this patient population because of its efficacy in delivery of nutritional substrate, its relatively low risk of complications, and its lower cost.[432, 433] Regional anesthetic and analgesic techniques can facilitate early enteral refeeding by minimizing postoperative ileus, making the procedures attractive considerations when designing postoperative therapy to accelerate rate of convalescence, minimize risk of complications, and minimize cost.

Regional Anesthesia and Nausea and Vomiting

Various factors may contribute to perioperative nausea and vomiting in the setting of regional anesthesia, including unopposed vagal activity, hypotension, hypoxemia, systemic medication (particularly opioids), and psychologic stimuli. Many clinicians think that spinal anesthesia poses the highest risk for nausea and vomiting among regional anesthetic procedures. For example, Bonica and coworkers[434] found a 21% incidence of emesis with spinal anesthesia and only an 8.8% incidence with local anesthetic block of the extremity. Other investigators[153, 435] have reported a similar incidence of nausea and vomiting associated with spinal anesthesia. In addition to the sources commonly proposed as causes of nausea and vomiting with spinal anesthesia, another possible cause is activation of cardiac vagal afferents by ventricular mechanoreceptors in response to decreased venous return, even in the setting of normal blood pressure (i.e., Bezold-Jarisch reflex).[436–438] The correlation of an increased risk of nausea and vomiting with high block levels and more extensive sympathectomy and vasodilation may be evidence of this cardiac mechanism of nausea and vomiting.[153, 155]

Influence of Regional Anesthesia on Perioperative Outcome

Many of the early proponents of regional anesthesia, such as Crile, Cushing, Halsted, Babcock, Jonnesco, and Matas, were surgeons who advocated local and regional anesthetic techniques to facilitate the operative procedure or improve the surgical outcome.[21, 439-446] Despite this initial enthusiasm, the use of regional anesthesia seemed to plateau or decline during the middle portion of this century, perhaps because the development and clinical use of neuromuscular relaxants allowed the anesthesiologist to provide the surgeon with excellent operating conditions during general anesthesia with greater ease and relatively less skill.[447] However, several publications[107, 111, 448-454] suggest that regional anesthetic and analgesic modalities may decrease postoperative pain and suffering, lessen perioperative morbidity and mortality, and accelerate convalescence, rekindling an interest in regional techniques. The influence of regional anesthesia on perioperative outcome depends on many factors, including the degree of patient debility and operative trespass, the anesthesiologist's comprehensive understanding of the patient's perioperative pathophysiology, and the anesthesiologist's knowledge of and skill in using the regional anesthetic and analgesic techniques available.

References

1. Koller C: On the use of cocaine for producing anaesthesia on the eye. Lancet 1884; 2: 990–992.
2. Corning JL: Spinal anaesthesia and local medication of the cord. N Y Med J 1885; 62: 483–485.
3. Goldan SO: Intraspinal cocainization for surgical anesthesia. Phila Med J 1900; 6: 850–857.
4. Matas R: Local and regional anesthesia with cocain and other analgesic drugs, including the subarachnoid method, as applied in general surgical practice. Phila Med J 1900; 6: 820–843.
5. Cushing H: On the avoidance of shock in major amputations by cocainization of large nerve-trunks preliminary to their division. With observations on blood-pressure changes in surgical cases. Ann Surg 1902; 36: 321–345.
6. Gray HT, Parsons L: Blood-pressure variations associated with lumbar puncture, and the induction of spinal anaesthesia. Q J Med 1912; 5: 339–367.
7. Crile GW: The kinetic theory of shock and its prevention through anoci-association (shockless operation). Lancet 1913; 2: 7–16.
8. Labat G: Circulatory disturbances associated with subarachnoid nerve-block. Long Island Med J 1927; 21: 573–579.
9. Koster H, Kasman LP: Spinal anaesthesia for the head, neck, and thorax: its relation to respiratory paralysis. Surg Gynecol Obstet 1929; 49: 617–630.
10. Glazer S, Portenoy RK: Systemic local anesthetics in pain control. J Pain Symptom Manage 1991; 6: 30–39.
11. Christie JM, Valdes C, Markowsky SJ: Neurotoxicity of lidocaine combined with mexiletine. Anesth Analg 1993; 77: 1291–1294.
12. Greene NM, Brull SJ: Physiology of Spinal Anesthesia, 4th ed. Baltimore, Williams & Wilkins, 1993.
13. Yaksh TL, Rudy TA: Analgesia mediated by a direct spinal action of narcotics. Science 1976; 192: 1357–1358.
14. Bernards CM, Hill HF: The spinal nerve root sleeve is not a preferred route for redistribution of drugs from the epidural space to the spinal cord. Anesthesiology 1991; 75: 827–832.
15. Bernards CM, Hill HF: Physical and chemical properties of drug molecules governing their diffusion through the spinal meninges. Anesthesiology 1992; 77: 750–756.
16. Bernards CM: Flux of morphine, fentanyl, and alfentanil through rabbit arteries in vivo. Evidence supporting a vascular route for redistribution of opioids between the epidural space and the spinal cord. Anesthesiology 1993; 78: 1126–1131.
17. Bromage PR, Joyal AC, Binney JC: Local anesthetic drugs: penetration from the spinal extradural space into the neuraxis. Science 1963; 140: 392–394.
18. Forbes AR, Roizen F: Does spinal anesthesia anesthetize the spinal cord? Anesthesiology 1978; 48: 440–445.
19. Lang E, Krainick JU, Gerbershagen HU: Spinal cord transmission of impulses during high spinal anesthesia as measured by cortical evoked potentials. Anesth Analg 1989; 69: 15–20.
20. Payne R: Subarachnoid injection of cocain as a general anesthetic for operation upon the head. Trans Am Laryngol Rhinol Otol Soc 1901; 7: 215–225.
21. Jonnesco T: Remarks on general spinal analgesia. Br Med J 1909; 2: 1396–1401.
22. Koster H: Spinal anesthesia, with special reference to its use in surgery of the head, neck and thorax. Am J Surg 1928; 5: 554–570.
23. Kozody R, Swartz J, Palahniuk RJ, et al: Spinal cord blood flow following subarachnoid lidocaine. Can Anaesth Soc J 1985; 32: 472–478.
24. Kozody R, Palahniuk RJ, Cuming MO: Spinal cord blood flow following subarachnoid tetracaine. Can Anaesth Soc J 1985; 32: 23–29.
25. Porter SS, Albin MS, Watson WA, et al: Spinal cord and cerebral blood flow responses to subarachnoid injection of local anesthetics with and without epinephrine. Acta Anaesthesiol Scand 1985; 29: 330–338.
26. Dohi S, Matsumiya N, Takeshima R, et al: The effects of subarachnoid lidocaine and phenylephrine on spinal cord and cerebral blood flow in dogs. Anesthesiology 1984; 61: 238–244.
27. Dohi S, Takeshima R, Naito H: Spinal cord blood flow during spinal anesthesia in dogs: the effects of tetracaine, epinephrine, acute blood loss, and hypercapnia. Anesth Analg 1987; 66: 599–606.
28. Kozody R, Palahniuk RJ, Wade JG, et al: The effect of subarachnoid epinephrine and phenylephrine on spinal cord blood flow. Can Anaesth Soc J 1984; 31: 503–508.
29. Kozody R, Ong B, Palahniuk RJ, et al: Subarachnoid bupivacaine decreases spinal cord blood flow in dogs. Can Anaesth Soc J 1985; 32: 216–222.
30. Tkachenko BI, Krasilnikov VG, Polenov SA, et al: Responses of resistance and capacitance vessels at various frequency electrical stimulation of sympathetic nerves. Experientia 1969; 25: 38–40.
31. Scheinberg P: Cerebral blood flow in vascular disease of the brain, with observations on the effects of stellate ganglion block. Am J Med 1950; 8: 139–147.
32. Harmel MH, Hafkenschiel JH, Austin GM, et al: The effect of bilateral stellate ganglion block on the cerebral circulation in normotensive and hypertensive patients. J Clin Invest 1949; 28: 415–418.
33. Kety SS, King BD, Horvath SM, et al: The effects of an acute reduction in blood pressure by means of differential spinal sympathetic block on the cerebral circulation of hypertensive patients. J Clin Invest 1950; 29: 402–407.
34. Kleinerman J, Sancetta SM, Hackel DB: Effects of high spinal anesthesia on cerebral circulation and metabolism in man. J Clin Invest 1958; 37: 285–293.
35. Guyton AC: Textbook of Medical Physiology, 8th ed, pp 648–658. Philadelphia, WB Saunders, 1991.
36. Huvos MC, Greene NM, Glaser GH: Electroencephalographic studies during acute subtotal sensory denervation in man. Yale J Biol Med 1962; 34: 592–597.
37. Cole DJ, Lin DM, Drummond JC, et al: Spinal tetracaine decreases central nervous system metabolism during somatosensory stimulation in the rat. Can J Anaesth 1990; 37: 231–237.
38. Wesolowski JA, Lema MJ: Phantom limb pain. Reg Anesth 1993; 18: 121–127.
39. Tucker GT, Mather LE: Clinical pharmacokinetics of local anaesthetics. Clin Pharmacokinet 1979; 4: 241–278.

40. Tucker GT: Safety in numbers: the role of pharmacokinetics in local anesthetic toxicity: the 1993 ASRA lecture. Reg Anesth 1994; 19: 155–163.
41. Reynolds F: Adverse effects of local anaesthetics. Br J Anaesth 1987; 59: 78–95.
42. Voulgaropoulos DS, Johnson MD, Covino BG: Local anesthetic toxicity. Semin Anesth 1990; 9: 8–15.
43. Modica PA, Tempelhoff R, White PF: Pro- and anticonvulsant effects of anesthetics (part II). Anesth Analg 1990; 70: 433–444.
44. Tanaka K, Yamasaki M: Blocking of cortical inhibitory synapses by intravenous lidocaine. Nature 1967; 209: 207–208.
45. Dohi S, Kitahata LM, Toyooka H, et al: An analgesic action of intravenously administered lidocaine on dorsal-horn neurons responding to noxious thermal stimulation. Anesthesiology 1979; 51: 123–126.
46. Woolf CJ, Wiesenfeld-Hallin Z: The systemic administration of local anaesthetics produces a selective depression of C-afferent fibre evoked activity in the spinal cord. Pain 1985; 23: 361–374.
47. Abram SE, Yaksh TL: Systemic lidocaine blocks nerve injury-induced hyperalgesia and nociceptor-driven spinal sensitization in the rat. Anesthesiology 1994; 80: 383–391.
48. Wallin G, Cassuto J, Högström S, et al: Effects of lidocaine infusion on the sympathetic response to abdominal surgery. Anesth Analg 1987; 66: 1008–1013.
49. Yukioka H, Hayashi M, Terai T, et al: Intravenous lidocaine as a suppressant of coughing during tracheal intubation in elderly patients. Anesth Analg 1993; 77: 309–312.
50. Warner LO, Rogers GL, Martino JD, et al: Intravenous lidocaine reduces the incidence of vomiting in children after surgery to correct strabismus. Anesthesiology 1988; 68: 618–621.
51. Cassuto J, Wallin G, Högström S, et al: Inhibition of postoperative pain by continuous low-dose intravenous infusion of lidocaine. Anesth Analg 1985; 64: 971–974.
52. Edmondson EA, Simpson RK Jr, Stubler DK, et al: Systemic lidocaine therapy for poststroke pain. South Med J 1993; 86: 1093–1096.
53. Maciewicz R, Chung RY, Strassman A, et al: Relief of vascular headache with intravenous lidocaine: clinical observations and a proposed mechanism. Clin J Pain 1988; 4: 11–16.
54. Kastrup J, Petersen P, Dejgård A, et al: Intravenous lidocaine infusion—a new treatment of chronic painful diabetic neuropathy? Pain 1987; 28: 69–75.
55. Giesbrecht GG: Human thermoregulatory inhibition by regional anesthesia. (Editorial.) Anesthesiology 1994; 81: 277–281.
56. Lopez M, Sessler DI, Walter K, et al: Rate and gender dependence of the sweating, vasoconstriction, and shivering thresholds in humans. Anesthesiology 1994; 80: 780–788.
57. Imrie MM, Hall GM: Body temperature and anaesthesia. Br J Anaesth 1990; 64: 346–354.
58. Sessler DI: Perianesthetic thermoregulation and heat balance in humans. FASEB J 1993; 7: 638–644.
59. Frank SM, Beattie C, Christopherson R, et al: Unintentional hypothermia is associated with postoperative myocardial ischemia. Anesthesiology 1993; 78: 468–476.
60. Glosten B, Sessler DI, Faure EA, et al: Central temperature changes are poorly perceived during epidural anesthesia. Anesthesiology 1992; 77: 10–16.
61. Sessler DI, Ponte J: Shivering during epidural anesthesia. Anesthesiology 1990; 72: 816–821.
62. Joris J, Ozaki M, Sessler DI, et al: Epidural anesthesia impairs both central and peripheral thermoregulatory control during general anesthesia. Anesthesiology 1994; 80: 268–277.
63. Kurz A, Sessler DI, Schroeder M, et al: Thermoregulatory response thresholds during spinal anesthesia. Anesth Analg 1993; 77: 721–726.
64. Sessler DI, Olofsson CI, Rubinstein EH: The thermoregulatory threshold in humans during nitrous oxide-fentanyl anesthesia. Anesthesiology 1988; 69: 357–364.
65. Washington DE, Sessler DI, Moayeri A, et al: Thermoregulatory responses to hyperthermia during isoflurane anesthesia in humans. J Appl Physiol 1993; 74: 82–87.
66. Ozaki M, Kurz A, Sessler DI, et al: Thermoregulatory thresholds during epidural and spinal anesthesia. Anesthesiology 1994; 81: 282–288.
67. Emerick TH, Ozaki M, Sessler DI, et al: Epidural anesthesia increases apparent leg temperature and decreases the shivering threshold. Anesthesiology 1994; 81: 289–298.
68. Hynson JM, Sessler DI, Glosten B, et al: Thermal balance and tremor patterns during epidural anesthesia. Anesthesiology 1991; 74: 680–690.
69. Holdcroft A, Hall GM, Cooper GM: Redistribution of body heat during anaesthesia. A comparison of halothane, fentanyl and epidural anaesthesia. Anaesthesia 1979; 34: 758–764.
70. Hendolin H, Lansimies E: Skin and central temperatures during continuous epidural analgesia and general anaesthesia in patients subjected to open prostatectomy. Ann Clin Res 1982; 14: 181–186.
71. Jenkins J, Fox J, Sharwood-Smith G: Changes in body heat during transvesical prostatectomy. A comparison of general and epidural anaesthesia. Anaesthesia 1983; 38: 748–753.
72. Frank SM, Beattie C, Christopherson R, et al: Epidural versus general anesthesia, ambient operating room temperature, and patient age as predictors of inadvertent hypothermia. Anesthesiology 1992; 77: 252–257.
73. Frank SM, Shir Y, Raja SN, et al: Core hypothermia and skin-surface temperature gradients: epidural versus general anesthesia and the effects of age. Anesthesiology 1994; 80: 502–508.
74. Raymond SA, Strichartz GR: The long and short of differential block. (Editorial.) Anesthesiology 1989; 70: 725–728.
75. Greene NM: Area of differential block in spinal anesthesia with hyperbaric tetracaine. Anesthesiology 1958; 19: 45–50.
76. Bromage PR: An evaluation of bupivacaine in epidural analgesia for obstetrics. Can Anaesth Soc J 1969; 16: 46–56.
77. Brull SJ, Greene NM: Zones of differential sensory block during extradural anaesthesia. Br J Anaesth 1991; 66: 651–655.
78. White JL, Stevens RA, Beardsley D, et al: Differential epidural block: does the choice of local anesthetic matter? Reg Anesth 1994; 19: 335–338.
79. Gasser HS, Erlanger J: The rôle of fibre size in the establishment of a nerve block by pressure or cocaine. Am J Physiol 1929; 88: 581–591.
80. Helrich M, Papper EM, Brodie BB, et al: The fate of intrathecal procaine and spinal fluid level required for surgical anesthesia. J Pharmacol Exp Ther 1950; 100: 78–82.
81. Fink BR: Mechanisms of differential axial blockade in epidural and subarachnoid anesthesia. Anesthesiology 1989; 70: 851–858.
82. Chamberlain DP, Chamberlain BDL: Changes in the skin temperature of the trunk and their relationship to sympathetic blockade during spinal anesthesia. Anesthesiology 1986; 65: 139–143.
83. Brull SJ, Greene NM: Time-courses of zones of differential sensory blockade during spinal anesthesia with hyperbaric tetracaine or bupivacaine. Anesth Analg 1989; 69: 342–347.
84. Hedenstierna G: Mechanisms of postoperative pulmonary dysfunction. Acta Chir Scand Suppl 1988; 550: 152–158.
85. Hedenstierna G: Gas exchange during anaesthesia. Br J Anaesth 1990; 64: 507–514.
86. Nunn JF: Effects of anaesthesia on respiration. Br J Anaesth 1990; 65: 54–62.
87. Lindberg P, Gunnarsson L, Tokics L, et al: Atelectasis and lung function in the postoperative period. Acta Anaesthesiol Scand 1992; 36: 546–553.
88. Hedenstierna G, Strandberg A, Brismar B, et al: Functional residual capacity, thoracoabdominal dimensions, and central blood volume during general anesthesia with muscle paralysis and mechanical ventilation. Anesthesiology 1985; 62: 247–254.
89. Wahba RW: Perioperative functional residual capacity. Can J Anaesth 1991; 38: 384–400.
90. Ford GT, Whitelaw WA, Rosenal TW, et al: Diaphragm function after upper abdominal surgery in humans. Am Rev Respir Dis 1983; 127: 431–436.
91. Fratacci MD, Kimball WR, Wain JC, et al: Diaphragmatic shortening after thoracic surgery in humans. Effects of mechanical ventilation and thoracic epidural anesthesia. Anesthesiology 1993; 79: 654–665.
92. Mankikian B, Cantineau JP, Bertrand M, et al: Improvement of diaphragmatic function by a thoracic extradural block after upper abdominal surgery. Anesthesiology 1988; 68: 379–386.
93. Pansard J-L, Mankikian B, Bertrand M, et al: Effects of thoracic

extradural block on diaphragmatic electrical activity and contractility after upper abdominal surgery. Anesthesiology 1993; 78: 63–71.

94. Burgess FW, Anderson DM, Colonna D, et al: Thoracic epidural analgesia with bupivacaine and fentanyl for postoperative thoracotomy pain. J Cardiothorac Vasc Anesth 1994; 8: 420–424.

95. Egbert LD, Tamersoy K, Deas TC: Pulmonary function during spinal anesthesia: the mechanism of cough depression. Anesthesiology 1961; 22: 882–885.

96. Moir DD: Ventilatory function during epidural analgesia. Br J Anaesth 1963; 35: 3–7.

97. Freund FG, Bonica JJ, Ward RJ, et al: Ventilatory reserve and level of motor block during high spinal and epidural anesthesia. Anesthesiology 1967; 28: 834–837.

98. Steinbrook RA, Concepcion M: Respiratory effects of spinal anesthesia: resting ventilation and single-breath CO_2 response. Anesth Analg 1991; 72: 182–186.

99. Ward RJ, Bonica JJ, Freund FG, et al: Epidural and subarachnoid anesthesia: cardiovascular and respiratory effects. JAMA 1965; 191: 275–278.

100. de Jong RH: Arterial carbon dioxide and oxygen tensions during spinal block. JAMA 1965; 191: 698–702.

101. Eisele J, Trenchard D, Burki N, et al: The effect of chest wall block on respiratory sensation and control in man. Clin Sci 1968; 35: 23–33.

102. Steinbrook RA, Topulos GP, Concepcion M: Ventilatory responses to hypercapnia during tetracaine spinal anesthesia. J Clin Anesth 1988; 1: 75–80.

103. McCarthy GS: The effect of thoracic epidural analgesia on pulmonary gas distribution and functional residual capacity and airway closure. Br J Anaesth 1976; 48: 243–248.

104. Sundberg A, Wattwil M, Arvill A: Respiratory effects of high thoracic epidural anaesthesia. Acta Anaesthesiol Scand 1986; 30: 215–217.

105. Harrop-Griffiths AW, Ravalia A, Browne DA, et al: Regional anaesthesia and cough effectiveness. A study in patients undergoing caesarean section. Anaesthesia 1991; 46: 11–13.

106. Hecker BR, Bjurstrom R, Schoene RB: Effect of intercostal nerve blockade on respiratory mechanics and CO_2 chemosensitivity at rest and exercise. Anesthesiology 1989; 70: 13–18.

107. Yeager MP, Glass DD, Neff RK, et al: Epidural anesthesia and analgesia in high-risk surgical patients. Anesthesiology 1987; 66: 729–736.

108. Hjortsø NC, Neumann P, Frøsig F, et al: A controlled study on the effect of epidural analgesia with local anaesthetics and morphine on morbidity after abdominal surgery. Acta Anaesthesiol Scand 1985; 29: 790–796.

109. Bredtmann RD, Herden HN, Teichmann W, et al: Epidural analgesia in colonic surgery: results of a randomized prospective study. Br J Surg 1990; 77: 638–642.

110. Seeling W, Bruckmooser K-P, Hüfner C, et al: Continuous thoracic epidural analgesia does not diminish postoperative complications after abdominal surgery in patients at risk. Anaesthetist 1990; 39: 33–40.

111. Tuman KJ, McCarthy RJ, March RJ, et al: Effects of epidural anesthesia and analgesia on coagulation and outcome after major vascular surgery. Anesth Analg 1991; 73: 696–704.

112. Jayr C, Thomas H, Rey A, et al: Postoperative pulmonary complications: epidural analgesia using bupivacaine and opioids versus parenteral opioids. Anesthesiology 1993; 78: 666–676.

113. Christopherson R, Beattie C, Frank SM, et al: Perioperative morbidity in patients randomized to epidural or general anesthesia for lower extremity vascular surgery. Anesthesiology 1993; 79: 422–434.

114. Sandler AN: Opioid-induced respiratory depression in the postoperative period. Anesthesiol Clin North Am 1989; 7: 193–210.

115. Bailey PL, Rhondeau S, Schafer PG, et al: Dose-response pharmacology of intrathecal morphine in human volunteers. Anesthesiology 1993; 79: 49–59.

116. Coda BA, Brown MC, Schaffer R, et al: Pharmacology of epidural fentanyl, alfentanil, and sufentanil in volunteers. Anesthesiology 1994; 81: 1149–1161.

117. Stenseth R, Sellevold O, Breivik H: Epidural morphine for postoperative pain: experience with 1085 patients. Acta Anaesthesiol Scand 1985; 29: 148–156.

118. Rawal N, Arnér RS, Gustafsson LL, et al: Present state of extradural and intrathecal opioid analgesia in Sweden. A nationwide follow-up survey. Br J Anaesth 1987; 59: 791–799.

119. Crews JC: Epidural opioid analgesia. Crit Care Clin 1990; 6: 315–342.

120. Ready LB, Loper KA, Nessly M, et al: Postoperative epidural morphine is safe on surgical wards. Anesthesiology 1991; 75: 452–456.

121. Riley RH: Respiratory arrest following interpleural block in a narcotized patient. (Letter to the editor.) Can J Anaesth 1990; 37: 487–488.

122. Cory P, Mulroy M: Postoperative respiratory failure following intercostal block. Anesthesiology 1981; 54: 418–419.

123. Hanks GW, Twycross RG, Lloyd JW: Unexpected complication of successful nerve block: morphine induced respiratory depression precipitated by removal of severe pain. Anaesthesia 1981; 36: 37–39.

124. McQuay H: Potential problems of using both opioids and local anaesthetic. (Letter to the editor.) Br J Anaesth 1988; 61: 121.

125. Inagaki Y, Mashimo T, Kuzukawa A, et al: Epidural lidocaine delays arousal from isoflurane anesthesia. Anesth Analg 1994; 79: 368–372.

126. Davies MJ, Scott DA, Cook PT: Continuous monitoring of arterial oxygen saturation with pulse oximetry during spinal anesthesia. Reg Anesth 1987; 12: 63–69.

127. Smith DC, Crul JF: Oxygen desaturation following sedation for regional analgesia. Br J Anaesth 1989; 62: 206–209.

128. Gross JB, Caldwell CB, Shaw LM, et al: The effect of lidocaine on the ventilatory response to carbon dioxide. Anesthesiology 1983; 59: 521–525.

129. Gross JB, Caldwell CB, Shaw LM, et al: The effect of lidocaine infusion on the ventilatory response to hypoxia. Anesthesiology 1984; 61: 662–665.

130. Johnson A, Löfström JB: Influence of local anesthetics on ventilation. Reg Anesth 1991; 16: 7–12.

131. Vrugt B, Aalbers R: Inflammation and bronchial hyperresponsiveness in allergic asthma and chronic obstructive pulmonary disease. Respir Med 1993; 87(Suppl B): 3–7.

132. Ingram RH Jr: Asthma and airway hyperresponsiveness. Annu Rev Med 1991; 42: 139–150.

133. Richardson JB: Nerve supply to the lungs. Am Rev Respir Dis 1979; 119: 785–802.

134. Barnes PJ: The role of neurotransmitters in bronchial asthma. Lung 1990; 168: 57–65.

135. de Jongste JC, Jongejan RC, Kerrebijn KF: Control of airway caliber by autonomic nerves in asthma and in chronic obstructive pulmonary disease. Am Rev Respir Dis 1991; 143: 1421–1426.

136. Black JL: Pharmacology of airway smooth muscle in chronic obstructive pulmonary disease and in asthma. Am Rev Respir Dis 1991; 143: 1177–1181.

137. Aviado DM: Regulation of bronchomotor tone during anesthesia. Anesthesiology 1975; 42: 68–80.

138. Mallampati SR: Bronchospasm during spinal anesthesia. Anesth Analg 1981; 60: 839–840.

139. Eldor J, Frankel DZN, Barav E, et al: Acute bronchospasm during epidural anesthesia in asthmatic patients. J Asthma 1989; 26: 15–16.

140. Barnes P, FitzGerald G, Brown M, et al: Nocturnal asthma and changes in circulating epinephrine, histamine, and cortisol. N Engl J Med 1980; 303: 263–267.

141. Shnider SM, Papper EM: Anesthesia for the asthmatic patient. Anesthesiology 1961; 22: 886–892.

142. McGough EK, Cohen JA: Unexpected bronchospasm during spinal anesthesia. J Clin Anesth 1990; 2: 35–36.

143. Morrow BC, Swan H: Regional techniques in the asthmatic patient. (Letter to the editor.) Anaesthesia 1993; 48: 1018–1019.

144. Zachariah M, Korula G, Nagamani S: Bronchospasm under spinal anaesthesia for transurethral resection of prostate. Anaesth Intensive Care 1992; 20: 363–365.

145. Wang CY, Ong GSY: Severe bronchospasm during epidural anaesthesia. Anaesthesia 1993; 48: 514–515.

146. Zucker-Pinchoff B, Ramanathan S: Anaphylactic reaction to epidural fentanyl. Anesthesiology 1989; 71: 599–601.

147. Stoelting RK: Allergic reactions during anesthesia. Anesth Analg 1983; 62: 341–356.
148. Groeben H, Schwalen A, Irsfeld S, et al: High thoracic epidural anesthesia does not alter airway resistance and attenuates the response to an inhalational provocation test in patients with bronchial hyperreactivity. Anesthesiology 1994; 81: 868–874.
149. Kingston HGG, Hirshman CA: Perioperative management of the patient with asthma. Anesth Analg 1984; 63: 844–855.
150. Slinger PD: Perioperative respiratory assessment and management. Can J Anaesth 1992; 39(5 Pt 2): R115–R131.
151. Goldan SO: Intraspinal cocainization from the anaesthetist's standpoint. N Y Med J 1900; 72: 1089–1091.
152. Cook PR, Malmqvist L-Å, Bengtsson M, et al: Vagal and sympathetic activity during spinal analgesia. Acta Anaesthesiol Scand 1990; 34: 271–275.
153. Carpenter RL, Caplan RA, Brown DL, et al: Incidence and risk factors for side effects of spinal anesthesia. Anesthesiology 1992; 76: 906–916.
154. McCrae AF, Wildsmith JAW: Prevention and treatment of hypotension during central neural block. Br J Anaesth 1993; 70: 672–680.
155. Tarkkila P, Isola J: A regression model for identifying patients at high risk of hypotension, bradycardia and nausea during spinal anesthesia. Acta Anaesthesiol Scand 1992; 36: 554–558.
156. Webb-Peploe MM, Shepherd JT: Veins and their control. N Engl J Med 1968; 278: 317–322.
157. Shimosato S, Etsten BE: The role of the venous system in cardiocirculatory dynamics during spinal and epidural anesthesia in man. Anesthesiology 1969; 30: 619–628.
158. Sancetta SM, Lynn RB, Simeone FA, et al: Studies of hemodynamic changes in humans following induction of low and high spinal anesthesia. I. General considerations of the problem. The changes in cardiac output, brachial arterial pressure, peripheral and pulmonary oxygen contents and peripheral blood flows induced by spinal anesthesia in humans not undergoing surgery. Circulation 1952; 6: 559–571.
159. Greene NM: Preganglionic sympathetic blockade in man: a study of spinal anesthesia. The Torsten Gordh lecture, 1980. Acta Anaesthesiol Scand 1981; 25: 463–469.
160. Pathak CL: The fallacy of the Bainbridge reflex. Am Heart J 1966; 72: 577–581.
161. Pathak CL: Autoregulation of chronotropic response of the heart through pacemaker stretch. Cardiology 1973; 58: 45–64.
162. Baron JF, Decaux-Jacolot A, Edouard A, et al: Influence of venous return on baroreflex control of heart rate during lumbar epidural anesthesia in humans. Anesthesiology 1986; 64: 188–193.
163. Bonica JJ, Kennedy WF Jr, Ward RJ, et al: A comparison of the effects of high subarachnoid and epidural anesthesia. Acta Anaesthesiol Scand Suppl 1966; 23: 429–437.
164. McLean APH, Mulligan GW, Otton P, et al: Hemodynamic alterations associated with epidural anesthesia. Surgery 1967; 62: 79–87.
165. Stanton-Hicks MD: Cardiovascular effects of extradural anesthesia. Br J Anaesth 1975; 47(Suppl): 253–261.
166. Wattwil M, Sundberg A, Arvill A, et al: Circulatory changes during high thoracic epidural anaesthesia—influence of sympathetic block and of systemic effect of the local anaesthetic. Acta Anaesthesiol Scand 1985; 29: 849–855.
167. Reiz S: Circulatory effects of epidural anesthesia in patients with cardiac disease. Acta Anaesthesiol Belg 1988; 39(Suppl 2): 21–27.
168. Mark JB, Steele SM: Cardiovascular effects of spinal anesthesia. Int Anesthesiol Clin 1989; 27: 31–39.
169. Bengtsson M: Changes in skin blood flow and temperature during spinal analgesia evaluated by laser Doppler flowmetry and infrared thermography. Acta Anaesthesiol Scand 1984; 28: 625–630.
170. Malmqvist LÅ, Bengtsson M, Björnsson G, et al: Sympathetic activity and haemodynamic variables during spinal analgesia in man. Acta Anaesthesiol Scand 1987; 31: 467–473.
171. Lundin S, Kirnö K, Wallin BG, et al: Effects of epidural anesthesia on sympathetic nerve discharge to the skin. Acta Anaesthesiol Scand 1990; 34: 492–497.
172. Kimura T, Goda Y, Kemmotsu O, et al: Regional differences in skin blood flow and temperature during total spinal anaesthesia. Can J Anaesth 1992; 39: 123–127.
173. Kennedy WF Jr, Bonica JJ, Akamatsu TJ, et al: Cardiovascular and respiratory effects of subarachnoid block in the presence of acute blood loss. Anesthesiology 1968; 29: 29–35.
174. Bonica JJ, Kennedy WF, Akamatsu TJ, et al: Circulatory effects of peridural block. III. Effects of acute blood loss. Anesthesiology 1972; 36: 219–227.
175. Graves CL, Underwood PS, Klein RL, et al: Intravenous fluid administration as therapy for hypotension secondary to spinal anesthesia. Anesth Analg 1968; 47: 548–556.
176. Edstrom HH, Blitt CD, Draper EM, et al: Hypotension in spinal anesthesia, comparison of tetracaine and bupivacaine. Reg Anesth 1986; 11: 139–142.
177. Venn PJ, Simpson DA, Rubin AP, et al: Effect of fluid preloading on cardiovascular variables after spinal anaesthesia with glucose-free 0.75% bupivacaine. Br J Anaesth 1989; 63: 682–687.
178. Carpenter RL, Caplan RA: Hypotension and spinal anesthesia. (Reply to letter to the editor.) Anesthesiology 1993; 78: 402–403.
179. Butterworth JF IV, Piccione W Jr, Berrizbeitia LD, et al: Augmentation of venous return by adrenergic agonists during spinal anesthesia. Anesth Analg 1986; 65: 612–616.
180. Miyabe M, Namiki A: The effect of head-down tilt on arterial blood pressure after spinal anesthesia. Anesth Analg 1993; 76: 549–552.
181. Tuvemo T, Willdeck-Lund G: Smooth muscle effects of lidocaine, prilocaine, bupivacaine and etidocaine on the human umbilical artery. Acta Anaesthesiol Scand 1982; 26: 104–107.
182. Norén H, Lindblom B, Källfelt B: Effects of bupivacaine and calcium antagonists on the rat uterine artery. Acta Anaesthesiol Scand 1991; 35: 77–80.
183. Blair MR: Cardiovascular pharmacology of local anaesthetics. Br J Anaesth 1975; 47(Suppl): 247–252.
184. Johns RA, DiFazio CA, Longnecker DE: Lidocaine constricts or dilates rat arterioles in a dose-dependent manner. Anesthesiology 1985; 62: 141–144.
185. Johns RA, Seyde WC, DiFazio CA, et al: Dose-dependent effects of bupivacaine on rat muscle arterioles. Anesthesiology 1986; 65: 186–191.
186. Johns RA: Local anesthetics inhibit endothelium-dependent vasodilation. Anesthesiology 1989; 70: 805–811.
187. Benowitz NL: Clinical pharmacology and toxicology of cocaine. Pharmacol Toxicol 1993; 72: 3–12.
188. Welder AA, Grammas P, Melchert RB: Cellular mechanisms of cocaine cardiotoxicity. Toxicol Lett 1993; 69: 227–238.
189. Lange RA, Cigarroa RG, Yancy CW Jr, et al: Cocaine-induced coronary-artery vasoconstriction. N Engl J Med 1989; 321: 1557–1562.
190. Hollander JE, Hoffman RS: Cocaine-induced myocardial infarction: an analysis and review of the literature. J Emerg Med 1992; 10: 169–177.
191. Chiu Y, Brecht K, Das Gupta D, et al: Myocardial infarction with topical cocaine anesthesia for nasal surgery. Arch Otolaryngol Head Neck Surg 1986; 112: 988–990.
192. Kennedy WF Jr, Bonica JJ, Ward RJ, et al: Cardiorespiratory effects of epinephrine when used in regional anesthesia. Acta Anaesthesiol Scand Suppl 1966; 23: 320–333.
193. Bonica JJ, Akamatsu TJ, Berges PU, et al: Circulatory effects of peridural block. II. Effects of epinephrine. Anesthesiology 1971; 34: 514–522.
194. Salevsky FC, Whalley DG, Kalant D, et al: Epidural epinephrine and the systemic circulation during peripheral vascular surgery. Can J Anaesth 1990; 37: 160–165.
195. Modig J: Influence of regional anesthesia, local anesthetics, and sympathicomimetics on the pathophysiology of deep vein thrombosis. Acta Chir Scand Suppl 1989; 550: 119–127.
196. Sharrock NE, Go G, Mineo R, et al: The hemodynamic and fibrinolytic response to low dose epinephrine and phenylephrine infusions during total hip replacement under epidural anesthesia. Thromb Haemost 1992; 68: 436–441.
197. Moore DC, Scurlock JE: Possible role of epinephrine in prevention or correction of myocardial depression associated with bupivacaine. Anesth Analg 1983; 62: 450–453.
198. Nadkarni AV, Tondare AS: Epinephrine and systemic local anes-

thetic toxicity. (Letter to the editor.) Anesth Analg 1984; 63: 702.

199. Toyoda Y, Kubota Y, Kubota H, et al: Prevention of hypokalemia during axillary nerve block with 1% lidocaine and epinephrine 1:100,000. Anesthesiology 1988; 69: 109–112.

200. Löfgren A, Hahn RG: Serum potassium levels after induction of epidural anaesthesia using mepivacaine with and without adrenaline. Acta Anaesthesiol Scand 1991; 35: 170–174.

201. Löfgren A, Hahn RG: Hypokalemia from intercostal nerve block. Reg Anesth 1994; 19: 247–254.

202. Hansen O, Johansson BW, Gullberg B: Metabolic, hemodynamic, and electrocardiographic responses to increased circulating adrenaline: effects of pretreatment with class 1 antiarrhythmics. Angiology 1991; 42: 990–1001.

203. Vitez TS, Soper LE, Wong KC, et al: Chronic hypokalemia and intraoperative dysrhythmias. Anesthesiology 1985; 63: 130–133.

204. McGovern B: Hypokalemia and cardiac arrhythmias. (Editorial.) Anesthesiology 1985; 63: 127–129.

205. Butterworth JF IV, Strichartz GR: Molecular mechanisms of local anesthesia: a review. Anesthesiology 1990; 72: 711–734.

206. Hondeghem LM: Antiarrhythmic agents: modulated receptor applications. Circulation 1987; 75: 514–520.

207. Clarkson CW, Hondeghem LM: Mechanism for bupivacaine depression of cardiac conduction: fast block of sodium channels during the action potential with slow recovery from block during diastole. Anesthesiology 1985; 62: 396–405.

208. Moller R, Covine BG: Cardiac electrophysiologic properties of bupivacaine and lidocaine compared with those of ropivacaine, a new amide local anesthetic. Anesthesiology 1990; 72: 322–329.

209. Kendig JJ: Clinical implications of the modulated receptor hypothesis: local anesthetics and the heart. (Editorial.) Anesthesiology 1985; 62: 382–384.

210. Reiz S, Nath S: Cardiotoxicity of local anaesthetic agents. Br J Anaesth 1986; 58: 736–746.

211. Buffington CW: The magnitude and duration of direct myocardial depression following intracoronary local anesthetics: a comparison of lidocaine and bupivacaine. Anesthesiology 1989; 70: 280–287.

212. Thomas RD, Behbehani MM, Coyle DE, et al: Cardiovascular toxicity of local anesthetics: an alternative hypothesis. Anesth Analg 1986; 65: 444–450.

213. Heavner JE: Cardiac dysrhythmias induced by infusion of local anesthetics into the lateral cerebral ventricle of cats. Anesth Analg 1986; 65: 133–138.

214. Bernards CM, Artru AA: Effect of intracerebroventricular picrotoxin and muscimol on intravenous bupivacaine toxicity. Evidence supporting central nervous system involvement in bupivacaine cardiovascular toxicity. Anesthesiology 1993; 78: 902–910.

215. Schwartz PJ: Sympathetic imbalance and cardiac arrhythmias. In Randall WC (ed): Nervous Control of Cardiovascular Function, pp 225–252. New York, Oxford University Press, 1984.

216. Galloway PA, Glass PS: Anesthetic implications of prolonged QT interval syndromes. Anesth Analg 1985; 64: 612–620.

217. Strickland RA, Stanton MS, Olsen KD: Prolonged QT syndrome: perioperative management. Mayo Clin Proc 1993; 68: 1016–1020.

218. Yanowitz F, Preston JB, Abildskov JA: Functional distribution of right and left stellate innervation to the ventricles: production of neurogenic electrocardiographic changes by unilateral alteration of sympathetic tone. Circ Res 1966; 18: 416–428.

219. Randall WC, Kaye MP, Hageman GR, et al: Cardiac dysrhythmias in the conscious dog after surgically induced autonomic imbalance. Am J Cardiol 1976; 38: 178–183.

220. Austoni P, Rosati R, Gregorini L, et al: Stellectomy and exercise in man. (Abstract.) Am J Cardiol 1979; 43: 399.

221. Moss AJ: Prolonged QT-interval syndromes. JAMA 1986; 256: 2985–2987.

222. Pfeiffer D, Fiehring H, Henkel HG, et al: Long QT syndrome associated with inflammatory degeneration of the stellate ganglia. Clin Cardiol 1989; 12: 222–224.

223. Stramba-Badiale M, Lazzarotti M, Schwartz PJ: Development of cardiac innervation, ventricular fibrillation, and sudden infant death syndrome. Am J Physiol 1992; 263: H1514–H1522.

224. Talman WT, Kelkar P: Neural control of the heart: central and peripheral. Neurol Clin 1993; 11: 239–256.

225. Kamarck T, Jennings JR: Biobehavioral factors in sudden cardiac death. Psychol Bull 1991; 109: 42–75.

226. Uchida Y, Ueda H: Non-uniform myocardial blood flow caused by stellate ganglion stimulation. Jpn Heart J 1975; 16: 162–173.

227. Schwartz PJ, Stone HL: Tonic influence of the sympathetic nervous system on myocardial reactive hyperemia and on coronary blood flow distribution in dogs. Circ Res 1977; 41: 51–58.

228. Tanaka H, Minagoe S-I, Kashima T, et al: Sympathetically induced atrial tachycardia. Successful treatment by left stellate ganglion block. J Electrocardiol 1978; 11: 403–406.

229. Grossman MA: Cardiac arrhythmias in acute central nervous system disease. Successful management with stellate ganglion block. Arch Intern Med 1976; 136: 203–207.

230. Schwartz PJ, Locati EH, Moss AJ, et al: Left cardiac sympathetic denervation in the therapy of congenital long QT syndrome. A worldwide report. Circulation 1991; 84: 503–511.

231. Otteni JC, Pottecher T, Bronner G, et al: Prolongation of the Q-T interval and sudden cardiac arrest following right radical neck dissection. Anesthesiology 1983; 59: 358–361.

232. Kashima T, Tanaka H, Minagoe S, et al: Electrocardiographic changes induced by the stellate ganglion block in normal subjects. J Electrocardiol 1981; 14: 169–174.

233. Gardner MJ, Kimber S, Johnstone DE, et al: The effects of unilateral stellate ganglion blockade on human cardiac function during rest and exercise. J Cardiovasc Electrophysiol 1993; 4: 2–8.

234. Crampton RS: Stellate ganglion block and stimulation in long QT syndrome, sympathetic dystrophy of the arm, and normals. In Schwartz PJ, Brown AM, Malliani A, et al (eds): Neural Mechanisms in Cardiac Arrhythmias, pp 55–74. New York, Raven Press, 1978.

235. Rogers MC, McPeek J, Battit G, et al: Lateralization of sympathetic control of the human sinus node. (Abstract.) Circulation 1975; 51–52(Suppl II): II-112.

236. Eckberg DL: Human sinus arrhythmia as an index of vagal cardiac outflow. J Appl Physiol 1983; 54: 961–966.

237. van Ravenswaaij-Arts CMA, Kollée LAA, Hopman JCW, et al: Heart rate variability. Ann Intern Med 1993; 118: 436–447.

238. Malik M, Camm AJ: Heart rate variability. Clin Cardiol 1990; 13: 570–576.

239. Kleiger RE, Stein PK, Bosner MS, et al: Time domain measurements of heart rate variability. Cardiol Clin 1992; 10: 487–498.

240. Ori Z, Monir G, Weiss J, et al: Heart rate variability: frequency domain analysis. Cardiol Clin 1992; 10: 499–537.

241. Kamath MV, Fallen EL: Power spectral analysis of heart rate variability: a noninvasive signature of cardiac autonomic function. Crit Rev Biomed Eng 1993; 21: 245–311.

242. Schwartz JB, Gibb WJ, Tran T: Aging effects on heart rate variation. J Gerontol 1991; 46: M99–M106.

243. Esler M: The autonomic nervous system and cardiac arrhythmias. Clin Auton Res 1992; 2: 133–135.

244. Lloyd R, Okada R, Stagg J, et al: The treatment of recurrent ventricular tachycardia with bilateral cervico-thoracic sympathetic-ganglionectomy. A report of two cases. Circulation 1974; 50: 382–388.

245. Vanoli E, Schwartz PJ: Sympathetic-parasympathetic interaction and sudden death. Basic Res Cardiol 1990; 85(Suppl 1): 305–321.

246. Ewing DJ: Heart rate variability: an important new risk factor in patients following myocardial infarction. Clin Cardiol 1991; 14: 683–685.

247. Casolo GC, Stroder P, Signorini C, et al: Heart rate variability during the acute phase of myocardial infarction. Circulation 1992; 85: 2073–2079.

248. Anema JR, Heijenbrok MW, Faes TJ, et al: Cardiovascular autonomic function in multiple sclerosis. J Neurol Sci 1991; 104: 129–134.

249. Malpas SC, Whiteside EA, Maling TJ: Heart rate variability and cardiac autonomic function in men with chronic alcohol dependence. Br Heart J 1991; 65: 84–88.

250. Leipzig TJ, Lowensohn RI: Heart rate variability in neurosurgical patients. Neurosurgery 1986; 19: 356–362.

251. Kuroiwa Y, Shimada Y, Toyokura Y: Postural hypotension and

low R-R interval variability in parkinsonism, spino-cerebellar degeneration, and Shy-Drager syndrome. Neurology 1983; 33: 463–467.

252. Pincus SM, Viscarello RR: Approximate entropy: a regularity measure for fetal heart rate analysis. Obstet Gynecol 1992; 79: 249–255.

253. Podrid PJ: Role of higher nervous activity in ventricular arrhythmia and sudden cardiac death: implications for alternative antiarrhythmic therapy. Ann N Y Acad Sci 1984; 432: 296–313.

254. Coumel P, Leenhardt A: Mental activity, adrenergic modulation, and cardiac arrhythmias in patients with heart disease. Circulation 1991; 83(Suppl II): II-58–II-70.

255. Frerichs RL, Campbell J, Bassell GM: Psychogenic cardiac arrest during extensive sympathetic blockade. Anesthesiology 1988; 68: 943–944.

256. Latson TW, Ashmore TH, Reinhart DJ, et al: Autonomic reflex dysfunction in patients presenting for elective surgery is associated with hypotension after anesthesia induction. Anesthesiology 1994; 80: 326–337.

257. Burgos LG, Ebert TJ, Asiddao C, et al: Increased intraoperative cardiovascular morbidity in diabetics with autonomic neuropathy. Anesthesiology 1989; 70: 591–597.

258. Fleisher LA, Pincus SM, Rosenbaum SH: Approximate entropy of heart rate as a correlate of postoperative ventricular dysfunction. Anesthesiology 1993; 78: 683–692.

259. Steinberg JS, Zelenkofske S, Wong S-C, et al: Value of the P-wave signal-averaged ECG for predicting atrial fibrillation after cardiac surgery. Circulation 1993; 88: 2618–2622.

260. Halliwill JR, Billman GE: Effect of general anesthesia on cardiac vagal tone. Am J Physiol 1992; 262: H1719–H1724.

261. Latson TW, McCarroll SM, Mirhej MA, et al: Effects of three anesthetic induction techniques on heart rate variability. J Clin Anesth 1992; 4: 265–276.

262. Kato M, Komatsu T, Kimura T, et al: Spectral analysis of heart rate variability during isoflurane anesthesia. Anesthesiology 1992; 77: 669–674.

263. Kimura T, Komatsu T, Hirabayashi A, et al: Autonomic imbalance of the heart during total spinal anesthesia evaluated by spectral analysis of heart rate variability. Anesthesiology 1994; 80: 694–698.

264. Eisenach JC, Tuttle R, Stein A: Is ST segment depression of the electrocardiogram during cesarean section merely due to cardiac sympathetic block? Anesth Analg 1994; 78: 287–292.

265. Fleisher LA, Frank SM, Shir Y, et al: Cardiac sympathovagal balance and peripheral sympathetic vasoconstriction: epidural versus general anesthesia. Anesth Analg 1994; 79: 165–171.

266. McCann RL, Clements FM: Silent myocardial ischemia in patients undergoing peripheral vascular surgery: incidence and association with perioperative cardiac morbidity and mortality. J Vasc Surg 1989; 9: 583–587.

267. Mangano DT, Hollenberg M, Fegert G, et al: Perioperative myocardial ischemia in patients undergoing noncardiac surgery. I. Incidence and severity during the 4 day perioperative period. J Am Coll Cardiol 1991; 17: 843–850.

268. Mangano DT, Wong MG, London MJ, et al: Perioperative myocardial ischemia in patients undergoing noncardiac surgery. II. Incidence and severity during the 1st week after surgery. J Am Coll Cardiol 1991; 17: 851–857.

269. Urmey WF, Lambert DH: Spinal anesthesia associated with reversal of myocardial ischemia. Anesth Analg 1986; 65: 908–910.

270. Blomberg S, Curelaru I, Emanuelsson H, et al: Thoracic epidural anaesthesia in patients with unstable angina pectoris. Eur Heart J 1989; 10: 437–444.

271. Vik-Mo H, Ottesen S, Renck H: Cardiac effects of thoracic epidural analgesia before and during acute coronary artery occlusion in open-chest dogs. Scand J Clin Lab Invest 1978; 38: 737–746.

272. Davis RF, DeBoer LW, Maroko PR: Thoracic epidural anesthesia reduces myocardial infarct size after coronary artery occlusion in dogs. Anesth Analg 1986; 65: 711–717.

273. Blomberg S, Emanuelsson H, Ricksten S-E: Thoracic epidural anesthesia and central hemodynamics in patients with unstable angina pectoris. Anesth Analg 1989; 69: 558–562.

274. Pasqualucci V, Moricca G, Solinas P: Intrathecal morphine for

the control of the pain of myocardial infarction. (Letter to the editor.) Anaesthesia 1981; 36: 68–69.

275. Skoeld M, Gillberg L, Ohlsson O: Pain relief in myocardial infarction after continuous epidural morphine analgesia. (Letter to the editor.) N Engl J Med 1985; 312: 650.

276. Toft P, Jorgensen A: Continuous thoracic epidural analgesia for the control of pain in myocardial infarction. Intensive Care Med 1987; 13: 388–389.

277. Yeager M: The role of regional anesthesia in improving surgical outcome, 1991 Review Course Lectures. International Anesthesia Research Society 65th Congress, San Antonio, Texas, 1991, pp 122–129.

278. Beattie WS, Buckley DN, Forrest JB: Epidural morphine reduces the risk of postoperative myocardial ischaemia in patients with cardiac risk factors. Can J Anaesth 1993; 40: 532–541.

279. VanHoutte PM: Platelets, endothelium-derived vasoactive factors, and coronary disease. (Editorial.) Cardiologia 1992; 37: 89–93.

280. Breslow MJ: The role of stress hormones in perioperative myocardial ischemia. Int Anesthesiol Clin 1992; 30: 81–100.

281. Slogoff S, Keats AS: Does perioperative myocardial ischemia lead to postoperative myocardial infarction? Anesthesiology 1985; 62: 107–114.

282. Slogoff S, Keats AS: Further observations on perioperative myocardial ischemia. Anesthesiology 1986; 65: 539–542.

283. Knight AA, Hollenberg M, London MJ, et al: Perioperative myocardial ischemia: importance of the preoperative ischemic pattern. Anesthesiology 1988; 68: 681–688.

284. Randall WC, Armour JA, Geis WP, et al: Regional cardiac distribution of the sympathetic nerves. Fed Proc 1972; 31: 1199–1208.

285. Sylvén C: Angina pectoris. Clinical characteristics, neurophysiological and molecular mechanisms. Pain 1989; 36: 145–167.

286. Meller ST, Gebhart GF: A critical review of the afferent pathways and the potential chemical mediators involved in cardiac pain. Neuroscience 1992; 48: 501–524.

287. Heusch G: Alpha-adrenergic mechanisms in myocardial ischemia. Circulation 1990; 81: 1–13.

288. Jonnesco T: Traitement chirurgical de l'angine de poitrine par la résection du sympathique cervico-thoracique. Presse Med 1921; 19: 193–194.

289. Leriche R, Fontaine R: The surgical treatment of angina pectoris: what it is and what it should be. Am Heart J 1928; 3: 649–671.

290. Heusch G, Deussen A, Thamer V: Cardiac sympathetic nerve activity and progressive vasoconstriction distal to coronary stenoses: feed-back aggravation of myocardial ischemia. J Auton Nerv Syst 1985; 13: 311–326.

291. Klassen GA, Bramwell RS, Bromage PR, et al: Effect of acute sympathectomy by epidural anesthesia on the canine coronary circulation. Anesthesiology 1980; 52: 8–15.

292. Tsuchida H, Omote T, Miyamoto M, et al: Effects of thoracic epidural anesthesia on myocardial pH and metabolism during ischemia. Acta Anaesthesiol Scand 1991; 35: 508–512.

293. Kock M, Blomberg S, Emanuelsson H, et al: Thoracic epidural anesthesia improves global and regional left ventricular function during stress-induced myocardial ischemia in patients with coronary artery disease. Anesth Analg 1990; 71: 625–630.

294. Blomberg S, Emanuelsson H, Kvist H, et al: Effects of thoracic epidural anesthesia on coronary arteries and arterioles in patients with coronary artery disease. Anesthesiology 1990; 73: 840–847.

295. Blomberg SG: Long-term home self-treatment with high thoracic epidural anesthesia in patients with severe coronary artery disease. Anesth Analg 1994; 79: 413–421.

296. Estrin JA, Emery RW, Leonard JJ, et al: The Bezold reflex: a special case of the left ventricular mechanoreceptor reflex. Proc Natl Acad Sci U S A 1979; 76: 4146–4150.

297. Abboud FM: Ventricular syncope: is the heart a sensory organ? (Editorial.) N Engl J Med 1989; 320: 390–392.

298. Milstein S, Buetikofer J, Lesser J, et al: Cardiac asystole: a manifestation of neurally mediated hypotension-bradycardia. J Am Coll Cardiol 1989; 14: 1626–1632.

299. Sharpey-Schafer EP, Hayter CJ, Barlow ED: Mechanism of acute hypotension from fear or nausea. Br Med J 1958; 2: 878–880.

300. Henry JP: On the triggering mechanism of vasovagal syncope. (Editorial.) Psychosom Med 1984; 46: 91–93.

301. Johnson AM: Aortic stenosis, sudden death, and the left ventricular barocceptors. Br Heart J 1971; 33: 1–5.

302. Nemerovski M, Shah PK: Syndrome of severe bradycardia and hypotension following sublingual nitroglycerin administration. Cardiology 1981; 67: 180–189.

303. Robertson D, Hollister AS, Forman MB, et al: Reflexes unique to myocardial ischemia and infarction. J Am Coll Cardiol 1985; 5(Suppl 6): 99B–104B.

304. Eckberg DL, White CW, Kioschos JM, et al: Mechanisms mediating bradycardia during coronary arteriography. J Clin Invest 1974; 54: 1455–1461.

305. Koren G, Weiss AT, Ben-David Y, et al: Bradycardia and hypotension following reperfusion with streptokinase (Bezold-Jarisch reflex): a sign of coronary thrombolysis and myocardial salvage. Am Heart J 1986; 112: 468–471.

306. Simpson RJ Jr, Podolak R, Mangano CA Jr, et al: Vagal syncope during recurrent pulmonary embolism. JAMA 1983; 249: 390–393.

307. Berk JL, Levy MN: Profound reflex bradycardia produced by transient hypoxia or hypercapnia in man. Eur Surg Res 1977; 9: 75–84.

308. Rørsgaard S, Secher NH: Slowing of the heart during hypotension in major abdominal surgery. Acta Anaesthesiol Scand 1986; 30: 507–510.

309. Sanders JS, Ferguson DW: Profound sympathoinhibition complicating hypovolemia in humans. Ann Intern Med 1989; 111: 439–441.

310. Caplan RA, Ward RJ, Posner K, et al: Unexpected cardiac arrest during spinal anesthesia: a closed claims analysis of predisposing factors. Anesthesiology 1988; 68: 5–11.

311. Mackey DC, Carpenter RL, Thompson GE, et al: Bradycardia and asystole during spinal anesthesia: a report of three cases without morbidity. Anesthesiology 1989; 70: 866–868.

312. Evans CH: Possible complications with spinal anesthesia: their recognition and the measures employed to prevent and to combat them. Am J Surg 1928; 5: 581–593.

313. Sise LF: Spinal anesthesia fatalities and their prevention. N Engl J Med 1929; 200: 1071–1074.

314. Babcock ME: Spinal anesthesia deaths: a survey. Anesth Analg 1932; 11: 184–188.

315. Kral VA: Neuropsychiatric sequelae of cardiac arrest during spinal anaesthesia: one year follow-up of a case. Can Med Assoc J 1951; 64: 138–142.

316. Naesh O, Friis JT, Hindberg I, et al: Platelet function in surgical stress. Thromb Haemost 1985; 54: 849–852.

317. Nielsen TH, Nielsen HK, Husted SE, et al: Stress response and platelet function in minor surgery during epidural bupivacaine and general anaesthesia: effect of epidural morphine addition. Eur J Anaesthesiol 1989; 6: 409–417.

318. Steele SM, Slaughter TF, Greenberg CS, et al: Epidural anesthesia and analgesia: implications for perioperative coagulability. (Editorial.) Anesth Analg 1991; 73: 683–685.

319. Qizilbash N, Jones L, Warlow C, et al: Fibrinogen and lipid concentrations as risk factors for transient ischaemic attacks and minor ischaemic strokes. Br Med J 1991; 303: 605–609.

320. Trip MD, Cats VM, van Capelle FJL, et al: Platelet hyperreactivity and prognosis in survivors of myocardial infarction. N Engl J Med 1990; 322: 1549–1554.

321. Meade TW, Ruddock V, Stirling Y, et al: Fibrinolytic activity, clotting factors, and long-term incidence of ischaemic heart disease in the Northwick Park Heart Study. Lancet 1993; 342: 1076–1079.

322. Hendolin H, Mattila MAK, Poikolainen E: The effect of lumbar epidural analgesia on the development of deep vein thrombosis of the legs after open prostatectomy. Acta Chir Scand 1981; 147: 425–429.

323. Rosenfeld BA, Beattie C, Christopherson R, et al: The effects of different anesthetic regimens on fibrinolysis and the development of postoperative arterial thrombosis. Anesthesiology 1993; 79: 435–443.

324. Prins MH, Hirsh J: A comparison of general anesthesia and regional anesthesia as a risk factor for deep vein thrombosis following hip surgery: a critical review. Thromb Haemost 1990; 64: 497–500.

325. Sorenson RM, Pace NL: Anesthetic techniques during surgical repair of femoral neck fractures. A meta-analysis. Anesthesiology 1992; 77: 1095–1104.

326. Cousins MJ, Wright CJ: Graft, muscle, skin blood flow after epidural block in vascular surgical procedures. Surg Gynecol Obstet 1971; 133: 59–64.

327. Modig J, Malmberg P, Karlström G: Effect of epidural versus general anaesthesia on calf blood flow. Acta Anaesthesiol Scand 1980; 24: 305–309.

328. Foate JA, Horton H, Davis FM: Lower limb blood flow during transurethral resection of the prostate under spinal or general anaesthesia. Anaesth Intensive Care 1985; 13: 383–386.

329. Perhoniemi V, Linko K: Effect of spinal versus epidural anaesthesia with 0.5% bupivacaine on lower limb blood flow. Acta Anaesthesiol Scand 1987; 31: 117–121.

330. Donadoni R, Baele G, Devulder J, et al: Coagulation and fibrinolytic parameters in patients undergoing total hip replacement: influence of the anaesthesia technique. Acta Anaesthesiol Scand 1989; 33: 588–592.

331. Borg T, Modig J: Potential anti-thrombotic effects of local anaesthetics due to their inhibition of platelet aggregation. Acta Anaesthesiol Scand 1985; 29: 739–742.

332. Henny CP, Odoom JA, ten Cate H, et al: Effects of extradural bupivacaine on the haemostatic system. Br J Anaesth 1986; 58: 301–305.

333. Odoom JA, Dokter PWC, Sturk A, et al: The influence of epidural analgesia on platelet function and correlation with plasma bupivacaine concentrations. Eur J Anaesthesiol 1988; 5: 305–312.

334. Schulze S: Humoral and neural mediators of the systemic response to surgery. Dan Med Bull 1993; 40: 365–377.

335. Shirasaka C, Tsuji H, Asoh T, et al: Role of the splanchnic nerves in endocrine and metabolic response to abdominal surgery. Br J Surg 1986; 73: 142–145.

336. Møller IW, Hjortsø E, Krantz T, et al: The modifying effect of spinal anaesthesia on intra- and postoperative adrenocortical and hyperglycaemic response to surgery. Acta Anaesthesiol Scand 1984; 28: 266–269.

337. Kehlet H: Surgical stress: the role of pain and analgesia. Br J Anaesth 1989; 63: 189–195.

338. Schulze S, Sommer P, Bigler D, et al: Effect of combined prednisolone, epidural analgesia, and indomethacin on the systemic response after colonic surgery. Arch Surg 1992; 127: 325–331.

339. Hosada R, Hattori M, Shimada Y: Favorable effects of epidural analgesia on hemodynamics, oxygenation and metabolic variables in the immediate post-anesthetic period. Acta Anaesthesiol Scand 1993; 37: 469–474.

340. O'Garra A: Interleukins and the immune system 2. Lancet 1989; 1: 1003–1005.

341. O'Garra A: Interleukins and the immune system 1. Lancet 1989; 1: 943–947.

342. Fong Y, Moldawer LL, Shires GT, et al: The biologic characteristics of cytokines and their implication in surgical injury. Surg Gynecol Obstet 1990; 170: 363–378.

343. Naito Y, Tamai S, Shingu K, et al: Responses of plasma adrenocorticotropic hormone, cortisol, and cytokines during and after upper abdominal surgery. Anesthesiology 1992; 77: 426–431.

344. Salo M: Effects of anaesthesia and surgery on the immune response. Acta Anaesthesiol Scand 1992; 36: 201–220.

345. Faist E, Ertel W, Cohnert T, et al: Immunoprotective effects of cyclooxygenase inhibition in patients with major surgical trauma. J Trauma 1990; 30: 8–17.

346. Hole A: Depression of monocytes and lymphocytes by stress-related humoral factors and anaesthetic-related drugs. Acta Anaesthesiol Scand 1984; 28: 280–286.

347. Weigent DA, Carr DJ, Blalock JE: Bidirectional communication between the neuroendocrine and immune systems. Common hormones and hormone receptors. Ann N Y Acad Sci 1990; 579: 17–27.

348. Blalock JE: Production of peptide hormones and neurotransmitters by the immune system. Chem Immunol 1992; 52: 1–24.

349. Przewlocki R, Hassan AH, Lason W, et al: Gene expression and localization of opioid peptides in immune cells of inflamed tissue: functional role in antinociception. Neuroscience 1992; 48: 491–500.

350. Levine JD, Coderre TJ, Basbaum AI: The peripheral nervous system and the inflammatory process. Pain Res Clin Manage 1988; 13: 33–43.
351. Kimball ES: Substance P, cytokines, and arthritis. Ann N Y Acad Sci 1990; 594: 293–308.
352. Kidd BL, Mapp PI, Blake DR, et al: Neurogenic influences in arthritis. Ann Rheum Dis 1990; 49: 649–652.
353. Pollock RE, Lotzová E, Stanford SD: Mechanism of surgical stress impairment of human perioperative natural killer cell cytotoxicity. Arch Surg 1991; 126: 338–342.
354. Pollock RE, Lotzová E, Stanford SD: Surgical stress impairs natural killer cell programming of tumor for lysis in patients with sarcomas and other solid tumors. Cancer 1992; 70: 2192–2202.
355. Lotzová E: Definition and functions of natural killer cells. Nat Immun 1993; 12: 169–176.
356. Garcia-Peñarrubia P, Koster FT, Kelley RO, et al: Antibacterial activity of human natural killer cells. J Exp Med 1989; 169: 99–113.
357. Whiteside TL, Herberman RB: The role of natural killer cells in human disease. Clin Immunol Immunopathol 1989; 53: 1–23.
358. Shavit Y, Depaulis A, Martin FC, et al: Involvement of brain opiate receptors in the immune-suppressive effect of morphine. Proc Natl Acad Sci U S A 1986; 83: 7114–7117.
359. Beilin B, Martin FC, Shavit Y, et al: Suppression of natural killer cell activity by high-dose narcotic anesthesia in rats. Brain Behav Immun 1989; 3: 129–137.
360. Liebeskind JC: Pain *can* kill. (Editorial.) Pain 1991; 44: 3–4.
361. Yeager MP, Colacchio TA: Effect of morphine on growth of metastatic colon cancer in vivo. Arch Surg 1991; 126: 454–456.
362. Page GG, Ben-Eliyahu S, Yirmiya R, et al: Morphine attenuates surgery-induced enhancement of metastatic colonization in rats. Pain 1993; 54: 21–28.
363. Mogil JS, Sternberg WF, Liebeskind JC: Studies of pain, stress, and immunity. In Chapman CR, Foley KM (eds): Current and Emerging Issues in Cancer Pain: Research and Practice, pp 31–47. New York, Raven Press, 1993.
364. Moore TC, Spruck CH, Leduc LE: Depression of lymphocyte traffic in sheep by anaesthesia and associated changes in efferent-lymph PGE₂ and antibody levels. Immunology 1988; 63: 139–143.
365. Stevenson GW, Hall SC, Rudnick S, et al: The effect of anesthetic agents on the human immune response. Anesthesiology 1990; 72: 542–552.
366. Markovic SN, Murasko DM: Inhibition of induction of natural killer activity in mice by general anesthesia (Avertin): role of interferon. Clin Immunol Immunopathol 1991; 60: 181–189.
367. Lockwood LL, Silbert LH, Laudenslager ML, et al: Anesthesia-induced modulation of in vivo antibody levels: a study of pentobarbital, chloral hydrate, methoxyflurane, halothane, and ketamine/xylazine. Anesth Analg 1993; 77: 769–774.
368. Markovic SN, Knight PR, Murasko DM: Inhibition of interferon stimulation of natural killer cell activity in mice anesthetized with halothane or isoflurane. Anesthesiology 1993; 78: 700–706.
369. Clark WR: Prevention of anesthesia-induced immunosuppression: a novel strategy involving interferons. (Editorial.) Anesthesiology 1993; 78: 627–628.
370. Lundy J, Lovett EJ III, Hamilton S, et al: Halothane, surgery, immunosuppression and artificial pulmonary metastases. Cancer 1978; 41: 827–830.
371. Radosevic-Stasic B, Cuk M, Mrakovcic-Sutic I, et al: Immunosuppressive properties of halothane anesthesia and/or surgical stress in experimental conditions. Int J Neurosci 1990; 51: 235–236.
372. Rem J, Brandt MR, Kehlet H: Prevention of postoperative lymphopenia and granulocytosis by epidural analgesia. Lancet 1980; 1: 283–284.
373. Hole A, Unsgaard G, Breivik H: Monocyte functions are depressed during and after surgery under general anaesthesia but not under epidural anaesthesia. Acta Anaesthesiol Scand 1982; 26: 301–307.
374. Whelan P, Morris PJ: Immunological responsiveness after transurethral resection of the prostate: general versus spinal anaesthetic. Clin Exp Immunol 1982; 48: 611–618.
375. Hole A, Unsgaard G: The effect of epidural and general anaesthesia on lymphocyte functions during and after major orthopaedic surgery. Acta Anaesthesiol Scand 1983; 27: 135–141.
376. Hole A: Pre- and postoperative monocyte and lymphocyte functions: effects of sera from patients operated under general or epidural anaesthesia. Acta Anaesthesiol Scand 1984; 28: 287–291.
377. Hole A: Pre- and postoperative monocyte and lymphocyte functions: effects of combined epidural and general anaesthesia. Acta Anaesthesiol Scand 1984; 28: 367–371.
378. Ryhänen P, Jouppila R, Lanning M, et al: Natural killer cell activity after elective cesarean section under general and epidural anesthesia in healthy parturients and their newborns. Gynecol Obstet Invest 1985; 19: 139–142.
379. Tønnesen E, Wahlgreen C: Influence of extradural and general anaesthesia on natural killer cell activity and lymphocyte subpopulations in patients undergoing hysterectomy. Br J Anaesth 1988; 60: 500–507.
380. Triulzi DJ, Heal JM, Blumberg N: Transfusion-induced immunomodulation and its clinical consequences. In Nance ST (ed): Transfusion Medicine in the 1990's, pp 1–33. Basel, S Karger, 1990.
381. van Twuyver E, Mooijaart RJ, ten Berge IJ, et al: Pretransplantation blood transfusion revisited. N Engl J Med 1991; 325: 1210–1213.
382. Schriemer PA, Longnecker DE, Mintz PD: The possible immunosuppressive effects of perioperative blood transfusion in cancer patients. Anesthesiology 1988; 68: 422–428.
383. Mezrow CK, Bergstein I, Tartter PI: Postoperative infections following autologous and homologous blood transfusions. Transfusion 1992; 32: 27–30.
384. Keith I: Anaesthesia and blood loss in total hip replacement. Anaesthesia 1977; 32: 444–450.
385. Valentin N, Lomholt B, Jensen JS, et al: Spinal or general anaesthesia for surgery of the fractured hip? A prospective study of mortality in 578 patients. Br J Anaesth 1986; 58: 284–291.
386. MacKenzie AR: Influence of anaesthesia on blood loss in transurethral prostatectomy. Scott Med J 1990; 35: 14–16.
387. Bonica JJ: Autonomic innervation of the viscera in relation to nerve block. Anesthesiology 1968; 29: 793–813.
388. Andrews PLR: Vagal afferent innervation of the gastrointestinal tract. Prog Brain Res 1986; 67: 65–86.
389. Iggo A: Afferent C-fibres and visceral sensation. Prog Brain Res 1986; 67: 29–36.
390. Procacci P, Zoppi M, Maresca M: Clinical approach to visceral pain. Prog Brain Res 1986; 67: 21–28.
391. Paintal AS: The visceral sensations—some basic mechanisms. Prog Brain Res 1986; 67: 3–19.
392. Jänig W, Morrison JFB: Functional properties of spinal visceral afferents supplying abdominal and pelvic organs, with special emphasis on visceral nociception. Prog Brain Res 1986; 67: 78–114.
393. Cervero F: Neurophysiology of gastrointestinal pain. Baillieres Clin Gastroenterol 1988; 2: 183–199.
394. Scratcherd T, Grundy D: The physiology of intestinal motility and secretion. Br J Anaesth 1984; 56: 3–18.
395. Treissman DA: Disruption of colonic anastomosis associated with epidural anesthesia. Reg Anesth 1980; 5: 22–23.
396. Bigler D, Hjortsø N-C, Kehlet H: Disruption of colonic anastomosis during continuous epidural analgesia: an early postoperative complication. Anaesthesia 1985; 40: 278–280.
397. Schnitzler M, Kilbride MJ, Senagore A: Effect of epidural analgesia on colorectal anastomotic healing and colonic motility. Reg Anesth 1992; 17: 143–147.
398. Aitkenhead AR, Wishart HY, Peebles Brown DA: High spinal nerve block for large bowel anastomosis: a retrospective study. Br J Anaesth 1978; 50: 177–183.
399. Worsley MH, Wishart HY, Peebles Brown DA, et al: High spinal nerve block for large bowel anastomosis: a prospective study. Br J Anaesth 1988; 60: 836–840.
400. Shandall A, Lowndes R, Young HL: Colonic anastomotic healing and oxygen tension. Br J Surg 1985; 72: 606–609.
401. Aitkenhead AR, Gilmour DG, Hothersall AP, et al: Effects of subarachnoid spinal nerve block and arterial Pco₂ on colon blood flow in the dog. Br J Anaesth 1980; 52: 1071–1077.

402. Johansson K, Ahn H, Lindhagen J, et al: Effect of epidural anaesthesia on intestinal blood flow. Br J Surg 1988; 75: 73–76.

403. Livingston EH, Passaro EP Jr: Postoperative ileus. Dig Dis Sci 1990; 35: 121–132.

404. Moss G, Regal ME, Lichtig L: Reducing postoperative pain, narcotics, and length of hospitalization. Surgery 1986; 99: 206–210.

405. Smith J, Kelly KA, Weinshilboum RM: Pathophysiology of postoperative ileus. Arch Surg 1977; 112: 203–209.

406. Woods JH, Erickson LW, Condon RE, et al: Postoperative ileus: a colonic problem? Surgery 1978; 84: 527–533.

407. Walus KM, Jacobson ED: Relation between small intestinal motility and circulation. (Editorial.) Am J Physiol 1981; 241: G1–G15.

408. Chou CC, Gallavan RH: Blood flow and intestinal motility. Fed Proc 1982; 41: 2090–2095.

409. Galligan JJ, Burks TF: Inhibition of gastric and intestinal motility by centrally and peripherally administered morphine. Proc West Pharmacol Soc 1982; 25: 307–311.

410. Kaufman PN, Krevsky B, Malmud LS, et al: Role of opiate receptors in the regulation of colonic transit. Gastroenterology 1988; 94: 1351–1356.

411. Golden RF, Mann FC: The effects of drugs used in anesthesiology on the tone and motility of the small intestine: an experimental study. Anesthesiology 1943; 4: 577–595.

412. Disbrow EA, Bennett HL, Owings JT: Effect of preoperative suggestion on postoperative gastrointestinal motility. West J Med 1993; 158: 488–492.

413. Thorén T, Wattwil M: Effects of gastric emptying of thoracic epidural analgesia with morphine or bupivacaine. Anesth Analg 1988; 67: 687–694.

414. Thorén T, Wattwil M, Järnerot G, et al: Epidural and spinal anesthesia do not influence gastric emptying and small intestinal transit in volunteers. Reg Anesth 1989; 14: 35–42.

415. Udassin R, Eimerl D, Schiffman J, et al: Epidural anesthesia accelerates the recovery of postischemic bowel motility in the rat. Anesthesiology 1994; 80: 832–836.

416. Markowitz J, Campbell WR: The relief of experimental ileus by spinal anesthesia. Am J Physiol 1927; 81: 101–106.

417. Ochsner A, Gage IM, Cutting RA: Comparative value of splanchnic and spinal analgesia in treatment of experimental ileus. Arch Surg 1930; 30: 802–831.

418. Rimbäck G, Cassuto J, Tollesson P-O: Treatment of postoperative paralytic ileus by intravenous lidocaine infusion. Anesth Analg 1990; 70: 414–419.

419. Rimbäck G, Cassuto J, Faxén A, et al: Effect of intra-abdominal bupivacaine instillation on postoperative colonic motility. Gut 1986; 27: 170–175.

420. Groudine S, Wilkins L: Epidural drugs also act systemically. (Letter to the editor.) Anesthesiology 1994; 81: 787.

421. Gelman S, Feigenberg Z, Dintzman M, et al: Electroenterography after cholecystectomy: the role of high epidural analgesia. Arch Surg 1977; 112: 580–583.

422. Nimmo WS, Littlewood DG, Scott DB, et al: Gastric emptying following hysterectomy with extradural analgesia. Br J Anaesth 1978; 50: 559–561.

423. Rawal N, Sjöstrand U, Christoffersson E, et al: Comparison of intramuscular and epidural morphine for postoperative analgesia in the grossly obese: influence on postoperative ambulation and pulmonary function. Anesth Analg 1984; 63: 583–592.

424. Wallin G, Cassuto J, Högström S, et al: Failure of epidural anesthesia to prevent postoperative paralytic ileus. Anesthesiology 1986; 65: 292–297.

425. Scheinen B, Asantila R, Orko R: The effect of bupivacaine and morphine on pain and bowel function after colonic surgery. Acta Anaesthesiol Scand 1987; 31: 161–164.

426. Wattwil M, Thorén T, Hennerdal S, et al: Epidural analgesia with bupivacaine reduces postoperative paralytic ileus after hysterectomy. Anesth Analg 1989; 68: 353–358.

427. Ahn H, Bronge A, Johansson K, et al: Effect of continuous postoperative epidural analgesia on intestinal motility. Br J Surg 1988; 75: 1176–1178.

428. Thorén T, Sundberg A, Wattwil M, et al: Effects of epidural bupivacaine and epidural morphine on bowel function and pain after hysterectomy. Acta Anaesthesiol Scand 1989; 33: 181–185.

429. Thörn S-E, Wattwil M, Näslund I: Postoperative epidural morphine, but not epidural bupivacaine, delays gastric emptying on the first day after cholecystectomy. Reg Anesth 1992; 17: 91–94.

430. Wattwil M: Postoperative pain relief and gastrointestinal motility. Acta Chir Scand Suppl 1989; 550: 140–145.

431. England DW, Davis IJ, Timmins AE, et al: Gastric emptying: a study to compare the effects of intrathecal morphine and I.M. papaveretum analgesia. Br J Anaesth 1987; 59: 1403–1407.

432. Anderson JD, Moore FA, Moore EE: Enteral feeding in the critically injured patient. Nutr Clin Pract 1992; 7: 117–122.

433. Moore FA, Feliciano DV, Andrassy RJ, et al: Early enteral feeding, compared with parenteral, reduces postoperative septic complications. The results of a meta-analysis. Ann Surg 1992; 216: 172–183.

434. Bonica JJ, Crepps W, Monk B, et al: Postanesthetic nausea, retching and vomiting: evaluation of cyclizine (Marezine) suppositories for treatment. Anesthesiology 1958; 19: 532–540.

435. Crocker JS, Vandam LD: Concerning nausea and vomiting during spinal anesthesia. Anesthesiology 1959; 20: 587–592.

436. Sleight P: Cardiac vomiting. Br Heart J 1981; 46: 5–7.

437. Abrahamsson H, Thorén P: Vomiting and reflex vagal relaxation of the stomach elicited from heart receptors in the cat. Acta Physiol Scand 1973; 88: 433–439.

438. Johannsen UJ, Summers R, Mark AL: Gastric dilation during stimulation of cardiac sensory receptors. Circulation 1981; 63: 960–964.

439. Pauchet V: Spinal anesthesia. Am J Surg 1920; 34: 1–5.

440. Lundy JS: Balanced anesthesia. Minn Med 1926; 9: 399–404.

441. Pitkin GP: Controllable spinal anesthesia. Am J Surg 1928; 5: 537–553.

442. Babcock WW: Spinal anesthesia: an experience of twenty-four years. Am J Surg 1928; 5: 571–576.

443. Sebrechts J: Spinal anaesthesia. Br J Anaesth 1934; 12: 4–27.

444. Matas R: Local and regional anesthesia: a retrospect and prospect. Am J Surg 1934; 25: 189–196; 362–379.

445. Adriani J: From Koller to Labat: a historic resumé. Reg Anesth 1980; 5: 3–7.

446. Fink BR: Leaves and needles: the introduction of surgical local anesthesia. Anesthesiology 1985; 63: 77–83.

447. Griffith HR, Johnson GE: The use of curare in general anesthesia. Anesthesiology 1942; 3: 418–420.

448. Mangano DT, Siliciano D, Hollenberg M, et al: Postoperative myocardial ischemia: therapeutic trials using intensive analgesia following surgery. Anesthesiology 1992; 76: 342–353.

449. Anand KJS, Hickey PR: Halothane-morphine compared with high-dose sufentanil for anesthesia and postoperative analgesia in neonatal cardiac surgery. N Engl J Med 1992; 326: 1–9.

450. Shir Y, Raja SN, Frank SM: The effect of epidural versus general anesthesia on postoperative pain and analgesic requirements in patients undergoing radical prostatectomy. Anesthesiology 1994; 80: 49–56.

451. Yeager MP: Regional anesthesia: testing whether it makes a difference. (Editorial.) J Clin Anesth 1990; 2: 67–70.

452. Brown DL, Mackey DC: Management of postoperative pain: influence of anesthetic and analgesic choice. Mayo Clin Proc 1993; 68: 768–777.

453. Kehlet H, Dahl JB: The value of "multimodal" or "balanced analgesia" in postoperative pain treatment. Anesth Analg 1993; 77: 1048–1056.

454. Kehlet H: Anesthetic technique and surgical convalescence. Acta Chir Scand Suppl 1988; 550: 182–191.

CHAPTER 23

Concurrent Medical Problems and Regional Anesthesia

Terese T. Horlocker, M.D.

Preexisting medical conditions may have a profound impact on anesthetic choice and perioperative management. Optimal management of regional anesthesia balances the pathophysiology of concurrent medical conditions, the cause and significance of physiologic responses to a regional block, the clinical pharmacology of local anesthetic agents, and the results of surgical outcome studies involving patients with preexisting medical conditions undergoing regional anesthesia. This chapter characterizes cardiovascular, pulmonary, hepatic, renal, hematologic, and neurologic disorders and discusses anesthetic management as it pertains to preoperative evaluation, regional anesthetic technique, selection of local anesthetic solution, and perioperative monitoring.

Cardiovascular Disease

Cardiovascular morbidity contributes significantly to surgical mortality. Identifying patients at increased risk for cardiac complications is a crucial step in the preoperative evaluation. Patients with ischemic or valvular heart disease, cardiomyopathy, congestive heart failure, and peripheral vascular disease require a thorough clinical history, physical examination, and selective testing to optimize their medical conditions before surgery. In high-risk patients, such as those with severe aortic stenosis or unstable angina, the potential risks and benefits of an invasive cardiac diagnostic procedure or coronary artery revascularization must be carefully considered before major noncardiac surgery.

Ischemic Cardiac Disease

The risk of perioperative myocardial infarction in cardiac patients undergoing noncardiac surgery has been well documented. In a combined series totaling more than 46,000 patients, the risk of perioperative myocardial infarction was 0.15% among patients without prior clinical evidence of coronary artery disease.[1-3] However, for patients with a prior myocardial infarction, the overall incidence of reinfarction during a major noncardiac operation varied from 2.8% to 17.7%.[1-4] The incidence of perioperative reinfarction is also inversely related to the time between the previous myocardial infarction and the surgical procedure. The reinfarction rate after a surgical procedure performed within 3 mo of a myocardial infarction is as high as 37%.[1] However, the reinfarction rate decreases dramatically if at least 6 mo elapse between the myocardial infarction and surgery. Rao and colleagues[5] reported significantly lower reinfarction rates and attributed the improved cardiac outcome to aggressive management of patients, including invasive perioperative hemodynamic monitoring.

General and regional anesthetic techniques did not significantly affect the reinfarction rate in the previously mentioned studies. However, later evidence[6-8] suggests that epidural anesthesia combined with postoperative epidural analgesia may improve outcome in patients with ischemic cardiac disease who undergo noncardiac surgery. Knowledge of the etiology and physiologic effects of neuraxial block is paramount to safe patient management and to understanding the indications and contraindications of neuraxial anesthesia in this patient population.

The effects of neuraxial block on the determinants of myocardial oxygen supply and demand have been extensively studied. Intrathecal or epidural administration of a local anesthetic results in sympathetic block. The hemodynamic effects depend on the location and extension of the block, use of epinephrine, presence of coronary artery disease, and intravascular volume status of the patient.

The sympathectomy associated with neuraxial block results in venous and arterial vasodilation.[9, 10] The venodilatory effect predominates, because 75% of the total blood volume is contained in the venous system. A reflex compensatory sympathetic response occurs in the nonanesthetized segments, sometimes resulting in vasoconstriction in the upper extremities, splanchnic vasculature, and coronary arteries. This redistribution of blood volume is often accompanied by a decrease in central venous pressure, with associated decreases in stroke volume and cardiac output.[11–13] Although moderate decreases in preload and afterload may lower myocardial oxygen demand and therefore be beneficial in patients with coronary artery disease, a substantial lowering of systemic blood pressure may decrease coronary perfusion pressure and blood flow.[14] In patients with a history of coronary artery disease, lumbar spinal or epidural anesthesia may improve or worsen cardiac function, as evaluated by echocardiography and radionuclide angiography.[12, 15]

Lumbar Epidural Anesthesia

Baron and coworkers[12] studied the influence of lumbar epidural anesthesia without cardiac sympathectomy on global and regional left ventricular function in 8 healthy patients and 10 patients with stable, mild effort-related angina. Radionuclide angiography was used to determine cardiac output, left ventricular ejection fraction, end-systolic and end-diastolic volumes, and left ventricular wall motion. Measurements were made before the block, after epidural block (10 mL of 0.5% bupivacaine, T-6 to T-10 sensory levels) and before volume loading, and after epidural block following volume loading (500 mL of lactated Ringer's solution). Eight of the 10 patients with a history of angina had hypokinetic myocardial segments before block. In these patients, epidural blocks before volume loading induced significant improvements in left ventricular ejection fraction and in regional wall motion. The improvement in ventricular wall function before volume loading was attributed to a decrease in afterload and an improved myocardial oxygen balance. No change in these variables was observed in normal subjects. After volume loading, left ventricular preload increased in all patients. In patients with a history of angina, the left ventricular ejection fraction significantly decreased, and in each of the eight patients with hypokinetic segments at baseline, at least one hypokinetic sector was identified. Throughout the surgical procedure, no patient with a history of angina complained of chest pain or exhibited electrocardio-graphic evidence of myocardial ischemia. The researchers concluded that a decrease in left ventricular loading induced by lumbar epidural anesthesia may improve left ventricular global and regional function in patients with a history of mild angina, as long as volume loading is limited.

These findings differ from those of Saada and colleagues,[15] who studied the effect of lumbar epidural block on myocardial wall motion by using continuous two-dimensional echocardiography in 5 healthy patients and 10 patients with documented coronary artery disease (including unstable angina). All healthy patients had normal preepidural echocardiograms, whereas baseline left ventricular regional wall motion abnormalities were present in 8 of 10 patients with a history of coronary artery disease. Epidural block was performed with 12.5 mL of 2% lidocaine, resulting in sensory block up to T-6 to T-12 sensory levels. In the healthy patients, segmental wall motion became hyperkinetic within 20 min after epidural injection and returned to preepidural levels at 60 min. However, induction of lumbar epidural anesthesia in patients with coronary artery disease had markedly different results. Ten minutes after epidural injection, segmental wall motion decreased in all 10 patients who had coronary artery disease. The hypokinesis was most severe from 10 to 20 min after epidural injection, and typically it occurred in and adjacent to segments with baseline abnormalities. Isolated segments often became hyperkinetic in patients with coronary artery disease. The wall motion abnormalities occurred simultaneously with significant decreases in blood pressure. There was no electrocardiographic evidence of myocardial ischemia; only one patient complained of angina. The researchers concluded that hemodynamic changes due to lumbar epidural anesthesia, particularly decreases in diastolic blood pressure, may impair myocardial perfusion in patients with coronary artery disease.

These studies indicate that the hemodynamic changes associated with lumbar epidural anesthesia are well tolerated in healthy patients. However, patients with coronary artery disease may have a limited adaptation to the decrease in venous return, and epidural use must be individualized. In these patients, significant decreases in systemic blood pressure may jeopardize myocardial oxygen supply despite a decrease in myocardial oxygen consumption. The compensatory sympathetic activation may induce tachycardia and coronary artery vasoconstriction.[16, 17] Myocardial ischemia also activates cardiac sympathetic afferents at a spinal level. This cardiocardiac spinal reflex has the potential to aggravate myocardial ischemia and is most effectively treated with cardiac sympathetic block.

Thoracic Epidural Anesthesia

Although lumbar spinal and epidural anesthesia may impair myocardial perfusion, thoracic epidural anesthesia, including block of the cardiac sympathetic efferents and afferents, may have beneficial effects on ischemic myocardium. Blomberg and associates[18] studied the effect of high thoracic epidural anesthesia (4 mL of 0.5%

bupivacaine, T-1 to T-8 segmental sensory block) on central hemodynamics in nine patients with unstable angina. The patients were also treated with calcium antagonists, β-blockers, and nitrates. During episodes of ischemic chest pain, thoracic epidural anesthesia relieved angina and decreased systolic blood pressure, heart rate, pulmonary artery and pulmonary capillary wedge pressures, without significant changes in cardiac output, coronary perfusion pressure, and systemic or pulmonary vascular resistances.

In a subsequent study, Blomberg and colleagues[17] examined the effect of high thoracic epidural anesthesia on the luminal diameter of normal and diseased portions of epicardial coronary arteries and coronary arterioles in patients with severe coronary artery disease. Thoracic epidural anesthesia increased the luminal diameter in stenotic segments of epicardial coronary arteries, but the diameter of nonstenotic segments remained unchanged. Regional cardiac block also caused no changes in coronary perfusion pressure, myocardial blood flow, or coronary venous oxygen content, indicating a lack of effect on coronary resistance vessels (coronary arterioles). Lessening of ST-segment depression was also observed in some patients.

High thoracic epidural anesthesia decreases the major determinants of myocardial oxygen consumption and may have antiischemic properties by favorably altering the myocardial oxygen supply and demand in ischemic cardiac segments. High thoracic epidural anesthesia can be used to control pain in patients with coronary artery disease and unstable angina or severe chest pain at rest.

Outcome Studies

There are few data supporting the intraoperative superiority of regional over general anesthetic technique with regard to cardiovascular outcome. However, there is evidence that epidural anesthesia with postoperative epidural analgesia may decrease cardiac morbidity. Yeager and coworkers[6] demonstrated a significant decrease in the incidence of congestive heart failure in high-risk patients receiving epidural anesthesia and analgesia compared with patients receiving general anesthesia and conventional parenteral opioid therapy. Perioperative anesthetic management allowed the dose, concentration, and type of epidural medications to be individualized.

Tuman and colleagues[7] similarly compared perioperative outcome after lower extremity vascular surgery in 80 patients who received general anesthesia combined with epidural anesthesia and analgesia or received general anesthesia with parenteral or oral administration of opioid (or both). Patients in both groups had major cardiac risk factors, such as prior myocardial infarction or history of congestive heart failure. The rates of cardiovascular, infectious (including pneumonia), and overall complications were significantly decreased in the epidural anesthesia and analgesia group (Table 23-1).

Anesthetic Management

Intraoperative myocardial ischemia occurs when myocardial oxygen delivery is inadequate relative to

Table 23-1 Effect of Epidural Anesthesia and Analgesia on Cardiopulmonary Outcome After Major Vascular Surgery

VARIABLE	PATIENTS	
	General Anesthesia	Combined General-Epidural Anesthesia
Patients, no.	40	40
Patient characteristics, %		
History of chronic obstructive pulmonary disease	8	8
History of angina	14	20
Ejection fraction <0.4	6	9
Congestive heart failure	1	4
Previous myocardial infarction*	10	19
Postoperative cardiopulmonary morbidity, no.		
Cardiovascular (total)*	11	4
Myocardial infarction	3	0
Congestive heart failure	4	2
Tachyarrhythmia*	11	3
Prolonged tracheal intubation	5	1
Pneumonia*	4	0

*$P < .05$.
Data from Tuman KJ, McCarthy RJ, March RJ, et al: Effects of epidural anesthesia and analgesia on coagulation and outcome after major vascular surgery. Anesth Analg 1991; 73: 696–704.

myocardial oxygen requirements (Table 23-2). Persistent tachycardia, hypotension, activation of the sympathetic nervous system, and arterial hypoxemia may occur with neuraxial block and may adversely affect this balance. Conversely, the decreases in preload and afterload associated with spinal or epidural anesthesia decrease oxygen requirements and are therefore advantageous. The effects of neuraxial block on left ventricular function in patients with coronary artery disease are controversial, and induction of spinal or epidural anesthesia in these patients carries the risk of worsening myocardial ischemia or the advantage of decreasing myocardial ischemic events.

Appropriate management of regional anesthesia in patients with coronary artery disease involves the thoughtful use of fluids given intravenously, vasopressors, and invasive monitoring. Patients undergoing regional anesthesia should be adequately sedated to decrease anxiety and the associated secretion of catecholamines. The use of epinephrine-containing local anesthetic solutions in patients with coronary artery disease is controversial, because epinephrine may cause vasodilation and cardiac stimulation. Patients should receive limited volume loading before induction of spi-

Table 23-2 Intraoperative Events That Affect Myocardial Oxygen Delivery and Myocardial Oxygen Requirements

DECREASED OXYGEN DELIVERY	INCREASED OXYGEN REQUIREMENTS
Tachycardia	Tachycardia
Increased preload	Increased afterload
Diastolic hypotension	Increased myocardial contractility
Coronary artery spasm	Systolic hypertension
Anemia	
Arterial hypoxemia	

nal or epidural anesthesia to avoid hypotension. Because most episodes of ischemia in the study by Saada and associates[15] occurred with significant decreases in blood pressure, immediate treatment of a decrease in diastolic blood pressure that exceeds 20% of baseline with fluids given intravenously or a sympathomimetic drug (or both) is advised. Even though intraoperative anesthetic technique (regional or general) may not affect cardiac outcome, the use of epidural anesthesia and analgesia with postoperative infusion of opioid or local anesthetic solutions significantly decreases the incidence of cardiac morbidity and is recommended in appropriate surgical procedures.

Valvular Cardiac Disease

Anesthetic management of the patient with valvular cardiac disease requires knowledge of the hemodynamic alterations associated with valvular dysfunction, the severity of the cardiac disease indicated by the functional classification (Table 23–3), and the cardiovascular modifications induced by neuraxial block. Preoperative history and physical examination are important in evaluating cardiac reserve and the presence of congestive heart failure. The electrocardiogram and chest radiograph may exhibit changes often accompanying valvular cardiac disease, such as ventricular hypertrophy, left atrial enlargement, and increased pulmonary vascularity. However, Doppler echocardiography is the most valuable laboratory test in evaluating valvular dysfunction and can be used to determine transvalvular pressure gradients, valvular orifice area, and cardiac valve regurgitation. Patients with valvular cardiac disease should receive antibiotic prophylaxis against the development of infective endocarditis.

Mitral Stenosis

Mitral stenosis is usually the result of rheumatic heart disease. Patients do not become symptomatic until 10 to 15 yr later, when the size of the normal mitral valve orifice (4 to 6 cm^2) has decreased 50%. A left atrial pressure of 25 mm Hg (normal, 5 mm Hg) is required to maintain cardiac output when the valve orifice is decreased to 1 cm^2. Without surgical intervention, right ventricular failure and pulmonary hypertension develop.

Management of anesthesia in patients with mitral stenosis includes maintaining cardiac output and

Table 23–4 Anesthetic Considerations for Patients With Mitral Stenosis

Maintain normal sinus rhythm.
Prevent rapid ventricular rates.
Minimize increases in central blood volume.
Avoid marked decreases in systemic vascular resistance.
Prevent increases in pulmonary artery pressure.
Avoid events such as hypoxemia that may exacerbate pulmonary hypertension.

avoiding events that may precipitate pulmonary hypertension or right ventricular failure (Table 23–4). Sinus tachycardia and atrial fibrillation with a rapid ventricular rate are poorly tolerated. Decreases in systemic vascular resistance are compensated for by increases in heart rate, which may result in decreased cardiac output. Because increases in central blood volume from overtransfusion, Trendelenburg position, or regressing sympathetic block may result in pulmonary hypertension and right-sided heart failure, the volume status of these patients must be closely monitored. Invasive monitoring of radial and pulmonary artery pressures and cardiac output may be necessary in patients with severe mitral stenosis.

The hemodynamic effects of spinal or epidural anesthesia, including a decrease in preload, slight decrease in afterload, and maintenance of contractility, should improve cardiac performance in patients with mitral stenosis. However, significant decreases in preload and afterload are poorly tolerated and result in a reduction in cardiac output. Consequently, if a regional anesthetic is indicated, a continuous technique may be preferred, to establish the spinal level slowly. Epinephrine is sometimes omitted from the local anesthetic solution because of the potential for tachycardia and vasodilation. During neuraxial block, blood pressure may be maintained with a sympathomimetic drug, such as phenylephrine or ephedrine, if necessary. Ephedrine increases myocardial contractility, but it may also result in tachycardia. Phenylephrine has no direct effect on heart rate, but the α-agonist effect may decrease left ventricular stroke volume. Postoperatively, pain, respiratory acidosis, and hypoxemia may increase heart rate and pulmonary vascular resistance.

Mitral Regurgitation

Mitral regurgitation may occur acutely with papillary muscle rupture or chronically in association with rheumatic heart disease. Chronic mitral regurgitation is usually well tolerated, and patients may remain asymptomatic for 30 to 40 yr. Mitral regurgitation increases volume work of the heart. Left atrial volume overload occurs as a fraction of the stroke volume is regurgitated from the left ventricle back through the incompetent mitral valve. A regurgitant fraction of 0.6 or greater is associated with congestive heart failure. The amount of regurgitant flow correlates with the intensity of the insufficiency murmur and the size of the v wave on the pulmonary artery occlusion pressure tracing. Mitral stenosis combined with mitral regurgitation increases

Table 23–3 New York Heart Association Classification of Patients With Heart Disease

CLASS	DESCRIPTION
I	No limitation of physical activity
II	Symptoms with ordinary physical activity
III	Symptoms with less than ordinary physical activity
IV	Symptoms at rest

Data from The Criteria Committee of the New York Heart Association: Nomenclature and Criteria for Diagnosis of Diseases of the Heart and Great Vessels, 8th ed. New York, New York Heart Association, 1979.

Table 23–5 Anesthetic Considerations for Patients With Mitral Regurgitation

Prevent peripheral vasoconstriction.
Avoid myocardial depressants.
Treat acute atrial fibrillation immediately.
Maintain a normal or slightly increased heart rate.
Monitor the size of the *v* wave and intensity of murmur as reflections of regurgitant flow.

the volume and the pressure work of the heart. In these patients, pulmonary hypertension and edema occur earlier than in patients with only mitral regurgitation.

Management of regional anesthesia in patients with mitral regurgitation includes maintaining cardiac output and forward flow through the regurgitant valve (Table 23–5). Because large increases in systemic vascular resistance can cause acute decompensation of the left ventricle, afterload reduction is recommended. Myocardial depressants are also poorly tolerated. Forward stroke volume may depend on heart rate, and bradycardia may result in acute overload of the left ventricle and increase in the regurgitant fraction. Maintenance of a normal to slightly increased heart rate is advocated. Atrial fibrillation can precipitate left ventricular decompensation and should be treated immediately.

The sympathectomy induced by regional anesthetic techniques helps reduce the regurgitant flow across the mitral valve. However, neuraxial block also increases venous capacitance and may require intravenous administration of fluids to maintain the filling volume of the enlarged left ventricle. The positive inotropic and chronotropic effects of ephedrine are useful in preventing and treating hypotension.

Mitral Valve Prolapse

Mitral valve prolapse is the most common congenital valvular lesion, occurring in 5% to 10% of the population. Most patients with mitral valve prolapse are asymptomatic, but 15% require medical management. Arrhythmias, particularly paroxysmal supraventricular tachycardia, are common.

Regional anesthetic management in asymptomatic patients with mitral valve prolapse may be approached in a routine manner. However, patients with evidence of mitral regurgitation require special considerations (Table 23–6). Decreases in left ventricular volume generally cause increased prolapse.

Table 23–6 Anesthetic Considerations for Patients With Mitral Valve Prolapse

Avoid decreases in preload.
Continue antiarrhythmic therapy.
With moderate to severe mitral valve prolapse–induced mitral insufficiency, apply the considerations listed for mitral regurgitation.
Avoid decreases in systemic vascular resistance.
Avoid sympathetic nervous system stimulation.

Anesthetic management consists of maintaining intravascular and intraventricular volume through intravenous administration of fluids and blood transfusion. A normal to slightly increased heart rate, prevention of peripheral vasoconstriction, and avoidance of myocardial depressants decrease the regurgitant fraction and enhance forward flow. Antiarrhythmics should also be continued perioperatively, and arrhythmias should be treated aggressively.

Regional anesthesia is often beneficial in patients with mitral valve prolapse. The sympathectomy prevents peripheral vasoconstriction and increases the forward flow of blood. Intravenous administration of fluids is required to maintain the filling volume of the enlarged left ventricle and to minimize the degree of prolapse.

Aortic Stenosis

Aortic stenosis usually results from progressive calcification and stenosis of a congenitally abnormal bicuspid valve or from rheumatic fever, often in association with mitral valve involvement. Patients are often asymptomatic for 30 yr, and then angina, dyspnea on exertion, and syncope develop. Surgical intervention is indicated when the valvular orifice is less than 1 cm² (normal, 2.5 to 3.5 cm²) or when the transvalvular pressure gradient is greater than 50 mm Hg. Patients with moderate to severe aortic stenosis often have angina, despite the absence of coronary artery disease, resulting from the increased myocardial oxygen consumption and decreased myocardial oxygen delivery to the hypertrophied left ventricle.

Management of regional anesthesia in patients with aortic stenosis includes maintaining cardiac output and coronary artery perfusion (Table 23–7). Preservation of normal sinus rhythm is necessary to maintain stroke volume. Increases in heart rate decrease the time available for diastolic filling and ventricular ejection, and bradycardia may result in acute volume overload of the left ventricle. Significant decreases in systemic vascular resistance may be associated with decreases in blood pressure and coronary blood flow, resulting in myocardial ischemia. Decreases in venous return are also poorly tolerated, because left ventricular stroke volume is maintained only if the end-diastolic volume is adequate.

Aortic stenosis may be associated with increased perioperative mortality, regardless of whether a general or regional anesthetic technique is used.[19] Spinal and epidural anesthesia are relatively contraindicated for patients with moderate to severe aortic stenosis, defined as a valvular orifice of less than 1 cm², with a transvalvular gradient of 30 to 50 mm Hg. The sympa-

Table 23–7 Anesthetic Considerations for Patients With Aortic Stenosis

Avoid decreases in systemic vascular resistance.
Avoid bradycardia.
Maintain venous return and left ventricular filling.
Maintain normal sinus rhythm.

thetic block and reduction in preload may produce a profound and irreversible decrease in cardiac output, blood pressure, and coronary artery perfusion. Cardiopulmonary resuscitation is extremely difficult in the presence of aortic stenosis with left ventricular hypertrophy. If a regional anesthetic is indicated, a continuous-catheter technique is recommended, with titration of the local anesthetic dose to minimize the sympathetic block. Adequate intravascular volume expansion must occur before induction of regional anesthesia. Systemic vascular resistance may be maintained with a vasoconstrictor such as phenylephrine, metaraminol, or ephedrine. The use of invasive monitoring, such as radial artery and pulmonary artery catheters, depends on the severity of the aortic stenosis.

Aortic Regurgitation

Aortic regurgitation usually becomes symptomatic 15 to 20 yr after an acute attack of rheumatic fever. Left ventricular overload and failure occur with chronic aortic regurgitation. Initially, the left ventricle tolerates the chronic increase in volume and develops eccentric hypertrophy while compliance increases. Eventually, left ventricular failure begins, forward stroke volume decreases, and pulmonary congestion and edema follow.

The anesthetic management of patients with aortic regurgitation is similar to that of patients with mitral regurgitation and involves maintaining cardiac output and forward flow through the regurgitant valve (Table 23–8). Increases in systemic vascular resistance and myocardial depressants may precipitate left ventricular failure. Bradycardia increases the duration of diastole and therefore the amount of blood regurgitated across the aortic valve. The heart rate should be maintained between 80 and 100 beats/min. As with mitral regurgitation, the intensity and duration of the murmur correlate with the amount of regurgitant flow and should be monitored.

Regional anesthesia may benefit patients with aortic regurgitation. The sympathectomy decreases peripheral vasoconstriction and enhances forward flow across the aortic valve. However, the accompanying increase in venous capacitance and decrease in preload require intravenous administration of fluids to maintain the filling volume of the enlarged left ventricle. Ephedrine is useful in treating hypotension because of its positive inotropic and chronotropic properties. Invasive monitoring of radial and pulmonary artery pressures and cardiac output may be necessary in patients with severe aortic regurgitation.

Table 23–8 Anesthetic Considerations for Patients With Aortic Regurgitation

Avoid marked increases in systemic vascular resistance.
Maintain a normal or slightly increased heart rate.
Avoid myocardial depressants.
Monitor the intensity of murmurs.

Table 23–9 Anesthetic Considerations for Patients With a Left-to-Right Shunt

Avoid increases in systemic vascular resistance.
Avoid marked increases in heart rate.
With pulmonary hypertension, avoid marked decreases in systemic vascular resistance.
With pulmonary hypertension, avoid further increases in pulmonary vascular resistance.

Congenital Cardiac Disease

Congenital cardiac disease is present in approximately 1% of neonates. The diagnosis is made in the first week of life in 50% of cases. Echocardiography is the initial diagnostic test recommended, and cardiac catheterization with angiography provides the definitive diagnosis. As in patients with valvular cardiac disease, management of regional anesthesia in patients with congenital cardiac disease requires thorough understanding of the cardiac defect. The major categories of congenital cardiac disease are left-to-right intracardiac shunt, right-to-left intracardiac shunt, congenital valvular lesions, and congenital vascular lesions. Only the more common congenital cardiac defects are discussed in this section.

Left-to-Right Intracardiac Shunts

Ventricular septal defect, atrial septal defect, and patent ductus arteriosus are associated with left-to-right intracardiac shunt. Significant hemodynamic changes are not present when these shunts are small, and patients with these cardiac lesions are managed without special anesthetic considerations. With larger defects, however, there is a marked increase in pulmonary blood flow and development of pulmonary hypertension. Chronic pulmonary hypertension eventually results in Eisenmenger syndrome, a bidirectional or right-to-left intracardiac shunt with peripheral cyanosis.

Management of regional anesthesia involves optimizing conditions that decrease the magnitude of the left-to-right shunt, such as avoiding tachycardia and increases in systemic vascular resistance (Table 23–9). This is possible with spinal or epidural block. However, in the presence of pulmonary hypertension and right ventricular compromise, decreases in systemic vascular resistance (as with regional anesthesia) or increases in pulmonary vascular resistance may lead to right-to-left shunting and hypoxemia. Neuraxial block usually is not recommended in these patients.

Right-to-Left Intracardiac Shunts

Tetralogy of Fallot is the most common cyanotic congenital cardiac defect. This anomaly is characterized by right ventricular outflow tract obstruction, ventricular septal defect, right ventricular hypertrophy, and an overriding aorta. Patients with tetralogy of Fallot are often able to improve arterial oxygenation by increasing systemic vascular resistance and therefore the magnitude of the right-to-left shunt by squatting. Episodes

Table 23–10 Anesthetic Considerations for Patients With Tetralogy of Fallot

Avoid decreases in systemic vascular resistance.
Avoid decreases in blood volume.
Avoid decreases in venous return.
Avoid myocardial depressants.

of hypercyanosis or "tet spells" can also occur. The proposed mechanism is a sudden decrease in pulmonary blood flow due to spasm of the infundibular muscle or decreased systemic vascular resistance. Treatment of a hypercyanotic spell induced by infundibular spasm consists of β-blockers, but intravenous administration of fluid or phenylephrine (or both) is used to treat a decrease in vascular resistance.

Patients with corrected tetralogy of Fallot can usually undergo regional anesthesia without special considerations, although the patient should be evaluated preoperatively for signs of right ventricular failure (Table 23–10). Patients with uncorrected tetralogy of Fallot do not tolerate decreases in preload or afterload. Decreases in systemic vascular resistance increase the right-to-left flow and hypoxemia. These patients are most often managed with general anesthesia or peripheral nerve blocks.

Hypertrophic Cardiomyopathy

The principal symptoms of hypertrophic cardiomyopathy with ventricular outflow obstruction are syncope, congestive heart failure, angina, and tachyarrhythmias. The degree of left ventricular outflow depends on myocardial contractility, preload, and afterload.

Anesthetic management of patients with hypertrophic cardiomyopathy is directed toward relieving the obstruction to left ventricular outflow; it includes medications and maneuvers that decrease myocardial contractility and increase preload and afterload (Table 23–11). Conversely, events that decrease preload and afterload, such as spinal or epidural anesthesia, increase left ventricular outflow obstruction. Neuraxial block is therefore relatively contraindicated in symptomatic patients. Regional anesthesia in patients with hypertrophic cardiomyopathy is conducted as for patients with aortic stenosis.

Table 23–11 Anesthetic Considerations for Patients With Hypertrophic Cardiomyopathy

Avoid decreases in blood volume and venous return.
Avoid or correct supraventricular tachycardia, atrial fibrillation, and atrial flutter.
Avoid decreases in systemic vascular resistance.
Avoid increases in myocardial contractility.
Treat ventricular compromise with phenylephrine, fluids given intravenously, and propranolol.

Pulmonary Disease

Postoperative pulmonary dysfunction is a major cause of surgical morbidity and mortality. Surgical procedures, especially involving the thorax and abdomen, result in marked alterations in respiratory mechanics. Regional anesthesia may additionally influence respiratory function. Central and peripheral nerve blocks may have significant effects on respiration, including altered pulmonary function, chest wall mechanics, gas exchange, and ventilatory control. Most of the respiratory changes associated with regional anesthesia are directly attributed to motor block of the muscles of respiration. Knowledge of the physiologic effects of abdominal, intercostal, and phrenic muscle paralysis is useful in the perioperative management of patients with preexisting pulmonary disease who receive regional anesthesia and analgesia.

Epidural and Spinal Anesthesia

Spinal and epidural anesthesia typically have similar effects on pulmonary function. However, epidural block with lower doses or concentrations of local anesthetics may result in a differential block, with impaired sensation and intact motor function of the muscles of respiration.[20] This was demonstrated in a study by Freund and colleagues,[21] who reported a 48% decrease in the expiratory reserve volume with spinal anesthesia, compared with a 21% decrease with similar epidural anesthesia sensory levels. Doses and concentrations of local anesthetics required for surgical anesthesia typically result in paralysis of the muscles of respiration in the blocked segments. Spinal anesthesia and epidural anesthesia typically produce similar effects on the respiratory system.

Thoracic levels of spinal or epidural anesthesia result in paralysis of the abdominal and chest wall muscles. Block of motor function up to the T-1 level leaves the patient dependent on diaphragmatic respiration and produces conditions similar to those in the quadriplegic patient. In this situation, isolated diaphragmatic motion expands only the lower rib cage, while the upper rib cage is passively pulled inward by decreasing pleural pressure. This movement characterizes the classic deformation of the rib cage during high levels of epidural or spinal anesthesia and in quadriplegia.[22, 23] However, even with complete chest wall paralysis, the preservation of diaphragmatic function maintains near-normal pulmonary function in most patients during quiet respiration.

Although spinal and epidural forms of anesthesia result in significant alterations in chest wall mechanics, conventional pulmonary function tests are relatively insensitive in detecting changes in lung volumes and pressures. Most studies[13, 24–26] report little or no effect on pulmonary function tests in patients undergoing spinal or epidural anesthesia. Urmey and McDonald[24] studied changes in the pulmonary function tests of 22 patients during lumbar epidural anesthesia with a mean sensory block at T-6. As expected, there was no significant decrease in the peak inspiratory flow rate because the main inspiratory muscles (diaphragm and accessory neck muscles) remained innervated during lumbar epidural anesthesia. However, there were significant decreases in the effort-dependent expiratory parameters, such as forced vital capacity and peak expiratory flow rate, which depend on intact expiratory musculature. Although the decreases in mean forced vital capacity (176 mL) and peak expiratory flow rate (0.34 L/s) were statistically significant, they represent only a modest decrease from baseline and were therefore of limited clinical importance. Similar clinically insignificant decreases in forced vital capacity and 1-s forced expiratory volume were reported during cervical and thoracic epidural anesthesia.[25, 26] The results suggest that conventional pulmonary function tests evaluate intrinsic pulmonary mechanics (airway conduction properties) rather than chest wall mechanics and are a relatively insensitive method of evaluating changes in respiratory effort in patients with high thoracic levels of epidural or spinal anesthesia.

In contrast to the minor changes in pulmonary function tests, spinal or epidural anesthesia results in a 50% decrease in maximum intrapleural and intra-abdominal pressures during forced exhalation.[27, 28] Turbulent pulmonary airflow produced by forceful contraction of the abdominal and chest wall muscles is attenuated by thoracoabdominal muscle paralysis during spinal or epidural anesthesia. The ability to cough may be compromised by regional anesthetic techniques. The effects of high levels of spinal or epidural anesthesia are important in patients with tracheal or bronchial secretions who depend on their ability to cough to maintain airway patency.

Minute ventilation, pulmonary shunt, pulmonary dead space, and the alveolar-arterial oxygen partial pressure gradient are unaffected during spinal and epidural anesthesia.[27, 29] Arterial blood gas tensions are typically unchanged in patients spontaneously breathing room air. However, decreases in oxygenation have been reported, presumably from variations in regional ventilation produced by changes in chest wall motion.[30, 31]

Control of ventilation is altered little by neuraxial block. Respiratory arrest during total spinal anesthesia is not a result of direct local anesthetic effects on the muscles of respiration or on the medullary respiratory center, but rather it results from hypoperfusion of the brain stem due to decreased cardiac output. Because sedation during regional anesthesia may cause respiratory depression and upper airway obstruction, intraoperative monitoring of the patient is important.

Outcome Studies

Several studies have examined the effect of spinal or epidural anesthesia on respiratory outcome in patients with preexisting pulmonary disease. Ravin[32] measured arterial blood gases during and after lower abdominal surgery in 20 patients with chronic obstructive pulmonary disease. There were no significant perioperative changes in mean blood gas tensions with general or spinal anesthesia. A study by Tarhan and coworkers[33] suggested a beneficial effect of spinal anesthesia in patients with lung disease. Of 585 patients with moderate to severe chronic lung disease, 464 received general anesthesia. Thirty-three of these patients died of respiratory complications within 9 wk after surgery. The remaining 121 patients received spinal or epidural anesthesia; none died of respiratory complications in the ensuing 9 wk. However, the surgical procedures were different for the groups. All thoracic and upper abdominal procedures were performed during general anesthesia, which may explain the increased mortality rate for the general anesthesia patients.

Epidural anesthesia and analgesia have also been shown to decrease pulmonary complications in high-risk patients. Although preoperative pulmonary status was not mentioned, Yeager and colleagues[6] reported a significant decrease in prolonged ventilation and reintubation in patients with a functioning epidural catheter postoperatively. Twenty percent of the patients studied by Tuman and associates[7] had a history of chronic obstructive pulmonary disease. The patients who received general anesthesia combined with epidural anesthesia and analgesia had fewer pulmonary infections than patients who received general anesthesia and on-demand narcotic analgesia (see Table 23–1). There was no difference in the incidence of respiratory failure between groups.

Brachial Plexus Block

Diaphragmatic paresis produced by motor block of phrenic nerve has long been considered a potential source of pulmonary complications after regional anesthesia. Although most clinicians caution against performing nerve blocks that would result in bilateral phrenic paresis, the actual risk of respiratory complications in patients with preexisting pulmonary disease after unilateral phrenic nerve block is unknown.

The incidence of ipsilateral hemidiaphragmatic paresis after supraclavicular brachial plexus block varied from 28% to 80%, depending on the volume of local anesthetic injected and the method of evaluating diaphragmatic motion.[34–36] Only recently have the incidence, onset, and duration of phrenic nerve paresis after interscalene brachial plexus block been established. Urmey and colleagues[37] studied 13 healthy patients who received interscalene blocks by using a paresthesia technique with 34 to 52 mL of 1.5% mepivacaine. Changes from normal (caudad) to paradoxical (cephalad) motion of the ipsilateral hemidiaphragm, as detected by ultrasonography, were seen in all patients within 5 min (and in 11 of 13 patients within 2 min) of anesthetic injection. The paradoxical hemidiaphragmatic excursion was present during forced sniff and, to a lesser extent, during quiet or deep breathing. On questioning, only 5 of the 13 patients noticed any change in respiration, although none was sedated. The respiratory changes were described as mild dyspnea or an alteration in normal breathing sensations. Diaphragmatic motion returned to normal in 10 of 11 patients between 3 and 4 h after injection and in the remaining patient by 5 h after injection.

In a subsequent study, Urmey and McDonald[38] evaluated the effect of hemidiaphragmatic paresis during interscalene brachial plexus block on pulmonary function and chest wall mechanics. Interscalene blocks were performed on eight patients by using a paresthesia technique with 45 mL of 1.5% mepivacaine. Large decreases in pulmonary function variables were measured in every patient. Forced vital capacity and 1-s forced expiratory volume both decreased 27%. Peak expiratory and maximum midexpiratory flow rates were also significantly decreased. In four additional patients, chest wall motion was studied by magnetometry. In all four patients, rib cage motion was more pronounced than abdominal motion after interscalene block, indicating heightened activity of intercostal and accessory muscles of respiration. These alterations in pulmonary function and chest wall mechanical motion are similar to those published in previous studies[39-41] on patients with hemidiaphragmatic paresis of pathologic or surgical cause.

These two studies[37, 38] suggest that ipsilateral hemidiaphragmatic paresis should be considered an expected consequence of routine interscalene brachial plexus anesthesia and not considered a complication. Interscalene block probably should not be performed in patients who are dependent on bilaterally intact diaphragmatic function and those who are unable to tolerate a 25% decrease in pulmonary function. This includes patients with preexisting contralateral hemidiaphragmatic paresis, severe chronic obstructive pulmonary disease, or even perhaps ankylosing spondylitis, in which rib cage motion is restricted.

Pneumothorax

Pneumothorax is a recognized complication of many regional anesthetic techniques (Table 23–12). Although pneumothorax may be associated with intercostal and supraclavicular brachial plexus blocks, it has also occurred with stellate ganglion block, interscalene brachial plexus block, and paravertebral somatic and sympathetic blocks. However, because the original reports are decades old and the incidence varies greatly among reports, the actual incidence of pneumothorax with a specific regional anesthetic technique is unknown.

The most common symptoms of a pneumothorax are sudden and severe chest pain accompanied by dyspnea. Routine postoperative chest radiographs after most regional blocks are not recommended because, depending on the amount of parenchymal trauma, the pneumothorax may not be evident for 6 to 12 h. It is acceptable to permit spontaneous resorption of the pneumothorax if the patient is asymptomatic or less than 20% of the lung is collapsed. Although the administration of supplemental oxygen accelerates spontaneous resorption by favoring the transfer of nitrogen out of the pleural space, positive pressure ventilation may increase the size of an asymptomatic pneumothorax and possibly result in a tension pneumothorax. Treatment of a clinically significant pneumothorax typically involves placement of a chest tube, although aspiration of the pleural space with a small-gauge catheter under radiographic guidance has also been described. Subsequent chest radiographs should be performed to ensure resolution.

Anesthetic Management

Regional anesthesia produces significant and predictable effects on respiration. The changes include altered pulmonary function, chest wall mechanics, gas exchange, and ventilatory control. However, the impact of regional anesthesia on respiratory function in patients with preexisting pulmonary disease remains controversial and largely unstudied.

Anesthetic management involves anticipating the effects of motor block on the respiratory musculature. The level of motor block with spinal or epidural anesthesia should be appropriate to the surgical procedure to minimize chest and abdominal wall paralysis and ensure adequate cough strength and clearance of secretions. High spinal levels of anesthesia may result in bronchospasm because of the unopposed parasympathetic tone of the bronchioles and should be minimized in patients with reactive airways. Patients at risk for respiratory failure with phrenic nerve paralysis or pneumothorax should be identified preoperatively, and the decision to proceed with regional anesthesia should be made on an individual basis. Patients unable to tolerate a 25% decrease in pulmonary function may benefit from an alternative anesthetic technique. Excessive sedation during regional anesthesia may cause respiratory depression and contribute to postoperative pulmonary complications, such as atelectasis and aspiration pneumonitis.

Supplemental oxygen should be administered to all patients who undergo regional anesthesia to minimize the effects of sedation and altered pulmonary mechanics. Adequate patient monitoring, including pneumography and pulse oximetry, is essential for prevention and early detection of critical events. Epidural analgesia may be continued postoperatively in an effort to decrease respiratory complications, including pneumonia.

Table 23–12 Reported Incidence of Pneumothorax After Various Nerve Blocks

NERVE BLOCK	INCIDENCE, %
Supraclavicular brachial plexus block	0.6–2
Stellate ganglion block	
Anterior approach	0.25
Anterolateral approach	0.5–8
Posterior approach	3–13
Thoracic paravertebral (somatic) block	0–6
Thoracic paravertebral (sympathetic) block	1.4–7.9

From Bridenbaugh PO: Complications of local anesthetic neural blockade. In Cousins MJ, Bridenbaugh PO (eds): Neural Blockade in Clinical Anesthesia and Management of Pain, 2nd ed, pp 695–717. Philadelphia, JB Lippincott, 1988.

Hepatic Disease

Liver disease, including cirrhosis, is the seventh leading cause of death in the United States. It is estimated that 5% to 10% of all patients with cirrhosis of the liver will have an operation in the last 2 yr of life. Patients in the early stages of liver disease respond to medications and anesthesia differently than those in end-stage liver failure. Preoperative criteria correlate with surgical risk and postoperative outcome of patients with cirrhosis undergoing major surgery.[42-44] The presence of any of the following four pathologic variables in a patient with liver disease constitutes high risk: prothrombin time increased more than 4 s above normal, increased plasma bilirubin concentration, decreased serum albumin concentration, or ascites. Increased concentrations of aminotransferases do not predict surgical risk but indicate that parenchymal damage has occurred.

Pathophysiology

Hepatic and extrahepatic complications of cirrhosis are often present in patients with progressive disease. Chronic portal vein hypertension produces hepatomegaly, ascites, and esophageal varices. Right-to-left intrapulmonary shunts develop in the presence of portal vein hypertension, leading to arterial hypoxemia. Impaired diaphragmatic motion from the accumulation of ascites and frequent pulmonary infections further contribute to low values for the partial pressure of arterial oxygen. A hyperdynamic circulation with high cardiac output occurs as a result of true shunts. However, alcoholic cardiomyopathy accompanied by congestive heart failure may also occur. Abnormal clotting often results from qualitative and quantitative platelet defects, decreased synthesis of coagulation factors, and increased consumption of coagulation factors.[45]

The hepatic blood supply is derived from the hepatic artery and the portal vein. Increased resistance to blood flow through the portal vein makes hepatocyte oxygenation dependent on hepatic artery blood flow. Because hepatic artery autoregulation is limited, hepatic blood flow depends on arterial blood pressure. Hepatic blood flow decreases during spinal anesthesia to the extent that arterial blood pressure decreases. The incidence and magnitude of postoperative hepatic complications are the same with spinal anesthesia as with general anesthesia in patients who have preexisting liver disease. Neuraxial block has not been demonstrated to represent an advantage or a disadvantage in this patient population. Theoretically, spinal or epidural anesthesia may be used to avoid halothane hepatitis in susceptible patients.

Local anesthetic solutions depend on the liver for metabolism. The plasma half-life of the esters is increased in patients with liver disease as a result of decreased synthesis of pseudocholinesterase. However, because red cell esterase activity is unchanged, local anesthetic systemic toxicity is not significantly increased. Amide metabolism is also altered because of considerable increases in the volume of distribution and half-life and a decrease in the rate of clearance of local anesthetics (Table 23–13). Patients with cirrhosis exhibit accumulations of amides and prolonged systemic effects, including those of local anesthetic systemic toxicity.

Anesthetic Management

Regional anesthetic management of the patient with preexisting liver disease involves correction of clotting abnormalities, maintenance of hepatic perfusion pressure, and close observation for signs and symptoms of local anesthetic systemic toxicity. The predisposition of cirrhotic patients for thrombocytopenia, hypoprothrombinemia, and disseminated intravascular coagulation places these patients at risk for spinal hematoma after neuraxial block. Evidence of a preoperative coagulopathy is a strong contraindication for spinal or epidural anesthesia, because clotting may further deteriorate postoperatively. However, peripheral nerve blocks may be performed safely and are an alternative to general anesthesia in these patients.

Arterial blood pressure should not decrease by more than 20% of baseline to ensure hepatic blood flow and hepatocyte oxygenation. Intravenous replacement of albumin may be valuable in decreasing third-space tissue losses and maintaining blood pressure. Local anesthetic doses and concentrations should be individualized to allow for the impaired clearance and prolonged systemic effects. Supplemental oxygen and judicious administration of sedatives aid in the prevention of systemic local anesthetic reactions.

Renal Disease

Chronic renal failure has many causes, including chronic glomerulonephritis, pyelonephritis, and diabetic nephropathy. The chronic and progressive loss of nephrons results in a decrease in glomerular filtration rate and renal reserve. Patients remain asymptomatic until 60% of the nephrons have ceased to function. Renal insufficiency occurs when only 10% to 40% of

Table 23–13 Lidocaine Disposition in Patients With Preexisting Cardiac, Renal, and Hepatic Disease

DISEASE STATUS	LIDOCAINE DISPOSITION		
	$T_{1/2}$, h	V_{ss}, L/kg	CL, mL/min/kg
Normal	1.8	1.32	10.0
Heart failure	1.9	0.88*	6.3*
Liver cirrhosis	4.9*	2.31*	6.0*
Renal failure	1.3	1.2	13.7

*Significant difference from normal subjects, $P < .05$. CL, clearance rate; $T_{1/2}$, elimination half-life; V_{ss}, volume of distribution.

Data from Thompson P, et al: Ann Intern Med 1973; 78: 499; table from Tucker GT, Mather LE: Properties, absorption, and disposition of local anesthetic agents. In Cousins MJ, Bridenbaugh PO (eds): Neural Blockade in Clinical Anesthesia and Management of Pain, 2nd ed, pp 47–110. Philadelphia, JB Lippincott, 1988.

nephrons are functioning. The loss of more than 90% of functioning nephrons results in uremia and renal failure.

Patients with renal failure often have associated medical conditions such as fluid and electrolyte imbalances, metabolic acidosis, chronic anemia, and coagulopathies. Although hypocalcemia, hyperphosphatemia, and hypermagnesemia occur in patients with renal failure, hyperkalemia is the most serious electrolyte abnormality. Cardiac conduction abnormalities accompanying hyperkalemia may lead to complete heart block or to ventricular fibrillation. Elective surgery should be postponed unless the plasma potassium concentration is less than 5.5 mEq/L.[46]

The loss of functioning nephrons decreases the kidney's ability to excrete hydrogen ions and results in a metabolic acidosis. Acidosis decreases myocardial contractility and responsiveness to catecholamines, although little clinical effect is noticed until the pH is below 7.2. Chronic anemia is a well-recognized complication of renal failure and is a result of decreased renal production of erythropoietin. Increased cardiac output and a shift in the oxyhemoglobin dissociation curve to the right compensate for the reduced oxygen-carrying capacity produced by chronic hemoglobin concentrations of 5 to 8 g/dL. Activation of the renin-angiotensin-aldosterone system and intravascular volume expansion result in hypertension in more than 80% of patients with end-stage renal disease and are risk factors for the development of stroke, myocardial infarction, and congestive heart failure. Patients with renal failure exhibit a qualitative platelet dysfunction induced by chronic uremia and the presence of a defective von Willebrand factor. The coagulopathy is not consistently improved with dialysis, but it has been treated successfully with desmopressin or cryoprecipitate. Chronic uremia also affects the central and peripheral nervous systems. Altered permeability of the blood-brain barrier exaggerates the effects of even small amounts of opioids and other central nervous system depressants. A sensory-motor polyneuropathy may develop, theoretically predisposing these patients to peripheral nerve injury after regional anesthesia, although this remains speculative.

Renal blood flow is autoregulated (much like cerebral blood flow) and maintained through a wide range in arterial blood pressures. Renal blood flow remains constant between mean arterial pressures ranging from 50 to 150 mm Hg. Activation of the sympathetic nervous system produces renal artery vasoconstriction and decreased renal blood flow despite maintenance of renal perfusion pressure within the autoregulated range. In the absence of renal artery vasoconstriction, renal blood flow and urine output are unaffected by neuraxial block, if the arterial blood pressure is maintained within autoregulatory limits. However, when spinal or epidural anesthesia is associated with significant hypotension, decreases in renal blood flow and urine output occur. Further compromise in renal blood flow may result from sympathetic nervous system stimulation and release of catecholamines.

The systemic disposition of local anesthetic solutions is not significantly altered by the presence of chronic renal failure (see Table 23–13). Ester hydrolysis is prolonged proportionately to the blood urea nitrogen value, apparently as a result of decreased pseudocholinesterase synthesis rather than inactivation or inhibition of the enzyme by uremic serum.[47, 48] Metabolism of the amides is unaffected by renal disease, because these drugs are eliminated almost entirely by the liver. However, in contrast to the parent drugs, polar metabolites may accumulate in patients with decreased renal function, although resulting plasma concentrations are not likely to cause systemic reactions.

Outcome Studies

Brachial plexus anesthesia is often used for the placement of a vascular shunt for chronic hemodialysis. Johnson and coworkers[49] studied the effect of anesthetic technique on morbidity and mortality in arteriovenous fistula placement in 469 dialysis-dependent patients. Preoperative anesthetic risk factors included hypertension (92%), coronary artery disease (86%), and previous myocardial infarction (42%). Local anesthesia was used in 54%, brachial plexus block in 33%, and general anesthesia in 13% of cases. A nonfatal perioperative cardiac complication (arrest or myocardial infarction) occurred in 1.5% of patients, and 2.1% of patients experienced a fatal cardiac event. Increased age and previous myocardial infarction were associated with an adverse outcome. However, the anesthetic technique was not a significant risk factor for increased postoperative morbidity and mortality.

Anesthetic Management

Intraoperative preservation of renal function in patients with renal insufficiency or renal failure depends on rational replacement of fluid and electrolytes and maintenance of adequate renal perfusion pressure. Patients with renal insufficiency require careful perioperative fluid management to maintain urine output. The balance between excessive and insufficient fluid administration in anuric patients is even more difficult. Patients with severe renal dysfunction are typically dialyzed before elective surgical procedures and arrive in the operating room with a contracted extracellular volume. Preoperative infusion of a balanced salt solution may be required to avoid hypotension associated with neuraxial block. Lactated Ringer's solution or other potassium-containing fluid should not be administered to dialysis-dependent patients. Noninvasive operations, such as placement of a vascular shunt for hemodialysis, require replacement of only insensible losses, but more extensive procedures may be associated with the loss of intravascular fluid to the interstitial space and with surgical blood loss. Blood transfusion may be necessary to increase oxygen-carrying capacity. Coagulation abnormalities should be evaluated before regional anesthesia is initiated.

Caution is advised in the administration of intraoperative sedatives. Uremia-induced disruption of the blood-brain barrier may intensify central nervous system effects of opioids and cause hypoventilation. Metabolic acidosis alone or combined with respiratory acidosis decreases the seizure threshold for local anesthetics. Patients with a preexisting peripheral neuropathy may be at increased risk for neurologic complications associated with regional anesthesia, although this is speculative. Continuation of supplemental oxygen postoperatively is recommended if the patient has significant anemia.

Disorders of Coagulation

Spinal hematoma is a rare and potentially catastrophic complication of spinal or epidural anesthesia. The actual incidence of neurologic dysfunction resulting from hemorrhagic complications associated with neuraxial block is unknown, but the incidence is probably less than 1 in 10,000 procedures.[50] Hemorrhage into the spinal canal most commonly occurs in the epidural space because of the prominent epidural venous plexus.

Although hemorrhagic complications can occur after virtually all regional anesthetic techniques, bleeding into the spinal canal is perhaps the most serious hemorrhagic complication associated with regional anesthesia because the spinal canal is a concealed and nonexpandable space. Spinal cord compression from spinal hematoma may result in neurologic ischemia and paraplegia. Spinal hematoma may result from vascular trauma caused by needle or catheter placement into the subarachnoid or epidural space. It also may be associated with neoplastic disease or preexisting vascular abnormalities. Of special interest to the anesthesiologist are the spinal hematomas that occur spontaneously, with or without antiplatelet or anticoagulation therapy. More than 100 spontaneous epidural hematomas have been reported, 25% of which were associated with anticoagulation therapy.[51]

In a review of the literature, Owens and colleagues[52] reported 34 cases of spinal hematoma after lumbar puncture, six of which involved the administration of an anesthetic. Fourteen of the patients had received anticoagulants, although only two patients were given anticoagulants before needle placement. Another two patients were treated with antiplatelet medications immediately before or after lumbar puncture. Eleven patients had evidence of coagulopathy or significant thrombocytopenia. In 27 (79%) of the 34 patients, the spinal hematomas associated with lumbar puncture occurred in patients with evidence of hemostatic abnormality.

To decrease the risk of spinal hematoma associated with neuraxial block, it is necessary to understand the mechanisms of blood coagulation, the pharmacologic properties of the anticoagulant and antiplatelet medications, and the clinical studies involving patients undergoing neuraxial block while receiving these medications. Although this section focuses mainly on neuraxial block and anticoagulants, the same principles apply to all regional anesthetic techniques.

Heparin Given Intravenously

Heparin is a complex polysaccharide that exerts its anticoagulant effect by accelerating the inhibition of activated coagulation factors by antithrombin III. There are at least six activated clotting factors that are inhibited by antithrombin III: thrombin; factors XIIa, XIa, Xa, and IXa; and kallikrein.[53] Heparin also potentiates the action of activated factor X inhibitors (anti-Xa).[54] The key position of factor X in the coagulation cascade enables it to generate thrombin through the intrinsic or extrinsic pathway (Fig. 23–1). Inhibitors of this enzyme's activation prevent thrombin formation.

Five minutes after intravenous injection of 10,000 U of heparin, coagulation time is prolonged two to four times the control level. Heparin has a half-life in circulating blood of 1.5 to 2 h.[53] Patients with acute thromboembolic disease may clear heparin even more rapidly. Within 4 to 6 h of the administration of a therapeutic dose of heparin, its effect has ceased. Intravenously administered heparin can be neutralized promptly by protamine.

In perhaps the most important study evaluating the safety of systemic heparinization and neuraxial block, Rao and El-Etr[55] reported 3164 patients who had continuous epidural anesthesia and 847 patients who had continuous spinal anesthesia for lower extremity vascular procedures. Patients with preexisting coagulation abnormalities, thrombocytopenia, or preoperative anticoagulation therapy were excluded. All catheters were placed through a 17-G Tuohy needle. In four patients, after insertion of the needle into the epidural space, blood was freely aspirated. The needle was withdrawn, and the patients were given general anesthesia the next day. Heparin was administered 50 to 60 min after catheter placement to maintain the activated clotting time at twice the baseline value. The heparin dose was repeated every 6 h after measurement of the activated clotting time throughout the period of anticoagulation therapy.

The catheters were removed the next day, 1 h before administration of the maintenance dose of heparin. No patient had signs or symptoms of epidural or subarachnoid hematoma, including the four patients who had traumatic needle placement and subsequently received a general anesthetic. Although the patients in this study safely underwent placement of indwelling epidural or spinal catheters followed by systemic heparinization, the heparin activity was closely monitored and the indwelling catheters were removed at a time when circulating heparin levels were relatively low. There also were no neurologic sequelae reported by Mathews and Abrams[56] in 40 cardiac surgical patients who received morphine intrathecally through a 20- to 25-G needle 50 min before complete heparinization and cardiopulmonary bypass.

Although the two previous studies suggest that neuraxial block followed by heparinization can be

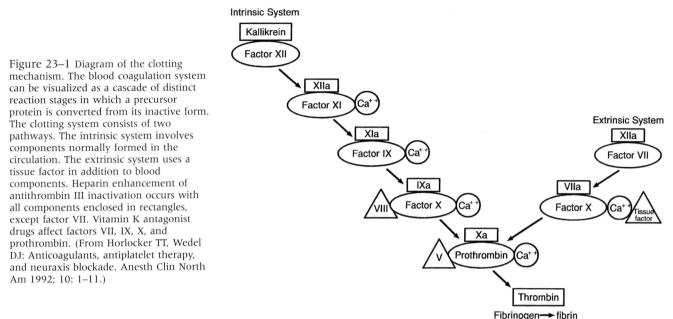

Figure 23–1 Diagram of the clotting mechanism. The blood coagulation system can be visualized as a cascade of distinct reaction stages in which a precursor protein is converted from its inactive form. The clotting system consists of two pathways. The intrinsic system involves components normally formed in the circulation. The extrinsic system uses a tissue factor in addition to blood components. Heparin enhancement of antithrombin III inactivation occurs with all components enclosed in rectangles, except factor VII. Vitamin K antagonist drugs affect factors VII, IX, X, and prothrombin. (From Horlocker TT, Wedel DJ: Anticoagulants, antiplatelet therapy, and neuraxis blockade. Anesth Clin North Am 1992; 10: 1–11.)

safely conducted, Ruff and Dougherty[57] reported spinal hematomas in 7 (2%) of 342 patients who underwent a diagnostic lumbar puncture with a 20-G needle. The patients presented with signs of cerebral ischemia, and after subarachnoid hemorrhage was eliminated as a possibility, the patients had anticoagulation therapy with intravenously administered heparin. The amount of heparin used and coagulation studies were not reported. Patients were followed neurologically. Paraparesis developed in five patients. There were also 18 patients with severe or radicular back pain lasting more than 48 h. Seven of these patients subsequently died of unrelated causes, and at autopsy, one patient had findings of chronic epidural hematoma and another showed an organized subdural hematoma. The researchers identified traumatic needle placement, initiation of anticoagulation within 1 h of lumbar puncture, and concomitant aspirin therapy as being risk factors in the development of spinal hematoma in patients who have received anticoagulation therapy.

The conflicting results of these studies and the rarity of this complication make it difficult to assess the relative risk and contributing variables for spinal hematoma associated with neuraxial block in patients who have received anticoagulation therapy. However, the factors contributing to increased risk in these patients appear to be preexisting coagulopathy or thrombocytopenia, concomitant aspirin therapy, traumatic or difficult needle placement, heparinization within 1 h of spinal or epidural puncture, and absence of monitoring the anticoagulant activity.[52, 55, 56]

Heparin Given Subcutaneously

Therapeutic use of subcutaneously administered low-dose heparin (5000 U every 8 to 12 h) is based on heparin-mediated inhibition of activated factor X. The inhibition of small amounts of activated factor X prevents amplification of the coagulation cascade (see Fig. 23–1). Smaller doses of heparin are therefore required when it is administered as prophylaxis rather than as treatment for thromboembolic disease. After intramuscular or subcutaneous injection of 5000 U of heparin, the maximum anticoagulation effect is observed in 40 to 50 min, and the system usually returns to baseline within 4 to 6 h.[58] The activated partial thromboplastin time may remain in the normal range and often is not monitored.[59] However, wide variations in individual patient responses to subcutaneous injection of heparin have been reported.[60]

The wide variation in response to subcutaneous injection of low-dose heparin makes it difficult to formulate a generalized recommendation regarding neuraxial block in these patients. Lowson and Goodchild[61] and Allemann and associates[62] reported no cases of spinal hematoma in a combined total of 204 epidural and 119 spinal anesthesias performed on patients who had received 5000 U of unfractionated heparin subcutaneously 2 h before needle placement. Spinal hematoma in patients who receive regional anesthesia in combination with low-dose heparin is extremely rare; there are only three reported cases in the literature.[63–65]

Low-Molecular-Weight Heparin

Unfractionated heparin is a heterogeneous mixture of polysaccharide chains that can be separated into fragments of various molecular weights. Because each low-molecular-weight heparin fractionation contains heparins of different molecular weights, each must be evaluated as a specific pharmacologic substance. Several low-molecular-weight heparin preparations (Fraxiparin, Fragmin, Logiparin, Sandoz) are in clinical use in Europe, but it remains in investigational status in the United States. Low-molecular-weight heparin exhibits a dose-dependent antithrombotic effect that is most accurately assessed by measuring the anti-Xa activity level. The advantages of low-molecular-weight heparin over unfractionated heparin include a higher and more predictable bioavailability after subcutaneous administration; a longer biologic half-life, which makes one injection per day sufficient; and a smaller impact on platelet function.[66]

In a review of the literature, Bergqvist and colleagues[67] identified 44 articles on low-molecular-weight heparin for thromboprophylaxis. If the studies in which the mode of anesthesia was described are combined, low-molecular-weight heparin was administered in conjunction with spinal or epidural anesthesia in 9013 patients. There are no reported cases of spinal hematoma with neurologic dysfunction in these patients. Although the actual number of patients who have received low-molecular-weight heparin in combination with neuraxial block is unknown, pharmaceutical companies estimate it to be at least 1,000,000 patients.[67] One case of spinal hematoma in a patient receiving low-molecular-weight heparin who underwent epidural catheter placement has been reported in the European literature. The patient had minimal bleeding during insertion of the catheter, and 3 h later, after the third injection of low-molecular-weight heparin, irreversible paraplegia developed. An epidural hematoma extending from T-9 to L-4 was evacuated without neurologic improvement.[68]

In April 1995, the package insert for Lovenox (enoxaparin sodium) was revised to include a warning that the drug be used with "extreme caution" in patients with indwelling intrathecal or epidural catheters.

Orally Administered Anticoagulants

Orally administered anticoagulants, including warfarin, exert their anticoagulant effect indirectly by interfering with the synthesis of the vitamin K-dependent clotting factors (VII, IX, X, and thrombin). The effects of warfarin are not apparent until a significant amount of biologically inactive factors is synthesized. Because factor VII has a relatively short half-life (6 to 8 h), the prothrombin time may be prolonged into the therapeutic range (1.5 to 2 times normal) in 24 to 36 h. However, because factor VII participates only in the extrinsic pathway, adequate anticoagulation is not achieved until the levels of biologically active factors II and X are sufficiently depressed, which requires 4 to 6 d because of their longer half-lives[53] (see Fig. 23–1). With initial high loading doses of warfarin (15 to 30 mg) for the first 2 to 3 d of therapy, the desired anticoagulant effect is achieved within 48 to 72 h.[54] Similarly, the anticoagulant effects persist for 4 to 6 d after termination of therapy, while new biologically active vitamin K factors are synthesized. In an emergent situation, the anticoagulant effects can be reversed by transfusing fresh frozen plasma and giving vitamin K injections.

Few data exist regarding the risk of spinal hematoma in patients with indwelling spinal or epidural catheters who subsequently receive anticoagulation therapy with warfarin. Odoom and Sih[69] performed 1000 continuous lumbar epidural anesthesia procedures in 950 patients undergoing vascular procedures who preoperatively received anticoagulants orally. The thrombotest, a test measuring factor IX activity, result was decreased and the activated partial thromboplastin time was prolonged in all patients before needle placement. Epidural catheters remained in place for 48 h postoperatively. The coagulation status at catheter removal was not described. There were no neurologic complications. Although the results of this study are reassuring, the obsolescence of the thrombotest as a measure of anticoagulation and the unknown coagulation status of the patients at catheter removal limit their usefulness.

The use of an indwelling epidural or intrathecal catheter and the timing of its removal in an anticoagulated patient are also controversial. Although the trauma of needle placement occurs with single injection and continuous-catheter techniques, the presence of an indwelling catheter could theoretically provoke additional injury to tissue and vascular structures. There were no reported spinal hematomas in 192 patients receiving postoperative epidural analgesia in conjunction with low-dose warfarin after total knee arthroplasty.[70] Patients received warfarin to prolong the prothrombin time to 15.0 to 17.3 s (normal, 10.9 to 12.8 s). Epidural catheters were left indwelling 37 ± 15 h (range, 13 to 96 h). Mean prothrombin time at epidural catheter removal was 13.4 ± 2 s (range, 10.6 to 25.8 s). This small sample begins to document the relative safety of low-dose warfarin anticoagulation in patients with an indwelling epidural catheter. However, there was great variability in the patient response to warfarin, and the researchers[70] recommended close monitoring of coagulation status to avoid excessive prolongation of the prothrombin time.

Thrombolytic Therapy

Thrombolytic agents actively dissolve fibrin clots that have already formed. Exogenous plasminogen activators, such as streptokinase and urokinase, dissolve the thrombus and affect circulating plasminogen, leading to decreased levels of plasminogen and fibrin. Recombinant tissue-type plasminogen activator, an endogenous agent, is more selective for fibrin and has less effect on circulating plasminogen levels.[71] Clot lysis leads to increased concentrations of fibrin degradation products, which themselves have an anticoagulant effect by inhibiting platelet aggregation. In addition to the fibrinolytic agent, these patients frequently receive heparin intravenously to maintain an activated partial thromboplastin time of 1.5 to 2 times normal.[72]

In a study[72] involving 290 patients with acute myocardial infarction who were treated with thrombolytic therapy using streptokinase or recombinant tissue-type plasminogen activator and subsequently with heparin therapy, fibrinogen and plasminogen were maximally depressed at 5 h after thrombolytic therapy and remained significantly depressed at 27 h. Hemorrhagic events occurred in 33% of the patients who received recombinant tissue-type plasminogen activator and 31% of the patients who received streptokinase. For more than 70% of the patients with hemorrhagic events in each group, the primary bleeding site was the catheterization or other puncture site. The researchers[72] recommended avoiding invasive procedures in patients receiving thrombolytic therapy.

Even though epidural or spinal needle and catheter placement with subsequent heparinization appears relatively safe, the risk of spinal hematoma in patients who receive thrombolytic therapy is less well defined. Two cases of spinal hematoma in patients with indwelling epidural catheters who received thrombolytic agents have been reported in the literature. Dickman and coworkers[73] reported a case in which a patient with femoral artery occlusion received an epidural anesthetic for surgical placement of an intra-arterial catheter for infusion of urokinase. Three hours postoperatively, the patient complained of back pain, which progressed to paraplegia despite discontinuation of the urokinase infusion. An emergency decompressive laminectomy was performed, and a large, solidified hematoma compressing the thecal sac was evacuated. The patient recovered full neurologic function within 3 d.

Onishchuk and Carlsson[74] reported a patient with superficial femoral artery occlusion who underwent epidural catheter placement for femoral-popliteal artery bypass. Blood was seen in the epidural catheter during placement. The patient received a bolus of 6300 U of heparin 90 min later, and a single bolus of urokinase was also injected intra-arterially during the surgical procedure. A heparin infusion of 1000 U/h was initiated and continued postoperatively for 24 h. The patient was taken to the recovery room and the epidural catheter was removed. On the fourth postoperative day, paraplegia developed. A magnetic resonance image revealed an epidural hematoma extending from T-10 to L-2. An emergency decompressive laminectomy was performed but produced no improvement. The researchers recommended that epidural anesthesia be avoided in patients who will receive thrombolytic therapy.

Antiplatelet Therapy

Antiplatelet therapy, including medications such as aspirin, naproxen, piroxicam, and dipyridamole, has been theorized to be a relative contraindication to neuraxial block by some researchers because of the associated prolongation of the bleeding time and theoretically greater risk of spinal hematoma formation.

Antiplatelet medications inhibit platelet cyclooxygenase and prevent the synthesis of thromboxane A_2. Thromboxane A_2 is a potent vasoconstrictor and facilitates secondary platelet aggregation and release reactions. Platelets from patients who have been taking these medications have normal platelet adherence to subendothelium and normal primary hemostatic plug formation. An adequate, although potentially fragile, clot may form. Although such plugs may be satisfactory hemostatic barriers for smaller vascular lesions, they may not ensure adequate perioperative hemostatic clot formation.

It has been suggested that the Ivy bleeding time is the most reliable predictor of abnormal bleeding in patients receiving antiplatelet drugs.[75] However, the "post-aspirin" bleeding time is not a reliable indicator of platelet function.[76, 77] Although the bleeding time may normalize within 3 d after aspirin ingestion, platelet function as measured by platelet response to adenosine diphosphate, epinephrine, and collagen may take as long as 1 wk to return to normal. There is no evidence to suggest that bleeding time can predict hemostatic compromise; studies[77, 78] have failed to show a correlation between aspirin-induced prolongation of the bleeding time and surgical blood loss. Measurement of an Ivy bleeding time before induction of spinal or epidural anesthesia may not identify the patients at increased risk for hemorrhagic complications and is clinically not indicated. Other nonsteroidal analgesics, such as naproxen, piroxicam, and ibuprofen, produce a short-term defect that normalizes within 3 d.[79] Platelet function in patients receiving antiplatelet medications should be assumed to be decreased for 1 wk with aspirin and 3 to 5 d with other nonsteroidal antiinflammatory drugs. Special platelet function assays are also available to monitor platelet aggregation and degranulation.

There has been one reported case of spontaneous epidural hematoma formation in the absence of spinal or epidural anesthesia in a patient with a history of aspirin ingestion.[80] The patient self-administered 1500 mg of aspirin in the form of an aspirin-containing antacid and a short time later complained of severe lower extremity weakness. A myelogram revealed complete epidural block at the T5-6 level. The cerebrospinal fluid was clear, although prolonged bleeding from the lumbar puncture site was observed after myelography. A laminectomy was performed, and the hematoma was removed. Neurologic function gradually improved.

The risk associated with administration of spinal or epidural anesthetics to a patient receiving antiplatelet medications remains controversial. Owens and colleagues[52] implicated antiplatelet therapy in 2 of the 34 cases of spinal hematoma occurring after attempted lumbar puncture. Horlocker and associates[81] retrospectively reported 1013 cases of spinal and epidural anesthesia in which antiplatelet drugs were taken by 39% of the patients, including 11% of patients who received multiple antiplatelet medications. Although no patient had signs of spinal hematoma, patients receiving antiplatelet medications showed a higher incidence of blood aspirated through the spinal or epidural needle or catheter.

This study was subsequently performed prospectively on an additional 1000 patients, 39% of whom reported preoperative antiplatelet therapy.[82] There were no spinal hematomas. Blood was seen during needle or catheter placement in 22% of patients, including 7% of patients with frank blood. Preoperative antiplatelet therapy was not a risk factor for bloody needle or catheter placement. However, many patient and anesthetic variables, including female sex, increased age, a history of excessive bruising or bleeding, continuous catheter technique, large-gauge needle, multiple needle passes, and difficult needle placement, were significant risk factors. The lack of correlation between antiplatelet medications and bloody needle or catheter placement (producing clinically insignificant collections of blood within the spinal canal) is strong evidence that preoperative antiplatelet therapy is not a significant risk factor for the development of neurologic dysfunction from spinal hematoma in patients who undergo spinal or epidural anesthesia while receiving these medications.

Anesthetic Management

The decision to perform neuraxial block on a patient receiving thrombolytic, anticoagulant, or antiplatelet medications should be made on an individual basis, weighing the small but definite risk of spinal hematoma with the benefits of regional anesthesia. Preoperatively, the patient's history should be reviewed for medical conditions associated with bleeding tendencies such as preeclampsia, severe liver disease, or recent chemotherapy, and the patient should be questioned about previous episodes of sustained bleeding after trauma or surgery. Because patients react to anticoagulants with different sensitivities, it may be useful to verify reversal of heparin or warfarin effects before performance of spinal or epidural block (Table 23–14).

The following statements, based on the pharmacology of anticoagulant, thrombolytic, and antiplatelet drugs as well as case reports and clinical studies involving patients undergoing neuraxial block while receiving these medications, can guide the clinician faced with this difficult decision.[83]

Except in extraordinary circumstances, the risk of spinal hematoma outweighs the potential benefits of neuraxial block in patients who have known coagulopathies or significant thrombocytopenia or who have received thrombolytic therapy within the previous 24 h. Although the data by Odoom and Sih[69] are reassuring, neuraxial block should also probably be avoided in patients who have had full anticoagulant therapy. Patients who have received only one or two doses of an orally administered anticoagulant (e.g., 5 to 10 mg warfarin) generally do not have an increased prothrombin time and may safely undergo regional anesthesia. Prothrombin time may be measured before needle placement.

Patients who have had full anticoagulant therapy with a continuous heparin infusion should have the infusion discontinued 4 to 6 h before needle or catheter placement, unless early normalization is verified by activated partial thromboplastin time. Although the anticoagulant effect of heparin given subcutaneously is typically less significant than that of heparin given intravenously, ideally, low-dose heparin given subcutaneously should also not be administered within 4 to 6 h of a spinal or epidural anesthetic to allow for normalization of the heparin effect.

Epidural or spinal anesthesia followed by systemic anticoagulation therapy with heparin or warfarin is probably safe, provided adequate precautions are taken.[55, 56, 70] Heparinization should not be initiated for at least 1 h after needle placement.[55-57] If needle placement is traumatic or difficult, the decision to proceed with surgery should be reevaluated.[55, 57] Patients receiving antiplatelet medications who will undergo subsequent heparinization appear to be at increased risk for spinal hematoma and should be followed closely.[57] The

Table 23–14 Pharmacologic Activities of Anticoagulants and Nonsteroidal Antiinflammatory Drugs

AGENT	EFFECT ON COAGULATION VARIABLES		TIME TO PEAK EFFECT	TIME TO NORMAL HEMOSTASIS AFTER THERAPY	COMMENTS
	PT	APTT			
Heparin					
Intravenous	↑	↑ ↑ ↑	Minutes	4–6 h	Monitor ACT, APTT; delay heparinization for 1 h after needle placement
Subcutaneous	↑	↑ ↑	40–50 min	4–6 h	APTT may remain normal; monitor anti-Xa activity
Warfarin	↑ ↑ ↑	↑	4–6 d (3 d with loading dose)	4–6 d	Monitor PT
Aspirin	—	—	Hours	7 d	Bleeding time not reliable predictor of platelet function
Other NSAIDs	—	—	Hours	1–4 d	Bleeding time not reliable predictor of platelet function
Thrombolytic agent	↑	↑	Minutes	1–2 d	Usually heparinized in addition; monitor closely

ACT, activated clotting time; APTT, activated partial thromboplastin time; NSAID, nonsteroidal antiinflammatory drug; PT, prothrombin time; ↑, clinically insignificant increase; ↑ ↑, possibly clinically significant increase; ↑ ↑ ↑, clinically significant increase.
Adapted from Horlocker TT: Central neural blockade for patients receiving anticoagulants. Clin Anesth Updates 1994; 5: 1–9.

activated partial thromboplastin time and prothrombin time should be monitored carefully to avoid excessive anticoagulation therapy.[55, 70]

Few data exist on the timing of spinal or epidural catheter removal in a patient who has had anticoagulant therapy. The most conservative practice is to remove an indwelling catheter under the same conditions in which placement is considered safe. Removal of an indwelling epidural catheter in a patient receiving heparin intravenously or subcutaneously should ideally occur 4 to 6 h after the last heparin dose, and anticoagulation should not be reinstituted for at least 1 h after catheter removal. In a patient with a perioperative coagulopathy such as diffuse intravascular coagulation or dilutional thrombocytopenia, every attempt should be made to normalize the coagulation status before catheter removal. If the coagulation defect is expected to be prolonged, the decision about when to remove the indwelling catheter should be made on an individual basis, taking into account the evolving coagulation status of the patient during the perioperative period.

Epidural and spinal anesthesia can be safely performed in a patient receiving antiplatelet therapy.[81, 82] Even though the platelet defect of most antiplatelet medications reverses in 3 to 5 d, the defect produced by aspirin is present for 1 wk.

Needle and catheter placement during neuraxial block should be as atraumatic as possible. Small-gauge needles and the midline approach may help decrease needle trauma; a paramedian or lateral approach may increase the risk of venous puncture. Epidural catheters should not be inserted more than 3 to 4 cm into the epidural space to minimize trauma to the epidural venous structures.

Short-acting local anesthetics should be used in patients at increased risk of spinal hematoma to allow their neurologic status to be evaluated immediately postoperatively. Likewise, an epidural block should be allowed to regress sufficiently to allow neurologic evaluation before initiating a continuous local anesthetic infusion for postoperative analgesia. A narcotic, rather than local anesthetic infusion, allows continuous monitoring of neurologic function and may be a more prudent choice in high-risk patients.

The patient should be monitored closely in the perioperative period for early signs of cord compression. If spinal hematoma is suspected, the treatment of choice is immediate decompressive laminectomy. Recovery is unlikely if surgical treatment is postponed for more than 12 h; only 45% of the patients in the series reported by Owens and colleagues[52] had partial or good recovery of neurologic function.

Neurologic Disease

Patients with preexisting neurologic disease present a unique challenge to the anesthesiologist. The cause of postoperative neurologic deficits is difficult to evaluate, because neural injury may occur as a result of surgical trauma, tourniquet pressure, prolonged labor, improper patient positioning, or anesthetic technique. Progressive neurologic diseases such as multiple sclerosis may coincidentally worsen perioperatively, independent of the anesthetic method. The most conservative legal approach is to avoid regional anesthesia in these patients. However, high-risk patients, including those with significant cardiopulmonary disease, may benefit medically from regional anesthesia and analgesia. The decision to proceed with a regional anesthesia in these patients should be made on a case-by-case basis. Meticulous regional anesthetic technique should be observed to minimize further neurologic injury.

Intracranial Tumors, Aneurysms, and Arteriovenous Malformations

Patients with preexisting intracranial masses and vascular lesions such as primary or metastatic brain tumors, saccular aneurysms, or arteriovenous malformations are at increased risk for neurologic compromise during spinal or epidural anesthesia. Alterations in intracranial pressure and mean arterial pressure associated with neuraxial block may result in subarachnoid hemorrhage, cerebral infarction, or cerebral herniation. Dural puncture is not recommended in patients with evidence of increased intracranial pressure such as cerebral edema, lateral shift of the midline structures, and obliteration of the fourth ventricle.[84] In patients with increased intracranial pressure, dural puncture causes an acute leakage of cerebrospinal fluid which decreases cerebrospinal fluid pressure and may produce cerebellar herniation. In patients with uncorrected vascular malformations, the decreased cerebrospinal fluid pressure increases the aneurysmal transmural pressure (mean arterial pressure-intracranial pressure) gradient and may result in subarachnoid hemorrhage.

Rupture of an occult arteriovenous malformation coincident with dural puncture during attempted epidural anesthesia has been reported.[85] Epidural and caudal anesthesia are also contraindicated in patients with increased intracranial pressure because of the risk of accidental dural puncture and because the intracranial pressure may be further increased by injection of local anesthetic solution into the epidural space. Patients with surgically repaired vascular malformations may undergo spinal or epidural anesthesia without increased risk of neurologic complications.

Epilepsy

Epilepsy is a recurrent seizure disorder that affects 0.5% to 1% of the population. Idiopathic epilepsy typically begins in childhood, but adult-onset seizure disorders represent intracranial pathologic conditions such as neoplasm, trauma, infection, or stroke. Seizure activity results from synchronous discharge of a group of neurons in the cerebral cortex. The neuronal hyperactivity may remain localized or may propagate to the thalamus and across to the contralateral hemisphere, resulting in generalized seizures. Epilepsy is treated with anticonvulsant medications; the choice of drug is determined primarily by the classification of the seizure disorder.

Central nervous system toxicity is a known complication of regional anesthesia. Most local anesthetic effects are believed to be dose-related, but a dichotomy of these effects on the brain is well documented. At low blood levels, local anesthetics are potent anticonvulsants, but at high levels, they act as convulsants.[86, 87] Intravenous infusion of lidocaine at 4 to 6 mg/kg in human volunteers produced initial depression of the electroencephalogram, with a slowing down or a decrease in the amplitude of the alpha waves. Higher doses of lidocaine (7 to 9 mg/kg) induced tonic-clonic convulsions and spike waves. After convulsions ceased, no electrical activity was found for 10 to 20 s, raising the possibility of neuronal hypoxia secondary to convulsive activity.[87] However, a subsequent study reported lidocaine-induced seizures resulted in only small increases in cerebral blood flow and metabolism, unlike the seizures associated with epilepsy.[86]

The initial state of central nervous system excitation elicited by local anesthetic agents is produced by a selective block of the inhibitory pathways in the cerebral cortex. Activity of the unopposed excitatory neurons leads to convulsions. Eventually, the inhibitory and excitatory pathways are blocked, resulting in generalized central nervous system depression. The central nervous system toxicity of specific local anesthetic solutions is primarily related to anesthetic potency, but it is also affected by rate of biotransformation and penetrability through the blood-brain barrier. The acid-base status of the patient also profoundly affects the central nervous system toxicity of local anesthetics. Hypercapnia and acidosis may decrease the convulsive threshold by 50%.

Many regional anesthetic techniques may be safely performed in patients with seizure disorders. Anesthetic management in the patient with epilepsy includes consideration of the cause and treatment of the seizure disorder as well as physiologic factors affecting local anesthetic central nervous system toxicity. Anticonvulsant medications should be identified. Measurement of serum anticonvulsant levels is useful to assess adequacy of treatment. Selection of a less potent and therefore less toxic local anesthetic is recommended. Local anesthetic blood levels should be minimized through the use of an appropriate dose and concentration of the local anesthetic, addition of vasoconstrictors, and slow and incremental injection (with frequent aspiration) through a short-bevel needle. A continuous catheter may be used if the regional anesthetic technique is associated with rapid uptake of local anesthetic solution, as with epidural or brachial plexus block.

The patient should be continuously monitored for early warning signs of local anesthetic systemic toxicity until the peak plasma concentration is achieved. Even small amounts of local anesthetics injected into the carotid, subclavian, or axillary arteries may result in seizures.[88] Administration of a benzodiazepine, such as midazolam or diazepam, increases the seizure threshold. However, if hypoventilation occurs from oversedation and results in hypercapnia and acidosis, it increases the likelihood of central nervous system side effects. Postoperative infusions must be carefully managed to avoid accumulation of local anesthetic. An opioid rather than a local anesthetic infusion may be a more prudent choice in these patients.

Chronic Disorders of Central and Peripheral Nerves

Patients with preexisting neurologic disorders of the central nervous system, such as multiple sclerosis or amyotrophic lateral sclerosis, and those with disorders of the peripheral nerves, such as lumbar radiculopathy, ancient poliomyelitis, and sensory-motor peripheral neuropathy, present potential management dilemmas for anesthesiologists. The presence of preexisting deficits, signifying chronic neural compromise, theoretically places these patients at increased risk for further neurologic injury. It is difficult to define the actual risk of neurologic complications in patients with preexisting neurologic disorders who receive regional anesthesia; no controlled studies have been performed, and accounts of complications have appeared in the literature as individual case reports. The decision to use regional anesthesia in these patients is determined on a case-by-case basis and involves understanding the pathophysiology of neurologic disorders, the mechanisms of neural injury associated with regional anesthesia, and the overall incidence of neurologic complications after regional techniques.

Neurologic injury directly related to regional anesthesia may be caused by trauma, neurotoxicity, and ischemia. Direct needle- or catheter-induced trauma rarely results in permanent neurologic injury. The overall incidence of persistent paresthesias has been estimated at 0.08% after spinal anesthesia and at 2% after brachial plexus block.[89, 90] It has been suggested that paresthesia techniques may be associated with a higher incidence of neurologic injury after brachial plexus block, but there are no conclusive data supporting that claim.[90, 91]

Needle-bevel configuration may influence the frequency and severity of peripheral nerve damage during regional anesthesia. In an in vitro study, Selander and coworkers[92] demonstrated an increased frequency in perineural injury when a long-beveled needle was used instead of a short-beveled needle. However, severity of neuronal injury was not evaluated. Rice and McMahon[93] assessed frequency and severity of neural trauma after nerve impalement by histologic and clinical methods and reported that injury produced by short-beveled needles was more severe, more frequent, and recovered more slowly than those produced by long-beveled needles. No human studies have been performed to determine which of these in vitro studies accurately predicts clinical outcome. However, these studies illustrate the importance of minimizing direct needle trauma during regional techniques, especially in patients at increased risk for neurologic complications.

Neurologic deficits after regional anesthesia may be a direct result of local anesthetic toxicity. Clinical and laboratory findings indicate that local anesthetic solutions are potentially neurotoxic.[94-96] It is generally agreed that local anesthetics administered in clinically appropriate doses and concentrations do not cause nerve damage.[97] However, prolonged exposure or high concentrations of local anesthetic solutions may result in permanent neurologic deficits. Maldistribution of local anesthetic within the cerebrospinal fluid has been implicated in the development of cauda equina syndrome after continuous spinal anesthesia.[98, 99] Patients with underlying nerve dysfunction may have a decreased requirement for local anesthetic and a decreased threshold for neurotoxicity.[96]

Neural ischemia may occur as a result of systemic or local vascular insufficiency. Systemic hypotension with or without a spinal anesthetic may produce spinal cord ischemia in the watershed areas between radicular vessels, resulting in flaccid paralysis of the lower extremities (anterior spinal artery syndrome). The use of local anesthetic solutions containing epinephrine or phenylephrine theoretically may result in local ischemia, especially in patients with microvascular disease,[100] but clinical data are lacking. Myers and Heckman[95] studied the effect of lidocaine with and without epinephrine on blood flow to nerves. Decreased rates of blood flow to nerves ranged from 19% for 1% lidocaine to 78% for 2% lidocaine with epinephrine. Epinephrine by itself also significantly decreased blood flow. Despite these laboratory results, large clinical studies have failed to identify the use of vasopressors as a risk factor for neurologic injury. Most cases of presumed vasopressor-induced neurologic deficits after spinal anesthesia have been single case reports, often with several other risk factors present.[101]

Although laboratory studies have identified multiple risk factors for the development of neurologic injury after regional anesthesia, clinical studies have not been performed to verify the results. Even less information is available for the variables affecting neurologic damage in patients with preexisting neurologic disease. However, several disorders of the central and peripheral nerves require further mention.

Multiple Sclerosis

Multiple sclerosis is a degenerative disease of the central nervous system, characterized by multiple sites of demyelination in the brain and spinal cord. The peripheral nerves are not involved. The course of the disease consists of exacerbations and remissions of symptoms, and the unpredictability in the patient's changing neurologic status must be appreciated when selecting an anesthetic technique. Stress, surgery, and fatigue have been implicated in the exacerbation of multiple sclerosis. Epidural and, more often, spinal anesthesia have been implicated in the relapse of multiple sclerosis, although the evidence is not strong.[102] The mechanism by which spinal anesthesia may exacerbate multiple sclerosis is unknown, but it may be direct local anesthetic toxicity.

Epidural anesthesia has been recommended over spinal anesthesia because the concentration of local anes-

thetic in the white matter of the spinal cord is one-fourth the level after epidural administration.[103] A dilute solution of local anesthetic with spinal or epidural anesthesia is also advised. Because multiple sclerosis is a disorder of the central nervous system, peripheral nerve blocks do not affect neurologic function and are considered appropriate anesthetic techniques.

Diabetes Mellitus

A substantial proportion of diabetic patients report clinical symptoms of a peripheral neuropathy. However, a subclinical peripheral neuropathy may be present before the onset of pain, paresthesia, or sensory loss and may remain undetected without electrophysiologic testing for slowing of nerve conduction velocity. The presence of underlying nerve dysfunction suggests that patients with diabetes may have a decreased requirement for local anesthetic. The diabetes-associated microangiopathy of nerve blood vessels decreases the rate at which local anesthetic uptake occurs from the site of administration, resulting in prolonged exposure to local anesthetic solutions. The combination of these two mechanisms may cause nerve injury with an otherwise safe dose of local anesthetic in diabetic patients.[104]

In a study examining the effect of local anesthetics on nerve conduction block and injury in diabetic rats, Kalichman and Calcutt[96] reported that the local anesthetic requirement is decreased and the risk of local anesthetic-induced nerve injury is increased in diabetes. These findings support the suggestions that diabetic patients may require less local anesthetic to produce anesthesia and that a reduction in dose may be necessary to prevent neural injury by doses considered safe in nondiabetic patients.

Anesthetic Management of Neurologic Disease

Progressive neurologic disease is considered by some to be a relative contraindication to regional anesthesia because of the difficulty in determining the cause of new neurologic deficits that appear perioperatively. There are no controlled clinical studies identifying regional anesthesia as a significant factor for increased risk of neurologic injury; only anecdotal reports are available. The medicolegal issue, however, remains, and if regional anesthesia is indicated for other preexisting medical conditions or by patient request, the patient should be informed of the risk of neurologic complications, including coincidental progression of preoperative deficits, associated with anesthesia and surgery. This discussion, along with preoperative neurologic status, should be fully documented in the patient's record.

Patients with preoperative neurologic deficits may undergo further nerve damage more readily from needle or catheter placement, local anesthetic systemic toxicity, and vasopressor-induced neural ischemia. Although the use of paresthesia techniques is not contraindicated, care should be taken to minimize needle trauma and intraneuronal injection. Dilute local anesthetic solutions should be used when feasible to decrease the risk of local anesthetic systemic toxicity.

The use of epinephrine-containing solutions is controversial. The potential risk of vasopressor-induced nerve ischemia must be weighed against the advantages of predicting local anesthetic intravascular injections, improved quality of block, and decreased blood levels of local anesthetics. Because epinephrine also prolongs the block and therefore neural exposure to local anesthetics, the appropriate concentration and dose of local anesthetic solutions must be considered. Patients with microvascular disease in combination with an underlying peripheral neuropathy, such as those with diabetes, may be most sensitive to the vasoconstrictive effects of epinephrine.

Efforts should also be made to decrease neural injury in the operating room through careful patient positioning. Postoperatively, these patients must be followed closely to detect potentially treatable sources of neurologic injury, including constrictive dressings, improperly applied casts, and increased pressure on neurologically vulnerable sites. New neurologic deficits should be evaluated promptly by a neurologist to document formally the patient's evolving neurologic status, arrange further testing, and provide long-term follow-up.

Epidural and Spinal Anesthesia After Major Spinal Surgery

Previous spinal surgery has been considered to represent a relative contraindication to the use of regional anesthesia. Many of these patients experience chronic back pain and are reluctant to undergo epidural or spinal anesthesia, fearing exacerbation of their preexisting back complaints. Several postoperative anatomic changes make needle or catheter placement more difficult and complicated after major spinal surgery. In a study[105] of 48 patients with chronic low back pain after spinal fusion, eight showed significant spinal stenosis on computed tomographic scans and required surgical decompression. The ligamentum flava may be injured during surgery, resulting in adhesions within or obliteration of the epidural space. The spread of epidural local anesthetic may be affected by adhesions, producing an incomplete or "patchy" block. Obliteration of the epidural space may increase the incidence of dural puncture and make subsequent placement of an epidural blood patch difficult. Needle placement in an area of the spine that has undergone bone grafting and posterior fusion is not possible with midline or lateral approaches; needle insertion can be accomplished at unfused segments only.

The guidelines for epidural anesthesia after spinal surgery are unclear. Daley and colleagues[106] reviewed the charts of 18 patients with previous Harrington rod instrumentation who underwent 21 attempts at epidural anesthesia for obstetric analgesia. Continuous lumbar epidural anesthesia was successfully established in 20 of 21 attempts, but only 10 procedures were performed easily on the first attempt. The remaining 11 patients required larger amounts of local anesthetics or complained of a patchy block or both. There was no correlation between the level of surgery and the ease of insertion or the quality of epidural anesthesia. There were no side effects except for low back pain in two patients with multiple attempts at catheter placement.

Crosby and Halpern[107] studied nine parturients with previous Harrington rod instrumentation who underwent epidural anesthesia for analgesia during labor and delivery. Five of the nine catheters were successfully placed on the first attempt. Four of the nine procedures were complicated and involved multiple attempts before successful insertion, traumatic catheter placement requiring a second insertion, inadequate epidural analgesia with subsequent dural puncture on a repeated attempt, or an inability to locate the epidural space despite attempts at two levels. Seven of the nine patients obtained satisfactory analgesia. There were no adverse sequelae related to the epidural insertion.

Hubbert[108] described attempted epidural anesthesia in 17 patients with Harrington rod instrumentation. Four of five patients with fusions terminating above the interspace between L-3 and L-4 had successful epidural placement. However, in 12 patients with fusions extending to the interspace between L-5 and S-1, six attempts were unsuccessful, five patients required multiple attempts, and one patient had a dural puncture after multiple attempts before success at epidural placement. A false loss of resistance was reported to have occurred frequently.

No studies have evaluated the complications and quality of spinal anesthesia in patients with previous spinal surgery. However, even though needle placement may be more difficult or traumatic in these patients, the spread of local anesthetic within the subarachnoid space and quality of block should not be affected. A spinal anesthetic may be more desirable after spinal surgery because the technique does not depend on a subjective loss of resistance; it instead has a definite end point: the presence of cerebrospinal fluid. A smaller needle may produce less trauma and decrease the incidence of postoperative low back pain.

Epidural anesthesia may be successfully performed in patients who have had previous spinal surgery, but successful catheter placement may be possible on the first attempt in only 50% of patients, even by an experienced anesthesiologist. Although adequate epidural anesthesia is eventually produced in 40% to 95% of patients, there appears to be a higher incidence of traumatic needle placement, unintentional dural puncture, and unsuccessful epidural needle or catheter placement, especially if spinal fusion extends to between L-5 and S-1. Spinal anesthesia may produce a more reliable block than epidural anesthesia, but this has not been studied. The presence of postoperative spinal stenosis or other degenerative changes in the spine or preexisting neurologic symptoms may make the use of regional anesthesia less effective in these patients.

References

1. Tarhan S, Moffitt EA, Taylor WF, et al: Myocardial infarction after general anesthesia. JAMA 1972; 220: 1451–1454.

2. von Knorring J: Postoperative myocardial infarction: a prospective study in a risk group of surgical patients. Surgery 1981; 90: 55–60.

3. Goldman L, Caldera DL, Southwick FS, et al: Cardiac risk factors and complications in non-cardiac surgery. Medicine (Baltimore) 1978; 57: 357–370.

4. Steen PA, Tinker JH, Tarhan S: Myocardial reinfarction after anesthesia and surgery. JAMA 1978; 239: 2566–2570.

5. Rao TL, Jacobs KH, El-Etr AA: Reinfarction following anesthesia in patients with myocardial infarction. Anesthesiology 1983; 59: 499–505.

6. Yeager MP, Glass DD, Neff RK, et al: Epidural anesthesia and analgesia in high-risk surgical patients. Anesthesiology 1987; 66: 729–736.

7. Tuman KJ, McCarthy RJ, March RJ, et al: Effects of epidural anesthesia and analgesia on coagulation and outcome after major vascular surgery. Anesth Analg 1991; 73: 696–704.

8. Christopherson R, Beattie C, Frank SM, et al: Perioperative morbidity in patients randomized to epidural or general anesthesia for lower extremity vascular surgery. Perioperative Ischemia Randomized Anesthesia Trial Study Group. Anesthesiology 1993; 79: 422–434.

9. Shimosato S, Etsten BE: The role of the venous system in cardiocirculatory dynamics during spinal and epidural anesthesia in man. Anesthesiology 1969; 30: 619–628.

10. Ottesen S: The influence of thoracic epidural analgesia on the circulation at rest and during physical exercise in man. Acta Anaesthesiol Scand 1978; 22: 537–547.

11. Bonica JJ, Berges PU, Morikawa K: Circulatory effects of peridural block. I. Effects of level of analgesia and dose of lidocaine. Anesthesiology 1970; 33: 619–626.

12. Baron JF, Decaux-Jacolot A, Edouard A, et al: Influence of venous return on baroreflex control of heart rate during lumbar epidural anesthesia in humans. Anesthesiology 1986; 64: 188–193.

13. Cousins MJ, Bromage PR: Epidural neural blockade. In Cousins MJ, Bridenbaugh PO (eds): Neural Blockade in Clinical Anesthesia and Management of Pain, 2nd ed, pp 253–360. Philadelphia, JB Lippincott, 1988.

14. Hackel DB, Sancetta SM, Kleinerman J: Effect of hypotension due to spinal anesthesia on coronary blood flow and myocardial metabolism in man. Circulation 1956; 13: 92–97.

15. Saada M, Duval AM, Bonnet F, et al: Abnormalities in myocardial segmental wall motion during lumbar epidural anesthesia. Anesthesiology 1989; 71: 26–32.

16. Brown BG, Lee AB, Bolson EL, et al: Reflex constriction of significant coronary stenosis as a mechanism contributing to ischemic left ventricular dysfunction during isometric exercise. Circulation 1984; 70: 18–24.

17. Blomberg S, Emanuelsson H, Kvist H, et al: Effects of thoracic epidural anesthesia on coronary arteries and arterioles in patients with coronary artery disease. Anesthesiology 1990; 73: 840–847.

18. Blomberg S, Emanuelsson H, Ricksten S-E: Thoracic epidural anesthesia and central hemodynamics in patients with unstable angina pectoris. Anesth Analg 1989; 69: 558–562.

19. O'Keefe JH Jr, Shub C, Rettke SR: Risk of noncardiac surgical procedures in patients with aortic stenosis. Mayo Clin Proc 1989; 64: 400–405.

20. Fink BR: Mechanism of differential epidural block. Anesth Analg 1986; 65: 325–329.

21. Freund FG, Bonica JJ, Ward RJ, et al: Ventilatory reserve and level of motor block during high spinal and epidural anesthesia. Anesthesiology 1967; 28: 834–837.

22. Urmey W, Loring S, Mead J, et al: Upper and lower rib cage deformation during breathing in quadriplegics. J Appl Physiol 1986; 60: 618–622.

23. Eisele J, Trenchard D, Burki N, et al: The effect of chest wall block on respiratory sensation and control in man. Clin Sci 1968; 35: 23–33.

24. Urmey WF, McDonald M: Changes in pulmonary function tests (PFT) during high-dose epidural anesthesia. (Abstract.) Anesthesiology 1990; 73: A1154.

25. Sundberg A, Wattwil M, Arvill A: Respiratory effects of high thoracic epidural anaesthesia. Acta Anaesthesiol Scand 1986; 30: 215–217.

26. Takasaki M, Takahashi T: Respiratory function during cervical and thoracic extradural analgesia in patients with normal lungs. Br J Anaesth 1980; 52: 1271–1276.

27. Bridenbaugh PO, Greene NM: Spinal (subarachnoid) neural blockade. In Cousins MJ, Bridenbaugh PO (eds): Neural Blockade in Clinical Anesthesia and Management of Pain, 2nd ed, pp 213–251. Philadelphia, JB Lippincott, 1988.

28. Egbert LD, Tamersoy K, Deas TC: Pulmonary function during spinal anesthesia: the mechanism of cough depression. Anesthesiology 1961; 22: 882–885.

29. Ciofolo MJ, Clergue F, Seebacher J, et al: Ventilatory effects of laparoscopy under epidural anesthesia. Anesth Analg 1990; 70: 357–361.

30. Fisher J, James ML: Blood gas changes during spinal and epidural analgesia. Anaesthesia 1969; 24: 511–520.

31. Yamakage M, Namiki A, Tsuchida H, et al: Changes in ventilatory pattern and arterial oxygen saturation during spinal anaesthesia in man. Acta Anaesthesiol Scand 1992; 36: 569–571.

32. Ravin MB: Comparison of spinal and general anesthesia for lower abdominal surgery in patients with chronic obstructive pulmonary disease. Anesthesiology 1971; 35: 319–322.

33. Tarhan S, Moffitt EA, Sessler AD, et al: Risk of anesthesia and surgery in patients with chronic bronchitis and chronic obstructive pulmonary disease. Surgery 1973; 74: 720–726.

34. Shaw WM: Paralysis of the phrenic nerve during brachial plexus anesthesia. Anesthesiology 1949; 10: 627–628.

35. Knoblanche GE: The incidence and aetiology of phrenic nerve blockade associated with supraclavicular brachial plexus block. Anaesth Intensive Care 1979; 7: 346–349.

36. Dhuner K-G, Moberg E, Önne L: Paresis of the phrenic nerve during brachial plexus block analgesia and its importance. Acta Chirurg Scand 1955; 109: 53–57.

37. Urmey WF, Talts KH, Sharrock NE: One hundred percent incidence of hemidiaphragmatic paresis associated with interscalene brachial plexus anesthesia as diagnosed by ultrasonography. Anesth Analg 1991; 72: 498–503.

38. Urmey WF, McDonald M: Hemidiaphragmatic paresis during interscalene brachial plexus block: effects on pulmonary function and chest wall mechanics. Anesth Analg 1992; 74: 352–357.

39. Arborelius M Jr, Lilja B, Senyk J: Regional and total lung function studies in patients with hemidiaphragmatic paralysis. Respiration 1975; 32: 253–264.

40. Fackler CD, Perret GE, Bedell GN: Effect of unilateral phrenic nerve section on lung function. J Appl Physiol 1967; 23: 923–926.

41. Gould L, Kaplan S, McElhinney AJ, et al: A method for the production of hemidiaphragmatic paralysis. Its application to the study of lung function in normal man. Am Rev Respir Dis 1967; 96: 812–814.

42. Child CG III, Turcotte JG: The liver and portal hypertension. Major Probl Clin Surg 1964; 1–85.

43. Pugh RN, Murray-Lyon IM, Dawson JL, et al: Transection of the oesophagus for bleeding oesophageal varices. Br J Surg 1973; 60: 646–649.

44. Garrison RN, Cryer HM, Howard DA, et al: Clarification of risk factors for abdominal operations in patients with hepatic cirrhosis. Ann Surg 1984; 199: 648–655.

45. Stoelting RK, Dierdorf SF: Anesthesia and Co-existing Disease, 3rd ed, pp 251–276. New York, Churchill Livingstone, 1993.

46. Stoelting RK, Dierdorf SF: Anesthesia and Co-existing Disease, 3rd ed, pp 289–312. New York, Churchill Livingstone, 1993.

47. Reidenberg MM, James M, Dring LG: The rate of procaine hydrolysis in serum of normal subjects and diseased patients. Clin Pharmacol Ther 1972; 13: 279–284.

48. Calvo R, Carlos R, Erill S: Procaine hydrolysis defect in uraemia does not appear to be due to carbamylation of plasma esterases. Eur J Clin Pharmacol 1983; 24: 533–535.

49. Johnson ME, Solomonson MD, Ilstrup D: Effect of anesthetic technique on morbidity and mortality in arteriovenous fistula creation. (Abstract.) Reg Anesth 1994; 19: S19.

50. Gustafsson H, Rutberg H, Bengtsson M: Spinal haematoma following epidural analgesia. Report of a patient with ankylosing spondylitis and a bleeding diathesis. Anaesthesia 1988; 43: 220–222.

51. Spurny OM, Rubin S, Wolff JW, et al: Spinal epidural hematoma during anticoagulant therapy. Arch Intern Med 1964; 114: 103–107.

52. Owens EL, Kasten GW, Hessel EA II: Spinal subarachnoid hematoma after lumbar puncture and heparinization: a case report, review of the literature, and discussion of anesthetic implications. Anesth Analg 1986; 65: 1201–1207.

53. Joist JH, Sherman LA (eds): Venous and Arterial Thrombosis: Pathogenesis, Diagnosis, Prevention, and Therapy, pp 159–172. New York, Grune & Stratton, 1979.

54. Linn BJ, Mazza JJ, Friedenberg WR: Treatment of venous thromboembolic disease. A pragmatic approach to anticoagulation and thrombolysis. Postgrad Med 1986; 79: 171–180.

55. Rao TL, El-Etr AA: Anticoagulation following placement of epidural and subarachnoid catheters: an evaluation of neurologic sequelae. Anesthesiology 1981; 55: 618–620.

56. Mathews ET, Abrams LD: Intrathecal morphine in open heart surgery. (Letter to the editor.) Lancet 1980; 2: 543.

57. Ruff RL, Dougherty JH Jr: Complications of lumbar puncture followed by anticoagulation. Stroke 1981; 12: 879–881.

58. Malinovsky NN, Kozlov VA: Anticoagulant and Thrombolytic Therapy in Surgery, pp 12–37. St. Louis, CV Mosby, 1979.

59. Ockelford P: Heparin 1986. Indications and effective use. Drugs 1986; 31: 81–92.

60. Poller L, Taberner DA, Sandilands DG, et al: An evaluation of APTT monitoring of low-dose heparin dosage in hip surgery. Thromb Haemost 1982; 47: 50–53.

61. Lowson SM, Goodchild CS: Low-dose heparin therapy and spinal anaesthesia. (Letter to the editor.) Anaesthesia 1989; 44: 67–68.

62. Allemann BH, Gerber H, Gruber UF: Perispinal anesthesia and subcutaneous administration of low-dose heparin-dihydergot for prevention of thromboembolism. [German] Anaesthesist 1983; 32: 80–83.

63. Darnat S, Guggiari M, Grob R, et al: A case of spinal extradural hematoma during the insertion of an epidural catheter. [French] Ann Fr Anesth Reanim 1986; 5: 550–552.

64. Dean WM, Woodside JR: Spinal hematoma compressing cauda equina. Urology 1979; 13: 575–577.

65. Metzger G, Singbartl G: Spinal epidural hematoma following epidural anesthesia versus spontaneous spinal subdural hematoma. Two case reports. Acta Anaesthesiol Scand 1991; 35: 105–107.

66. Andersson LO: Prevention and treatment of thrombosis by low molecular weight heparins. Drug Des Deliv 1989; 5: 1–11.

67. Bergqvist D, Lindblad B, Matzsch T: Low molecular weight heparin for thromboprophylaxis and epidural/spinal anaesthesia—is there a risk? Acta Anaesthesiol Scand 1992; 36: 605–609.

68. Tryba M: Hemostatic requirements for the performance of regional anesthesia. Workshop on hemostatic problems in regional anesthesia. [German] Reg Anaesth 1989; 12: 127–131.

69. Odoom JA, Sih IL: Epidural analgesia and anticoagulant therapy. Experience with one thousand cases of continuous epidurals. Anaesthesia 1983; 38: 254–259.

70. Horlocker TT, Wedel DJ, Schlichting JL: Postoperative epidural analgesia and oral anticoagulant therapy. Anesth Analg 1994; 79: 89–93.

71. Hirsch DR, Goldhaber SZ: Bleeding time and other laboratory tests to monitor the safety and efficacy of thrombolytic therapy. Chest 1990; 97(Suppl 4): 124S–131S.

72. Rao AK, Pratt C, Berke A, et al: Thrombolysis in Myocardial Infarction (TIMI) Trial—phase I: hemorrhagic manifestations and changes in plasma fibrinogen and the fibrinolytic system in patients treated with recombinant tissue plasminogen activator and streptokinase. J Am Coll Cardiol 1988; 11: 1–11.

73. Dickman CA, Shedd SA, Spetzler RF, et al: Spinal epidural hematoma associated with epidural anesthesia: complications of systemic heparinization in patients receiving peripheral vascular thrombolytic therapy. Anesthesiology 1990; 72: 947–950.

74. Onishchuk JL, Carlsson C: Epidural hematoma associated with epidural anesthesia: complications of anticoagulant therapy. Anesthesiology 1992; 77: 1221–1223.

75. Rapaport SI: Preoperative hemostatic evaluation: which tests, if any? Blood 1983; 61: 229–231.

76. Hindman BJ, Koka BV: Usefulness of the post-aspirin bleeding time. Anesthesiology 1986; 64: 368–370.

77. Rodgers RP, Levin J: A critical reappraisal of the bleeding time. Semin Thromb Hemost 1990; 16: 1–20.

78. Ferraris VA, Swanson E: Aspirin usage and perioperative blood loss in patients undergoing unexpected operations. Surg Gynecol Obstet 1983; 156: 439–442.

79. Cronberg S, Wallmark E, Soderberg I: Effect on platelet aggregation of oral administration of 10 non-steroidal analgesics to humans. Scand J Haematol 1984; 33: 155–159.

80. Locke GE, Giorgio AJ, Biggers SL Jr, et al: Acute spinal epidural hematoma secondary to aspirin-induced prolonged bleeding. Surg Neurol 1976; 5: 293–296.

81. Horlocker TT, Wedel DJ, Offord KP: Does preoperative antiplatelet therapy increase the risk of hemorrhagic complications associated with regional anesthesia? Anesth Analg 1990; 70: 631–634.

82. Horlocker TT, Wedel DJ, Offord KP, et al: Preoperative antiplatelet drugs do not increase the risk of spinal hematoma associated with regional anesthesia. (Abstract.) Reg Anesth 1994; 19: 8.

83. Horlocker TT: Coagulation problems. In Wedel DJ (ed): Orthopedic Anesthesia, pp 55–68. New York, Churchill Livingstone, 1993.

84. Gower DJ, Baker AL, Bell WO, et al: Contraindications to lumbar puncture as defined by computed cranial tomography. J Neurol Neurosurg Psychiatry 1987; 50: 1071–1074.

85. Wedel DJ, Mulroy MF: Hemiparesis following dural puncture. Anesthesiology 1983; 59: 475–477.

86. Sakabe T, Maekawa T, Ishikawa T, et al: The effects of lidocaine on canine cerebral metabolism and circulation related to the electroencephalogram. Anesthesiology 1974; 40: 433–441.

87. Usubiaga JE, Wikinski J, Ferrero R, et al: Local anesthetic-induced convulsions in man—an electroencephalographic study. Anesth Analg 1966; 45: 611–620.

88. Perkins WJ Jr, Lanier WL, Sharbrough FW: Cerebral and hemodynamic effects of lidocaine accidentally injected into the carotid arteries of patients having carotid endarterectomy. Anesthesiology 1988; 69: 787–790.

89. Phillips OC, Ebner H, Nelson AT, et al: Neurologic complications following spinal anesthesia with lidocaine: a prospective review of 10,440 cases. Anesthesiology 1969; 30: 284–289.

90. Selander D, Edshage S, Wolff T: Paresthesiae or no paresthesiae? Nerve lesions after axillary blocks. Acta Anaesthesiol Scand 1979; 23: 27–33.

91. Plevak DJ, Linstromberg JW, Danielson DR: Paresthesia vs nonparesthesia—the axillary block. (Abstract.) Anesthesiology 1983; 59: A216.

92. Selander D, Dhuner KG, Lundborg G: Peripheral nerve injury due to injection needles used for regional anesthesia. An experimental study of the acute effects of needle point trauma. Acta Anaesthesiol Scand 1977; 21: 182–188.

93. Rice AS, McMahon SB: Peripheral nerve injury caused by injection needles used in regional anaesthesia: influence of bevel configuration, studied in a rat model. Br J Anaesth 1992; 69: 433–438.

94. Schneider M, Ettlin T, Kaufmann M, et al: Transient neurologic toxicity after hyperbaric subarachnoid anesthesia with 5% lidocaine. Anesth Analg 1993; 76: 1154–1157.

95. Myers RR, Heckman HM: Effects of local anesthesia on nerve blood flow: studies using lidocaine with and without epinephrine. Anesthesiology 1989; 71: 757–762.

96. Kalichman MW, Calcutt NA: Local anesthetic-induced conduction block and nerve fiber injury in streptozotocin-diabetic rats. Anesthesiology 1992; 77: 941–947.

97. Selander D: Neurotoxicity of local anesthetics: animal data. Reg Anesth 1993; 18(Suppl 6): 461–468.

98. Rigler ML, Drasner K, Krejcie TC, et al: Cauda equina syndrome after continuous spinal anesthesia. Anesth Analg 1991; 72: 275–281.

99. Drasner K: Models for local anesthetic toxicity from continuous spinal anesthesia. Reg Anesth 1993; 18(6 Suppl): 434–438.

100. Bromage PR: "Paraplegia following epidural analgesia": a misnomer. (Letter to the editor.) Anaesthesia 1976; 31: 947–949.

101. Kane RE: Neurologic deficits following epidural or spinal anesthesia. Anesth Analg 1981; 60: 150–161.

102. Crawford JS, James FM III, Nolte H, et al: Regional analgesia for patients with chronic neurological disease and similar conditions. Anaesthesia 1981; 36: 821.

103. Warren TM, Datta S, Ostheimer GW: Lumbar epidural anesthesia in a patient with multiple sclerosis. Anesth Analg 1982; 61: 1022–1023.

104. Selander D: Nerve toxicity of local anaesthetics. In Löfstrom JB, Sjöstrand U (eds): Local Anaesthesia and Regional Blockade: Pharmacology, Physiology, and Clinical Effects, pp 77–97. Amsterdam, Elsevier, 1988.

105. Laasonen EM, Soini J: Low-back pain after lumbar fusion. Surgical and computed tomographic analysis. Spine 1989; 14: 210–213.

106. Daley MD, Rolbin SH, Hew EM, et al: Epidural anesthesia for obstetrics after spinal surgery. Reg Anesth 1990; 15: 280–284.

107. Crosby ET, Halpern SH: Obstetric epidural anaesthesia in patients with Harrington instrumentation. Can J Anaesth 1989; 36: 693–696.

108. Hubbert CH: Epidural anesthesia in patients with spinal fusion. (Letter to the editor.) Anesth Analg 1985; 64: 843.

CHAPTER 24

Acute Complications and Side Effects of Regional Anesthesia

Mercedes Concepcion, M.D.

When all in the world understands beauty to be beautiful, then ugliness exists; when all understands goodness to be good, then evil exists.

Lao Tzu

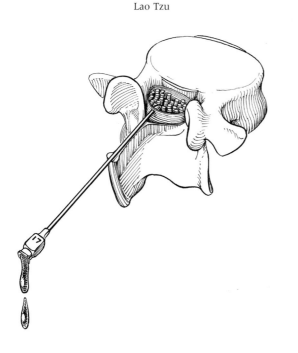

Eastern mystics teach the individuality of all things, but at the same time, they recognize the existence of differences and contrast within each individual unity. Good and bad and pleasure and pain are not absolute independent categories, but rather there are two sides to the same reality. Regional anesthesia must be understood as a concept in which opposites exist. Its beneficial effects include excellent surgical anesthesia and pain relief for acute postoperative pain and chronic pain syndromes. However, the various regional anesthetic techniques may be associated with potential complications.

The popularity of regional anesthesia is the result of several factors, including the development of newer local anesthetic drugs, a better understanding of the physiologic effects of regional anesthesia, and increased teaching of different techniques. Another important factor in the increased use of regional anesthesia is the seemingly minimal effect of regional anesthesia on the functions of various organ systems. However, regional anesthesia is not devoid of profound physiologic effects or of potential significant complications.

The complications of regional anesthesia were readily recognized when local anesthetics were first used and became more evident when spinal anesthesia was introduced into clinical practice. For an interesting historical review of complications, the reader is referred to *Complications of Regional Anesthesia: Past and Present* by Vandam.[1]

Understanding the mechanisms of potential complications and side effects allows the anesthesiologist to feel more confident with the techniques and to be prepared to treat complications as they arise. The acute complications and side effects of regional anesthesia can be divided into two categories: those resulting from the local anesthetic drugs and those related to the specific techniques.

Drug-Related Complications

Systemic Toxic Responses

Under clinical conditions, the systemic toxic responses to local anesthetic drugs result from unintentional intravascular injections of the drug or administration of excessive amounts of local anesthetic. After an intravascular injection, local anesthetic systemic toxicity is directly related to the inherent anesthetic potency of the drug. For example, bupivacaine, one of the most potent local anesthetic agents, is one of the most potentially toxic after an unintentional intravascular injection.

Toxicity secondary to extravascular administration of large doses of local anesthetics is related to the pharmacokinetic properties of the drug. Blood concentration of the local anesthetic depends on the site of injection, amount of drug administered, drug distribution, and drug degradation. Another factor affecting blood concentration is the drug itself. For example, at equal doses, prilocaine results in significantly lower blood levels of drug than lidocaine.[2, 3] This difference between the two amides may reflect a more rapid metabolism and a larger volume of distribution for prilocaine. Chloroprocaine, which undergoes rapid hydrolysis, theoretically exhibits the least toxicity after administration of a large amount of drug. In contrast, drugs with a slow rate of metabolism, such as tetracaine and bupivacaine, are potentially the most toxic when excessive doses are administered.

Local anesthetic systemic toxicity essentially involves the central nervous system (CNS) and the cardiovascular system. Although local anesthetic blood concentrations that result in toxic effects have been established for most local anesthetics, these values are only guides to local anesthetic use. Table 24–1 shows the dose of local anesthetic drug required to produce signs of CNS toxic reactions in animals and humans. Caution must be exercised because of considerable individual variation. For example, in a case reported by Hasselstrom and Mogensen,[4] convulsions and loss of consciousness occurred at a bupivacaine plasma level of 1.1 μg/mL, which is lower than the plasma level usually considered to produce CNS toxicity.

Central Nervous System Toxic Responses

Manifestations of CNS toxic responses to local anesthetics are related to blood levels of the drug. Initially, there is an excitatory phase, thought to result from block of inhibitory pathways in the amygdala. This inhibition allows facilitatory neurons to function unopposed.[5] With an increase in blood and brain levels of local anesthetic, inhibitory and facilitatory pathways are inhibited, resulting in CNS depression.

The initial symptoms of CNS toxic responses include lightheadedness and dizziness, frequently associated with difficulty in focusing and tinnitus. Shivering, muscle twitching, and tremors are early signs of CNS toxic responses. Tremors initially involve the facial musculature and distal parts of the extremities. At high blood and brain levels, generalized tonic-clonic convulsions

Table 24–2 Signs and Symptoms of Local Anesthetic Toxicity in the Central Nervous System

	TOXICITY IN THE CENTRAL NERVOUS SYSTEM	
PHASE	**Signs and Symptoms**	**Mechanism**
Excitatory	Muscle twitching, tremors, tonic-clonic convulsions	Block of inhibitory pathways
Depression	Drowsiness, unconsciousness, respiratory arrest	Block of inhibitory and facilitatory pathways

occur.[6] Table 24–2 shows the signs and symptoms of local anesthetic toxicity in the CNS.

When excessively high doses of local anesthetic have been used, CNS depression may occur without a preceding excitatory phase. This may occur when other CNS depressant drugs, such as sedatives, have been used.

CNS effects of local anesthetics are influenced by a patient's acid-base status. Animal studies[6] have demonstrated that the convulsive threshold of local anesthetics is inversely proportional to the Pa_{CO_2}. An increase in Pa_{CO_2} or a decrease in pH lowers the convulsive threshold. The effects of hypercapnia on cerebral blood flow could explain this. Increased Pa_{CO_2} increases cerebral blood flow, which may lead to increased local anesthetic uptake by the brain. Plasma protein binding also is decreased in the presence of acidosis or hypercapnia (or both), which results in an increased free drug level.[7] Heavner and associates,[8] using lightly anesthetized pigs, demonstrated that severe hypoxemia enhances bupivacaine toxicity in the CNS and cardiovascular system. In this investigation, animals exposed to low F_{IO_2} developed arrhythmias before seizures occurred.

Cardiovascular Systemic Toxic Responses

The cardiovascular system is thought to be more resistant than the CNS to the effects of local anesthetic drugs. CNS toxic responses usually occur at lower blood levels than cardiovascular system toxic re-

Table 24–1 Threshold for Production of Toxic Reactions in the Central Nervous System by Various Local Anesthetic Agents

AGENT	CONVULSIVE THRESHOLD IN MONKEYS		DOSE FOR CONVULSIVE THRESHOLD IN CATS, mg/kg	DOSE FOR THE THRESHOLD OF CNS SYMPTOMS IN HUMANS, mg/kg		
	Dose, mg/kg	Arterial Blood Level, μg/mL		1	2	3
Procaine			50	18–55	19.2	
Chloroprocaine					22.8	
Lidocaine	14–22	18–26	22	6–9	6.4	>4
Mepivacaine	18	22	21		9.8	
Prilocaine	18	20	35			>6
Bupivacaine	4.3	4.5–5.5	5.8			1.6
Etidocaine	5.4	4.3				3.4
Tetracaine					2.5	

CNS, central nervous system.
From Covino BG, Vassallo HG: Local Anesthetics: Mechanisms of Action and Clinical Use, p 126. New York, Grune & Stratton, 1976. By permission of WB Saunders Company.

sponses. However, local anesthetic levels associated with the onset of convulsions and circulatory collapse (circulatory collapse–CNS ratio) differ for the various local anesthetic agents. For example, potent local anesthetics such as bupivacaine and etidocaine exhibit a lower circulatory collapse–CNS ratio than other less potent amino-amides (Fig. 24–1).

Local anesthetic toxicity in the cardiovascular system results from drug effects on smooth muscle and cardiac muscle. Local anesthetics affect the electrical and the mechanical activities of the heart. Initially, the cardiovascular system toxic responses are manifested by hypertension and tachycardia, possibly the result of sympathetic discharge during the excitatory phase of CNS toxic responses. With increasing blood levels of local anesthetic, the initial phase is followed by myocardial depression, moderate hypotension, and decreased cardiac output. As the severity of toxicity progresses, there is peripheral vasodilatation, profound hypotension, conduction defects, sinus bradycardia, and ventricular arrhythmias, ultimately followed by cardiovascular collapse. Table 24–3 summarizes the symptoms of cardiovascular system toxic responses.

Inhibition of sodium channels in cardiac membranes decreases the maximal rate of depolarization (V_{max}) of Purkinje fibers and ventricular muscle and decreases the action potential duration and effective refractory period.[9–11] At high blood levels, local anesthetics prolong conduction time, and at even higher levels, these drugs depress spontaneous pacemaker activity.[6]

In addition to the electrophysiologic effects, local anesthetics exhibit a negative inotropic action on myocardial contractility. Tanz and colleagues,[12] examining the effects of lidocaine and bupivacaine on the isolated guinea pig heart, reported significant decreases in heart rate, coronary artery blood flow, and myocardial O_2 consumption. Although these changes were present with both drugs, the effects were consistently greater with bupivacaine. The investigators concluded that re-

Table 24–3 Signs and Symptoms of Local Anesthetic–Induced Toxic Reactions in the Cardiovascular System

PHASE	SIGNS AND SYMPTOMS
Initial events	Tinnitus, lightheadedness, confusion, circumoral numbness
Excitation phase	Tonic-clonic convulsions
Depression phase	Unconsciousness, generalized central nervous system depression, respiratory arrest

From Covino BG: Pharmacology of local anesthetic agents. In Rogers MC, Tinker JH, Covino BG, et al (eds): Principles and Practice of Anesthesiology, vol II, pp 1235–1257. St. Louis, Mosby–Year Book, 1993.

ductions in coronary blood flow and myocardial O_2 consumption were directly related to the negative inotropic and chronotropic effects of the local anesthetics.

The severity and characteristics of cardiac toxic reactions differ among the various local anesthetic agents. For example, depression of the V_{max} of Purkinje fibers and ventricular muscle is of significantly greater magnitude with bupivacaine than with lidocaine. Recovery from lidocaine is rapid and complete, but recovery from bupivacaine is slow, resulting in incomplete recovery of V_{max} between action potentials.[9–11]

Some local anesthetics exhibit a greater arrhythmogenic potential. Although arrhythmias rarely occur with lidocaine, mepivacaine, and tetracaine, severe cardiac arrhythmias may occur with bupivacaine and etidocaine and, to a lesser extent, with ropivacaine. This arrhythmogenic activity of potent local anesthetics has been demonstrated in several animal species.[13–17] Severe cardiac arrhythmias have been reported[18] in humans after unintentional intravascular injection of bupivacaine and etidocaine.

The arrhythmogenic activity and myocardial depressing activity of bupivacaine have been the subject of extensive investigation. Several mechanisms have been proposed to explain bupivacaine's cardiotoxic effect: direct myocardial depression, secondary to block of sodium channels; depression of atrioventricular node conduction; and depression of myocardial contractility.[12, 19, 20]

Animal studies[14, 21] have shown that toxic doses of bupivacaine induce ventricular arrhythmias. In animals treated with toxic doses of bupivacaine, ventricular arrhythmias, tachycardia, or fibrillation developed. In contrast, none of the animals receiving lidocaine had ventricular arrhythmias. Progressive hypotension, bradycardia, respiratory arrest, and cardiovascular collapse were the cause of death in these animals.

The primary mechanism of bupivacaine's cardiotoxic effect appears to be depression of cardiac conduction resulting from the block of sodium channels. However, all local anesthetics depress cardiac conduction by the same mechanism. Why are there differences in the severity of toxic reactions?

In an attempt to elucidate the underlying mechanism of bupivacaine toxicity, several investigators have conducted studies using numerous animal species. Clarkson and Hondeghem[11] conducted electrophysiologic

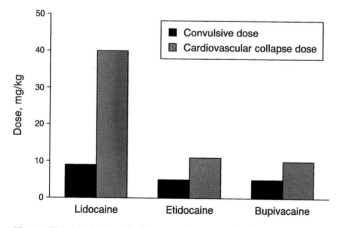

Figure 24–1 Relationships between doses of lidocaine, bupivacaine, and etidocaine that cause toxic responses in the central nervous system and doses that produce cardiovascular collapse. (From Covino BG: Pharmacology of local anesthetic agents. In Rogers MC, Tinker JH, Covino BG, et al [eds]: Principles and Practice of Anesthesiology, vol II, pp 1235–1257. St. Louis, Mosby–Year Book, 1993.)

studies of the effects of bupivacaine and lidocaine on the guinea pig ventricular muscle. The results showed that block development and recovery are different with the two drugs. Although lidocaine rapidly blocks inactivated and open sodium channels during the action potential, a bupivacaine block develops slowly at low concentrations but rapidly at higher concentrations. Recovery from a bupivacaine block is significantly slower than from lidocaine. The researchers stated that "lidocaine blocks channels in a fast-in-fast-out fashion." In contrast, bupivacaine could be considered to block "sodium channels in a slow-in-slow-out manner (at low concentrations) or in a fast-in-slow-out manner" at higher concentrations. Bupivacaine was more potent in depressing V_{max} in ventricular muscle, resulting in slowed conduction of action potentials. This effect is manifested in the electrocardiogram by a prolonged PR interval and a widened QRS complex. The slow conduction may cause unidirectional block and reentry arrhythmias, such as ectopic ventricular beats and ventricular tachycardias. The differences in the ability of bupivacaine and lidocaine to produce toxic cardiac responses may be attributed to differences in the affinity of binding and kinetics of these drugs at the level of the sodium channels.

Kasten[15] reported that the effects of various local anesthetic agents on the effective refractory period temporal dispersion in anesthetized dogs were remarkably different. After burst ventricular pacing, most of the dogs given bupivacaine and etidocaine developed polymorphic ventricular tachycardia similar to torsades de pointes. These arrhythmias were also occasionally seen with mepivacaine. The differences in the incidence of this type of arrhythmia with the various drugs may be explained by the magnitude with which each drug prolonged the effective refractory period temporal dispersion.

An investigation conducted by de la Coussaye and coworkers[22] used high-resolution ventricular epicardial mapping of rabbit heart. Bupivacaine significantly prolonged the ventricular effective refractory period and slowed longitudinal and transverse conduction velocities in a dose- or use-dependent manner, leading to reentry ventricular arrhythmias. Epicardial mapping also showed that tachycardia was consistently the result of "reentry of the impulse around an arc of functional conduction block."[22]

It has been proposed that high concentrations of local anesthetics in the CNS may contribute to local anesthetic toxicity in the cardiovascular system. Two groups of investigators conducted studies[23–25] to determine the role of the CNS in mediating bupivacaine cardiotoxic effects. The results of these investigations support the role of the CNS in cardiac toxic reactions. Direct application of local anesthetics within vasomotor and cardioactive regions of the rat medulla leads to hypotension, bradycardia, and ventricular arrhythmias. By using equal numbers of molecules of lidocaine and bupivacaine, Thomas and colleagues[23] demonstrated that bupivacaine is two to four times more potent than lidocaine in producing these arrhythmias. However, the site and mechanisms of action appeared to be the

same for both drugs. In a somewhat similar investigation, Bernards and Artru[24, 25] demonstrated that administration of bupivacaine into the cerebral ventricles resulted in hypertension and ventricular arrhythmias, both of which were terminated by midazolam administration.

Most bupivacaine-related cardiovascular complications in humans occurred after the use of bupivacaine in pregnant patients, suggesting that pregnant patients were more susceptible to the toxic effects of bupivacaine. Morishima and associates[26] reported that the dose of bupivacaine resulting in cardiovascular collapse was significantly lower in pregnant than in nonpregnant ewes. Similar studies[27, 28] conducted with other local anesthetics (mepivacaine, lidocaine) reported no differences in the dose required to produce cardiovascular collapse in pregnant and nonpregnant sheep. This suggests that pregnant animals are more sensitive to the toxic effects of bupivacaine. It has become accepted that peripheral nerves from pregnant animals and pregnant patients are more sensitive to the blocking effects of local anesthetics.[29, 30] It appears that hormonal changes in pregnancy may alter membrane excitability in nerve and heart.

The basic mechanism for bupivacaine-induced cardiotoxic effects may not be completely elucidated, but existing data strongly support several mechanisms:

1. Bupivacaine markedly depresses the rapid phase of depolarization (V_{max}) of the cardiac action potential.
2. Depressed V_{max} results in slowed conduction of potentials, which leads to unidirectional block and development of reentry ventricular arrhythmias.
3. The recovery phase of sodium channels is prolonged after bupivacaine block.
4. Bupivacaine significantly increases the effective refractory period, leading to polymorphic undulant ventricular tachycardias similar to torsades de pointes.
5. Bupivacaine cardiotoxic responses may be partially mediated by the CNS.

To minimize these severe, potentially fatal complications, incremental, slow injection of local anesthetics is recommended. Frequent aspirations alert the anesthesiologist to intravascular injections, and the anesthesiologists should maintain verbal contact with the patient while performing the block. Recommended doses of local anesthetics should not be exceeded. However, systemic absorption of local anesthetics varies with the site of injection, and this should be taken into consideration in determining the total dose of local anesthetic to be injected. Monitoring is essential while performing any technique of regional anesthesia. Resuscitation equipment and drugs should be immediately available.

Miscellaneous Toxic Responses

Although local anesthetic toxicity mostly affects the cardiovascular system and CNS, other local and less severe systemic toxic effects may occur. Major systemic toxic effects are primarily related to the local anesthetic concentration in brain and myocardial tissue, although toxic reactions can result from metabolites of the local anesthetic agent.

Prilocaine, for example, is a safe amino-amide local anesthetic with relatively low potency for toxic reactions. However, when used in amounts exceeding 600 mg, one of its metabolites, hydroxylated *o*-toluidine, reduces oxyhemoglobin, resulting in the formation of methemoglobin. The amount of methemoglobin necessary to produce cyanosis is at least 1.5 g/dL. This corresponds to oxyhemoglobin reduction of 10% or greater. Methemoglobinemia is clinically manifested by cyanosis of mucous membranes and nail beds, and it is easily treated with the intravenous administration of methylene blue.

In most patients, methemoglobinemia has little clinical significance, but in the presence of anemia or congestive heart failure, minimal reduction of oxyhemoglobin may decrease the O_2 carrying capacity and exert deleterious effects on the patient's condition.

Local Toxicity

Histologic studies have shown that skeletal tissue is particularly sensitive to irritation by local anesthetic agents.[31-33] Reversible myotoxic effects have been reported in animals and humans from bupivacaine and other local anesthetics.[31-34]

In humans, myotoxic effects have been reported after injection of trigger points,[35] retrobulbar block,[36] and continuous brachial plexus block.[37] Biopsy of the affected muscle has shown muscle fiber degeneration, with occasional areas of necrosis. Inflammatory changes are present, with infiltrates of neutrophils, granulocytes, and significant amounts of eosinophils. Concomitantly, regenerating muscle fibers are also found.[32] Bupivacaine myotoxic reactions occur early. Within 15 min of injection into muscle tissue or adjacent tissue, muscle fiber damage can be demonstrated.[38]

Local anesthetic toxicity in muscle is dose dependent, and it increases with repeated injections.[39] Other factors that may worsen these effects include the simultaneous use of epinephrine, steroids, or both agents.[38, 40] After exposure to local anesthetics is terminated, regeneration of muscle fibers can be demonstrated in 4 days.[32]

Allergy

Allergic reactions, hypersensitivity, and anaphylactic reactions to local anesthetics have been reported occasionally.

The amino-ester local anesthetics are the compounds most commonly implicated in these reactions. Amino-esters are derivatives of *p*-aminobenzoic acid, which is known to be highly allergenic. The relative frequency of allergic reaction reports is not surprising. In contrast, allergic reactions to amino-amides are relatively uncommon, although several reports[41-46] of allergy to these compounds have appeared in the literature.

The mechanism involved in these allergic reactions is poorly understood. It has been proposed that allergy associated with amino-amide local anesthetics is immunologically mediated. An example of this type of reaction is the case reported by Brown and associates.[46] Two minutes after the intradermal injection of 0.2 mL of 0.5% bupivacaine, severe symptoms developed, including a tight feeling in the throat, urticaria of the upper extremities and trunk, and visual difficulties. These signs and symptoms were associated with a generalized unwell feeling. The systemic reaction was associated with a dramatic decrease in plasma concentration of C4 complement, although no antibodies to the local anesthetic were identified. Similarly, in the case reported by Tannenbaum and colleagues,[45] complement component levels were markedly decreased and remained low for several hours. Immune complexes and antibodies could not be demonstrated. However, total hemolytic activity levels varied, with the hemolytic activity of C4 and C2 decreased. It was postulated that an endogenous complement abnormality present in the patient contributed to the anaphylactic reaction.

Stefanini and Hoffman[47] reported a case of acute thrombocytopenic purpura that developed after the use of lidocaine. It appeared that thrombocytopenia was related to the presence of a specific antibody predominantly mediated by immunoglobulin M. The antibody's action was lytic. The investigators postulated that it coupled to the drug, forming an antigen-antibody complex that then fixed to and lysed platelets. The reaction was reproducible with a minimal dose of lidocaine.

Other investigators[48] proposed a direct histamine release induced by local anesthetic as the major contributing factor in adverse reactions to local anesthetics.

Patch and prick tests as well as intradermal testing have been recommended for patients with an unclear history of local anesthetic allergy. These tests have limitations. In one study,[49] 104 persons with positive patch tests were subjected to prick and intradermal testing. All prick tests were negative, and only 14 patients had positive reactions to intradermal testing. Eleven of these reactions were positive to ester-type local anesthetics, one to the amide butanilicaine, and two to both types of local anesthetic.

The lymphocyte transformation test has also been used to diagnose local anesthetic allergy. Using the lymphocyte transformation test, Sabbah[50] reported that the incidence of allergic reactions to procaine was three times as great as that to lidocaine.

Allergic reactions to local anesthetics may occur with amino-ester and amino-amide drugs. Allergy to amino-esters is probably related to *p*-aminobenzoic acid, a highly allergenic substance, but allergy to amino-amides is probably immunologically mediated.

Different modes of testing have been suggested for patients with unclear histories of response to local anesthetics, although the limitations to their significance must be appreciated. Patch testing, intradermal testing, and the lymphocyte transformation test have confirmed that these allergic reactions are more common with ester-type local anesthetics.

Technique-Related Complications and Side Effects

Neuraxial Blocks

Complications or side effects of neuraxial blocks include those related to spinal, epidural, and caudal anesthesia. Some of the complications discussed are common to all techniques. These include hypotension, epidural hematoma, and epidural abscess.

Complications of Spinal Anesthesia

Complications of spinal anesthesia can be considered in two categories: minor side effects and major complications.

Post-dural puncture headache (PDPH) and backache are transient, minor complications. Physiologic alterations resulting from high cephalad spread of anesthesia with extensive sympathetic block could also be in this category. Hypotension is the prototype of these physiologic responses. If treated promptly, it has no significant implications; however, profound hypotension inadequately treated can lead to major complications.

The incidence of side effects in spinal anesthesia and the risk factors involved were prospectively studied by Carpenter and associates.[51] The researchers examined the incidence of minor side effects (Table 24–4) and reported that some risk factors could be identified for each of these side effects. For example, nausea was more prevalent in patients with high sensory block and in the presence of hypotension. Nausea also occurred more frequently in patients with a baseline heart rate of at least 60 beats/min. In contrast, bradycardia occurring during spinal anesthesia was more prevalent in patients with a baseline heart rate of less than 60 beats/min. Other risk factors for bradycardia included American Society of Anesthesiologists' physical status I patients and sensory block level higher than T-5.

Carpenter and colleagues demonstrated that patients who developed hypotension had a significantly higher incidence of other side effects, such as nausea. In patients who experienced multiple side effects, hypotension generally occurred earlier than other side effects.

Major complications occur much less frequently and blur the line between acute and chronic. These include meningitis, isolated nerve injury, and major neurologic dysfunction such as cauda equina syndrome.

Table 24–4 Incidence of Minor Side Effects from Spinal Anesthesia

SIDE EFFECT	INCIDENCE, %
Hypotension (SBP < 90 mm Hg)	33
Nausea	18.4
Bradycardia (HR < 50 beats/min)	13.1
Vomiting	6.8
Arrhythmia	2.1

HR, heart rate; SBP, systolic blood pressure.
Data from Carpenter RL, Caplan RA, Brown DL, et al: Incidence and risk factors for side effects of spinal anesthesia. Anesthesiology 1992; 76: 906–916.

Hypotension. Hypotension is a predictable physiologic response to spinal or epidural anesthesia. The underlying mechanism of arterial hypotension after neuraxial block is the block of preganglionic sympathetic fibers. The degree of hypotension depends on the extent of the sympathetic block. It has been universally taught that sympathetic block extends two segments above the sensory anesthesia level.[52] However, studies have shown significant variability. Although Chamberlain and Chamberlain[53] reported that sympathetic block extended as much as six segments above sensory block, Malmqvist and colleagues[54] reported low or no sympathetic block. The variability of reported sympathetic block levels probably results from different methods used to measure sympathetic activity.

Spinal anesthesia limited to the lumbar and sacral segments causes little or no change in blood pressure. A block that extends to the low thoracic to midthoracic level may result in a moderate decrease in blood pressure. A more extensive block, generally one extending above T-5, may lead to profound hypotension. However, in an individual patient, it is difficult to predict the degree of hypotension on the basis of spinal block level. These individual variations may reflect differences in sympathetic block level, and the degree of sympathetic tone before induction of spinal anesthesia plays an important role in the incidence and magnitude of hypotension.[55] For example, in a healthy normovolemic patient, spinal anesthesia levels even to midthoracic dermatomes may cause no changes in blood pressure or only mild hypotension. In contrast, the same level of block results in severe hypotension in an individual who is hypovolemic or with an obstruction to venous return and who requires high sympathetic tone to maintain arterial pressure.

Changes in blood pressure are related to changes in vascular resistance, cardiac output, or both circumstances. Peripheral vascular resistance is determined by arterial tone, which is regulated by sympathetic innervation. (Local metabolism also plays a role in vascular resistance.) The block of arterial vasoconstrictors results in arterial dilation and loss of arterial tone. However, after a sympathetic block, arterial tone is not completely lost; significant residual tone remains. Arterial dilation is not uniform, even within sympathetically blocked regions. Vasodilation of the blocked area triggers a compensatory vasoconstriction of nonblocked regions. This event explains the low incidence of hypotension in spinal anesthesia extending only to the low thoracic segments. As the block extends higher, leading to vasodilation of a greater area, the ability to compensate with vasoconstriction decreases.

In addition to the effect on arterial tone, a sympathetic block affects venous tone to a greater extent. The tone of capacitance vessels depends on an intact sympathetic nervous system. Sympathetic block abolishes venous tone, leading to the inability of veins to constrict. Venodilation results in increased capacitance, and because of the inability of capacitance vessels to constrict, venous return decreases. Because preload is a major determinant of cardiac output, the decreased venous return leads to decreased cardiac output.

In the presence of a high spinal block affecting the cardiac sympathetics (T-1 to T-5), heart rate is moderately affected, with reductions of 5% to 25%.[56] The greatest decrease in heart rate is thought to occur as a reflex response to the decreased cardiac preload. The limited bradycardia resulting from spinal anesthesia plays only a small role in producing hypotension. However, if parasympathetic tone is clinically activated, a vasovagal response develops with bradycardia, which may lead to temporary cardiac arrest.[54, 57] Although few data exist to demonstrate a reduction in contractility by spinal anesthesia, a block of cardioaccelerators may result in the reduction of myocardial contractility.

Factors contributing to hypotension include decreased arterial tone, leading to a moderate decrease in vascular resistance; increased venous capacitance and decreased venous tone, resulting in decreased venous return that leads to decreased cardiac output; and block of cardiac sympathetics, resulting in bradycardia, which may contribute to hypotension. Other factors may play a role in the development of hypotension. The patient's physical condition is an important factor. In the presence of hypovolemia, spinal anesthesia may lead to profound cardiovascular depression. This is related to the increased sympathetic tone present in patients with hypovolemia. Sympathetic block in these patients may result in severe hypotension. In the presence of mechanical obstruction to venous return, as in a pregnant patient, further decreases in venous return secondary to sympathetic block are poorly tolerated. The incidence of hypotension and the magnitude of blood pressure decrease are greater in elderly patients, especially in those with coronary artery disease, than in young, healthy patients.

The patient's position affects the degree of hypotension. Head-up position or lowering the legs, as during arthroscopic surgery of the knee, may result in hypotension secondary to venous pooling.

Neurologic Complications. Neurologic complications of spinal anesthesia include minor complications such as persistent postoperative paresthesias and major, devastating complications such as adhesive arachnoiditis and cauda equina syndrome. Fortunately, these major complications are rare (see Chapter 25).

Trauma to the Spinal Cord or a Spinal Nerve Root. Direct trauma to the spinal cord may result in severe neurologic deficit. Performing the lumbar puncture below the L-2 level minimizes the potential of injury to the spinal cord. Direct injury to a spinal nerve, although rare, is possible. Vandam and Dripps,[58] in their classic review of 10,096 cases of spinal anesthesia, concluded that neurologic complication resulting from direct trauma was more likely to occur after multiple attempts to achieve a lumbar puncture.

An intraneural injection disrupts the nerve fibers, and the intraneural injection of local anesthetic into a spinal nerve may spread the local anesthetic along the nerve root to the spinal cord, damaging the cell bodies.[56] Pain during needle insertion or during injection is the presenting symptom. Intraneural injection is followed by paresthesias or hypalgesia in the nerve root distribution. Occasionally, a burning sensation is also present in the area supplied by the injured nerves. Generally, this kind of injury resolves in weeks to several months.

Meningitis. Septic meningitis secondary to introduction of bacteria into the subarachnoid space is unlikely. In the rare cases of septic meningitis, the most commonly found organisms have been *Staphylococcus aureus*, coliforms, and pseudomonads.[59] Before the advent of disposable needles and equipment, aseptic meningitis was the most likely form of meningitis after spinal anesthesia. Contamination with a chemical irritant such as detergents used to clean syringes and needles or the unintentional injection of a chemical irritant is presumed to be the cause of aseptic meningitis. Fever, stiff neck, and signs of meningeal irritation occurring 24 to 48 h after spinal anesthesia are the most frequent signs and symptoms at presentation. Cerebrospinal fluid pressure is increased, and cerebrospinal fluid analysis reveals normal glucose and protein concentrations, with high counts of polymorphonuclear cells. Cultures have negative results for bacteria. A case of prolonged diabetes insipidus in a patient who presented with aseptic meningitis after spinal anesthesia was reported by Garfield and coworkers.[60] In that case, remnants of detergent used to clean a glass syringe were presumed to be the causal agent. Meningitis should be rare if appropriate aseptic technique, disposable equipment, and local anesthetics without preservative are used.

Cardiac Arrest. In the American Society of Anesthesiologists' Closed Claims Study, Caplan and colleagues[61] reported 14 cases of sudden, unexpected cardiac arrests during spinal anesthesia. Most cases were in young healthy persons. Of the 14 cases, 6 patients died in hospital, and of the 8 survivors, only 1 patient recovered meaningful neurologic function. In some of these cases, intraoperative sedation was probably excessive. Cyanosis, hypotension, and bradycardia heralded the cardiac arrest. The researchers hypothesized that unrecognized respiratory insufficiency may have been a factor in approximately half of the cases. Bradycardia during spinal anesthesia has been recognized for many years and has been attributed to sympathetic block and to decreased venous return.[62] It develops slowly and usually to only a moderate degree.[63]

In 1989, Mackey and associates[64] reported one case of profound bradycardia and two cases of asystole during spinal anesthesia. Immediately before the bradycardia or asystole, these patients were hemodynamically stable, had no signs of hypoxemia, and had received little sedation. All three cases had propitious outcomes. Mackey and colleagues[64] speculated that in cases of significant bradycardia and asystole associated with spinal anesthesia, a paradoxical Bezold-Jarisch reflex should be considered. The investigators suggested that paradoxical stimulation of ventricular receptors may occur during hypovolemia, resulting in a paradoxical Bezold-Jarisch reflex.

Preexisting conditions also may predispose the patient to profound bradycardia and asystole, which may be associated with spinal anesthesia. For example, a preexisting autonomic imbalance or dysfunction could predispose the patient to this complication. Asystole has also been reported during spinal anesthesia in a patient with sick sinus syndrome.[65]

Prompt recognition of progressive bradycardia during spinal anesthesia and adequate treatment cannot be overemphasized. In a letter to the editor, Brown and coworkers[66] outlined treatment for progressive bradycardia: atropine and ephedrine or epinephrine (or both) should be used promptly if profound bradycardia develops during spinal anesthesia.

After the report by Caplan and colleagues,[61] vigilance during spinal anesthesia was emphasized by various investigators.[66-68] Adequate monitoring and constant vigilance during regional anesthesia are as important as during general anesthesia.

Inadequate Spinal Anesthesia. Inadequate spinal anesthesia is generally attributed to errors of technique[69-71] or to inactive local anesthetic.[72] A report by Cohen and Knight[73] attributed the inadequate spinal anesthetic to high alkalinity of the cerebrospinal fluid. In a report of five cases of inadequate spinal anesthesia, Schmidt and associates[74] were able to demonstrate that technical difficulties, errors, or inactive lidocaine was not responsible for the failure of spinal anesthesia in their cases. A subarachnoid catheter demonstrated free aspiration of cerebrospinal fluid before and after the injection of lidocaine. The lidocaine assay of cerebrospinal fluid from four of these patients revealed adequate levels to produce anesthesia. In four of the five patients, subsequent injection of bupivacaine resulted in adequate spinal anesthesia. The researchers suggested that some patients may have resistance to a specific local anesthetic agent or to various local anesthetics. Schmidt and colleagues[74] also suggested that this may be a "temporary resistance because of physicochemical changes."

Complications of Epidural Anesthesia

The complications associated with epidural anesthesia can be divided into drug-related complications and technique-related complications. Epidural block also can be associated with neurologic complications. Minor neurologic complications, such as trauma to a spinal root, may result in a temporary neurologic deficit. However, other complications, such as an epidural hematoma, not treated appropriately may lead to permanent deficit. Fortunately, the incidence of these major, sometimes catastrophic complications is extremely low.

Drug-Related Complications. Complications may result from systemic absorption of local anesthetic or from unintentional intravascular injection. Relatively large volumes of local anesthetics are required to provide adequate epidural anesthesia. The amount required depends on the site of injection and the extent of the surgical procedure. The greatest volume of local anesthetic is required for caudal blocks and lumbar epidural blocks, but a thoracic epidural block to provide segmental anesthesia generally requires lower doses.

Systemic toxicity during epidural block may result from an unintentional intravascular injection or from significant systemic absorption. The epidural space con-

tains widespread venous plexuses; systemic absorption of drugs injected into the epidural space can be significant. The epidural veins can be penetrated by an epidural needle or catheter, with the potential for an unrecognized intravascular injection of local anesthetic.

Several factors influence the blood and tissue levels of local anesthetics. These include the rate of absorption, drug redistribution, metabolism, and excretion. After epidural injection of local anesthetics, drug plasma levels are significantly lower than after an intravenous injection. Figure 24–2 demonstrates the blood levels of local anesthetic after a fast and a slow intravenous injection and after injection of local anesthetic in the epidural space. An unintentional intravascular injection of local anesthetic during an epidural block results in blood levels similar to those obtained with a fast intravenous injection.

To prevent high drug concentration in plasma, several measures have been recommended: epidural placement in a segmental space close to the site of incision, if not at the center of the incision, which avoids the need for large volumes of local anesthetic to obtain adequate anesthesia; the use of a test dose with an epinephrine-containing local anesthetic; titration of drug during injection; and the use of only the concentration and volume required for the operation planned.

Technique-Related Complications

Hypotension. Hypotension is the most frequent cardiovascular side effect of epidural anesthesia. It should be considered a physiologic response rather than a complication. The mechanisms responsible for hypotension discussed under spinal anesthesia are also applicable to hypotension with epidural anesthesia.

The addition of light general anesthesia to spinal or epidural anesthesia alters the cardiovascular response to the block. General anesthesia usually increases the magnitude of hypotension, presumably by further decreasing peripheral resistance. However, the induction of light general anesthesia has the advantage of sup-

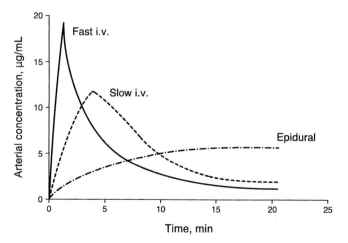

Figure 24–2 Relationships among arterial concentrations of local anesthetic after rapid intravenous, slow intravenous, and epidural administration. (From Covino BG, Scott DB: Handbook of Epidural Anaesthesia and Analgesia, p 133. Orlando, FL, Grune & Stratton, 1985. By permission of Mediglobe SA.)

pressing vagal hyperactivity. It must be emphasized that hypotension is only a sign. If hypotension is treated promptly and adequately, it seldom leads to a poor outcome.

Subarachnoid Air Injection. Air, isotonic saline, or a combination of both is frequently used to identify the epidural space by the loss of resistance technique.

Several cases of sudden headache during epidural placement have been reported. It was thought that unintentional subarachnoid injection of air was the cause of the headache. In only one case was the dural puncture recognized; in two cases, intracranial air was demonstrated radiographically.[75–77]

An early frontal headache while an epidural block is being performed may represent a warning symptom of dural penetration by the epidural needle or by the force generated by the injection of air when it enters the epidural space. This forced air injection may separate dural fibers, allowing air to enter the subarachnoid space.[77]

Dural Puncture. Because cerebrospinal fluid flows freely through the epidural needle, a dural puncture is easy to diagnose. PDPH is likely to occur. A high incidence of headache, 50% to 70% in young patients, has been reported after dural puncture with a large epidural needle.[57] However, some investigators have reported the absence of PDPH after continuous spinal anesthesia with an 18-G epidural needle.[78, 79]

High Block or Total Spinal Block. Unintentional subarachnoid injection of a large dose of local anesthetic intended for epidural anesthesia results in high or total spinal block. Although a feared complication of epidural anesthesia, a high block or total spinal block is self-limiting and seldom leads to adverse sequelae if treated appropriately. A profound motor and sensory block developing soon after an intended epidural injection should alert the anesthesiologist that a subarachnoid injection has occurred. A block at a high dermatomal level develops rapidly. If the block spreads to the upper cervical dermatomes, respiratory insufficiency and respiratory arrest ensue secondary to diaphragmatic paralysis. Because the spinal subarachnoid and the cerebral subarachnoid spaces communicate freely, if a relatively high concentration of local anesthetic reaches the cranium, total neural paralysis leads to loss of consciousness, respiratory arrest, and hypotension.

If subarachnoid penetration is suspected, even in the absence of free-flowing cerebrospinal fluid, a test dose of 3 to 4 mL of a rapid-onset local anesthetic should be used, allowing adequate time to produce an effect.

If this dramatic situation occurs, oxygenation must be maintained, first by mask, followed by tracheal intubation until spontaneous respiration resumes. Supportive therapy to maintain hemodynamic stability includes fluids and vasopressor agents.

Subdural Injection. It is reportedly relatively easy to inject local anesthetics intended for epidural anesthesia or to place an epidural catheter into the subdural space. The subdural space is a potential space between the dura and the arachnoid. Local anesthetics injected into this space spread with ease and are separated from the spinal cord and the spinal nerves by only the thin arachnoid and pia mater.[57]

The block that results from a subdural injection develops faster than an epidural block, but it takes longer than a subarachnoid block. An extensive and profound proximal sensory block, occasionally sparing distal dermatomes, and a weak or absent motor block of the lower extremities are characteristic of subdural block. Unilateral blocks also may develop.

Several cases of subdural injection have been reported.[80] Some have shown evidence of a mixed epidural-subdural block. The incidence of this complication has been reported to be 0.3% to 0.8%.[81, 82] If such a block develops, a subdural block is suggested. The definite diagnosis is made by the injection of radiopaque dye. Radiographs show a thin film of contrast medium spreading cephalad for a variable number of segments. This could be unilateral, but more typically, it is bilateral, producing the characteristic railroad track image of a subdural injection.[80]

Neurologic Complications. Epidural anesthesia may be associated with relatively minor or with severe, potentially devastating neurologic complications. This was discussed under spinal anesthesia, and the mechanism and presentation are similar. Table 24–5 presents a summary of the neurologic complications, clinical presentations, and outcomes that may be associated with epidural anesthesia.

Space-occupying lesions include epidural hematoma and epidural abscess. Entry into epidural veins is common while performing an epidural block. Dawkins[81] reported an incidence of 2.3% for blood vessel puncture and found this to be the most common complication of epidural and caudal blocks. Horlocker and coworkers[83] reported a 4.5% incidence for 805 patients given 1013 spinal or epidural anesthetics.

It is easier to understand the frequency of blood vessel puncture if the anatomy of the epidural space, which contains a rich vascular plexus, is considered. The lateral position of the larger epidural veins may increase the incidence of blood vessel puncture when the paramedian approach is used. In a healthy patient, bleeding caused by entering an epidural vein should be minimal and of short duration.[84] However, in patients with clotting disorders or those on anticoagulant therapy, bleeding may persist, and an epidural hematoma may form. If the clotting study results are abnormal, the indication for epidural anesthesia must be compelling if the technique is used. Epidural hematoma is rare if the coagulation profile is normal.

Spontaneous epidural hematomas do occur, and they have been reported even in patients with normal coagulation. For example, Lerner and colleagues[85] reported an epidural hematoma in a patient with normal coagulation. They attributed the hematoma to repeated lumbar dural punctures. Delayed epidural hematomas have also been reported after regional blocks. In one case, the location of the epidural clot higher than the point of needle entry and the delayed (72 h) appearance of neurologic signs suggested a spontaneously occurring epidural hematoma.[8?] Epidural hematoma, although rare, is a serious complication that, if unrecognized,

Table 24–5 Summary of Various Types of Neurologic Damage After Epidural Block

PATHOLOGY	CAUSE	ONSET	CLINICAL FEATURES	OUTCOME
Spinal nerve neuropathy	Trauma (needle, catheter, injection)	0–2 d	Pain during insertion of needle or catheter; pain on injection; paresthesia, pain, and numbness over distribution of spinal nerve	Recovery 1–12 wk
Anterior spinal artery syndrome	Arteriosclerosis hypotension	Immediate	Postoperative painless paraplegia	Painless paraplegia
Adhesive arachnoiditis	Irritant injectant	0–7 d	Pain on injection; variable degree of neurologic deficit; often progressive with pain and paraplegia	May progress to severe disability with pain and paralysis
Space-occupying lesion (hematoma or abscess)	Hypocoagulation Bacteremia	0–2 d	Severe backache postoperatively with progressive paraplegia	Requires immediate surgery, otherwise paraplegia

From Covino BG, Scott DB: Handbook of Epidural Anaesthesia and Analgesia, p 165. Orlando, FL, Grune & Stratton, 1985. By permission of Mediglobe SA.

leads to catastrophic outcome. As Bridenbaugh[87] pointed out, "The real risk in using these techniques is less in the occurrence than in the failure to diagnose and treat accurately and quickly."

The typical symptoms are persistent, moderate to severe back pain, occasionally radiating to the legs; numbness; and weakness of the lower extremities, progressing to complete paresis. Hematoma formation occurs dorsal to the dural sac and may extend over several spinal segments. Spinal cord compression syndrome may be more significant in the thoracic or lumbar areas.

In a patient who has undergone epidural or spinal anesthesia, an epidural hematoma may not produce back pain. Failure of a block to resolve at the expected time or an increase in intensity and level of the block (or both) requires immediate evaluation for hematoma formation. A high-quality magnetic resonance image should clarify the diagnosis. If an epidural hematoma is present, an urgent laminectomy to evacuate the hematoma is mandatory. Surgical intervention within 6 to 8 h provides greater chance for neurologic recovery. Late intervention often leads to permanent neurologic dysfunction.

Epidural abscess is thought to occur in the presence of bacteremia with colonization of an epidural hematoma. Use of contaminated equipment and injection of contaminated drugs are rare and should not occur when careful attention to asepsis is undertaken while performing the block. Epidural abscess formation has also been reported after multiple spinal anesthetics.[88]

Epidural abscess can be superficial or follow the needle tract. Patients who have abscesses along the needle tract present with fever, local tenderness, and signs of superficial infection that rarely lead to neurologic deficits. Antibiotics and occasionally surgical drainage are all that is required. In contrast, the patient with abscess formation in the epidural space presents with fever, leukocytosis, back pain radiating to the legs, and progressive neurologic deficit. S. aureus has been the most commonly found organism.[89]

An epidural hematoma often develops immediately after the epidural block. In contrast, an epidural abscess has a slower course, manifesting 2 to 3 days after the block. As with epidural hematoma, if an epidural abscess is suspected, time-efficient evaluation and surgical interaction are required to maximize neurologic recovery.

Miscellaneous Complications. Several cases of Horner's syndrome have been reported after epidural anesthesia in the obstetric population.[89–91] Pupillary constriction has also been reported after thoracic epidural block. Following the observation of a high incidence of miosis, Mohan and Potter[92] observed 20 consecutive pregnant patients with caudal epidural analgesia for labor and delivery. In most patients, miosis, ptosis, or both conditions developed, sometimes unilaterally and occasionally bilaterally. Anhidrosis of one side of the face was also reported. The researchers concluded that this self-limiting side effect was caused by the rapid and widespread action of epidurally injected local anesthetics in the pregnant patient, resulting in block of preganglionic sympathetic fibers supplying the pupils. These fibers are thought to arise from the gray column of the first and second thoracic segments, leaving the cord by the upper thoracic nerves.[93] High thoracic levels of anesthesia would explain this side effect.

Most back pain during epidural anesthesia develops by the same mechanism as that of spinal anesthesia. However, severe back pain after epidural anesthesia with the new formulation of 2-chloroprocaine has been reported. It was presumed that the back pain resulted from large volumes of anesthetic, leading to leakage of the anesthetic solution along the dural sleeves, causing paraspinous muscle irritation. Other proposed etiologic factors include the preservative ethylenediaminetetraacetic acid (EDTA), local infiltration with chloroprocaine, and low pH.[94, 95]

Complications of Peripheral Nerve Blocks

A block of peripheral nerves is performed for various surgical procedures. These blocks often require multiple injections and the use of relatively large volumes of local anesthetics.

With the exception of intercostal nerve block, systemic absorption of local anesthetic after a peripheral nerve block is generally slow and high plasma levels are usually not a clinical problem. However, peripheral nerves are typically close to major blood vessels, and the potential for an intravascular injection always exists. Local anesthetic systemic toxicity after peripheral nerve blocks may be secondary to an unintentional intravascular injection or to injection of an excessive amount of local anesthetic.

Intercostal nerve block is associated with the highest systemic absorption compared with all other regional anesthetic techniques. Nerve block at the neck area can also lead to local anesthetic toxicity as a result of the high vascularity of the area.

In addition to the potential for vascular injection, peripheral nerve blocks may be associated with trauma to nerve fibers from the needle, resulting in postoperative neuropathy. Hematoma formation, infection, prolonged analgesia, temporary muscle damage, and spasm due to myotoxicity of local anesthetic may be associated with peripheral nerve blocks.

Complications of Head and Neck Blocks

Many surgical procedures of the head and neck can be successfully performed with regional anesthesia. Certain areas are especially suitable for regional anesthetic techniques, such as ophthalmic surgery; plastic surgery of the face, ear, and nose; maxillofacial surgery; and dental extraction. With all these techniques, unintentional intravascular injection of local anesthetics leading to systemic toxicity is always a possibility of which the anesthesiologist should be aware.

The type of head surgery for which regional anesthesia is most commonly performed is ophthalmic surgery. Ophthalmic regional anesthesia offers several advantages. Most patients requiring eye surgery are elderly and have significant associated systemic disease and multiple organ involvement. Regional anesthesia may be preferable in these kinds of patients; it provides adequate surgical conditions, with a smooth postoperative course, rapid recovery, early ambulation, and early hospital dismissal. However, ophthalmic anesthesia can be associated with complications.

Complications of Retrobulbar Blocks

The potential complications of retrobulbar block are listed in Table 24–6.

Intravascular Injection. Intravascular injection of local anesthetics leads to systemic toxicity. Intravascular injection can occur into the retinal vein, which empties into the cavernous sinus or into the ophthalmic artery. Small amounts of local anesthetic injected into these vessels are sufficient to elicit signs of systemic toxicity. Aldrete and associates[96] have postulated that injection of local anesthetic into an artery with reversed arterial flow could be a pathway for early and rapid toxicity in the CNS. Meyers and coworkers[97] reported a case of immediate onset of convulsions after a retrobulbar block.

Symptoms of intravascular injection include mental status changes and convulsions. Loss of consciousness

Table 24–6 Complications of Retrobulbar Block

SYSTEMIC COMPLICATIONS
Intravascular injection
Brain-stem anesthesia
Local toxicity (myotoxicity)
Allergy
Oculocardiac reflex
OCULAR COMPLICATIONS
Retrobulbar hemorrhage
Optic nerve injury
Central retinal artery occlusion
Globe perforation
Contralateral amaurosis
Contralateral extraocular akinesia

and cardiorespiratory depression may follow. Frequent aspirations before and during injection should be done in an attempt to prevent this complication.

Brain-Stem Anesthesia. Small amounts of local anesthetics injected into the optic nerve sheath may spread along the optic nerve into the midbrain. This leads to midbrain anesthesia involving cranial nerves, respiratory centers, or both.

For a series of 6000 retrobulbar blocks, Nicoll and colleagues[98] reported that the incidence of CNS involvement was 0.27%. A similar incidence was reported by Ahn and Stanley.[99] However, Lombardi[100] reported 2% incidence for 150 cases, indicating that perhaps midbrain anesthesia occurs with greater frequency than that reported in the previous series.

Wang and associates[101] demonstrated the connection between the optic nerve sheath and the subarachnoid space. Injecting methylene blue into the optic nerve sheath of a cadaver's orbit, these investigators showed that the dye tracked along the optic nerve sheath into the chiasmatic cistern of the subarachnoid space in the midcranial fossa. They also demonstrated that the pressure required to inject into the nerve sheath was significantly greater than that required to inject into the retrobulbar adipose tissue. Any increase in resistance to injection during a retrobulbar block injection may indicate injection into the sheath, and repositioning the needle tip is recommended.

Symptoms of midbrain anesthesia include dysphagia, contralateral ocular muscle paresis, and loss of vision. Drowsiness, loss of consciousness, and apnea may also occur, although convulsions do not. Symptoms occur within 10 min of the injection. Respiratory arrest may ensue, and if not treated promptly, it may lead to catastrophic consequences.

Injection of local anesthetics into the nerve sheath tracking down the chiasm may also lead to contralateral optic nerve dysfunction and partial contralateral akinesia.[102, 103]

If the eye is elevated and adducted, the optic nerve, ophthalmic artery, and orbital vein are in close contact with the retrobulbar block needle. Nerve damage, intravascular injection, or both may be more likely.[104, 105] The retrobulbar block in an awake patient is best performed with the patient looking straight ahead.[106] This eye position maximizes the distance between the optic nerve and the tip of the needle, decreasing the possibilities of nerve injury and injection of local anesthetics into the nerve sheath.

Allergy Myotoxicity. As with other regional techniques, this complication may be associated with ophthalmic anesthesia. Several patients have had clinical courses suggesting myotoxicity.

Oculocardiac Reflex. The oculocardiac reflex may be elicited by traction on the extraocular muscles or conjunctiva, pressure on the globe, or hematoma. The most common manifestation of the trigeminovagal reflex is bradycardia, but other arrhythmias may occur. If the block is adequate, manipulation of the eye does not elicit the reflex. However, when incomplete anesthesia is obtained, the reflex may occur during manipulation of the eye.

Retrobulbar Hemorrhage. Hemorrhage is the most common complication of retrobulbar block.[106] Symptoms and signs include pain, increased intraocular pressure, decreased visual acuity, hemorrhage, and proptosis. Although uncommon, permanent blindness may occur, secondary to optic nerve compression or ischemia.

Optic Nerve Injury. Injury to the optic nerve may occur as the result of direct needle injury or intraneural injection of local anesthetic. This injury is most likely to occur when the patient is directed to look upward and nasally, because in this position, the nerve lies in proximity to the needle tip. This injury is associated with nerve and retina edema and vitreous hemorrhage. It may lead to severe loss of vision.

Globe Perforation. Perforation of the globe is a rare complication that can also be associated with peribulbar injection of local anesthetics. This injury is more likely to occur in the myopic eye because of the greater anteroposterior diameter of the eye.

Central Retinal Artery Occlusion. Compression of the central retinal artery may be caused by direct injury to the vessel, retrobulbar hemorrhage, or by the bolus of local anesthetic injected. The addition of epinephrine to the local anesthetic could have an additional effect by causing retinal artery spasm.

Deep Cervical Plexus Blocks

Intravascular injection may occur. Spinal or epidural anesthesia, cervical plexalgia, phrenic nerve block, and Horner's syndrome are potential side effects of cervical plexus blocks. To minimize these potential side effects, deep needle insertion should be avoided; a caudad direction is recommended, frequent aspirations for cerebrospinal fluid or blood should be performed, and a 1-mL test dose should be injected to ascertain appropriate position and lack of systemic effects.[107]

Intercostal Nerve Blocks

One complication of intercostal nerve block is local anesthetic systemic toxicity. The intercostal space is supplied by a rich vascular network, and intravascular injection could easily occur. The high metabolic activity of the intercostal muscle leads to greater absorption of local anesthetic, which leads to a high plasma level. The result is higher blood levels that peak sooner than if the same amount of local anesthetic was injected in any other peripheral area. A second complication is pneumothorax. The incidence of pneumothorax is relatively low, less than 1%, and in most cases, it can be treated with simple pleural catheter aspiration and observation. A remote but potential complication associated with intercostal nerve block is spinal anesthesia. Dye studies have proved that in some cases the dura extends along the intercostal nerve for a variable distance. Local anesthetic injected could enter into the subarachnoid space. Unexplained, profound hypotension during and after intercostal block may indicate the development of spinal anesthesia and warrants immediate attention.[107]

Attention to technical details of the technique decreases the potential for pneumothorax. Frequent aspirations to prevent intravascular injection and immediately available resuscitative equipment are warranted.

Brachial Plexus Blocks

Possibly the most common peripheral technique of regional anesthesia is the brachial plexus block. Several of these approaches—interscalene and subclavian perivascular or supraclavicular—are performed in the neck area. Figure 24–3 demonstrates the anatomy of the area where these blocks are performed and suggests the anatomic reasons accounting for complications associated with these blocks.

Interscalene Block. Table 24–7 summarizes the potential complications associated with interscalene nerve block.

Needle A in Figure 24–3 shows the direction of needle insertion for interscalene block. The needle is advanced slightly mesiad, caudad, and dorsad, as described by Winnie.[108] If the needle is directed too medially, injection of local anesthetic into the subarachnoid or epidural space could occur, resulting in total spinal or high epidural anesthesia.

A needle insertion too deep in the interscalene groove may easily lead to injection into the vertebral artery. Minimal amounts of local anesthetic (0.5 mL) injected into the vertebral artery result in high CNS concentration and lead to toxic responses in the CNS. Other possible intravascular injections are into the carotid artery and the external jugular vein.

Phrenic nerve block is the most common side effect of an interscalene block. The phrenic nerve derives from C-3 to C-5. Winnie[108] demonstrated that injection of local anesthetic by the interscalene approach to the brachial plexus may cause sensory anesthesia of the

Table 24–7 Complications of Interscalene Block

COMPLICATION	PATHOPHYSIOLOGIC EFFECT
Total spinal epidural anesthesia	Hypotension, respiratory impairment
Intravascular injection	Systemic toxicity
Phrenic nerve block	Decreased ventilatory capacity
Laryngeal nerve block	Hoarseness
Stellate ganglion block	Horner's syndrome
Pneumothorax	Dyspnea

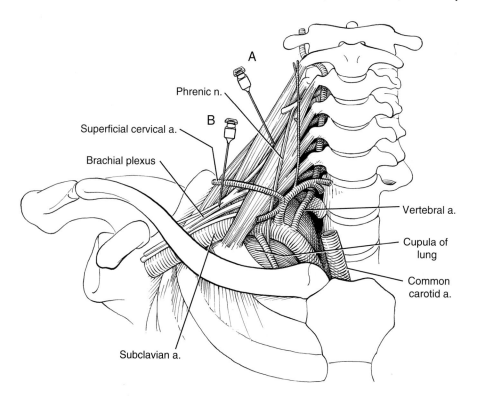

Figure 24–3 Anatomic relationship of neck area and needle placement for (A) interscalene block and (B) subclavian perivascular technique. a., artery; n., nerve.

Phrenic n.

Superficial cervical a.

Brachial plexus

Vertebral a.

Cupula of lung

Common carotid a.

Subclavian a.

brachial plexus roots and of C-4 and frequently extending to C-3. The frequency of phrenic nerve block after interscalene block has been reported to be between 23% and 100%. Urmey and colleagues[109] demonstrated a 100% incidence of phrenic nerve block. In a subsequent investigation, Urmey and McDonald[110] again reported 100% incidence of phrenic nerve block after interscalene block. These investigators also studied the incidence of alterations in routine pulmonary function tests associated with the unilateral hemidiaphragmatic paresis caused by the phrenic nerve block. They demonstrated that forced vital capacity and forced expiratory volume at 1 s were decreased by 27% and 26%, respectively. Peak expiratory and maximum midexpiratory flow rate were also significantly decreased. These changes were apparent 5 min after the injection.

Laryngeal nerve block may result from an interscalene block, producing hoarseness, but no treatment is required. Pneumothorax may also occur.

Supraclavicular or Subclavian Perivascular Block. Needle B in Figure 24–3 represents the needle direction for the subclavian perivascular technique. In the classic approach or Winnie's modification, the needle is directed caudad. The proximity of the pleural apex can be appreciated in Figure 24–3.

The incidence of pneumothorax has been reported to be between 0.5% and 6% with the classic approach. With the subclavian perivascular technique, as described by Winnie, the plexus is approached somewhat higher in the interscalene groove; the incidence of pneumothorax may be lower.[111]

Pneumothorax after supraclavicular block is usually delayed hours after the block. The patient may complain of shortness of breath and pain on expiration. If

a pneumothorax is suspected, a chest radiograph can confirm the diagnosis. Pneumothorax of 10% to 20% usually does not require chest tube insertion. Patient observation is warranted in the event that the pneumothorax becomes larger and evacuation is required.

Other complications of brachial plexus block include neuropathy and hematoma formation. Hematoma in the axillary area usually has few clinical implications, but a neck hematoma, if large, could lead to airway impairment.

Neuropathy After Peripheral Nerve Block. Another potential problem with peripheral nerve block is the development of postoperative neuropathy; however, regional blocks are not the cause of all neuropathies after their use. A logical and systematic approach to determining the cause of a neuropathy is necessary if we are to understand the incidence and origin of neuropathy after peripheral block. Although there are many editorials and reports about avoiding paresthesia as a means of decreasing the incidence of postoperative neuropathy, no conclusive data support the concept that elicitation of mild paresthesia is accompanied by an increased incidence of postoperative neuropathy.[112–115]

Intravenous Regional Anesthesia

The most likely side effect of this otherwise safe technique is a high blood concentration of local anesthesia leading to systemic toxicity. High blood levels can result from a malfunction of the tourniquet or after unintentional tourniquet release.

Conclusions

Properly performed regional anesthesia is a safe and valuable form of anesthesia. Many of the potential side effects or complications associated with regional anesthesia can be minimized by appropriate patient selection and preoperative evaluation. The appropriate choice of technique and local anesthetic agent that together provide adequate anesthesia can prevent the use of excessive amounts of local anesthetic, decreasing the potential for toxic reactions.

In 1961, Greene[116] speculated that the lower incidence of complications after spinal anesthesia probably resulted from the lower concentration of local anesthetic used. This statement is as important now as it was more than 30 years ago. Studies showing neurotoxicity of local anesthetics[117-119] may be associated with increased concentrations of local anesthetics warrant the use of the lowest effective local anesthetic concentration.

Intraoperative management of patients during regional anesthesia should include appropriate hemodynamic and respiratory monitoring, and resuscitative equipment should be available. Awareness of the possible side effects and complications associated with the technique and prompt recognition and management of these changes increase the probability of a successful outcome.

References

1. Vandam LD: Complications of regional anesthesia: past and present. Semin Anesth 1990; 9: 26–31.
2. Scott DB, Cousins MJ: Clinical pharmacology of local anesthetic agents. In Cousins MJ, Bridenbaugh PO (eds): Neural Blockade in Clinical Anesthesia and Management of Pain, pp 86–121. Philadelphia, JB Lippincott, 1980.
3. Bader AM, Concepcion M, Hurley RJ, et al: Comparison of lidocaine and prilocaine for intravenous regional anesthesia. Anesthesiology 1988; 69: 409–412.
4. Hasselstrom LJ, Mogensen T: Toxic reaction of bupivacaine at low plasma concentration. Anesthesiology 1984; 61: 99–100.
5. Wagman IH, De Jong RH, Prince DA: Effects of lidocaine on the central nervous system. Anesthesiology 1967; 28: 155–172.
6. Covino BG: Pharmacology of local anesthetic agents. In Rogers MC, Tinker JH, Covino BG, et al (eds): Principles and Practice of Anesthesiology, pp 1235–1257. St. Louis, Mosby–Year Book, 1993.
7. Englesson S: The influence of acid-base changes on central nervous system toxicity of local anaesthetic agents. I. An experimental study in cats. Acta Anaesthesiol Scand 1974; 18: 79–87.
8. Heavner JE, Dryden CF Jr, Sanghani V, et al: Severe hypoxia enhances central nervous system and cardiovascular toxicity of bupivacaine in lightly anesthetized pigs. Anesthesiology 1992; 77: 142–147.
9. Lynch C III: Depression of myocardial contractility in vitro by bupivacaine, etidocaine, and lidocaine. Anesth Analg 1986; 65: 551–559.
10. Moller RA, Covino BG: Cardiac electrophysiologic effects of lidocaine and bupivacaine. Anesth Analg 1988; 67: 107–114.
11. Clarkson CW, Hondeghem LM: Mechanism for bupivacaine depression of cardiac conduction: fast block of sodium channels during the action potential with slow recovery from block during diastole. Anesthesiology 1985; 62: 396–405.
12. Tanz RD, Heskett T, Loehning RW, et al: Comparative cardiotoxicity of bupivacaine and lidocaine in the isolated perfused mammalian heart. Anesth Analg 1984; 63: 549–556.
13. de Jong RH, Ronfeld RA, DeRosa RA: Cardiovascular effects of convulsant and supraconvulsant doses of amide local anesthetics. Anesth Analg 1982; 61: 3–9.
14. Feldman HS, Arthur GR, Covino BG: Comparative systemic toxicity of convulsant and supraconvulsant doses of intrave-
nous ropivacaine, bupivacaine, and lidocaine in the conscious dog. Anesth Analg 1989; 69: 794–801.
15. Kasten GW: High serum bupivacaine concentrations produce rhythm disturbances similar to torsades de pointes in anesthetized dogs. Reg Anesth 1986; 11: 20–26.
16. Kotelko DM, Shnider SM, Dailey PA, et al: Bupivacaine-induced cardiac arrhythmias in sheep. Anesthesiology 1984; 60: 10–18.
17. Sage D, Feldman H, Arthur G, et al: The cardiovascular effects of convulsant dose of lidocaine and bupivacaine in the conscious dog. Reg Anesth 1985; 10: 175–183.
18. Albright GA: Cardiac arrest following regional anesthesia with etidocaine or bupivacaine. (Editorial.) Anesthesiology 1979; 51: 285–287.
19. Wojtczak JA, Pratilas V, Griffin RM, et al: Cellular mechanisms of cardiac arrhythmias induced by bupivacaine. (Abstract.) Anesthesiology 1984; 61: A37.
20. Morishima HO, Pedersen H, Finster M, et al: Is bupivacaine more cardiotoxic than lidocaine? (Abstract.) Anesthesiology 1983; 59: A409.
21. Nancarrow C, Rutten AJ, Runciman WB, et al: Myocardial and cerebral drug concentrations and the mechanisms of death after fatal intravenous doses of lidocaine, bupivacaine, and ropivacaine in the sheep. Anesth Analg 1989; 69: 276–283.
22. de la Coussaye JE, Brugada J, Allessie MA: Electrophysiologic and arrhythmogenic effects of bupivacaine. A study with high-resolution ventricular epicardial mapping in rabbit hearts. Anesthesiology 1992; 77: 132–141.
23. Thomas RD, Behbehani MM, Coyle DE, et al: Cardiovascular toxicity of local anesthetics: an alternative hypothesis. Anesth Analg 1986; 65: 444–450.
24. Bernards CM, Artru AA: Hexamethonium and midazolam terminate dysrhythmias and hypertension caused by intracerebroventricular bupivacaine in rabbits. Anesthesiology 1991; 74: 89–96.
25. Bernards CM, Artru AA: Effect of intracerebroventricular picrotoxin and muscimol on intravenous bupivacaine toxicity. Evidence supporting central nervous system involvement in bupivacaine cardiovascular toxicity. Anesthesiology 1993; 78: 902–910.
26. Morishima HO, Pedersen H, Finster M, et al: Bupivacaine toxicity in pregnant and nonpregnant ewes. Anesthesiology 1985; 63: 134–139.
27. Morishima HO, Finster M, Arthur GR, et al: Pregnancy does not alter lidocaine toxicity. Am J Obstet Gynecol 1990; 162: 1320–1324.
28. Santos AC, Pedersen H, Harmon TW, et al: Does pregnancy alter the systemic toxicity of local anesthetics? Anesthesiology 1989; 70: 991–995.
29. Datta S, Lambert DH, Gregus J, et al: Differential sensitivities of mammalian nerve fibers during pregnancy. Anesth Analg 1983; 62: 1070–1072.
30. Butterworth JF IV, Walker FO, Lysak SZ: Pregnancy increases median nerve susceptibility to lidocaine. Anesthesiology 1990; 72: 962–965.
31. Brun A: Effect of procaine, Carbocaine and Xylocaine on cutaneous muscle in rabbits and mice. Acta Anaesthesiol Scand 1959; 3: 59–73.
32. Yagiela JA, Benoit PW, Buoncristiani RD, et al: Comparison of myotoxic effects of lidocaine with epinephrine in rats and humans. Anesth Analg 1981; 60: 471–440.
33. Pere P, Watanabe H, Pitkanen M, et al: Local myotoxicity of bupivacaine in rabbits after continuous supraclavicular brachial plexus block. Reg Anesth 1993; 18: 304–307.
34. Pizzolato P, Renegar OJ: Histopathologic effects of long exposure to local anesthetics on peripheral nerves. Anesth Analg 1959; 38: 138–141.
35. Paris WCV, Dettbarn WD: Muscle atrophy following bupivacaine trigger point injection. Anesth Rev 1989; 16: 50–53.
36. Rainin EA, Carlson BM: Postoperative diplopia and ptosis. A clinical hypothesis based on the myotoxicity of local anesthetics. Arch Ophthalmol 1985; 103: 1337–1339.
37. Hogan Q, Dotson R, Erickson S, et al: Local anesthetic myotoxicity: a case and review. Anesthesiology 1994; 80: 942–947.
38. Benoit PW: Reversible skeletal muscle damage after administra-

tion of local anesthetics with and without epinephrine. J Oral Surg 1978; 36: 198–201.

39. Kytta J, Heinonen E, Rosenberg PH, et al: Effects of repeated bupivacaine administration on sciatic nerve and surrounding muscle tissue in rats. Acta Anaesthesiol Scand 1986; 30: 625–629.

40. Guttu RL, Page DG, Laskin DM: Delayed healing of muscle after injection of bupivacaine and steroid. Ann Dent 1990; 49: 5–8.

41. Thomas AD, Caunt JA: Anaphylactoid reaction following local anaesthesia for epidural block. Anaesthesia 1993; 48: 50–52.

42. Bonnet MC, du Cailar G, Deschodt J: Anaphylaxis caused by lidocaine [French]. Ann Fr Anesth Reanim 1989; 8: 127–129.

43. Curley RK, Macfarlane AW, King CM: Contact sensitivity to the amide anesthetics lidocaine, prilocaine, and mepivacaine. Case report and review of the literature. Arch Dermatol 1986; 122: 924–926.

44. Kennedy KS, Cave RH: Anaphylactic reaction to lidocaine. Arch Otolaryngol Head Neck Surg 1986; 112: 671–673.

45. Tannenbaum H, Ruddy S, Schur PH: Acute anaphylaxis associated with serum complement depletion. J Allergy Clin Immunol 1975; 56: 226–234.

46. Brown DT, Beamish D, Wildsmith JA: Allergic reaction to an amide local anaesthetic. Br J Anaesth 1981; 53: 435–437.

47. Stefanini M, Hoffman MN: Studies on platelets: XXVIII: Acute thrombocytopenic purpura due to lidocaine (Xylocaine)-mediated antibody. Report of a case. Am J Med Sci 1978; 275: 365–371.

48. Fulcher DA, Katelaris CH: Anaphylactoid reactions to local anaesthetics despite IgE deficiency: a case report. Asian Pac J Allergy Immunol 1990; 8: 133–136.

49. Ruzicka T, Gerstmeier M, Przybilla B, et al: Allergy to local anesthetics: comparison of patch test with prick and intradermal test results. J Am Acad Dermatol 1987; 16: 1202–1208.

50. Sabbah A: A study of allergy to local anesthetics using the lymphoblast transformation test. [French] Ann Anesthesiol Fr 1976; 17: 281–284.

51. Carpenter RL, Caplan RA, Brown DL, et al: Incidence and risk factors for side effects of spinal anesthesia. Anesthesiology 1992; 76: 906–916.

52. Greene NM: Area of differential block during spinal anesthesia with hyperbaric tetracaine. Anesthesiology 1958; 19: 45–50.

53. Chamberlain DP, Chamberlain BD: Changes in the skin temperature of the trunk and their relationship to sympathetic blockade during spinal anesthesia. Anesthesiology 1986; 65: 139–143.

54. Malmqvist LA, Bengtsson M, Bjornsson G, et al: Sympathetic activity and haemodynamic variables during spinal analgesia in man. Acta Anaesthesiol Scand 1987; 31: 467–473.

55. Mark JB, Steele SM: Cardiovascular effects of spinal anesthesia. Int Anesthesiol Clin 1989; 27: 31–39.

56. Vandam L: Neurological sequelae of spinal and epidural anesthesia. Int Anesthesiol Clin 1986; 24: 231–255.

57. Covino BG: Complications of epidural anesthesia. In Covino BG, Scott DB (eds): Handbook of Epidural Anesthesia and Analgesia, chap 6. Orlando, FL, Grune & Stratton, 1985.

58. Vandam LD, Dripps RD: Long-term follow-up of patients who received 10,098 spinal anesthetics: syndrome of decreased intracranial pressure (headache and ocular and auditory difficulties). JAMA 1956; 161: 586–591.

59. Wedel DJ: Complications. In Raj PP (ed): Clinical Practice of Regional Anesthesia, pp 511–526. New York, Churchill Livingstone, 1991.

60. Garfield JM, Andriole GL, Vetto JT, et al: Prolonged diabetes insipidus subsequent to an episode of chemical meningitis. Anesthesiology 1986; 64: 253–254.

61. Caplan RA, Ward RJ, Posner K, et al: Unexpected cardiac arrest during spinal anesthesia: a closed claims analysis of predisposing factors. Anesthesiology 1988; 68: 5–11.

62. Greene NM: Physiology of Spinal Anesthesia, 3rd ed. Baltimore, Williams & Wilkins, 1981.

63. Thompson KW: Fatalities from spinal anesthesia. Anesth Analg 1934; 13: 75–79.

64. Mackey DC, Carpenter RL, Thompson GE, et al: Bradycardia and asystole during spinal anesthesia: a report of three cases without morbidity. Anesthesiology 1989; 70: 866–868.

65. Cohen LI: Asystole during spinal anesthesia in a patient with sick sinus syndrome. Anesthesiology 1988; 68: 787–788.

66. Brown DL, Carpenter RL, Moore DC, et al: Cardiac arrest during spinal anesthesia, III. (Letter to the editor.) Anesthesiology 1988; 68: 971–972.

67. Keats AS: Anesthesia mortality—a new mechanism. (Editorial.) Anesthesiology 1988; 68: 2–4.

68. Anonymous: Cardiac arrest during spinal anesthesia. (Letter to the editor.) Anesthesiology 1988; 68: 970–974.

69. Covino BG, Scott DB, Lambert DH (eds): Handbook of Spinal Anaesthesia and Analgesia, pp 149–162. Philadelphia, WB Saunders Co, 1994.

70. Munhall RJ, Sukhani R, Winnie AP: Incidence and etiology of failed spinal anesthetics in a university hospital: a prospective study. Anesth Analg 1988; 67: 843–848.

71. Levy JH, Islas JA, Ghia JN, et al: A retrospective study of the incidence and causes of failed spinal anesthetics in a university hospital. Anesth Analg 1985; 64: 705–710.

72. Sinclair DM: Failure of 4 successive spinal anaesthetics. (Letter to the editor.) S Afr Med J 1973; 47: 1984.

73. Cohen EN, Knight RT: Hydrogen ion concentration of the spinal fluid and its relation to spinal anesthetic failures. Anesthesiology 1947; 8: 594–600.

74. Schmidt SI, Moorthy SS, Dierdorf SF, et al: A series of truly failed spinal anesthetics. J Clin Anesth 1990; 2: 336–338.

75. Abram SF, Cherwenka RW: Transient headache immediately following epidural steroid injection. Anesthesiology 1979; 50: 461–462.

76. Ahlering JR, Brodsky JB: Headache immediately following attempted epidural analgesia in obstetrics. (Letter to the editor.) Anesthesiology 1980; 52: 100–101.

77. Diaz JM, Prevost M: Subarachnoid air injection during epidural anesthesia. Anesth Rev 1982; 9: 27–30.

78. Denny N, Masters R, Pearson D, et al: Postdural puncture headache after continuous spinal anesthesia. Anesth Analg 1987; 66: 791–794.

79. Kallos T, Smith TC: Continuous spinal anesthesia with hypobaric tetracaine for hip surgery in lateral decubitus. Anesth Analg 1972; 51: 766–773.

80. Collier CB: Accidental subdural block: four more cases and a radiographic review. Anaesth Intensive Care 1992; 20: 215–225.

81. Dawkins CJ: An analysis of the complications of extradural and caudal block. Anaesthesia 1969; 24: 554–563.

82. Lubenow T, Keh-Wong E, Kristof K, et al: Inadvertent subdural injection: a complication of an epidural block. Anesth Analg 1988; 67: 175–179.

83. Horlocker TT, Wedel DJ, Offord KP: Does preoperative antiplatelet therapy increase the risk of hemorrhagic complications associated with regional anesthesia? Anesth Analg 1990; 70: 631–634.

84. Cousins MJ, Bromage PR: Epidural neural blockade. In Cousins MJ, Bridenbaugh PO (eds): Neural Blockade in Clinical Anesthesia and Management of Pain, 2nd ed, pp 253–360. Philadelphia, JB Lippincott, 1988.

85. Lerner SM, Gutterman P, Jenkins F: Epidural hematoma and paraplegia after numerous lumbar punctures. Anesthesiology 1973; 39: 550–551.

86. Ganjoo P, Singh AK, Mishra VK, et al: Postblock epidural hematoma causing paraplegia. Case report. Reg Anesth 1994; 19: 62–65.

87. Bridenbaugh PO: Complications of local anesthetic neural blockade. In Cousins MJ, Bridenbaugh PO (eds): Neural Blockade in Clinical Anesthesia and Management of Pain, 2nd ed, p 701. Philadelphia, JB Lippincott, 1988.

88. Beaudoin MG, Klein L: Epidural abscess following multiple spinal anaesthetics. Anaesth Intensive Care 1984; 12: 163–164.

89. Mamourian AC, Dickman CA, Drayer BP, et al: Spinal epidural abscess: three cases following spinal epidural injection demonstrated with magnetic resonance imaging. Anesthesiology 1993; 78: 204–207.

90. Zoellner PA, Bode ET: Horner's syndrome after epidural block in early pregnancy. Reg Anesth 1991; 16: 242–244.

91. McLean APH, Mulligan GW, Otton P, et al: Hemodynamic alterations associated with epidural anesthesia. Surgery 1967; 62: 79–87.

92. Mohan J, Potter JM: Pupillary constriction and ptosis following caudal epidural analgesia. Anaesthesia 1975; 30: 769–773.

93. Warwick R, Williams PL: Gray's Anatomy, 35th ed, p 1129. Edinburgh, Longman, 1973.

94. Stevens RA, Chester WL, Artuso JD, et al: Back pain after epidural anesthesia with chloroprocaine in volunteers: preliminary report. Reg Anesth 1991; 16: 199–203.

95. Stevens RA, Urmey WF, Urquhart BL, et al: Back pain after epidural anesthesia with chloroprocaine. Anesthesiology 1993; 78: 492–497.

96. Aldrete JA, Romo-Salas F, Arora S, et al: Reverse arterial blood flow as a pathway for central nervous system toxic responses following injection of local anesthetics. Anesth Analg 1978; 57: 428–433.

97. Meyers EF, Ramirez RC, Boniuk I: Grand mal seizures after retrobulbar block. Arch Ophthalmol 1978; 96: 847.

98. Nicoll JM, Acharya PA, Ahlen K, et al: Central nervous system complications after 6000 retrobulbar blocks. Anesth Analg 1987; 66: 1298–1302.

99. Ahn JC, Stanley JA: Subarachnoid injection as a complication of retrobulbar anesthesia. Am J Ophthalmol 1987; 103: 225–230.

100. Lombardi G: Radiology in Neuro-Ophthalmology, pp 6–8. Baltimore, Williams & Wilkins, 1967.

101. Wang BC, Bogart B, Hillman DE, et al: Subarachnoid injection—a potential complication of retrobulbar block. Anesthesiology 1989; 71: 845–847.

102. Follette JW, LoCascio JA: Bilateral amaurosis following unilateral retrobulbar block. (Letter to the editor.) Anesthesiology 1985; 63: 237–238.

103. Friedberg HL, Kline OR Jr: Contralateral amaurosis after retrobulbar injection. Am J Ophthalmol 1986; 101: 688–690.

104. Drysdale DB: Experimental subdural retrobulbar injection of anesthetic. Ann Ophthalmol 1984; 16: 716–718.

105. Unsold R, Stanley JA, DeGroot J: The CT-topography of retrobulbar anesthesia. Anatomic-clinical correlation of complications and suggestion of a modified technique. Albrecht Von Graefes Arch Klin Exp Ophthalmol 1981; 217: 125–136.

106. Raj PP, Gesund P, Phero J, et al: Rationale and choice for surgical procedures. In Raj PP (ed): Clinical Practice of Regional Anesthesia, pp 197–269. New York, Churchill Livingstone, 1991.

107. Raj PP, Pai U, Rawal N: Techniques of regional anesthesia in adults. In Raj PP (ed): Clinical Practice of Regional Anesthesia, pp 271–363. New York, Churchill Livingstone, 1991.

108. Winnie AP: Plexus Anesthesia, vol I. Perivascular Techniques of Brachial Plexus Block, pp 167–180. Philadelphia, WB Saunders Co, 1983.

109. Urmey WF, Talts KH, Sharrock NE: One hundred percent incidence of hemidiaphragmatic paresis associated with interscalene brachial plexus anesthesia as diagnosed by ultrasonography. Anesth Analg 1991; 72: 498–503.

110. Urmey WF, McDonald M: Hemidiaphragmatic paresis during interscalene brachial plexus block: effects on pulmonary function and chest wall mechanics. Anesth Analg 1992; 74: 352–357.

111. Winnie AP: Plexus Anesthesia, vol I. Perivascular Techniques of Brachial Plexus Block, pp 145–163. Philadelphia, WB Saunders Co, 1983.

112. Selander D, Edshage S, Wolff T: Paresthesiae or no paresthesiae? Nerve lesions after axillary blocks. Acta Anaesthesiol Scand 1979; 23: 27–33.

113. Brown DL: Atlas of Regional Anesthesia, pp 9–21. Philadelphia, WB Saunders Co, 1992.

114. Plevak DJ, Linstromberg JW, Danielson DR: Paresthesia vs nonparesthesia—the axillary block. (Abstract.) Anesthesiology 1983; 59: A216.

115. Selander D: Axillary plexus block: paresthetic or perivascular. (Editorial.) Anesthesiology 1987; 66: 726–728.

116. Greene NM: Neurological sequelae of spinal anesthesia. Anesthesiology 1961; 22: 682–698.

117. Lambert LA, Lambert DH, Strichartz GR: Irreversible conduction block in isolated nerve by high concentrations of local anesthetics. Anesthesiology 1994; 80: 1082–1093.

118. Myers RR, Kalichman MW, Reisner LS, et al: Neurotoxicity of local anesthetics: altered perineurial permeability, edema, and nerve fiber injury. Anesthesiology 1986; 64: 29–35.

119. Barsa J, Batra M, Fink BR, et al: A comparative in vivo study of local neurotoxicity of lidocaine, bupivacaine, 2-chloroprocaine, and a mixture of 2-chloroprocaine and bupivacaine. Anesth Analg 1982; 61: 961–967.

CHAPTER 25

Delayed Complications and Side Effects of Regional Anesthesia

Kenneth Drasner, M.D., Jeffrey L. Swisher, M.D.

After these experiments on our own bodies we both went to dinner without any physical complaints. We drank wine and smoked several cigars. I went to bed at 11 o'clock and slept well throughout the night. I woke up, feeling refreshed and well the following morning and went for a walk for one hour. Towards the end of this walk I noticed a slight headache, which increased during the course of the day while I did my usual work. Towards 3 p.m. my face turned pale, the pulse was rather faint but remained regular and was about 70 beats per minute. Furthermore, I had the feeling of a very strong pressure in my head and felt a little dizzy when I rose quickly from my chair. All these symptoms disappeared as soon as I lay down horizontally, but they returned when I got up. In the late afternoon I had therefore to go to bed and had to stay in bed for 9 days, since all the described symptoms returned on getting up.

August Bier, *Experiments with the cocainisation of the spinal cord*, 1899

Delayed complications and side effects have been, and continue to be, a factor impacting the use of regional anesthesia. Thus, an appreciation of complications associated with regional anesthesia is a prerequisite to rational selection and appropriate application of these techniques. This chapter focuses on the infrequent major and the frequent minor complications—there are no frequent major complications, and infrequent minor complications are, by definition, of little clinical significance.

Major Complications of Neuraxial Block

Serious delayed complications after spinal or epidural anesthesia may be divided into the following general categories: (1) chemical toxicity as a result of dose-related effects of injected agents; (2) immunologic reaction to injected substances; (3) infection as a result of a break in sterile technique or contamination of the epidural or intrathecal space with an infectious agent present in blood or other tissue space; (4) direct trauma to neurologic or vascular structures from needles or catheters; (5) indirect trauma from compression owing to bleeding or infection (e.g., epidural hematoma or abscess); (6) ischemia resulting from thrombosis, spasm, or disruption of vascular structures or from alteration in blood flow; and (7) unrelated injury secondary to positioning or the surgical procedure.

Chemical Toxicity

Durocaine

Although sporadic reports of neurologic injury associated with spinal anesthesia suggested that local anesthetics, per se, might be neurotoxic, the relative infrequency of injury led some[1] to conclude that the tissues of affected patients were particularly "sensitive" to these agents. In 1937, Ferguson and Watkins[2] challenged this view, reporting 14 cases of cauda equina syndrome associated with the use of "heavy" Durocaine, an anesthetic formulation containing 10% procaine, 15% ethanol, glycerin, and gum acacia or gliadin. Experimental studies in cats[3] demonstrated that 10% procaine alone induced similar injury, whereas vehicle components did not. Ferguson and Watkins concluded "this is not in the nature of an idiosyncrasy, but that in the concentration employed the drug itself has a toxicity but little short of that which would produce paralysis in a high percentage of cases."

The Chloroprocaine Controversy

Sporadic cases of neurologic injury after spinal or epidural anesthesia continued to occur. However, concern that clinically used anesthetic agents might induce predictable injury dissipated until nearly half a century later when several cases of severe neurologic damage were associated with presumed intrathecal injection of

Table 25–1 Continuous Spinal Anesthesia Guidelines for Anesthetic Administration

1. Insert catheter just far enough to confirm and maintain placement.
2. Use the lowest effective concentration of local anesthetic.
3. Place a limit on the amount of local anesthetic to be used.
4. Administer a test dose, and assess the extent of block.
5. If maldistribution is suspected, use maneuvers to increase the spread of local anesthetic (e.g., change the patient's position, alter the lumbosacral curvature, switch to a local anesthetic solution with a different baricity).
6. If well-distributed sensory anesthesia is not achieved before the dose limit is reached, abandon the technique.

Adapted from Rigler ML, Drasner K, Krejcie TC, et al: Cauda equina syndrome after continuous spinal anesthesia. Anesth Analg 1991; 72: 275–281.

an intended epidural dose of chloroprocaine.[4] Unlike the injuries associated with Durocaine, the circumstances of these patients and the experimental studies that followed failed to clearly identify chloroprocaine as the specific causative agent. First, the clinical circumstances varied considerably and only for some patients was there strong evidence for intrathecal injection.[5–7] Second, some patients' care was complicated by significant hypotension and a need for resuscitation, which might have contributed to injury.[5, 6] Third, the administration of relatively large volumes of fluid into the subarachnoid space generated speculation that increased subarachnoid pressure might have impaired perfusion of neural tissue.[8] Fourth, the pattern of injury varied widely. Finally, all of the reported cases occurred after 1976, yet the formulation of chloroprocaine had not changed since 1971.

Animal experiments provided conflicting evidence regarding chloroprocaine neurotoxicity. Although some studies[9, 10] suggested that chloroprocaine had greater intrinsic neurotoxicity than other anesthetic agents, other studies[11, 12] did not. Using rabbit isolated vagus nerves, Gissen[8] found that exposure to the commercial solution of 3% chloroprocaine (containing 0.2% sodium bisulfite and with a pH of approximately

3) produced an irreversible block, but exposure to the same solution buffered to a pH of 7.3 resulted in complete recovery. Additional experiments indicated that irreversible block resulted from the combination of bisulfite and a low pH, suggesting that liberation of sulfur dioxide might be the cause of injury. Data from some in vivo studies[12, 13] were consistent with this mechanism, whereas data from other studies[14] sharply conflicted. Although significant disagreement persisted, the prevailing conclusion was that chloroprocaine per se was not neurotoxic or, at least, no more neurotoxic than other available anesthetic agents.[8, 15] Concern about local anesthetic toxicity again subsided, but not for long.

Continuous Spinal Anesthesia

In 1991, Rigler et al[16] reported four cases of the cauda equina syndrome that occurred with a continuous spinal technique. In three of these cases, 5% lidocaine with 7.5% dextrose was administered through a 28-G catheter; in the remaining patient, 0.5% tetracaine with 5% dextrose was administered through a 20-G "epidural" catheter. The evidence that these injuries resulted from a direct effect of the local anesthetic is substantial.

In all four cases, the initial dose of anesthetic produced a restricted block, and the total dose of anesthetic required to achieve surgical anesthesia exceeded that commonly used with a single-injection technique. These circumstances led us to conclude that the combination of maldistribution and the relatively high dose of anesthetic resulted in exposure of the nerve roots of the cauda equina to a toxic concentration of anesthetic and to suggest guidelines for the administration of anesthetic through an indwelling subarachnoid catheter (Table 25–1). Within a year, eight additional cases were reported[17]—all consistent with this etiology.

Studies performed with models of the subarachnoid space support this etiology for injury. Administration of hyperbaric local anesthetic through a sacrally directed catheter produces a restricted distribution,[18–21] and relatively high concentrations can be achieved with clini-

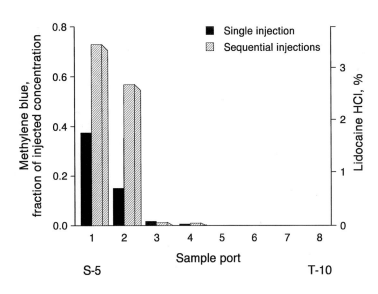

Figure 25–1 Effect of three sequential injections through a sacrally directed 28-G catheter on distribution of a lidocaine-dye mixture. Two experiments are compared. In the first, 1 mL of lidocaine-dye mixture (4.76% lidocaine hydrochloride) was injected over 60 s; in the second, three sequential 1-mL injections (5 min apart) were made with the catheter in the same fixed position. (From Rigler ML, Drasner K: Distribution of catheter-injected local anesthetic in a model of the subarachnoid space. Anesthesiology 1991; 75: 684–692.)

cally administered doses (Fig. 25–1).[19, 20] Several factors appear to affect distribution, including catheter size, tip configuration, tip position, injection rate, and injection velocity.[19–21]

In vitro and in vivo animal studies provide further evidence for local anesthetic neurotoxicity as the etiology of injury. Using the "sucrose gap" method to study the effect of anesthetic concentration on reversibility of regional block, Lambert et al[22] observed that exposure of desheathed sciatic nerves of bullfrogs to 5% lidocaine with 7.5% glucose for 15 min results in persistent block; neither 3-h wash nor overnight soak resulted in recovery. In contrast, 1.5% lidocaine (with or without dextrose) had no apparent irreversible effect. Additional studies performed in the same laboratory by Bainton and Strichartz[23] demonstrated progressive nonreversible loss of impulse activity with increasing concentrations of lidocaine, beginning at approximately 1%. However, the absolute concentration for conduction failure in vitro must be interpreted with caution—differences exist between an irreversible conduction block and neurotoxic injury and between a desheathed amphibian nerve segment lacking a cell body and devoid of a blood supply and a mammalian cauda equina. Nonetheless, the results leave open the possibility that brief exposure to concentrations of lidocaine well below those achieved in in vitro spinal canal models might induce persistent loss of function.

That deficits may occur with intrathecal administration of lidocaine at concentrations currently used for spinal anesthesia has been demonstrated by in vivo studies[24, 25] using chronic indwelling catheters in rats (Fig. 25–2). Catheters were placed distal to the conus medullaris, and anesthetic was administered by continuous infusion to encourage restricted distribution and selective exposure of the cauda equina. Sensory impairment (e.g., lack of response to a heat stimulus applied to the tail) persisted 4 days after infusion of 5% lidocaine with 7.5% glucose. These findings support the hypothesis that the clinical injuries after continuous spinal anesthesia were the direct consequence of local anesthetic administered at a relatively high dose and in a relatively restricted distribution.

Withdrawal of Microcatheters

In May 1992, the Food and Drug Administration withdrew approval for small-bore catheters (27-G and smaller) and issued a bulletin[17] to all health care providers to alert them to "a serious hazard associated with continuous spinal anesthesia." This alert focused on the risk associated with microcatheters, stating that they had "received 11 reports of cauda equina syndrome in which small-bore catheters were used to deliver 5% lidocaine with 7.5% glucose to the intrathecal space. This compares with only one reported case of cauda equina syndrome associated with the use of large-bore catheters since 1984." That 11 of the 12 reports of cauda equina syndrome involved small-bore catheters may, in fact, indicate a higher incidence of injury with these devices. Alternatively, it may simply reflect relatively greater usage of small catheters or reporting bias. More importantly, a clear upper limit that defines a safe catheter size cannot exist; maldistribution can occur with catheters of any size or configuration. In a subarachnoid model, administration of anesthetic through any sacrally directed catheter can produce a relatively restricted distribution, and, clinically, maldistribution has been documented[26] with catheters as large as 3.5 F.

Repeat Single-Injection Spinal Anesthesia

Maldistribution is not restricted to continuous spinal anesthesia—it can, and does, occur with single-injection spinal anesthesia, and it is an important cause for failure to achieve adequate sensory block, i.e., a "failed" spinal block.[27] As with the continuous technique, there is the potential (albeit less than with a catheter in fixed position) for a similar restricted distribution of anesthetic with repeat injection. Thus, neurotoxic concentrations might be achieved within the subarachnoid space. Review of the closed claims database appears to support this concern[27]: of 308 claims for nerve damage, 5 claims for cauda equina syndrome

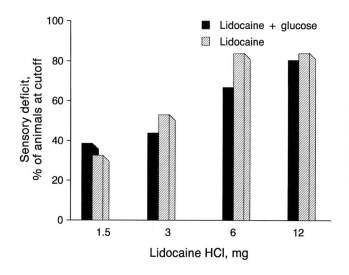

Figure 25–2 The percentage of animals failing to respond to a heat stimulus 4 days after infusion of 5% lidocaine with 7.5% glucose or 5% lidocaine alone. The two solutions produced similar, dose-dependent sensory impairment. (From Sakura S, Chan VWS, Ciriales R, et al: The addition of 7.5% glucose does not alter the neurotoxicity of 5% lidocaine administered intrathecally in the rat. Anesthesiology 1995; 82: 236–240.)

were found; 3 involved a subarachnoid block, 2 of which occurred with repeat injection after an inadequate spinal block (unfortunately, documentation for the third case was insufficient to determine whether a repeat injection was made). Consequently, management of an inadequate spinal block should include assessment of the likelihood of technical error and adjustment of dose for the repeat injection (Table 25–2). Recent events also suggest that relatively high doses of anesthetic should be avoided when a restricted distribution is deliberately sought (e.g., saddle block).

5% Lidocaine With 7.5% Dextrose

Our review of the cases of cauda equina syndrome associated with continuous spinal anesthesia led to our recommending that anesthetics be administered at the lowest effective concentration.[16] This recommendation was based on data suggesting that injury was, to some extent, concentration-dependent[12, 28, 29] and that the concentrations used in these cases, i.e., 5% lidocaine and 0.5% tetracaine, exceeded those required for adequate sensory block. The eight additional cases reported[17] to the Food and Drug Administration associated with the use of 5% lidocaine and 7.5% glucose and the reports[30] of transient neurologic symptoms after single injection of this same solution have generated further concern about administration of lidocaine as a 5% solution.

Although anesthetic concentration can be decreased without loss of efficacy, the extent to which reduction within the clinically relevant range decreases neurotoxic risk remains to be determined. Surprisingly, preliminary in vivo data[31] suggest that the toxicity of a dose of lidocaine may be equivalent whether the anesthetic is administered as a 5% or a 2% solution. Furthermore, that major neurologic injuries have occurred after intrathecal administration of intended epidural doses of 2% lidocaine indicates that modest reduc-

tion in concentration does not completely eliminate risk.[32, 33]

Existing data suggest that commonly used concentrations of glucose do not contribute to neurotoxicity. In vitro, anesthetic-induced, irreversible conduction failure is not altered by the presence of 7.5% glucose.[22] Moreover, when administered intrathecally in rats, 5% lidocaine, with and without glucose, induces similar, dose-dependent alteration in sensory function (Fig. 25–2).[25]

With respect to major neurologic injury, lidocaine has a remarkable safety record. In addition to large prospective studies,[34] the rarity of reported injury despite millions of administrations attests to the drug's overall safety. Nonetheless, reports of permanent injury and transient neurologic symptoms indicate the need for reevaluation of the relative toxicity of this and other commonly used anesthetics. Studies performed by Sakura et al[35] indicated that local anesthetic neurotoxicity does not result from sodium channel blockade per se, suggesting that there may be differences in neurotoxic potential among anesthetics and that the development of better local anesthetics is a realistic goal.

Immunologic Reaction

Arachnoiditis

Adhesive arachnoiditis is a sterile, inflammatory process, which actually affects all of the meningeal components. Intense connective tissue proliferation leads to adhesion of the nerve roots, restrictive bands enmeshing the spinal cord and cauda equina, and, at times, complete obliteration of substantial portions of the subarachnoid space. A wide variety of circumstances (e.g., trauma, surgery, infection, tumor, or intrathecal administration of various compounds) have been associated with arachnoiditis and thereby implicated as potential causes. Whether, in fact, they are causal and the mechanism by which the reaction is induced remains obscure; indeed, in some cases, no specific etiology can be identified, the disorder being termed "idiopathic primary adhesive arachnoiditis."

Of importance for spinal and epidural anesthesia, arachnoiditis has been attributed to contamination of anesthetic solution by detergents, chemicals used for sterilization, and preservatives and other vehicle components and to anesthetic agents per se.[6, 36–38] Symptom onset may be immediate or delayed for months after an event. The diagnosis can be made by myelography, computed tomography, or magnetic resonance imaging, the last two being preferable because arachnoiditis has been reported after intrathecal administration of contrast material. Clumping and displacement of the nerve roots are the most characteristic imaging findings. In some patients, the disorder results in progressive motor and sensory loss, leading to paraplegia, quadriplegia, and death. There is no effective treatment. Fortunately, modern technique, possibly including the use of disposable equipment, improved pharmaceutical practice, and more limited vehicle

---

Table 25–2 Spinal Anesthesia Guidelines for Anesthetic Administration After a "Failed Spinal"

1. Aspiration of CSF should be attempted immediately before and after injection of local anesthetic.
2. Sacral dermatomes should always be included in an evaluation of the presence of a spinal block.
3. If CSF is aspirated after anesthetic injection, it should be assumed that the local anesthetic has been delivered into the subarachnoid space; total anesthetic dosage should be limited to the maximum dose a clinician would consider reasonable to administer in a single injection.
4. If an injection is repeated, the technique should be modified to avoid reinforcing the same restricted distribution (e.g., alter the patient's position, use an anesthetic with a different baricity, straighten the lumbosacral curvature).
5. If CSF cannot be aspirated after injection, repeat injection of a full dose of local anesthetic should not be considered unless careful sensory examination (conducted after sufficient time for development of sensory anesthesia) reveals no evidence of block.

CSF, cerebrospinal fluid.
Modified from Drasner K, Rigler ML: Repeat injection after a "failed spinal": at times, a potentially unsafe practice. (Letter to the editor.) Anesthesiology 1991; 75: 713–714.

components, has made this complication extremely rare.

Aseptic Meningitis

Aseptic meningitis after spinal anesthesia likely results from injection of an irritant into the subarachnoid space. Similar to arachnoiditis, the incidence of this complication has decreased to near zero with modern technique. Patients present with fever, headache, and stiff neck, requiring that infection be eliminated as a possibility. Examination of cerebrospinal fluid is diagnostic, showing an increased number of cells but, as the name suggests, normal glucose values and no organisms. The prognosis is uniformly good.

Infection

Infection in the epidural or intrathecal space may occur as a result of a break in sterile technique or from contamination with an infectious agent present in blood or other tissue space. The former should be completely preventable. If reasonable precautions are used, the risk of the latter should be relatively small.

Epidural Abscess

Epidural abscess is a rare infection; the diagnosis accounted for fewer than 1 in 10,000 admissions in two retrospective studies of tertiary care centers.[39, 40] Moreover, epidural abscess generally develops after bacteremia or from extension of bone, soft tissue, or skin infection; rarely is epidural anesthesia implicated (in the two above-mentioned studies, only 1 of 74 documented cases was preceded by an epidural anesthetic). Similarly, large retrospective reviews[41] of epidural anesthesia attest to the rarity of this complication.

An epidural abscess can result in devastating sequelae that may be averted by early, comprehensive treatment. Patients generally present with fever (57% to 95%) and back pain (89% to 100%).[39, 40] Symptoms classically progress in four phases: spinal ache, root pain, weakness, and paralysis,[42] with outcome related to the severity of the neurologic impairment before treatment (Fig. 25–3) and postsurgical improvement dependent on the duration of deficit before operation.[40] Reviewing a 12-year experience at New York Hospital, Danner and Hartman[40] found that of seven patients with preoperative weakness or paralysis for 1.5 days or less, all had some recovery after operation compared with only 2 of 11 patients with impairment for 1.5 days or more.

Most investigators classify abscess as acute or chronic from the duration of symptoms or surgical findings.[40] When symptoms have been present for less than 2 weeks, pus is generally observed at operation, whereas granulation tissue is seen in the majority of chronic cases. Patients who have anesthetic- or catheter-related infections generally present early and the infection progresses rapidly; however, cases of infection occurring more than 1 month after a procedure have also been reported.[43] *Staphylococcus aureus* remains the most

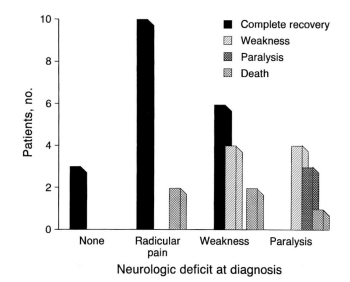

Figure 25–3 Outcome versus initial neurologic deficit in 35 cases of spinal epidural abscess. (Redrawn from Danner RL, Hartman BJ: Update of spinal epidural abscess: 35 cases and review of the literature. Rev Infect Dis 1987; 9: 265–274. The University of Chicago, publisher.)

common organism isolated. Often, there is a history of significant back trauma, suggesting that hematoma formation may be causal, providing a nidus for infection. Weakness or paralysis may develop suddenly despite previous slow progression or stability of symptoms. Because loss of neurologic function may be irreversible, most authorities recommend early surgical intervention.[40]

Long-term catheterization for management of cancer pain is associated with a higher incidence of infection. Du Pen et al[44] studied 350 terminally ill patients and identified 15 cases of epidural space infection. However, these infections were detected at an early stage—none of the patients demonstrated fever, increased leukocyte count, meningism, or neurologic signs of cord or root compression—probably as a result of continuous patient follow-up. Consequently, all were managed effectively with removal of the catheter and antibiotic therapy; none required decompressive surgery.

Management of the Febrile Patient

Although data do not exist, common sense dictates that spinal or epidural needles should not be passed through areas of known or suspected infection. The decision to administer a spinal or an epidural anesthetic to a febrile patient requires more informed judgment. There is both experimental and clinical evidence to suggest that lumbar puncture performed during a period of bacteremia might cause meningitis. Using cisternal puncture in rats, Carp and Bailey[45] found that meningitis developed in 12 of 40 rats undergoing puncture during bacteremia. In contrast, a similar group of bacteremic animals not undergoing puncture did not develop meningitis; animals undergoing puncture in the absence of bacteremia also did not develop meningitis. Perhaps most importantly, these investigators also found that prior treatment with a single dose of an effective antibiotic eliminated risk.

Clinical studies have reported inconsistent data. Teele et al[46] conducted a retrospective review of 277 children with bacteremia and found that meningitis developed in 7 of 46 who had a negative result of diagnostic lumbar puncture but in only 2 of the 231 who did not undergo lumbar puncture. Of note, meningitis occurred only in infants younger than age 1 year and in only 2 of 17 treated with antibiotics. However, caution must be exercised when extrapolating from lumbar puncture performed because meningitis is suspected to dural puncture or epidural catheterization for anesthetic administration. Moreover, other investigators[47] have not found that diagnostic lumbar puncture was associated with subsequent meningitis.

Case reports[48] of meningitis occurring after spinal anesthesia during possible bacteremia have been published. Similarly, apparent bacteremia has been associated with subsequent epidural abscess.[49] However, considering the number of procedures performed on patients at risk, these appear to be extraordinarily rare. Consequently, we believe that fever alone should not be considered a contraindication to spinal or epidural anesthesia. The decision should rest on assessment of the patient's condition, predisposing factors, current therapy, and the indication for the technique.

Hematoma

Bleeding in the epidural or subarachnoid space as a result of disruption of a blood vessel by a needle or catheter can result in spinal cord compression or ischemia or both. Morbidity may range from mild sensory or motor deficit in the lower body to quadriplegia and death.[50–52] Initial signs or symptoms of a neuraxial hematoma may vary; in a review by Vandermeulen and colleagues[52] of published reports, the chief complaint was muscle weakness in 46%, back pain with a radicular component in 38%, and sensory deficit in 14%. As with abscess, delay in diagnosis and therapy was correlated with worse neurologic outcome (Fig. 25–4).[52] Consequently, if a hematoma is suspected, immediate radiologic examination and neurosurgical consultation are critical. Magnetic resonance imaging is the preferred diagnostic modality.

Historically, hematoma has been a rare complication. In a retrospective review by Tryba[53] of spinal and epidural anesthetics, only three symptomatic hematomas were identified among 1.5 million anesthetic procedures. According to Vandermeulen et al,[52] only 61 anesthetic-related cases have been reported since 1909. However, risk of this complication may now be greater as a result of changes in anesthetic and surgical practice—specifically, increased use of combined regional-general anesthesia, postoperative epidural analgesia, and perioperative anticoagulant therapy. More comprehensive use of regional anesthetic techniques stems largely from studies demonstrating beneficial effects for patients undergoing vascular and orthopedic

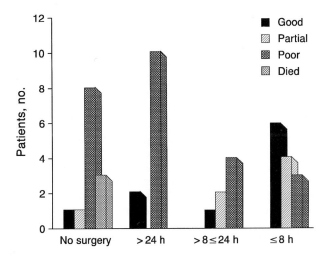

Figure 25–4 Neurologic recovery from epidural hematoma as a function of time to surgical intervention. (Data from Vandermeulen EP, Van Aken H, Vermylen J: Anticoagulants and spinal-epidural anesthesia. Anesth Analg 1994; 79: 1165–1177.)

procedures[54–56]—populations most likely to receive various regimens of antiplatelet, thrombolytic, or anticoagulative therapy.

Coagulopathy and Hemostatic Disorders

Severe hemostatic or coagulative disorders such as disseminated intravascular coagulation preclude neuraxial blocks. Neuraxial techniques also are relatively contraindicated in the presence of preexisting coagulopathy or hemostatic disorders such as hemophilia, idiopathic thrombocytopenic purpura, or von Willebrand's disease. The extent to which mild to moderate alterations in coagulation or platelet activity contraindicate neuraxial block remains controversial.

One of the more common neuraxial anesthetic-coagulation-related dilemmas faced by anesthesiologists is whether to perform spinal or epidural anesthesia in a patient with preeclampsia. Approximately 7% of all pregnancies are complicated by this disorder, of which approximately 10% to 30% may develop thrombocytopenia; disorders of coagulation also occur.[57] Because regional analgesia and anesthesia are of potential benefit to these patients, the clinician must consider how to assess risk of bleeding and decide what is an acceptable risk.

To determine practice patterns for management of regional anesthesia in the preeclamptic patient, Voulgaropoulos and Palmer[58] surveyed the 113 anesthesiology residency programs in the United States; the data analyzed were from 74 programs. The investigators asked which screening tests were required for mild and severe preeclampsia under two hypothetical degrees of operative urgency. In the urgent setting, approximately 30% of programs required a platelet count and less than 20% required a prothrombin time and partial thromboplastin time (PT/PTT) or a bleeding time for patients with mild preeclampsia compared with approximately 75% of programs that required a platelet count and 35% to 40% that required additional studies in the presence of severe preeclampsia. Screening was more thorough in the elective setting, with approximately 60% of programs obtaining platelet counts and 25% obtaining PT/PTT or bleeding times for the mildly preeclamptic patient and 100% obtaining platelet counts and 60% to 75% obtaining a PT/PTT or a bleeding time in the patient with severe disease.

In a survey of obstetric units covering 22% of all deliveries in the United Kingdom, Barker and Callander[59] found significant variability in coagulation tests ordered: practice ranged from full coagulation screening of all patients to only limited testing (e.g., only a platelet count or PT for severe disease). The investigators, therefore, conducted a retrospective study of 434 coagulation screens ordered for preeclamptic patients being evaluated for epidural analgesia. They found platelet counts of less than 150×10^4 cells/L present in 28% of cases. Significant thrombocytopenia (platelet counts less than 100×10^4 cells/L) was observed only with severe disease. They also found that patients with coagulation abnormalities always had a decreased platelet count. These authors concluded that coagulation testing should be limited to severely preeclamptic patients and first-line testing should be limited to a platelet count.

Some studies have documented functional platelet abnormalities in nonthrombocytopenic patients with preeclampsia.[60, 61] However, in other studies,[57, 62] platelet dysfunction, abnormal fibrinogen level, or prolonged PT or PTT has not occurred in the absence of thrombocytopenia. Overall, few clinicians would hesitate to perform a regional anesthetic in the patient with a platelet count exceeding 100×10^4 cells/L, providing support for the use of a platelet count alone for initial screening. The incidence of thrombocytopenia (platelet count $\leq 150 \times 10^4$ cells/L) is approximately 8% in normal parturients.[63]

There is no clear consensus for the management of the patient with more significant thrombocytopenia. Some investigators[62] advocate measuring bleeding times for patients with platelet counts between 50×10^4 cells/L and 100×10^4 cells/L. However, meta-analysis by Rodgers and Levin[64] of 862 published papers failed to support bleeding time as a clinically useful tool (i.e., it is not clear that this test changes in advance of significant bleeding or that bleeding from the skin can predict bleeding elsewhere). Thromboelastography, a relatively simple test that provides a global assessment of hemostatic function, may prove to be a more useful clinical tool. However, at the present time, the data are inadequate to rely on this measurement. Moreover, the decision to place a catheter must consider the inherent uncertainty of the disorder's clinical progression.

Heparin and Low-Molecular-Weight Heparin

Preoperative administration of low-dose heparin significantly decreases risk of postoperative deep venous thrombosis.[65] A potential problem with this form of therapy is interpatient variability in anticoagulation effect. Additionally, standard laboratory tests of heparin anticoagulation may be unreliable during low-dose prophylaxis.[66] Either unfractionated heparin or low-molecular-weight heparin may be given prophylactically. Low-molecular-weight heparin may replace unfractionated heparin for deep venous thrombosis prophylaxis because it offers the following advantages: near 100% bioavailability at low doses, longer half-life, more predictable dose-response function, lower cost, and probable decreased hemorrhagic and thrombotic ratio.[67] Although large-scale reviews[68, 69] suggest lack of neurologic risk, several of the 61 cases of hematoma reviewed by Vandermeulen et al[52] involved prophylactic administration of heparin. And, of note, the package insert for Lovenox (enoxaparin sodium) was revised in April, 1995 to include a warning that the drug should be used with "extreme caution" in patients with indwelling intrathecal or epidural catheters.

Small to intermediate incremental doses are used during peripheral vascular procedures, and full heparinization is used for larger vascular and coronary bypass procedures. Rao and El-Etr[70] prospectively studied the risk of maintaining an epidural or spinal catheter after heparinization in 4011 patients undergoing peripheral vascular operations. Patients were excluded if blood was aspirated during catheter placement, and heparinization was monitored by measurement of activated clotting times every 6 h postoperatively. Catheters were removed the day after operation, 1 h before administration of the next maintenance dose of heparin. The lack of symptomatic hematoma was attributed to rigorous patient selection, atraumatic technique, close monitoring of the activated clotting times, and timing of catheter removal. However, extrapolation of these results to routine clinical practice requires adherence to these authors' protocol, including a 24-h delay if frank blood is aspirated. This may impose an unacceptable limitation on most clinical practices because the incidence of aspiration of blood generally exceeds that observed by these investigators (<1:1000).

Although heparin has been administered without ill effect to patients receiving regional anesthesia, a 1981 nonanesthetic study by Ruff and Dougherty[71] reported a surprisingly high rate of complications associated with heparin therapy after diagnostic lumbar puncture for acute cerebral ischemia. Two groups of 342 patients were compared: the first group received heparin for anticoagulation after the lumbar puncture; the second did not. Spinal hematomas developed in seven of the patients who received heparin (five with paraparesis, two with severe back pain). The risk of symptomatic hematoma was increased by a traumatic lumbar puncture, initiation of anticoagulation within 1 h of lumbar puncture, or aspirin treatment before the lumbar puncture.

Warfarin Compounds

Preoperative prophylaxis with vitamin K antagonists (e.g., warfarin) may also prevent postoperative deep venous thrombosis.[72] Warfarin is generally administered once a day throughout the perioperative period to maintain prothrombin time at 1.3 to 1.5 times control. In a study examining the risks of warfarin prophylaxis in 950 patients receiving a total of 1000 continuous lumbar anesthetics, Odoom and Sih[73] found no evidence of epidural hematoma or neurologic complications.

Postoperative warfarin therapy has been studied retrospectively in 188 patients recovering from total knee replacement with epidural anesthesia. Horlocker et al[74] found no evidence of symptomatic hematoma, despite 13 instances of bloody aspirate during epidural catheterization and concurrent administration of nonsteroidal anti-inflammatory drugs in 36 of 188 patients. Catheters were removed postoperatively according to patient analgesic requirements. Horlocker et al[74] noted that warfarin had a highly variable dose-response effect, and they recommended close continuous monitoring of prothrombin time in patients with indwelling epidural catheters.

Nonsteroidal Anti-inflammatory Drugs

The lack of reported complications despite frequent (and often unrecognized) use of nonsteroidal anti-inflammatory drugs by the general population suggests that these drugs do not significantly increase risk of neuraxial hematoma. However, the safety of these agents has not been adequately demonstrated. Benzon and associates[75] prospectively studied 87 patients undergoing 246 epidural or spinal anesthetic procedures who had received aspirin preoperatively and found no evidence of neurologic complications. However, some procedures were delayed until the bleeding time normalized or was considered acceptable. In a retrospective review of 1013 epidural or spinal anesthetic procedures by Horlocker et al,[76] the incidence of aspiration of blood from the epidural or spinal needle was significantly greater in patients receiving antiplatelet medication. Whether such bleeding indicates increased risk of clinically significant hemorrhage is not known. In contrast, preliminary data from a prospective study[77] of 934 patients undergoing 1000 neuraxial blocks at the same institution found no neurologic complications or evidence of increased bleeding associated with preoperative use of nonsteroidal anti-inflammatory drugs. However, the combination of a nonsteroidal anti-inflammatory drug and anticoagulant therapy has been associated with increased risk in medical patients undergoing diagnostic lumbar punctures.[71]

Conclusion

Despite retrospective and prospective studies demonstrating negative results, the high number of patients required to document safety precludes definitive statements regarding risk. Although hematoma has been reported rarely, the majority of cases have been associated with anticoagulant or fibrinolytic therapy.[52] Thus, thoughtful balancing of risk and benefit is required when the perioperative management includes drugs known to increase the risk of bleeding.

Minor Complications or Side Effects of Neuraxial Block

Post–Dural Puncture Headache

It is remarkable that, nearly a century after Bier's description of a post–dural puncture headache (PDPH), this complication remains one of the most significant factors limiting the use of spinal anesthesia. Indeed, the Medline database contains more than 661 articles pertaining to PDPH published between 1985 and 1995. Although headache has commonly accompanied the technique, it was not until the late 1940s (when increased experience, use of vasopressors, and standardization of technique made serious cardiorespiratory and neurologic complications rare events) that attention became focused on this less morbid, but far more common, adverse outcome. Many theorized on the origin of PDPH, including Labat,[78] who believed that headache was due to increased cerebrospinal fluid (CSF) pressure "incidental to inadequate withdrawal of cerebrospinal fluid" and prescribed repeat dural puncture and withdrawal of 15 to 20 mL of CSF for refractory cases. However, it became generally accepted that loss of CSF decreases the volume or pressure in the thecal sac, establishing the goal of prevention of spinal headache as minimizing the loss of CSF and the goal of treatment as restoration of the normal volume and pressure relationship within the subarachnoid space.

Although the brain itself is insensitive to noxious stimuli, the structures that surround the brain, i.e., the meninges and the blood vessels, are richly innervated by nociceptive fibers. CSF loss causes these supporting structures of the brain and brain stem to stretch, presumably activating stretch-sensitive nociceptors (Fig. 25–5). Pain may also result from distension of the blood vessels, which, because of the fixed volume of the skull, must compensate for the loss of CSF volume (Monro-Kellie doctrine). Consistent with this etiology, maneuvers that further increase intracranial blood volume (e.g., jugular venous compression or Valsalva maneuver) typically exacerbate the headache.

Onset

Typically, headache evolves between 24 and 48 h after dural puncture; however, PDPH also may occur immediately after dural puncture or days to weeks after the procedure.[79] In the series by Vandam and Dripps[79] of 10,098 spinal anesthetic procedures, 59% of patients in whom PDPH developed experienced PDPH within the first 48 h, but in two patients PDPH did not develop until 5 months after spinal anesthesia.

Postural Component

Vandam and Dripps[79] reported an 11% incidence of spinal headache that was "postural in nature, appearing with the assumption of the erect position and usually relieved by recumbency." Indeed, exacerbation of headache by sitting or standing is so typical of PDPH that most studies classify headache based on the presence or absence of a postural effect.

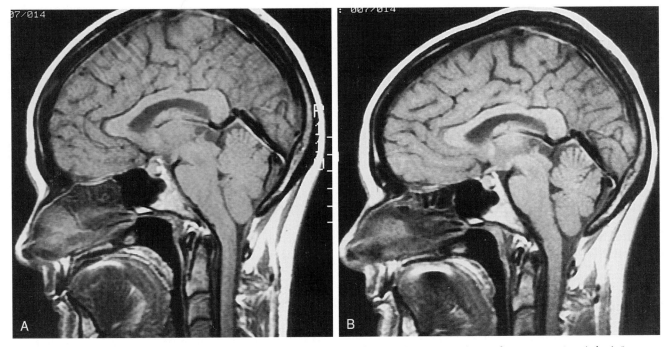

Figure 25–5 *A*, Anatomy of a "low-pressure" headache. T1-weighted sagittal magnetic resonance image demonstrates "ptotic brain" manifested as tonsillar herniation below the foramen magnum, forward displacement of the pons, absence of suprasellar cistern, kinking of the chiasm, and fullness of the pituitary gland. *B*, Comparable image of the same patient after epidural blood patch and resolution of symptoms demonstrates normal anatomy.

To minimize loss of CSF and promote patient comfort, the strategy of maintaining patients in a recumbent position was introduced into clinical practice; some early practitioners advocated transporting patients from the operating room in the Trendelenburg position and maintaining this position for up to 24 h. However, although intuitively appealing, most controlled studies have failed to demonstrate significant benefit from bed rest.[80, 81]

Quality

PDPH pain is generally dull or throbbing. Typically, the pain is occipital, frontal, or a combination of both: the incidence of each has been reported to be approximately 25%. The majority of cases are accompanied by nuchal pain and stiffness, and, in approximately one third of cases, by back pain.[82]

Associated Symptoms and Complications

Associated symptoms and complications include nausea; vomiting; anorexia; malaise; and ocular, auditory, and vestibular dysfunction. Subdural hematoma may occur and, although rare, is the most feared complication associated with PDPH.

Visual Disturbance. Vandam and Dripps[79] reported a 0.4% incidence of ocular findings manifested by diplopia, blurred vision, photophobia, or "spots." These symptoms are believed to result from stretch of the cranial nerves, most commonly the sixth, as the brain descends because of the loss of CSF.

Hearing Loss. Loss of CSF volume may decrease intralabyrinthine pressure,[83] with symptomatic hearing loss occurring in approximately 0.4% of cases.[79] However, studies applying sensitive measures of auditory function document that subtle changes postoperatively are quite common, even in the older patient population. Using pure tone audiometry, Wang and coworkers[84] found a 42% incidence of minor hearing loss postoperatively when spinal anesthesia was performed with a 22-G needle. These same investigators failed to detect impairment in a comparable group of surgical patients given epidural anesthesia, providing evidence that dysfunction results from CSF loss.

Subdural Hematoma. Hematoma is believed to result from tearing of the bridging veins secondary to the caudal displacement of the brain. Vulnerability to tearing may also be enhanced by vessel engorgement. A 1991 literature review by Vos et al[85] identified 47 cases of subdural hematoma after lumbar puncture, 35 of which were associated with spinal or epidural anesthesia. Five of these 35 patients died, and four had only partial recovery of neural function. This poor outcome warrants a caution—subdural hematoma should be considered whenever headache is refractory, loses its postural component, or returns after resolution. In addition, the significance of this complication argues for early treatment of PDPH with an epidural blood patch; however, whether this decreases risk remains unproved.

To minimize the problem of PDPH, the clinician should first identify those at greatest risk and modify anesthetic technique accordingly. Second, measures may be taken to decrease CSF loss, restore CSF pressure and volume relationships, relieve the vascular component of pain, and, finally, treat symptomatic pain with adjunct medications.

Identification of Those at Risk

The reported rate of PDPH may range from 0%[86] to 41%[87] with spinal anesthesia, and it may be as high as 85% after unintended dural puncture during performance of an epidural block.[88] This wide range is due to multiple patient-related, technique-related, and study design-related factors. Patient variables known to influence the development of PDPH include age, sex, body habitus, pregnancy, and history of previous PDPH. Younger people are, in general, at greater risk; women may be at greater risk than men, and gravid women appear to be at greatest risk.[79]

Age. Age is clearly one of the most important factors determining risk of PDPH. Children appear to be at low risk.[89] However, after puberty, risk initially increases dramatically and then decreases with advancing age.[79, 81] Although it has never been established why advanced age affords protection against PDPH, some have speculated that the elderly have an increased pain threshold, a progressive decrease in sensitivity of neural elements, or a decrease in elasticity of the cerebral vasculature.[79] Factors that might contribute to the high frequency of headache in gravid women include increased intra-abdominal pressure causing greater loss of CSF through the dural puncture, and dehydration secondary to blood loss, diuresis, and lactation.

Sex. Traditionally, it was believed that women were at higher risk for PDPH than men.[79] However, Lybecker et al[81] have challenged this perception. Using multivariate analysis of 1021 spinal anesthetic procedures, these investigators failed to find a significant association between sex and incidence of headache. Additionally, they pointed out that prior studies used bivariate analysis and questioned whether the positive correlation between sex and headache might be due to inclusion of obstetric cases and study of a female patient population of younger age.

Prior History of PDPH. Several studies[81] have documented increased risk in patients with a prior history of PDPH. This may reflect susceptibility to headache rather than relative CSF hypotension; experimental alteration of CSF volume in patients has identified various thresholds for headache provocation.[90] Of note, psychologic factors do not appear to be important—in 100 patients given general anesthesia who were unaware that they had also received spinal anesthesia, Vandam and Dripps[79] found an incidence of headache similar to that in patients given only spinal anesthesia.

Modification of Equipment and Technique

Attempts to decrease the incidence of PDPH have included modification of the equipment and technique used in performing lumbar puncture and the development of measures to prevent headache after dural puncture has occurred.

Needle Size. Because the incidence of PDPH increases with needle size, one strategy for decreasing PDPH has been to develop needles of increasingly smaller diameter. This has practical limitations, because ease of use also decreases with decreasing diameter. In addition to the problems encountered manipulating a fine needle, slow flow of CSF can make confirmation of subarachnoid placement difficult. For example, it may take up to 15 s for CSF to reach the hub of a 26-G needle.[91]

Needle Design. Traditional beveled or cutting needles (e.g., Quincke) produce relatively large tears in the fibrous connective tissue of the dura. Modification of the tip to a conical shape or pencil point (e.g., Whitacre or Sprotte) permits separation of the fibers, producing less tear and a smaller hole for a given diameter needle.[92] These modifications appear to decrease the incidence of PDPH.[86, 93]

Direction of Bevel. Orientation of the bevel of a cutting needle along the longitudinal plane results in a lower incidence of PDPH.[91, 94] Some in vitro studies also demonstrate slower transdural leak with this orientation.[92] These findings are consistent with the traditional perception that the dural fibers run longitudinally, a view that has been challenged.[95]

Approach. Some have suggested that the oblique angle of dural penetration occurring with a paramedian approach may create a flap valve that would tend to close when fluid pressure is applied to the arachnoidal surface. Data from in vitro studies of flow across human dura appear to support this concept: the mean leak rates observed when a 25-G needle penetrated the dura at a 90°, 60°, and 30° angle were 3.3, 2.5, and 0.3 mL/min, respectively. Some leak was present during a 1-min observation with all punctures made at 90° and 60° but not in 4 of the 10 punctures performed at 30°.[92]

Other Minor Complications or Side Effects

Pain in the back, buttock, or lower extremity also frequently follows spinal or epidural anesthesia. Four etiologic factors have been suggested: patient positioning, direct needle trauma, localized musculoskeletal reaction, and local anesthetic toxicity.

Patient Positioning

Postoperative back pain is not unique to regional anesthesia, occurring in approximately 20% of patients without a prior history of backache who are given general anesthesia.[96] That the incidence correlates with time on the operating table suggests that backache may result from stretching of the vertebral column and the lumbosacral ligaments secondary to prolonged immobility and relaxation of the paraspinous muscles.

Direct Needle Trauma

Although postoperative back pain frequently occurs with general anesthesia, there may be a higher incidence after neuraxial block in select patient groups.[97, 98] Pain at the site of injection may occur in nearly one half of patients receiving spinal[99] or epidural[97] anesthesia: the actual incidence varies depending, in part, on how aggressively symptoms are sought. In addition, pain may be more frequent with an epidural than with a spinal technique. For example, a prospective comparison reported an incidence of post–lumbar puncture back pain of 11% and 31% after spinal and epidural anesthesia (without chloroprocaine), respectively.[100] Although postpuncture back pain generally is a minor, self-limiting side effect, it may have clinical significance—in the preceding study, it was the most frequently cited reason for patient refusal to have a similar anesthetic in the future.

Localized Musculocutaneous Reaction

As a result of concern that sodium bisulfite might be neurotoxic, a new formulation of 2-chloroprocaine (Nesacaine-MPF [methylparaben-free], Astra Pharmaceuticals) was introduced into clinical practice in 1987. This formulation contains the preservative disodium ethylenediaminetetraacetic acid (EDTA), a chelator of heavy metals. Shortly after introduction of this new anesthetic formulation, Fibuch and Opper[101] reported that epidural administration resulted in a 40% incidence of severe paralumbar pain in patients undergoing outpatient surgery. The authors postulated that the expected binding of calcium lowered the tissue concentration, inducing muscle spasm and pain. The anecdotal report of successful treatment with intravenous administration of calcium[102] and preliminary animal data demonstrating tetanic muscle contraction after epidural administration of EDTA[103] are consistent with the theory that pain results from hypocalcemic tetany of the paraspinous muscles.

The association between back pain and epidural administration of Nesacaine-MPF has been confirmed by others.[104–107] In a study[104] investigating thermal regulation, severe back pain was observed in 4 of 5 volunteers receiving Nesacaine-MPF but in none of 10 receiving lidocaine and in none of 4 receiving saline. In another study,[106] 10 volunteers receiving three sequential escalating epidural doses of Nesacaine-MPF reported back pain that increased in severity after resolution of each block. More recently, Stevens et al[107] presented convincing evidence that severe back pain after epidurally administered Nesacaine-MPF is, in fact, caused by EDTA and that symptoms can be minimized by restricting the total volume to 25 mL or less. These investigators found a similar incidence of localized superficial back pain with epidural administration of five different anesthetic solutions, but a higher incidence of deep aching burning pain in patients receiving high volumes of Nesacaine-MPF (Table 25–3). The pH of the solution per se did not appear to be a factor, although alkalization did produce a modest reduction in severity.

Local Anesthetic Toxicity

Local anesthetic toxicity also has been implicated as a potential source of postoperative back pain. Schneider et al[30] reported on four patients in whom pain in the buttock or lower back developed, radiating to the dorsolateral thighs and calves following recovery from spinal anesthesia. All four cases had common characteristics: (1) onset 1 to 20 h postoperatively, after com-

plete recovery from anesthesia; (2) neurologic examination that was either normal or positive only for dysesthesia; and (3) resolution of symptoms within 7 days. In addition, all four cases occurred with 5% lidocaine in 7.5% dextrose and with the patient operated on in the lithotomy position. The authors postulated that pain or dysesthesia resulted from a direct neurotoxic effect of the local anesthetic solution. In addition, they suggested that the lithotomy position produced stretching of the cauda equina, resulting in an increased vulnerability of the sacral roots and an enhancement of toxicity.

The report[108] of six similar cases provided further evidence for an association between 5% lidocaine in 7.5% dextrose and transient pain and dysesthesia. Additionally, data from a prospective study[109] indicated a 37% incidence of transient neurologic symptoms (defined as pain or dysesthesia developing after recovery from the anesthetic and resolving in 72 h) in patients given 5% lidocaine compared with an incidence of less than 1% in patients given bupivacaine, including those undergoing operation in the lithotomy position. However, several factors limit interpretation of these data, including lack of randomization, nonuniformity of the surgical procedures, nonequivalent doses of anesthetic, and use of only a single formulation of lidocaine. (In fact, anecdotal reports of apparent transient toxicity after administration of 2% lidocaine raise doubt whether this side effect is restricted to one particular anesthetic formulation.[109a]) Clearly, the etiology of this side effect, its significance, and factors that affect it have yet to be defined. In addition to the inherent importance of this side effect, it is critical to determine if, in fact, these transient symptoms represent the lower end of a spectrum of toxicity. If so, these could be used as a surrogate end point for more serious injury, providing an invaluable tool for evaluating the safety of anesthetic agents and techniques; nevertheless, this link remains speculative.

Complications of Peripheral Nerve Block

Injury due to peripheral block is reported infrequently. However, damage to a peripheral nerve can be relatively minor and onset of symptoms may be delayed. Thus, injury may be unappreciated or unreported. Conversely, damage to a nerve occurring from other causes such as patient positioning or surgical trauma might be mistakenly attributed to the anesthetic. A 1990 review[110] of the American Society of Anesthesiologists' closed claims database disclosed 227 claims for anesthesia-related nerve injury, but only 82 cases, or 36%, involved a regional anesthetic. Moreover, the mechanism of injury was apparent in only 5 of 77 of the ulnar nerve injuries and 15 of 53 claims involving the brachial plexus. Thus, every attempt should be made to establish the cause of injury before ascribing fault to the anesthetic technique.

Although many factors may affect the risk of peripheral nerve injury, the needle used and the method selected to locate the nerve remain the most controversial.

Table 25–3 Effect of Anesthetic Solution on Back Pain*

| | | PATIENTS, % | | | |
| | | Type 1 | | Type 2 | |
GROUP	ANESTHETIC SOLUTION VOLUME (INITIAL/SUPPLEMENTAL)	Immediate	24 h	Immediate	24 h
1	2% lidocaine HCl (30 mL/10 mL)	15	30	5	0
2	3% chloroprocaine w/EDTA (15 mL/5 mL)	5	30	10	5
3	3% chloroprocaine w/EDTA (30 mL/10 mL)	25	10	50	60
4	3% chloroprocaine (w/o EDTA) w/metabisulfite (30 mL/10 mL)	35	35	10	15
5	3% chloroprocaine w/EDTA pH adjusted (30 mL/10 mL)	20	30	25	30
	P	NS	NS	.0032†	<.0001‡

*Type 1 = localized superficial pain confined to the area of needle insertion. Type 2 = deep, aching, or burning pain confined to the lumbar area but diffuse in location.
†Group 3 differs significantly from groups 1, 2, and 4.
‡Group 3 differs significantly from groups 1, 2, and 4; group 5 differs significantly from group 1.
EDTA, ethylenediaminetetraacetic acid; w/, with; w/o, without.
Data from Stevens RA, Urmey WF, Urquhart BL, et al: Back pain after epidural anesthesia with chloroprocaine. Anesthesiology 1993; 78: 492–497.

Choice of needle may play a role in production of nerve injury. Selander et al[111] examined the acute effects of injecting rabbit sciatic nerves in vitro and in situ and found that 45° short-beveled needles produced damage less frequently than 14° long-beveled needles. Additionally, injections made parallel to nerve fibers generally produced less damage than injections made with the bevel perpendicular to the nerve axis. More recent studies by Rice and McMahon[112] do not support an advantage for short-beveled needles. Using sciatic nerve injection in the rat, these investigators examined both immediate and long-term histologic and physiologic effects of short-beveled (27°) and long-beveled (12°) needles. The frequency, severity, and time course of intrafascicular injury were greater with short-beveled than with long-beveled needles. Similarly, behavioral changes observed with the short-beveled needle were more severe and persisted longer than those resulting from injections with long-beveled needles. Like Selander and colleagues,[111] these investigators also found less damage when injection was made with the bevel oriented parallel to the nerve fiber. However, the relative size of these experimental species and the lack of information regarding clinical incidence of nerve penetration with different needles require large-scale clinical study to firmly establish optimal configuration for minimizing nerve damage.

Intrafascicular injection induces trauma, and the resultant increase in intraneural pressure may induce ischemia and potentiate neural toxicity. Consequently, intraneural injection should be avoided. Therefore, if significant pain occurs with injection, the block needle should be repositioned before administering additional anesthetic because the pain may signify intraneural injection. Because paresthesias indicate that the needle is near or in contact with the nerve, some investigators suggest that a nonparesthetic technique may reduce the risk of neural injury. To investigate this possiblity, Selander et al[113] prospectively studied 533 patients undergoing hand surgery with an axillary block. In 290 patients, the axillary block was performed with a paresthesia technique; in 243 patients, the axillary block

was completed using transmitted arterial pulsation to establish proximity to the plexus. Unintentional paresthesias occurred in 40% of the latter group. Postoperative neural injury attributed to the block occurred in eight patients in the first group and in two patients in the second group; in both these patients, unintentional paresthesia had been elicited. Although the authors of the study concluded that searching for paresthesia increases the risk of postanesthetic neurologic sequelae, the incidence of nerve injury in the two groups did not differ significantly. Further, the study was conducted in two hospitals, with blocks performed with a paresthesia technique in one hospital and a nonparesthesia technique in the other (Selander D: Personal communication, 1986). In addition, all the patients in the first group received an epinephrine-containing solution, compared with only 48% in the second group, and all patients who experienced neuropathies received epinephrine. This may impact the result because, in an in vitro rabbit model, adding epinephrine to anesthetic solution increased pathologic change in the nerves.[114] Conversely, there are clinical data for a series of patients receiving epinephrine for a large number of peripheral blocks that suggest that its use is acceptable.[115] In any event, existing clinical data have not established that using a nonparesthetic technique or avoiding epinephrine decreases risk of neural injury.

References

1. Brock S, Bell A, Davison C: Nervous complications following spinal anesthesia: a clinical study of seven cases, with tissue study in one instance. JAMA 1936; 106: 441–446.
2. Ferguson FR, Watkins KH: Paralysis of the bladder and associated neurological sequelae of spinal anaesthesia (cauda equina syndrome). Br J Surg 1937; 25: 735–752.
3. Macdonald AD, Watkins KH: Experimental investigation into cause of paralysis following spinal anaesthesia. Br J Surg 1938; 25: 879–883.
4. Covino BG, Marx GF, Finster M, et al: Prolonged sensory/motor deficits following inadvertent spinal anesthesia. (Editorial.) Anesth Analg 1980; 59: 399–400.
5. Ravindran RS, Bond VK, Tasch MD, et al: Prolonged neural blockade following regional analgesia with 2-chloroprocaine. Anesth Analg 1980; 59: 447–451.

6. Reisner LS, Hochman BN, Plumer MH: Persistent neurologic deficit and adhesive arachnoiditis following intrathecal 2-chloroprocaine injection. Anesth Analg 1980; 59: 452–454.

7. Moore DC, Spierdijk J, vanKleef JD, et al: Chloroprocaine neurotoxicity: four additional cases. Anesth Analg 1982; 61: 155–159.

8. Gissen AJ: Toxicity of local anaesthetics in obstetrics II: chloroprocaine—research and clinical aspects. Clin Anaesthesiol 1986; 4: 101–108.

9. Ravindran RS, Turner MS, Muller J: Neurologic effects of subarachnoid administration of 2-chloroprocaine-CE, bupivacaine, and low pH normal saline in dogs. Anesth Analg 1982; 61: 279–283.

10. Barsa J, Batra M, Fink BR, et al: A comparative in vivo study of local neurotoxicity of lidocaine, bupivacaine, 2-chloroprocaine, and a mixture of 2-chloroprocaine and bupivacaine. Anesth Analg 1982; 61: 961–967.

11. Rosen MA, Baysinger CL, Shnider SM, et al: Evaluation of neurotoxicity after subarachnoid injection of large volumes of local anesthetic solutions. Anesth Analg 1983; 62: 802–808.

12. Ready LB, Plumer MH, Haschke RH, et al: Neurotoxicity of intrathecal local anesthetics in rabbits. Anesthesiology 1985; 63: 364–370.

13. Wang BC, Hillman DE, Spielholz NI, et al: Chronic neurological deficits and Nesacaine-CE—an effect of the anesthetic, 2-chloroprocaine, or the antioxidant, sodium bisulfite? Anesth Analg 1984; 63: 445–447.

14. Kalichman MW, Powell HC, Reisner LS, et al: The role of 2-chloroprocaine and sodium bisulfite in rat sciatic nerve edema. J Neuropathol Exp Neurol 1986; 45: 566–575.

15. Covino BG: Toxicity of local anesthetic agents. Acta Anaesthesiol Belg 1988; 39(3 Suppl 2): 159–164.

16. Rigler ML, Drasner K, Krejcie TC, et al: Cauda equina syndrome after continuous spinal anesthesia. Anesth Analg 1991; 72: 275–281.

17. Benson JS: FDA Safety Alert: Cauda equina syndrome associated with the use of small-bore catheters in continuous spinal anesthesia. Rockville, MD, Food and Drug Administration, May 29, 1992.

18. Lambert DH, Hurley RJ: Cauda equina syndrome and continuous spinal anesthesia. Anesth Analg 1991; 72: 817–819.

19. Rigler ML, Drasner K: Distribution of catheter-injected local anesthetic in a model of the subarachnoid space. Anesthesiology 1991; 75: 684–692.

20. Ross BK, Coda B, Heath CH: Local anesthetic distribution in a spinal model: a possible mechanism of neurologic injury after continuous spinal anesthesia. Reg Anesth 1992; 17: 69–77.

21. Robinson RA, Stewart SF, Myers MR, et al: In vitro modeling of spinal anesthesia. A digital video image processing technique and its application to catheter characterization. Anesthesiology 1994; 81: 1053–1060.

22. Lambert LA, Lambert DH, Strichartz GR: Irreversible conduction block in isolated nerve by high concentrations of local anesthetics. Anesthesiology 1994; 80: 1082–1093.

23. Bainton CR, Strichartz GR: Concentration dependence of lidocaine-induced irreversible conduction loss in frog nerve. Anesthesiology 1994; 81: 657–667.

24. Drasner K, Sakura S, Chan VW, et al: Persistent sacral sensory deficit induced by intrathecal local anesthetic infusion in the rat. Anesthesiology 1994; 80: 847–852.

25. Sakura S, Chan VW, Ciriales R, et al: The addition of 7.5% glucose does not alter the neurotoxicity of 5% lidocaine administered intrathecally in the rat. Anesthesiology 1995; 82: 236–240.

26. Mörch ET, Rosenberg MK, Truant AT: Lidocaine for spinal anesthesia: a study of the concentration in the spinal fluid. Acta Anaesthesiol Scand 1957; 1: 105–115.

27. Drasner K, Rigler ML: Repeat injection after a "failed spinal": at times, a potentially unsafe practice. (Letter to the editor.) Anesthesiology 1991; 75: 713–714.

28. Myers RR, Kalichman MW, Reisner LS, et al: Neurotoxicity of local anesthetics: altered perineurial permeability, edema, and nerve fiber injury. Anesthesiology 1986; 64: 29–35.

29. Kalichman MW, Powell HC, Myers RR: Quantitative histologic analysis of local anesthetic-induced injury to rat sciatic nerve. J Pharmacol Exp Ther 1989; 250: 406–413.

30. Schneider M, Ettlin T, Kaufmann M, et al: Transient neurologic toxicity after hyperbaric subarachnoid anesthesia with 5% lidocaine. Anesth Analg 1993; 76: 1154–1157.

31. Sakura S, Chan V, Ciriales R, et al: Intrathecal infusion of lidocaine in the rat results in dose-dependent, but not concentration-dependent, sacral root injury. (Abstract.) Anesthesiology 1993; 79: A851.

32. Drasner K, Rigler ML, Sessler DI, et al: Cauda equina syndrome following intended epidural anesthesia. Anesthesiology 1992; 77: 582–585.

33. Cheng AC: Intended epidural anesthesia as possible cause of cauda equina syndrome. Anesth Analg 1994; 78: 157–159.

34. Phillips OC, Ebner H, Nelson AT, et al: Neurologic complications following spinal anesthesia with lidocaine: a prospective review of 10,440 cases. Anesthesiology 1969; 30: 284–289.

35. Sakura S, Bollen AW, Ciriales R, et al: Local anesthetic neurotoxicity does not result from blockade of voltage-gated sodium channels. Anesth Analg 1995; 81: 338–346.

36. Winkelman NW: Neurologic symptoms following accidental intraspinal detergent injection. Neurology 1952; 2: 284–291.

37. Kennedy F, Effron AS, Perry G: The grave spinal cord paralyses caused by spinal anesthesia. Surg Gynecol Obstet 1950; 91: 385–398.

38. Cope RW: The Woolley and Roe case: Woolley and Roe versus ministry of health and others. Anaesthesia 1954; 9: 249–270.

39. Baker AS, Ojemann RG, Swartz MN, et al: Spinal epidural abscess. N Engl J Med 1975; 293: 463–468.

40. Danner RL, Hartman BJ: Update on spinal epidural abscess: 35 cases and review of the literature. Rev Infect Dis 1987; 9: 265–274.

41. Kane RE: Neurologic deficits following epidural or spinal anesthesia. Anesth Analg 1981; 60: 150–161.

42. Heusner AP: Nontuberculous spinal epidural infections. N Engl J Med 1948; 239: 845–854.

43. Strong WE: Epidural abscess associated with epidural catheterization: a rare event? Report of two cases with markedly delayed presentation. Anesthesiology 1991; 74: 943–946.

44. Du Pen SL, Peterson DG, Williams A, et al: Infection during chronic epidural catheterization: diagnosis and treatment. Anesthesiology 1990; 73: 905–909.

45. Carp H, Bailey S: The association between meningitis and dural puncture in bacteremic rats. Anesthesiology 1992; 76: 739–742.

46. Teele DW, Dashefsky B, Rakusan T, et al: Meningitis after lumbar puncture in children with bacteremia. N Engl J Med. 1981; 305: 1079–1081.

47. Shapiro ED, Aaron NH, Wald ER, et al: Risk factors for development of bacterial meningitis among children with occult bacteremia. J Pediatr 1986; 109: 15–19.

48. Berman RS, Eisele JH: Bacteremia, spinal anesthesia, and development of meningitis. Anesthesiology 1978; 48: 376–377.

49. Crawford JS: Some maternal complications of epidural analgesia for labour. Anaesthesia 1985; 40: 1219–1225.

50. Owens EL, Kasten GW, Hessel EA II: Spinal subarachnoid hematoma after lumbar puncture and heparinization: a case report, review of the literature, and discussion of anesthetic implications. Anesth Analg 1986; 65: 1201–1207.

51. McQuarrie IG: Recovery from paraplegia caused by spontaneous spinal epidural hematoma. Neurology 1978; 28: 224–228.

52. Vandermeulen EP, Van Aken H, Vermylen J: Anticoagulants and spinal-epidural anesthesia. Anesth Analg 1994; 79: 1165–1177.

53. Tryba M: Etat de l'hemostase et anesthesie locoregionale. (French.) Ann Fr Anesth Reanim 1990; 9: 375–377.

54. Tuman KJ, McCarthy RJ, March RJ, et al: Effects of epidural anesthesia and analgesia on coagulation and outcome after major vascular surgery. Anesth Analg 1991; 73: 696–704.

55. Yeager MP, Glass DD, Neff RK, et al: Epidural anesthesia and analgesia in high-risk surgical patients. Anesthesiology 1987; 66: 729–736.

56. Rosenfeld BA, Beattie C, Christopherson R, et al: The effects of different anesthetic regimens on fibrinolysis and the development of postoperative arterial thrombosis. Anesthesiology 1993; 79: 435–443.

57. Leduc L, Wheeler JM, Kirshon B, et al: Coagulation profile in severe preeclampsia. Obstet Gynecol 1992; 79: 14–18.

58. Voulgaropoulos DS, Palmer CM: Coagulation studies in the pre-eclamptic parturient: a survey. J Clin Anesth 1993; 5: 99–104.

59. Barker P, Callander CC: Coagulation screening before epidural analgesia in pre-eclampsia. Anaesthesia 1991; 46: 64–67.

60. Kelton JG, Hunter DJ, Neame PB: A platelet function defect in preeclampsia. Obstet Gynecol 1985; 65: 107–109.

61. Ramanathan J, Sibai BM, Vu T, et al: Correlation between bleeding times and platelet counts in women with preeclampsia undergoing cesarean section. Anesthesiology 1989; 71: 188–191.

62. Schindler M, Gatt S, Isert P, et al: Thrombocytopenia and platelet functional defects in pre-eclampsia: implications for regional anaesthesia. Anaesth Intensive Care 1990; 18: 169–174.

63. Burrows RF, Kelton JG: Incidentally detected thrombocytopenia in healthy mothers and their infants. N Engl J Med 1988; 319: 142–145.

64. Rodgers RP, Levin J: A critical reappraisal of the bleeding time. Semin Thromb Hemost 1990; 16: 1–20.

65. Sharnoff JG, DeBlasio G: Prevention of fatal postoperative thromboembolism by heparin prophylaxis. Lancet 1970; 2: 1006–1007.

66. Cooke ED, Lloyd MJ, Bowcock SA, et al: Monitoring during low-dose heparin prophylaxis. (Letter to the editor.) N Engl J Med 1976; 294: 1066–1067.

67. Cosmi B, Hirsh J: Low molecular weight heparins. Curr Opin Cardiol 1994; 9: 612–618.

68. Schwander D, Bachmann F: Heparine et anesthesies medullaires: analyse de decision. (French.) Ann Fr Anesth Reanim 1991; 10: 284–296.

69. Bergqvist D, Lindblad B, Matzsch T: Low molecular weight heparin for thromboprophylaxis and epidural/spinal anaesthesia—is there a risk? Acta Anaesthesiol Scand 1992; 36: 605–609.

70. Rao TL, El-Etr AA: Anticoagulation following placement of epidural and subarachnoid catheters: an evaluation of neurologic sequelae. Anesthesiology 1981; 55: 618–620.

71. Ruff RL, Dougherty JH Jr: Complications of lumbar puncture followed by anticoagulation. Stroke 1981; 12: 879–881.

72. Stow PJ, Burrows FA: Anticoagulants in anaesthesia. Can J Anaesth 1987; 34: 632–649.

73. Odoom JA, Sih IL: Epidural analgesia and anticoagulant therapy. Experience with one thousand cases of continuous epidurals. Anaesthesia 1983; 38: 254–259.

74. Horlocker TT, Wedel DJ, Schlichting JL: Postoperative epidural analgesia and oral anticoagulant therapy. Anesth Analg 1994; 79: 89–93.

75. Benzon H, Brunner E, Vaisrub N: Bleeding time and nerve blocks after aspirin. Reg Anesth 1984; 9: 86–89.

76. Horlocker TT, Wedel DJ, Offord KP: Does preoperative antiplatelet therapy increase the risk of hemorrhagic complications associated with regional anesthesia? Anesth Analg 1990; 70: 631–634.

77. Horlocker T, Wedel D, Offord K, et al: Preoperative anti-platelet drugs do not increase the risk of spinal hematoma associated with regional anesthesia. (Abstract.) Reg Anesth 1994; 19(Suppl): 8.

78. Labat G: Regional Anesthesia: Its Technic and Clinical Application. Philadelphia, WB Saunders Co, 1922.

79. Vandam LD, Dripps RD: Long-term follow-up of patients who received 10,098 spinal anesthetics: syndrome of decreased intracranial pressure (headache and ocular and auditory difficulties). JAMA 1956; 161: 586–591.

80. Carbaat PA, van Crevel H: Lumbar puncture headache: controlled study on the preventive effect of 24 hours' bed rest. Lancet 1981; 2: 1133–1135.

81. Lybecker H, Moller JT, May O, et al: Incidence and prediction of postdural puncture headache. A prospective study of 1021 spinal anesthesias. Anesth Analg 1990; 70: 389–394.

82. Abouleish E, Vega S, Blendinger I, et al: Long-term follow-up of epidural blood patch. Anesth Analg 1975; 54: 459–463.

83. Hughson W: Note on relationship of cerebrospinal and intralabyrinthine pressures. Am J Physiol 1932; 101: 396–407.

84. Wang LP, Fog J, Bove M: Transient hearing loss following spinal anaesthesia. Anaesthesia. 1987; 42: 1258–1263.

85. Vos PE, de Boer WA, Wurzer JA, et al: Subdural hematoma after lumbar puncture: two case reports and review of the literature. Clin Neurol Neurosurg 1991; 93: 127–132.

86. Cesarini M, Torrielli R, Lahaye F, et al: Sprotte needle for intrathecal anaesthesia for caesarean section: incidence of postdural puncture headache. Anaesthesia 1990; 45: 656–658.

87. Greene BA: A 26 gauge lumbar puncture needle: its value in the prophylaxis of headache following spinal analgesia for vaginal delivery. Anesthesiology 1950; 11: 464–469.

88. Brownridge P: The management of headache following accidental dural puncture in obstetric patients. Anaesth Intensive Care 1983; 11: 4–15.

89. Bolder PM: Postlumbar puncture headache in pediatric oncology patients. Anesthesiology 1986; 65: 696–698.

90. Fay T: New test for diagnosis of certain headaches: the cephalalgiogram. Dis Nerv System 1940; 1: 312–315.

91. Cruickshank RH, Hopkinson JM: Fluid flow through dural puncture sites. An in vitro comparison of needle point types. Anaesthesia 1989; 44: 415–418.

92. Ready LB, Cuplin S, Haschke RH, et al: Spinal needle determinants of rate of transdural fluid leak. Anesth Analg 1989; 69: 457–460.

93. Buettner J, Wresch KP, Klose R: Postdural puncture headache: comparison of 25-gauge Whitacre and Quincke needles. Reg Anesth 1993; 18: 166–169.

94. Mihic D: Postspinal headache and relationship of needle bevel to longitudinal dural fibers. Reg Anesth 1985; 10: 76–81.

95. Dittmann M, Schafer HG, Ulrich J, et al: Anatomical re-evaluation of lumbar dura mater with regard to postspinal headache. Effect of dural puncture. Anaesthesia 1988; 43: 635–637.

96. Middleton MJ, Bell CR: Postoperative backache: attempts to reduce incidence. Anesth Analg 1965; 44: 446–448.

97. Rickford JK, Speedy HM, Tytler JA, et al: Comparative evaluation of general, epidural and spinal anaesthesia for extracorporeal shockwave lithotripsy. Ann R Coll Surg Engl 1988; 70: 69–73.

98. Dahl JB, Schultz P, Anker-Moller E, et al: Spinal anaesthesia in young patients using a 29-gauge needle: technical considerations and an evaluation of postoperative complaints compared with general anaesthesia. Br J Anaesth 1990; 64: 178–182.

99. Mayer DC, Quance D, Weeks SK: Headache after spinal anesthesia for cesarean section: a comparison of the 27-gauge Quincke and 24-gauge Sprotte needles. Anesth Analg 1992; 75: 377–380.

100. Seeberger MD, Lang ML, Drewe J, et al: Comparison of spinal and epidural anesthesia for patients younger than 50 years of age. Anesth Analg 1994; 78: 667–673.

101. Fibuch EE, Opper SE: Back pain following epidurally administered Nesacaine-MPF. Anesth Analg 1989; 69: 113–115.

102. Dirks WE Jr: Treatment of Nesacaine-MPF–induced back pain with calcium chloride. (Letter to the editor.) Anesth Analg 1990; 70: 461–462.

103. Wang BC, Li D, Hiller JM, et al: Epidural EDTA induces tetanic contractions in rats. (Abstract.) Anesth Analg 1991; 72: S312.

104. Hynson JM, Sessler DI, Glosten B: Back pain in volunteers after epidural anesthesia with chloroprocaine. Anesth Analg 1991; 72: 253–256.

105. Levy L, Randel GI, Pandit SK: Does chloroprocaine (Nesacaine MPF) for epidural anesthesia increase the incidence of backache? (Letter to the editor.) Anesthesiology 1989; 71: 476.

106. Stevens RA, Chester WL, Artuso JD, et al: Back pain after epidural anesthesia with chloroprocaine in volunteers: preliminary report. Reg Anesth 1991; 16: 199–203.

107. Stevens RA, Urmey WF, Urquhart BL, et al: Back pain after epidural anesthesia with chloroprocaine. Anesthesiology 1993; 78: 492–497.

108. Snyder R, Hui G, Flugstad P, et al: More cases of possible neurologic toxicity associated with single subarachnoid injections of 5% hyperbaric lidocaine. (Letter to the editor.) Anesth Analg 1994; 78: 411.

109. Hampl K, Schneider M, Ummenhofer W, et al: Transient neurologic symptoms after spinal anesthesia. Anesth Analg 1995; 81: 1148–1153.

109a. Fenerty J, Sonner J, Sakura S, et al: Transient radicular pain following spinal anesthesia: review of the literature and report of a case involving 2% lidocaine. Int J Obstet Anesth 1996; 5: 32–35.

110. Kroll DA, Caplan RA, Posner K, et al: Nerve injury associated with anesthesia. Anesthesiology 1990; 73: 202–207.

111. Selander D, Dhuner KG, Lundborg G: Peripheral nerve injury due to injection needles used for regional anesthesia. An experimental study of the acute effects of needle point trauma. Acta Anaesthesiol Scand 1977; 21: 182–188.

112. Rice AS, McMahon SB: Peripheral nerve injury caused by injection needles used in regional anaesthesia: influence of bevel configuration, studied in a rat model. Br J Anaesth 1992; 69: 433–438.

113. Selander D, Edshage S, Wolff T: Paresthesiae or no paresthesiae? Nerve lesions after axillary blocks. Acta Anaesth Scand 1979; 23: 27–33.

114. Selander D, Brattsand R, Lundborg G, et al: Local anaesthetics: importance of mode of application, concentration and adrenaline for the appearance of nerve lesions: an experimental study of axonal degeneration and barrier damage after intrafascicular injection or topical application of bupivacaine (Marcain). Acta Anaesth Scand 1979; 23: 127–136.

115. Moore DC, Bridenbaugh LD, Thompson GE, et al: Bupivacaine: a review of 11,080 cases. Anesth Analg 1978; 57: 42–48.

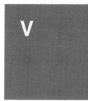

Regional Anesthesia and Analgesia in Practice

Surgery and Subspecialties

CHAPTER 26

Neurosurgery

Anne C.P. Lui, M.D., Kevin J. Nolan, M.D.

Regional anesthesia and neurosurgery may appear incompatible at first glance. Procedures on the cranium were performed long before general anesthesia was developed. Trephination dates back to the Neolithic period (about 7000 BC to 3000 BC). Bur holes for evacuation of a hematoma can be drilled during local anesthesia. Stereotactic biopsy of brain tumors seldom requires general anesthetics. Craniotomy involving mapping of the cerebral cortex necessitates the cooperation of an awake patient. Surgical procedures on the spinal column are easily performed with regional anesthesia. Most peripheral nerve operations can be performed with local or regional techniques. In neurovascular surgery, the benefits of carotid endarterectomy are becoming better defined together with renewed interest in regional anesthesia for this procedure.

Craniotomy

The precise localization of neurologic function in areas of the brain was demonstrated in humans by Penfield and Rasmussen, who performed craniotomy with local anesthesia in epileptic patients.[1] They carefully noted the sensations produced in their patients by stimulation of various areas of the exposed cerebral cortex. These observations allowed determination of the site from which the seizure originated and permitted its surgical excision with minimal damage to surrounding structures. Modifications of these techniques are still used to guide surgical removal of epileptogenic

foci. These same principles can be applied to the surgical removal of nonepileptic lesions in or near important functional areas of the brain.[2] Tumors or arteriovenous malformations near the speech center represent examples of such a challenge; the ability to perform a neurologic examination of the patient during the actual operation can guide the surgeon in the stepwise removal of the lesion.

Advantages of Regional Anesthesia for Craniotomy

Evaluation of an awake patient permits accurate localization of areas on the cerebral cortex at risk during operation. This avoids many of the difficulties inherent in using arbitrary values and reference points derived from preoperative electroencephalogram, computed tomography, or population data. Furthermore, the reference points are often poorly defined and remote from the surgical site after the patient is positioned and draped. The surgeon can confidently determine the location of a particular function by using the awake patient's responses for guidance and modify the surgical procedure to the individual patient's anatomy rather than rely on uncertain measurements. During local anesthesia and appropriate sedation, the patient's verbal or motor response can be monitored. If required, specialized cortical surface electrodes can be used with minimal interference from the effects of drugs.

Disadvantages of Regional Anesthesia for Craniotomy

Conversion to general anesthesia may be necessary if any of the following develop: frequent seizures, intense anxiety, excessive bleeding, or marked swelling of the brain. The anesthesiologist should be prepared to provide a safe induction of general anesthesia in a patient in the lateral position, distressed by a complication, and with the brain exposed.

Archer et al[3] reviewed 354 cases of craniotomy in awake patients for treatment of intractable epilepsy and documented the incidence of complications. Seizures developed in 16%, nausea and vomiting in 8%, excessive sedation in 3%, conversion to general anesthesia in 2%, local anesthetic systemic toxicity in 2%, and serious brain swelling in 1.4% of the cases.

Anesthesia for Craniotomy in Awake Patients

Manninen and Contreras[4] and Geevarghese and Garretson[5] have written excellent reviews of craniotomy in the awake patient. Anesthesia for the procedure is achieved by a field block of the scalp (Fig. 26–1) with a 25-G Quincke-type spinal needle. A long-acting local anesthetic agent, such as 0.25% bupivacaine with added epinephrine 1:200,000, is recommended to decrease surgical bleeding from the scalp. This solution is injected in the subcutaneous tissue superficial to the epicranial aponeurosis where the nerves and blood vessels are located. Local anesthetic is also injected into the temporal muscle. The analgesia can last up to 8 h. Because of difficulty in performing this block without producing discomfort, pretreatment is suggested with small doses of propofol (0.3 to 0.5 mg/kg) or alfentanil (3 to 5 µg/kg) given intravenously. The dura mater is pain-sensitive at the base of the skull along the middle meningeal artery. Small amounts of local anesthetic (0.25 to 0.5 mL) can be injected around this artery. Subarachnoid injection should be avoided.

This technique is used in combination with intravenously administered sedatives and analgesics. The drug combination has evolved over the years from a combination of neuroleptic agents (droperidol and opioid)[6] through neuroleptic agents and hypnotics[3] to current combinations of short-acting sedative-hypnotics (propofol) and opioids (alfentanil).[7]

Monitoring includes electrocardiography, pulse oximetry, noninvasive blood pressure recording, and end-tidal carbon dioxide measured through nasal prongs. Supplemental oxygen is administered, and maintenance fluids are given intravenously. When intravenous administration of fluids is kept to a minimum, a urinary catheter is often unnecessary.

Clinical Note: *Careful attention to appropriate sedation and positioning is a prerequisite to success. Heavy sedation may hinder recording of epileptiform activity on the electroencephalogram or interfere with the intraoperative neurologic examination. Judicious use of short-acting sedatives or opioids is certainly acceptable during phases of the procedure that are potentially painful or frightening. For example, the patient may experience pain during the field block of the scalp or may be alarmed by the noise and vibration associated with the drilling of the cranium. A calm and reassuring anesthesiologist is the best anxiolytic for these patients. This is as important to the success of craniotomy in the awake patient as is the skillful performance of the nerve block.*

The operative procedure typically lasts several hours. Surgical intermission should be planned to allow the patient to move and relieve muscle strain. Ice chips are useful for wetting the patient's mouth. A thick foam mattress or circulating mattress is recommended to optimize patient comfort. Positioning aids should be added to maintain the patient's lateral position. A soft doughnut-shaped headrest should be used to avoid pressure on the ear. The surgical drapes should be arranged to ensure easy access to the patient (Fig. 26–2). Awake patients undergoing craniotomy often become diaphoretic and warm as the operation proceeds. A light sheet over the patient usually suffices. Music is helpful during periods when the patient's attention is not required. The operating room environment should be quiet, and personnel must perform their tasks with an etiquette appropriate to an awake patient.

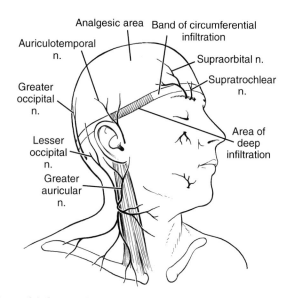

Figure 26–1 Nerve block for craniotomy. The anterior part of the scalp is innervated by the supratrochlear, frontal, zygomaticotemporal, and auriculotemporal nerves. The posterior part is innervated by the great auricular, lesser occipital, and greater occipital nerves. n., nerve.

Analgesic area
Band of circumferential infiltration
Auriculotemporal n.
Supraorbital n.
Supratrochlear n.
Greater occipital n.
Area of deep infiltration
Lesser occipital n.
Greater auricular n.

Spinal Column

Surgical procedures involving the posterior approach to the lower spinal column can be performed during

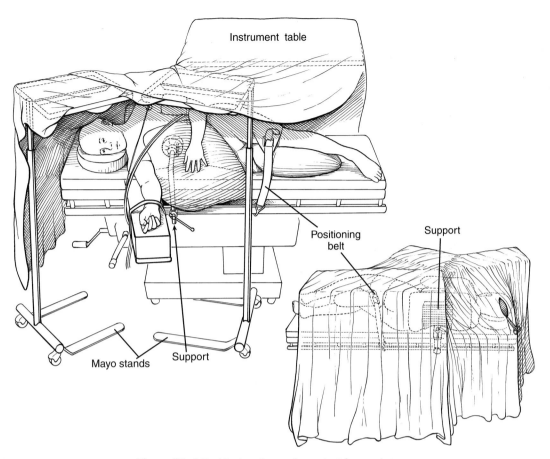

Figure 26–2 Positioning the awake patient for craniotomy.

regional anesthesia. Operation involving the cervical spine is better tolerated during general anesthesia, although a discussion on airway blocks for patients with an unstable cervical spine is included here.

Lumbar Spine Surgery

Back surgery is frequently performed during general anesthesia; regional anesthesia is seldom considered as an option. Interestingly, as early as 1922, Labat[8] described a paraspinal block combined with application to the dura of cotton pads soaked in local anesthetic for operations on the spine. Palmer[9] suggested that hypobaric dibucaine injected intrathecally was suitable for back operation but warned that the patient first should be placed prone to bathe the dorsal sensory nerves and then placed supine to bathe the anterior motor nerves.

By 1992, titles such as "Rekindle an Old Technique: Spinal Anesthesia for Lumbar Laminectomies"[10] reminded practitioners that the types of back operation amenable to regional anesthesia include lumbar disk surgery (unilateral, bilateral, multilevel), facetectomy, decompressive laminectomy, and spinal fusion. The authors of this paper studied 140 patients who presented for back surgery, and they found that spinal block was ideal for patients when general anesthesia was relatively contraindicated. Their series included 12 re-

vision operations as well as 14 obese patients who tolerated the prone position. More than 9000 disk operations were performed during spinal anesthesia at the Hartford Hospital with no serious neurologic complications attributable to the anesthetic method.[11]

A retrospective study[12] on epidural anesthesia in 1322 patients (994 patients undergoing single-level lumbar disk surgery; 261, multilevel lumbar disk surgery; and 67, decompressive laminectomies for neoplasms, with 31 of the 67 at the thoracic level) demonstrated a success rate of 94% (i.e., considered adequate by surgeon and patient without adjuvant local anesthetic or analgesic given intravenously). Spread of local anesthetic in the epidural space may be limited by mechanical occlusion by the protruding disk or tumor or by fibrosis of the epidural space after an inflammatory reaction.

There are many advantages to regional anesthesia for back operation. Some authors[11] believe that mortality is decreased in patients undergoing back operation with spinal anesthetic. In instances in which there is significant risk of complication with intubation, such as in cervical cord dysfunction and temporomandibular joint dysfunction, neuraxial block provides an alternative. Airway obstruction seldom occurs in the prone position because the tongue is displaced anteriorly.

The brachial plexus is susceptible to injury with the patient in the prone position. The nerve roots may be stretched when the head is turned. The plexus may be compressed between the clavicle and the first rib. The shoulder may also be displaced posteriorly, stretching the plexus over the head of the humerus or compressing the ulnar nerve at the cubital tunnel. The awake patient may be better able to detect pressure paresthesias, and neurologic deficits can be avoided by repositioning the arm.

Positive pressure ventilation may cause epidural vein distension, which increases the likelihood of surgical bleeding and compromises surgical exposure. During neuraxial anesthesia, the patient breathes spontaneously and bleeding at the surgical site may be less. Muscle relaxation from the spinal anesthetic also allows for atraumatic retraction and good surgical exposure. Although all these potential advantages appear to be true intuitively, there has been no prospective randomized study on back operations comparing the outcomes between general anesthesia and regional anesthesia. For patients who prefer not to have general anesthesia, such as those predisposed to severe postoperative nausea and vomiting, neuraxial block is the ideal anesthesia. This anesthetic technique is contraindicated in patients with total myelographic block in the presence of arachnoiditis.

Surgeons unfamiliar with regional anesthesia for back operation are skeptical initially. What are the implications for the surgeons? Historically, back operation done with spinal anesthesia was performed with the patient in the lateral decubitus position. The prone position is equally well tolerated by the awake patient. What about transverse myelitis and adhesive arachnoiditis that may affect the outcome of the operation? These complications are rare, although renewed interest in the neurotoxicity of local anesthetic and the cauda equina syndrome suggests prudent selection of the type and dose of local anesthetic.[13] Are patients with preexisting neurologic deficit more susceptible to local anesthetic neurotoxicity? There are no data on this issue, although Silver's group[11] reported no neurologic morbidity attributable to spinal anesthetic. Urinary retention is not uncommon and is often resolved with a single passage of the urinary catheter, with minimal consequences. The incidence of post–dural puncture headache appears to be 10 times lower than usual, perhaps as a result of the presence of blood in the surgical site serving as an epidural "autopatch."[11] The restrictive respiratory defect in the morbidly obese may be exacerbated in the prone position on a frame that compresses the wide abdominal girth. There are no published recommendations of the limit a patient can tolerate the prone position without respiratory compromise. A trial of positioning the unanesthetized patient on the frame is helpful when in doubt.

Clinical Note: *Neuraxial block is generally well accepted by patients, surgeons, and anesthesiologists. The key to success is good communication among all three parties regarding the nature and duration of the operation. The patient must be psychologically prepared and accepting of the prone position. The patient is often intimidated by the appearance of the frame, only to discover that the position is much more comfortable than it appears (Fig. 26–3). Soft pillows for the head, music via earphones, and appropriate sedation provide a pleasant environment. Head movement translates into lumbar "earthquakes" under the magnification of the operating microscope, and patients should be reminded not to move without warning. The abdomen must be free of compression to allow for ease of respiration. Choose the local anesthetic to match the duration of operation, and remember that motor block improves exposure.*

The block is best performed one level above the surgical site, where the spinous interspace is often the narrowest. For spinal anesthesia, isobaric bupivacaine gives ideal segmental spread in the vicinity of the operation. Although rare, the possibility exists of a motor block without sensory block when hyperbaric local anesthetic pools in the anterior part of the spinal cord when the patient is in the prone position. When hyperbaric solution is used, place the patient supine to bathe the dorsal roots and check for the onset of sensory block before turning the patient prone, as recommended by Palmer.[9] Additional anesthesia can be administered by simply passing a sterile syringe with local anesthetic attached to a spinal needle to the surgeon for repeat subarachnoid block. Isobaric or hypobaric local anesthetic is preferred (e.g., about 5 mg of bupivacaine). Epidural anesthesia is achieved after the 3-mL test dose of 2% lidocaine with epinephrine plus 5-mL incremental aliquots of local anesthetic injected via the Tuohy needle until a total of 15 to 20 mL is injected. No catheter is inserted, in order to avoid foreign matter in the surgical site. The patient is then placed prone. If analgesia regresses before the completion of the operation, an additional dose of spinal anesthetic can be administered.

Unstable Cervical Spine

The technique of choice for intubating the patient who has an unstable cervical spine remains controver-

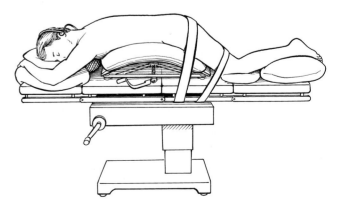

Figure 26–3 Positioning the awake patient for back operation.

sial.[14] If a fiberoptic technique in an awake patient is selected, the airway must be anesthetized after the patient is adequately sedated. Various blocks for upper airway anesthesia have been well described,[15] but these do not provide anesthesia below the vocal cords. A cough in reaction to the placement of the tracheal tube has the potential to precipitate or exacerbate neurologic deficits and must be avoided. Transtracheal injection of local anesthetic in itself is frequently accompanied by coughing and is not ideal for someone with an unstable cervical spine. Nebulized 4% lidocaine is effective for anesthetizing the airway above and below the vocal cords.[16]

The following technique provides excellent analgesia for fiberoptic bronchoscopy, especially in the patient whose neck is immobilized by a collar or halo device. Approximately 4 mL of 4% lidocaine is placed in a de Vilbiss atomizer (Fig. 26–4). The patient is instructed to open the mouth and extend the tongue while taking long, deep breaths. The spray is coordinated with inhalation, and the nozzle tip is advanced toward the pharynx. After several breaths, the pharynx is anesthetized enough to allow careful advancement of the nozzle tip such that it is pointing downward toward the larynx.[17] Inspiration draws the spray below the vocal cords. It is important to perform this technique slowly and gently. To test the adequacy of the anesthesia and at the same time supplement any inadequate block, cotton balls soaked in lidocaine gel are gently slid into the posterior pharynx, along the base and the lateral aspect of the tongue, aiming for the piriform fossae. The fiberoptic bronchoscope can then be inserted. When the vocal cords are visualized, 2 mL of 2% lidocaine is injected past the cords via the bronchoscope's injection port. With adequate anesthesia of the airway and sedation

in the awake patient, the patient will also be able to tolerate prone positioning while awake with good control of the neck alignment. The neurologic status can then be reexamined after positioning before induction of general anesthesia.

Peripheral Nerve Procedures

Most peripheral nerve procedures can be performed during local anesthetic infiltration. Regional techniques for the two most common entrapment neuropathies are described.

Carpal Tunnel Syndrome

Carpal tunnel syndrome is the most common entrapment neuropathy in humans and requires surgical decompression in many patients. This procedure can be performed during local anesthetic infiltration, intravenous regional anesthesia, or axillary block. All three techniques are well accepted by the patient, with surgical preference often a major consideration. Some surgeons believe that local infiltration does not always provide adequate analgesia for an exquisitely sensitive nerve during the decompression procedure. Others believe that tourniquet placement is contraindicated because the nerve is already ischemic. Avoiding the tourniquet allows for better hemostasis because the veins or arteries are coagulated or ligated when they are first encountered. At our institution, median neurolysis is performed during intravenous regional anesthesia by using a double tourniquet set at 200 mm Hg, with good results perhaps because the procedure lasts only 15 min and ischemic consequences are minimal. Tourniquet pain is seldom a problem. The local anesthetic dose can be halved when the tourniquet is placed on the forearm. In cases in which this procedure requires more operating time, the axillary approach to the brachial plexus block is the technique of choice and provides excellent intraoperative analgesia without the need for a tourniquet. Special attention must be paid to block the musculocutaneous, median, and ulnar nerves to ensure analgesia at the surgical site.

Ulnar Nerve Entrapment

Ulnar nerve entrapment at the elbow is the second most common entrapment neuropathy. Various surgical procedures are used. An in situ decompression within the cubital tunnel can be performed by using an 8- to 10-cm incision behind the medial epicondyle during local infiltration. Another method involves medial epicondylectomy in which the epicondyle and 2 to 5 cm of the supracondylar ridge are removed. A third method involves the transposition of the nerve from the subcutaneous tissue to an intramuscular position. Whatever the surgical technique used, the regional anesthetic technique of choice is the supraclavicular approach to the brachial plexus block combined with

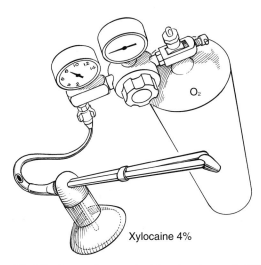

Xylocaine 4%

Figure 26–4 Equipment for anesthetizing the airway. de Vilbiss atomizer is shown; note that the nozzle can swivel downward to deliver solution into the larynx. The oxygen tubing is attached at one end to an oxygen source with a flow rate of approximately 8 to 10 L/min and to the de Vilbiss atomizer at the other end. A 0.5- to 1-cm hole is cut in the side of the oxygen tubing (outlined in black for clarity) near its attachment to the de Vilbiss atomizer. The hole can be occluded with the index finger to initiate nebulization in synchrony with inspiration.

intercostobrachial nerve block. The aim is to provide analgesia to the cutaneous area of the surgical site (medial cutaneous nerves of the arm and forearm, with their origins in the medial cord of the brachial plexus, and the intercostobrachial nerve) as well as to the deeper soft tissues and osseous innervation of the medial supracondyle and epicondyle (C-6 and C-7 roots). Combined axillary and interscalene brachial plexus block has also been shown[18] in 18 patients to be a reliable method of anesthesia for elbow surgery.

Clinical Note: *The medial aspect of the arm is innervated by the medial cutaneous nerve of the arm or the intercostobrachial nerve, or frequently a combination of both nerves. An intercostobrachial nerve block is, therefore, crucial to ensure analgesia to the surgical site. The medial cutaneous nerve of the forearm can be blocked proximal to the cord level of the brachial plexus (supraclavicular approach) or as the nerve courses along the medial aspect of the axillary artery (axillary approach).*

Neurovascular Procedures

Carotid Endarterectomy

Atherosclerotic disease of the carotid artery can produce symptoms in two ways: thrombotic or embolic. The resultant cerebral ischemia may be transient or permanent. Transient ischemic attacks last less than 1 day. Reversible ischemic neurologic deficits last up to 7 days. A common finding is a history of cerebrovascular events preceding the event that precipitated carotid endarterectomy. In one study,[19] 60% of the patients under consideration for carotid endarterectomy had a previous transient ischemic attack and 28% had a prior stroke.

Carotid endarterectomy has been the subject of much controversy[20] since its introduction in 1954.[21] It was not until 1991 that the first controlled multicenter studies were reported[19, 22, 23] that confirmed the procedure's long-term benefit in patients with symptomatic disease.

The goal of carotid endarterectomy is to prevent development of permanent neurologic deficit. Yet the operation itself carries a risk of irreversible cerebral damage. Emboli may be released during carotid angiography, surgical manipulation of the diseased artery, or shunt insertion or removal. Ischemic infarction of neurons may arise from a state of low cerebral blood flow during carotid occlusion or from systemic hypotension. Rarely, restoration of flow in a previously stenosed carotid artery may lead to profoundly hyperemic cerebral vessels and possible hemorrhagic infarction.[24]

Patients presenting for carotid endarterectomy have a high incidence of medical problems: 61% hypertension, 25% stable angina pectoris, 18% prior myocardial infarction, 16% peripheral vascular disease, 33% tobacco smokers, 21% diabetes mellitus, and 25% hyperlipidemia.[22] Perioperative morbidity includes myocardial infarction, congestive heart failure, dysrhythmia, respiratory failure, and sudden death.

Regional Anesthesia

Carotid endarterectomy can be performed during regional anesthesia. This does not mean that regional anesthesia is superior to general anesthesia. The choice of anesthesia has not yet been shown to affect patient outcome. There are advantages and disadvantages with regional anesthesia for this surgical procedure.

The major advantage is the ability to assess the neurologic state of the awake patient. Although various electrophysiologic methods may be used to determine changes in neuronal function in an asleep patient, they require experienced personnel to interpret the findings. In addition, an awake patient can report the onset of angina, but silent myocardial ischemia is asymptomatic.

Some evidence[25] suggests that blood pressure is more stable in the perioperative period in individuals receiving regional anesthesia. A smooth transition can be made to the chosen regimen of postoperative analgesia. Certain postoperative complications are better managed during local anesthesia. Early exploration of wound hematoma can often be performed before the block regresses and with no additional drugs required. Postoperative confusion is more likely to be a sign of cerebral ischemia and unlikely to be related to anesthesia.

There are several disadvantages to regional anesthesia. The surgical, anesthesia, and nursing staff must be able to perform their tasks in the presence of an awake patient. The patient needs to be calm and cooperative for carotid endarterectomy to be performed during regional anesthesia. There is a limit to the amount of sedation that the patient can receive without impairment of neurologic status. Regional anesthesia precludes the potential benefit from decreased cerebral metabolic rate during general anesthesia—a maneuver that may decrease neuronal ischemia. Complications from the regional anesthesia—e.g., injection of local anesthetic into the vertebral artery, hematoma from needle trauma, and paralysis of the diaphragm[26]—may deter the uninitiated.

There are two regional anesthesia techniques often used for patients undergoing carotid endarterectomy: cervical epidural anesthesia and cervical plexus block.[27] The general approach to the patient is the same for both techniques. Several extra steps are recommended when performing the cervical plexus block for carotid endarterectomy.

Cervical Plexus Block

The incision for a carotid endarterectomy is at the anterior border of the sternocleidomastoid muscle from the mastoid process to a point two thirds the distance to the sternoclavicular joint. The operation is well tolerated by using the deep cervical nerve block of C-2, C-3, and C-4, which form the lesser auricular nerve, transverse cutaneous nerve, and supraclavicular nerves that supply the area of the surgical site. At our institution, we routinely add several steps to the block to ensure patient comfort and intraoperative hemodynamic stability. One hour before the patient's arrival in the operating room, 5 to 10 g of EMLA (eutectic mixture of local anesthetics) cream (a topical analgesic cream consisting of a mixture of 25 mg lidocaine and 25 mg prilocaine per gram of cream) is applied to the surgical site (Fig. 26–5) and covered with an occlusive dressing to provide 3-mm-deep cutaneous analgesia with minimal levels of systemic local anesthetic (less than 10% absorbed). This improves patient comfort during the deep cervical block. In addition to the deep cervical block, a superficial cervical block is performed. Finally, the muscle belly of the sternocleidomastoid is infiltrated with 5 mL of local anesthetic just proximal to where it divides into its sternal and clavicular heads in order to minimize discomfort (often reported as a "stiff neck" intraoperatively) as the muscle is retracted laterally for surgical exposure. Intraoperatively, the carotid sinus is infiltrated with local anesthetic to minimize hypotension, bradycardia, and nausea.

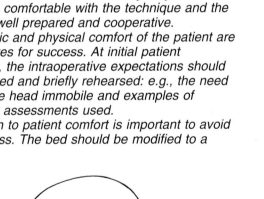

Clinical Note: *Regional anesthesia should be selected for carotid endarterectomy only when the surgeon is comfortable with the technique and the patient is well prepared and cooperative. Psychologic and physical comfort of the patient are prerequisites for success. At initial patient evaluation, the intraoperative expectations should be explained and briefly rehearsed: e.g., the need to keep the head immobile and examples of neurologic assessments used.*

Attention to patient comfort is important to avoid restlessness. The bed should be modified to a

lounge-chair position. Surgical draping must be designed to avoid claustrophobia and facilitate eye contact between the patient and anesthesia personnel.

Neurologic deficits that develop may be profound and of sudden onset. They can involve apnea, loss of consciousness, or severe motor deficit. A definite plan of action for these complications must be agreed on among surgical and anesthesia team members before their occurrence.

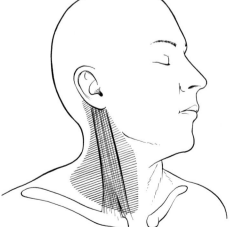

Figure 26–5 Preoperative application of EMLA (eutectic mixture of local anesthetics) cream for carotid endarterectomies. Shaded area indicates where EMLA cream should be applied.

References

1. Kandel ER, Jessell TM: Touch. In Kandel ER, Schwartz JH, Jessell TM (eds): Principles of Neural Science, 3rd ed, pp 367–384. New York, Elsevier Science Publishing, 1991.
2. Girvin JP: Resection of intracranial lesions under local anesthesia. Int Anesthesiol Clin 1986; 24(3): 133–155.
3. Archer DP, McKenna JM, Morin L, et al: Conscious-sedation analgesia during craniotomy for intractable epilepsy: a review of 354 consecutive cases. Can J Anaesth 1988; 35: 338–344.
4. Manninen P, Contreras J: Anesthetic considerations for craniotomy in awake patients. Int Anesthesiol Clin 1986; 24(3): 157–174.
5. Geevarghese KP, Garretson HD: "Alert" anesthesia in craniotomy. Int Anesthesiol Clin 1977; 15(3): 231–252.
6. Tasker RR, Marshall BM: Analgesia for surgical procedures performed on conscious patients. Can Anaesth Soc J 1965; 12: 29–33.
7. Welling EC, Donegan J: Neuroleptanalgesia using alfentanil for awake craniotomy. Anesth Analg 1989; 68: 57–60.
8. Labat G: Regional Anesthesia: Its Technic and Clinical Application. Philadelphia, WB Saunders Co, 1922.
9. Palmer LA: Spinal anesthesia. In Southworth JL, Hingson RA (eds): Conduction Anesthesia: Clinical Studies of George P. Pitkin, pp 726–824. Philadelphia, JB Lippincott, 1946.
10. Thiagarajah S, Bergland R: Rekindle an old technique: spinal anesthesia for lumbar laminectomies. (Letter to the editors.) J Neurosurg Anesthesiol 1992; 4: 221.
11. Silver DJ, Dunsmore RH, Dickson CM: Spinal anesthesia for lumbar disc surgery: review of 576 operations. Anesth Analg 1976; 55: 550–554.
12. Rifat K, Morniroli J, Orselli A, et al: Peridural anesthesia in disk hernia. (French.) Schweiz Rundsch Med Prax 1987; 76: 928–930.
13. Schneider M, Ettlin T, Kaufmann M, et al: Transient neurologic toxicity after hyperbaric subarachnoid anesthesia with 5% lidocaine. Anesth Analg 1993; 76: 1154–1157.
14. Crosby ET, Lui A: The adult cervical spine: implications for airway management. Can J Anaesth 1990; 37: 77–93.
15. Benumof JL: Management of the difficult adult airway. With special emphasis on awake tracheal intubation. Anesthesiology 1991; 75: 1087–1110.
16. Bourke DL, Katz J, Tonneson A: Nebulized anesthesia for awake endotracheal intubation. Anesthesiology 1985; 63: 690–692.
17. Benumof JL: Anesthesia for Thoracic Surgery, p 330. Philadelphia, WB Saunders Co, 1987.
18. Urmey WF: Combined axillary-interscalene (AXIS) brachial plexus block for elbow surgery. (Abstract.) Reg Anesth 1993; 18(2S): 88.
19. Mayberg MR, Wilson SE, Yatsu F, et al: Carotid endarterectomy and prevention of cerebral ischemia in symptomatic carotid stenosis. Veterans Affairs Cooperative Studies Program 309 Trialist Group. JAMA 1991; 266: 3289–3294.
20. Winslow CM, Solomon DH, Chassin MR, et al: The appropriateness of carotid endarterectomy. N Engl J Med 1988; 318: 721–727.
21. Eastcott HHG, Pickering GW, Rob CG: Reconstruction of internal carotid artery in a patient with intermittent attacks of hemiplegia. Lancet 1954; 2: 994–996.
22. North American Symptomatic Carotid Endarterectomy Trial Collaborators: Beneficial effect of carotid endarterectomy in symp-

tomatic patients with high-grade carotid stenosis. N Engl J Med 1991; 325: 445–453.

23. European Carotid Surgery Trialists' Collaborative Group: MRC European Carotid Surgery Trial: interim results for symptomatic patients with severe (70–99%) or with mild (0–29%) carotid stenosis. Lancet 1991; 337: 1235–1243.

24. Sundt TM Jr, Sharbrough FW, Piepgras DG, et al: Correlation of cerebral blood flow and electroencephalographic changes during carotid endarterectomy: with results of surgery and hemodynamics of cerebral ischemia. Mayo Clin Proc 1981; 56: 533–543.

25. Cirone R, Sullivan P, Posner M, et al: Regional vs general anaesthesia for carotid endarterectomy surgery. (Abstract.) Can J Anaesth 1994; 41(5 part II): A37.

26. Castresana MR, Masters RD, Castresana EJ, et al: Incidence and clinical significance of hemidiaphragmatic paresis in patients undergoing carotid endarterectomy during cervical plexus block anesthesia. J Neurosurg Anesthesiol 1994; 6: 21–23.

27. Peitzman AB, Webster MW, Loubeau JM, et al: Carotid endarterectomy under regional (conductive) anesthesia. Ann Surg 1982; 196: 59–64.

CHAPTER 27

Ophthalmology and Otorhinolaryngology

Robert S. Neill, M.D.

The simultaneous publication of these papers, "On the Use of Cocaine for Producing Anaesthesia on the Eye" by Carl Koller of Vienna, Austria, and "Value of Hydrochlorate of Cocaine in Ophthalmic Surgery" by J. Crawford Renton of Glasgow, Scotland, in the *Lancet* of December 6, 1884, demonstrates the rapidity with which the experimental observations of Carl Koller, first reported to the Vienna Royal Imperial Society of Physicians on October 17, 1884, spread and were accepted into clinical practice. Renton concluded his communication with the comment, "Its value in preventing pain during an operation and keeping the eye soothed for some time after cannot fail to conduce to good results in ophthalmic surgery"—an early recommendation for regional anesthesia for postoperative analgesia. The drug and the technique have survived the intervening century unchanged, further confirmation of the seminal nature of Koller's original observation.

The 1910 Ether Anniversary address to the Massachusetts General Hospital[1] is another milestone in the history of regional anesthesia of the head and neck. In it, Crile introduced his concept of anociassociation in which the patient was protected from noxious input by "a combination of special management of patients (applied psychology), morphine, inhalation anesthesia and local anesthesia." Of his experience of operating on patients with Graves disease he said, "There is scarcely a change in the pulse, the respiration or in the nervous state at the close of the operation. Against the effect of the inflowing stimuli from the wound after the cocaine has worn off I know no remedy. . . . Since the adoption of this new method (anociassociation) my operative results have been so vastly improved that I now regard no case of Graves disease as inoperable, at least to the extent of making a double ligation."

Labat's classic text *Regional Anesthesia,*[2] first published in 1922, has a foreword written by William J. Mayo in which he stated that regional anesthesia has come to stay. However, he continued that in order to overcome certain inherent defects, it is necessary in certain cases and desirable in many to use some form of general anesthesia with the regional anesthesia. This comprehensive text includes several chapters describing techniques and indications for such major interventions in the head and neck as partial glossectomy and laryngectomy. Labat emphasized the importance of relief of anxiety and apprehension by the careful application of the practices of patient management described by Crile.

This concept was further developed by Lundy. In 1926, he described[3] "balanced anesthesia," a term he used for a combination of agents—such as premedication, regional anesthesia, and general anesthesia with one or more agents—so that pain relief was obtained by a nice balance of agents and techniques.

The development of safe and routine tracheal intubation together with the introduction of neuromuscular blocking agents and powerful short-acting opioids altered this concept of balanced anesthesia and relegated regional nerve block to a lesser role.[4]

Regional nerve block anesthesia retained its popularity in ophthalmology, otorhinolaryngology, and maxillofacial surgery for many procedures, minor and major, in which general anesthesia was not required or was contraindicated.[5-8] Nicoll and colleagues[9] and Hamilton and associates[10] have published large series on patients undergoing cataract extraction during regional anesthesia, and other investigators[11] have stressed the benefits of this technique of anesthesia in these patients. Rubin[12] and Nicoll and coworkers[9] have emphasized the importance of anesthetic input in the management of these patients—preoperative assessment, choice of anesthetic management, and intraoperative monitoring—if optimum operating conditions with minimal complications are to be achieved.

Rubin[12] concluded his editorial "Anaesthesia for Cataract Surgery—Time for Change?" with the statement,

"It would be to the detriment of our patients and specialty if anaesthetists are not involved" [in cataract surgery]. Why would this be a detriment in cataract surgery only? A reappraisal of the role of regional nerve block in all areas of head and neck surgery is overdue. A reappraisal might possibly lead to a return to the original concepts of Crile and Lundy for the provision of "balanced" anesthesia.[1, 3]

Innervation and Physiologic Responses

A large proportion of the nerve supply to the head and neck is of a specialized sensory or secretomotor nature, with no relevance to regional anesthesia. Another distinctive feature is the almost complete separation of motor and sensory function, permitting intraoral anesthesia without loss of control of the airway muscles. At most other sites, motor block is induced in combination with any sensory block. For example, during cataract surgery the branches of the facial nerve supplying the orbicularis oculus muscle should be blocked to decrease the risk of iris or vitreous prolapse.

Research[13] into the effects of postoperative pain has shown a definite relationship between severe unrelieved pain and morbidity and mortality. The adverse physiologic effects of this unrelieved pain can be prevented by effective analgesia. Tissue trauma evokes nociceptive afferent activity that affects spinal segments above and below the point of entry of the pain stimulus, with action potentials also propagating antidromically into the surrounding vascular bed. A complex neurohumoral response is initiated, creating hyperalgesia, which intensifies as the increased efferent sympathetic activity releases norepinephrine to further sensitize receptors. This increased sensitivity is further compounded by the release of local vasoactive substances: bradykinin, serotonin, and prostaglandin E. A vicious circle of nociceptor activity is now established and results in vasoconstriction, edema, and tissue acidosis. Anesthesia of the regional nerve supply blocks either or both afferent and efferent limbs of the reflex sympathetic arc and limits the magnitude of the response to pain and surgical trauma.[14, 15]

Patient Groups in Which Regional Nerve Block Is of Potential Benefit

Outpatient Surgery

Uncomplicated dental surgery is most frequently performed using regional anesthesia, supplemented if required by intravenous administration of sedatives. Nerve block or infiltration of local anesthetic has been demonstrated to decrease the incidence of arrhythmias during halothane–nitrous oxide–oxygen anesthesia.[16, 17] Patients also exhibited more rapid recovery with enhanced postoperative analgesia.

Hundreds of thousands of cataract extractions have been performed since 1884, in a wide variety of locations and patients, using virtually the same method as Koller used. Increasingly, in developed countries the procedure is centered on outpatient facilities, mimicking the traveling "eye camps" of India.[11, 12, 18]

Corrective plastic surgery in the head and neck is another area in which outpatient surgery and regional anesthesia are compatible. Blepharoplasty, face-lift, rhinoplasty, and correction of prominent ears have all been performed using nerve block, supplemented by intravenous administration of sedatives. Attwood and Evans[19] described the use of such a technique for correction of prominent ears in a group of patients in whom 20% were younger than age 13 years. The majority were in favor of regional anesthesia, and 30% found they "enjoyed" the experience. The author's own series confirmed these observations in a similar group of patients, the youngest of whom was age 8 years.

An investigation[20] into perioperative complications conducted by the Federal Ambulatory Surgery Association showed that the lowest incidence of complications (1/275) occurred when unsupplemented regional anesthesia was the method used. Addition of sedatives significantly increased complications to the rate associated with general anesthesia (1/120).

Poor-Risk Patients

Conflicting views have been expressed on the benefits gained by use of regional anesthesia. Backer and colleagues[21] reported no myocardial reinfarction after 288 ophthalmic procedures during local anesthesia in 195 patients with a history of myocardial infarction. Local anesthesia was also found to prevent the increase in norepinephrine and glucose concentrations found with general anesthesia and was associated with greater cardiovascular stability.[22, 23] General anesthesia has a significantly higher risk of producing nausea and vomiting, both undesirable after cataract surgery.[24] Memory and cognitive function showed no significant difference after local and general anesthesia, and no difference has been found in morbidity rates or mortality.[25]

Ophthalmic surgeons can perform the majority of their operations with local anesthesia; however, the cooperation of an anesthesiologist familiar with these techniques can broaden the choice of methods available. Careful sedation and monitoring can improve the patient's prognosis.[12] More efficient use of time with increased throughput can be achieved if both surgeon and anesthesiologist can perform the regional nerve blocks.[9, 10] Similar considerations apply to middle ear operations, e.g., stapedectomy, when these are performed using regional anesthesia.

Airway Abnormalities

Patients presenting for major head and neck operations frequently have severe airway abnormalities: congenital, traumatic, or neoplastic. Some may be of such severity that tracheal intubation or tracheostomy should be performed before induction of general anesthesia.[26] This may be accomplished by a combination of regional nerve block and topical anesthesia with a short-duration agent to decrease the time to return of laryngeal reflexes.[27] Proximal block of the trigeminal nerve with a long-duration agent ensures postoperative analgesia with decreased dependence on opioid analgesics in those patients in whom the airways may be at risk after major facial operation.[4]

Intractable Pain

Neurolysis of the trigeminal nerve at the foramen ovale or cervical plexus at the appropriate transverse process can relieve the pain from inoperable tumors or recurrence of disease. After a successful block, patients have a decreased dependence on potent opioid analgesics with an improvement in quality of life.[28–32]

Analgesia With Reduction in Opioid Requirements

Nerve blocks provided the analgesic component of balanced anesthesia, as originally described.[3] Used in this manner, the residual effects of the local anesthetic agent extend into the immediate postoperative period, ensuring a quiet recovery with adequate time to create effective postoperative analgesia.

Currently available local anesthetic drugs with prolonged activity have the potential for further advances in both quality of analgesia and independence from opioid analgesia.[33] Great auricular nerve block with such an agent significantly decreases the requirements for postoperative analgesia and the incidence of nausea and vomiting after surgical correction of prominent ears in children and adults, irrespective of the use of general anesthesia.[34, 35]

Similar benefits may be gained by the use of infraorbital, mental, and palatal nerve blocks in children requiring cleft lip and palate or cleft rhinoplasty surgery, especially if tongue flaps are required to close the palatal defect. In these circumstances, it is mandatory to maintain efficient pharyngeal and laryngeal reflexes, at the same time ensuring that pain and associated crying do not increase venous pressure and increase the risk of hemorrhage from the operative site. The residual analgesia from a comprehensive regional nerve block is often successful in controlling pain and discomfort at this crucial period without use of potentially depressant doses of opioids (Neill RS, 1992: unpublished data).

Alternative to Induction of Hypotensive Anesthesia

Surgical requests for decrease in bleeding at operative sites by the use of induced hypotension often conflict with the anesthesiologist's assessment of the potential risk to the patient. In head and neck surgery, regional nerve block using small amounts of local anes-

thetic plus a vasoconstrictor has been shown to decrease bleeding. Major eyelid surgery can be undertaken in elderly poor-risk patients with excellent operating conditions if appropriate nerve blocks are used in association with minimal sedation.[36] Dacryocystorhinostomy, rhinoplasty, septal resection, and rhinophyma reduction are procedures associated with considerable hemorrhage unless preventive measures are taken. The author's own experience suggests that comprehensive regional nerve blocks produce operating conditions similar to those obtained with profound induced hypotension.[37]

Autonomic Block

Reconstruction of the defects produced by excision of intraoral and laryngeal tumors frequently involves free tissue transfer.[38] Survival of the transposed tissue depends on the rapid establishment of arterial input and venous drainage through the microanastomosis. Meticulous surgical anastomosis is undoubtedly the most important determinant of success or failure, but the effects of arousal from anesthesia, postoperative pain, and blood volume replacement must not be ignored.[39] Rapid arousal may trigger a vasoconstrictor response, and unresolved postoperative pain may initiate a profound physiologic stress response with deleterious effects on the microcirculation of the transposed flap. In reconstructive surgery of the head and neck, a combination of trigeminal nerve blocks with cervical plexus and stellate ganglion blocks will ensure a pain-free arousal from anesthesia and prevent a sympathetically induced vasoconstrictor response at the site of the microanastomosis[40] (Fig. 27–1).

Incorporation Into Anesthetic Practice

Regional nerve block may be used as the sole anesthetic procedure, perhaps supplemented by careful intravenous administration of sedatives or as a component of balanced general anesthesia when it is essential or requested by the patient. In both situations, meticulous attention must be paid to preoperative assessment, intraoperative monitoring, and postoperative care if favorable results are to be ensured. Before each surgical procedure, the appropriate combination of nerve blocks and volumes and concentrations of local anesthetic agents must be determined and followed by a sympathetic, detailed explanation to the patient of the procedures involved before any invasive approach is made.

Branches of the trigeminal nerve may be blocked proximally at the pterygoid plate or distally as they emerge from the bony foramina of the skull. The deep branches of the cervical plexus can be blocked at the transverse process; the superficial branches of the cervical plexus can be blocked at the posterior border of the sternocleidomastoid muscle (Fig. 27–2).

Young children are not suitable subjects for unsupplemented nerve block anesthesia but benefit from its use in combination with general anesthesia. Older chil-

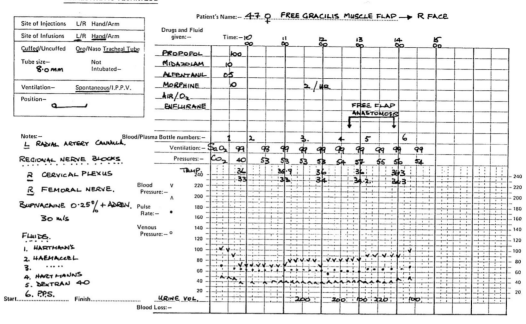

Figure 27–1 Anesthetic record of a 47-year-old woman undergoing a free gracilis muscle flap during a combined regional and general anesthetic. This combination allowed minimal hemodynamic changes.

dren are often prepared to have quite extensive procedures performed during nerve block anesthesia if they are handled gently and sympathetically. Some have even stated that they "enjoyed" the experience and would be willing to have it repeated.[19]

Drugs and Equipment

Self-aspirating dental cartridge syringes fitted with 27- or 30-G needles have proved more versatile than disposable equivalents and are recommended for all distal blocks and local infiltration. Cartridges containing different strengths of local anesthetic agent and vasoconstrictor drug are universally available. Lidocaine 2% with epinephrine 1/80,000 has been used as the standard solution and has provided consistently rapid onset of intense anesthesia.

Proximal blocks intended for prolonged analgesia are most satisfactorily produced with bupivacaine, again readily available in different concentrations with or without added epinephrine. Manufacturers in the United Kingdom recommend a maximum dose of bupivacaine of 2 mg/kg in any 4-h period, thus allowing 25 to 30 mL of 0.5% solution for a 65- to 70-kg adult.

Such small volumes can lead to incomplete blocks; dilution to increase the volume can have the same effect. Moore and associates[41] reported a series of more than 11,000 patients in whom much larger dosing regimens were used. Only 15 patients exhibited local anesthetic systemic toxic effects resulting from unintentional intravascular injection or absorption. The author's own study[42] using higher than recommended dosages of 0.5% bupivacaine for major head and neck surgery produced venous plasma levels in the range of 3.0 to 6.5 µg/mL, but no signs of cardiovascular or

central nervous system local anesthetic systemic toxicity were detected. Subsequently, 0.375% bupivacaine has been used alone for cranial nerve blocks and with added vasoconstrictor for cervical plexus block. With this combination, total and free venous plasma levels were recorded at 15 min as 2.5 µg/mL ± 0.9 (total) and 91 ng ± 53 (free) and at 60 min as 1.98 µg/mL ± 0.45 (total) and 60.8 ng ± 40 (free). These values are lower than those reported by Denson and associates[43] as causing signs of central nervous system local anesthetic systemic toxicity.

Clinical Examples

The following clinical examples demonstrate the use of distal and proximal nerve blocks as the sole anesthetic in sedated patients or as a component of balanced general anesthesia.

Ear Surgery

Figure 27–3 demonstrates a technique of nerve block anesthesia suitable for a range of surgical procedures on the ear—e.g., correction of prominent ears or excision of tumors (from wedge resection to amputation of the pinna). Great auricular, auriculotemporal, and auricular branches of the vagus (Arnold's) nerve blocks are combined with areas of local infiltration to induce hemostasis. In children, postoperative analgesia with decreased nausea and vomiting can be provided if these nerve blocks are performed after induction of general anesthesia.

Eye Surgery

A 66-year-old woman presented with a penetrating basal cell carcinoma of the medial canthus of the right

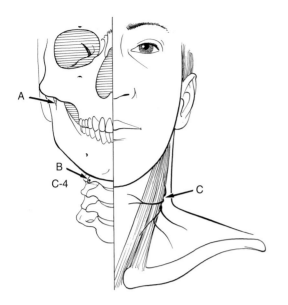

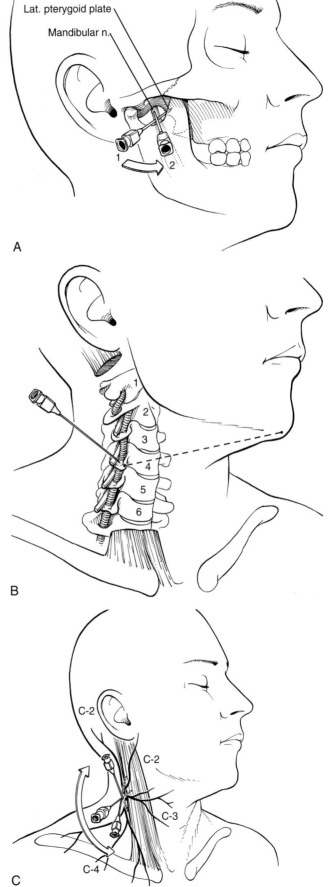

Figure 27–2 Head and neck regional anesthetic options. *A,* Peripterygoid trigeminal blocks (mandibular and maxillary). *B,* Deep cervical plexus block. *C,* Superficial cervical plexus block. Lat., lateral; n., nerve.

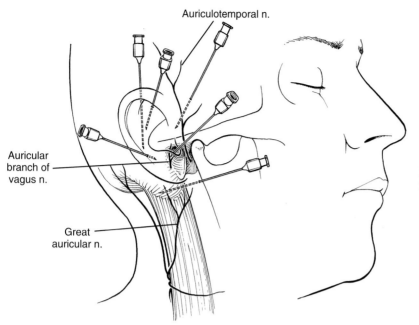

Auriculotemporal n.

Auricular branch of vagus n.

Great auricular n.

Figure 27–3 Regional block of the ear shows the nerves of importance and locations of needle insertion for these nerves. n., nerve.

eye (Fig. 27–4; see Color Plate 9). Excision of the tumor with reconstruction by using a forehead rotation flap was scheduled. A combination of bilateral supraorbital, supratrochlear, infratrochlear, and right infraorbital nerve blocks formed the basis of the anesthesia. Conjunctival anesthesia was achieved with tetracaine (amethocaine) ophthalmic drops; the boundaries of the flap were infiltrated with dilute lidocaine and epinephrine to improve hemostasis. Light sedation produced with benzodiazepine and opioid combination given intravenously ensured that the patient had no memory of the operative procedure. If full-thickness excision of either eyelid is required, a small amount of anesthetic should be injected into the "gray" margin because this is anesthetized by neither the infraorbital nerve block nor the conjunctival drops.

Lip Surgery I

A 72-year-old man presented with a large squamous cell carcinoma of the lower lip (Fig. 27–5; see Color Plate 9) associated with many years of pipe smoking. Excision of two thirds of the lower lip with reconstruction using Karapandicz rotation flaps was scheduled. Anesthesia was provided by bilateral blocks of the mandibular and maxillary branches of the trigeminal nerve by the peripterygoid approach, supplemented by local infiltration of 0.125% lidocaine and epinephrine with minimal intravenous administration of sedative. Airway reflexes were present and active throughout the procedure.

Lip Surgery II

A 78-year-old man presented for reconstruction of a defect of the upper lip (Fig. 27–6; see Color Plate 10) after serial excisions for squamous cell carcinoma. Regional nerve block anesthesia was provided by using bilateral mental and infraorbital nerve blocks with infil-

tration of the lateral commissure to anesthetize terminal branches of the buccal nerve.

Facial Surgery

A woman in the sixth decade of life presented with a penetrating basal cell carcinoma of the right cheek (Fig. 27–7, p. 493 and Color Plate 10). Excision and reconstruction using a glabellar flap were planned. Regional nerve block anesthesia was provided by a combination of bilateral supraorbital, supratrochlear, and infratrochlear nerve blocks to permit elevation of the flap and block of the right infraorbital nerve and zygomatic branch of the facial nerve to permit excision of the tumor.

Nasal Surgery

A 47-year-old man with a history of severe, chronic obstructive pulmonary disease and emphysematous bullae formation presented for assessment of suitability for forehead rhinoplasty (Fig. 27–8; see Color Plate 11). Previous operation had resulted in a large nasal defect concealed by a plastic prosthesis, which the patient wished to dispense with. General anesthesia on two previous occasions had resulted in severe coughing during recovery, with the development of spontaneous pneumothoraces. He requested that regional nerve block anesthesia be used if at all possible. Bilateral supraorbital, supratrochlear, infratrochlear, and infraorbital nerve blocks were combined with right external nasal nerve block, nasal packing with cocaine 10% solution, and local infiltration with 0.125% lidocaine and epinephrine 1/400,000. The patient remained responsive, cooperative, and talkative throughout the procedure despite generous administration of sedatives intravenously. In the postoperative phase, he had minimal recollection of events during the 2.5-h operation.

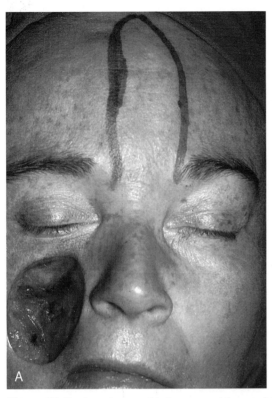
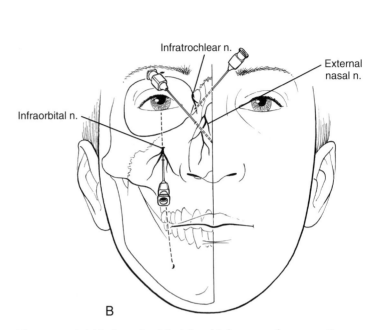

Figure 27–7 Bilateral supraorbital, supratrochlear, and infratrochlear nerve (n.) blocks and a right infraorbital nerve and a zygomatic branch of the facial nerve block, with sedation, used to prepare a patient for creation of a glabellar flap. *A,* Preoperative photograph (see Color Plate 10). *B,* Regional blocks used for this procedure.

As Component of Balanced Anesthesia

A 44-year-old man presented for wide excision of buccal squamous cell carcinoma, radical neck dissection, and reconstruction using a free radial forearm flap (Fig. 27–9; see Color Plate 11). After induction of general anesthesia and bilateral trigeminal nerve blocks at the pterygoid plate, left deep cervical plexus and brachial plexus and right superficial cervical plexus blocks were performed to constitute the analgesia component of balanced general anesthesia.

Clinical Notes: *Successful regional nerve block anesthesia depends on a secure knowledge of anatomy, with an innovative approach to anesthesia. Ability to relate sympathetically to patients is of paramount importance to surgeon and anesthesiologist, who must both maintain a calm demeanor and a flexible response if and when trouble occurs. Conversion to general anesthesia does not necessarily imply failure.*

The learning process should be conducted during general anesthesia, until confidence is developed and surgeons' irritation at delay is minimized. Surgical colleagues have been known to request the use of regional anesthesia for certain procedures because of the improved operating conditions.

Published guidelines on dosage of local anesthetic agents have a rigidity, which if interpreted literally could preclude effective regional blocks. Individual situations should be assessed in the light of previous experience and the pharmacokinetics and pharmacodynamics of the sites of the regional nerve block. Larger than recommended doses have been used with no ill effects, provided the anesthesiologist is alert to the possibility of toxic responses and equipped to treat any eventuality.

References

1. Crile GW: Phylogenetic association in relation to certain medical problems. Boston Med Surg J 1910; 163: 893–904.
2. Labat G: Regional Anesthesia: Its Technique and Clinical Application. Philadelphia, WB Saunders Co, 1922.
3. Lundy JS: Balanced anesthesia. Minn Med 1926; 9: 399–404.
4. Murphy TM: Somatic blockade of head and neck. In Cousins MJ, Bridenbaugh PO (eds): Neural Blockade in Clinical Anesthesia and Management of Pain, 2nd ed, pp 533–558. Philadelphia, JB Lippincott, 1988.
5. Allen ED, Elkington AR: Local anaesthesia and the eye. Br J Anaesth 1980; 52: 689–694.
6. Jahrsdoerfer RA: Anesthesia in otologic surgery. Otolaryngol Clin North Am 1981; 14: 699–704.
7. Martof AB: Anesthesia of the teeth, supporting structures, and oral mucous membrane. Otolaryngol Clin North Am 1981; 14: 653–668.
8. Stromberg BV: Regional anesthesia in head and neck surgery. Clin Plast Surg 1985; 12: 123–136.
9. Nicoll JM, Acharya PA, Ahlen K, et al.: Central nervous system

complications after 6000 retrobulbar blocks. Anesth Analg 1987; 66: 1298–1302.

10. Hamilton RC, Gimbel HV, Strunin L: Regional anaesthesia for 12,000 cataract extraction and intraocular lens implantation procedures. Can J Anaesth 1988; 35: 615–623.

11. Wong DHW: Regional anaesthesia for intraocular surgery. Can J Anaesth 1993; 40: 635–657.

12. Rubin AP: Anaesthesia for cataract surgery—time for change? (Editorial.) Anaesthesia 1990; 45: 717–718.

13. Cousins M: Acute and postoperative pain. In Wall PD, Melzack R (eds): Textbook of Pain, 2nd ed, pp 284–305. Edinburgh, Churchill Livingstone, 1989.

14. Hannington-Kiff JG: Pain: sympathetic maintenance and central nervous sensitization. In Kaufman L (ed): Anaesthesia: Review 9, pp 112–126. Edinburgh, Churchill Livingstone, 1992.

15. Kehlet H: Modification of responses to surgery by neural blockade: clinical implications. In Cousins MJ, Bridenbaugh PO (eds): Neural Blockade in Clinical Anesthesia and Management of Pain, 2nd ed, pp 145–188. Philadelphia, JB Lippincott, 1988.

16. Plowman PE, Thomas WJ, Thurlow AC: Cardiac dysrhythmias during anaesthesia for oral surgery. The effect of local blockade. Anaesthesia 1974; 29: 571–575.

17. Rashad A, el-Attar A: Cardiac dysrhythmias during oral surgery: effect of combined local and general anaesthesia. Br J Oral Maxillofac Surg 1990; 28: 102–104.

18. Feitl ME, Krupin T: Neural blockade for ophthalmologic surgery. In Cousins MJ, Bridenbaugh PO (eds): Neural Blockade in Clinical Anesthesia and Management of Pain, 2nd ed, pp 577–592. Philadelphia, JB Lippincott, 1988.

19. Attwood AI, Evans DM: Correction of prominent ears using Mustarde's technique: an out-patient procedure under local anaesthetic in children and adults. Br J Plast Surg 1985; 38: 252–258.

20. White PF: Outpatient anesthesia. In Miller RD (ed): Anesthesia, 3rd ed, vol 2, pp 2025–2059. New York, Churchill Livingstone, 1990.

21. Backer CL, Tinker JH, Robertson DM, et al.: Myocardial reinfarction following local anesthesia for ophthalmic surgery. Anesth Analg 1980; 59: 257–262.

22. Barker JP, Vafidis GC, Robinson PN, et al.: Plasma catecholamine response to cataract surgery: a comparison between general and local anaesthesia. Anaesthesia 1991; 46: 642–645.

23. Barker JP, Robinson PN, Vafidis GC, et al.: Local analgesia prevents the cortisol and glycaemic responses to cataract surgery. Br J Anaesth 1990; 64: 442–445.

24. Lynch S, Wolf GL, Berlin I: General anesthesia for cataract surgery: a comparative review of 2217 consecutive cases. Anesth Analg 1974; 53: 909–913.

25. O'Sullivan G, Kerr-Muir M, Lim M, et al.: Day-case ophthalmic surgery: general or local anaesthesia? (Letter to the editor.) Anaesthesia 1990; 45: 885–886.

26. Murrin KR: Awake intubation. In Latto IP, Rosen M (eds): Difficulties in Tracheal Intubation, pp 90–98. London, Baillière Tindall, 1985.

27. Gotta AW, Sullivan CA: Anaesthesia of the upper airway using topical anaesthetic and superior laryngeal nerve block. Br J Anaesth 1981; 53: 1055–1058.

28. Moore DC: Regional Block: A Handbook for Use in the Clinical Practice of Medicine and Surgery, 4th ed, p 93. Springfield, IL, Charles C Thomas, 1965.

29. Lipton S: Pain relief in active patients with cancer: the early use of nerve blocks improves the quality of life. BMJ 1989; 298: 37–38.

30. Carron H: Control of pain in the head and neck. Otolaryngol Clin North Am 1981; 14: 631–652.

31. Cousins MJ, Dwyer B, Gibb D: Chronic pain and neurolytic neural blockade. In Cousins MJ, Bridenbaugh PO (eds): Neural Blockade in Clinical Anesthesia and Management of Pain, 2nd ed, pp 1053–1084. Philadelphia, JB Lippincott, 1988.

32. Neill RS: Terminal care of intraoral cancer. Eur J Pain 1992; 13: 8–11.

33. Neill RS: Head and neck. In Nimmo WS, Robotham DJ, Smith G (eds): Anaesthesia, 2nd ed, vol 2, pp 1524–1536. London, Blackwell Scientific Publications, 1994.

34. Blogg CE: Anaesthesia for plastic surgery. In Nimmo WS, Robotham DJ, Smith G (eds): Anaesthesia, 2nd ed, vol 2, pp 1037–1041. London, Blackwell Scientific Publications, 1994.

35. Neill RS: Head and neck and airway. In Wildsmith JAW, Armitage EN (eds): Principles and Practice of Regional Anaesthesia, 2nd ed, pp 203–211. Edinburgh, Churchill Livingstone, 1993.

36. Neill RS: Regional analgesia combined with intravenous sedation in major eyelid surgery: an alternative to induced hypotension. Br J Plast Surg 1983; 36: 29–35.

37. Neill RS: Head and neck surgery. In Henderson JJ, Nimmo WS (eds): Practical Regional Anaesthesia, pp 165–183. Oxford, Blackwell Scientific Publications, 1983.

38. Soutar DS, Scheker LR, Tanner NS, et al.: The radial forearm flap: a versatile method for intra-oral reconstruction. Br J Plast Surg 1983; 36: 1–8.

39. Vance JP: General anaesthesia for microvascular surgery. In Soutar DS (ed): Microvascular Surgery and Free Tissue Transfer, pp 12–16. London, Edward Arnold, 1993.

40. Neill RS: Regional anaesthesia for microvascular surgery. In Soutar DS (ed): Microvascular Surgery and Free Tissue Transfer, pp 17–25. London, Edward Arnold, 1993.

41. Moore DC, Bridenbaugh LD, Thompson GE, et al.: Bupivacaine: a review of 11,080 cases. Anesth Analg 1978; 57: 42–53.

42. Neill RS, Watson R: Plasma bupivacaine concentrations during combined regional and general anaesthesia for resection and reconstruction of head and neck carcinomata. Br J Anaesth 1984; 56: 485–492.

43. Denson DD, Myers JA, Hartrick CT, et al.: The relationship between free bupivacaine concentration and central nervous system toxicity. (Abstract.) Anesthesiology 1984; 61: A211.

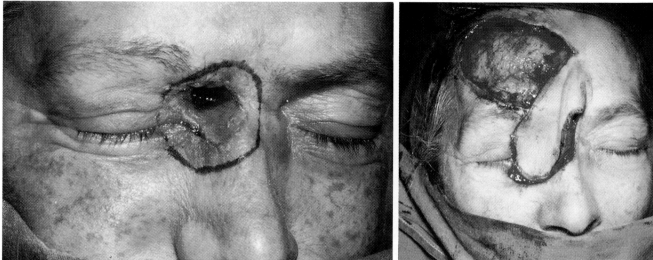

Figure 27–4 Bilateral supraorbital, supratrochlear, and infratrochlear nerve blocks, coupled with right infraorbital conjunctival drops and minimal infiltration of the flap, were used with minimal sedation to perform a rotation flap in a patient with a penetrating periorbital basal cell carcinoma. *A*, Preoperative photograph. *B*, Rotation flap creation.

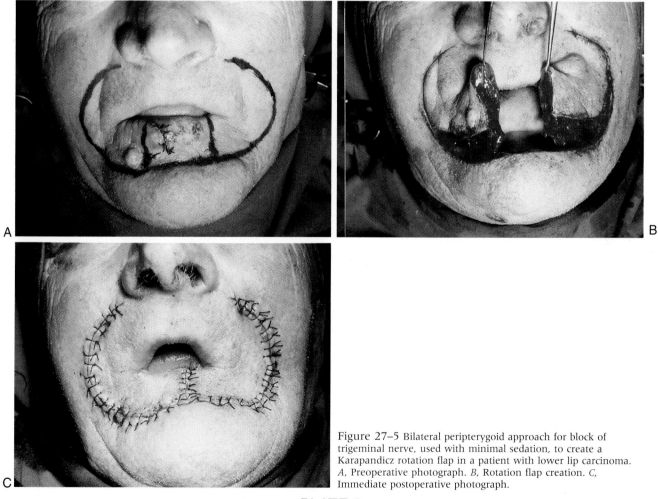

Figure 27–5 Bilateral peripterygoid approach for block of trigeminal nerve, used with minimal sedation, to create a Karapandicz rotation flap in a patient with lower lip carcinoma. *A*, Preoperative photograph. *B*, Rotation flap creation. *C*, Immediate postoperative photograph.

PLATE 9

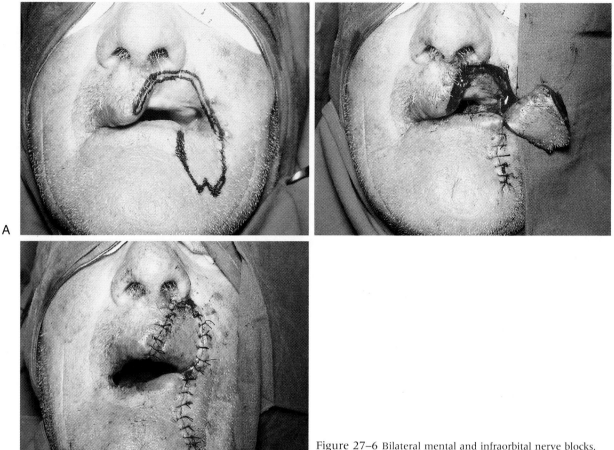

Figure 27–6 Bilateral mental and infraorbital nerve blocks, with minimal sedation, used to create an Abbe flap in a patient with a perioral defect. *A,* Preoperative photograph. *B,* Abbe flap creation. *C,* Immediate postoperative photograph.

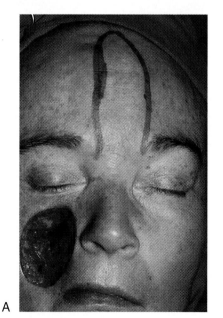

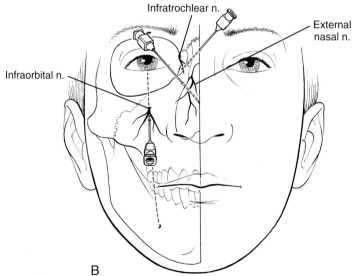

Figure 27–7 Bilateral supraorbital, supratrochlear, and infratrochlear nerve (n.) blocks and a right infraorbital nerve and a zygomatic branch of the facial nerve block, with sedation, used to prepare a patient for creation of a glabellar flap. *A,* Preoperative photograph. *B,* Regional blocks used for this procedure.

PLATE 10

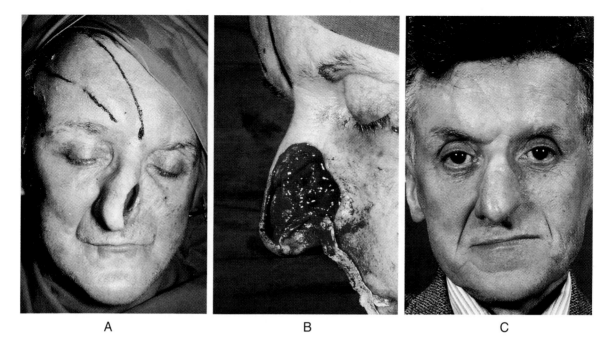

Figure 27–8 Regional anesthesia (bilateral supraorbital, supratrochlear, infratrochlear, and infraorbital nerve blocks with right external nasal nerve block and nasal packing with cocaine and infiltration with lidocaine and epinephrine) used as sole anesthetic to create a glabellar flap to provide coverage for a nasal reconstruction defect. The patient had severe obstructive airway disease and had experienced two spontaneous pneumothoraces after previous use of general anesthetics. The patient requested regional block. A, Preoperative photograph. B, Intraoperative lateral view. C, Postoperative result.

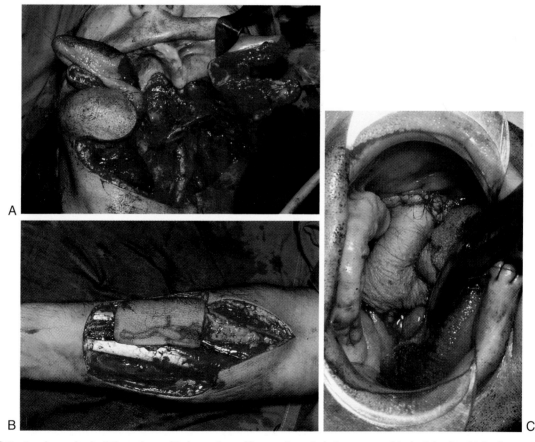

Figure 27–9 Regional anesthesia (bilateral mandibular and maxillary and cervical plexus nerve blocks [plus brachial]) for partial glossectomy and creation of free radial forearm flap in a patient with squamous cell carcinoma. The patient requested regional block. A, Intraoperative view. B, Forearm flap ready for transfer. C, Postoperative intraoral result.

PLATE 11

CHAPTER 28

General Surgery and Trauma

Way Yin, M.D.

Regional anesthetic techniques have found widespread application for procedures performed in the traditional operating room environment and in other areas of the hospital, such as the emergency department and the intensive care unit. The proliferation of acute pain services in many hospitals may further extend the availability of regional anesthetic techniques to patients who previously would not have had access to these specialized modalities of analgesia.

Regional anesthesia and analgesia result in many favorable physiologic effects in the perioperative period and appear to decrease morbidity and mortality when used in certain high-risk patient populations.[1-3] Regional anesthesia blunts the hormonal response to surgical stress,[4] reduces the hypercoagulable state after operation,[2, 5] and often provides perioperative analgesia superior to other modalities of pain relief. Preincisional use of regional blocks may even exert analgesic effects long after the cessation of regional block.[6-10] In many situations, the benefits of regional anesthesia and analgesia may be combined with those of general anesthesia to provide renewed meaning to the phrase "balanced anesthesia." This chapter reviews regional anesthetic applications for general surgical procedures and highlights regional anesthetic considerations for traumatic injuries. Application of regional anesthetic techniques for analgesia in the emergency department and intensive care unit settings is explored. Specific regional block techniques are described in detail elsewhere in this textbook and are reviewed only where applicable in this chapter. Owing to the tremendous variety of potential procedures in the general surgeon's repertoire and the myriad combinations of regional techniques applicable to various traumatic injuries, an in-depth analysis of regional anesthesia for general surgery and trauma will be forsaken in favor of a more focused approach highlighting specific examples of regional anesthesia for certain general surgical procedures and for certain classes of traumatic injuries.

Regional Anesthesia in General Surgery

The majority of general surgical procedures are amenable to some form of regional technique used as a stand-alone anesthetic, as a complement to a general anesthetic, or for postoperative analgesia. Regional anesthesia, especially peripheral regional block, is effective in blocking somatic pain. Although many general surgical procedures involve intraoperative visceral stimulation, most postoperative pain is usually due to the incision. For example, both open cholecystectomy and inguinal herniorrhaphy may involve various degrees of intraoperative visceral and peritoneal stimulation. Although regional anesthetic techniques may be used as stand-alone anesthesia in these operations, visceral impulses conducted via autonomic afferent fibers may not be so reliably blocked as those conducted via dermatomal somatic afferents. However, appropriate peripheral regional block (e.g., interpleural or intercostal block for cholecystectomy and inguinal field block for herniorrhaphy) performed for these procedures may provide complete postoperative analgesia. Regional anesthesia may be used intraoperatively to decrease general anesthetic requirements and to provide complete, or nearly complete, postoperative analgesia in the early postoperative period.

Application of regional anesthesia in the perioperative period has been clearly demonstrated to decrease postoperative pain for many procedures compared with general anesthesia alone,[6-11] and techniques involving either peripheral or neuraxial block can provide superior postoperative analgesia compared with parenterally administered opioids or other modalities of postoperative pain control. The analgesic effects of preincisional block may also outlast the estimated duration of regional block.[6-10] Decreased postoperative opioid requirements, with corresponding minimization of opioid-associated side effects such as respiratory depression, somnolence, nausea, and emesis, may increase patient satisfaction and speed recovery. Unlike opioid analgesic regimens, regional anesthesia with local anesthetic agents is not associated with delays in gastric emptying or small bowel transit times.[12]

Local anesthesia has been associated with greater intraoperative and postoperative hemodynamic stability compared with general anesthesia[13] and, when applicable, can provide an attractive alternative in situations in which hemodynamic lability may increase perioperative risk. Regional anesthesia also provides an alternative for patients who are, for one reason or another, reluctant to undergo general anesthesia, and it may allow patients to feel a greater sense of control over the course of their medical management. Regional blocks used for certain procedures are associated with shorter recovery room stays and may contribute to overall cost savings by obviating the need for general anesthesia in these circumstances.[14] The use of peripheral regional block has also been correlated with a decreased incidence of postoperative nausea, emesis, and urinary retention[13, 15, 16] as well as a lower incidence of unintentional hypothermia compared with general anesthesia.[17]

Regional Anesthesia for General Surgical Procedures by Anatomic Region

Head and Neck

Superficial general surgical procedures involving the head and neck may be performed with various regional techniques. Procedures such as sebaceous cyst excision, scar revisions, excisional biopsies, and lymph node biopsies, although often performed during local anesthesia, may in many situations be amenable to simple regional or field blocks. This can decrease the overall amount of local anesthetic required to perform the procedure and minimize the number of injections required to obtain anesthesia. Figure 28–1 illustrates the cutaneous innervation of the head and neck, which is

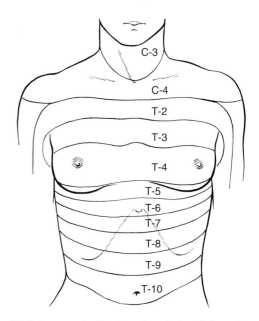

Figure 28–2 Sensory distribution of cervical and thoracic dermatomes. The C-4 dermatome abuts the T-2 dermatome, whereas the T-4 dermatome is typically thought to provide sensation to the dermatome at nipple level and the T-10 dermatome similarly is located at the level of the umbilicus.

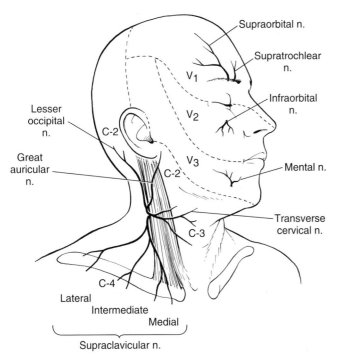

Figure 28–1 Cutaneous innervation of the head and neck. The innervation is via the trigeminal for face and superficial cervical plexus and other upper cervical nerve roots for the neck. n., nerve.

supplied by branches from the trigeminal nerve and superficial cervical plexus. The cutaneous distribution of the terminal branches of the trigeminal nerve (Fig. 28–1) is effectively blocked at their point of origin from the facial bones and mandible. Where procedures are likely to involve midline structures of the face, bilateral block of the appropriate trigeminal branches is recommended, because the distributions of these nerves may cross the midline.

Surgery for procedures involving structures in the neck was believed by many to be a contraindication for regional techniques. However, a growing body of experience with thyroid, parathyroid, and carotid artery surgery has renewed awareness of the potential benefits of performing these procedures during regional block.[13] These advantages include continuous neurologic monitoring during the procedure, a more stable intraoperative hemodynamic profile,[13] decreased postoperative nausea and emesis,[13] less postoperative hypoxemia during the immediate postoperative period, and a high degree of patient acceptance and satisfaction.[18, 19] In special situations, regional or local anesthesia may represent the only feasible method of anesthesia. For example, Manoppo[20] described the use of local anesthesia for the successful resection of a huge goiter (75 × 60 × 45 cm) in a patient with airway compromise who was unable to sit or stand and able to breathe only in the prone position.

The sensory innervation of the neck is supplied by branches of the superficial cervical plexus (see Figs. 28–1 and 28–2). Superficial cervical plexus block provides excellent analgesia for most neck procedures and, in conjunction with small amounts of directed local anesthesia, can provide anesthesia for procedures ranging from the excision of small skin lesions to carotid endarterectomy and thyroidectomy. Block of the superficial cervical plexus (Fig. 28–3) is easily performed with a 22- to 25-G, 2.5-in spinal needle and control syringe.

Deep cervical plexus block may be used to provide anesthesia for operations involving deeper structures in the neck, such as carotid endarterectomy. The anatomy of the deep cervical plexus and its relationships with the transverse processes of the cervical vertebrae and vertebral artery are illustrated in Figure 28–4. Side effects of deep cervical plexus block include block of adjacent or nearby structures such as the phrenic nerve, stellate ganglion, and recurrent laryngeal nerve, leading to ipsilateral diaphragmatic palsy, Horner's syndrome, and hoarseness, respectively. Because of these side effects, bilateral deep cervical plexus blocks are not routinely performed. Potential major complications of the block involve unintentional intravascular, epidural, or subarachnoid injection. If the anesthesiologist is un-

familiar with this block, superficial cervical plexus block and directed injections of local anesthetic by the surgeon may be preferable to the potential complications of improperly performed deep cervical plexus block. Cervical epidural anesthesia may also be used for operations in the head and neck region,[21] although relatively few studies have been published for its use in general surgical procedures in this region.

Operations in the Trunk

In contrast to the extremities, where cutaneous innervation is defined in relation to the distribution of peripheral nerves, sensory innervation of the thorax and abdomen follows a segmental, or dermatomal, pattern defined by the distribution of the thoracic spinal, or intercostal, nerves (see Fig. 28–2). These nerves exit the spinal cord, course along the inferior interior margin of the ribs, and give rise to posterior, lateral, and anterior cutaneous branches (Fig. 28–5). The proximal portion of each intercostal nerve lies in close proximity to the chain of sympathetic ganglia in the paravertebral space.

Superficial or minor surgical procedures of the truncal area, such as excision of superficial lesions, central venous catheter placement, minor incision and drainage procedures, and excisional breast biopsies, may be performed during local, intercostal, or field block (Fig. 28–6). For example, a combination of intercostal (T-2 to T-4) and superficial cervical plexus block has been described as providing complete anesthesia for the placement of cardiac pacemakers.[22] More involved surgical procedures, such as mastectomy, may be performed during several regional techniques. Regional anesthesia for breast operations can offer an attractive alternative to general anesthesia; however, many patients undergoing breast operation are often understandably anxious, and careful patient selection and appropriate use of sedatives intraoperatively are needed. Figure 28–7 depicts the technique of breast block, which may be used for procedures ranging from excisional biopsies of breast masses to simple mastectomy.

Alternative regional techniques to provide anesthesia for breast operation include intercostal nerve blocks of T-3 through T-7,[23] thoracic epidural anesthesia,[24] and interpleural anesthesia.[25, 26] Although regional techniques have been associated with less nausea and better analgesia postoperatively compared with general anesthesia,[23] techniques of intercostal block are associated with the highest serum levels of local anesthetic of any regional technique. The risk of pneumothorax with intercostal and interpleural anesthesia and of hypotension and bradycardia with thoracic epidural anesthesia[24] needs to be balanced with expected benefits.

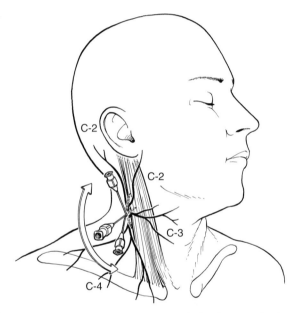

Figure 28–3 Superficial cervical plexus block. The superficial cervical plexus arises from beneath the belly of the sternocleidomastoid muscle at its posterior border, sending sensory branches in a fan-like manner over the superficial portion of the muscle. Block of the plexus is most easily achieved at its point of emergence from this posterior border. A 22- to 25-G, 2.5-in needle with a "ring" or "control" syringe facilitates aspiration and injection. The needle is placed through the skin at the posterior border of the sternocleidomastoid muscle, midway between the jugular notch and the mastoid process. The needle is advanced along the posterior border of the muscle, first toward the clavicular insertion and then toward the mastoid process. To detect unintentional vascular puncture of the external jugular vein or other vascular structures, aspiration with the ring syringe is performed while the needle is advanced, and 3 to 5 mL of local anesthetic is deposited as the needle is slowly withdrawn along the posterior edge of the muscle. Caution should be exercised to avoid penetration below or medial to the posterior border of the muscle; unintentional puncture of the carotid artery, internal jugular vein, or other vascular structures in the neck may result. Before removal of the needle, a further 3 to 5 mL of local anesthetic may be deposited at the midpoint of the muscle, where the plexus branches forth. Because the superficial cervical plexus provides no motor innervation to the neck or shoulder region, 0.25% bupivacaine or 1% lidocaine provides sufficient sensory block.

Intra-abdominal Procedures

Although many intra-abdominal operations may be performed during neuraxial block, the majority of up-

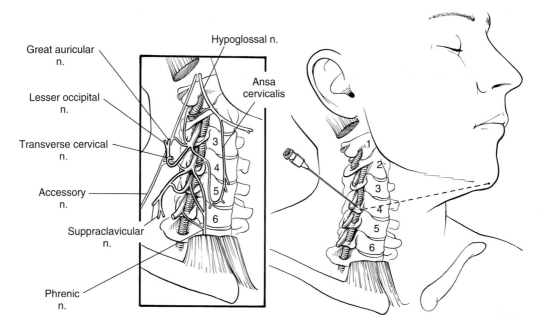

Figure 28–4 Deep cervical plexus block. Landmarks for the deep cervical plexus block include the transverse process of C-6 (Chassaignac's tubercle) and the inferior border of the mastoid process. A line connecting these points is drawn; the transverse process of C-4 usually lies on this line at the level of the mental process of the mandible. The remaining distance from the transverse process of C-4 to the mastoid process is divided in thirds to identify the approximate locations of the transverse processes of C-3 and C-2. A 22-G, 1.5- to 2-in short-bevel needle is inserted at the level of the transverse process of C-4, aiming slightly caudally and ventrally to minimize unintentional puncture of the dural cuff. Once the transverse process of the vertebra is identified, the needle may be walked slightly caudad to identify the caudal extent of the transverse process, then cephalad to identify the sulcus of the transverse process in which the nerve (n.) root lies. Particular attention to aspiration before injection is required because of the close proximity of the vertebral artery; intra-arterial injection of less than a milliliter of local anesthetic can cause local anesthetic systemic toxicity. After a negative aspiration for blood or cerebrospinal fluid, 3 to 4 mL of local anesthetic is injected into the sulcus; the procedure is then repeated for the transverse processes of C-3 and C-2. (Alternatively, a single-shot technique may be used, in which 8 to 10 mL of local anesthetic is injected at the level of C-4; this volume often is sufficient to result in rostral spread of the local anesthetic along the plexus to block the nerve roots of C-3 and C-2.) When properly performed, brachial plexus block *should not* result (C-5 to T-1). Deep cervical plexus block frequently results in ipsilateral phrenic nerve, recurrent laryngeal nerve, and stellate ganglion block. For these reasons, bilateral deep cervical plexus block is not routinely performed.

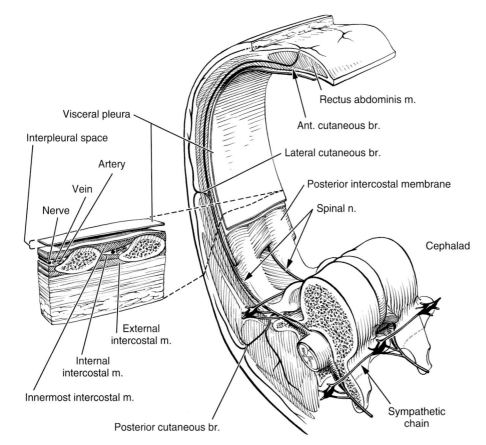

Figure 28–5 Anatomy of the intercostal nerves shows the groove in rib containing the intercostal nerve (n.), artery, and vein as well as branching points of the important intercostal nerves—i.e., posterior cutaneous, lateral cutaneous, and anterior (Ant.) cutaneous branch (br.)—and the proximity of sympathetic chain to the proximal intercostal nerve. m., muscle.

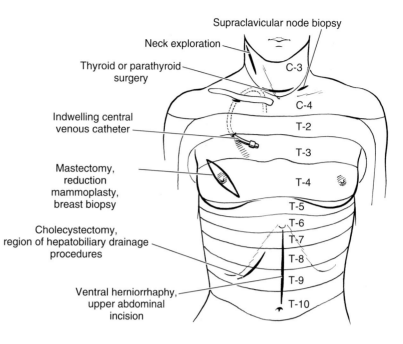

Figure 28–6 Dermatomes involved in neck, truncal, and upper abdominal incisions. The operations identified in the illustration are common and allow band-like segmental anesthesia for the superficial procedures to be adequate. For the intra-abdominal procedures, diaphragmatic irritation demands a higher dermatomal level to maintain patient comfort.

per abdominal procedures and other major intra-abdominal procedures are performed during general anesthesia. Subcostal and upper midline incisions are associated with decreases in respiratory compliance,[27] and block of the intercostal muscles, in conjunction with intra-abdominal retraction of upper abdominal contents, may impair diaphragmatic excursion and hamper adequate gas exchange in the spontaneously breathing patient.

Alterations in respiratory mechanics in upper abdominal operations[28] are greater than those seen in lower abdominal procedures.[29] Upper abdominal operation is also associated with a higher incidence of postoperative respiratory complications than is lower abdominal operation.[28] The postoperative impairment of pulmonary function caused by upper abdominal incisions[30, 31] can be diminished with epidural,[32, 33] intercostal, and interpleural analgesia.[34, 35] Postoperative epidural analgesia has been associated with lower rates of pulmonary complication compared with parenteral opioid analgesia after major intra-abdominal operation in high-risk patients.[1, 3] Regional analgesia can also decrease the side effects of equianalgesic regimens of parenteral opioids, such as excessive sedation or hypoventilation, and may speed the recovery of bowel motility after operation. Although epidural techniques can provide effective analgesia for virtually any procedure below the neck, alternative modes of regional analgesia and anesthesia such as intercostal[36] and interpleural[26, 34, 35, 37] block have proved effective for procedures involving subcostal incisions (such as cholecystectomy) or procedures of the flank (such as nephrectomy and percutaneous drainage procedures of the biliary and renal systems).[26, 34, 35, 37]

Interpleural techniques are a relatively recent development in regional anesthesia. Local anesthetic instilled into the pleural space is absorbed across the parietal pleura, blocking conduction at the level of the intercostal nerves and sympathetic chain.[38] Interpleural analgesia has been used in various acute and chronic pain situations and can provide near-complete analgesia after subcostal incision. A modification of the "falling-column" technique of interpleural block described by Ben-David and Lee[39] is illustrated in Figure 28–8. This technique has been advocated for its simplicity and relatively unequivocal end point—i.e., when the interpleural space has been reached, the negative pressure in this potential space causes the column of saline to fall. The original method involved the use of a well-lubricated air-filled syringe.[26, 40] Entry into the interpleural space results in the plunger of the syringe being drawn downward by the negative pressure. Another technique relying on loss of resistance may be less sensitive, because the sensation of loss of resistance can be encountered in the intercostal space and in the interpleural space[41] and has been associated with the highest frequency of pneumothorax and displaced catheters (including catheters placed into the parenchyma of the lung).[42, 43] In a retrospective review, Strømskag et al[41] attempted to assign a frequency to the complications associated with interpleural techniques, including pneumothorax (overall incidence 2%; small pneumothoraces may be due to 10 to 20 mL of air entrained into the interpleural space during catheter placement); signs of systemic toxicity (1.3%); pleural effusion (0.4%); infection; Horner's syndrome; catheter displacement; transient phrenic nerve palsy[44]; and unilateral bronchospasm.[45] The authors concluded, however, that if performed correctly and with care, the procedure "is so safe that it can be used routinely for pain treatment."[41]

Use of epidural, intercostal, or interpleural analgesia in conjunction with general anesthesia can decrease general anesthetic requirements in intra-abdominal procedures and provides excellent analgesia in the postoperative period. Continuous infusion techniques

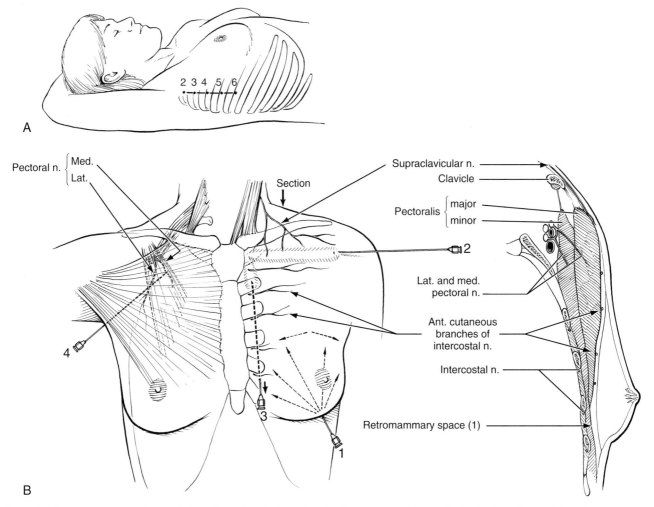

Figure 28–7 Breast block. *A*, The block is performed with the patient in the supine position, with the ipsilateral arm abducted at the shoulder and hand held above or tucked under the head. *B*, Sequential block of the sensory nerves (n.) supplying the breast is performed with a 22-G, 3.5- to 5-in needle. The anterior (Ant.) and lateral (Lat.) cutaneous branches of the intercostal nerves from T-2 through T-5 are blocked with a fan-like distribution of local anesthetic placed in the retromammary space through a single needle puncture just inferior to the lower margin of the breast at the anterior axillary line *(1)*. Care should be taken to ensure needle placement superficial to the pectoralis muscles but deep to the tissue of the breast. Block of the descending branches of the supraclavicular nerves, arising from the superficial cervical plexus, is performed with a subcutaneous wheal of local anesthetic deposited below the clavicle, extending from the sternal border laterally toward the axilla *(2)*. Cutaneous fibers from the anterior cutaneous branches of the intercostal nerves supplying the medial (Med.) aspect of the breast are blocked with a subcutaneous wheal of anesthetic deposited just lateral to the sternum *(3)*. Finally, branches of the pectoralis nerves, arising from the brachial plexus, are blocked by injection of local anesthetic into the substance of the pectoralis muscles at a point just inferior to the clavicle at its midpoint *(4)*. The total volume of local anesthetic used usually approaches 60 mL, and use of 0.25% to 0.375% bupivacaine with 5 μg/mL epinephrine is recommended. Attention should be paid to careful aspiration before injection to avoid unintentional intravascular injection. The placement of the needle should always be parallel to the axis of the ribs to avoid entry into the pleural space.

of epidural analgesia using dilute solutions of local anesthetic with opioid in conjunction with general anesthesia minimize hemodynamic changes from sympathectomy as a result of excessive administration of volatile agent or high concentration of local anesthetic. The anesthetic synergy between low-dose inhalational agent and dilute local anesthetic-opioid combinations administered through epidural infusion can be dramatic. One method of providing a combined general–epidural infusion anesthetic is presented below.

After placement of a catheter in the thoracic or lumbar epidural space has been confirmed, administration of a bolus of 15 to 20 mL of dilute local anesthetic-opioid combination (such as 1/16% or 1/8% bupiva-

caine with 2 to 4 μg/mL fentanyl) results in differential sensory block detectable by changes in temperature sensation. No motor block should be observed. After the desired dermatomal level of block has been achieved, an epidural infusion of the solution is immediately begun at approximately two thirds the initial volume (in mL/h) required to attain the desired level. Induction of general anesthesia is then performed, with muscle relaxation maintained by intravenous administration of muscle relaxant. Typically, maintenance of anesthesia for operation can be accomplished with 0.5 minimum alveolar concentration doses of volatile agent and the epidural infusion. Reaction to surgical stimulation is treated preferentially with additional bo-

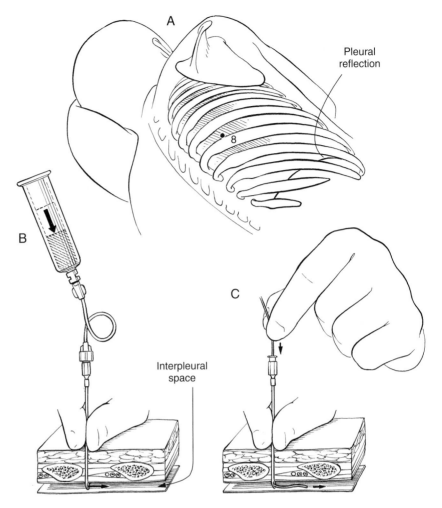

Figure 28–8 Interpleural block. The patient assumes the lateral position, with the operative side uppermost. The catheter may be placed in different interspaces, depending on the desired result; however, the seventh intercostal interspace has been selected for this illustration. Following aseptic skin preparation, aseptic technique is observed. *A,* The rostral edge of the eighth rib is identified lateral to the paraspinous muscles, approximately 8 to 10 cm lateral to the spine. After a wheal of local anesthetic is injected into the skin and periosteum of the eighth rib, an 18-G Touhy or other blunt-tipped epidural needle is inserted perpendicular to the width of the rib, and the tip is walked off the rostral edge of the rib. A syringe filled with saline (with the plunger removed) is connected via a length of intravenous extension tubing to the hub of the needle. The needle is then advanced deep to the rostral edge of the rib toward the pleural cavity. Perforation of the intercostal membrane usually yields a distinct "pop." *B,* Entrance into the interpleural space is evident when the column of fluid in the syringe begins to fall and may be felt as a "click" or heard as a small "pop." *C,* An epidural catheter is threaded 5 to 6 cm into the interpleural space. The catheter should be threaded without delay, because air will be entrained into the interpleural space through the needle. Before injection of medication, the aspiration should be performed to detect unintentional intravascular cannulation, and a test dose of local anesthetic containing epinephrine may be administered to further identify intravascular injection. If air is entrained during the threading of the catheter, aspiration of the catheter may be effective in removing some of the air.

luses of epidural solution or by increasing the inspired concentration of volatile agent; occasionally, intravenous administration of opioids is required. Caution should be exercised when stimulating areas not covered by the epidural block (such as the trachea), because the dose of volatile anesthetic may be insufficient to block movement or hemodynamic responses to these stimuli. When significant changes in patient position are anticipated after the induction of general anesthesia, use of laryngotracheal anesthesia eliminates the response to tracheal stimulation caused by tracheal tube movement during the positioning phase. The author and colleagues have used this technique successfully in procedures ranging from thoracoabdominal aortic aneurysm repair and other major intra-abdominal or thoracic procedures to major open reduction and internal fixation procedures of the pelvis and acetabulum. Advantages of this type of dilute local anesthetic–opioid epidural infusion combination with general anesthesia compared with opioid or volatile anesthetic–based techniques include rapid emergence from general anesthesia, early extubation, and excellent postoperative analgesia, which can be provided by various epidural analgesic regimens. The use of dilute local anesthetic concentrations in the epidural infusion also diminishes the likelihood of hemodynamically significant sympathectomy developing intraoperatively or postoperatively. Furthermore, this method incorporates preemptive analgesia (balanced anesthesia) concepts effectively.

Herniorrhaphy

A procedure that is particularly amenable to regional anesthesia and analgesia is inguinal herniorrhaphy. Appropriate techniques of regional block include neuraxial (spinal or epidural) block, inguinal field block, local anesthesia, and local anesthetic irrigation of the wound.[46] Block of afferent nociceptive signals from the surgical site decreases postoperative analgesic requirements and may have a preemptive analgesic effect manifested by decreased long-term pain. The use of local or regional field blocks has been associated with a lower incidence of urinary retention compared with general or spinal anesthesia,[15, 16] and use of regional or local anesthesia has been advocated to decrease costs associated with general anesthesia and recovery room time.[14] Unlike spinal anesthesia, local or regional field block is not associated with hypotension.[47] In the pediatric population, caudal anesthesia, local wound infiltration, and ilioinguinal and iliohypogastric nerve block have all been demonstrated to decrease postoperative pain compared with placebo or general anesthesia alone.[48-51] Regional anesthesia may also represent an attractive alternative to general anesthesia in former premature infants who may be at risk for apneic spells.[52-54]

Preoperative ilioinguinal and iliohypogastric nerve blocks have been used in conjunction with spinal anesthesia to provide long-term postoperative analgesia superior to spinal block alone.[55] The anatomy and distribution of the nerves supplying sensation to the groin are depicted in Figures 28–9 and 28–10. Block of the ilioinguinal and iliohypogastric nerves is easily performed, and in conjunction with block of the terminal fibers of the anterior branches of the intercostal nerves from T-10 to T-12, it composes the inguinal field block (Fig. 28–11).

Regional Anesthesia for Trauma

Background

In the United States, accidental injury remains the leading cause of death during the first three decades of life and is responsible for more productive years lost than any other single disease process.[56] Provision of comprehensive support for operative procedures and postinjury analgesia in the trauma patient presents unique challenges to the anesthesiologist. The evaluation and initial treatment of the traumatized patient are often performed under time pressure, and even in large trauma centers, these procedures may be chaotic. In the attempt to identify and immediately treat life-threatening injuries, other injuries or conditions may

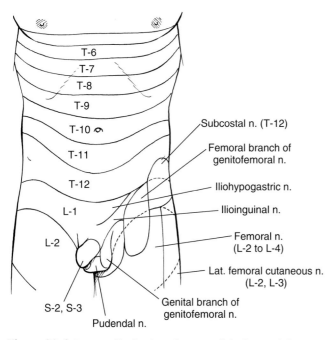

Figure 28–9 Sensory distribution of nerves of the lower abdomen and groin. For effective anesthesia for inguinal operation, consideration needs to be given to blocking all the nerves identified, although in individual patients the surgical procedure dictates which nerves should be blocked. Lat., lateral; n., nerve.

be overlooked, only to surface as sources of potential morbidity or mortality later in the patient's hospital course. The delayed expression of occult injuries may lead to confusion in diagnosis and treatment and forces physicians involved in the care of the trauma patient to remain ever vigilant. Trauma anesthesiologists frequently are placed in situations in which management of a critically ill patient must proceed with a minimum of preoperative historical and diagnostic information, and they must learn to quickly evaluate and identify special problems associated with trauma in order to prevent morbidity associated with multisystem injuries, occult insults, and metabolic derangements. Although a detailed review of anesthesia for major trauma is beyond the scope of this chapter, the following priorities must always be considered in evaluation and treatment of any victim of trauma: (1) preservation of life, (2) preservation of limb, (3) preservation of function, (4) avoidance of complications, and (5) avoidance of diagnostic delay.[57]

When called to evaluate the trauma victim for pain control or before a planned operative procedure, it is imperative that the anesthesiologist be able to stratify the level of injury and impairment sustained and be aware of the implications of any pharmacologic or invasive interventions on subsequent diagnosis and treatment. An example involves the treatment of acute pain in the trauma patient. The treatment of injury-related pain is often assigned a lower management priority during the initial stages of evaluation and treatment in the victim of trauma. Although treatment of anxiety and pain is certainly laudable, well-intentioned but injudicious use of hypnotic or analgesic agents may hamper the diagnostic abilities of the trauma surgeon, especially early in the hospital course of the patient. Hypnotic and analgesic agents may also depress airway reflexes, depress respiratory drive, exacerbate hypoxemia, cause hypotension in the hypovolemic patient, obfuscate changes in mental status from head injury or metabolic derangements, and mask pain on physical examination, which may delay diagnosis and treatment. Anesthesiologists must coordinate their interventions with those of the surgeon to optimize care. Stratification of the severity of injury sustained by the victim of trauma therefore impacts directly and indirectly on the options available for anesthesia and analgesia. Operative procedures in patients who have sustained significant injury to multiple organ systems; who have suffered significant hemorrhage; who are in shock; who are undergoing emergent or urgent procedures involving the cranial, chest, abdominal, or pelvic cavities; or who are to undergo complex or prolonged reparative procedures usually warrant general anesthesia with levels of invasive monitoring and support appropriate to each clinical situation. In cases in which preservation of life or limb depends on urgent or emergent surgical therapy, the implementation of regional anesthetic techniques for control of anticipated postoperative pain must not delay therapeutic surgical intervention.

In patients who have been identified as candidates for regional anesthesia or analgesia, other factors may

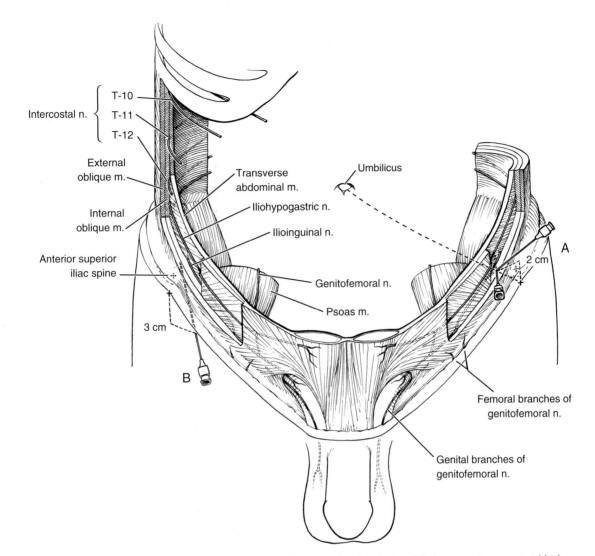

Figure 28–10 Ilioinguinal and iliohypogastric nerve block. Two techniques of ilioinguinal and iliohypogastric nerve (n.) block are illustrated. The ilioinguinal and iliohypogastric nerves lie deep to the internal and external oblique muscles (m.), respectively, at the approximate level of the anterior superior iliac spine. Block of these nerves is most easily performed near the easily identifiable landmark of the anterior superior iliac spine. *A*, A point is identified approximately 2 cm inferior and medial to the anterior superior iliac spine. Following aseptic skin preparation, a wheal of local anesthetic is deposited in the dermis at this point, and a 22-G, 2-in short-bevel needle is directed in a slightly posterior direction to pass just medial to the anterior superior iliac spine. The needle is advanced through the external and internal oblique muscles (which may be identified by a subtle click), and after negative aspiration, 5 to 8 mL of local anesthetic is deposited as the needle is withdrawn to the skin. The needle is aimed slightly medially, and the procedure is repeated. *B*, An alternative method may be easier to perform in obese patients. A point is identified 3 cm medial and inferior to the anterior superior iliac spine. Following aseptic skin preparation, a wheal of local anesthetic is deposited at this point. A 22-G, 3.5-in needle is introduced in a cephalolateral direction, contacting the inner surface of the ilium just deep to the anterior superior iliac spine. After negative aspiration, 6 to 10 mL of local anesthetic is slowly injected as the needle is withdrawn to the skin. The needle is then redirected at a steeper angle, penetrating the layers of the external and internal oblique muscles, and another 6 to 10 mL of local anesthetic is injected. Ilioinguinal and iliohypogastric blocks are easily performed and may be expected to result in pure sensory anesthesia. However, several case reports have been published in which block of these nerves has resulted in unintentional femoral nerve motor block, especially in children.

be present that militate against safe implementation of regional block. Contraindications to regional anesthesia in the trauma patient are no different than those encountered in the elective setting. Some conditions that are found in trauma victims that may affect the decision to proceed with general anesthesia instead of a regional technique are summarized in Table 28–1. Caution must be exercised before proceeding with a neuraxial technique that may result in hemodynamically significant sympathectomy in the patient who is already hypovolemic or who has a history of unex-

plained hypotension. The anesthesiologist must also be aware of situations in which regional anesthesia or analgesia may mask underlying pathologic features or confuse diagnosis. For example, a peripheral regional block may mask the pain indicative of a developing compartment syndrome; neuraxial analgesia may mask pain associated with developing peritonitis; and, in the case of neurologic injury involving an extremity, it may be difficult to determine if the changes are a result of the injury, the operation, or the block itself.

The decision to proceed with regional anesthesia or

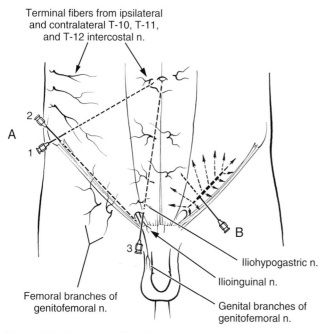

Terminal fibers from ipsilateral
and contralateral T-10, T-11,
and T-12 intercostal n.

Femoral branches of
genitofemoral n.

Iliohypogastric n.

Ilioinguinal n.

Genital branches of
genitofemoral n.

Figure 28–11 Inguinal field block. A, After ilioinguinal and iliohypogastric nerve (n.) block (see Fig. 28–10), the terminal cutaneous branches of intercostal nerves T-10 to T-12 are blocked with a 22- to 25-G, 3.5- to 5-in needle inserted just above the anterior superior iliac spine (1). The needle is advanced subcutaneously, with continuous aspiration, toward the umbilicus. Approximately 6 to 10 mL of local anesthetic is then deposited as the needle is slowly withdrawn. The femoral cutaneous branches of the genitofemoral nerve are blocked by redirecting the needle subcutaneously along the inguinal ligament toward the pubic tubercle (2). An additional 6 to 10 mL of local anesthetic is injected as the needle is slowly withdrawn. Finally, the terminal cutaneous fibers from the contralateral intercostal branches of T-10 to T-12 are blocked by injecting 6 to 10 mL of local anesthetic subcutaneously from the umbilicus to the level of the external inguinal ring (3). B, An alternative method of local infiltration along the proposed incision line. A 22- to 25-G, 2- to 3.5-in needle is used to inject local anesthetic into the subcutaneous tissues in a fan-like manner above and below the proposed incision line.

analgesia in the trauma patient must be considered in light of the level of severity of injury, the applicability of the regional technique to the injury sustained, the possible side effects of the block and their impact on further management of the patient's injuries, and the risk-to-benefit ratio of the block itself. For example, a patient with an open fracture of the olecranon requiring open reduction and internal fixation who also has a rib fracture on the ipsilateral side, but no pneumothorax on initial chest radiograph, a full stomach, a history of poorly controlled asthma, but no other apparent injury may be strongly considered for brachial plexus block instead of general anesthesia. However, if the supraclavicular route of brachial plexus anesthesia is chosen, the anesthesiologist must be aware that although the chosen block may be the ideal block for the procedure,[58] if a pneumothorax were to develop in this patient, the cause would be difficult to determine, at least initially. Because immediate or delayed pneumothorax may complicate both rib fracture and supraclavicular block (pneumothorax incidence of 0.5% to 6% with supraclavicular block), an argument could be

made that supraclavicular block should not be performed in this setting. A counterargument may also be made that if the practitioner is cognizant of the most likely complications of the chosen regional procedure (in this case, pneumothorax) and actively looks for evidence of this complication, this may actually allow earlier diagnosis and treatment of the problem regardless of cause.

Regional anesthesia may play an important role in disaster or other mass casualty situations in which physician resources may be maximally extended through the use of peripheral, plexus, or neuraxial block. The use of these techniques may allow a limited number of anesthesiologists to attend to a larger number of victims and allow anesthesiologists to focus on those patients requiring additional resuscitation or general anesthesia.[59] Although the safety of spinal anesthesia for wartime casualties has not always enjoyed the best reputation, advances in the understanding of the pathophysiology of hypovolemic shock and fluid management have led several authors[60, 61] to endorse the use of spinal anesthesia in the management of injuries of the lower extremities and perineum, but they caution against its use in intra-abdominal procedures. There are fewer studies available describing the efficacy of plexus or peripheral regional blocks in the wartime setting, but the personnel, analgesic, and hemodynamic advantages of regional block demonstrated in the civilian setting may well transfer to treatment units near the battlefield.[62] The use of Kevlar body armor has created a fundamental shift in the injury patterns experienced by today's soldier. Casualty data from the United States' involvement in the Somalia conflict reveal that 60% to 80% of incapacitating injuries sustained now involve the extremities rather than truncal body cavities. Although data are lacking, this shift in injury pattern could highlight regional anesthetic advantages in the acute or subacute treatment of these casualties.

Emergency Department Procedures

Regional block can improve patient satisfaction for many common emergency department procedures. Al-

Table 28–1 Conditions That May Be Present in the Trauma Patient That May Swing Decision Toward General Rather Than Regional Anesthesia

Alcohol or drug intoxication
Mental incompetence
Belligerent or uncooperative patient
Inability to obtain informed consent
Patient refusal of regional anesthesia
History of unexplained hemodynamic instability
Incomplete evaluation in emergency department
Patient younger than age of consent and without legal guardian
Multisystem injuries
Airway trauma or edema
Coagulopathy
Severe hypothermia
Anticipated large volume blood loss during operative procedure
Significant or unexplained hypoxemia or hypoventilation

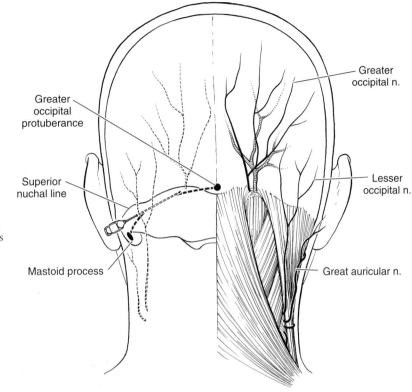

Figure 28–12 Posterior cutaneous innervation of the neck and scalp. The great auricular nerve (n.) and lesser occipital nerve are distal branches of the superficial cervical plexus, whereas the greater occipital nerve is primarily formed from the C-2 root. The superior nuchal line allows superficial infiltration to block both greater and lesser occipital nerves (for example, if a posterior scalp procedure is planned).

though local anesthetic solutions with epinephrine are frequently used to provide local anesthesia and wound hemostasis in the treatment of many lacerations involving vascular cutaneous areas, peripheral and field blocks can provide superior anesthesia for the irrigation and closure of many of these injuries where infiltration of local anesthetic agents would otherwise cause soft tissue distortion, compromising optimal cosmetic closure. These benefits may be most apparent in injuries to the face, ears, or other cosmetically important areas.

Figures 28–1 and 28–12 illustrate the peripheral cutaneous innervation of the scalp and face. Appropriate nerve blocks of the head and neck region are determined by the location of the injury. Injuries near the midline may necessitate bilateral blocks, because cutaneous innervation may cross the midline in the face and scalp. Repair of lacerations or injuries of the ear may be performed during regional block of the ear (Fig. 28–13). The great auricular and lesser occipital branches of the superficial cervical plexus may be blocked by subcutaneous infiltration of local anesthetic anterior to the mastoid process, extending over the upper portion of the sternocleidomastoid muscle. The auriculotemporal branch of the trigeminal nerve, supplying sensation to the superior two thirds of the anterior surface of the ear, may be blocked by infiltrating local anesthetic along the anterior aspect of the auricle, forward of the external auditory meatus. Because the auriculotemporal nerve lies near branches of the facial nerve, partial facial nerve block (cranial nerve VII), resulting in paresis of ipsilateral facial musculature, may result from auriculotemporal nerve block. If unintentional facial nerve block occurs, the ipsilateral eye

should be protected from corneal abrasion until motor function returns.

Regional anesthesia techniques may also be used to provide anesthesia for the removal of foreign bodies, minor incision and drainage procedures, and repair of lacerations involving the distal extremities or digits. For example, the incision and drainage of paronychia can

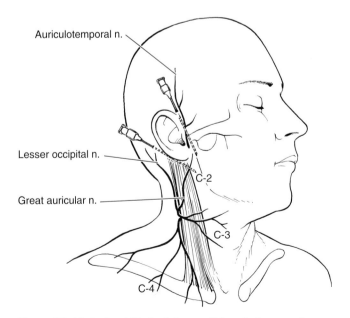

Figure 28–13 Regional block of the ear. This technique requires block of branches of the superficial cervical plexus as well as a branch of the trigeminal nerve (n.) and the auriculotemporal nerve.

be accomplished painlessly with digital or wrist or ankle block. Digital block has been shown[63] to provide better anesthesia and to be better tolerated than local infiltration for the suturing of digital lacerations. The débridement and irrigation of deeper puncture wounds of the plantar aspect of the foot can be accomplished with block of the tibial nerve at the level of the ankle (with sural and saphenous nerve block if the injury is on the lateral or medial midfoot region, respectively). Débridement procedures involving large abraded areas on an extremity can be performed with peripheral plexus block, which also provides the patient with analgesia after the procedure that is superior to other modalities. Epinephrine-containing local anesthetic solutions should not be used for digital blocks and offer no advantage when used for ankle or wrist blocks.

Many orthopedic procedures performed in the emergency department can be made less painful through the use of regional anesthetics. Intravenous regional anesthetic techniques, hematoma blocks, and plexus blocks have been used successfully to facilitate orthopedic examination and closed reduction of extremity fractures or dislocations.[64–67] For example, analgesia for the manipulation of Colles fracture can be achieved with hematoma block,[67, 68] intravenous regional block,[64, 65] and plexus or peripheral nerve blocks.[65, 67] The simplicity, relative effectiveness, and low serum local anesthetic levels[68] attained in hematoma block make it an attractive technique of analgesia for manipulation of distal extremity fractures. Hematoma block is performed with aseptic technique after sterile preparation of the skin overlying the fracture. A 22-G, 1.5- to 2-in needle is attached to a ring syringe containing 1% to 2% lidocaine. The needle is inserted into the fracture site, and aspiration of blood from the fracture hematoma confirms placement of the needle in the fracture. Following aspiration, 6 to 10 mL of lidocaine is injected. Although concern may be raised over the injection of material into a previously closed fracture site, hematoma block has not been associated with an increased incidence of osteomyelitis.[69] Hematoma block may be particularly helpful in the pediatric patient, who may otherwise be an unsuitable candidate for plexus block. Peripheral regional block may also be used to provide analgesia in the patient with an extremity injury who is awaiting operation, without incurring the potentially undesirable side effects of anxiolytic or opioid medications. Plexus block has also been used to provide prolonged sympathectomy after ischemic events involving the upper extremity.

Selected regional blocks may also improve patient tolerance of otherwise painful invasive procedures performed in the emergency department, such as tube thoracostomy. Intercostal block of the ribs above and below the insertion site of the thoracostomy tube can provide superior analgesia compared with local infiltration (although the pleural component of pain on insertion will not be blocked and is perhaps best treated with the judicious administration of parenteral medications). Interpleural administration of local anesthetic into the chest tube itself or via an interpleural catheter can also decrease the discomfort of this pleural irritation.[70, 71]

Analgesia in the Intensive Care Unit

Regional techniques can provide superb analgesia for several traumatic injuries treated in a nonoperative fashion, while often minimizing potentially undesirable effects of anxiolytics and narcotic analgesics.

Nonoperatively treated chest injuries are most frequently caused by blunt trauma. Damage to the rib cage in the form of multiple rib fractures, severe contusion, costochondral dislocations, or flail chest combined with pulmonary parenchymal contusion may lead to progressive pulmonary deterioration, especially in the elderly, obese, or debilitated patient. The injury may cause decreases in chest wall compliance and altered chest wall mechanics, thereby increasing the work of breathing. Ventilatory compromise from these alterations in function is compounded by the severe pain associated with these types of injuries, which all too frequently lead to a downward spiral of hypoventilation, decreased functional residual capacity, atelectasis and lobar collapse, increased shunt fraction, poor pulmonary toilet, hypoxemia, and pneumonia and culminate in tracheal intubation or tracheostomy, prolonged mechanical ventilation, and an increase in morbidity and mortality.[72]

Therapy is for the underlying pulmonary injury and relieving the pain associated with chest trauma in order to restore pulmonary function while avoiding respiratory depression, if possible. Parenterally administered opioids, although effective analgesics, may exacerbate respiratory depression in this clinical situation.

Continuous or intermittent intercostal,[73–75] paravertebral,[76–78] interpleural,[79] and epidural[77, 80, 81] analgesia have all been demonstrated to provide effective analgesia and improve pulmonary function in patients with multiple rib fractures. Interpleural analgesia, a technique described relatively recently,[26] has found diverse applications in chronic and acute pain settings and provides excellent analgesia for unilateral chest injuries. In one clinical trial, application of interpleural analgesia for flail chest produced significant improvements in pulmonary mechanics and gas exchange in patients in whom parenteral opioid therapy had failed and who otherwise would have required intubation and mechanical ventilation.[79] (An interesting case in which an interpleural catheter was used to manage rib fracture pain in conjunction with continuous suprascapular nerve block for scapular fracture has been described by Breen and Haigh.[82]) Placement of an interpleural catheter is relatively simple and does not require multiple-level injections. Figure 28–8 diagrams the placement of an interpleural catheter by a modification of the falling-column technique of Ben-David and Lee.[39] Dosing with 20 mL of 0.5% bupivacaine solution with 5 µg/mL epinephrine can provide analgesia for an average of 8 h, whereas the same volume of 0.25% solution with 5 µg/mL epinephrine provides analgesia for about 4 to 5 h.[83] Continuous infusions of

0.25% bupivacaine solutions at rates of 8 to 15 mL/h may also be used. At Wilford Hall Medical Center, Lackland Airforce Base, Texas, interpleural analgesia has been used successfully in the ward setting by the surgical and anesthesia services and has provided excellent analgesia for patients with multiple rib fractures (and other patients with subcostal incisions) who previously had or otherwise would have required care in an intensive care unit. In patients with bilateral chest injuries, the technique of choice for pain control is thoracic or lumbar epidural infusions of dilute local anesthetic-opioid combinations (typically 1/16% bupivacaine with 2 to 5 µg/mL fentanyl at 8 to 15 mL/h). Epidurally administered opioids and combined dilute local anesthetic-opioid provide excellent analgesia and can improve pulmonary function in patients after blunt chest injury or thoracotomy.[84-86]

Although neuraxial techniques, including epidurally administered opioids, can decrease the undesirable effects of equianalgesic regimens of parenterally administered opioids on ventilation and level of consciousness, both may mask the physical signs of underlying or developing abnormality. As an example, Pond et al[87] described a case in which interpleural analgesia masked the pain from delayed traumatic splenic rupture. The practitioner must be aware that analgesic interventions may be incompatible with diagnostic methods dependent on serial physical examination, and definitive diagnosis may require more invasive (e.g., diagnostic peritoneal lavage) or expensive (e.g., computed tomographic scan) interventions if these analgesic methods are used.

Regional Anesthesia for Traumatic Injuries Requiring Operative Therapy

The use of regional anesthesia in operative procedures performed on the victim of trauma affords significant advantages compared with general anesthesia in certain circumstances. In selected patients with isolated injuries to an extremity, a regional anesthetic may be the anesthetic of choice, providing rapid preoperative pain relief, superb operating conditions, and excellent postoperative analgesia. After injury, increases in sympathetic tone may cause delays in gastric emptying, and all victims of trauma should be considered at high risk for aspiration of residual gastric contents. Regional anesthesia obviates the need for airway manipulation and may provide an added margin of safety for those patients undergoing procedures amenable to peripheral or plexus block. In patients who have lost consciousness or when there is concern over the possibility of head injury, regional techniques allow the physician to monitor the patient's neurologic status continuously, possibly saving the patient from more invasive and indirect monitoring methods (such as ventriculostomy or other intracranial pressure monitors). In patients with significant coexisting disease, regional anesthesia may also provide a more hemodynamically stable anesthetic course and avoid airway manipulations that may exacerbate underlying pulmonary processes (such as asthma). Extremity block can

also decrease the likelihood of unintentional intraoperative hypothermia by preserving, to a greater extent than possible with general anesthesia, intrinsic thermoregulatory mechanisms.[17] The use of continuous, or catheter-mediated, regional anesthesia techniques allows intermittent or continuous infusions of local anesthetics for prolonged analgesia and sympathectomy, desirable effects in the patient undergoing arterial repair, digital or limb reimplantation, or free-flap procedures.[88-91]

Operative Procedures in the Head and Neck

Most cases of facial injuries requiring acute operative intervention are managed with general anesthesia. Although most areas of the head and neck are accessible to nerve block, the nature of acute injuries to the head and neck, potential distortion of anatomy, presence of residual gastric contents, and relative inaccessibility of the airway during operation favor general anesthesia in these cases. Frequently, however, patients require operative reduction and internal fixation of facial fractures after treatment of the acute injury. In this setting, several procedures are amenable to regional blocks. Patients who are most likely to benefit from nerve block include those undergoing repair of mandibular and maxillary fractures. Block of the maxillary or mandibular branches of the trigeminal nerve (or both) in conjunction with a "light" general anesthetic affords several advantages. With successful block of the involved nerves, anesthesia can be performed with little or no narcotic supplementation and with amnestic or "tube-tolerating" doses of volatile agent. Because these patients are most often stabilized with intermaxillary fixation, an anesthetic that allows the patient to emerge rapidly, is devoid of sedative and respiratory-depressant side effects, and affords analgesia has obvious advantages in the early postoperative stages, allowing the patient to be extubated earlier, perhaps with a greater margin of safety. The profound analgesia afforded by these blocks is impressive, and the duration of the blocks approaches 12 h or more if 0.5% bupivacaine with 5 µg/mL epinephrine is used.

Operations in the Thorax and Abdomen

The majority of operations performed in the chest and abdomen necessitated by traumatic injury should be performed during general anesthesia for several reasons. Although many procedures can be performed in the abdomen during regional block, the nature of traumatic injuries to these major body cavities is often complex, especially those caused by high-velocity missiles and blunt trauma. Consequently, the potential for significant blood loss, prolonged reparative maneuvers, and large intravascular volume fluid shifts is high. When these problems are combined with the other concurrent problems frequently encountered in trauma patients, the prudent course is nearly always that of definitive airway management with a tracheal tube and general anesthesia.

Considerations of postoperative analgesia with regional techniques (epidural, intercostal, interpleural) definitely have a place in the overall anesthetic management plan but must not delay surgical intervention for urgent indications in the trauma patient. The risk involved in placing catheters for postoperative pain management must also be considered in light of transient coagulation disorders that often occur in the trauma patient. Although superb postoperative analgesia may be afforded by neuraxial or other techniques[92] for post-thoracotomy or major intra-abdominal procedures, placement and dosing of these catheters may best be timed after the acute postoperative phase—after metabolic, coagulopathic, and toxic derangements have been reversed.

Operations in the Extremities

The bulk of the procedures that are amenable to regional anesthesia or analgesia involve operations to restore function or to preserve viability of the extremities after injury. Regional anesthesia may be used in the immediate postinjury setting to provide preoperative analgesia and intraoperative anesthesia, to provide anesthesia in procedures of an urgent nature (such as reduction and fixation of open extremity fractures), and to perform procedures several days after acute injury. Regional anesthesia may also be used to facilitate orthopedic examination, and specialized techniques using catheters can be used to provide prolonged postoperative analgesia and sympathectomy in patients who require multiple débridements or dressing changes or who have had arterial repairs, microvascular reanastomoses, or digital reimplantation.[88–91]

Although catheters have been placed to block nerves of the brachial plexus above[88, 90] and below the clavicle,[89, 91, 93] the axillary approach is relatively easily and quickly performed.[93] However, because the axillary catheter technique fails to provide adequate surgical *anesthesia* in the radial nerve distribution in 20% to 30% of patients[94] and because microvascular and digital reimplantation operations are typically prolonged procedures, the author and colleagues prefer to use the technique predominantly to provide postoperative sympathectomy and *analgesia,* in conjunction with a general anesthetic intraoperatively.

Prolonged analgesia for an extremity may delay the clinical diagnosis of postoperative complications resulting from a compartment syndrome or vascular insufficiency. Coordination with the orthopedic or vascular surgeon must be done for appropriate postoperative monitoring if regional techniques are used for anesthesia or analgesia in patients at risk of compartment syndrome developing, such as those suffering from both bone fractures of the forearm associated with significant soft tissue injury, high-grade tibial plateau fractures, and midshaft fractures of the lower extremity below the knee.

Lower Extremity Blocks

Fractures and other injuries of the lower extremities resulting from trauma are common and particularly amenable to regional techniques. Various techniques have been used for the relief of pain and to provide anesthesia for intraoperative fixation of lower extremity fractures, which may vary tremendously from nondisplaced femoral neck fractures in the elderly, treated with percutaneous pin fixation, to complicated tibial plateau fractures requiring knee arthrotomy and prolonged reduction and fixation maneuvers. Several techniques may be used to provide analgesia and anesthesia for these operations; the choice depends on the type and location of the fracture(s), degree of difficulty anticipated with reduction and fixation, and degree of coexisting injury or disease.

Virtually any lower extremity procedure may be accomplished with neuraxial block. Subarachnoid block has been used extensively in operations for hip fracture in the elderly, with some demonstrable advantages over general anesthesia including a decreased incidence of deep vein thrombosis, a clearer postoperative mental status, and an avoidance of early postoperative hypoxemia associated with general anesthesia.[95, 96] However, the incidence of hypotension requiring vasopressor in this patient population can approach 70% with subarachnoid block,[97] and the duration of postoperative analgesia is relatively short lived. Epidural anesthesia may allow greater control of the rostral spread of block and permits continuing postoperative analgesia via continuous infusions or repeated boluses of local anesthetic, opioids, or a combination of both. In institutions in which postoperative support for epidural (or continuous subarachnoid) analgesia is unavailable or limited, femoral nerve block may be used to provide postoperative analgesia. Three approaches are the femoral nerve block at the level of the inguinal ligament; "3 in 1," or "triple" nerve block modification of the femoral nerve block (femoral, lateral femoral cutaneous, and obturator nerves)[98, 99]; and psoas compartment block.[100, 101]

Femoral block has been used successfully to provide analgesia for femoral shaft fractures in children[102] and can be used to provide analgesia for intermedullary fixation of femur fractures in adults. Continuous femoral nerve block may also be used to provide excellent analgesia and muscle relaxation for procedures involving the repair of torn or ruptured quadriceps or patellar tendons (placement of femoral nerve catheters is technically not difficult and can be used to provide prolonged quadriceps motor block, minimizing the stress on a fresh surgical repair of these structures). In conjunction with sciatic nerve block, femoral nerve block can provide anesthesia and analgesia for open-knee procedures and repair of tibial plateau fractures, although failure to adequately block the median obturator nerve of the knee may result in the failure of femoral-sciatic block to provide stand-alone anesthesia for these and other open-knee procedures.

Sciatic nerve block, with or without femoral nerve block, can be used to provide prolonged relief of pain associated with distal lower extremity fractures, especially fractures of the ankle bones, midfoot, and calcaneus. Caution should be exercised before proceeding with sciatic block when shaft fractures of the tibia and fibula are present, because postoperative analgesia for these procedures may delay the clinical diagnosis of a compartment syndrome. Although the author and associates prefer the posterior approach to sciatic nerve block, the nerve may also be blocked in the popliteal fossa.

Summary

Techniques of regional anesthesia and analgesia can play an important role in the overall anesthetic management of many patients undergoing general surgical procedures as well as those who have sustained trauma. Regional anesthesia and analgesia play major roles in preemptive analgesic regimens, which may also include preoperative administration of opioids and nonsteroidal anti-inflammatory drugs. These techniques can be applied to most operations performed by the general surgeon and may decrease postoperative pain well beyond the duration of the original block. Some of the advantages offered by regional techniques in the elective setting include minimizing the effects of the surgical stress response, decreasing postoperative pain, improving postoperative pulmonary function, decreasing recovery room stays, decreasing postoperative nausea, and decreasing the incidence of postoperative urinary retention. Although the role of regional anesthesia and analgesia in decreasing perioperative morbidity and mortality needs further focus, the benefits afforded by regional techniques may be extended to most patients with little or no added risk.

Regional anesthesia and analgesia can also provide significant benefit to patients suffering traumatic injury. Meticulous evaluation of patients, proper selection of patients, appropriate choice of anesthetic technique, and frequent communication with the trauma surgeon are essential if complications unique to the trauma setting are to be avoided. The benefits of regional anesthesia and analgesia may also be extended to other patients, improving the quality of analgesia for procedures performed in the emergency department and intensive care unit. Regional techniques may be of special benefit to patients who suffer from blunt chest injury or who have severe orthopedic pain from multiple fractures. Catheter-mediated peripheral techniques may also be used to provide prolonged analgesia and sympathectomy for patients who have had peripheral vascular accidents.

References

1. Yeager MP, Glass DD, Neff RK, et al: Epidural anesthesia and analgesia in high-risk surgical patients. Anesthesiology 1987; 66: 729–736.
2. Christopherson R, Beattie C, Frank SM, et al: Perioperative morbidity in patients randomized to epidural or general anesthesia for lower extremity vascular surgery. Perioperative Ischemia Randomized Anesthesia Trial Study Group. Anesthesiology 1993; 79: 422–434.
3. Tuman KJ, McCarthy RJ, March RJ, et al: Effects of epidural anesthesia and analgesia on coagulation and outcome after major vascular surgery. Anesth Analg 1991; 73: 696–704.
4. Kehlet H: Surgical stress: the role of pain and analgesia. Br J Anaesth 1989; 63: 189–195.
5. Rosenfeld BA, Beattie C, Christopherson R, et al: The effects of different anesthetic regimens on fibrinolysis and the development of postoperative arterial thrombosis. Perioperative Ischemia Randomized Anesthesia Trial Study Group. Anesthesiology 1993; 79: 435–443.
6. Tverskoy M, Cozacov C, Ayache M, et al: Postoperative pain after inguinal herniorrhaphy with different types of anesthesia. Anesth Analg 1990; 70: 29–35.
7. Jebeles JA, Reilly JS, Gutierrez JF, et al: The effect of pre-incisional infiltration of tonsils with bupivacaine on the pain following tonsillectomy under general anesthesia. Pain 1991; 47: 305–308.
8. Ringrose NH, Cross MJ: Femoral nerve block in knee joint surgery. Am J Sports Med 1984; 12: 398–402.
9. Rademaker BM, Sih IL, Kalkman CJ, et al: Effects of interpleurally administered bupivacaine 0.5% on opioid analgesic requirements and endocrine response during and after cholecystectomy: a randomized double-blind controlled study. Acta Anaesthesiol Scand 1991; 35: 108–112.
10. Tuffin JR, Cunliffe DR, Shaw SR: Do local analgesics injected at the time of third molar removal under general anaesthesia reduce significantly post operative analgesic requirements? A double-blind controlled trial. Br J Oral Maxillofac Surg 1989; 27: 27–32.
11. McQuay HJ, Carroll D, Moore RA: Postoperative orthopaedic pain—the effect of opiate premedication and local anaesthetic blocks. Pain 1988; 33: 291–295.
12. Thorén T, Wattwil M, Järnerot G, et al: Epidural and spinal anesthesia do not influence gastric emptying and small intestinal transit in volunteers. Reg Anesth 1989; 14: 35–42.
13. Bergenfelz A, Algotsson L, Ahren B: Surgery for primary hyperparathyroidism performed under local anaesthesia. Br J Surg 1992; 79: 931–934.
14. Behnia R, Hashemi F, Stryker SJ, et al: A comparison of general versus local anesthesia during inguinal herniorrhaphy. Surg Gynecol Obstet 1992; 174: 277–280.
15. Young DV: Comparison of local, spinal, and general anesthesia for inguinal herniorrhaphy. Am J Surg 1987; 153: 560–563.
16. Finley RK Jr, Miller SF, Jones LM: Elimination of urinary retention following inguinal herniorrhaphy. (With discussion.) Am Surg 1991; 57: 486–489.
17. Frank SM, Beattie C, Christopherson R, et al: Epidural versus general anesthesia, ambient operating room temperature, and patient age as predictors of inadvertent hypothermia. Anesthesiology 1992; 77: 252–257.
18. Hochman M, Fee WE Jr: Thyroidectomy under local anesthesia. Arch Otolaryngol Head Neck Surg 1991; 117: 405–407.
19. Chapuis Y, Icard P, Fulla Y, et al: Parathyroid adenomectomy under local anesthesia with intra-operative monitoring of UcAMP and/or 1-84 PTH. World J Surg 1992; 16: 570–575.
20. Manoppo AE: Resection of an unusually large goitre. Br J Surg 1977; 64: 158–159.
21. Wittich DJ Jr, Berny JJ, Davis RK: Cervical epidural anesthesia for head and neck surgery. Laryngoscope 1984; 94: 615–619.
22. Raza SM, Vasireddy AR, Candido KD, et al: A complete regional anesthesia technique for cardiac pacemaker insertion. J Cardiothorac Vasc Anesth 1991; 5: 54–56.
23. Atanassof PG, Alon E, Pasch T, et al: Intercostal nerve block for minor breast surgery. Reg Anesth 1991; 16: 23–27.
24. Jarosz J, Pihowicz A, Towpik E: The application of continuous thoracic epidural anaesthesia in outpatient oncological and reconstructive surgery of the breast. Eur J Surg Oncol 1991; 17: 599–602.
25. Schlesinger TM, Laurito CE, Baughman VL, et al: Interpleural bupivacaine for mammography during needle localization and breast biopsy. Anesth Analg 1989; 68: 394–395.
26. Reiestad F, Strømskag KE: Interpleural catheter in the management of postoperative pain. A preliminary report. Reg Anesth 1986; 11: 89–91.
27. Larsson A, Jonmarker C, Werner O: Lung mechanics during upper abdominal surgery. Acta Chir Scand 1989; 155: 329–332.
28. Ford GT, Rosenal TW, Clergue F, et al: Respiratory physiology in upper abdominal surgery. Clin Chest Med 1993; 14: 237–252.
29. Dureuil B, Cantineau JP, Desmonts JM: Effects of upper or lower abdominal surgery on diaphragmatic function. Br J Anaesth 1987; 59: 1230–1235.

30. Ford GT, Whitelaw WA, Rosenal TW, et al: Diaphragm function after upper abdominal surgery in humans. Am Rev Respir Dis 1983; 127: 431–436.

31. Parfrey PS, Harte PJ, Quinlan JP, et al: Pulmonary function in the early postoperative period. Br J Surg 1977; 64: 384–389.

32. Bigler D, Dirkes W, Hansen R, et al: Effects of thoracic paravertebral block with bupivacaine versus combined thoracic epidural block with bupivacaine and morphine on pain and pulmonary function after cholecystectomy. Acta Anaesthesiol Scand 1989; 33: 561–564.

33. Spence AA, Logan DA: Respiratory effects of extradural nerve block in the postoperative period. Br J Anaesth 1975; 47 Suppl: 281–283.

34. VadeBoncouer TR, Riegler FX, Gautt RS, et al: A randomized, double-blind comparison of the effects of interpleural bupivacaine and saline on morphine requirements and pulmonary function after cholecystectomy. Anesthesiology 1989; 71: 339–343.

35. Frenette L, Boudreault D, Guay J: Interpleural analgesia improves pulmonary function after cholecystectomy. Can J Anaesth 1991; 38: 71–74.

36. Moore DC: Intercostal nerve block for postoperative somatic pain following surgery of thorax and upper abdomen. Br J Anaesth 1975; 47 (Suppl): 284–286.

37. Trivedi NS, Robalino J, Shevde K: Interpleural block: a new technique for regional anaesthesia during percutaneous nephrostomy and nephrolithotomy. Can J Anaesth 1990; 37: 479–481.

38. Riegler FX, VadeBoncouer TR, Pelligrino DA: Interpleural anesthetics in the dog: differential somatic neural blockade. Anesthesiology 1989; 71: 744–750.

39. Ben-David B, Lee E: The falling column: a new technique for interpleural catheter placement. (Letter to the editor.) Anesth Analg 1990; 71: 212.

40. Kvalheim L, Reiestad F: Interpleural catheter in the management of postoperative pain. (Abstract.) Anesthesiology 1984; 61 Suppl: A231.

41. Strømskag KE, Minor B, Steen PA: Side effects and complications related to interpleural analgesia: an update. Acta Anaesthesiol Scand 1990; 34: 473–477.

42. Gomez MN, Symreng T, Johnson B, et al: Intrapleural bupivacaine for intraoperative analgesia—a dangerous technique? (Abstract.) Anesth Analg 1988; 67 Suppl: S78.

43. Symreng T, Gomez MN, Johnson B, et al: Intrapleural bupivacaine—technical considerations and intraoperative use. J Cardiothorac Anesth 1989; 3: 139–143.

44. Lauder GR: Interpleural analgesia and phrenic nerve paralysis. Anaesthesia 1993; 48: 315–316.

45. Shantha TR: Unilateral bronchospasm after interpleural analgesia. Anesth Analg 1992; 74: 291–293.

46. Spittal MJ, Hunter SJ: A comparison of bupivacaine instillation and inguinal field block for control of pain after herniorrhaphy. Ann R Coll Surg Engl 1992; 74: 85–88.

47. Bigler D, Hjortso NC, Edstrom H, et al: Comparative effects of intrathecal bupivacaine and tetracaine on analgesia, cardiovascular function and plasma catecholamines. Acta Anaesthesiol Scand 1986; 30: 199–203.

48. Langer JC, Shandling B, Rosenberg M: Intraoperative bupivacaine during outpatient hernia repair in children: a randomized double blind trial. J Pediatr Surg 1987; 22: 267–270.

49. Cross GD, Barrett RF: Comparison of two regional techniques for postoperative analgesia in children following herniotomy and orchidopexy. Anaesthesia 1987; 42: 845–849.

50. Hinkle AJ: Percutaneous inguinal block for the outpatient management of post-herniorrhaphy pain in children. Anesthesiology 1987; 67: 411–413.

51. Fell D, Derrington MC, Taylor E, et al: Paediatric postoperative analgesia: a comparison between caudal block and wound infiltration of local anaesthetic. Anaesthesia 1988; 43: 107–110.

52. Webster AC, McKishnie JD, Watson JT, et al: Lumbar epidural anaesthesia for inguinal hernia repair in low birth weight infants. Can J Anaesth 1993; 40: 670–675.

53. Peutrell JM, Hughes DG: Epidural anaesthesia through caudal catheters for inguinal herniotomies in awake ex-premature babies. Anaesthesia 1993; 48: 128–131.

54. Warner LO, Teitelbaum DH, Caniano DA, et al: Inguinal herniorrhaphy in young infants: perianesthetic complications and associated preanesthetic risk factors. J Clin Anesth 1992; 4: 455–461.

55. Bugedo GJ, Carcamo CR, Mertens RA, et al: Preoperative percutaneous ilioinguinal and iliohypogastric nerve block with 0.5% bupivacaine for post-herniorrhaphy pain management in adults. Reg Anesth 1990; 15: 130–133.

56. Committee on Trauma Research, Commission of Life Sciences, National Research Council and Institute of Medicine: Injury in America: A Continuing Public Health Problem, pp 18–36. Washington, DC, National Academic Press, 1985.

57. Mackersie RC, Karagianes TG: Pain management following trauma and burns. Crit Care Clin 1990; 6: 433–449.

58. Lanz E, Theiss D, Jankovic D: The extent of blockade following various techniques of brachial plexus block. Anesth Analg 1983; 62: 55–58.

59. Whiffler K, Leiman BC: The application of regional anaesthesia in a disaster situation. S Afr Med J 1983; 63: 409–410.

60. Bion JF: An anaesthetist in a camp for Cambodian refugees. Anaesthesia 1983; 38: 798–801.

61. Bion JF: Isobaric bupivacaine for spinal anaesthesia in acute war injuries. Anaesthesia 1984; 39: 554–559.

62. Thompson GE: Anesthesia for battle casualties in Vietnam. JAMA 1967; 201 (Suppl): 215–219.

63. Robson AK, Bloom PA: Suturing of digital lacerations: digital block or local infiltration? Ann R Coll Surg Engl 1990; 72: 360–361.

64. Colizza WA, Said E: Intravenous regional anesthesia in the treatment of forearm and wrist fractures and dislocations in children. Can J Surg 1993; 36: 225–228.

65. Hunter JB, Scott MJ, Harries SA: Methods of anaesthesia used for reduction of Colles' fractures. BMJ 1989; 299: 1316–1317.

66. Abbaszadegan H, Jonsson U: Regional anesthesia preferable for Colles' fracture: controlled comparison with local anesthesia. Acta Orthop Scand 1990; 61: 348–349.

67. Haasio J: Cubital nerve block vs haematoma block for the manipulation of Colles' fracture. Ann Chir Gynaecol 1990; 79: 168–171.

68. Meinig RP, Quick A, Lobmeyer L: Plasma lidocaine levels following hematoma block for distal radius fractures. J Orthop Trauma 1989; 3: 187–191.

69. Johnson PQ, Noffsinger MA: Hematoma block of distal forearm fractures: is it safe? Orthop Rev 1991; 20: 977–979.

70. Knottenbelt JD, James MF, Bloomfield M: Intrapleural bupivacaine analgesia in chest trauma: a randomized double-blind controlled trial. Injury 1991; 22: 114–116.

71. Engdahl O, Boe J, Sandstedt S: Interpleural bupivacaine for analgesia during chest drainage treatment for pneumothorax: a randomized double-blind study. Acta Anaesthesiol Scand 1993; 37: 149–153.

72. Trinkle JK, Richardson JD, Franz JL, et al: Management of flail chest without mechanical ventilation. Ann Thorac Surg 1975; 19: 355–363.

73. Bridenbaugh PO, DuPen SL, Moore DC, et al: Postoperative intercostal nerve block analgesia versus narcotic analgesia. Anesth Analg 1973; 52: 81–85.

74. Pedersen VM, Schulze S, Hoier-Madsen K, et al: Air-flow meter assessment of the effect of intercostal nerve blockade on respiratory function in rib fractures. Acta Chir Scand 1983; 149: 119–120.

75. O'Kelly E, Garry B: Continuous pain relief for multiple fractured ribs. Br J Anaesth 1981; 53: 989–991.

76. Sabanathan S, Mearns AJ, Bickford Smith PJ, et al: Efficacy of continuous extrapleural intercostal nerve block on postthoracotomy pain and pulmonary mechanics. Br J Surg 1990; 77: 221–225.

77. Richardson J, Sabanathan S, Eng J, et al: Continuous intercostal nerve block versus epidural morphine for postthoracotomy analgesia. Ann Thorac Surg 1993; 55: 377–380.

78. Gilbert J, Hultman J: Thoracic paravertebral block: a method of pain control. Acta Anaesthesiol Scand 1989; 33: 142–145.

79. Rocco A, Reiestad F, Gudman J, et al: Intrapleural administration of local anesthetics for pain relief in patients with multiple rib fractures: preliminary report. Reg Anesth 1987; 12: 10–14.

80. Mackersie RC, Shackford SR, Hoyt DB, et al: Continuous epidural fentanyl analgesia: ventilatory function improvement with routine use in treatment of blunt chest injury. J Trauma 1987; 27: 1207–1212.

81. Rankin AP, Comber RE: Management of fifty cases of chest injury with a regimen of epidural bupivacaine and morphine. Anaesth Intensive Care 1984; 12: 311–314.

82. Breen TW, Haigh JD: Continuous suprascapular nerve block for analgesia of scapular fracture. Can J Anaesth 1990; 37: 786–788.

83. Strømskag KE, Reiestad F, Holmqvist EL, et al: Intrapleural administration of 0.25%, 0.375%, and 0.5% bupivacaine with epinephrine after cholecystectomy. Anesth Analg 1988; 67: 430–434.

84. Katz J, Kavanagh BP, Sandler AN, et al: Preemptive analgesia: clinical evidence of neuroplasticity contributing to postoperative pain. Anesthesiology 1992; 77: 439–446.

85. Swenson JD, Hullander RM, Bready RJ, et al: A comparison of patient controlled epidural analgesia with sufentanil by the lumbar versus thoracic route after thoracotomy. Anesth Analg 1994; 78: 215–218.

86. Brodsky JB, Chaplan SR, Brose WG, et al: Continuous epidural hydromorphone for postthoracotomy pain relief. Ann Thorac Surg 1990; 50: 888–893.

87. Pond WW, Somerville GM, Thong SH, et al: Pain of delayed traumatic splenic rupture masked by intrapleural lidocaine. Anesthesiology 1989; 70: 154–155.

88. Manriquez RG, Pallares V: Continuous brachial plexus block for prolonged sympathectomy and control of pain. Anesth Analg 1978; 57: 128–130.

89. Rosenblatt R, Pepitone-Rockwell F, McKillop MJ: Continuous axillary analgesia for traumatic hand injury. Anesthesiology 1979; 51: 565–566.

90. Vatashsky E, Aronson HB: Continuous interscalene brachial plexus block for surgical operations on the hand. (Letter to the editor.) Anesthesiology 1980; 53: 356.

91. Tuominen M, Rosenberg PH, Kalso E: Blood levels of bupivacaine after single dose, supplementary dose and during continuous infusion in axillary plexus block. Acta Anaesthesiol Scand 1983; 27: 303–306.

92. Chan VW, Chung F, Cheng DC, et al: Analgesic and pulmonary effects of continuous intercostal nerve block following thoracotomy. Can J Anaesth 1991; 38: 733–739.

93. Selander D: Catheter technique in axillary plexus block: presentation of a new method. Acta Anaesthesiol Scand 1977; 21: 324–329.

94. Baranowski AP, Pither CE: A comparison of three methods of axillary brachial plexus anaesthesia. Anaesthesia 1990; 45: 362–365.

95. Covert CR, Fox GS: Anaesthesia for hip surgery in the elderly. Can J Anaesth 1989; 36: 311–319.

96. Sorenson RM, Pace NL: Anesthetic techniques during surgical repair of femoral neck fractures: a meta-analysis. Anesthesiology 1992; 77: 1095–1104.

97. Van Gessel EF, Forster A, Gamulin Z: Surgical repair of hip fractures using continuous spinal anesthesia: comparison of hypobaric solutions of tetracaine and bupivacaine. Anesth Analg 1989; 68: 276–281.

98. Hood G, Edbrooke DL, Gerrish SP: Postoperative analgesia after triple nerve block for fractured neck of femur. Anaesthesia 1991; 46: 138–140.

99. Coad NR: Post-operative analgesia following femoral-neck surgery—a comparison between 3 in 1 femoral nerve block and lateral cutaneous nerve block. Eur J Anaesthesiol 1991; 8: 287–290.

100. Ben-David B, Lee E, Croitoru M: Psoas block for surgical repair of hip fracture: a case report and description of a catheter technique. Anesth Analg 1990; 71: 298–301.

101. Farny J, Girard M, Drolet P: Posterior approach to the lumbar plexus combined with a sciatic nerve block using lidocaine. Can J Anaesth 1994; 41: 486–491.

102. Ronchi L, Rosenbaum D, Athouel A, et al: Femoral nerve blockade in children using bupivacaine. Anesthesiology 1989; 70: 622–624.

CHAPTER 29

Cardiothoracic and Vascular Surgery

Mark P. Yeager, M.D., Mary P. Fillinger, M.D.,
Johan Lundberg, M.D., Ph.D.

Patients who require cardiothoracic and vascular surgery are at increased risk of perioperative morbidity because they frequently have chronic, even life-threatening diseases and because they often undergo surgery that causes significant impairment of already limited organ function. Regional anesthesia and analgesia may have particular benefit for these patients. For example, regional techniques have a design advantage when administered before operation for control of the many neural and endocrine responses to surgical trauma. Many intravenous or inhalational agents are titrated to effect only after the surgical stimulus. Neuraxial administration of opioids, with or without a combination of local anesthetics, has expanded the capability of anesthesiologists to control perioperative pain and thereby influence postoperative events. Finally, the introduction and widespread acceptance of continuous catheter techniques for epidural or spinal anesthesia and analgesia have made these techniques attractive options for intraoperative and postoperative care. Continuous catheter techniques automatically extend the practice of anesthesia into the postoperative period when most surgical morbidity occurs. Just how much these new treatment options have changed clinical practice and surgical outcome is difficult to measure, but expanded

use of regional techniques appears to represent a lasting shift in modern anesthetic practice.

Effects of Regional Anesthesia on Cardiovascular Function in Cardiothoracic and Vascular Patients

The most common complications after cardiothoracic and vascular operation are myocardial ischemia or infarction, pulmonary dysfunction, renal failure, and intestinal ischemia. Choice of anesthetic technique may affect surgical outcome for these patients by maintaining and protecting the cardiovascular system, maintaining pulmonary function, or reducing thromboembolic events. For these reasons, regional anesthesia is often added to general anesthesia during cardiothoracic and vascular surgery.[1-17] The goal of regional block during cardiac and vascular surgery is to protect the heart from adverse hemodynamic reflexes, improve cardiovascular compliance, inhibit afferent surgical stimuli, decrease the neurohormonal stress response, and improve surgical outcome. This may require dermatomal anesthesia that not only blocks the surgical field but also interrupts sympathetic innervation to the adrenals, the vasculature, and the heart. Any one or a combination of these factors may have a major influence on circulatory performance during regional anesthesia.

Circulatory Effects of Regional Anesthesia

The cardiovascular response to a regional anesthetic is a reflection of block of the afferent nervous system, extent of efferent sympathetic block, and preexisting sympathetic nervous discharge. Sympathetic nerves originate from the T-1 to L-2 spinal segments (Fig. 29–1). Each spinal nerve root gives off efferent branches via the sympathetic chain to adjacent spinal levels cephalad and caudad to the exit site from the vertebral column. Within the sympathetic chain, upper spinal segments originating from T-1 to T-4 form the cardiac accelerator nerves that modulate myocardial contractility and heart rate. Preganglionic sympathetic innervation of the adrenals (approximately T-5 to T-11) controls adrenal medullary release of epinephrine into the circulation. A regional block in the lower part of the body decreases perfusion pressure as a result of arterial vasodilatation and increased venous capacitance. This results in decreased cardiac filling with lower heart rate and cardiac output. Upper extremity vasoconstriction can compensate for some of these effects. When a dermatomal block extends into the upper thoracic region and involves the cardiac sympathetic efferents, the effect is a further reduction in cardiac performance with lower heart rate, cardiac output, and myocardial contractility and a decrease in intrathoracic venous filling and systemic vascular resistance.[5, 17–20] If the regional block is limited to the upper thoracic region, the vascular system can compensate for block of the cardioaccelerator nerves by systemic vasoconstriction in the lower parts of the body and a decrease in venous capacitance to maintain cardiac output and mean arterial pressure.[17, 21]

In patients with coronary artery disease, echocardiographic studies demonstrate that induction of lumbar epidural anesthesia may transiently induce myocardial ischemia, probably owing to decreased coronary perfusion pressure.[22] This finding points out the importance of maintaining systemic arterial pressure within the patient's normal limits in order to avoid myocardial ischemia. If lumbar epidural anesthesia is administered without a volume load to patients with a history of angina pectoris, it may improve ejection fraction and wall motion abnormalities,[23] although subsequent volume loading may minimize these benefits (Fig. 29–2). However, when thoracic epidural anesthesia is induced during general anesthesia, no signs of increased echocardiographic wall motion abnormalities are observed in patients with coronary artery disease despite a decrease in perfusion pressure.[24] In this situation, cardiac sympathectomy may protect the myocardium via coronary vasodilatation[25–27] or a favorable redistribution of intracoronary blood flow or both.[28, 29]

Dermatomal and Sympathetic Block

Sympathetic efferent denervation often does not correlate with the area of sensory block during epidural or spinal anesthesia.[30–32] A partial sympathetic block can exceed the sensory level (differential block).[31–33] Although spinal anesthesia may cause a more widespread sympathetic block,[33] some investigators believe sympathetic block is more profound during epidural anesthesia.[32] Defalque[34] compared the hemodynamic effects of epidural and spinal anesthesia and observed a 10% greater decrease in systolic pressure during epidural anesthesia despite similar levels of sensory analgesia. However, Kennedy et al[35, 36] found that arterial pressure decreases more during spinal anesthesia at a T-1 level than during epidural anesthesia at the same

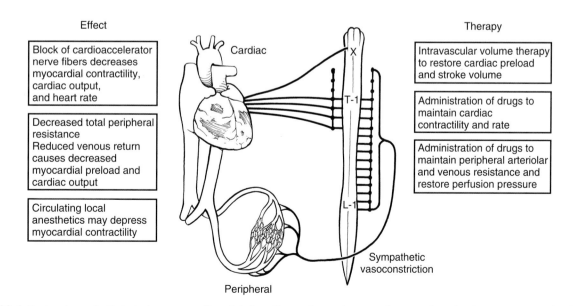

Figure 29–1 Regional anesthetic techniques may affect global cardiovascular performance by several mechanisms. Treatment should be managed according to each physiologic alteration as well as the patient's ability to tolerate changes in cardiovascular performance and myocardial oxygen supply.

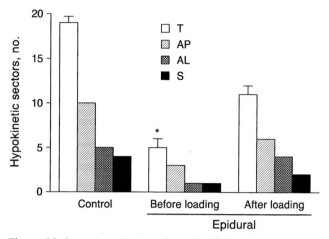

Figure 29–2 Number of echocardiographically hypokinetic sectors (T, total; AP, apicoposterior; AL, anterolateral; S, septal) in group 2 patients at control measurement, during epidural block before volume loading, and after volume loading. Significant change from control: *$P < .01$. (Redrawn from Baron JF, Coriat P, Mundler O, et al: Left ventricular global and regional function during lumbar epidural anesthesia in patients with and without angina pectoris. Influence of volume loading. Anesthesiology 1987; 66: 621–627.)

level. A slower onset of block during epidural anesthesia may allow compensatory mechanisms to be mobilized, and higher blood levels of lidocaine may also offset some of the hypotension induced by the block. The combination of spinal and epidural anesthesia may be the most effective way of blocking afferent neural activity.[37]

Thoracic epidural anesthesia extending from T-1 to L-3 in awake patients and in anesthetized patients during aortic surgery causes a marked decrease in plasma norepinephrine and epinephrine levels in parallel with a decrease in mean arterial pressure, cardiac output, heart rate, and systemic vascular resistance.[5, 6] The level of block is important in this regard. Pflug and Halter[38] found that spinal anesthesia with an upper level at T-2 to T-6 caused suppression of plasma catecholamines and mean arterial pressure whereas no changes in these variables were observed during spinal anesthesia at a T-9 to T-12 dermatomal level.

Factors That Modify the Circulatory Effects of Regional Anesthesia

Choice of local anesthetic may affect the circulatory response to regional anesthesia. Stevens and colleagues[39] evaluated healthy volunteers during lumbar anesthesia with sensory levels up to T-1 achieved by 3% 2-chloroprocaine, 2% lidocaine, and 0.75% bupivacaine. Beardsley et al[40] then assessed the impact of the block on plasma catecholamines and hemodynamics during a cold pressor test as a measure of the degree of sympathetic nervous activity. The authors found that 3% 2-chloroprocaine and 0.75% bupivacaine caused an incomplete sympathetic block, whereas patients receiving 2% lidocaine did not respond to the cold pressor test. In another study, 2% mepivacaine was more

effective than 0.5% bupivacaine as an agent to attenuate sympathetic nervous activity during epidural anesthesia.[32] High blood levels of lidocaine may induce increases in heart rate and cardiac output that may offset vasodilating effects of neuraxial block and result in no change in arterial pressure.[18] If epinephrine is added to lidocaine, cardiac output increases further, whereas systemic vascular resistance decreases more than when plain lidocaine is used.[41]

With increasing age, basal plasma catecholamine levels increase,[42, 43] which implies that older individuals are more dependent on sympathetic activity for cardiovascular function. The circulatory response to regional anesthesia may therefore be more profound in elderly patients. Goertz and associates[44] did not observe any alterations in mean arterial pressure during thoracic epidural anesthesia from T-1 to L2-3 in healthy, middle-aged patients who received either 0.25% or 0.5% bupivacaine. These findings are in contrast to the hemodynamic and plasma catecholamine changes found in elderly patients receiving thoracic epidural anesthesia.[5] Mean arterial pressure and plasma catecholamine levels decreased markedly during T-1 to L-3 thoracic epidural anesthesia with 2% mepivacaine in awake elderly patients despite premedication. When a similar thoracic epidural block is induced during general anesthesia in patients with increased plasma catecholamine levels, the circulatory changes and plasma catecholamine decreases are even more pronounced.[6, 45]

The balance between cardiac accelerator nerves and vagal activity can be altered by sympathetic nerve block during high spinal or epidural anesthesia. Resultant vagal dominance, especially in combination with hypovolemia, may lead to hypotension with severe bradycardia and, on rare occasions, vagal arrest.[46] By use of 0.4 mg atropine during high spinal anesthesia, heart rate may increase at the expense of a diminished stroke volume that leaves cardiac output and mean arterial pressure unaltered.[47] Atropine given during high regional anesthesia may also eliminate nausea caused by unopposed vagal activity.

Induction of spinal and epidural anesthesia decreases preload and afterload as a result of increased venous capacitance and redistribution of blood volume in skeletal muscle, skin, and gastrointestinal tract.[20] Arndt and coworkers[19] found that lumbar epidural anesthesia to the T-4 to T-5 level increased blood volume in the denervated legs approximately 10% while decreasing blood volume by 8% in the thorax, 5% in the splanchnic vasculature, and 10% in the unblocked arms. Overall decreases in regional blood volumes corresponded to a 500- to 600-mL sequestration of blood in the legs. Endocrine homeostasis may partially counteract these effects. A 30° head-up tilt in elderly men does not alter plasma renin, vasopressin, and catecholamines before epidural anesthesia,[48] whereas the same maneuver during a lumbar epidural block causes an increase in vasopressin and renin at the same time mean arterial pressure and plasma norepinephrine are decreased by the epidural block. High epidural anesthesia combined with a specific vasopressin receptor blocker induced a 35% decrease in mean arterial pressure compared with a 14% decrease in perfusion pressure caused by epidural anesthesia alone. Thus, the cardiovascular system may rely on increased vasopressin levels to counteract decreased cardiac filling and arterial hypotension caused by an extensive epidural anesthesia.[49]

Hypertensive patients may have higher plasma catecholamine levels as a reflection of sympathetic activity.[43] Dagnino and Prys-Roberts[50] compared untreated hypertensive patients receiving lumbar epidural anesthesia with treated hypertensive patients and found marked decreases in mean arterial pressure (42%) and heart rate in the untreated group. Hypertensive patients also experience a greater decrease in arterial pressure during induction of lumbar epidural anesthesia for hip arthroplasty.[51] Interestingly, Stenseth et al[16] found that patients receiving therapy with β-adrenergic blockers who were scheduled for aortocoronary bypass did not show signs of myocardial depression and manifested only a slight decrease in mean arterial pressure, even when a widespread thoracic epidural anesthetic was induced.

The combination of regional and general anesthesia has gained widespread acceptance, especially during major surgical procedures. When this technique is used, systemic hypotension and decreased systemic vascular resistance and venous return are probably the most common side effects with low levels of sensory block. When higher (thoracic) levels of sensory anesthesia are achieved, an additional decrease in cardiac performance is caused by decreased myocardial contractility, decreased cardiac loading conditions, and unopposed vagal activity. When thoracic epidural anesthesia is added to general anesthesia, it induces decreases in mean arterial pressure, cardiac output, and heart rate.[6, 24, 45] However, in patients with documented coronary artery disease, the frequency of segmental wall motion abnormalities is not altered when thoracic epidural anesthesia is added to general anesthesia.[24]

Regional Anesthesia During Aortic Surgery

The combination of general and epidural anesthesia has been reported as a useful technique during abdominal aortic surgery to control hemodynamic function, attenuate the stress response, and provide postoperative pain relief. Use of a combined technique may result in greater hemodynamic stability, with maintenance of cardiac output and systemic vascular resistance during aortic cross-clamping compared with general anesthesia alone.[2, 52-54] As a result of a decrease in preload and afterload conditions, cross-clamping of the aorta may even be associated with augmented myocardial performance, with increases in cardiac output.[2] However, the addition of epidural anesthesia to general anesthesia during aortic surgery does not seem to decrease myocardial ischemia measured by new segmental wall motion abnormalities during cross-clamping.[55] Patients who have received a combined anesthetic experience hypotension and decreases in systemic vascular resistance after declamping, and, despite volume replacement, these patients often need inotropic or vasopres-

sor support, whereas systemic pressure in patients who have received general anesthesia alone may recover spontaneously.[3] If volume replacement during cross-clamping increases left ventricular filling pressures about 3 to 4 mm Hg above baseline values, the risk of hypotension after aortic declamping is minimized.[1]

Hypotension is a major concern when regional anesthesia is used during aortic surgery. If a hypodynamic circulation is sustained in this population, it could jeopardize circulation to vascular regions with impaired arterial inflow and evoke tissue hypoxia and reductive metabolism.[6] Inotropic or vasoactive agents can counteract hypotension and even improve systemic and regional hemodynamics during aortic surgery.[2, 5, 6, 54] As an alternative, a weaker solution of local anesthetic agent, such as 0.25% bupivacaine, may be used to minimize hypotension and excessive fluid load during aortic surgery,[3, 4] although the nerve block may then be less effective. Despite a decrease in arterial perfusion pressure after thoracic epidural anesthesia, the coronary circulation shows only moderate decreases in coronary sinus blood flow, with lower oxygen and lactate utilization associated with a decrease in cardiac work.[56]

Epidural and spinal anesthesia can decrease renal blood flow owing to a reduction in mean arterial pressure,[57-59] although renal function is not significantly altered if perfusion pressure is maintained.[60, 61] Epidural anesthesia does not prevent a deterioration in renal function and blood flow during aortic cross-clamping,[60-62] whereas epidural and spinal anesthesia will either increase[63, 64] or decrease[35, 58, 59, 65] intestinal blood flow, depending on the change in mean arterial pressure. Superior mesenteric artery blood flow increases if the arterial pressure is maintained with dopamine after thoracic epidural anesthesia for aortic surgery,[66] and infrarenal cross-clamping and declamping further increase intestinal blood flow (Fig. 29–3).[6] In contrast, a decrease in intestinal blood flow during and after cross-clamping is seen with general anesthesia alone.[62, 67]

After operation, the potential benefits of epidural anesthesia include a decrease in thromboembolic events via modification of hypercoagulability[68] and an increased lower extremity blood flow.[69, 70] Plasma norepinephrine levels, as an indicator of postsurgical stress, are attenuated in patients receiving bupivacaine-fentanyl for thoracic epidural anesthesia[15] or morphine epidurally (Fig. 29–4).[10] Oxygen uptake after aortic surgery is increased as much as threefold after general anesthesia, with compensatory increases in cardiac work.[71] Although epidural anesthesia blocks sympathetic outflow, improves myocardial function, and is reported to maintain perioperative body temperature,[72] thoracic epidural anesthesia when used without inotropic support does not improve and may even impair systemic oxygen supply-demand ratio after aortic surgery.[8]

Managing the Hemodynamic Effects of Regional Anesthesia in Patients With Cardiovascular Disease

The risk of inducing circulatory depression during regional anesthesia, with or without general anesthe-

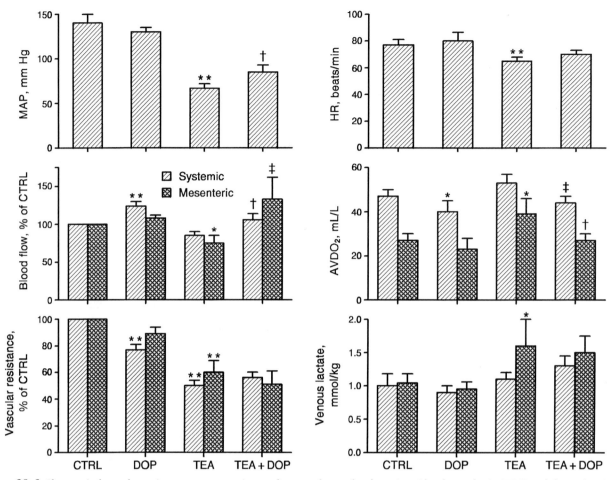

Figure 29–3 Changes in hemodynamics, oxygen extraction, and venous lactate by thoracic epidural anesthesia (TEA) and dopamine (DOP) 4 μg/kg/min during laparotomy in humans. * and ** = significant change in relation to control (CTRL); † and ‡ = significant change in relation to TEA ($P < .05$ and $P < .01$, respectively). AVDO$_2$, arteriovenous oxygen difference; HR, heart rate; MAP, mean arterial pressure. (Redrawn from Lundberg J, Lundberg D, Norgren L, et al: Intestinal hemodynamics during laparotomy: effects of thoracic epidural anesthesia and dopamine in humans. Anesth Analg 1990; 71: 9–15.)

sia, raises the question of risk versus benefit for surgical procedures in patients with known cardiovascular disease. In a patient with arteriosclerotic disease, the overriding clinical goal is to prevent ischemic events and maintain blood flow to the heart, kidneys, gastrointestinal system, spinal cord, brain, and extremities. Volume treatment and pharmacotherapy both counteract hypodynamic circulatory states during regional anesthesia, although there are advantages and disadvantages with both approaches.

Volume Replacement

The cardiovascular changes seen during regional anesthesia can, in part, be treated by intravascular volume replacement. Increases in circulating blood volume of approximately 400 mL (range, 0 to 1100 mL) have been shown[16] to maintain central venous pressure at the preinduction level during T-1 to T-12 thoracic epidural anesthesia. However, despite restoration of cardiac filling, mean arterial pressure is usually not normalized by this treatment during an extensive re-

gional block. The finding of decreased segmental wall motion during lumbar epidural anesthesia in patients with coronary artery disease indicates that mean arterial pressure should be maintained.[22] If a similar block is established without a prophylactic volume load, a paradoxic echocardiographic improvement in left ventricular performance has been observed.[23] However, after a subsequent 500-mL volume load, hypokinetic sectors returned. This finding suggests that volume preload should be carefully monitored during lumbar epidural anesthesia in patients with cardiovascular disease. An alternative approach to avoid a volume load is hypertonic saline.[73] The extra sodium load with this treatment is transient, and serum sodium levels usually remain normal. Colloid solutions such as 5% albumin[74] and dextran 70[75–77] can also limit total volume.

Vasoactive Medications

Intravenous administration of boluses of ephedrine, 5 to 15 mg, are probably the most commonly used pharmacologic intervention to treat hypotension dur-

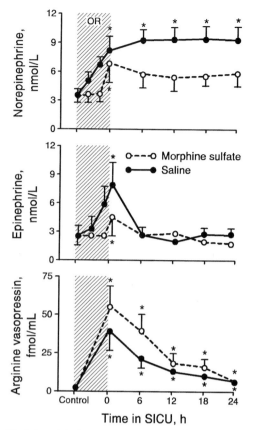

Figure 29–4 Arterial plasma concentrations of norepinephrine (top), epinephrine (center), and arginine vasopressin (bottom) before induction of anesthesia (control); at two points during operation; and 0, 6, 12, 18, and 24 h after aortic surgery. OR, operating room (shaded area); SICU, surgical intensive care unit. *$P < .05$ compared with preinduction value. Data are mean ± SE (vertical bars). (Redrawn from Breslow MJ, Jordan DA, Christopherson R, et al: Epidural morphine decreases postoperative hypertension by attenuating sympathetic nervous system hyperactivity. JAMA 1989; 261: 3577–3581. Copyright 1989, American Medical Association.)

ing regional anesthesia.[47, 78–80] Ephedrine can also be administered prophylactically: 12.5 to 25 mg subcutaneously,[78] 37.5 mg intramuscularly,[81] or continuous intravenous infusion with an initial rate of 1 to 5 mg/min.[82, 83] The mixed α- and β-adrenergic properties of ephedrine, characterized by a normalization of perfusion pressure and restoration of cardiac output and systemic vascular resistance, usually do not cause hypertension or marked increases in heart rate.[47, 78] As an unanticipated side effect, restoration of hemodynamics during epidural anesthesia may actually increase the plasma level of a local anesthetic agent, even to toxic levels.[84] Prophylactic administration of ephedrine is useful during subarachnoid anesthesia, especially in high-risk patients because of a higher incidence of hypotension compared with healthy patients.[81] Echocardiographic studies during combined thoracic and general anesthesia for aortic surgery demonstrate that ephedrine maintains left ventricular function without increasing heart rate compared with phenylephrine.[54] However, ephedrine may induce reversible segmental

wall motion abnormalities during thoracic epidural anesthesia combined with general anesthesia when systemic pressure decreases more than 30% in patients at risk of myocardial ischemia.[24]

Dopamine has dose-dependent dopaminergic and β$_1$- and α-adrenergic properties that make it a suitable agent for cardiovascular support during extensive regional block and prolonged operation. Regional anesthesia alters the hemodynamic properties of dopamine such that a low dose markedly improves mean arterial pressure and cardiac output and slightly augments a lowered systemic vascular resistance (Fig. 29–5).[5, 6, 45, 64, 85, 86] An infusion rate of 2 to 8 μg/kg/min is usually sufficient to normalize cardiovascular function. Dopamine is known to induce tachycardia at higher infusion rates, which may limit its use in patients with coronary artery disease. If dopamine is combined with a volume load during thoracic epidural anesthesia and infused at 2 to 8 μg/kg/min, the heart rate typically remains at 50 to 75 beats/min,[5] which may decrease the risk of myocardial ischemia. At an infusion rate of 4 μg/kg/min, dopamine markedly increases intestinal blood flow despite moderate increases in systemic perfusion pressure. When an infrarenal aortic cross-clamp is applied, intestinal blood flow increases further and remains above control levels after removal of the clamp.[6, 66]

Dobutamine produces a different hemodynamic pattern than dopamine during regional anesthesia. Before total spinal anesthesia was induced in dogs on cardiopulmonary bypass with constant flow, dobutamine (1 to 50 μg/kg/min) decreased mean arterial pressure; during spinal block, dobutamine had no significant effect on mean arterial pressure.[85] Venous capacitance decreased in a dose-related fashion in both instances. Dobutamine restores myocardial blood flow during thoracic epidural anesthesia[87] and, when 1 to 3 μg/kg/min dobutamine is used in conjunction with epidural anesthesia reaching at least T-4, arterial pressure and cardiac output markedly increase, and heart rate and cardiac filling pressures do not show any remarkable changes.[88]

Epinephrine is often used as an adjunct to local anesthetics to limit the vascular uptake of local anesthetic agent and to improve the regional quality of the block. Besides these desired effects, systemic absorption of epinephrine leads to additional cardiovascular changes—increases in cardiac performance and decreases in perfusion pressure and vascular resistance.[36, 41, 57, 89] Renal plasma flow and hepatic blood flow may decrease owing to a decrease in perfusion pressure.[35, 36] Low-dose intravenous epinephrine for cardiovascular support during regional blocks has been proposed. During hypotensive epidural anesthesia, <0.1 μg/kg/min of epinephrine maintains cardiac output at preblock levels and mean arterial pressure between 50 and 60 mm Hg in elderly patients (Fig. 29–6).[9, 90]

Despite a marked increase in arterial pressure, norepinephrine causes no change in cardiac index or stroke volume during thoracolumbar epidural anesthesia.[17] The increase in systemic vascular resistance is even more marked than when norepinephrine is ad-

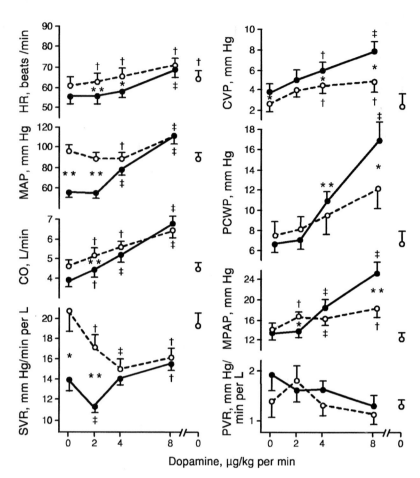

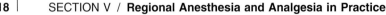

Dopamine, μg/kg per min

Figure 29–5 Changes in heart rate (HR), mean arterial pressure (MAP), cardiac output (CO), systemic vascular resistance (SVR), central venous pressure (CVP), pulmonary capillary wedge pressure (PCWP), mean pulmonary artery pressure (MPAP), and pulmonary vascular resistance (PVR) by dopamine before (dashed line) and during (solid line) thoracic epidural analgesia (TEA). Values are mean and 1 SEM. The last point is the postinfusion control value obtained before TEA. * and ** = significant differences before and during TEA ($P < .05$ and $P < .01$, respectively). † and ‡ = significant change in comparison with the measurement without dopamine. (Redrawn from Lundberg J, Norgren L, Thomson D, et al: Hemodynamic effects of dopamine during thoracic epidural analgesia in man. Anesthesiology 1987; 66: 641–646.)

Figure 29–6 Hemodynamic changes after epidural injection of 0.75% bupivacaine plain 25 mL in six patients receiving low-dose epinephrine (solid circles) and in nine patients receiving phenylephrine (open circles) by intravenous infusions (mean and SD). *P < .05; †P = .05; **P < .01. CO, cardiac output; HR, heart rate; MAP, mean arterial pressure; PADP, pulmonary artery diastolic pressure. (Redrawn from Sharrock NE, Go G, Mineo R: Effect of i.v. low-dose adrenaline and phenylephrine infusions on plasma concentrations of bupivacaine after lumbar extradural anaesthesia in elderly patients. Br J Anaesth 1991; 67: 694–698. Published by BMJ Publishing Group.)

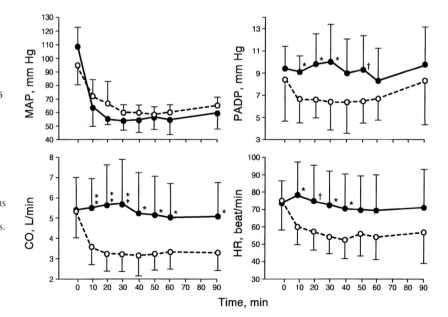

Time, min

ministered during a limited thoracic epidural block. Experimental findings during extensive thoracic epidural anesthesia show that an infusion rate of 0.1 to 0.5 μg/kg/min restores mean arterial pressure without any significant changes in cardiac output.[91] Equipressor infusion rates of dopamine in the same study increased cardiac output and myocardial contractility at markedly lower plasma norepinephrine levels.

Use of a pure α₁-adrenergic agonist such as phenylephrine can support coronary perfusion pressure during extensive regional block.[92, 93] However, one report[94] of patients with advanced cardiovascular disease indicated that the incidence of myocardial ischemia increases markedly in patients who receive phenylephrine for pressure support during carotid endarterectomy. This finding may limit use of phenylephrine in the same patient population during other procedures performed with epidural anesthesia. When phenylephrine is infused at 20 to 60 μg/min during combined general and thoracic epidural anesthesia for abdominal aortic surgery, arterial pressure is restored but cardiac index and ejection fraction are compromised.[54] Even in healthy middle-aged patients, a phenylephrine bolus of 1 μg/kg caused transient impairment of left ventricular function with increased end-systolic wall stress and decreased fractional diameter and circumferential fiber shortening during thoracic epidural anesthesia (compared with lumbar epidural anesthesia).[43] Phenylephrine (<0.5 μg/kg/min) paradoxically did not decrease renal blood flow.[9] When phenylephrine is added to the local anesthetic agent for epidural anesthesia, it may preserve mean arterial pressure but cardiac output decreases and central venous pressure increases, while the plasma level of local anesthetic agent is not decreased.[89] This is similar to what is observed when phenylephrine is administered by infusion (see Fig. 29–6).[95] On the basis of current knowledge, during epidural block, phenylephrine should be used with caution in patients with signs of coronary artery disease, but it is still useful during regional blocks in other patient categories.

Thoracic Surgery: Regional Techniques

Proponents of regional anesthesia and analgesia argue that use of regional techniques allows for a comfortable, responsive patient who is able to breathe deeply and cough effectively without a requirement for large systemic doses of opioids that may result in sedation and respiratory depression. These effects may be particularly desirable for patients who undergo thoracic surgery.

Effects of Regional Techniques on Pulmonary Function

Patients who undergo major vascular and cardiothoracic surgery have a restrictive pattern of postoperative pulmonary function characterized by decreases in functional residual capacity and vital capacity.[96 – 101] Vital capacity is normally decreased to approximately 40% to 50% of preoperative values but may be decreased to as low as 25% of the preoperative level. Decreases in postoperative functional residual capacity to 70% to 80% of preoperative values are common and lead to small airway closure, atelectasis, ventilation-perfusion mismatch, and impaired gas exchange, sometimes with hypercapnia and hypoxemia. Flow rates also decrease to 40% to 60% of baseline values after upper abdominal (including abdominal aortic) and thoracic surgery.[15, 102, 103] These abnormalities may persist for 2 to 3 weeks. Pain, preexisting disease, diaphragmatic dysmotility, surgical incision and local surgical trauma, cardiopulmonary bypass, and residual effects of general anesthesia (respiratory depressants, muscle relaxants) all contribute to postoperative pulmonary dysfunction.[96, 97, 104]

Epidural anesthesia to the T-4 sensory level with 1.5% lidocaine in patients free of cardiopulmonary disease does not cause derangement of ventilatory capacity, functional residual capacity, or alveolar gas exchange.[105] In contrast, some investigators have found that thoracic epidural block causes modest reductions in vital capacity, 1-s forced expiratory volume, peak expiratory flow rate, and mid-expiratory flow rate.[106 – 108] These changes may be related to the degree of spread of the thoracic epidural block.[109] Phrenic nerve denervation secondary to lower cervical epidural block may result in diaphragmatic dysfunction, whereas abdominal muscle weakness from lower thoracic or upper abdominal block may result in impaired expiratory function and cough. Lower chest wall and upper abdominal muscle paralysis from intercostal nerve block appears to be well tolerated in healthy subjects. Except for a minimal decrease in peak expiratory flow rate, Hecker et al[110] did not find clinically significant deleterious effects on respiratory function after intercostal nerve block, even at the extremes of ventilatory demand.

Using indirect methods to assess postoperative diaphragmatic function, some investigators have found partial restoration of diaphragmatic shortening with intercostal nerve block and thoracic epidural analgesia after upper abdominal surgery.[111 – 113] However, Fratacci et al[114] implanted sonomicrometry crystals and electromyogram electrodes on the costal diaphragm of six patients undergoing thoracotomy and found that thoracic epidural analgesia did not reverse the impairment of diaphragmatic shortening after thoracotomy despite measurable increases in tidal volume, forced vital capacity, and maximal inspiratory pressure.

Theoretically, decreases in expiratory flow rates after motor block of the chest wall and upper abdominal musculature may precipitate respiratory failure in patients with borderline pulmonary function. Harrop-Griffiths and associates[115] noted that patients with significant chronic obstructive pulmonary disease had a decreased ability to clear secretions after extensive thoracic epidural block to T-12. In contrast, Tarhan et al[116] demonstrated that regional anesthesia improved postoperative pulmonary outcome in patients with chronic obstructive pulmonary disease compared with those receiving general anesthesia. Other investigators[102] have reported safe epidural administration of low concentrations of bupivacaine (<0.25%) for postoperative analgesia without deleterious effects. It may be prudent to limit the extent and intensity of epidural block in patients with preexisting pulmonary disease.

Epidural and Intrathecal Techniques

Several analgesic agents have been used for epidural and subarachnoid analgesia, including opioids, local anesthetics, combinations of opioids and local anesthetics, and clonidine (Table 29–1).[99, 101–103, 117–132] Although the optimum combination has not been fully defined, a combination of local anesthetics and opioids may prove most effective. Intermittent spinal administration of opioids and local anesthetics provides effective intraoperative anesthesia and postoperative analgesia.[103–120] However, a high incidence of systemic side effects may be associated with these agents after intermittent administration,[121] and rare, but potentially serious, complications can occur (Fig. 29–7). In order to decrease these side effects and achieve greater versatility, continuous spinal administration of opioids and local anesthetics through indwelling epidural and, more recently, intrathecal catheters has become popular. Use of patient-controlled epidural analgesia to deliver on-demand supplements may further improve postoperative analgesia.

Effective epidural analgesia for post-thoracotomy pain has been achieved with both lumbar and thoracic epidural catheters.[101, 102, 118, 122] Local anesthetic infusions are delivered optimally through epidural catheters placed near the center of the required dermatomal bands (midthoracic region) for post-thoracotomy analgesia. Although thoracic epidural catheters are technically more difficult to place than lumbar catheters, provision of segmental anesthesia and analgesia should lower the risk of local anesthetic systemic toxicity and avoid unnecessary block of the lumbosacral region. Pain secondary to regression of a block can be over-

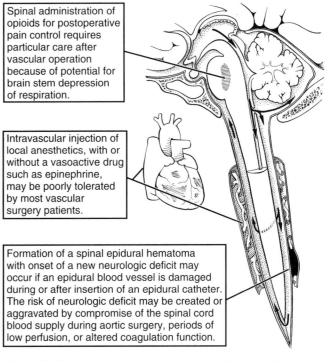

Spinal administration of opioids for postoperative pain control requires particular care after vascular operation because of potential for brain stem depression of respiration.

Intravascular injection of local anesthetics, with or without a vasoactive drug such as epinephrine, may be poorly tolerated by most vascular surgery patients.

Formation of a spinal epidural hematoma with onset of a new neurologic deficit may occur if an epidural blood vessel is damaged during or after insertion of an epidural catheter. The risk of neurologic deficit may be created or aggravated by compromise of the spinal cord blood supply during aortic surgery, periods of low perfusion, or altered coagulation function.

Figure 29–7 Rare but potentially serious complications of spinal analgesic techniques include central respiratory depression from opioids, intravascular injection of local anesthetics or epinephrine, and spinal or epidural hematoma formation.

come by increasing the infusion rate or by adding an opioid to the infusion.

Post-thoracotomy analgesia by epidural administration of hydrophilic opioids, usually morphine, is equally effective when administered via the lumbar or the thoracic route.[101, 123] The hydrophilic nature of morphine allows cephalad migration in the cerebrospinal fluid, with coverage of more spinal cord segments. Lipophilic opioids, such as fentanyl and sufentanil, have a more rapid onset, higher receptor affinity, and possibly a decreased risk of causing delayed respiratory depression. The optimum epidural catheter site for administration of lipophilic opioids is controversial, as is their mode of action. Some investigators[122, 124] have recommended that the epidural catheter be preferentially placed in the midthoracic region to provide segmental anesthesia and analgesia, decrease opioid requirements, and keep systemic opioid effects to a minimum. Others[125–127] have found no clinical advantage of thoracic over lumbar epidural administration of lipophilic opioids. It may be that the mechanism of action of lipophilic epidural opioids is predominantly via systemic absorption,[128] although arbitrary dosing regimens confound this issue.

Even though spinal administration of opioids and local anesthetics for thoracic surgery may decrease intraoperative volatile agent requirements,[99] most of the investigations with regional techniques for thoracic surgery have concentrated on postoperative effects. Post-thoracotomy analgesia from intermittent and continuous epidural infusions of morphine or fentanyl has been reported to be superior to analgesia provided by

Table 29–1 Intraspinal Administration of Opioids for Post-thoracotomy Pain*

DRUG	SINGLE DOSE	INFUSION	ONSET, min	DURATION, h
Epidural				
Morphine	1–6 mg	0.1–1.0 mg/h	30	6–24
Meperidine	20–150 mg	2–20 mg/h	5	6–8
Fentanyl	25–150 μg	25–100 μg/h	5	3–6
Sufentanil	10–60 μg	10–50 μg/h	5	2–4
Subarachnoid				
Morphine	0.1–0.3 mg		15	8–24
Fentanyl	5–25 μg		5	3–6

*Doses must be carefully adjusted for patient age and catheter position (epidural). Duration of analgesia varies—tends to increase with dose and patient age. For accuracy and convenience of administration, adjust concentration to allow approximately 10 mL/h for infusion. For infusion with bupivacaine, use 0.0625% bupivacaine solution.

From Stevens DS, Edwards WT: Management of pain after thoracic surgery. In Kaplan JA (ed): Thoracic Anesthesia, 2nd ed, pp 563–591. New York, Churchill Livingstone, 1991.

either intramuscular or intravenous administration of morphine.[101-117] El-Baz and colleagues[118] demonstrated that continuous epidural infusion of morphine at 0.1 mg/h provided effective analgesia in the majority of post-thoracotomy patients while avoiding major systemic side effects from intermittent epidural injections.

Logas and coworkers[117] randomized 53 patients scheduled to undergo thoracotomy to receive continuous intraoperative anesthesia and postoperative analgesia from epidural infusions of morphine 0.1 mg/mL, bupivacaine 0.1%, bupivacaine 0.1% and morphine 0.1 mg/mL in combination, or saline. A fifth group of patients received morphine 0.1 mg/kg intramuscularly as needed for postoperative pain. Analgesia from opioids given intramuscularly was inferior to that of the continuous epidural administration of morphine or the combination of bupivacaine plus morphine. The epidural combination of bupivacaine plus morphine provided better analgesia than the epidural administration of bupivacaine alone. Addition of bupivacaine to morphine given epidurally made no significant difference in terms of analgesia, total opioid requirements, or the incidence of nausea and pruritus after thoracotomy. In another study,[129] the addition of bupivacaine 0.1% to fentanyl (10 µg/mL) given epidurally likewise did not improve post-thoracotomy analgesia compared with epidural infusion of fentanyl alone. George et al[102] demonstrated that 0.2% bupivacaine combined with thoracic epidural administration of fentanyl did improve postoperative analgesia without causing hypotension. Epidural local anesthetics alone provide excellent post-thoracotomy analgesia but may be associated with side effects of hypotension and motor weakness.[130] Finally, epidural analgesia is not always effective in relieving the ipsilateral shoulder pain after thoracotomy. Ipsilateral stellate ganglion block has been reported to be effective in decreasing this pain.[131]

Compared with systemic administration of opioids, reports of beneficial effects from regional analgesia on indices of pulmonary function have varied. Bromage and colleagues[103] and Shulman and associates[101] reported that epidural administration of opioids to patients undergoing thoracotomy resulted in a significant improvement in pulmonary function compared with intravenous administration of opioids. In contrast, post-thoracotomy patients who had received superior analgesia from morphine given intrathecally had no difference in results of pulmonary function tests during the first and second postoperative days compared with patients who received meperidine intravenously.[99] When compared with patients receiving morphine intravenously, cryoanalgesia, or interpleural analgesia, patients receiving intermittent lumbar epidural injection of morphine had better analgesia but showed no difference in prevention of postoperative pulmonary dysfunction.[132]

Side effects associated with neuraxial administration of opioids include early and delayed respiratory depression, central narcosis, nausea, vomiting, pruritus, and urinary retention. Depending on the agent used, respiratory depression from opioid given neuraxially peaks at 5 to 10 h and may persist for up to 24 h. Frequent vital sign checks by personnel trained to recognize and treat this potentially life-threatening complication may minimize risks in patients receiving neuraxial opioids. Side effects associated with epidural administration of local anesthetics include hypotension and bradycardia secondary to sympathectomy-induced peripheral vasodilation and block of the cardiac sympathetic nerves T-1 to T-4 and unwanted motor weakness.

Intercostal Nerve Blocks

Intercostal nerve block can be provided by several techniques, including separate injections of individual intercostal nerves in their respective intercostal spaces, percutaneous jet injection of local anesthetic near intercostal nerves, and continuous intercostal infusion.[133-139] Paravertebral and interpleural analgesia may also be variations of intercostal nerve block.[140] Intrathoracic cryoanalgesia of intercostal nerves at the end of thoracic surgery is another method of providing pain relief.[132, 141] For intermittent separate injection of intercostal nerves, a long-acting agent such as bupivacaine is desirable. Bupivacaine 0.375% to 0.5% is preferable when intercostal nerve block is used as an adjunct to general anesthesia. Concentrations of bupivacaine from 0.1% to 0.25% result in less motor block and less total mass of drug. Epinephrine 1:200,000 is added to decrease local anesthetic systemic absorption, prolong duration of effect on intercostal nerves, and attenuate the systemic cardiovascular side effects of local anesthetics. Injection of a total of 3 to 5 mL of local anesthetic is used per nerve. The insertion site for intercostal catheters is 7 cm from the midline[140] along the inferior border of the angle of the chosen rib. Catheters have been placed in the intercostal space for continuous intercostal analgesia for up to 6 days.[142] Twenty milliliters of bupivacaine 0.25% to 0.5% with epinephrine 1:200,000 may be given as an initial bolus injection, with subsequent infusions of bupivacaine 0.25% with epinephrine 1:200,000 at an initial rate of 10 mL/h.[143] The insertion site for paravertebral catheters is 3 to 4 cm from the midline at the inferior border of the chosen rib. One 15-mL injection of local anesthetic is reportedly effective in covering four intercostal spaces.[144] Dosing and agents used for the paravertebral approach to intercostal nerve block are similar to those used for continuous intercostal catheters except for initial infusion rates of 5 mL/h.

Intercostal nerve block with local anesthetics is a safe and effective means of achieving effective post-thoracotomy analgesia without central respiratory depression. Sabanathan et al[138] randomized 56 patients undergoing thoracotomy to receive continuous intercostal catheter infusions of either bupivacaine or saline in a masked (double-blind) study design. Analgesia was better in the bupivacaine group, and there were no complications related to the infusions. Continuous intercostal block significantly decreased the early loss of postoperative pulmonary function. In their series, maximal decrease of forced vital capacity, 1-s forced expiratory volume, and peak expiratory flow rate at 24 h was 56%, 60%, and 57%, respectively, of preoperative control values in the bupivacaine group versus 25%, 30%, and 32%, respectively, in the control group. Restoration of respiratory function was also faster in the bupivacaine group. Other investigators[139] have found no difference in pulmonary function for post-thoracotomy patients who received bupivacaine intercostally compared with saline intercostally or opioids intramuscularly. Continuous extrapleural intercostal block is as effective as lumbar epidural administration of morphine in decreasing post-thoracotomy pain and restoring pulmonary function without unwanted opioid side effects.[135] Although early studies[145] showed cryoanalgesia to be effective for post-thoracotomy pain management, later studies[141] demonstrated that addition of cryoanalgesia to conventional pain regimens provided no significant decrease in either postoperative pain or analgesic requirements. Cardiovascular effects from intercostal nerve block with bupivacaine are negligible when total dosage of local anesthetic is within recommended ranges. However, peripheral vasodilation, bradycardia, and cardiac depression may result in the presence of high serum concentrations of local anesthetics. Systemic absorption of epinephrine may also result in β-adrenergic effects. These effects may have deleterious consequences in patients who have ischemic heart disease or who are catecholamine-sensitive. An upper limit has been suggested for the dose of epinephrine—0.2 mg.[140]

Pneumothorax can complicate intercostal nerve block, with a reported incidence ranging from less than 0.1% to 2% in some studies to 19% in others.[146] Most pneumothoraces are asymptomatic and detected on follow-up chest radiographs. Treatment of pneumothorax ranges from observation for asymptomatic lesions to needle aspiration or thoracostomy tube placement for more clinically significant abnormalities. Because of minimal interference with pulmonary function, intercostal nerve blocks have been used in patients with coexisting pulmonary disease to provide effective analgesia. However, the benefits of intercostal nerve block must be weighed against the risk of pneumothorax or loss of expiratory muscle tone in patients with borderline pulmonary function. Local anesthetic systemic blood concentrations are higher after intercostal nerve block (compared with epidural, caudal, sciatic-femoral, and brachial plexus nerve blocks).[147] Neuraxial spread of local anesthetics resulting in subarachnoid or epidural anesthesia after paravertebral block is possible because the paravertebral space communicates medially with the epidural space. Profound hypotension, presumably as a result of unintentional epidural or spinal block, has been reported[148] after surgeon-performed intrathoracic intercostal nerve block. Formation of a flank hematoma has also been reported[149] with continuous intercostal analgesia. Problems associated with cryoanalgesia of intercostal nerves include the development of long-term neuralgias necessitating chronic analgesic treatments and the potential for cold damage to the surrounding tissues.

Interpleural Analgesia

Introduction of a catheter into the space between the parietal and visceral pleura to administer local an-

esthesia for perioperative analgesia was first described in 1984 by Kvalheim and Reiestad.[150] The mechanism of action of interpleural anesthetics is not entirely clear. Diffusion of interpleural local anesthetic to block intercostal nerves, splanchnic nerves, epidural space, or spinal nerves has been proposed as a possible mechanism. The usual recommended drug regimen is 20 to 30 mL of bupivacaine 0.25% to 0.5% as intermittent injections every 4 to 6 h.[143] The addition of epinephrine 1:200,000 may decrease mean peak plasma levels of bupivacaine.[151] High plasma concentrations of local anesthetic can occur with both bupivacaine and lidocaine.[152, 153]

Reports of the efficacy of interpleural analgesia are conflicting. Preoperative interpleural administration of sufentanil, 50 μg, was shown[154] to be as effective as interpleural administration of 0.5% bupivacaine with epinephrine in decreasing intraoperative analgesic requirements. In contrast, bupivacaine given interpleurally did not decrease intraoperative isoflurane requirements.[155] Postoperative analgesia appears to be unpredictable after this technique, with reported efficacy ranging from effective to inadequate.[151, 153] Advocates of interpleural analgesia argue that success in achieving adequate analgesia depends on correct catheter placement, proper patient positioning, and prevention of local anesthetic loss via thoracostomy drainage tubes. Discrepancies in the efficacy of interpleural analgesia among studies may be a result of failure to achieve any or all of these conditions. Except for a modest, nonsustained improvement in forced vital capacity noted in one study,[153] interpleural analgesia has not been shown to offer any advantage in terms of restoration of pulmonary function compared with intravenous[132] or intramuscular[156] administration of opioids. Interpleural analgesia is associated with a 2% incidence of pneumothorax. Local anesthetic systemic toxicity, infection, iatrogenic pleural effusions, and Horner's syndrome have also been reported[157] after use of this technique.

Cardiac Surgery: Regional Techniques

Advocates of regional techniques suggest that the benefits seen during noncardiac surgery may also be provided for cardiac surgical patients (Table 29–2). Use of epidural and intrathecal techniques for intraoperative anesthesia (combined with general anesthesia) or postoperative analgesia (or both) has been described in patients with normal to moderately impaired left ventricular function (ejection fraction > 40%) undergoing coronary artery bypass graft surgery. Neuraxial administration of opioids,[100, 158–164] local anesthet-

Table 29–2 Benefits of Regional Anesthesia for Cardiac Surgery

Good postoperative analgesia
Early awakening
Hemodynamic stability
Early extubation
Attenuation of the perioperative stress response

ics,[16, 165, 166] and opioids combined with local anesthetics[167–169] has been described. The use of continuous intercostal analgesia after cardiac surgery has also been reported.[149] Opioids or local anesthetics (or both) given epidurally have been administered via the caudal, lumbar, or thoracic routes. In the literature, timing of epidural catheter placement for cardiac surgery ranges from 1[158] to 24 h[16, 165, 167–169] before heparinization and 20 to 24 h[100] after operation. Coagulation status was normal before catheter placement in all of these studies. Rosen and Rosen[164] administered morphine as a caudal epidural single shot to pediatric patients at the end of uncomplicated cardiac surgery when the activated clotting time was within 10% of control and when there was no clinical evidence of coagulopathy or neurologic sequelae. The trend toward same-day admission of cardiac surgical patients does not allow catheter placement far in advance of heparinization, and even when epidural catheters are placed hours before heparinization, catheters may still migrate. Ruff and Dougherty[170] found that delaying anticoagulation for at least 1 h after lumbar puncture could decrease the risk of spinal hematoma development.

Liem and colleagues[167] reported on 54 patients with normal to moderately impaired left ventricular function undergoing coronary artery bypass grafting who were randomized to receive high thoracic epidural analgesia with bupivacaine 0.375% plus sufentanil 5 μg/mL combined with a light general anesthetic of midazolam and nitrous oxide or a general anesthetic consisting of high-dose sufentanil (mean total 15 μg/kg) with midazolam. They found that 5 of 27 patients in the general anesthetic group required dopamine to treat a low cardiac index, compared with 0 of 27 patients in the thoracic epidural analgesia group (*P* < .05). Patients in the general anesthetic group also required significantly more sodium nitroprusside to treat hypertension. No patient in the thoracic epidural analgesia group exhibited electrocardiographic evidence of prebypass myocardial ischemia, whereas four patients in the general anesthetic group had ischemia. The authors concluded that hemodynamic stability was at least as good or better in the thoracic epidural analgesia group. Coronary artery bypass grafting during thoracic epidural analgesia combined with general anesthesia is well tolerated by patients on chronic therapy with β-adrenergic blockers.

Stenseth and coworkers[16] investigated the influence of thoracic epidural block alone and in combination with general anesthesia on cardiovascular function and myocardial metabolism in patients receiving therapy with β-adrenergic blockers and undergoing coronary artery bypass grafting. Eighteen patients with left ventricular ejection fraction greater than 0.5 received a T-1 to T-12 epidural block and were subsequently randomized into a low-dose fentanyl (5 μg/kg) or higher-dose fentanyl (30 μg/kg) group as part of their general anesthetic. Crystalloid was infused to maintain filling pressures at the preinduction level. Induction of epidural analgesia in well-sedated patients who had received β-adrenergic blockers did not result in clinically significant cardiovascular effects. Subsequent induction of general anesthesia was also without problem except for an increase in heart rate and coronary vascular resistance in the low-dose fentanyl group and minor myocardial depression in the high-dose fentanyl group.

Casey and associates[162] randomized 40 patients scheduled for coronary artery bypass grafting to receive either intrathecal administration of morphine 0.02 mg/kg or isotonic saline after induction of general anesthesia. General anesthesia consisted of 40 μg/kg fentanyl with enflurane supplementation. The investigators found that addition of morphine given intrathecally did not improve hemodynamic stability or decrease enflurane requirements during operation. Vanstrum et al[161] confirmed this finding in another randomized, prospective, masked (double-blind) study. In their study, the addition of 0.5 mg morphine given intrathecally to a sufentanil (7 μg/kg), diazepam, and isoflurane general anesthetic did not result in a difference in the numbers of patients requiring either isoflurane supplementation or vasodilator drugs.

The first reported use of postoperative regional analgesia for cardiac surgery was published by Mathews and Abrams in 1980.[159] They presented retrospective data on intrathecal administration of morphine in 40 patients undergoing coronary artery bypass grafting. All patients were pain-free during the first 27 h postoperatively and had satisfactory recoveries. Since then, two randomized, masked (double-blind) trials using standardized general anesthetics have reported conflicting outcomes. Casey and associates[162] found no difference in postoperative analgesic, sedative, or vasodilator requirements, whereas Vanstrum et al[161] found no difference in quality of analgesia, but patients receiving 0.5 mg morphine intrathecally required significantly less supplemental morphine given intravenously during the first 24 h postoperatively and also required less sodium nitroprusside during the first 24 h. Liem et al[167] found that patients receiving thoracic epidural analgesia with a light general anesthetic had significantly better analgesia and sedation scores for the first 72 h postoperatively compared with patients who received high-dose sufentanil general anesthetic with intermittent intravenous administration of opioid. Fitzpatrick and Moriarty[160] randomized 44 patients undergoing coronary artery bypass grafting during a primary inhalation general anesthetic to receive either 30 mg morphine intravenously or 1 to 2 mg morphine intrathecally. The patients who received morphine intrathecally as a supplement had a significantly better quality of analgesia and required significantly less supplemental postoperative analgesics than the group given morphine intravenously.

The addition of morphine given epidurally to a primary inhalation general anesthetic for open heart surgery has been studied in adults and in children. El-Baz and Goldin[158] were the first to publish a prospective, randomized study of postoperative analgesia in 30 patients who received an epidural infusion of morphine at 0.1 mg/h compared with a control group of 30 patients who received morphine intravenously at 2 mg/2 h and on demand. Effective analgesia with minimal side effects was achieved in 80% of patients receiving morphine epidurally compared with only 50% of patients receiving postoperative morphine intravenously. Although patients in the epidural group required occasional analgesic supplementation intravenously, the mean dose of morphine used in this group of patients was significantly lower than that used in the control group. These findings were confirmed by Rosen and Rosen[164] in pediatric patients randomized to single-shot, caudal epidural administration of morphine 0.075 mg/kg at the end of cardiac surgical procedures. The treated patients had significantly lower pain scores and used significantly less morphine given intravenously than patients who did not receive morphine epidurally.

Cardiac surgical patients receiving high-dose opioid general anesthetic supplemented with morphine given intrathecally showed no difference in extubation times.[161, 162] However, supplementation of inhalation or light general anesthetic techniques with neuraxial local anesthetics (with or without opioids) does allow for earlier extubation compared with patients who receive inhalation or high-dose opioid techniques followed by postoperative analgesia with opioid given intravenously.[158, 160, 168] Liem et al[168] reported the postoperative use of an epidural infusion of 0.125% bupivacaine with 1:100,000 sufentanil and found that patients who received epidural analgesia awoke sooner, resumed spontaneous respiration more quickly, were extubated earlier, and had significantly better partial pressure of alveolar oxygen with less respiratory depression for the first 72 h than did patients in a general anesthetic only group. Joachimsson and associates[165] demonstrated that cardiac surgery patients receiving thoracic epidural anesthesia with 0.5% bupivacaine plus intraoperative general anesthesia with enflurane were extubated within the first 2 h postoperatively after rewarming without increasing metabolic or ventilatory requirements.

Liem and colleagues[168] and Vanstrum and coworkers[161] reported that patients who underwent coronary artery bypass grafting during neuraxial analgesia had improved postoperative hemodynamic stability, as demonstrated by decreased requirements for postoperative cardiac medications compared with a control group. However, cardiac outcomes (myocardial infarction, death) were not different between groups in these two studies, perhaps because of small group sizes. Surprisingly, patients who received thoracic epidural analgesia plus general anesthesia for coronary artery bypass grafting have had no difference in fluid retention compared with patients who received general anesthetic only.[166] Finally, continuous epidural infusions of opioids with and without local anesthetics have been associated with a decrease in postoperative surgical stress, as reflected by serum cortisol, β-endorphin, and epinephrine levels.[158, 169] Etiology of the stress response inhibition by regional analgesia is multifactorial; the inhibition might be caused by local anesthetic-induced sympathectomy, pain relief, or earlier extubation.

In summary, the quality of analgesia afforded by regional techniques, an associated hemodynamic sta-

bility, earlier awakening, earlier extubation, and attenuation of the perioperative stress response may all improve outcomes after cardiac surgery. However, reports of use of regional anesthesia and analgesia for cardiac surgery are few and it is not known whether the addition of regional techniques to a standardized general anesthetic confers additional intraoperative or postoperative benefits compared with general anesthetic alone.

Carotid Surgery: Regional Techniques

There is no consensus regarding the ideal regional anesthetic technique for carotid endarterectomy. Deep and superficial cervical plexus block (Fig. 29–8),[171–180] cervical epidural block,[181–183] and local anesthetic infiltration[184–188] have all been used successfully for carotid endarterectomy. Light sedation, consisting of incremental doses of small amounts of a benzodiazepine and an opioid, such as midazolam and fentanyl, is generally used to maintain a cooperative but coherent patient during the procedure. The advantages of regional anesthesia for carotid artery surgery include functional intraoperative monitoring of neurologic status, fewer cardiopulmonary complications,[171, 173, 175, 178] and decreased hospital costs.[171, 173, 177, 187] Myocardial infarction is the leading cause of mortality after carotid endarterectomy, with a reported incidence of perioperative myocardial infarction ranging from 0% to 35%.[189] The incidence of perioperative stroke ranges from 3% to 6%.[171] Thus, the goals of successful anesthetic management include prevention of cardiac and cerebral ischemia.

Perioperative strokes associated with carotid endarterectomy are a result of cerebral ischemia, thromboembolic phenomena, or reperfusion injury.[174] Of patients who undergo carotid endarterectomy, 10% to 24% experience temporary cerebral ischemia as a result of cross-clamping of the carotid artery.[174, 179] Insertion of an intraluminal carotid artery shunt is one method to protect the brain, but placement of a shunt is not benign. Shunts make operation technically more difficult and have complications, including microembolization, intimal dissection, and thrombosis within the shunt.[174] Direct neurologic evaluation of an awake patient, electroencephalographic monitoring, and internal carotid artery back pressure (stump pressure) all assess cerebral perfusion during carotid endarterectomy, whereas regional cerebral blood flow, jugular venous oxygen saturation, and somatosensory-evoked potentials are used less often.

A significant decrease in intraoperative shunting during carotid endarterectomy occurs when direct neurologic assessment during regional anesthesia is used.[171, 178] Evans et al[186] studied the optimal cerebral monitor during 134 carotid artery procedures during local anesthesia. Neurologic assessment of the awake patient, electroencephalographic monitoring, and stump pressures were evaluated. The decision to insert a shunt was based solely on the development of a neurologic deficit during cross-clamping. Thirteen pa-

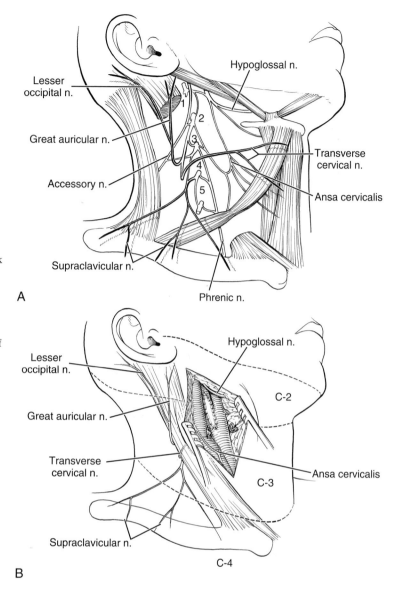

Figure 29–8 *A,* Functional anatomy of the cervical plexus–ventral rami of C-1 to C-5. *B,* Cervical plexus block for carotid endarterectomy. Cutaneous analgesia of the neck from the mandible to the clavicle (anteriorly and laterally) can be achieved by local anesthetic block of the superficial cervical plexus at the midpoint of the posterior border of the sternocleidomastoid muscle. Deep cervical plexus block of C-2 to C-4 provides profound relaxation and anesthesia of the muscles and other deep structures of the neck within this distribution. n., nerve.

tients (9.7%) had shunts placed to reverse neurologic deficits with cross-clamping. Of these patients, four had no electroencephalographic changes. On the other hand, significant electroencephalographic changes were found in 13 of 121 patients who did not have neurologic changes. Stump pressures proved to be unreliable in terms of sensitivity and specificity. The authors concluded that carotid artery clamping in the awake patient was the most reliable indicator for shunt placement. A collaborative, prospective study of 1200 carotid endarterectomies during local anesthesia by Hafner and Evans[185] confirmed these findings. In this series, 9% of patients (113 of 1200) required shunting based on new neurologic deficits during cross-clamping, whereas 86% of patients (343 of 401) with stump pressures less than 50 mm Hg would have been shunted unnecessarily. Again, assessment of the awake patient was the most reliable indicator of the need for shunting.

Evaluation of neurologic function during regional anesthesia may also identify patients at greater risk of

permanent neurologic dysfunction developing. Davies and associates[179] found that patients who had intraoperative neurologic changes with carotid artery cross-clamping had a sixfold increase in the incidence of postoperative stroke compared with patients who had no intraoperative changes (increased risk from 1.1% to 6.6%). Identification of this high-risk group may allow institution of therapy to improve outcome, such as admission to an intensive care unit, thrombolytic therapy, or early surgical exploration.

Several retrospective reviews of carotid endarterectomy during regional anesthesia have evaluated cardiovascular effects. Prough and coworkers[176] reviewed 185 carotid procedures performed during superficial cervical block on 153 patients. No patient sustained a perioperative myocardial infarction. Lee and colleagues[180] reported that after 305 carotid endarterectomies during superficial cervical plexus block, none of the 280 patients had a perioperative myocardial infarction within the first 30 postoperative days. Allen et al[171] retrospectively analyzed data on 584 consecutive patients undergoing 679 carotid endarterectomies during either cervical plexus block or general anesthesia. They found that regional anesthesia was associated with a significant reduction in operative time, use of a carotid artery shunt, and postoperative cardiopulmonary complications. Nine patients in the general anesthesia group had a myocardial infarction, compared with two in the regional anesthesia group. It appears that regional anesthesia for carotid endarterectomy is safe in patients with coronary artery disease and may even be associated with a lower risk of myocardial infarction compared with general anesthesia.

Reports of perioperative hemodynamics during carotid endarterectomy with regional anesthesia vary. Muskett and coworkers[173] found no significant difference between regional and general anesthesia groups in terms of perioperative blood pressures or need for intravenous pressor or antihypertensive medications. Forssell et al[184] found higher intraoperative blood pressures in a local anesthesia group, compared with a general anesthesia group, in a randomized, prospective study of 101 carotid endarterectomies. Takolander and associates[172] also reported that local anesthesia was associated with a hypertensive blood pressure response whereas general anesthesia frequently was associated with a hypotensive response in their series of 75 carotid endarterectomies. They found the hypertensive response exhibited by the local anesthesia group was associated with higher arterial plasma catecholamine concentrations. Awake patients having an operation may experience emotional stress that is not blocked by the regional anesthesia. In contrast, Corson et al[175] found that perioperative blood pressure was unstable significantly longer in a general anesthesia group (mean, 24.6 h) compared with the regional anesthesia group (mean, 2.1 h). Vasoactive drugs were also required for significantly longer periods in the general anesthesia group (mean, 12.6 h compared with 3.6 h). Finally, Goeau-Brissonniere and colleagues[188] compared the effects of cervical plexus block with cervical epidural block in a series of 85 carotid endarterectomies. The only difference between the groups in terms of perioperative events and analgesia was that intraoperative hypotension was significantly more frequent in the epidural anesthesia group. In their series, Bonnet et al[181] found that patients receiving cervical epidural block for carotid endarterectomy had a 10.9% incidence of hypotension and a 2.8% incidence of bradycardia requiring treatment.

Several studies have evaluated the cost-effectiveness of carotid endarterectomy performed during regional anesthesia. Godin et al[177] prospectively studied 100 patients receiving either general anesthesia ($n = 50$) or cervical plexus block ($n = 50$). Patients in the regional anesthesia group saved 54.5% in total hospital room costs alone, without an increase in mortality or morbidity rates. The decreased requirement for intensive care unit time and shorter postoperative hospitalization, resulting in cost savings, have been confirmed in studies by Muskett et al,[173] Gabelman and associates,[187] and Allen and coworkers.[171] Patients who required a second carotid endarterectomy for contralateral disease

almost universally chose to repeat the regional anesthetic.

Complications of regional anesthesia for carotid endarterectomy are rare but serious. Injection into the vertebral artery may result in seizures or loss of consciousness. Intrathecal injection with resultant total spinal anesthetic and direct cord trauma are possible complications. Unilateral phrenic nerve block or bilateral phrenic nerve block from epidural injection may result in respiratory insufficiency and the need for assisted ventilation. Epidural block may also result in hypotension and bradycardia associated with impairment in baroreceptor sensitivity. In addition, a criticism of using regional anesthesia for carotid endarterectomy is the possibility of inducing a general anesthetic under less than optimum conditions if the patient becomes neurologically unstable during the procedure. Factors other than technical facility with regional blocks are required to ensure a successful regional anesthetic for carotid endarterectomy: proper patient selection, surgeon acceptance of an awake patient, and good communication between surgeon and anesthesiologist. Patients selected for awake carotid endarterectomy should be cooperative and capable of understanding potential intraoperative events. Patients with difficult anatomy—i.e., short, thick necks or distal carotid artery lesions—may be hard to manage with a regional technique.

Abdominal Aortic and Lower Extremity Vascular Surgery: Regional Techniques

Intrathecal Techniques

Although spinal anesthesia can be used to supplement general anesthesia for intra-abdominal vascular surgery, it has several drawbacks. First, a relatively rapid onset of sympathetic block with local anesthetics may create a more profound hypotension. Second, for the block to provide effective anesthesia, it must reach a sensory dermatomal level that may be difficult to attain with accuracy. Finally, continuously placed spinal catheters are not yet widely accepted as a technique for repetitive dosing of medications into the subarachnoid space in these patients. These factors act to limit use of spinal anesthesia for procedures that may require prolonged operating times and also limit use of spinal techniques for postoperative analgesia after intra-abdominal procedures.

In contrast to intra-abdominal surgery, spinal anesthesia is often an excellent option for infrainguinal vascular surgery. Because blood flow to the affected extremity is usually limited, hemodynamic instability may be minimal if the block does not progress cephalad to the extent required for intra-abdominal surgery. Cook et al[190] randomized 101 patients to receive either general anesthesia with thiopental, fentanyl, nitrous oxide, oxygen, and muscle relaxant or a hyperbaric spinal anesthetic with dibucaine and epinephrine. Not surprisingly, the incidence of intraoperative hypotension was greater in the spinal anesthesia group (72%)

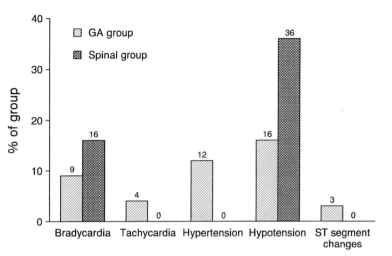

Figure 29–9 Intraoperative hemodynamics during general (GA) or spinal anesthesia for lower extremity revascularization. Bradycardia and hypotension were more common in the group who received spinal anesthesia, whereas hypertension and tachycardia were observed exclusively in patients who received general anesthesia. Numbers are numbers of patients. (Redrawn from Cook PT, Davies MJ, Cronin KD, et al: A prospective randomised trial comparing spinal anaesthesia using hyperbaric cinchocaine with general anaesthesia for lower limb vascular surgery. Anaesth Intensive Care 1986; 14: 373–380.)

compared with the general anesthesia group (31%), whereas hypertension was observed exclusively in the group that received general anesthesia (Fig. 29–9). Bradycardia was also more common in the group that received regional anesthesia (16%) compared with the general anesthesia group (9%). This study points out the potential advantage of regional techniques for control of the rate-pressure product as well as the possible disadvantages of hypotension with decreased arterial perfusion pressure.

Spinal analgesia for pain control after major intra-abdominal vascular surgery does not have the same limitations as spinal anesthesia. Spinal analgesic agents, especially opioids given spinally, have been effectively used for control of pain after intra-abdominal vascular surgery. An agent such as morphine with low lipophilicity can provide effective pain control of sufficient duration to be clinically useful but without hemodynamic effects. Intrathecal administration of morphine for abdominal aortic surgery improves the quality of analgesia in the early postoperative period. Davis[191] compared the hemodynamic effects of 600 μg morphine given intrathecally before abdominal aortic surgery with the effects of intravenous administration of opioids. In this study of 25 patients, no significant differences were found between study groups with regard to intraoperative pulse, blood pressure, or rate-pressure product. However, there was a clear improvement in early postoperative pain control and a decrease in opioid usage in patients who received morphine intrathecally (Fig. 29–10). Patients who received morphine intrathecally required virtually no opioids systemically during the first 24 h postoperatively, and a higher percentage of these patients were free of pain during the first 24 h postoperatively. This finding is significant because the early postoperative period tends to be a time of instability after abdominal aortic surgery and consistent pain control during emergence is a valuable and important intervention.

Epidural Techniques

Compared with spinal anesthesia, epidural anesthesia has been more extensively studied as a technique to care for patients who require both intra-abdominal and infrainguinal vascular surgery. Epidural anesthesia can control the neuroendocrine response to major operation, limit use of opioids, and improve the quality of postoperative pain control. The principal advantages of epidural anesthesia compared with spinal anesthesia include the ability to titrate medications through a catheter, to change or modify medication, and to continue medication administration for hours or days after operation during the time when patients are at highest risk of morbidity.

Even if an epidural catheter is used for postoperative analgesia only, it is more easily inserted before induction when the patient is able to cooperate with positioning and to report pain or paresthesia. Although the interspace chosen for insertion depends on the patient's anatomy, the goal should be to locate the catheter as close to the incisional dermatomes as possible. This usually means catheter placement in the low thoracic region for abdominal aortic surgery to afford optimal

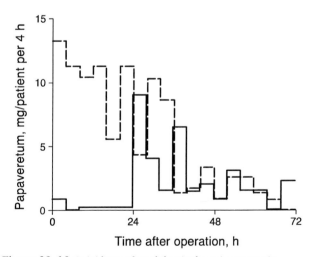

Figure 29–10 Opioid use after abdominal aortic surgery in patients who received 0.8 mg preoperative morphine intrathecally (solid line) compared with a similar group of patients who received no morphine intrathecally (dashed line). (Redrawn from Davis I: Intrathecal morphine in aortic aneurysm surgery. Anaesthesia 1987; 42: 491–497.)

pain control while minimizing the effects of a sympathetic block and the requirement for larger doses and volumes of local anesthetic. A retroperitoneal approach to the aorta, which may have some advantages with regard to surgery and surgical recovery,[192] should not prevent use of an epidural catheter.

One of the primary considerations with use of epidural anesthesia during major vascular surgery is the effects on cardiovascular function. These may be due to a direct effect of circulating local anesthetics, to indirect effects secondary to diminished catecholamine circulation, or to alterations in reflex neural control of cardiovascular function. Epidural anesthesia should be initiated with small increments of local anesthetic to help minimize unwanted cardiovascular effects. One useful technique to minimize hemodynamic alterations is to establish a band of sensory analgesia with local anesthetic before induction to ensure that the catheter is functioning; then, proceed with induction of general anesthesia and complete the administration of local anesthetic after general anesthesia induction. There are other maneuvers that may avoid or attenuate large fluctuations in cardiovascular performance. Awareness of patients at risk is the first step. Many vascular surgery patients have either untreated or poorly treated hypertension that places them at risk for hemodynamic instability during anesthesia induction. Patients should take their regularly scheduled antihypertensive medications the morning of the procedure. β-Adrenergic blockers or adrenergic blocking drugs[193] can help control the hyperdynamic response to anesthesia induction.

Hypotension may also be a problem. Vascular surgical patients often do not tolerate routine induction doses of agents such as thiopental without hypotension developing. If another drug that routinely causes tachycardia (e.g., pancuronium) is also administered, this can create a dangerous combination of tachycardia and hypotension with a high likelihood of inducing myocardial ischemia. Thiopental should be titrated in small increments and used for amnesia, not as a complete induction agent. Supplemental doses of a rapid-acting, potent opioid, such as fentanyl, sufentanil, or alfentanil, before or during induction help create an adequate anesthetic depth without necessitating prolonged postoperative mechanical ventilation. Etomidate is a useful alternative to thiopental because it causes less cardiovascular depression. Although it does inhibit adrenal steroid genesis, this is transient if the drug is used for induction only.[194]

Maintenance of adequate intravascular volume is important for patients who receive epidural anesthesia during abdominal aortic surgery because hemodynamic stability is improved with volume loading.[1, 195, 196] However, surgeons and intensivists who provide postoperative care for vascular surgery patients have justifiable concerns regarding large-volume crystalloid infusions and their potential cardiopulmonary effects after operation. For this reason, it seems reasonable to try to limit crystalloid replacement by using catecholamine infusions to maintain perfusion pressure and cardiac output, as long as the effects of vasopressors are carefully monitored and adjusted. The issue of whether crystalloid or colloid is the preferred solution for intravascular volume replacement remains unresolved. Interest has focused on the use of hypertonic saline as a potential resuscitation fluid during abdominal aortic surgery.[197, 198] This approach may allow for some limitation of total crystalloid infusion, although the role of hypertonic solutions during epidural anesthesia and abdominal aortic procedures has not been defined. During peritoneal exploration, some patients appear to undergo release of vasoactive mediators from the mesenteric circulation.[199] This can result in significant hypotension that may be more severe during epidural anesthesia.[4] It is difficult to predict which patients will manifest the reaction, but it can result in profound hypotension that requires vigorous treatment with fluids, vasopressors, or both.

Epidural anesthesia is widely used for infrainguinal vascular surgery.[200] With continuous catheter techniques, a relatively low epidural block can be maintained with excellent anesthetic results and minimal hemodynamic disturbance. One difficulty with this technique is the occasional prolonged operative procedure. Although these patients are often elderly and require only minimal sedation, they may become difficult to manage during prolonged procedures. A propofol infusion can be useful in this situation because of its short duration of action that allows for rapid titration to the desired effect. A loading dose is generally unnecessary if the patient is already sedated, and infusions are usually effective at doses of 25 to 50 μg/kg/min.

Epidural analgesia is an excellent pain control technique after major vascular procedures. Although early studies evaluated single injections of opioids, usually morphine,[10, 201] continuous infusions minimize gaps in analgesic coverage and decrease the need for repetitive dosing. Infusions also minimize side effects such as local anesthetic–induced vasodilation and opioid-induced respiratory depression, both of which can result from bolus dosing. There is some experimental and clinical evidence that early, prophylactic administration of analgesic agents helps prevent creation of neuroexcitatory circuits—the preemptive analgesia hypothesis.[202] Regardless of whether or not excitation circuits exist acutely, continuous pain control creates a smoother emergence from anesthesia with less hemodynamic disturbance. The use of combination mixtures of dilute local anesthetics, usually bupivacaine, with opioids, either fentanyl or morphine, provides effective analgesia. Epidural administration of fentanyl has the advantage of rapid onset and less cephalad migration in the cerebrospinal fluid. Probably the easiest technique for avoidance of gaps in postoperative analgesia is to initiate an analgesic infusion near the end of the operative procedure, although if preemptive concepts are adhered to, the infusion may be more effective if initiated before the surgical incision.

Clinical Effects and Outcomes After Abdominal Aortic Surgery

Epidural anesthesia during abdominal aortic procedures clearly decreases the determinants of myocardial oxygen consumption, which may be beneficial in patients with symptomatic coronary artery disease. However, it is important to remember that these same factors also determine global cardiac performance or cardiac output. Decreased cardiac performance with epidural anesthesia during abdominal aortic surgery has been documented.[8] This effect can be used to benefit patients at risk of myocardial ischemia, but it may be necessary to compensate for decreased cardiac performance with vasoactive medications.

Does epidural anesthesia have a favorable effect on cardiac events during or after abdominal aortic procedures? Reiz et al[203] studied this question in a group of patients scheduled for abdominal aortic procedures, all of whom had suffered a recent myocardial infarction. Patients were randomized to either a combined technique of epidural anesthesia with light general anesthesia or a general anesthetic. The study evaluated various indicators of myocardial ischemia and found that the group receiving epidural anesthesia had a markedly decreased incidence of ischemia during operation. Most episodes of ischemia in the epidural treatment group occurred during tracheal intubation and extubation (Table 29–3). This study showed that thoracic epidural anesthesia can have an independent and favorable effect on myocardial ischemia during abdominal aortic surgery. The study also raises the important question of what the ischemia incidence would be in a control group treated by protocol for control of cardiac function with use of nitrates or β-blockers. It appears that epidural anesthesia is one way to control myocardial ischemia during abdominal aortic procedures, although there are other techniques or approaches that may be just as beneficial.

In order to study the effect of epidural anesthesia on postoperative cardiac morbidity, Baron et al[13] studied 173 patients scheduled for abdominal aortic procedures who were randomized to either general anesthesia or

Table 29–4 Mortality and Major Postoperative Cardiac Morbidity

OUTCOME	NUMBER OF PATIENTS*	
	Group 1	Group 2
Mortality	4	3
Cardiac complications†	22	19
Myocardial infarction	5	5
Congestive heart failure	7	5
Prolonged myocardial ischemia	16	16
Ventricular tachyarrhythmia	0	1

*Group 1, general anesthesia; group 2, thoracic epidural anesthesia in combination with light general anesthesia.
†Number of patients with at least one cardiac complication.
Data from Baron JF, Bertrand M, Barré E, et al.: Combined epidural and general anesthesia versus general anesthesia for abdominal aortic surgery. Anesthesiology 1991; 75: 611–618.

combined epidural anesthesia and general anesthesia. Patients in both groups had a careful preoperative cardiac evaluation, and the groups were comparable. After operation, the incidence of cardiac events was the same in both groups (Table 29–4). Importantly, postoperative analgesia was not controlled by protocol in this study, so that a potential independent effect of epidural analgesia was not evaluated. The conclusion from these studies is that intraoperative use of epidural anesthesia during abdominal aortic surgery does not appear to have an independent effect on cardiac morbidity that is superior to other treatment options, as long as careful attention is paid to myocardial function during and after operation.

The question of how use of epidural analgesia after abdominal aortic surgery may contribute to postoperative recovery and morbidity is complicated because of the many contributing variables. An early outcome study[204] of epidural anesthesia and epidural analgesia in a group of high-risk surgical patients, about half of whom underwent abdominal aortic surgery, found a decrease in the incidence of cardiac complications, especially congestive heart failure, in the patient group managed with epidural anesthesia and analgesia (Table 29–5). Because the data from Baron et al[13] strongly suggest that intraoperative use of epidural anesthesia

Table 29–3 Effect of Thoracic Epidural Anesthesia on Incidence of Intraoperative Myocardial Ischemia

VARIABLE	NLA (n = 22)		ED + LIGHT BALANCED ANESTHESIA* (n = 23)	
	No.	%	No.	%
Mean pulmonary arteriolar occlusion pressure ≥ 18 mm Hg	16	73	4	17
Decrease in coronary vascular resistance by ≥ 25%	13	59	3	13
Increase in myocardial oxygen consumption ≥ 25%	22	100	1	4
Hypoxanthine production	9	41	1	4
ST-T segment depression ≥ 1 mm	11	50	3	13
Ventricular arrhythmias	8	36	2	8

*All $P < .001$ compared with NLA.
ED, epidural; NLA, neuroleptanesthesia.
From Reiz S, Bålfors E, Sørensen MB, et al.: Coronary hemodynamic effects of general anesthesia and surgery: modification by epidural anesthesia in patients with ischemic heart disease. Reg Anesth 1982; 7(Suppl): S8–S18.

Table 29–5 Overall Morbidity From Cardiac Complications

COMPLICATION	NUMBER OF PATIENTS*	
	Group I	Group II
Myocardial infarction	0	3
Congestive heart failure	1	10
Ventricular tachyarrhythmia	1	0
Supraventricular tachyarrhythmia	2†	4
Angina	0	1
Heart block	0	1

*Group I, epidural anesthesia and analgesia; group II, general anesthesia and standard analgesia.
†One of these complications was in a patient with a nonfunctioning epidural catheter.
Data from Yeager MP, Glass DD, Neff RK, et al.: Epidural anesthesia and analgesia in high-risk surgical patients. Anesthesiology 1987; 66: 729–736.

does not affect postoperative cardiac morbidity, it may be that these results were due primarily to postoperative epidural analgesia. This was a relatively small study and not specifically limited to abdominal aortic surgery patients. In another study,[68] 80 patients undergoing major vascular operations were randomized to either general anesthesia and systemic analgesia with opioids or epidural anesthesia and postoperative epidural analgesia. The investigators found a significant decrease in cardiovascular morbidity after operation in the patients who received epidural anesthesia and analgesia (Table 29–6). In this study, the decreased incidence of cardiac events was also associated with a decrease in postoperative hypercoagulability assessed by thromboelastography, which suggests that enhanced platelet aggregation may contribute to cardiac complications after major operation. This study suggested that effective epidural analgesia after high-risk operation, especially vascular surgery, may have a measurable effect on postoperative cardiac complications, although further clinical studies are still needed.

There is evidence that use of epidural analgesia after intra-abdominal operation can improve postoperative pulmonary function.[112, 205, 206] Although use of epidural or spinal anesthesia may have some benefits as a result of limitation of sedative medications during operation, this effect is likely to be transient. Regional analgesia not only improves pulmonary function in the early postoperative period but also can return pulmonary function to normal earlier.[206] Epidural analgesia with local anesthetic improves diaphragmatic function after abdominal aortic procedures, even when patients have received systemic analgesia with opioids titrated to effective pain relief.[112] The question of whether or not these effects translate into fewer postoperative complications has not been settled completely. Several studies[205] have reported fewer postoperative pulmonary complications after major operation when epidural analgesia is used for postoperative pain control. However, this has not been a consistent finding. For example, Jayr and associates[207] studied 153 patients after major abdominal surgery and found no effect of epidural

anesthesia and analgesia on postoperative pulmonary complications. One explanation for this finding may be that the study participants had a relatively low mean age of 55 to 60 years and a relatively low incidence of preexisting respiratory disease. It appears that epidural anesthesia and analgesia may be effective in decreasing postoperative pulmonary complications, but only in patients at high risk of postoperative pulmonary dysfunction.

Finally, regional techniques can alter the neuroendocrine response to major operation. This is a well-documented effect that is slowly making the transition from an interesting phenomenon with uncertain implications to a consistent finding with documented clinical benefits. For example, Breslow et al[10] reported that a single epidural injection of morphine before abdominal aortic surgery resulted in less adrenergic activity, as reflected by lower norepinephrine blood levels and a decreased mean arterial pressure after operation, with diminished requirement for vasodilator therapy to control blood pressure. Decreased cardiac demand translates into diminished myocardial oxygen consumption and decreased cardiac morbidity, as has been reported.[68, 204, 208] Similarly, epidural analgesia may help control the hypercoagulability that follows vascular operation, with a resultant decrease in postoperative thromboembolic events.[209, 210]

Clinical Effects and Outcomes After Infrainguinal Revascularization

Lower extremity revascularization is performed almost exclusively in patients with a high incidence of coexistent diseases.[211] Spinal anesthesia may have some benefits for this patient group. Cook and coworkers[190] showed that patients who underwent lower extremity revascularization during spinal anesthesia had less blood loss (560 mL) than those who received general anesthesia (790 mL). The incidence of postoperative events was similar in the two groups with regard to reoperative complications, death, and myocardial infarction. However, patients who received spinal anesthesia had significantly fewer chest infections (16%) compared with patients who received general anesthesia (35%). This study demonstrates the safety of spinal anesthesia for lower extremity vascular procedures and the potential to diminish the incidence of postoperative chest infections, although the mechanism for the latter effect is unclear.

Use of epidural anesthesia for lower extremity vascular operation was examined in the Perioperative Ischemia Randomized Anesthesia Trial study.[209, 212] This study evaluated 100 patients scheduled to undergo lower extremity revascularization. Patients were randomized to receive either general anesthesia and postoperative systemic analgesia with opioids or epidural anesthesia during operation followed by postoperative epidural analgesia with fentanyl. An important part of this study was careful attention to hemodynamic stability in the perioperative period by using a hemodynamic algorithm to maintain heart rate and blood pressure

Table 29–6 Postoperative Cardiovascular Morbidity and Mortality

COMPLICATION	NUMBER OF PATIENTS		P
	GEN (*n* = 40)	GEN-EPI (*n* = 40)	
Vascular occlusions*	9	1	0.007
Vascular graft failure	8	1	0.013
Deep venous thrombosis	1	0	0.314
Total complications	52	13	0.011
≥1 complication	18	8	0.017
≥2 complications	11	3	0.019

*Number of patients with one or more complications within category. GEN, general anesthesia and standard analgesia; GEN-EPI, combined general-epidural anesthesia and epidural analgesia.

Data from Tuman KJ, McCarthy RJ, March RJ, et al.: Effects of epidural anesthesia and analgesia on coagulation and outcome after major vascular surgery. Anesth Analg 1991; 73: 696–704.

within defined limits. The primary study end point was cardiac morbidity. Cardiac morbidity was assessed as cardiac death, myocardial infarction, or unstable angina. Myocardial ischemia was detected by continuous electrocardiographic monitoring and serial evaluation of cardiac enzymes. The study found no difference in the incidence of postoperative cardiac events or death. However, the investigators also studied the perioperative coagulation profile of study patients. Vascular surgery patients are known to be hypercoagulable,[210] and operation further increases coagulability as part of the stress response.[213, 214] Patients who received epidural anesthesia and analgesia had a diminution in the surgical stress response assessed by cortisol and catecholamine measurements and were also less hypercoagulable in the early postoperative period. This correlated with a decrease in the incidence of postoperative thrombotic events of all types, especially lower extremity graft failure (Fig. 29–11). There is experimental evidence to support this finding. Cousins and Wright[69] demonstrated many years ago that epidural anesthesia increases lower extremity blood flow after revascularization, presumably as a result of redistribution. In addition, attenuation of the hypercoagulable state may be beneficial in a graft with tenuous flow. Finally, avoidance of positive pressure ventilation, which impairs systemic venous return, may also be a factor.[215]

Spinal or Epidural Hematoma

Several reports[216, 217] of epidural hematomas after regional anesthesia and anticoagulation have appeared in the literature. The fact that these events appear only as case reports makes it practically impossible to study

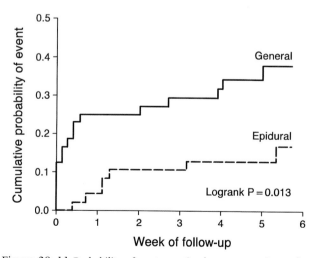

Figure 29–11 Probability of postoperative lower extremity graft failure (regrafting, thrombectomy, amputation) after operation performed during general anesthesia with intraoperative positive pressure ventilation and postoperative systemic narcotic analgesia or during epidural anesthesia with postoperative epidural analgesia. (From Christopherson R, Beattie C, Frank SM, et al: Perioperative morbidity in patients randomized to epidural or general anesthesia for lower extremity vascular surgery. Anesthesiology 1993; 79: 422–434.)

or document the safety or danger of any particular aspect of patient care, such as transient heparinization or differences in patient characteristics. The likelihood of observing an event is so low that formal study is difficult. However, several factors deserve mention. First, the incidence of spinal or epidural hematoma after regional anesthesia for abdominal aortic hematoma is clearly quite low. Series of several thousand patients have reported no hematomas.[1, 4, 8, 10, 12, 13, 68, 69, 200, 201, 204, 212, 218–221] This puts epidural hematomas in the category of other rare but serious reactions to anesthetics, such as allergic reactions, atypical reactions, and failed intubations, all of which have potentially serious sequelae. In this light, use of epidural anesthesia and analgesia is no different than any other anesthetic technique—it has rare, but serious, complications. Second, if a regional technique is to be used before or during heparin anticoagulation, it may be prudent to monitor the coagulation status of the patient using the activated clotting time or some other measure of procoagulant inhibition. Although this does not guarantee a hematoma will not form, the largest study[219] of regional techniques for vascular surgery with anticoagulation used activated clotting time monitoring during the period of heparinization. Third, practitioners who use epidural analgesia after vascular surgery should have a well-developed system for monitoring patients after operation.

Symptoms of spinal cord compression are most likely to appear after operation and should be detected as soon as possible so that the diagnosis can be made and treatment initiated. The use of dilute concentrations of local anesthetics, usually combined with an opioid, has the advantage of not obscuring sensory-motor findings characteristic of cord compression and not delaying diagnosis. Higher concentrations of local anesthetics may result in sensory-motor deficits that could make the diagnosis difficult. Also, spinal cord perfusion pressure should be maintained, especially during aortic cross-clamping when spinal arterial inflow may be restricted. Although the spinal cord blood supply is usually not compromised during infrarenal abdominal aortic procedures, the origin of this blood supply is rarely known and should be presumed to be at risk. This means maintenance of arterial perfusion pressure and also that practitioners should avoid bolus injections of drugs through an epidural catheter during the period of cross-clamping. Bolus injections transiently increase cerebrospinal fluid pressure[222] and may increase venous pressure of vessels draining the cord, thereby compromising spinal cord perfusion pressure.[223, 224] Finally, early diagnosis is important. The exact diagnostic technique used (myelography, computed tomography, magnetic resonance imaging) may not be as important as making an early diagnosis that leads to early treatment.

References

1. Lunn JK, Dannemiller FJ, Stanley TH: Cardiovascular responses to clamping of the aorta during epidural and general anesthesia. Anesth Analg 1979; 58: 372–376.

2. Reiz S, Nath S, Pontén E, et al: Effects of thoracic epidural block and the beta-1-adrenoreceptor agonist prenalterol on the cardiovascular response to infrarenal aortic cross-clamping in man. Acta Anaesthesiol Scand 1979; 23: 395–403.

3. Seeling W, Ahnefeld FW, Rosenberg G, et al: Aortofemoral bifurcation bypass—effect of anesthesia procedure (NLA, thoracic continuous catheter peridural anesthesia) on circulation, respiration and metabolism. Hemodynamic changes caused by peridural anesthesia and anesthesia induction. (German.) Anaesthesist 1985; 34: 217–228.

4. Seeling W, Ahnefeld FW, Grünert A, et al: Aortofemoral bifurcation bypass. Effect of the anesthesia procedure (NLA, thoracic continuous catheter peridural anesthesia) on circulation, respiration and metabolism. Homeostasis and oxygen transport. (German.) Anaesthesist 1986; 35: 80–92.

5. Lundberg J, Norgren L, Thomson D, et al: Hemodynamic effects of dopamine during thoracic epidural analgesia in man. Anesthesiology 1987; 66: 641–646.

6. Lundberg J, Lundberg D, Norgren L, et al: Intestinal hemodynamics during laparotomy: effects of thoracic epidural anesthesia and dopamine in humans. Anesth Analg 1990; 71: 9–15.

7. Stelzner J, Reinhart K, Föhring U, et al: The effect of thoracic peridural analgesia on the cortisol and glucose response in surgery of the abdominal aorta. (German.) Reg Anaesth 1988; 11: 16–20.

8. Reinhart K, Foehring U, Kersting T, et al: Effects of thoracic epidural anesthesia on systemic hemodynamic function and systemic oxygen supply-demand relationship. Anesth Analg 1989; 69: 360–369.

9. Zayas VM, Blumenfeld JD, Bading B, et al: Adrenergic regulation of renin secretion and renal hemodynamics during deliberate hypotension in humans. Am J Physiol 1993; 265: F686–F692.

10. Breslow MJ, Jordan DA, Christopherson R, et al: Epidural morphine decreases postoperative hypertension by attenuating sympathetic nervous system hyperactivity. JAMA 1989; 261: 3577–3581.

11. Her C, Kizelshteyn G, Walker V, et al: Combined epidural and general anesthesia for abdominal aortic surgery. J Cardiothorac Anesth 1990; 4: 552–557.

12. Mason RA, Newton GB, Cassel W, et al: Combined epidural and general anesthesia in aortic surgery. J Cardiovasc Surg (Torino) 1990; 31: 442–447.

13. Baron JF, Bertrand M, Barré E, et al: Combined epidural and general anesthesia versus general anesthesia for abdominal aortic surgery. Anesthesiology 1991; 75: 611–618.

14. Kataja J: Thoracolumbar epidural anaesthesia and isoflurane to prevent hypertension and tachycardia in patients undergoing abdominal aortic surgery. Eur J Anaesthesiol 1991; 8: 427–436.

15. George KA, Chisakuta AM, Gamble JA, et al: Thoracic epidural infusion for postoperative pain relief following abdominal aortic surgery: bupivacaine, fentanyl or a mixture of both? Anaesthesia 1992; 47: 388–394.

16. Stenseth R, Berg EM, Bjella L, et al: The influence of thoracic epidural analgesia alone and in combination with general anesthesia on cardiovascular function and myocardial metabolism in patients receiving beta-adrenergic blockers. Anesth Analg 1993; 77: 463–468.

17. McLean APH, Mulligan GW, Otton P, et al: Hemodynamic alterations associated with epidural anesthesia. Surgery 1967; 62: 79–87.

18. Bonica JJ, Berges PU, Morikawa K: Circulatory effects of peridural block. I. Effects of level of analgesia and dose of lidocaine. Anesthesiology 1970; 33: 619–626.

19. Arndt JO, Höck A, Stanton-Hicks M, et al: Peridural anesthesia and the distribution of blood in supine humans. Anesthesiology 1985; 63: 616–623.

20. Stanton-Hicks M, Höck A, Stuhmeier KD, et al: Venoconstrictor agents mobilize blood from different sources and increase intrathoracic filling during epidural anesthesia in supine humans. Anesthesiology 1987; 66: 317–322.

21. Otton PE, Wilson EJ: The cardiocirculatory effects of upper thoracic epidural analgesia. Can Anaesth Soc J 1966; 13: 541–549.

22. Saada M, Duval AM, Bonnet F, et al: Abnormalities in myocar-

dial segmental wall motion during lumbar epidural anesthesia. Anesthesiology 1989; 71: 26–32.

23. Baron J-F, Coriat P, Mundler O, et al: Left ventricular global and regional function during lumbar epidural anesthesia in patients with and without angina pectoris. Influence of volume loading. Anesthesiology 1987; 66: 621–627.

24. Saada M, Catoire P, Bonnet F, et al: Effect of thoracic epidural anesthesia combined with general anesthesia on segmental wall motion assessed by transesophageal echocardiography. Anesth Analg 1992; 75: 329–335.

25. Blomberg S, Emanuelsson H, Ricksten SE: Thoracic epidural anesthesia and central hemodynamics in patients with unstable angina pectoris. Anesth Analg 1989; 69: 558–562.

26. Blomberg S, Emanuelsson H, Kvist H, et al: Effects of thoracic epidural anesthesia on coronary arteries and arterioles in patients with coronary artery disease. Anesthesiology 1990; 73: 840–847.

27. Kock M, Blomberg S, Emanuelsson H, et al: Thoracic epidural anesthesia improves global and regional left ventricular function during stress-induced myocardial ischemia in patients with coronary artery disease. Anesth Analg 1990; 71: 625–630.

28. Klassen GA, Bramwell RS, Bromage PR, et al: Effect of acute sympathectomy by epidural anesthesia on the canine coronary circulation. Anesthesiology 1980; 52: 8–15.

29. Davis RF, DeBoer LW, Maroko PR: Thoracic epidural anesthesia reduces myocardial infarct size after coronary artery occlusion in dogs. Anesth Analg 1986; 65: 711–717.

30. Lund C, Selmar P, Hansen OB, et al: Effect of epidural bupivacaine on somatosensory evoked potentials after dermatomal stimulation. Anesth Analg 1987; 66: 34–38.

31. Malmqvist L-Å, Bengtsson M, Björnsson G, et al: Sympathetic activity and haemodynamic variables during spinal analgesia in man. Acta Anaesthesiol Scand 1987; 31: 467–473.

32. Malmqvist L-Å, Tryggvason B, Bengtsson M: Sympathetic blockade during extradural analgesia with mepivacaine or bupivacaine. Acta Anaesthesiol Scand 1989; 33: 444–449.

33. Chamberlain DP, Chamberlain BD: Changes in the skin temperature of the trunk and their relationship to sympathetic blockade during spinal anesthesia. Anesthesiology 1986; 65: 139–143.

34. Defalque RJ: Compared effects of spinal and extradural anesthesia upon the blood pressure. Anesthesiology 1962; 23: 627–630.

35. Kennedy WF Jr, Everett GB, Cobb LA, et al: Simultaneous systemic and hepatic hemodynamic measurements during high spinal anesthesia in normal man. Anesth Analg 1970; 49: 1016–1024.

36. Kennedy WF Jr, Everett GB, Cobb LA, et al: Simultaneous systemic and hepatic hemodynamic measurements during high peridural anesthesia in normal man. Anesth Analg 1971; 50: 1069–1077.

37. Dirkes WE, Rosenberg J, Lund C, et al: The effect of subarachnoid lidocaine and combined subarachnoid lidocaine and epidural bupivacaine on electrical sensory thresholds. Reg Anesth 1991; 16: 262–264.

38. Pflug AE, Halter JB: Effect of spinal anesthesia on adrenergic tone and the neuroendocrine responses to surgical stress in humans. Anesthesiology 1981; 55: 120–126.

39. Stevens RA, Artuso JD, Kao TC, et al: Changes in human plasma catecholamine concentrations during epidural anesthesia depend on the level of block. Anesthesiology 1991; 74: 1029–1034.

40. Beardsley DJ, White JL, Teague PA, et al: Effect of local anesthetic choice upon plasma catecholamine concentration during epidural anesthesia. (Abstract.) Anesth Analg 1993; 76: S14.

41. Bonica JJ, Akamatsu TJ, Berges PU, et al: Circulatory effects of peridural block. II. Effects of epinephrine. Anesthesiology 1971; 34: 514–522.

42. Engquist A, Fog-Möller F, Christiansen C, et al: Influence of epidural analgesia on the catecholamine and cyclic AMP responses to surgery. Acta Anaesthesiol Scand 1980; 24: 17–21.

43. Goldstein DS, Lake CR, Chernow B, et al: Age-dependence of hypertensive-normotensive differences in plasma norepinephrine. Hypertension 1983; 5: 100–104.

44. Goertz AW, Seeling W, Heinrich H, et al: Effect of phenyleph-

rine bolus administration on left ventricular function during high thoracic and lumbar epidural anesthesia combined with general anesthesia. Anesth Analg 1993; 76: 541–545.

45. Lundberg J, Lundberg D, Norgren L, et al: Dopamine counteracts hypertension during general anesthesia and hypotension during combined thoracic epidural anesthesia for abdominal aortic surgery. J Cardiothorac Anesth 1990; 4: 348–353.

46. Bonica JJ, Kennedy WF, Akamatsu TJ, et al: Circulatory effects of peridural block: 3. Effects of acute blood loss. Anesthesiology 1972; 36: 219–227.

47. Ward RJ, Kennedy WF, Bonica JJ, et al: Experimental evaluation of atropine and vasopressors for the treatment of hypotension of high subarachnoid anesthesia. Anesth Analg 1966; 45: 621–629.

48. Ecoffey C, Edouard A, Pruszczynski W, et al: Effects of epidural anesthesia on catecholamines, renin activity, and vasopressin changes induced by tilt in elderly men. Anesthesiology 1985; 62: 294–297.

49. Peters J, Schlaghecke R, Thouet H, et al: Endogenous vasopressin supports blood pressure and prevents severe hypotension during epidural anesthesia in conscious dogs. Anesthesiology 1990; 73: 694–702.

50. Dagnino J, Prys-Roberts C: Studies of anaesthesia in relation to hypertension. VI: Cardiovascular responses to extradural blockade of treated and untreated hypertensive patients. Br J Anaesth 1984; 56: 1065–1073.

51. Sharrock NE, Mineo R, Urquhart B: Haemodynamic effects and outcome analysis of hypotensive extradural anaesthesia in controlled hypertensive patients undergoing total hip arthroplasty. Br J Anaesth 1991; 67: 17–25.

52. Reiz S, Häggmark S, Rydvall A, et al: Beta-blockers and thoracic epidural analgesia. Cardioprotective and synergistic effects. Acta Anaesthesiol Scand 1982; 76(Suppl): 54–61.

53. Gold MS, Rizzuto C, DeCrosta D: Effect of epidural/general vs general anesthesia on catecholamine levels and hemodynamics during abdominal aortic cross-clamping. (Abstract.) Anesthesiology 1992; 77: A97.

54. Samain E, Coriat P, Le Bret F, et al: Ephedrine vs phenylephrine for hypotension due to thoracic epidural anesthesia associated with general anesthesia; effects on left ventricular function. (Abstract.) Anesthesiology 1990; 73: A82.

55. Yeager MP, Dodds TM, Burns AK, et al: Effect of epidural anesthesia on hemodynamics and ventricular wall motion during aortic surgery. (Abstract.) Anesthesiology 1993; 79: A74.

56. Reiz S, Nath S, Rais O: Effects of thoracic epidural block and prenalterol on coronary vascular resistance and myocardial metabolism in patients with coronary artery disease. Acta Anaesthesiol Scand 1980; 24: 11–16.

57. Kennedy WF Jr, Sawyer TK, Gerbershagen HY, et al: Systemic cardiovascular and renal hemodynamic alterations during peridural anesthesia in normal man. Anesthesiology 1969; 31: 414–421.

58. Sivarajan M, Amory DW, Lindbloom LE, et al: Systemic and regional blood-flow changes during spinal anesthesia in the rhesus monkey. Anesthesiology 1975; 43: 78–88.

59. Sivarajan M, Amory DW, Lindbloom LE: Systemic and regional blood flow during epidural anesthesia without epinephrine in the rhesus monkey. Anesthesiology 1976; 45: 300–310.

60. Gamulin Z, Forster A, Morel D, et al: Effects of infrarenal aortic cross-clamping on renal hemodynamics in humans. Anesthesiology 1984; 61: 394–399.

61. Gamulin Z, Forster A, Simonet F, et al: Effects of renal sympathetic blockade on renal hemodynamics in patients undergoing major aortic abdominal surgery. Anesthesiology 1986; 65: 688–692.

62. Gelman S, Patel K, Bishop SP, et al: Renal and splanchnic circulation during infrarenal aortic cross-clamping. Arch Surg 1984; 119: 1394–1399.

63. Johansson K, Ahn H, Lindhagen J, et al: Effect of epidural anaesthesia on intestinal blood flow. Br J Surg 1988; 75: 73–76.

64. Lundberg J, Biber B, Delbro D, et al: Effects of dopamine on intestinal hemodynamics and motility during epidural analgesia in the cat. Acta Anaesthesiol Scand 1989; 33: 487–493.

65. Greitz T, Andreen M, Irestedt L: Effects of dihydroergotamine on haemodynamics and oxygen consumption in the dog during

high epidural block with special reference to the splanchnic region. Acta Anaesthesiol Scand 1983; 27: 385–390.

66. Lundberg J: Intestinal blood flow and systemic hemodynamics during thoracic epidural anesthesia combined with dopamine infusion. Effects of infrarenal aortic crossclamping and declamping. (Abstract.) Anesthesiology 1992; 77: A878.

67. Fry RE, Huber PJ, Ramsey KL, et al: Infrarenal aortic occlusion, colonic blood flow, and the effect of nitroglycerin afterload reduction. Surgery 1984; 95: 479–486.

68. Tuman KJ, McCarthy RJ, March RJ, et al: Effects of epidural anesthesia and analgesia on coagulation and outcome after major vascular surgery. Anesth Analg 1991; 73: 696–704.

69. Cousins MJ, Wright CJ: Graft, muscle, skin blood flow after epidural block in vascular surgical procedures. Surg Gynecol Obstet 1971; 133: 59–64.

70. Shimosato S, Etsten BE: The role of the venous system in cardiocirculatory dynamics during spinal and epidural anesthesia in man. Anesthesiology 1969; 30: 619–628.

71. Viale JP, Annat GJ, Ravat FM, et al: Oxygen uptake and mixed venous oxygen saturation during aortic surgery and the first three postoperative hours. Anesth Analg 1991; 73: 530–535.

72. Frank SM, Beattie C, Christopherson R, et al: Epidural versus general anesthesia, ambient operating room temperature, and patient age as predictors of inadvertent hypothermia. Anesthesiology 1992; 77: 252–257.

73. Veroli P, Benhamou D: Comparison of hypertonic saline (5%), isotonic saline and Ringer's lactate solutions for fluid preloading before lumbar extradural anaesthesia. Br J Anaesth 1992; 69: 461–464.

74. Mathru M, Rao TL, Kartha RK, et al: Intravenous albumin administration for prevention of spinal hypotension during cesarean section. Anesth Analg 1980; 59: 655–658.

75. Otesen S, Renck H, Jynge P: Cardiovascular effects of epidural analgesia. II. Haemodynamic alterations secondary to lumbar epidural analgesia and their modification by plasma expansion and adrenaline administration. An experimental study in the sheep. Acta Anaesthesiol Scand Suppl 1978; 69: 17–31.

76. Greitz T, Andreen M, Irestedt L: Effects of prenalterol and volume loading with dextran on haemodynamics and oxygen consumption in dogs during high epidural block with special reference to the splanchnic region. Acta Anaesthesiol Scand 1985; 29: 37–44.

77. Wennberg E, Frid I, Haljamäe H, et al: Colloid (3% Dextran 70) with or without ephedrine infusion for cardiovascular stability during extradural caesarean section. Br J Anaesth 1992; 69: 13–18.

78. Engberg G, Wiklund L: The circulatory effects of intravenously administered ephedrine during epidural blockade. Acta Anaesthesiol Scand Suppl 1978; 66: 27–36.

79. Taivainen T: Comparison of ephedrine and etilefrine for the treatment of arterial hypotension during spinal anaesthesia in elderly patients. Acta Anaesthesiol Scand 1991; 35: 164–169.

80. Goertz AW, Hübner C, Seefelder C, et al: The effect of ephedrine bolus administration on left ventricular loading and systolic performance during high thoracic epidural anesthesia combined with general anesthesia. Anesth Analg 1994; 78: 101–105.

81. Hemmingsen C, Poulsen JA, Risbo A: Prophylactic ephedrine during spinal anaesthesia: double-blind study in patients in ASA groups I–III. Br J Anaesth 1989; 63: 340–342.

82. Kang YG, Abouleish E, Caritis S: Prophylactic intravenous ephedrine infusion during spinal anesthesia for cesarean section. Anesth Analg 1982; 61: 839–842.

83. Gajraj NM, Victory RA, Pace NA, et al: Comparison of an ephedrine infusion with crystalloid administration for prevention of hypotension during spinal anesthesia. Anesth Analg 1993; 76: 1023–1026.

84. Mather LE, Tucker GT, Murphy TM, et al: Hemodynamic drug interaction: peridural lidocaine and intravenous ephedrine. Acta Anaesthesiol Scand 1976; 20: 207–210.

85. Butterworth JF IV, Austin JC, Johnson MD, et al: Effect of total spinal anesthesia on arterial and venous responses to dopamine and dobutamine. Anesth Analg 1987; 66: 209–214.

86. Lundberg J, Biber B, Henriksson B-Å, et al: Effects of thoracic epidural anesthesia and adrenoceptor blockade on the cardio-

vascular response to dopamine in the dog. Acta Anaesthesiol Scand 1991; 35: 359–365.

87. Kitahata H, Shinohara S: Hemodynamic effects of dobutamine, dopamine and methoxamine during thoracic epidural anesthesia in dogs with coronary stenosis. (Japanese.) Masui 1989; 38: 216–228.

88. Kajimoto Y, Nishimura N: Metaraminol and dobutamine for the treatment of hypotension associated with epidural block. Resuscitation 1984; 12: 47–51.

89. Stanton-Hicks M, Berges PU, Bonica JJ: Circulatory effects of peridural block. IV. Comparison of the effects of epinephrine and phenylephrine. Anesthesiology 1973; 39: 308–314.

90. Sharrock NE, Mineo R, Urquhart B: Hemodynamic response to low-dose epinephrine infusion during hypotensive epidural anesthesia for total hip replacement. Reg Anesth 1990; 15: 295–299.

91. Lundberg J, Biber B, Martner J, et al: Dopamine or norepinephrine infusion during thoracic epidural anesthesia? Differences in hemodynamic effects and plasma norepinephrine levels. (Abstract.) Anesthesiology 1991; 75: A740.

92. Butterworth JF IV, Piccione W Jr, Berrizbeitia LD, et al: Augmentation of venous return by adrenergic agonist during spinal anesthesia. Anesth Analg 1986; 65: 612–616.

93. Sipes SL, Chestnut DH, Vincent RD Jr, et al: Which vasopressor should be used to treat hypotension during magnesium sulfate infusion and epidural anesthesia? Anesthesiology 1992; 77: 101–108.

94. Smith JS, Roizen MF, Cahalan MK, et al: Does anesthetic technique make a difference? Augmentation of systolic blood pressure during carotid endarterectomy: effects of phenylephrine versus light anesthesia and of isoflurane versus halothane on the incidence of myocardial ischemia. Anesthesiology 1988; 69: 846–853.

95. Sharrock NE, Go G, Mineo R: Effect of i.v. low-dose adrenaline and phenylephrine infusions on plasma concentrations of bupivacaine after lumbar extradural anaesthesia in elderly patients. Br J Anaesth 1991; 67: 694–698.

96. Craig DB: Postoperative recovery of pulmonary function. Anesth Analg 1981; 60: 46–52.

97. Sydow FW: The influence of anesthesia and postoperative analgesic management of lung function. Acta Chir Scand Suppl 1989; 550: 159–168.

98. Wahl GW, Swinburne AJ, Fedullo AJ, et al: Effect of age and preoperative airway obstruction on lung function after coronary artery bypass grafting. Ann Thorac Surg 1993; 56: 104–107.

99. Neustein SM, Cohen E: Intrathecal morphine during thoracotomy, Part II: Effect on postoperative meperidine requirements and pulmonary function tests. J Cardiothorac Vasc Anesth 1993; 7: 157–159.

100. Robinson RJ, Brister S, Jones E, et al: Epidural meperidine analgesia after cardiac surgery. Can Anaesth Soc J 1986; 33: 550–555.

101. Shulman M, Sandler AN, Bradley JW, et al: Postthoracotomy pain and pulmonary function following epidural and systemic morphine. Anesthesiology 1984; 61: 569–575.

102. George KA, Wright PM, Chisakuta A: Continuous thoracic epidural fentanyl for post-thoracotomy pain relief: with or without bupivacaine? Anaesthesia 1991; 46: 732–736.

103. Bromage PR, Camporesi E, Chestnut D: Epidural narcotics for postoperative analgesia. Anesth Analg 1980; 59: 473–480.

104. Hachenberg T, Tenling A, Nyström SO, et al: Ventilation-perfusion inequality in patients undergoing cardiac surgery. Anesthesiology 1994; 80: 509–519.

105. Wahba WM, Craig DB, Don HF, et al: The cardio-respiratory effects of thoracic epidural anaesthesia. Can Anaesth Soc J 1972; 19: 8–19.

106. Sundberg A, Wattwil M, Arvill A: Respiratory effects of high thoracic epidural anaesthesia. Acta Anaesthesiol Scand 1986; 30: 215–217.

107. Takasaki M, Takahashi T: Respiratory function during cervical and thoracic extradural analgesia in patients with normal lungs. Br J Anaesth 1980; 52: 1271–1276.

108. Sjogren S, Wright B: Respiratory changes during continuous epidural blockade. Acta Anaesthesiol Scand Suppl 1972; 46: 27–49.

109. O'Connor CJ: Thoracic epidural analgesia: physiologic effects and clinical applications. J Cardiothorac Vasc Anesth 1993; 7: 595–609.

110. Hecker BR, Bjurstrom R, Schoene RB: Effect of intercostal nerve blockade on respiratory mechanics and CO_2 chemosensitivity at rest and exercise. Anesthesiology 1989; 70: 13–18.

111. Bromage PR: Spirometry in assessment of analgesia after abdominal surgery: a method of comparing analgesic drugs. Br Med J 1955; 2: 589–593.

112. Manikian B, Cantineau JP, Bertrand M, et al: Improvement of diaphragmatic function by a thoracic extradural block after upper abdominal surgery. Anesthesiology 1988; 68: 379–386.

113. Pansard JL, Mankikian B, Bertrand M, et al: Effects of thoracic extradural block on diaphragmatic electrical activity and contractility after upper abdominal surgery. Anesthesiology 1993; 78: 63–71.

114. Fratacci M-D, Kimball WR, Wain JC, et al: Diaphragmatic shortening after thoracic surgery in humans. Effects of mechanical ventilation and thoracic epidural anesthesia. Anesthesiology 1993; 79: 654–665.

115. Harrop-Griffiths AW, Ravalia A, Browne DA, et al: Regional anaesthesia and cough effectiveness. A study in patients undergoing caesarean section. Anaesthesia 1991; 46: 11–13.

116. Tarhan S, Moffitt EA, Sessler AD, et al: Risk of anesthesia and surgery in patients with chronic bronchitis and chronic obstructive pulmonary disease. Surgery 1973; 74: 720–726.

117. Logas WG, el-Baz N, el-Ganzouri A, et al: Continuous thoracic epidural analgesia for postoperative pain relief following thoracotomy: a randomized prospective study. Anesthesiology 1987; 67: 787–791.

118. El-Baz NM, Faber LP, Jensik RJ: Continuous epidural infusion of morphine for treatment of pain after thoracic surgery: a new technique. Anesth Analg 1984; 63: 757–764.

119. Rostaing S, Bonnet F, Levron JC, et al: Effect of epidural clonidine on analgesia and pharmacokinetics of epidural fentanyl in postoperative patients. Anesthesiology 1991; 75: 420–425.

120. Modig J, Paalzow L: A comparison of epidural morphine and epidural bupivacaine for postoperative pain relief. Acta Anaesthesiol Scand 1981; 25: 437–441.

121. Bromage PR, Camporesi EM, Durant PA, et al: Nonrespiratory side effects of epidural morphine. Anesth Analg 1982; 61: 490–495.

122. Hurford WE, Dutton RP, Alfille PH, et al: Comparison of thoracic and lumbar epidural infusions of bupivacaine and fentanyl for post-thoracotomy analgesia. J Cardiothorac Vasc Anesth 1993; 7: 521–525.

123. Fromme GA, Steidl LJ, Danielson DR: Comparison of lumbar and thoracic epidural morphine for relief of postthoracotomy pain. Anesth Analg 1985; 64: 454–455.

124. Benzon HT: Post-thoracotomy epidural analgesia: lumbar or thoracic placement? (Editorial.) J Cardiothorac Vasc Anesth 1993; 7: 515–516.

125. Guinard J-P, Mavrocordatos P, Chiolero R, et al: A randomized comparison of intravenous versus lumbar and thoracic epidural fentanyl for analgesia after thoracotomy. Anesthesiology 1992; 77: 1108–1115.

126. Swenson JD, Hullander RM, Bready RJ, et al: A comparison of patient controlled epidural analgesia with sufentanil by the lumbar versus thoracic route after thoracotomy. Anesth Analg 1994; 78: 215–218.

127. Coe A, Sarginson R, Smith MW, et al: Pain following thoracotomy. A randomised, double-blind comparison of lumbar versus thoracic epidural fentanyl. Anaesthesia 1991; 46: 918–921.

128. Sandler AN, Stringer D, Panos L, et al: A randomized, double-blind comparison of lumbar epidural and intravenous fentanyl infusions for postthoracotomy pain relief. Analgesic, pharmacokinetic, and respiratory effects. Anesthesiology 1992; 77: 626–634.

129. Badner NH, Komar WE: Bupivacaine 0.1% does not improve post-operative epidural fentanyl analgesia after abdominal or thoracic surgery. Can J Anaesth 1992; 39: 330–336.

130. Conacher ID, Paes ML, Jacobson L, et al: Epidural analgesia following thoracic surgery. A review of two years' experience. Anaesthesia 1983; 38: 546–551.

131. Garner L, Coats RR: Ipsilateral stellate ganglion block effective

for treating shoulder pain after thoracotomy. Anesth Analg 1994; 78: 1195–1196.

132. Miguel R, Hubbell D: Pain management and spirometry following thoracotomy: a prospective, randomized study of four techniques. J Cardiothorac Vasc Anesth 1993; 7: 529–534.

133. Moore DC, Bridenbaugh LD: Intercostal nerve block in 4333 patients: indications, technique, and complications. Anesth Analg 1962; 41: 1–11.

134. Seddon SJ, Clayton KC: Intercostal nerve block by jet injection. Anaesthesia 1984; 39: 484–486.

135. Richardson J, Sabanathan S, Eng J, et al: Continuous intercostal nerve block versus epidural morphine for postthoracotomy analgesia. Ann Thorac Surg 1993; 55: 377–380.

136. Mozell EJ, Sabanathan S, Mearns AJ, et al: Continuous extrapleural intercostal nerve block after pleurectomy. Thorax 1991; 46: 21–24.

137. Eng J, Sabanathan S: Site of action of continuous extrapleural intercostal nerve block. Ann Thorac Surg 1991; 51: 387–389.

138. Sabanathan S, Mearns AJ, Bickford-Smith PJ, et al: Efficacy of continuous extrapleural intercostal nerve block on postthoracotomy pain and pulmonary mechanics. Br J Surg 1990; 77: 221–225.

139. Deneuville M, Bisserier A, Regnard JF, et al: Continuous intercostal analgesia with 0.5% bupivacaine after thoracotomy: a randomized study. Ann Thorac Surg 1993; 55: 381–385.

140. Thompson GE, Hecker BR: Peripheral-nerve blocks for management of thoracic surgical patients. In Gravlee GP, Rauck RL (eds): Pain Management in Cardiothoracic Surgery, pp 25–56. Philadelphia, JB Lippincott, 1993.

141. Roxburgh JC, Markland CG, Ross BA, et al: Role of cryoanalgesia in the control of pain after thoracotomy. Thorax 1987; 42: 292–295.

142. O'Kelly E, Garry B: Continuous pain relief for multiple fractured ribs. Br J Anaesth 1981; 53: 989–991.

143. Ferrante FM: Thoracic anesthesia and analgesia. Soc Cardiovasc Anesth 16th Annu Meeting 1994; 44–47.

144. Eason MJ, Wyatt R: Paravertebral thoracic block—a reappraisal. Anaesthesia 1979; 34: 638–642.

145. Nelson KM, Vincent RG, Bourke RS, et al: Intraoperative intercostal nerve freezing to prevent postthoracotomy pain. Ann Thorac Surg 1974; 18: 280–285.

146. Moore DC: Intercostal nerve block for postoperative somatic pain following surgery of thorax and upper abdomen. Br J Anaesth 1975; 47(Suppl): 284–286.

147. Tucker GT, Moore DC, Bridenbaugh PO, et al: Systemic absorption of mepivacaine in commonly used regional block procedures. Anesthesiology 1972; 37: 277–287.

148. Benumof JL, Semenza J: Total spinal anesthesia following intrathoracic intercostal nerve blocks. Anesthesiology 1975; 43: 124–125.

149. Baxter AD, Jennings FO, Harris RS, et al: Continuous intercostal blockade after cardiac surgery. Br J Anaesth 1987; 59: 162–166.

150. Kvalheim L, Reiestad F: Interpleural catheter in the management of postoperative pain. (Abstract.) Anesthesiology 1984; 61: A231.

151. Kambam JR, Hammon J, Parris WC, et al: Intrapleural analgesia for post-thoracotomy pain and blood levels of bupivacaine following intrapleural injection. Can J Anaesth 1989; 36: 106–109.

152. McIlvaine WB, Knox RF, Fennessey PV, et al: Continuous infusion of bupivacaine via intrapleural catheter for analgesia after thoracotomy in children. Anesthesiology 1988; 69: 261–264.

153. Raffin L, Fletcher D, Sperandio M, et al: Interpleural infusion of 2% lidocaine with 1:200,000 epinephrine for postthoracotomy analgesia. Anesth Analg 1994; 79: 328–334.

154. Haak-van der Lely F, van Kleef JW, Burm AG, et al: Preoperative interpleural administration of sufentanil or bupivacaine reduces intraoperative intravenous sufentanil requirements during thoracotomy. J Cardiothorac Vasc Anesth 1993; 7: 526–528.

155. Symreng T, Gomez MN, Johnson B, et al: Intrapleural bupivacaine—technical considerations and intraoperative use. J Cardiothorac Anesth 1989; 3: 139–143.

156. Rose U, Attar Z: Interpleurales Bupivacain und parenterales

Opioid zur postoperativen Analgesie. Eine vergleichende Studie. Anaesthesist 1992; 41: 53–57.

157. Strømskag KE, Hauge O, Steen PA: Distribution of local anesthetics injected into the interpleural space, studied by computerized tomography. Acta Anaesthesiol Scand 1990; 34: 323–326.

158. el-Baz N, Goldin M: Continuous epidural infusion of morphine for pain relief after cardiac operations. J Thorac Cardiovasc Surg 1987; 93: 878–883.

159. Mathews ET, Abrams LD: Intrathecal morphine in open heart surgery. (Letter to the editor.) Lancet 1980; 2: 543.

160. Fitzpatrick GJ, Moriarty DC: Intrathecal morphine in the management of pain following cardiac surgery. A comparison with morphine i.v. Br J Anaesth 1988; 60: 639–644.

161. Vanstrum GS, Bjornson KM, Ilko R: Postoperative effects of intrathecal morphine in coronary artery bypass surgery. Anesth Analg 1988; 67: 261–267.

162. Casey WF, Wynands JE, Ralley FE, et al: The role of intrathecal morphine in the anesthetic management of patients undergoing coronary artery bypass surgery. J Cardiothorac Anesth 1987; 1: 510–516.

163. Aun C, Thomas D, St John-Jones L, et al: Intrathecal morphine in cardiac surgery. Eur J Anaesthesiol 1985; 2: 419–426.

164. Rosen KR, Rosen DA: Caudal epidural morphine for control of pain following open heart surgery in children. Anesthesiology 1989; 70: 418–421.

165. Joachimsson PO, Nyström SO, Tyden H: Early extubation after coronary artery surgery in efficiently rewarmed patients: a postoperative comparison of opioid anesthesia versus inhalational anesthesia and thoracic epidural analgesia. J Cardiothorac Anesth 1989; 3: 444–454.

166. Rein KA, Stenseth R, Myhre HO, et al: The influence of thoracic epidural analgesia on transcapillary fluid balance in subcutaneous tissue. A study in patients undergoing aortocoronary bypass surgery. Acta Anaesthesiol Scand 1989; 33: 79–83.

167. Liem TH, Booij LH, Hasenbos MA, et al: Coronary artery bypass grafting using two different anesthetic techniques: Part 1: Hemodynamic results. J Cardiothorac Vasc Anesth 1992; 6: 148–155.

168. Liem TH, Hasenbos MA, Booij LH, et al: Coronary artery bypass grafting using two different anesthetic techniques: Part 2: Postoperative outcome. J Cardiothorac Vasc Anesth 1992; 6: 156–161.

169. Liem TH, Booij LH, Gielen MJ, et al: Coronary artery bypass grafting using two different anesthetic techniques: Part 3: Adrenergic responses. J Cardiothorac Vasc Anesth 1992; 6: 162–167.

170. Ruff RL, Dougherty JH Jr: Complications of lumbar puncture followed by anticoagulation. Stroke 1981; 12: 879–881.

171. Allen BT, Anderson CB, Rubin BG, et al: The influence of anesthetic technique on perioperative complications after carotid endarterectomy. J Vasc Surg 1994; 19: 834–843.

172. Takolander R, Bergqvist D, Hulthén UL, et al: Carotid artery surgery. Local versus general anaesthesia as related to sympathetic activity and cardiovascular effects. Eur J Vasc Surg 1990; 4: 265–270.

173. Muskett A, McGreevy J, Miller M: Detailed comparison of regional and general anesthesia for carotid endarterectomy. Am J Surg 1986; 152: 691–694.

174. Peitzman AB, Webster MW, Loubeau JM, et al: Carotid endarterectomy under regional (conductive) anesthesia. Ann Surg 1982; 196: 59–64.

175. Corson JD, Chang BB, Shah DM, et al: The influence of anesthetic choice on carotid endarterectomy outcome. Arch Surg 1987; 122: 807–812.

176. Prough DS, Scuderi PE, Stullken E, et al: Myocardial infarction following regional anaesthesia for carotid endarterectomy. Can Anaesth Soc J 1984; 31: 192–196.

177. Godin MS, Bell WH III, Schwedler M, et al: Cost effectiveness of regional anesthesia in carotid endarterectomy. Am Surg 1989; 55: 656–659.

178. Becquemin JP, Paris E, Valverde A, et al: Carotid surgery. Is regional anesthesia always appropriate? J Cardiovasc Surg (Torino) 1991; 32: 592–598.

179. Davies MJ, Mooney PH, Scott DA, et al: Neurologic changes

during carotid endarterectomy under cervical block predict a high risk of postoperative stroke. Anesthesiology 1993; 78: 829–833.

180. Lee KS, Davis CH Jr, McWhorter JM: Low morbidity and mortality of carotid endarterectomy performed with regional anesthesia. J Neurosurg 1988; 69: 483–487.

181. Bonnet F, Derosier JP, Pluskwa F, et al: Cervical epidural anaesthesia for carotid artery surgery. Can J Anaesth 1990; 37: 353–358.

182. Pluskwa F, Derosier JP, Bonnet F, et al: Cervical epidural anesthesia in carotid artery surgery. (French.) Presse Med 1989; 18: 927–931.

183. Pluskwa F, Bonnet F, Touboul C, et al: Carotid endarterectomy under cervical epidural anesthesia. Analysis of neurologic manifestations. (French.) Ann Fr Anesth Reanim 1988; 7: 36–41.

184. Forssell C, Takolander R, Bergqvist D, et al: Local versus general anaesthesia in carotid surgery. A prospective, randomised study. Eur J Vasc Surg 1989; 3: 503–509.

185. Hafner CD, Evans WE: Carotid endarterectomy with local anesthesia: results and advantages. J Vasc Surg 1988; 7: 232–239.

186. Evans WE, Hayes JP, Waltke EA, et al: Optimal cerebral monitoring during carotid endarterectomy: neurologic response under local anesthesia. J Vasc Surg 1985; 2: 775–777.

187. Gabelman CG, Gann DS, Ashworth CJ Jr, et al: One hundred consecutive carotid reconstructions: local versus general anesthesia. Am J Surg 1983; 145: 477–482.

188. Goeau-Brissonniere O, Bacourt F, Renier JF, et al: Carotid surgery under locoregional anesthesia. (French.) Presse Med 1989; 18: 1831–1835.

189. Youngberg JA: Pro: regional anesthesia is preferable to general anesthesia for carotid artery surgery. J Cardiothorac Anesth 1987; 1: 479–482.

190. Cook PT, Davies MJ, Cronin KD, et al: A prospective randomised trial comparing spinal anaesthesia using hyperbaric cinchocaine with general anaesthesia for lower limb vascular surgery. Anaesth Intensive Care 1986; 14: 373–380.

191. Davis I: Intrathecal morphine in aortic aneurysm surgery. Anaesthesia 1987; 42: 491–497.

192. Sicard GA, Freeman MB, VanderWoude JC, et al: Comparison between the transabdominal and retroperitoneal approach for reconstruction of the infrarenal abdominal aorta. J Vasc Surg 1987; 5: 19–27.

193. Pasternack PF, Imparato AM, Baumann FG, et al: The hemodynamics of beta-blockade in patients undergoing abdominal aortic aneurysm repair. Circulation 1987; 76: III1–7.

194. Fragen RJ, Shanks CA, Molteni A, et al: Effects of etomidate on hormonal responses to surgical stress. Anesthesiology 1984; 61: 652–656.

195. Whittemore AD, Clowes AW, Hechtman HB, et al: Aortic aneurysm repair. Reduced operative mortality associated with maintenance of optimal cardiac performance. Ann Surg 1980; 192: 414–421.

196. Hesdorffer CS, Milne JF, Meyers AM, et al: The value of Swan-Ganz catheterization and volume loading in preventing renal failure in patients undergoing abdominal aneurysmectomy. Clin Nephrol 1987; 28: 272–276.

197. Shackford SR, Sise MJ, Fridlund PH, et al: Hypertonic sodium lactate versus lactated Ringer's solution for intravenous fluid therapy in operations on the abdominal aorta. Surgery 1983; 94: 41–51.

198. Auler JO Jr, Pereira MH, Gomide-Amaral RV, et al: Hemodynamic effects of hypertonic sodium chloride during surgical treatment of aortic aneurysms. Surgery 1987; 101: 594–601.

199. Hudson JC, Wurm WH, Kane FR, et al: Prostacyclin mediates vasodilation in the blush syndrome during aortic surgery. (Abstract.) Anesthesiology 1988; 69: A131.

200. Bunt TJ, Manczuk M, Varley K: Continuous epidural anesthesia for aortic surgery: thoughts on peer review and safety. Surgery 1987; 101: 706–714.

201. Raggi R, Dardik H, Mauro AL: Continuous epidural anesthesia and postoperative epidural narcotics in vascular surgery. Am J Surg 1987; 154: 192–197.

202. Woolf CJ, Chong MS: Preemptive analgesia—treating postoperative pain by preventing the establishment of central sensitization. Anesth Analg 1993; 77: 362–379.

203. Reiz S, Bålfors E, Sørensen MB, et al: Coronary hemodynamic effects of general anesthesia and surgery: modification by epidural analgesia in patients with ischemic heart disease. Reg Anesth 1982; 7(Suppl): S8–S18.

204. Yeager MP, Glass DD, Neff RK, et al: Epidural anesthesia and analgesia in high-risk surgical patients. Anesthesiology 1987; 66: 729–736.

205. Grass JA: Surgical outcome: regional anesthesia and analgesia versus general anesthesia. Anesth Rev 1993; 20: 117–125.

206. Rawal N, Sjostrand U, Christoffersson E, et al: Comparison of intramuscular and epidural morphine for postoperative analgesia in the grossly obese: influence on postoperative ambulation and pulmonary function. Anesth Analg 1984; 63: 583–592.

207. Jayr C, Thomas H, Rey A, et al: Postoperative pulmonary complications. Epidural analgesia using bupivacaine and opioids versus parenteral opioids. Anesthesiology 1993; 78: 666–676.

208. Beattie WS, Buckley DN, Forrest JB: Epidural morphine reduces the risk of postoperative myocardial ischaemia in patients with cardiac risk factors. Can J Anaesth 1993; 40: 532–541.

209. Rosenfeld BA, Beattie C, Christopherson R, et al: The effects of different anesthetic regimens on fibrinolysis and the development of postoperative arterial thrombosis. Anesthesiology 1993; 79: 435–443.

210. Donaldson MC, Weinberg DS, Belkin M, et al: Screening for hypercoagulable states in vascular surgical practice: a preliminary study. J Vasc Surg 1990; 11: 825–831.

211. Hertzer NR: Fatal myocardial infarction following lower extremity revascularization. Two hundred seventy-three patients followed six to eleven postoperative years. Ann Surg 1981; 193: 492–498.

212. Christopherson R, Beattie C, Frank SM, et al: Perioperative morbidity in patients randomized to epidural or general anesthesia for lower extremity vascular surgery. Anesthesiology 1993; 79: 422–434.

213. Flinn WR, McDaniel MD, Yao JS, et al: Antithrombin III deficiency as a reflection of dynamic protein metabolism in patients undergoing vascular reconstruction. J Vasc Surg 1984; 1: 888–895.

214. Freyburger G, Janvier G, Dief S, et al: Fibrinolytic and hemorrheologic alterations during and after elective aortic graft surgery: implications for postoperative management. Anesth Analg 1993; 76: 504–512.

215. Hodgson DC: Venous stasis during surgery. Anaesthesia 1964; 19: 96–99.

216. Kane RE: Neurologic deficits following epidural or spinal anesthesia. Anesth Analg 1981; 60: 150–161.

217. Skouen JS, Wainapel SF, Willock MM: Paraplegia following epidural anesthesia. A case report and a literature review. Acta Neurol Scand 1985; 72: 437–443.

218. Baron HC, LaRaja RD, Rossi G, et al: Continuous epidural analgesia in the heparinized vascular surgical patient: a retrospective review of 912 patients. J Vasc Surg 1987; 6: 144–146.

219. Rao TL, El-Etr AA: Anticoagulation following placement of epidural and subarachnoid catheters: an evaluation of neurologic sequelae. Anesthesiology 1981; 55: 618–620.

220. Odoom JA, Sih IL: Epidural analgesia and anticoagulant therapy. Experience with one thousand cases of continuous epidurals. Anaesthesia 1983; 38: 254–259.

221. Cunningham FO, Egan JM, Inahara T: Continuous epidural anesthesia in abdominal vascular surgery. A review of 100 consecutive cases. Am J Surg 1980; 139: 624–627.

222. Paul DL, Wildsmith JA: Extradural pressure following the injection of two volumes of bupivacaine. Br J Anaesth 1989; 62: 368–372.

223. Wadouh F, Lindemann EM, Arndt CF, et al: The arteria radicularis magna anterior as a decisive factor influencing spinal cord damage during aortic occlusion. J Thorac Cardiovasc Surg 1984; 88: 1–10.

224. Griffiths IR, Pitts LH, Crawford RA, et al: Spinal cord compression and blood flow. I. The effect of raised cerebrospinal fluid pressure on spinal cord blood flow. Neurology 1978; 28: 1145–1151.

CHAPTER 30

Gynecology and Urology

F. Kayser Enneking, M.D.

Gynecologic and urologic procedures run the gamut from minor evaluations during anesthesia to major operations involving substantial physiologic trespass. Regional anesthesia is used in most of these procedures as the sole anesthetic, as a complement to a light general anesthetic or as a means of providing postoperative pain control. Familiarity with the extent of block provided by each of the various regional techniques enables the anesthesiologist to gauge the degree of sedation required during these procedures.

Neuraxial block (subarachnoid, epidural, and caudal anesthesia) is the primary regional anesthetic technique used for gynecologic and urologic procedures, but several other blocks may be used in conjunction. These include inguinal, penile, paracervical, and pudendal nerve blocks. This chapter describes the anatomy of the regions of interest, the rationale for choosing regional anesthesia, and the applications of each of the blocks. The goal is to guide the anesthesiologist in evaluating and incorporating regional techniques into daily practice.

Neuroanatomic Considerations of Regional Anesthesia

When planning regional anesthesia for gynecologic and urologic procedures, the somatic and autonomic innervation of the organ system must be considered. The somatic innervation of the pelvic region is readily visualized as a series of peripheral nerves and two small plexuses; the anatomy is straightforward and amenable to peripheral nerve blocks. Autonomic innervation is less readily visualized, because it is composed of a web of plexuses (Fig. 30–1). The celiac plexus is composed of visceral afferent and efferent fibers from the T-5 to T-12 nerve roots. It also carries parasympathetic input from cranial and sacral areas. The lumbar sympathetic chain is located close to the celiac plexus but is not considered a part of it. Some celiac plexus fibers contribute to the aortic, renal, and hypogastric plexuses that innervate the viscera, including the urogenital organs.[1] Because of this interwoven autonomic innervation, sensation from manipulation of the peritoneum

or viscera, which often accompanies gynecologic and urologic procedures, may be difficult to block despite adequate somatic block.

Somatic innervation of the skin, subcutaneous tissues, fascia, and muscles of the anterolateral abdominal wall is provided by branches of the inferior intercostal nerves (T-7 to T-11), the subcostal nerve (T-12), the ilioinguinal nerve (L-1), and the iliohypogastric nerve (L-1) (Fig. 30–1).

The lumbar plexus is formed by the ventral primary rami of L-1 to L-3 and the superior branch of the ventral primary ramus of L-4. Frequently, there is also a contribution from the subcostal nerve (T-12). The lumbar plexus gives rise to the obturator nerve (L-2 to L-4), the femoral nerve (L-2 to L-4), the ilioinguinal nerve (L-1), the iliohypogastric nerve (L-1), the genitofemoral nerve (L-1 to L-2), and the lateral femoral cutaneous nerve (L-2 to L-3). This plexus provides cutaneous innervation for the groin, the scrotum or labia majora, the suprapubic area, and the gluteal region. The lumbar plexus supplies sensory innervation for the anterolateral portion of the thigh through the lateral femoral cutaneous nerve and for the anteromedial portion of the thigh through the obturator nerve, and it supplies motor innervation to many lower extremity muscles. When performing peripheral nerve blocks for perineal and groin anesthesia, this relationship must be remembered. Patients often have difficulty walking after a block of the nerves in the lumbar plexus as a result of the accompanying motor block.

The sacral plexus has contributions from L-4 to S-4 nerve roots. This plexus gives rise to the sciatic nerve (L-4 to S-3), the pudendal nerve (S-2 to S-4), the superior gluteal nerve (L-4 to S-1), and various other nerves supplying pelvic and lower extremity musculature. The sacral plexus, by means of the pudendal nerve, provides cutaneous sensation for the external genitalia and motor function to the muscles of the perineum.

The principal frustration with regional anesthesia for gynecologic and urologic surgery is the occasional inability to completely block the autonomic response that occurs with visceral manipulation. Although the exact mechanism is not completely clear, its consequences

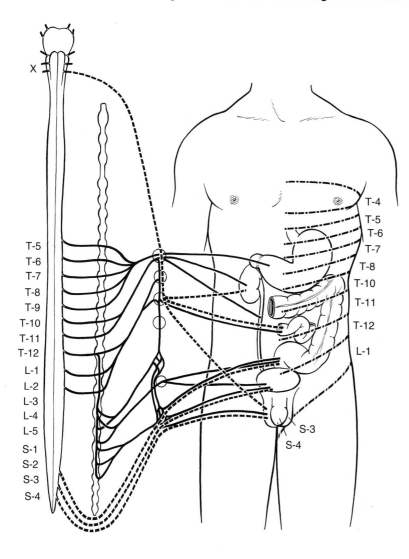

Figure 30–1 Somatic and autonomic innervation of the abdominal and pelvic regions. *Solid line,* sympathetic innervation; *dashed line,* parasympathetic innervation.

are well described. The hemodynamic response to mesenteric traction has been described as a uniform decrease in mean arterial blood pressure secondary to a marked systemic vasodilation, accompanied by a compensatory increase in cardiac output.[2] Associated with these hemodynamic effects, peritoneal or abdominal visceral manipulation can cause nausea, bradycardia, and colicky, poorly localized pain despite a dense, high (T-4) somatic block.[3]

This response may be attenuated by the neuraxial administration of opioids or by intraperitoneal lavage with a dilute solution of local anesthetics.[4–8] The dermatomal level required for the block of the autonomic and somatic innervation is shown in Figure 30–2. Because of their retroperitoneal location, manipulation of the kidneys may not elicit the hemodynamic response associated with peritoneal manipulation. But because of the kidneys' proximity to the diaphragm, a block to the cervical level may be required to prevent referred pain to the shoulder mediated through the phrenic nerve (C-3 to C-5), which innervates the diaphragm. The sensation of bladder fullness is carried by sensory fibers accompanying the sympathetic and parasympathetic nerves from the T-9 to L-2 segments. Bladder procedures require a block to at least this level. Affer-

ent impulses from the dome of the uterus also require block to the T-10 dermatomal level. The gonads are innervated by nerves from the aortic plexus to as high as the T-10 level. A dense block to at least the T-10 level is required for operations on the testes and the ovaries.

Rationale for Using Regional Anesthesia

Many gynecologic and urologic procedures are advantageously performed with regional anesthesia (Table 30–1). For procedures with a chance for perforation of a viscus, such as dilation and curettage of the uterus, regional anesthesia may be the anesthetic of choice. Perforation of the bladder or uterus intraoperatively is manifested with extremely sharp, colicky, or cramping pain. The pain may be abdominal if the perforation is extraperitoneal or referred to the shoulder if the perforation is intraperitoneal. If a procedure is performed during regional anesthesia and an acute persistent pain occurs, the surgeon should be informed immediately. If the procedure is performed during general anesthesia, the surgeon must infer perforation from an

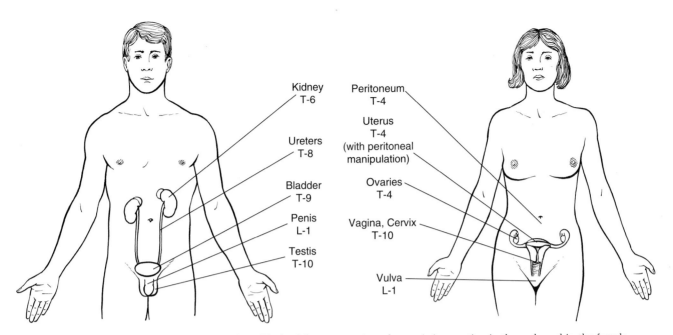

Figure 30–2 Dermatomal level required for a block of the autonomic and somatic innervation in the male and in the female.

incomplete return of the irrigating solution or from an unusual depth of sounding of the uterus.

Another advantage of regional anesthesia is the ability to follow the patient's mental status. This is particularly useful information during a transurethral resection of the prostate. During this procedure, large volumes of hyposmotic irrigating fluid can be resorbed by or infused into the open venous sinuses. Frequently, the first sign of "transurethral resection of the prostate syndrome," which is characterized by hyponatremia, fluid overload, and serum hyposmolality, is a change in the patient's mental status. If mental status changes occur, the surgeon is informed, blood is sent for hematologic and electrolyte analysis, and the resection is terminated as rapidly as possible. Transurethral resection of the prostate syndrome occurring during procedures with general anesthesia may not be noticed until the later and more ominous signs of electrocardiographic changes occur.

Several studies have compared the intraoperative blood loss and transfusion requirements associated with genital and urologic surgery performed during regional anesthesia with those during general anesthesia. Lower estimated blood loss and transfusion requirements have been demonstrated repeatedly for

Table 30–1 Advantages of Regional Anesthesia for Urologic and Genital Surgery

Intraoperative detection of bladder or uterine perforation
Intraoperative assessment of mental status
Decreased blood loss
Decreased transfusion requirements
Improved postoperative pain control
Decreased length of hospital stay
Fewer unanticipated hospital admissions after outpatient surgery
Decreased incidence of postoperative emesis

transurethral resection of the prostate, open prostatectomy, cesarean section, and vaginal procedures during regional anesthesia.[9–14] The proposed mechanisms for decreasing intraoperative blood loss when regional anesthesia is used include lower mean arterial blood pressure; spontaneous ventilation instead of intermittent positive pressure ventilation, resulting in lower intrathoracic and therefore pelvic venous pressures; hemodilution from volume loading before administration of regional anesthesia; and venous pooling and decreased venous tone in sympathectomized capacitance blood vessels, resulting in diminished venous blood and venous pressure available for loss.[10, 11, 15] It is easy to envision that any of these factors singly or in combination may lead to diminished blood loss during procedures with regional anesthesia. This is a major advantage and should be discussed with the patient when deciding on anesthetic management.

Postoperative deep venous thrombosis can lead to fatal pulmonary embolus or thrombophlebitis after major gynecologic and urologic procedures. The routine use of intermittent-compression stockings and subcutaneous administration of heparin decrease the incidence of these complications.[16, 17] Regional anesthesia may offer additional benefit by preventing intraoperative formation of deep venous thrombosis. Hendolin and colleagues[14] reported a nearly 40% decrease in calf thrombus formation in patients receiving epidural anesthesia for open prostatectomy compared with patients receiving general anesthesia. Mechanisms proposed for this decrease include increased regional blood flow that accompanies local anesthetic-induced sympathectomy, the inhibition of platelet aggregation by local anesthetics, and the local anesthetic-induced interference with the clotting cascade.[15, 18] This decrease in deep venous thrombosis has also been shown in orthopedic patients undergoing open hip procedures.[19]

The ability to provide continued neuraxial analgesia in the form of local anesthetics, opioids, or both is another considerable benefit for patients receiving lumbar epidural blocks. Patients undergoing major intra-abdominal or radical pelvic procedures for gynecologic malignancies had improved postoperative pain control if they received opioids epidurally rather than parenterally.[20, 21] However, the choice of intraoperative anesthetic technique and its effect on postoperative pain is still not completely understood.

Shir and colleagues[22] reported the postoperative pain scores and opioid usage of patients undergoing radical prostatectomy. The patients were divided into three groups on the basis of their intraoperative anesthetic management: epidural, epidural combined with general anesthesia, or general anesthesia only. All patients received the same epidurally administered local anesthetic and opioid by means of a patient-controlled device for postoperative pain management. Patients anesthetized with only bupivacaine (0.5%) through a lumbar epidural block had a significantly diminished demand for epidural analgesics postoperatively compared with those who received a general anesthetic or a combined general-epidural anesthetic (Fig. 30–3). The patients in the epidural only group had a mean sensory level of T-6 at the conclusion of the operation. Patients in the combined general-epidural group had a T-10 sensory level. The investigators speculated that the higher sensory level in the epidural-only group may have more completely blocked the afferent impulses from initiating the pain cycle than the lower sensory block or no block at all. This concept is in agreement with studies of preemptive analgesia in which the degree of postoperative pain was often dramatically influenced by the intraoperative anesthetic management.[23–25] The management of acute postoperative pain is beyond the scope of this chapter but should be considered when formulating an anesthetic plan.

The use of regional anesthesia during the intraoperative and postoperative periods may decrease the length of stay in the hospital. De Leon-Casasola and colleagues[26] prospectively studied 462 consecutive cancer patients undergoing major abdominal and thoracic procedures. They found that patients receiving combined epidural and general anesthesia followed by epidural administration of opioid analgesia averaged 11 days in the hospital and those receiving general anesthesia and intravenous administration of opioid analgesia averaged 17 days. This trend has also been demonstrated in patients undergoing donor nephrectomy. With combined epidural and general anesthesia and epidural analgesia, patients were dismissed from the hospital sooner than with general anesthesia and intravenous analgesia.[27] These observations are encouraging. The economic benefit of regional anesthesia and analgesia needs to be explored further.

Neuraxial Blocks

Neuraxial block refers to block of the spinal cord nerve roots by subarachnoid, epidural, or caudal routes. The major advantages and disadvantages of these three techniques are listed in Table 30–2. Prominent factors to consider are the dermatomal extent of block required for the procedure, the duration of the procedure, the intraoperative positioning of the patient, the need for postoperative neuraxial analgesia, and the patient's coexisting medical conditions.

Subarachnoid Block

Subarachnoid block has been the mainstay of regional anesthesia since early in the 20th century. The technique is predictable and provides a reliable means of intense anesthesia and analgesia with few side effects. Because of the small amount of drug required, it is popular for pregnant patients and for those at the extremes of age. For gynecologic and urologic procedures, subarachnoid block provides the best sacral nerve root block of any of the neuraxial blocks. The extent of the block can be manipulated by the choice of drug, the baricity of the solution, the position of the

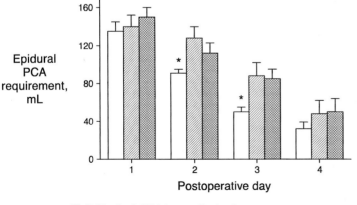

Figure 30–3 Analgesic requirements after three different anesthetic techniques for radical prostatectomy. PCA, patient-controlled analgesia; $*P < .01$ for the second postoperative day and $P < .005$ for the third postoperative day.

□ Epidural only T-6 intraoperative level
▨ General only
▩ Combined general epidural with T-10 intraoperative level

Table 30–2 Advantages and Disadvantages of Various Neuraxial Blocks

BLOCK	ADVANTAGES	DISADVANTAGES
Spinal	Intense, dense anesthesia Variable height and duration with lumbar approach Excellent sacral coverage Rapid onset	PDPH Backache Usually single-shot technique; does not allow for supplementation
Continuous spinal	Intense, dense anesthesia Height of block controlled better than single shot or epidural Fewer hemodynamic changes	Allegation of increased risk of cauda equina syndrome Large dural puncture may increase incidence of PDPH Backache
Epidural	Continuous technique possible Segmental anesthesia and analgesia Low risk of PDPH	Backache Greater mass of local anesthetic required Sacral sparing
Caudal	Lowest risk of PDPH Good sacral coverage	Occasional unfavorable anatomy in adults May require painful periosteal scraping Relative contraindication for prolonged catheter technique because of proximity to anus

PDPH, post-dural puncture headache.

patient, and the mass of drug administered. Because this is not an exact science, a block occasionally has much greater or much less spread than normally predicted. This variability of spread and the inability to supplement single-shot spinal anesthesia cause most anesthesiologists to choose a longer-acting agent and a larger dose than if a continuous-infusion technique were used. This tendency and the fact that the drug is delivered as a single bolus may result in greater hemodynamic changes with single-shot than with continuous-infusion neuraxial techniques.

The predominant reason that spinal anesthesia is not more widely practiced is the development of post-dural puncture headache, a complication that has been repeatedly studied and reviewed. The reported incidence of post-dural puncture headache varies tremendously (Table 30–3). With optimal conditions, such as a small needle, pencil-point bevel, and single dural pass, the incidence is probably no greater than 5% among young female patients and should be less for other patient groups.[35, 36] Post-dural puncture headache can be readily treated with hydration, caffeine, oral analgesics, and if

Table 30–3 Factors Influencing and Not Influencing the Incidence of Post-dural Puncture Headache

Factors Influencing the Incidence of PDPH
  Needle gauge ($\downarrow$ incidence with $\uparrow$ gauge)[28]
  Age ($\downarrow$ incidence with $\uparrow$ age)[28]
  Sex (female > male)[28]
  Number of dural punctures ($\uparrow$ incidence with $\uparrow$ passes)[29]
  Needle design (cutting bevel > pencil-point bevel > dilating
    bevel)[28]
  Needle position (bevel perpendicular > bevel parallel with cutting
    bevel)[30]
  Immediate blood patch ($\downarrow$ incidence)[31]
  Saline epidural infusion ($\downarrow$ incidence)[31]

Factors Not Influencing the Incidence of PDPH
  Early ambulation or length of recumbency
  Outpatient surgery[32]
  Intrathecal administration of opioids[33]
  Catheter techniques for continuous infusion[34]
  Pregnancy[28]

PDPH, post-dural puncture headache.

these conservative measures fail, epidural blood patch. For many patients, this is an acceptable low-risk complication compared with the sore throat, nausea, and vomiting associated with general anesthesia.

Continuous-infusion spinal techniques allow a precise block level to be achieved slowly. This may be an ideal technique for medically compromised patients in whom minimal hemodynamic derangements are the goal for the anesthetic. In the current regulatory environment, continuous spinal anesthesia should be done by using a large "epidural" catheter rather than a spinal microcatheter to maximize mixing of the local anesthetic with the cerebrospinal fluid.[37] This admonition largely limits the use of this technique to elderly patients at lower risk of post-dural puncture headache developing or to younger patients who have received a "wet tap" during attempted epidural placement.

To minimize the development of cauda equina syndrome, a maximum dose of local anesthetic should be determined before initiation of the block. If the block is focal, more local anesthetic should not be administered. Rigler and coworkers[37] suggested maneuvers such as changing the patient's position, decreasing the lumbar lordosis, changing the baricity of the local anesthetic, and manipulating the catheter to improve the distribution of the local anesthetic in the cerebrospinal fluid. With these caveats in mind, continuous spinal anesthesia is an excellent technique. It provides dense anesthesia and superb analgesia with the most precision and control of any of the neuraxial blocks.

Epidural Anesthesia

For patients undergoing major surgical interventions, such as radical prostatectomy or pelvic exenteration, my preferred regional technique is an epidural block. This block provides segmental anesthesia and analgesia that can be manipulated by the choice of anesthetic or opioid and by the level of catheter placement. During these procedures, anticipation of significant blood loss, intravascular fluid shifts, extreme lithotomy or Trendelenburg positioning, extended surgical time, and other factors may necessitate combining the epidural with a general anesthetic. The surgical management of these major procedures is facilitated by hypotension, which decreases the blood in the field, and by the bowel contraction resulting from sympathectomy that leaves parasympathetic activity uninhibited.

The anesthetic management requires meticulous volume replacement and judicious use of vasoactive drugs to maintain the desired hemodynamics. Invasive monitoring should not be minimized because the patient is "only" having an epidural block. Some anesthesiologists are uncomfortable managing a sympathectomized patient in the setting of major blood loss and fluid shifts. A continuous infusion of short-acting local anesthetic (2% lidocaine) allows rapid dissipation of the block if the need arises. However, allowing the block to dissipate may counter some of the previously mentioned benefits of the regional technique by allowing afferent impulses to be sensed centrally.

Lumbar epidural anesthesia has also been used in most minor urologic and gynecologic procedures, including laparoscopic procedures. Bridenbaugh and Soderstrom[38] compared epidural anesthesia with general tracheal anesthesia for laparoscopic tubal ligation in more than 200 patients. All patients had satisfactory anesthesia. They found no impairment of ventilation, as measured by arterial blood gases, during the period of pneumoperitoneum, with the patients spontaneously breathing during epidural anesthesia. Four patients in the epidural group had postanesthesia nausea and vomiting, compared with 38 in the general anesthesia group. This probably contributed to patients in the general anesthesia group being dismissed from the recovery unit an average of more than 1 h later than the epidural anesthesia patients.

Caudal Anesthesia

Caudal anesthesia is an excellent technique for providing dense sacral anesthesia without performing a dural puncture. However, with the advent of small-gauge spinal needles, the indications for caudal anesthesia have dwindled a bit. The technique may be technically challenging in adults because there is considerable variation in sacral anatomy and a somewhat ill-defined end point. As many as 7% of patients lack a patent sacral hiatus, the typical needle entry site for caudal anesthesia.[39] Chan and colleagues[40] studied 53 patients undergoing minor gynecologic procedures during caudal anesthesia. They defined three end points to successful identification of the caudal epidural space: a positive "give" when the needle penetrated the sacrococcygeal membrane; a loss of resistance to air when the needle was in the epidural space; and the "whoosh" test, consisting of a characteristic noise auscultated in the thoracolumbar region when 2 to 3 mL of air was injected into the caudal extradural space. They found the predictive value of a positive and a negative result of the whoosh test to be almost 100%, significantly better than either of the other predictive

tests. Perhaps the whoosh test will renew some interest in caudal anesthesia for adults.

In children, caudal anesthesia is a popular method for providing postoperative pain relief after hernia repair and minor urologic procedures.[41] Hannallah and colleagues[42] could not demonstrate any difference in postoperative pain scores after orchiopexy in children who had caudal analgesia and those who had ilioinguinal and iliohypogastric nerve block. Patients in both of the block groups had lower pain scores than the no-analgesia-block group; however, no other differences were found in the postoperative course. Blocks were placed at the end of the procedure, while the patient was still receiving general anesthesia. The investigators alluded to the possibility that, if the blocks had been placed before operation, a difference may have been detected between groups, as has been demonstrated in other studies.[23-25] This is a valid point that needs further investigation. The value of preemptive analgesia is easily proven experimentally, but clinical applicability remains to be proven conclusively for many types of surgical patients. Nevertheless, I am convinced that we see its impact in practice every day.

Peripheral Nerve Blocks

Moving away from neuraxial blocks frees the anesthesiologist from the worries of wet taps, post-dural puncture headache, central nervous system injury, and the hemodynamic changes associated with sympathectomy. However, the trade-off made in choosing a more peripheral site for regional block is the greater risk of an incomplete block. The overlap of peripheral innervation and arborizing nerves make surgical anesthesia difficult to achieve with a single percutaneous injection. As Bridenbaugh stated, "It is easier to hit the trunk of a tree than to touch each of its branches" (L.D. Bridenbaugh: Personal communication, 1995). With this in mind, the application of peripheral nerve blocks for gynecologic and urologic surgery should be undertaken with the need for supplementation and sedation planned for in advance.

Inguinal Block

The inguinal block provides anesthesia to the inguinal canal, excluding the contents of the spermatic cord, and is used most often for inguinal herniorrhaphy. Hannallah and associates[42] compared inguinal block with caudal block for relief of postoperative pain in children undergoing orchiopexy and found the two to be equivalent. This is surprising because the spermatic cord requires a T-10 level to block testicular pain. They surmised that the local anesthetic administered in the inguinal block may have bathed the spermatic cord or that testicular manipulation did not contribute much to pain after orchiopexy in children. In either case, this is a satisfactory means of providing pain relief after orchiopexy or anesthesia for inguinal herniorrhaphy.

The inguinal block is a field block of the iliohypogastric and ilioinguinal nerves. The landmarks for this block are the inguinal ligament and the anterior superior iliac spine (Fig. 30–4). In adults, after identifying the anterosuperior iliac spine, a point is marked 3 cm medial and 3 cm inferior to the anterosuperior iliac spine, just above the inguinal ligament. A 22-G, 8-cm needle is introduced at this point and directed cephalad until bone is contacted. The local anesthetic is then administered as the needle is slowly withdrawn. This procedure is repeated with the needle angled slightly more cephalad to ensure penetration of all three muscle layers: the external and internal obliques and the transverse muscle of the abdomen.

To block the iliohypogastric nerve and other cutaneous nerves, a skin wheal is made from the puncture site of the ilioinguinal nerve block to the umbilicus. An additional skin wheal is then raised from the umbilicus to the pubis. A total of 30 to 40 mL of local anesthetic should be used in performing this block in adults; in children, 10 mL may be sufficient. Remember that local anesthetic supplementation will be required to anesthetize the spermatic cord during the dissection. The maximum dose of local anesthetic should be calculated ahead of time to minimize local anesthetic toxicity. As with all field blocks, this block should be given sufficient "soak time" before surgical manipulation. At the conclusion of the operation, the motor strength of the quadriceps muscle should be tested before ambulation. Occasionally, the femoral nerve is anesthetized

with this technique, especially if supplementation of the anesthesia of the genital branch of the genital-femoral nerve has been performed intraoperatively.

Penile Block

The penile block is predominantly used for circumcision. It is also useful for any other operation that is restricted to the body of the penis, such as placement of a penile prosthesis or excision of penile cancer. Regional anesthesia for penile operations is relatively uncomplicated and easy to perform. The dorsal nerves of the penis, branches of the pudendal nerves, emerge from under the pubis in a triangular area bounded superiorly by Buck's fascia, posteriorly by the pubis, and inferiorly by the crura. They are blocked by depositing local anesthetic deep to the Buck's fascia at the base of the penis (Fig. 30–5).

The needle puncture sites are at the 10 o'clock and 2 o'clock positions at the base of the penis. The needle strikes the pubis and is then walked off in a caudal direction until bone is no longer contacted. A distinct "pop" may be felt by the anesthesiologist as the tough fascial layer is pierced. The local anesthetic is deposited deep to the fascia. These steps are repeated on the other side to block these bilateral nerves. Additional infiltration may be required if the dorsal nerves have branched early. The undersurface of the penis and the

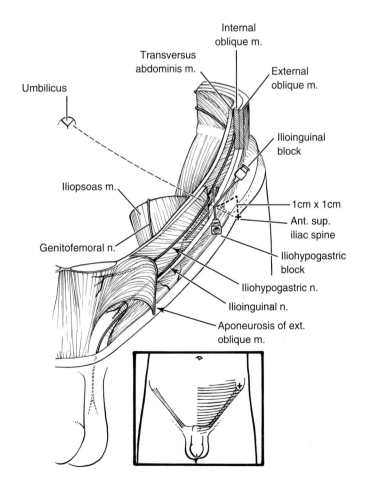

Figure 30–4 Landmarks for an inguinal block of the iliohypogastric and ilioinguinal nerves are the inguinal ligament and the anterosuperior iliac spine. Ant., anterior; sup., superior; ext., external; m., muscle; n., nerve. (Inset modified from Eltherington L, Chase R: Neural blockade for plastic surgery. In Cousins MJ, Bridenbaugh PO [eds]: Neural Blockade in Clinical Anesthesia and Management of Pain, 2nd ed, pp 635–661. Philadelphia, JB Lippincott, 1988.)

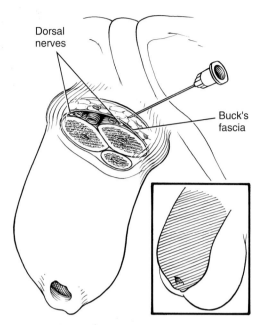

Figure 30–5 Penile nerve block shows points of injection at the 10 o'clock and 2 o'clock positions at the base of the penis. Buck's fascia must be pierced for the anesthetic to reach the nerve. A skin wheal in a triangular shape around the base of the penis completes the block.

frenulum are blocked by injecting superficial skin wheals in a triangular shape, with the pubic tubercles and a point just inferior to the undersurface of the penis on the scrotum as the triangle's corners (Fig. 30–5). The penile urethra is not blocked with this procedure.

A penile block is an effective means of providing anesthesia or postoperative analgesia after any penile procedure. The Buck's fascia must be pierced for the anesthetic to reach the nerve, and only non–epinephrine-containing solutions should be used.

Pudendal Nerve Block

Analogous to the penile block, the pudendal nerve block (Fig. 30–6) can provide anesthesia for many minor gynecologic surgeries. The pudendal nerve is formed from the lumbosacral plexus, with contributions from S-2 to S-4. It lies close to the internal pudendal artery, posterior to the sacrospinous ligament. A pudendal nerve block can provide anesthesia for cervical cerclage, marsupialization of Bartholin duct cysts, or other minor vaginal procedures.[43, 44] Successful block of the pudendal nerve bilaterally provides anesthesia to the lower third of the vagina and to the posterior two thirds of the vulva (Fig. 30–5). Leg strength should be assessed before the patient is dismissed.

Pudendal nerve blocks are usually approached transvaginally, although a transperitoneal approach has been described. Because this is a nonvisualized needle puncture in an area susceptible to unintentional needle placement into the rectum, bladder, bowel, or uterine

artery, the use of a shielded needle is recommended. A shielded or guided needle does not allow the needle to penetrate beyond a certain distance. The shielded needle is introduced through the vagina and punctures the lateral vaginal wall at the juncture of the ischial spine and the sacrospinous ligament. The sacrospinous ligament causes considerable resistance as the needle passes through it. When a loss of resistance occurs, the anesthesiologist should aspirate gently before injecting the local anesthetic.

Paracervical Block

The paracervical block is most commonly thought of in terms of obstetric anesthesia and fetal bradycardia. Despite a report[45] of 182 deliveries facilitated by using this technique, it has a limited role in obstetric anesthesia. However, like the pudendal nerve block, it may play a role in minor gynecologic surgeries. The paracervical block provides anesthesia and analgesia to the lower third of the uterus, including the cervix. Hasham and colleagues[46] performed paracervical blocks using a dilute solution of bupivacaine for analgesia after laser ablation of the endometrium. They found that hospital admission was required in 14 of 30 patients in a placebo group, but as a result of the improved analgesia, only 4 of 30 patients who received paracervical block required hospital admission. Paracervical block is probably most commonly used for anesthesia for dilatation and evacuation of the uterus. Judicious use of supplemental sedation should be planned for ahead of time, especially for a patient distraught over a lost pregnancy.

The technique for paracervical block involves bilateral injections into the lateral fornices of the vagina. A shielded needle is used to prevent injection deeper than 5 to 7 mm.[47] The needle is guided with the index and middle fingers to positions between the 3 and 4 o'clock positions and the 8 and 9 o'clock positions. The local anesthetic is injected, 10 mL to each side, with careful aspiration before and during the administration.

Special Considerations With Regional Anesthesia: Outpatient Surgery

Regional anesthesia in gynecologic and urologic patients can arguably be the technique of choice in a busy outpatient practice that requires rapid onset and dissipation of the anesthetic, with minimal side effects. Gold and associates[48] studied almost 10,000 ambulatory patients and found the three variables independently associated most with hospital admission were general anesthesia, postoperative emesis, and lower abdominal and urologic procedures. Other studies[49, 50] also cited pain as the major reason for unplanned postoperative admissions. Because of the high likelihood of unplanned hospital admission among gynecologic and urologic patients and to facilitate turnover, regional anesthesia with sedation should be considered as a primary anesthetic option for many of these patients. However, this cannot be accomplished efficiently with-

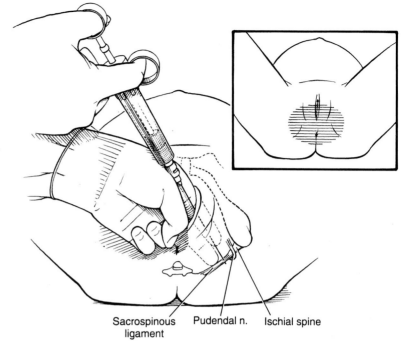

Figure 30–6 Pudendal nerve (n.) block in a female patient. Transvaginal technique. Inset, Area anesthetized. (Redrawn from Bonica JJ: Principles and Practice of Obstetric Analgesia and Anesthesia, vol 1, p 493. Philadelphia, FA Davis, 1967. Inset redrawn from Brownridge P, Cohen SE: Neural blockade for obstetrics and gynecologic surgery. In Cousins MJ, Bridenbaugh PO [eds]: Neural Blockade in Clinical Anesthesia and Management of Pain, 2nd ed, pp 593–634. Philadelphia, JB Lippincott, 1988.)

Sacrospinous ligament   Pudendal n.   Ischial spine

out a well-organized system for administering the blocks before entry into the operating suite to provide time for the agent to take effect and facilitate turnover.

The choice of local anesthetic influences the length of stay in the outpatient facility. Various local anesthetic solutions have been described for use in the outpatient setting, including epidurally administered 1.5% to 2.0% lidocaine, 2% mepivacaine, and 0.125% bupivacaine given intrathecally.[51–53] An effective solution for use in the outpatient setting was described by Liew and colleagues.[54] They reported on 30 patients receiving subarachnoid administration of 0.5% lidocaine (plain) who underwent minor outpatient gynecologic operation. Using 5 mL of this hypobaric solution, they achieved operative anesthesia for all patients and at least a T-10 sensory level in all but two patients. They observed a mean onset time of less than 8 min for effective anesthesia and a mean duration of the sensory block of 32.5 min; moreover, all patients had complete return of motor function within 1 h after receiving the spinal block. With the advent of small-gauge, pencil-point needles, the incidence of the most bothersome side effect of spinal anesthesia, post-dural puncture headache, is exceedingly low.

Nerve Injuries in Gynecologic and Urologic Surgery

Gynecologic surgery and urologic surgery share a common position—dorsal lithotomy. This position is notorious for stretching the femoral nerve and for compressing the peroneal nerve. Frequently, regional anesthetic techniques are blamed for injuries that are the result of positioning and other causes. Care must be taken to ensure that the peroneal nerve is not com-

pressed between the stirrup holder and the fibular head. To avoid stretching the femoral nerve around the inguinal ligament, the leg should be angled no more than 90° to the pelvis when supported in the stirrups.

Meticulous positioning cannot prevent all nerve injuries. Kvist-Poulsen and Borel[55] prospectively studied the incidence of femoral neuropathy after elective total abdominal hysterectomy. They found the overall incidence of postoperative femoral neuropathy was 12% of 147 patients studied. The highest incidence of femoral neuropathy was associated with the use of a large Balfour self-retaining retractor. This supports the findings of the closed claim studies[56] that showed only 28% of all lumbosacral nerve root damage could be identified as being related to anesthesia. All of the mechanisms of intraoperative nerve damage are not understood, and they are not all related to regional anesthesia.

Conclusion

If the patient or the surgeon is unwilling to participate in regional anesthesia, the technique is not likely to be a success. In this case, there are a few options involving the use of local anesthetics that can be suggested. During tubal ligation, etidocaine can be applied topically by direct visualization to the banded portion of the fallopian tube. This has decreased pain scores and the incidence of postoperative emesis.[57] Topical application of benzocaine can be used for several minor vaginal procedures. In one study,[58] pain was decreased during the procedure, and compliance with return visits was 83% for the treated group compared with 36% in a control group. Instillation of 80 mL of dilute local anesthetic intraperitoneally at the start of ambulatory laparoscopy has significantly decreased postoperative scapular pain for 48 h.[59] These are but a few of the many easy ways to introduce surgeons and patients to the advantages of local anesthetics. A few specific points are also useful:

1. Any regional technique works better if it is performed outside of the operating room and allowed setup before the surgical preparation.

2. Opioids (12.5 μg of fentanyl and 0.25 mg of morphine sulfate) added to spinal local anesthetics provide a denser block of visceral pain and prolong the surgical sensory block.

3. Pneumothorax can occur during nephrectomy and may be aggravated by spontaneous ventilation.

4. Preemptive analgesia is possible to achieve anytime before the patient awakens, but it is probably most effective if done before incision, even if the patient is receiving general anesthesia.

5. Diaphragmatic irritation requires a cervical level for complete block, but the surgeon can inject some local anesthetic (10 mL of 0.25% bupivacaine) on the diaphragm to quiet referred shoulder pain.

References

1. Berger JJ: Genitourinary surgery. In Kirby RR, Gravenstein N (eds): Clinical Anesthesia Practice, pp 1234–1245. Philadelphia, WB Saunders Co, 1994.

2. Seltzer JL, Ritter DE, Starsnic MA, et al: The hemodynamic response to traction on the abdominal mesentery. Anesthesiology 1985; 63: 96–99.

3. Alahuhta S, Kangas-Saarela T, Hollmen AI, et al: Visceral pain during caesarean section under spinal and epidural anaesthesia with bupivacaine. Acta Anaesthesiol Scand 1990; 34: 95–98.

4. Halonen PM, Paatero H, Hovorka J, et al: Comparison of two fentanyl doses to improve epidural anaesthesia with 0.5% bupivacaine for caesarean section. Acta Anaesthesiol Scand 1993; 37: 774–779.

5. Courtney MA, Bader AM, Hartwell B, et al: Perioperative analgesia with subarachnoid sufentanil administration. Reg Anesth 1992; 17: 274–278.

6. Connelly NR, Dunn SM, Ingold V, et al: The use of fentanyl added to morphine-lidocaine-epinephrine spinal solution in patients undergoing cesarean section. Anesth Analg 1994; 78: 918–920.

7. Capogna G, Celleno D, Tomassetti M: Maternal analgesia and neonatal effects of epidural sufentanil for cesarean section. Reg Anesth 1989; 14: 282–287.

8. Thompson GE, Moore DC: Celiac plexus, intercostal, and minor peripheral blockade. In Cousins MJ, Bridenbaugh PO (eds): Neural Blockade in Clinical Anesthesia and Management of Pain, 2nd ed, pp 503–530. Philadelphia, JB Lippincott, 1988.

9. Peters CA, Walsh PC: Blood transfusion and anesthetic practices in radical retropubic prostatectomy. J Urol 1985; 134: 81–83.

10. Abrams PH, Shah PJ, Bryning K, et al: Blood loss during transurethral resection of the prostate. Anaesthesia 1982; 37: 71–73.

11. Andrews WW, Ramin SM, Maberry MC, et al: Effect of type of anesthesia on blood loss at elective repeat cesarean section. Am J Perinatol 1992; 9: 197–200.

12. Gilstrap LC III, Hauth JC, Hankins GD, et al: Effect of type of anesthesia on blood loss at cesarean section. Obstet Gynecol 1987; 69: 328–332.

13. Moir DD: Blood loss during major vaginal surgery. A statistical study of the influence of general anaesthesia and epidural analgesia. Br J Anaesth 1968; 40: 233–240.

14. Hendolin H, Mattila MA, Poikolainen E: The effect of lumbar epidural analgesia on the development of deep vein thrombosis of the legs after open prostatectomy. Acta Chir Scand 1981; 147: 425–429.

15. Modig J: Influence of regional anesthesia, local anesthetics, and sympathicomimetics on the pathophysiology of deep vein thrombosis. Acta Chir Scand Suppl 1989; 550: 119–127.

16. Coe NP, Collins RE, Klein LA, et al: Prevention of deep vein thrombosis in urological patients: a controlled, randomized trial of low-dose heparin and external pneumatic compression boots. Surgery 1978; 83: 230–234.

17. Collins R, Scrimgeour A, Yusuf S, et al: Reduction in fatal pulmonary embolism and venous thrombosis by perioperative administration of subcutaneous heparin. Overview of results of randomized trials in general, orthopedic, and urologic surgery. N Engl J Med 1988; 318: 1162–1173.

18. Borg T, Modig J: Potential anti-thrombotic effects of local anaesthetics due to their inhibition of platelet aggregation. Acta Anaesthesiol Scand 1985; 29: 739–742.

19. Modig J, Borg T, Karlstrom G, et al: Thromboembolism after total hip replacement: role of epidural and general anesthesia. Anesth Analg 1983; 62: 174–180.

20. Rapp SE, Ready LB, Greer BE: Postoperative pain management in gynecology oncology patients utilizing epidural opiate analgesia and patient-controlled analgesia. Gynecol Oncol 1989; 35: 341–344.

21. Blythe JG, Hodel KA, Wahl TM, et al: Continuous postoperative epidural analgesia for gynecologic oncology patients. Gynecol Oncol 1990; 37: 307–310.

22. Shir Y, Raja SN, Frank SM: The effect of epidural versus general anesthesia on postoperative pain and analgesic requirements in patients undergoing radical prostatectomy. Anesthesiology 1994; 80: 49–56.

23. Tverskoy M, Cozacov C, Ayache M, et al: Postoperative pain after inguinal herniorrhaphy with different types of anesthesia. Anesth Analg 1990; 70: 29–35.

24. Ejlersen E, Andersen HB, Eliasen K, et al: A comparison between preincisional and postincisional lidocaine infiltration and postoperative pain. Anesth Analg 1992; 74: 495–498.

25. Bugedo GJ, Carcamo CR, Mertens RA, et al: Preoperative percutaneous ilioinguinal and iliohypogastric nerve block with 0.5% bupivacaine for post-herniorrhaphy pain management in adults. Reg Anesth 1990; 15: 130–133.

26. De Leon-Casasola OA, Parker BM, Lema MJ, et al: Epidural analgesia versus intravenous patient-controlled analgesia—differences in the postoperative course of cancer patients. Reg Anesth 1994; 19: 307–315.

27. Dixon CL, Sefton W, Gravenstein N: Epidural analgesia after donor nephrectomy decreases duration of hospitalization. (Abstract.) Reg Anesth 1992; 17(Suppl): 75.

28. Morewood GH: A rational approach to the cause, prevention and treatment of postdural puncture headache. Can Med Assoc J 1993; 149: 1087–1093.

29. Harrison DA, Langham BT: Spinal anaesthesia for urological surgery. A survey of failure rate, postdural puncture headache and patient satisfaction. Anaesthesia 1992; 47: 902–903.

30. Mihic DN: Postspinal headache and relationship of the needle bevel to the longitudinal dural fibers. Reg Anesth 1985; 10: 76–81.

31. Trivedi NS, Eddi D, Shevde K: Headache prevention following accidental dural puncture in obstetric patients. J Clin Anesth 1993; 5: 42–45.

32. Kang SB, Goodnough DE, Lee YK, et al: Comparison of 26- and 27-G needles for spinal anesthesia for ambulatory surgery patients. Anesthesiology 1992; 76: 734–738.

33. Devcic A, Sprung J, Patel S, et al: PDPH in obstetric anesthesia: comparison of 24-gauge Sprotte and 25-gauge Quincke needles and effect of subarachnoid administration of fentanyl. Reg Anesth 1993; 18: 222–225.

34. Norris MC, Leighton BL: Continuous spinal anesthesia after unintentional dural puncture in parturients. Reg Anesth 1990; 15: 285–287.

35. Brattebo G, Wisborg T, Rodt SA, et al: Intrathecal anaesthesia in patients under 45 years: incidence of postdural puncture symptoms after spinal anaesthesia with 27G needles. Acta Anaesthesiol Scand 1993; 37: 545–548.

36. Corbey MP, Berg P, Quaynor H: Classification and severity of postdural puncture headache. Comparison of 26-gauge and 27-gauge Quincke needle for spinal anaesthesia in day-care surgery in patients under 45 years. Anaesthesia 1993; 48: 776–781.

37. Rigler ML, Drasner K, Krejcie TC, et al: Cauda equina syndrome after continuous spinal anesthesia. Anesth Analg 1991; 72: 275–281.

38. Bridenbaugh LD, Soderstrom RM: Lumbar epidural block anesthesia for outpatient laparoscopy. J Reprod Med 1979; 23: 85–86.

39. Willis RJ: Caudal epidural anesthesia. In Cousins MJ, Bridenbaugh PO (eds): Neural Blockade in Clinical Anesthesia and Management of Pain, 2nd ed, pp 361–383. Philadelphia, JB Lippincott, 1988.

40. Chan SY, Tay HB, Thomas E: "Whoosh" test as a teaching aid in caudal block. Anaesth Intensive Care 1993; 21: 414–415.

41. Bramwell RG, Bullen C, Radford P: Caudal block for postoperative analgesia in children. Anaesthesia 1982; 37: 1024–1028.

42. Hannallah RS, Broadman LM, Belman AB, et al: Comparison of caudal and ilioinguinal/iliohypogastric nerve blocks for control of post-orchiopexy pain in pediatric ambulatory surgery. Anesthesiology 1987; 66: 832–834.

43. McCulloch B, Bergen S, Pielet B, et al: McDonald cerclage under pudendal nerve block. Am J Obstet Gynecol 1993; 168: 499–502.

44. Downs MC, Randall HW Jr: The ambulatory surgical management of Bartholin duct cysts. J Emerg Med 1989; 7: 623–626.

45. Goins JR: Experience with mepivacaine paracervical block in an obstetric private practice. Am J Obstet Gynecol 1992; 167: 342–345.

46. Hasham F, Mooney P, Garry R, et al: Bupivacaine paracervical block following ablation of the endometrium. Br J Obstet Gynaecol 1993; 100: 788–789.

47. Brownridge P, Cohen SE: Neural blockade for obstetrics and gynecologic surgery. In Cousins MJ, Bridenbaugh PO (eds): Neural Blockade in Clinical Anesthesia and Management of Pain, 2nd ed, pp 593–634. Philadelphia, JB Lippincott, 1988.

48. Gold BS, Kitz DS, Lecky JH, et al: Unanticipated admission to the hospital following ambulatory surgery. JAMA 1989; 262: 3008–3010.

49. Meeks GR, Waller GA, Meydrech EF, et al: Unscheduled hospital admission following ambulatory gynecologic surgery. Obstet Gynecol 1992; 80: 446–450.

50. Meridy HW: Criteria for selection of ambulatory surgical patients and guidelines for anesthetic management: a retrospective study of 1553 cases. Anesth Analg 1982; 61: 921–926.

51. Aribarg A: Epidural analgesia for laparoscopy. J Obstet Gynaecol Br Commonw 1973; 80: 567–568.

52. Sarma VJ, Lundstrom J: Epidural anaesthesia for day care surgery. A retrospective study. Anaesthesia 1989; 44: 683–685.

53. Tay DH, Tay SM, Thomas E: High-volume spinal anaesthesia. A dose-response study of bupivacaine 0.125%. Anaesth Intensive Care 1992; 20: 443–447.

54. Liew QY, Tay DH, Thomas E: Lignocaine 0.5% for spinal anaesthesia in gynaecological day surgery. Anaesthesia 1994; 49: 633–636.

55. Kvist-Poulsen H, Borel J: Iatrogenic femoral neuropathy subsequent to abdominal hysterectomy: incidence and prevention. Obstet Gynecol 1982; 60: 516–520.

56. Kroll DA, Caplan RA, Posner K, et al: Nerve injury associated with anesthesia. Anesthesiology 1990; 73: 202–207.

57. Baram D, Smith C, Stinson S: Intraoperative topical etidocaine for reducing postoperative pain after laparoscopic tubal ligation. J Reprod Med 1990; 35: 407–410.

58. Rabin JM, Spitzer M, Dwyer AT, et al: Topical anesthesia for gynecologic procedures. Obstet Gynecol 1989; 73: 1040–1044.

59. Narchi P, Benhamou D, Fernandez H: Intraperitoneal local anaesthetic for shoulder pain after day-case laparoscopy. Lancet 1991; 338: 1569–1570.

CHAPTER 31
Orthopedics

Alison Albrecht, M.D., Denise J. Wedel, M.D.

Orthopedic surgery carries with it particular anesthetic and surgical considerations. Patients undergoing orthopedic procedures often have coexisting medical problems that may complicate perioperative management. Common medical problems in the orthopedic population include heart disease, diabetes, and rheumatoid arthritis. Postoperative anesthetic management has expanded to assist with improving pain control and limb and digit salvage. In light of these considerations, in this chapter orthopedic anesthesia is discussed in relation to surgical site, with specific attention to management of pediatric and orthopedic trauma patients.

Lower Extremity Procedures

Total Hip Arthroplasty

Total hip arthroplasty can safely and reliably be performed during neuraxial block. Multiple studies[1-4] indicate that total hip arthroplasty completed during regional anesthesia is associated with decreased intraoperative blood loss and decreased incidence of deep venous thrombosis. The explanation for these differences is not known but may relate to redistribution of blood flow and rheologic changes. Induced hypotension has been used in an effort to decrease intraoperative blood loss and the need for blood transfusions.[5] Controversy still exists as to the efficacy of this technique. One investigation reemphasizes the importance of appropriate surgical hemostasis and decreased operating times, as opposed to induced decreases in blood pressure.[6]

Patients undergoing total hip arthroplasty are positioned laterally for the surgical procedure. The regional anesthetic of choice can be performed before or after the patient is positioned for operation. Subarachnoid and epidural blocks provide appropriate surgical anesthesia, and if an indwelling catheter is placed, postoperative pain management can be provided.

Knee Procedures

Total knee arthroplasty is performed on patients with joint space destruction related to osteoarthritis, rheumatoid arthritis, trauma, or other disease states. Joint replacement involves reconstruction using prosthetic devices to simulate the femoral, tibial, fibular, and, occasionally, patellar articulations. The site of this operation lends itself to regional anesthesia. Neuraxial block, lumbar plexus block, and individual nerve blocks are applicable.

Subarachnoid and epidural blocks are efficient and reliable methods of regional anesthesia for total knee arthroplasty. Subarachnoid block involves instilling local anesthetic into the cerebrospinal fluid to directly anesthetize the appropriate nerve roots. This block is established rapidly and reliably. Repeat administration at intervals can be achieved via an indwelling catheter. Epidural block is achieved by injecting local anesthetic into the epidural space, which is most often identified by a loss of resistance as the needle passes through the ligamentum flavum. The anesthetic agent diffuses to the nerve roots and results in conduction block. This block takes somewhat longer to be established than the subarachnoid block. Administration of anesthetic via an indwelling catheter ensures an adequate duration of anesthesia.

Lower extremity nerve blocks for total knee arthroplasty involve blocking the four major nerves at their characteristic peripheral locations (femoral, lateral femoral cutaneous, obturator, and sciatic nerves). The femoral nerve is blocked inferior to the inguinal ligament and immediately lateral to the femoral artery. The lateral femoral cutaneous nerve is anesthetized as it emerges from the fascia lata inferomedial to the anterior superior iliac spine. The obturator nerve is blocked as it emerges via the obturator canal. A suggested alternative to these individual blocks is the "three-in-one" block.[7] This block theoretically anesthetizes the femoral, lateral femoral cutaneous, and obturator nerves by infiltrating a larger volume (>24 mL) of local anesthetic via the femoral canal. The sciatic nerve is blocked individually either by the classic approach of Labat (posterior)[8] or by the anterior[9] or lithotomy approach. Blocking the individual nerves is an alternative to neuraxial block and likely results in fewer hemodynamic changes. Larger volumes of local anesthetic are required for peripheral nerve blocks of the lower extremity. However, the risk of systemic toxicity is not proportionally increased because of the decreased uptake of local anesthetic from the peripheral sites compared with an epidural block. Individual nerve blocks may be more difficult to learn, and the success rate reflects the anesthesiologist's experience. Lower extremity blocks may interfere with early mobilization after operation.

Amputations of the extremities are performed in order to return the affected extremity to functional use. An amputation may become necessary if there is irreparable loss of blood supply to the extremity. Additionally, if the limb is a threat to survival, is functionally limited, or is involved with a malignant process, the limb must be removed. Conditions that may predispose to amputation include congenital anomalies, tumor, nerve injuries, infection, trauma, and peripheral vascular disease.[10] Tourniquets are often used to improve surgical conditions and prevent the spread of infection or malignancy. The level of the amputation is mandated by the extent of the disease. All diseased or necrotic tissue needs to be resected to a margin where perfusion is adequate to promote healing. Postoperatively, many amputees may experience phantom limb sensation, phantom pain syndrome, or neuroma development. Some investigators[11, 12] suggest that the occurrence of phantom pain can be decreased with the use of preoperative, intraoperative, and postoperative regional block.

Below-the-knee amputations are the most frequently performed amputations. The advantage of these procedures is that the function of the knee is retained. Most patients tolerate below-the-knee prostheses with little or no functional impairment. Intraoperative management consists of neuraxial block or lower extremity nerve blocks, with care taken to provide tourniquet analgesia.

Above-the-knee amputations are the second most frequently performed amputations. These procedures do not retain the knee function and consequently are not as functional as below-the-knee amputations. The most important functional concern with above-the-knee amputations is to retain an appropriate stump length so that the leverage of the proximal lower extremity is retained. The friction-driven knee extends 8 in. above the prosthetic joint. Therefore, the amputation must occur 8 in. proximal to the knee to ensure equal limb length. Too long a stump results in that extremity being longer than the native leg. Too short a stump impairs the patient's mobility as a result of inadequate muscular strength of the extremity. Above-the-knee amputations are most often performed during neuraxial block to ensure anesthesia of the proximal limb. Overall, lower extremity amputations and the subsequent prosthetic devices are well tolerated.

Anterior cruciate ligament repairs are increasing in frequency as arthroscopic techniques become more refined. The anterior cruciate ligament provides the knee with anterior and posterior stability. In addition, it prevents hyperextension and excessive rotation of the knee. Damage to the anterior cruciate ligament does not usually occur as an isolated injury; meniscal tears are often found as concurrent injuries. Anesthesia is required in these patients to facilitate the examination of the affected joint and to allow arthroscopic or open repair. Neuraxial block and peripheral nerve blocks can be used for these procedures. Furthermore, diagnostic arthroscopy can be performed using local infiltration of the incision site followed by direct instillation of local anesthetic via the irrigating solution. Postoperatively, injection of local anesthetic or opioid into the joint space can provide adequate analgesia for a prolonged period.

Ankle and Foot Procedures

Surgical procedures on the ankle and foot can be completed by using regional anesthesia. The block to be used depends on the surgical site. Ankle procedures, such as joint reconstruction, are well suited to subarachnoid or peripheral nerve blocks. Peripheral nerve blocks can be completed at the groin or knee, depending on where the tourniquet will be placed.

Foot procedures such as distal amputations or débridements can be effectively completed during ankle block.[13] Owing to the distal site of this block, epinephrine-containing local anesthetic solutions should not be used. Ankle blocks have the advantage of being easy to perform and reliable in onset. Because small doses of local anesthetic are used at this peripheral location, local anesthetic systemic toxicity is not of particular concern. However, if bilateral ankle blocks are to be completed, care should be taken to calculate the maximum dose of local anesthetic.

Upper Extremity Procedures

Shoulder Procedures

Total shoulder arthroplasty procedures have been increasing in frequency and success in recent years. There are particular positioning concerns for the patient undergoing this and other shoulder procedures. In many cases, the patient is positioned sitting partially upright in the "beach chair" position. The hips and knees are flexed, and the patient is placed in a slight Trendelenburg position to improve venous return. The patient is then shifted laterally toward the edge of the table to allow unimpeded rotation of the extremity. The hips and chest are secured to avoid any further movement. The nonoperative arm is positioned in the lap, padded at all pressure points, and secured in such a way that there is no traction on the brachial plexus. The shoulders are elevated from the surface of the table with additional padding. The occiput is elevated to return the head to a neutral position. The head is then rotated away from the surgical site; care is taken to avoid excessive traction on the brachial plexus. When the head is properly positioned, it is secured with chin and forehead straps to avoid further movement (Fig. 31–1).

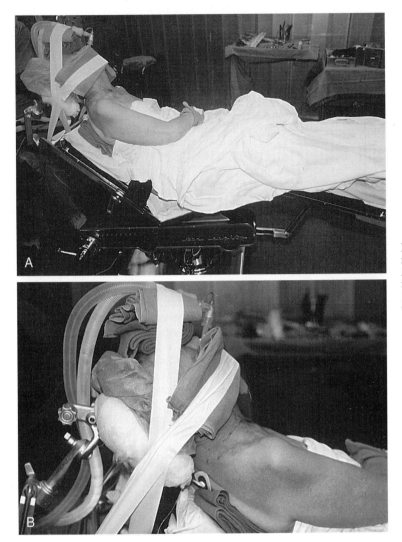

Figure 31–1 *A,* Position of patient for total shoulder repair, illustrating the semisitting position of the patient. *B,* Note the immobility of the head and neck. (*A* and *B* from Elliott BA: Positioning and monitoring. In Wedel DJ [ed]: Orthopedic Anesthesia, pp 99–128. New York, Churchill Livingstone, 1993.)

With the patient in the beach chair position, the surgical site (i.e., the shoulder) is superior to the level of the heart. When the operative site is 5 cm or more above the heart, there is the potential for air entrainment into the wound and, consequently, the systemic circulation.[14] Air that is entrained may embolize in the pulmonary circulation, resulting in pulmonary vasoconstriction and ventilation-perfusion mismatch. When significant amounts of air enter the systemic circulation, interstitial pulmonary edema and decreased cardiac output result from elevated pulmonary vascular resistance and intracardiac outflow obstruction. Additionally, this air may embolize paradoxically to the cerebral and coronary circulation via a patent foramen ovale.

Venous air embolism can be detected by mass spectrometry, precordial Doppler echocardiography, and transesophageal echocardiography, although the last two are rarely used in shoulder surgery. Physical findings, including profound hypotension and the classic "mill wheel" murmur, are late and often terminal events. With the initial detection of entrained air, nitrous oxide should be discontinued and the patient should receive 100% oxygen to avoid expansion of the entrained bubbles. If a right atrial catheter is in place, it should be aspirated in an attempt to remove air from the circulation. Furthermore, attempts should be made to prevent further entrainment by flooding the surgical field with saline and repositioning the patient with the heart superior to the surgical site.

Total shoulder arthroplasty can be completed during regional or general anesthesia. If a general anesthetic is provided, the interscalene brachial plexus block is ideally suited for intraoperative and postoperative analgesia.[15] Some investigators suggest the block should be performed postoperatively if there is a risk of intraoperative brachial plexus injury, in order that neurologic function may be assessed before the block. Others believe a preoperative interscalene block is not contraindicated in this setting. Regional anesthesia may be provided for this procedure with the additional block of the cervical plexus. With the interscalene approach to the brachial plexus, the ipsilateral phrenic nerve is predictably anesthetized.[16] For this reason, bilateral interscalene blocks are contraindicated and unilateral blocks should be performed with caution in patients with significant respiratory compromise. Other complications or side effects associated with this block include injection of local anesthetic into the vertebral artery, subarachnoid or epidural injection, recurrent laryngeal nerve block, and stellate ganglion block.

The rotator cuff of the shoulder consists of the supraspinatus, infraspinatus, teres minor, and subscapularis muscles. Injury to this muscle group can lead to the development of the supraspinatus syndrome. This can be caused by any of several lesions that directly or indirectly affect the supraspinatus tendon. This type of injury is characterized by pain, muscle spasm, limited range of motion, muscle atrophy, and tenderness over the insertion of the rotator muscles. The supraspinatus syndrome may involve any of the multiple structures of the shoulder, and anesthesia is often required to facilitate diagnosis.[17] When fibrous ankylosis of the shoulder (frozen shoulder) occurs, anesthesia is required to allow assessment of the joint and manipulation, which improves the range of motion of the shoulder. Evaluation of the drop sign is important in determining the extent of a rotator cuff tear. This test consists of infiltrating the subdeltoid region of the affected extremity with local anesthetic to assess the patient's ability to abduct the arm. If a patient cannot abduct the arm after the local anesthetic injection, the diagnosis of a complete rotator cuff tear is confirmed. Arthroscopy is often required to evaluate primary versus secondary rotator cuff injuries. For diagnostic or therapeutic assessment of the rotator cuff, regional or general anesthesia can be provided. Interscalene brachial plexus block provides the most reliable anesthesia for these procedures and rarely requires augmentation with a deep cervical plexus block. Postoperative assessment of neurologic function is delayed after regional anesthesia.

Elbow Procedures

Total elbow arthroplasty is becoming increasingly successful in the management of joint space disruption related to arthritic conditions and trauma of the elbow. Regional anesthesia is well suited to this surgical approach if the brachial plexus is blocked at a location proximal enough to reliably include the axillary and musculocutaneous nerves. For this reason, the axillary approach to the brachial plexus is not the most efficacious route. The infraclavicular and supraclavicular approaches are the most reliable alternatives. The infraclavicular approach involves injecting local anesthetic in the proximal axilla.[18] This approach is associated with a decreased risk of pneumothorax compared with the supraclavicular approach. The supraclavicular approach to the brachial plexus can be performed by using the midpoint of the clavicle and the first rib as landmarks. This block has been modified in the "perivascular" approach by blocking the plexus higher in the interscalene groove—a technique that claims a lower incidence of pneumothorax. Finally, the plexus can be accessed by using the "plumb-bob" technique. The plumb-bob technique is reported[19] to be associated with a decreased risk of pneumothorax and may be easier to master.

Brachial Plexus Catheters

Indwelling brachial plexus catheters are useful for replantation procedures of the upper extremity[20] and postoperative analgesia.[21] Any approach can be used; however, the axillary, infraclavicular, and interscalene approaches are most commonly used for catheter placement. When approaching the brachial plexus from any of these locations, either a nerve stimulator or the paresthesia technique can be used. The needle gauge must be large enough to accommodate the passage of a medium-gauge catheter. For the axillary approach, the catheter should be inserted approximately 7 cm. With the interscalene and infraclavicular approaches, 3 to 4 cm is sufficient. Figure 31–2 radiographically demonstrates an axillary catheter in proper position. The complications associated with brachial plexus catheter placement are the same as those associated with brachial plexus block. Interscalene catheters are difficult to secure and are often dislodged with typical patient head and neck movement. Additionally, these catheters, as with any foreign bodies, can predispose the patient to infection. The bacteriostatic properties of local anesthetics likely assist in decreasing the risk of infection. There has been a case report of Horner's syndrome associated with proximal migration of an axillary catheter and cephalad spread of local anesthetic.[22]

Hand Procedures

Minor hand procedures such as carpal tunnel release and wound débridements are well suited to regional

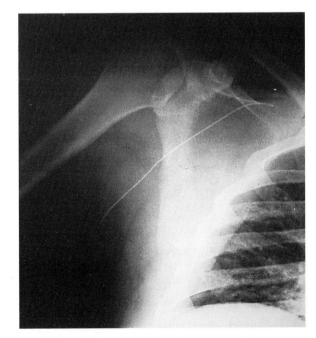

Figure 31–2 Axillary catheter in place. (From Lamer TJ: Postoperative analgesia. In Wedel DJ [ed]: Orthopedic Anesthesia, pp 363–384. New York, Churchill Livingstone, 1993.)

anesthetic techniques. Patients undergoing these procedures may have their regional anesthesia performed with short- to medium-acting local anesthetics. These patients have shorter recovery times and are dismissed from the outpatient unit sooner than those undergoing general anesthesia.[23, 24]

Procedures involving the distal forearm and hand can be effectively managed with axillary brachial plexus block.[25] Anesthetizing the brachial plexus at the axilla provides adequate analgesia at the wrist, forearm, and hand. The only exception is the distribution of the musculocutaneous nerve. This nerve exits the axillary sheath in the proximal axilla, and local anesthetic injected at this level does not reliably block it. For this reason, the musculocutaneous nerve should be blocked separately at the level of the axilla or at the antecubital fossa, if sensory anesthesia in its distribution is not present at completion of the axillary block. Additionally, if a tourniquet is used, the intercostobrachial cutaneous nerve (a branch of T-2) must be anesthetized.

The Bier block or intravenous regional block is another alternative for procedures on the upper extremity. The utility of this anesthetic may be limited by tourniquet pain related to the duration of operation. Use of a double tourniquet may partially alleviate this problem. When tourniquet pain begins, the more distal cuff is inflated and the proximal cuff is deflated to relieve the discomfort. Because this block is associated with a rapid termination of effect, additional analgesia may be required once the tourniquet is deflated.

The nerves that innervate the hand can also be blocked peripherally at the wrist or elbow. This involves injecting small amounts of local anesthetic near the median, radial, and ulnar nerves. Epinephrine-containing solutions should not be used at the wrist because of the peripheral location of this block. It must also be remembered that there is no provision for tourniquet analgesia with these blocks.

Joint replacement procedures on the hand and wrist are becoming increasingly popular. These procedures can easily be performed with regional anesthetic techniques. Tourniquets are frequently used with these procedures, and analgesia for tourniquet pain must be provided. Postoperatively, analgesia for range of motion exercises can be provided via indwelling brachial plexus catheters with continuous or bolus administration of local anesthetics, opioids, or combinations of both.

Spine Procedures

Degenerative disk disease refers to herniation of the nucleus pulposus through a fractured anulus fibrosus. This expulsion of disk material can result in neurologic sequelae if either the spinal cord or nerve root is involved. Initially, pain is related to stretching of the posterior spinal ligament. Without intervention, the associated nerve root compression may lead to progressive numbness, weakness, and hyporeflexia. The entire vertebral column can be involved, but most commonly disk herniation is seen in the lumbar and cervical regions. The C5-6 and C6-7 interspaces are the most frequently involved cervical segments. The L4-5 and L5-S1 interspaces are frequently involved in the lumbar region. The lumbar spine is involved six times more often than the cervical spine. Initially, a trial of bed rest and brief immobilization is warranted. If symptoms persist or increase, surgical repair via laminectomy may be warranted.

Spondylolisthesis describes the movement of one vertebral body on another and is caused by long-term intervertebral instability. At the site of displacement, the facet joints and anulus fibrosus demonstrate severe degeneration. This disease is also most commonly seen in the lumbar spine; the cervical spine is occasionally involved. Symptoms initially include back pain with or without leg pain. These symptoms may progress to pain with walking that is relieved when sitting or supine. This presentation indicates spinal stenosis that requires surgical intervention. Posterior fusion using iliac crest bone grafts to stabilize the weakened intervertebral segment is the surgical procedure of choice.

Patients with multiple levels of instability or severe instability related to vertebral fracture require stabilization with prosthetic stabilization devices. Placement of these devices may involve significant amounts of blood loss, depending on the number of vertebrae to be fused. Patients undergoing multilevel fusions are at risk for spinal cord injury and possible paraplegia. Three tests have been devised that can evaluate spinal cord compromise: the wake-up test, somatosensory-evoked potentials, and motor-evoked potentials. The wake-up test involves arousing the patients after instrumentation but before closure to assess their ability to move all extremities. When care is taken to provide adequate analgesia and warn patients preoperatively about the procedure, most patients tolerate this test quite well.[26]

Somatosensory-evoked potentials involve monitoring the cortical response to repetitive peripheral stimuli to ensure spinal cord integrity.[27] The main pitfall with this type of monitoring is that the anterior spinal cord, which provides motor function, is not monitored. Therefore, the risk of paraplegia still exists—a theoretic concern substantiated by a case report.[28] Additionally, somatosensory-evoked potentials are influenced by opioids, inhalational agents, and nitrous oxide, confounding the interpretation of potentials.[29] Studies[30] indicated that 0.75% minimum alveolar concentration of a potent inhalational agent with 60% nitrous oxide did not adversely affect interpretation.

Motor-evoked potentials provide direct monitoring of the motor system. By using transcranial electrical or magnetic stimulation of the motor cortex, corticospinal responses can be measured at the lateral columns of the spinal cord, epidural space, or peripheral muscles. This monitoring device allows assessment of motor function intraoperatively. Motor-evoked potentials involve the monitoring of electrical impulses that are quite small. As a result, these electrical potentials are sensitive to a wide variety of anesthetic agents. Currently, it appears that fentanyl has no effect on the latency or amplitude of the motor-evoked potentials.[31] Etomidate increases latency without affecting amplitude.[32] Ketamine,[33] nitrous oxide,[31] halothane,[34] and isoflurane[35] all increase latency and decrease the amplitude of the motor-evoked potentials. This sensitivity to anesthetics can be circumvented by monitoring repetitive stimulation as opposed to single twitches. Motor-evoked potentials are useful for detecting spinal cord injury in the descending motor tracts that may go unnoticed when somatosensory-evoked potentials are used.[36]

General anesthesia and regional anesthesia are applicable to back surgery. Spinal anesthesia with hypobaric local anesthetic solutions and epidural anesthesia have been used successfully for these procedures.[37] Operation in the lumbar region is better suited to regional anesthesia than procedures on the cervical and thoracic vertebrae. The high level of spinal anesthesia required for these operative sites would lead to respiratory and hemodynamic compromise. Most back surgery is completed during general anesthesia to ensure airway patency and patient comfort in the prone position.

Pediatric Orthopedic Procedures

Pediatric patients present with a wide variety of orthopedic pathologic findings, including congenital disorders, tumors, and traumatic injuries. Anesthetic care of pediatric patients has its own unique considerations that are fully outlined in textbooks relating to pediatric anesthesia. In this chapter, the particular concerns in anesthetizing pediatric orthopedic patients are considered.

Orthopedic procedures on the lower extremity are well suited to regional anesthesia. Sedation of the patient before the performance of the chosen regional technique can simplify its execution. Spinal, caudal, and epidural blocks are safe and effective in children provided that anatomic differences from the adult are remembered.[38, 39] Sciatic and femoral nerve blocks are useful for providing analgesia of the affected extremity and are useful when combined with significant sedation or a light general anesthetic.[40] Additionally, ankle and knee blocks are practical and effective for postoperative analgesia.

Procedures on the upper extremity can be performed with any of the techniques previously described for adults. However, the axillary and interscalene approaches to the brachial plexus[41] and the intravenous regional (Bier) block are most frequently used. With adequate sedation, pediatric patients tolerate these blocks. Older pediatric patients may tolerate the paresthesia technique more readily. In the younger patients, the sheath or transarterial approach seems better tolerated. Regardless of technique, the superficial position of the brachial plexus and relative lack of subcutaneous tissue in this population need to be considered.

The intravenous regional block is especially useful in the pediatric population, particularly for short procedures such as fracture reduction.[42] Adequate sedation combined with local anesthetic eutectic creams for the initial intravenous catheter placement improve patient tolerance of the block. Owing to the size of the upper extremity in pediatric patients, placement of a double tourniquet may not be possible, and tourniquet pain may become problematic. The integrity of the tourniquet used must be ensured before initiation of the block. With an optimally functioning tourniquet available, the institution of the block can proceed as previously described. Figure 31–3 demonstrates the proper setup for the intravenous regional block.

Trauma

Management of trauma patients requires a coordinated multidisciplinary approach to evaluate the extent of injuries and prioritize their treatment. After life-threatening injuries are addressed, orthopedic injuries may be stabilized. Immediate surgical intervention is required for some orthopedic injuries. Fracture immobilization leads to decreased pain and blood loss. Additionally, the risk of fat embolism and secondary injury as a result of bone fragments is decreased. Delayed repair of open injuries greatly increases the risk of infection. Similarly, delaying closed reductions of fractures may make the reduction difficult or impossible because of developing edema.

Trauma patients have delayed gastric emptying as a result of the traumatic event and subsequent pain. These patients must be considered to have full stomachs, and this condition may not improve even if sur-

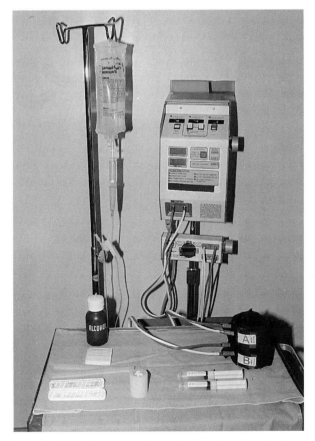

Figure 31–3 Bier block setup for fractured radius in pediatric patient.

gery is delayed 6 to 8 h. The cervical spine of trauma patients should be evaluated for evidence of instability and to prevent further neurologic injury. These factors play an important role in determining the anesthetic. The ability to safely secure the airway must be carefully evaluated before embarking on either regional or general anesthesia.

The patient sustaining a hip fracture will likely be elderly and often debilitated with significant coexisting disease. Careful preoperative evaluation is required to determine whether preexisting medical disorders are under adequate control and to determine if preoperative medications will alter the anesthetic plan. Once the patient has been fully evaluated, the choice of anesthetic technique can be made.

Regional anesthetic techniques applicable to patients with hip fractures include the neuraxial blocks. Block selection is determined after consideration of the patient's hemodynamic status, preexisting medical conditions, and mental status. Indwelling epidural catheters may be of significant benefit for postoperative pain control.

Patients with hip fractures often have significant pain before fixation. Positioning for regional anesthesia can, therefore, be difficult. Small, incremental doses of sedatives and analgesics can greatly improve the patient's tolerance of position changes. Additionally, adequate traction on the involved extremity decreases the degree of discomfort with movement. A paramedian approach is often required in these patients owing to their decreased ability to reduce lumbar lordosis in light of their pain. If a hyperbaric or hypobaric subarachnoid block is placed with the patient on the fracture table, altering the level of the block is difficult because most fracture tables do not allow motion about the horizontal axis. Femoral nerve block has also been used for pain relief in these cases.

With the anesthesia underway, the complex process of positioning can begin. Optimal positioning is a compromise between ideal surgical exposure and optimal physiologic function of the major organ systems. The fracture table is commonly used for fractures of the hip and femur. The fracture table allows greater ease of manipulation and traction of the involved extremity. It also allows greater freedom of access for radiographic evaluation.

The fracture table has three basic components. First, the main body provides support for the head and torso. Next is the sacral platform with a vertical perineal post that provides stabilization of the pelvis. Finally, there is a footrest to provide traction on the fracture and a stirrup to support the contralateral leg. The perineal post should be removed before moving the patient to the fracture table to avoid having to lift the patient over the post. When in place, the perineal post should fit snugly against the perineum without undue compression of the pudendal nerve; male genitalia should also be free from compression. The contralateral leg in its stirrup holder can be abducted to be excluded from the radiographic field; however, care must be taken to avoid common peroneal nerve compression. The contralateral arm is padded to avoid ulnar nerve com-

pression and is secured in the patient's lap or on an arm board. The ipsilateral arm can be positioned in an overhead sling, with care taken to avoid brachial plexus injury. The patient can also be positioned laterally on the fracture table. All the same positioning concerns for a supine patient apply to the patient in the lateral position. The main difference for lateral placement involves the pelvic rest, which is a large "C"-shaped support used to secure the superior thigh and anterior superior iliac crest of the superior hip. Before surgical draping, a quick review of nerve compression points can minimize postoperative complications. Examples of patient positioning on the fracture table are shown in Figure 31–4.

Patients who have sustained an ankle fracture that cannot be reduced externally require open reduction and internal fixation of the involved joint. For open fractures, delaying the repair beyond 6 h can preclude primary wound closure, and healing will have to occur by secondary intent. Regional anesthetic techniques are well suited to this peripheral location. Neuraxial block can be used for ankle repair; however, the epidural block may not reliably involve the low lumbar and sacral dermatomes of the ankle. For this reason, the subarachnoid block is the more reliable choice. Peripheral nerve blocks at the groin or popliteal fossa are also effective, although they may impair neurologic assessment postoperatively.

Of particular importance, in patients with traumatic injuries, are those individuals with amputation of digits or extremities. Patients with clean guillotine-type cuts have the greatest chance of successful replantation.[43] Conversely, those with multiple levels of amputation, crush injuries, or avulsion injuries are less suitable candidates. The patient with a warm ischemia time of greater than 10 h is less likely to have a successful replantation.[43]

Often these patients require prolonged surgical repair. Regional anesthetic techniques are well suited to these procedures because of the improved blood flow that occurs with sympathetic block. However, few patients can tolerate remaining immobile for the duration of the surgical procedure. For this reason, combined anesthesia techniques are often useful. Light general anesthesia provides patient comfort, and regional anesthesia optimizes graft survival.

Replantation of structures of the lower extremities can be completed with an indwelling epidural catheter. This can be the sole method of intraoperative anesthesia or may be combined with a general anesthetic. In either case, the sympathectomy provided improves peripheral blood flow, facilitating the anastomosis of severed vessels and improving the chances that adequate blood flow will be restored.

Special Considerations

The Cast Room

The cast room is of particular significance in orthopedic anesthesia because of the typically brief duration of

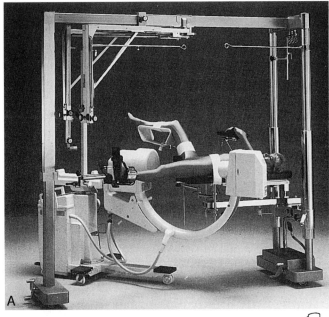

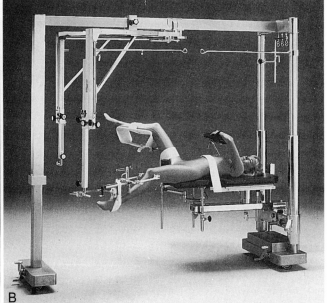

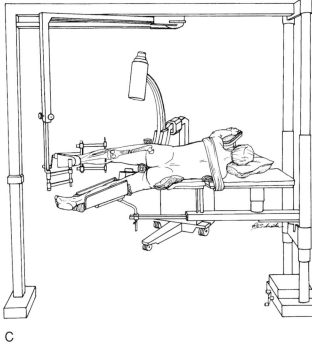

Figure 31–4 Position of patient on the fracture table. *A* and *B*, Supine positioning. *C*, Lateral positioning. (*A* and *B* from Elliott BA: Positioning and monitoring. In Wedel DJ [ed]: Orthopedic Anesthesia, pp 99–128. New York, Churchill Livingstone, 1993. [Courtesy of Midmark Corporation, Versailles, OH.] *C* from Day LJ: Unusual positions: orthopedics: surgical aspects. In Martin TJ [ed]: Positioning in Anesthesia and Surgery, 2nd ed, pp 223–231. Philadelphia, WB Saunders Co, 1987.)

treatment at this location. Anesthesia intervention may be required for cases involving a patient who is severely distressed or in pain. Therefore, the cast room should be fully equipped for general or regional anesthesia. This includes, but is not limited to, a reliable oxygen supply, airway equipment, suction, and appropriate monitoring devices. An anesthetic, regional or general, should not be undertaken in a location that lacks appropriate resuscitation equipment.

Radial fractures come to the attention of anesthesia personnel in those patients who have a marked displacement of the fragments or in patients with severe pain. For some patients, analgesics and amnestic agents may be all that is necessary to facilitate the reduction.

Patients who require general anesthesia need tracheal intubation to secure patency of their airway in the acute trauma setting. Alternatively, a regional anesthetic provides analgesia for the manipulation without excessive sedation. Patients often require analgesics to tolerate positioning of the extremity before initiation of the regional block. The axillary brachial plexus and Bier blocks are both well suited to reduction of radial head fractures. Bier blocks offer the advantage of rapid offset of anesthesia, allowing earlier neurologic assessment and the ability to eliminate the possibility of ischemia due to the cast. Adequate analgesia in these patients may well make the difference between closed and open reduction.

Other cases of particular interest in the cast room include joint dislocations. These injuries are often painful, with the discomfort substantially relieved after repair of the dislocation. Shoulder and hip dislocations are often seen in the cast room. Patients require analgesia and sedation to tolerate the brief procedure. Often muscle relaxation is necessary to allow successful relocation. A general anesthetic with intubation or regional anesthesia with motor block can be used. However, regional anesthesia offers certain advantages, particularly the avoidance of airway manipulation. The choice, of course, has to be individualized.

Tourniquet Pain

Tourniquets are often used in orthopedic surgery to decrease blood loss and improve visualization of the surgical site. With the advent of tourniquet use by orthopedic surgeons, anesthesiologists noted tourniquet pain. This pain is characterized as a dull, aching sensation that may be difficult for patients to localize. Typically, the pain begins 45 to 60 min after inflation of the tourniquet and persists until the tourniquet has been deflated for at least 10 to 15 min. The pain is thought to result from ischemia and local tissue acidosis, but the full etiology is yet to be determined.[44–47] The pain is mediated via unmyelinated C fibers and may be so severe as to necessitate a general anesthetic. During general anesthesia for procedures involving a thigh tourniquet, hypertension develops 45 to 60 min after tourniquet inflation. This hypertensive response is not seen during subarachnoid block and is only occasionally seen with epidural blocks. This physiologic response is believed to represent underlying tourniquet pain.[48] Neuraxial block appears to be effective in avoiding this response.

Methyl Methacrylate

Methyl methacrylate is an acrylic bone cement used for arthroplastic procedures. This cement is used primarily to distribute the forces of the prosthesis evenly. It has also been used for prosthetic testicles, cranioplasty, encapsulation of cerebral aneurysms, and prosthetic middle ear ossicles. Some patients demonstrate profound hypotension during insertion of the cement, particularly with the large volumes used for arthroplasty.[49] This is believed to be due to absorption of the volatile monomer of methyl methacrylate, embolization of air and bone marrow, lysis of blood cells and marrow induced by the exothermic reaction, and conversion of methyl methacrylate to methacrylic acid. Mixing according to instructions decreases the amount of volatile monomer. Adequate hydration minimizes the hypotension that occurs with cementing. Increasing the inspired oxygen concentration before insertion decreases the magnitude of the subsequent hypoxemia. Vigilance on the part of the anesthesiologist is of particular importance at this time during the procedure.

Fat Embolism

The fat embolism syndrome has been found to occur in up to 15% of patients with fractures of the pelvis or long bones. The characteristic features of this syndrome include increased temperature, tachypnea, and tachycardia.[50] Adult respiratory distress syndrome occasionally accompanies fat embolism, leading to hypoxemia and subsequent clouded sensorium. Petechiae occur early but may escape observation because they resolve quickly. Supportive care, often including mechanical ventilation, is used in these patients.

Summary

Orthopedic anesthesia is a challenging area of anesthesia care. The patient population often encompasses the extremes of age. This diverse group of patients often has a complex array of coexisting diseases. Additionally, in the context of acute trauma, a once straightforward case becomes far more intriguing. As the frequency of outpatient procedures increases, we are further challenged to provide safe, effective anesthesia care with minimal side effects. With these added demands, regional anesthetic and analgesic techniques are becoming increasingly popular among anesthesiologists, surgeons, and patients. Although outcome improvements are difficult to demonstrate, there are significant theoretic advantages to regional anesthetic procedures in orthopedic patients.

References

1. Tuman KJ, McCarthy RJ, March RJ, et al: Effects of epidural anesthesia and analgesia on coagulation and outcome after major vascular surgery. Anesth Analg 1991; 73: 696–704.
2. Modig J, Borg T, Karlstrom G, et al: Thromboembolism after total hip replacement: role of epidural and general anesthesia. Anesth Analg 1983; 62: 174–180.
3. Wille-Jorgensen P, Christensen SW, Bjerg-Nielsen A, et al: Prevention of thromboembolism following elective hip surgery. The value of regional anesthesia and graded compression stockings. Clin Orthop 1989; 247: 163–167.
4. Keith I: Anaesthesia and blood loss in total hip replacement. Anaesthesia 1977; 32: 444–450.
5. Sharrock NE, Mineo R, Urquhart B: Haemodynamic effects and outcome analysis of hypotensive extradural anaesthesia in controlled hypertensive patients undergoing total hip arthroplasty. Br J Anaesth 1991; 67: 17–25.
6. Lennon RL, Hosking MP, Gray JR, et al: The effects of intraoperative blood salvage and induced hypotension on transfusion requirements during spinal surgical procedures. Mayo Clin Proc 1987; 62: 1090–1094.
7. Winnie AP, Ramamurthy S, Durrani Z: The inguinal paravascular technic of lumbar plexus anesthesia: the "3-in-1 block." Anesth Analg 1973; 52: 989–996.
8. Labat G: Regional Anesthesia: Its Technic and Clinical Application. Philadelphia, WB Saunders Co, 1922.
9. Beck GP: Anterior approach to sciatic nerve block. Anesthesiology 1963; 24: 222–224.
10. Tooms RE: General principles of amputations. In Crenshaw AH (ed): Campbell's Operative Orthopaedics, 8th ed, vol 2, pp 677–687. St Louis, Mosby–Year Book, 1992.
11. Bach S, Noreng MF, Tjellden NU: Phantom limb pain in amputees during the first 12 months following limb amputation, after preoperative lumbar epidural blockade. Pain 1988; 33: 297–301.

12. Fisher A, Meller Y: Continuous postoperative regional analgesia by nerve sheath block for amputation surgery—a pilot study. Anesth Analg 1991; 72: 300–303.
13. Schurman DJ: Ankle-block anesthesia for foot surgery. Anesthesiology 1976; 44: 348–352.
14. Cucchiara RF: Safety of the sitting position. (Letter to the editor.) Anesthesiology 1984; 61: 790.
15. Winnie AP: Interscalene brachial plexus block. Anesth Analg 1970; 49: 455–466.
16. Urmey WF, Talts KH, Sharrock NE: One hundred percent incidence of hemidiaphragmatic paresis associated with interscalene brachial plexus anesthesia as diagnosed by ultrasonography. Anesth Analg 1991; 72: 498–503.
17. Crenshaw AH Jr: Shoulder and elbow injuries. In Crenshaw AH (ed): Campbell's Operative Orthopaedics, 8th ed, vol 3, pp 1733–1766. St Louis, Mosby–Year Book, 1992.
18. Raj PP, Montgomery SJ, Nettles D, et al: Infraclavicular brachial plexus block—a new approach. Anesth Analg 1973; 52: 897–904.
19. Brown DL, Cahill DR, Bridenbaugh LD: Supraclavicular nerve block: anatomic analysis of a method to prevent pneumothorax. Anesth Analg 1993; 76: 530–534.
20. Matsuda M, Kato N, Hosoi M: Continuous brachial plexus block for replantation in the upper extremity. Hand 1982; 14: 129–134.
21. Gaumann DM, Lennon RL, Wedel DJ: Continuous axillary block for postoperative pain management. Reg Anesth 1988; 13: 77–82.
22. Lennon RL, Gammel S: Horner's syndrome associated with brachial plexus anesthesia using an axillary catheter. (Letter to the editor.) Anesth Analg 1992; 74: 311.
23. Bridenbaugh LD: Regional anaesthesia for outpatient surgery—a summary of 12 years' experience. Can Anaesth Soc J 1983; 30: 548–552.
24. Allen HW, Mulroy MF, Fundis K, et al: Regional versus propofol general anesthesia for outpatient hand surgery. (Abstract.) Anesthesiology 1993; 79: A1.
25. DeJong RH: Axillary block of the brachial plexus. Anesthesiology 1961; 22: 215–225.
26. Dorgan JC, Abbott TR, Bentley G: Intra-operative awakening to monitor spinal cord function during scoliosis surgery. Description of the technique and report of four cases. J Bone Joint Surg Br 1984; 66: 716–719.
27. Grundy BL: Intraoperative monitoring of sensory-evoked potentials. Anesthesiology 1983; 58: 72–87.
28. Ginsburg HH, Shetter AG, Raudzens PA: Postoperative paraplegia with preserved intraoperative somatosensory evoked potentials. Case report. J Neurosurg 1985; 63: 296–300.
29. Grundy BL, Brown RH, Berilla JA: Fentanyl alters somatosensory cortical evoked potentials. (Abstract.) Anesth Analg 1980; 59: 544–545.
30. Pathak KS, Ammadio M, Kalamchi A, et al: Effects of halothane, enflurane, and isoflurane on somatosensory evoked potentials during nitrous oxide anesthesia. Anesthesiology 1987; 66: 753–757.
31. Zentner J, Kiss I, Ebner A: Influence of anesthetics—nitrous oxide in particular—on electromyographic response evoked by transcranial electrical stimulation of the cortex. Neurosurgery 1989; 24: 253–256.
32. Ghaly RF, Stone JL, Kartha RK, et al: The effect of etomidate on transcranial magnetic-induced motor evoked potentials in primates. (Abstract.) Anesthesiology 1990; 73: A746.
33. Ghaly RF, Stone JL, Aldrete JA, et al: Effects of incremental ketamine hydrochloride doses on motor evoked potentials (MEPs) following transcranial magnetic stimulation: a primate study. J Neurosurg Anesthesiol 1990; 2: 79–85.
34. Haghighi SS, Madsen R, Green KD, et al: Suppression of motor evoked potentials by inhalation anesthetics. J Neurosurg Anesthesiol 1990; 2: 73–78.
35. Haghighi SS, Green KD, Oro JJ, et al: Depressive effect of isoflurane anesthesia on motor evoked potentials. Neurosurgery 1990; 26: 993–997.
36. Lesser RP, Raudzens P, Luders H, et al: Postoperative neurological deficits may occur despite unchanged intraoperative somatosensory evoked potentials. Ann Neurol 1986; 19: 22–25.
37. Tetzlaff JE, Yoon HJ, O'Hara J, et al: Influence of anesthetic technique on the incidence of deep venous thrombosis after elective lumbar spine surgery. Reg Anesth 1994; 19: S28.
38. Yaster M, Maxwell LG: Pediatric regional anesthesia. Anesthesiology 1989; 70: 324–338.
39. Dalens B: Regional anesthesia in children. Anesth Analg 1989; 68: 654–672.
40. Wedel DJ: Femoral and lateral femoral cutaneous nerve block for muscle biopsies in children. (Abstract.) Reg Anesth 1989; 14: S63.
41. Wedel DJ, Krohn JS, Hall JA: Brachial plexus anesthesia in pediatric patients. Mayo Clin Proc 1991; 66: 583–588.
42. Gingrich TF: Intravenous regional anesthesia of the upper extremity in children. JAMA 1967, May 1; 200: 135.
43. Beatty ME, Smith AA: Hand and microvascular surgery. Evolution to present practice. J Fla Med Assoc 1989; 76: 592–594.
44. Hagenouw RR, Bridenbaugh PO, van Egmond J, et al: Tourniquet pain: a volunteer study. Anesth Analg 1986; 65: 1175–1180.
45. Chabel C, Russell LC, Lee R: Tourniquet-induced limb ischemia: a neurophysiologic animal model. Anesthesiology 1990; 72: 1038–1044.
46. MacIver MB, Tanelian DL: Activation of C fibers by metabolic perturbations associated with tourniquet ischemia. Anesthesiology 1992; 76: 617–623.
47. Crews JC, Cahall MA: An investigation of the neurophysiologic mechanisms of tourniquet pain: single unit spinal cord recording of nociresponsive neurons. Reg Anesth 1994; 19: S19.
48. Kaufman RD, Walts LF: Tourniquet-induced hypertension. Br J Anaesth 1982; 54: 333–336.
49. Ellis RH, Mulvein J: The cardiovascular effects of methylmethacrylate. J Bone Joint Surg Br 1974; 56: 59–61.
50. Gurd AR: Fat embolism: an aid to diagnosis. J Bone Joint Surg Br 1970; 52: 732–737.

CHAPTER 32

Pediatrics

Jeremy M. Geiduschek, M.D.

Regional anesthesia and analgesia have been stable components of the anesthesiologist's repertoire in caring for pediatric patients. There are many advantages to using regional anesthesia either alone or in conjunction with general anesthesia. The dose requirements for volatile agents are decreased, and often less cardiovascular depression occurs with a combined general plus regional technique than if volatile agents are used alone. Regional anesthesia produces muscle relaxation and facilitates immobilization of limbs without necessarily depressing respiration. Regional anesthesia decreases the stress response to operation and may decrease undesirable reflexes such as laryngospasm or vagally mediated bradycardia.[1-3] Emergence from regional anesthesia is more rapid, as is the potential to decrease postoperative nausea, vomiting, and recovery times. The persistence of regional block into the early postoperative period also produces excellent analgesia and decreases the need for opioids.

There are four major areas in which the approach to regional anesthesia differs between children and adults: (1) the psychology of how the option of regional anesthesia is presented; (2) the maturation of the autonomic nervous system with age; (3) the ability to assess success or failure of the regional technique; and (4) the pharmacokinetics and pharmacodynamics of local anesthetics in infants, children, and adolescents.

Many children are apprehensive in a hospital setting, and any discussion of the use of needles only heightens their anxiety. Because the expectation of most children and their families usually is that children will be "asleep" for their operation, it is important to discuss clearly the advantages of using regional techniques in conjunction with general anesthesia, or many families will consider it an unnecessary increase in anesthetic risk and will question its use.[4] Children older than age 3 years are able to comprehend the connection between needles and painful experiences. Therefore, when discussing regional anesthesia, it is important to reassure children that they will not feel anything painful and that the procedure will be accomplished after they are "asleep."

The hemodynamic response to sympathectomy from either epidural or spinal block is less pronounced in children than in adults. The usual decreases in blood pressure and heart rate that are seen in adults with sympathectomy are not routine side effects in children younger than age 5 years. In children from age 5 to 8 years the response to sympathectomy varies, whereas in children older than age 8 years decreases in heart rate and blood pressure are typical[5, 6] (Fig. 32–1). Several explanations have been offered for these differences, although none have been proved. Systemic vascular resistance is lower in infants and young children compared with adults, suggesting less sympathetic input to vascular tone.[7] However, there is plenty of evidence demonstrating the presence of intact reflexes involving the sympathetic nervous system in term and preterm neonates.[8, 9] In infants and younger children, there is a relatively smaller proportion of the total blood volume in the lower extremities. It has been demonstrated in infants receiving caudal anesthesia that brachial artery resistance increases and upper extremity blood flow decreases, while femoral blood flow remains unchanged. Cardiac index, heart rate, mean

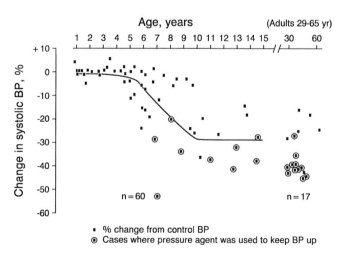

Figure 32–1 Of 60 patients younger than age 15 years who received spinal anesthesia, no significant change in blood pressure (BP) from baseline was noted in children younger than age 5 years. Eight patients between ages 6 and 15 years had a significant enough decrease in BP to warrant the intravenous use of ephedrine. square = maximal percent change in BP after spinal anesthesia. circled square = a case in which a pressor agent was administered to prevent a further decrease in BP. (From Dohi S, Naito H, Takahashi T: Age-related changes in blood pressure and duration of motor block in spinal anesthesia. Anesthesiology 1979; 50: 319–323.)

arterial pressure, and systolic and diastolic blood pressure also remain unchanged. These results suggest that hemodynamic stability results from a redistribution of blood flow away from the upper extremities where sympathetic tone remains intact.[10] (Failure of this redistribution with complete sympathectomy has not been demonstrated.) As a consequence, intravenous administration of large volumes of fluids before performing a spinal or epidural block is not necessary in children younger than age 5 years.

Assessment of the extent of regional block is difficult when regional anesthesia is used in conjunction with general anesthesia. Typically, one has to monitor for stability of vital signs while decreasing the level of volatile anesthetics below the minimum alveolar concentration of a potent inhaled agent. After emergence from general anesthesia, inability to move the blocked extremity is good evidence of a successful regional block. Assessment of block level in the awake preverbal child is also difficult. Use of a safety pin to determine the dermatome distribution of anesthesia only causes anxiety or crying, and light touch or cold versus warm discrimination often yields ambiguous results.[11] The author's preference is to assume that if the child appears comfortable, regional anesthesia has been successful; if the child is in distress, assessing the degree of block is secondary to using other means to comfort the child.

There are several factors that lead to differences in pharmacokinetics of local anesthetics in children. Volume of distribution varies with age (and the presence of coexisting disease).[12] Infants have a higher volume of distribution compared with older children and adults, which may result from a greater total body water content and less fat than older children and adults.[13] The expected consequence of this would be that a dose of local anesthetic given on a per weight basis would result in lower systemic local anesthetic concentrations. However, maximum serum or plasma concentrations are affected by many factors, including time to peak absorption, which depends on the vascularity at the site of local anesthetic deposition; cardiac output; presence of added epinephrine; age of the patient; and possibly the presence of right-to-left intravascular shunts.[14] A summary of available pharmacokinetic data for commonly used local anesthetics in pediatric regional anesthesia is presented in Table 32–1.[15–27]

Amide local anesthetics are highly protein-bound, and the amount of protein binding dictates the free fraction of local anesthetic capable of diffusing through membranes to cause neural block or toxic side effects.[12, 28] Infants younger than age 2 months have lower levels of α_1-acid glycoprotein and have a significantly higher free fraction of bupivacaine than older infants after caudal injection.[17] Plasma concentrations resulting in local anesthetic systemic toxicity have not been established for children. For adults, serum concentrations of bupivacaine greater than 2 μg/mL and of lidocaine greater than 5 to 10 μg/mL are sufficient in some patients to result in systemic toxicity.[29] Because there are several factors in infants and young children that

appear to place them at higher risk of systemic toxicity, recommended doses of local anesthetics are conservative in this chapter. In addition, an intravascular injection of local anesthetic, even if the dose is within the recommended range, may still result in systemic toxic reactions. Recommended doses to avoid toxic local anesthetic levels are as follows: bupivacaine (0.25% to 0.5%), 2 mg/kg; bupivacaine (0.25% to 0.5% with epinephrine 5 μg/mL), up to 4 mg/kg (except for intercostal block [3 mg/kg]); lidocaine (0.5% to 2%), 5 mg/kg; and lidocaine (0.5% to 2% with epinephrine 5 μg/mL), up to 7 mg/kg.

Ester local anesthetics are metabolized by plasma cholinesterase. The level of this enzyme is decreased in infants until age 6 months.[30] Theoretically this may lead to prolongation of regional block, but it has not been demonstrated clinically. In one study,[31] continuous caudal anesthesia with 3% 2-chloroprocaine was used for inguinal herniorrhaphy on former premature infants without any evidence of toxicity or prolonged blocks. Also, infants younger than age 3 months have decreased methemoglobin reductase (NADH methemoglobin diaphorase). In these patients, fetal hemoglobin may have an increased susceptibility to oxidation.[32–34] This leads to an increased risk of methemoglobinemia developing and would be a relative contraindication to the use of prilocaine in this age group.[35]

The remainder of the chapter focuses on the more frequently performed types of regional anesthesia in children.

Spinal Anesthesia

Spinal anesthesia in children has become increasingly popular since reports by Gregory and Steward[36–38] documenting that former premature infants were at increased risk of postoperative apnea after general anesthesia. Since then, many authors[39–41] have demonstrated prospectively an increased risk of apnea in this population. There is some evidence that when spinal anesthesia is used for herniorrhaphy in the former premature infant, there is a lower incidence of postoperative apnea compared with the use of general anesthesia. If the patient receiving regional anesthesia also requires intravenous administration of sedatives, any benefit is minimized.[42]

Spinal anesthesia has been administered to children for various surgical procedures since early in this century.[43–46] The author's preference is to use spinal anesthesia for procedures below the umbilicus in the former premature infant (e.g., inguinal herniorrhaphy or circumcision).

All medications and equipment should be prepared and easily accessible before positioning the patient. The author uses hyperbaric tetracaine with epinephrine. Other authors' recommendations[11, 45–50] for doses and expected duration of block for other local anesthetics are shown in Table 32–2. Tetracaine 1% (1 mL) is mixed with 1 mL of 10% dextrose. For infants younger than age 2 months, 0.5 mg/kg of tetracaine is used (i.e., 0.1 mL/kg of the 0.5% tetracaine solution). For

Table 32–1 Local Anesthetic Pharmacokinetics in Pediatric Regional Anesthesia

SITE	AGE RANGE OR MEAN ± SD, yr	LOCAL ANESTHETIC CONC, %	DOSE, mg/kg	SAMPLE SOURCE	SAMPLING SITE	C max,* µg/mL† (range)	T max,‡ min† (range)	Vd(ss),§ L/kg†	ELIMINATION HALF-LIFE, min†	CLEARANCE, mL/kg per min†	AUTHOR
Caudal	4.84 ± 1.63	Bupivacaine 0.2	2	Plasma	Venous	0.57 ± 0.17	29 ± 7.9	2.7 ± 0.2	277 ± 34	10 ± 0.7	Stow et al[15]
	5.5–10	Bupivacaine 0.25	2.5	Plasma	Venous	1.25 ± 0.09	29 ± 3.1				Ecoffey et al[16]
	1–6 mo	Bupivacaine 0.5	2.5	Serum	Venous	0.97 ± 0.42	28 ± 13	3.9 ± 2	462 ± 144	7.1 ± 3.2	Mazoit et al[17]
	2.4 ± 0.7	Bupivacaine 0.5 + epi 5 µg/mL	3.7	Blood	Venous	0.65 ± 0.08	30				Takasaki[18]
	1.8–8.5	Lidocaine 0.5	5	Plasma	Venous	2 ± 0.6	30	2.23 ± 0.8	103	13.6 ± 3.6	Yaster et al[19]
	3.5–9	Lidocaine 1	5	Plasma	Venous	2.05 ± 0.08 (1.6–2.5)	28.2 ± 2.9 (15–40)	3.05 ± 0.4	155 ± 32	15.4 ± 1.2	Ecoffey et al[20]
	2.6 ± 0.5	Lidocaine 1.5 + epi 5 µg/mL	11	Blood	Venous	2.19 ± 0.27	30				Takasaki[18]
Axillary	2–13	Bupivacaine 0.33	2	Plasma	Venous	1.35 ± 0.37	22 ± 8				Campbell et al[21]
	1.9–14.8	Bupivacaine 0.5	3	Plasma	Venous	1.84 ± 0.45	22 ± 8				Campbell et al[21]
Penile	1–3 d	Lidocaine 1	2.3	Plasma	Capillary	0.51 ± 0.17 (0.1–1.6)	60				Maxwell et al[22]
	4–10.5	Bupivacaine 0.5	0.5	Serum	Venous	0.27 ± 0.09 (0.13–0.35)	23 ± 5				Sfez et al[23]
	3–10.8	Bupivacaine 0.25 + lidocaine 1	0.25 (B) 1 (L)	Serum	Venous	0.09 ± 0.04(B) (0.06–0.16)(B) 0.36 ± 0.08(L) (0.23–0.47)(L)	27 ± 19 (B) 27 ± 18 (L)				Sfez et al[23]
Ilioinguinal and iliohypogastric	1.08–10	Bupivacaine 0.25 or 0.5	2	Plasma	Venous	1.35 ± 0.35 (0.91–2.29)	26 ± 10 (10–40)				Epstein et al[24]
	5.21 ± 1.64	Bupivacaine 0.5	1.25	Plasma	Venous	0.79 ± 0.38	22.3 ± 10.9				Stow et al[15]
Femoral	2–10	Bupivacaine 0.5	2	Plasma	Venous	0.89 ± 0.37 (0.44–1.52)	24.4 ± 12.6	3.51 ± 1.82	165 ± 71	17.5 ± 10.8	Ronchi et al[25]
Intercostal	1–28 d	Bupivacaine 0.25	1.5	Blood	Arterial	0.82 ± 0.56 (0.39–1.86)		2.56 ± 0.76	132 ± 59	16.93 ± 9.32	Bricker et al[26]
	1–6 mo	Bupivacaine 0.25	1.5	Blood	Arterial	0.91 ± 0.27 (0.44–1.33)		2.17 ± 0.71	102 ± 39	15.71 ± 6.99	Bricker et al[26]
	0.42–14.58	Bupivacaine 0.5 + epi 5 µg/mL	2	Blood	Arterial	0.77 ± 0.25 (0.55–1.23)					Rothstein et al[27]
	2.42–16	Bupivacaine 0.5 + epi 5 µg/mL	3	Blood	Arterial	1.37 ± 0.23 (1.05–1.65)		2.8 ± 0.8	147 ± 80	16 ± 7.4	
	0.42–10.92	Bupivacaine 0.5 + epi 5 µg/mL	4	Blood	Arterial	1.87 ± 0.53 (1.03–3.20)					

*C max = peak plasma concentrations.
†Mean ± SD.
‡T max = time to peak plasma concentrations.
§Vd(ss) = volume of distribution at steady state.
B, bupivacaine; conc, concentration; epi, epinephrine; L, lidocaine.

Table 32–2 Subarachnoid Anesthesia in Infants and Children

AUTHOR	AGE	CASES, no.	ANESTHETIC	ANESTHETIC DOSE, mg/kg	DURATION OF BLOCK, min
Berkowitz and Greene[11]	<13 yr	350	1% tetracaine + 5% procaine (1:1) or 0.5% dibucaine + 5% procaine (1:1)	0.2/1.0 tetracaine/procaine 0.11/1 dibucaine/procaine	Not stated
Gouvela[47]	3 mo–11 yr	50	5% lidocaine + dextrose + 0.05–0.1 mg epinephrine	1.6–2 (age < 3 yr) 0.8–1.5 (age > 3 yr)	Not stated
Melman et al[45]	Up to 15 yr	42	5% hyperbaric lidocaine + epinephrine*	1.5–2.5	Not stated
Blaise and Roy[48]	7 wk–9 yr	25	1% tetracaine (isobaric)	0.4–0.5 (age < 3 mo) 0.3–0.4 (age 3–24 mo) 0.2–0.3 (age >24 mo)	Not stated
Abajian et al[49]	"Infants"	57	1% tetracaine + 10% dextrose (1:1)	0.22–0.32	50–135
	"Infants"	16	1% tetracaine + 10% dextrose (1:1) + epinephrine 0.020 mg	0.22–0.32	80–145
Blaise and Roy[46]	7 wk–13 yr	30	0.75% hyperbaric bupivacaine or 1% tetracaine	Bupivacaine 0.3–0.4 (age < 24 mo) 0.3 (age > 24 mo) Tetracaine 0.4–0.5 (age < 3 mo) 0.3–0.4 (age 3–24 mo) 0.2–0.3 (age > 24 mo)	Up to 70
Mahe and Ecoffey[50]	1.5–5 mo	16	0.5% bupivacaine (isobaric)	1.25 mg (weight < 2 kg) 3.75 mg (weight 2–5 kg) 5 mg (weight > 5 kg)	70
	1–5 mo	12	0.5% bupivacaine (isobaric) + epinephrine 1:200,000†	1.25 mg (weight < 2 kg) 3.75 mg (weight 2–5 kg) 5 mg (weight > 5 kg)	80

*Specifics of epinephrine dosing not stated.
†Article does not specify how epinephrine dose was determined to result in a concentration of 1:200,000.

infants ages 2 to 6 months, 0.4 mg/kg, and for 6- to 12-month-old infants, 0.3 mg/kg of tetracaine is used. The dose requirements based on body weight are much higher in infants than in adults. It is unclear why this difference exists, although it has been suggested that infants and toddlers have a higher volume of cerebrospinal fluid per unit of body weight than older children and adults.[47]

A 1-mL (i.e., tuberculin) syringe is flushed with epinephrine 1:1000. The anesthetic dose is then drawn into the syringe. A typical tuberculin syringe has approximately 0.05 mL of dead space in the hub. A separate syringe with 1% lidocaine is prepared to provide cutaneous anesthesia. Intravenous access may be established before or after administering spinal medication. In infants, volume loading is not needed in advance, assuming that the infant has not been fasted for more than 6 h. Reports vary on the use of an anticholinergic agent. The author prefers to start an intravenous catheter and administer 0.02 mg/kg of glycopyrrolate before performing the dural puncture. Also, if the infant has been fasting more than 6 h, the author prefers to administer 10 mL/kg of fluid intravenously in advance. Electrocardiogram leads and pulse oximeter probe are applied to the patient. An assistant is responsible for positioning the patient and ensuring airway patency.

The procedure can be accomplished with the patient either sitting or in the lateral decubitus position. Care must be taken to keep the neck extended when the spine is flexed to avoid partial airway obstruction and the potential for arterial desaturation.[51, 52] The skin over the lumbar spine is prepared in an aseptic manner. Lidocaine 1% is used to raise a skin wheal. Lumbar puncture can be performed at the L4-5 or L5-S1 interspace in the midline by using a 22- or 25-G, 1-in. spinal needle with stylet. The anatomy of the sacrum and spinal canal varies with age (Fig. 32–2). At birth, the dural sac terminates at the S-3 level and the spinal

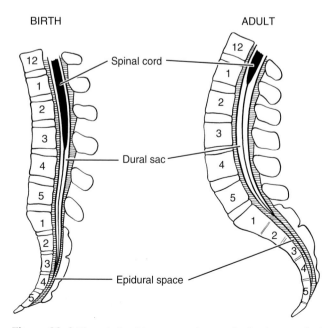

Figure 32–2 The relationships among the vertebral column, spinal cord, and dural sac vary with age.

cord at L-3. In an adult, they terminate at S-2 and L-1, respectively. A low approach is used to decrease the risk of spinal cord injury with needle insertion. A needle with stylet should be used to avoid the risk of epidermoid tumor formation.[53–55] In patients younger than age 1 year, the dura should be punctured 1 to 2 cm from the skin surface. A distinct "pop" may not be appreciated. Cerebrospinal fluid flow should be present after removal of the stylet. Continuous cerebrospinal fluid flow does not need to be tested for by rotating the spinal needle through 360°. The tuberculin syringe is attached to the needle hub, and the local anesthetic is injected over 5 s. Cerebrospinal fluid does not need to be aspirated at the end of the injection.

The grounding pad for the electrocautery unit is applied to the posterior of the patient, and the patient is quickly placed in the supine position. Provide the infant with a pacifier and a quiet environment and the infant usually falls asleep. Application of the pulse oximeter probe and noninvasive blood pressure cuff to the anesthetized lower extremities decreases the amount of stimulation the infant receives. Placement of the intravenous catheter in the lower extremity is also ideal but not always feasible. Loose soft restraints are applied to the wrists so that the infant cannot reach onto the sterile field. Care must be taken not to elevate the lower extremities because this may contribute to an undesirable high sensory and motor block.[56] Even though anesthesia of the T-4 dermatome may be appreciated, it is not unusual during spinal anesthesia for the infant to cry or become agitated when traction is applied to the peritoneum during herniorrhaphy. If the amount of traction cannot be decreased, local anesthetic may be infiltrated into the wound.

Sedation may increase the risk of postoperative apnea but nevertheless may be necessary. Incremental doses of sodium thiopental (0.5 mg/kg given intravenously), nitrous oxide (30% to 50%), or halothane (<0.5%) may be administered. The expected duration of a tetracaine with epinephrine subarachnoid block is from 80 to 145 min.[49] Regardless of whether or not supplemental sedatives or anesthetics are administered, any patient considered at risk for postoperative apnea is admitted to the hospital for overnight observation and continuous cardiorespiratory monitoring.

Epidural Anesthesia

Caudal Anesthesia

Caudal anesthesia is frequently the most used pediatric regional anesthesia technique. A caudal block is simple to perform and is useful for many procedures below the diaphragm. There are several large series[57–59] demonstrating the safety of caudal anesthesia in pediatric patients. There also have been reports[57, 60–63] of life-threatening complications, including regurgitation and aspiration, seizures, total spinal anesthesia, ventricular tachycardia, and cardiovascular collapse. Caudal anesthesia is usually used in conjunction with general anesthesia or deep sedation, although it also can be used

in the conscious infant considered to be at risk of postoperative apnea after general anesthesia.[31, 64, 65] For procedures of short duration, a single dose of local anesthetic usually suffices. For procedures scheduled for more than 2 h, a caudal catheter is usually placed to allow additional doses of local anesthetic to be administered. If a catheter is not used, the caudal epidural block can be repeated at the conclusion of the surgical procedure to provide postoperative analgesia.

The block is usually performed in a heavily sedated or anesthetized child in the lateral decubitus position with hips and knees flexed. Typically, the upper leg is flexed slightly more than the lower leg. Classically, the sacral hiatus is located at the apex of an equilateral triangle in which the base is formed with the posterior superior iliac spines (Fig. 32–3). The hiatus is a gap shaped like an inverted "V" and results from failure of posterior fusion of the fifth sacral vertebral arch. The hiatus is covered with a membrane attached to the sacral and coccygeal cornua (the sacrococcygeal ligament). In infants and children, the hiatus is shallow and lies close to the skin surface. With aging, a presacral fat pad develops, increasing the distance between the hiatus and skin surface.

The gluteal crease and buttocks are prepared and draped in sterile fashion from the coccyx to the level of the posterior superior iliac spines. The author prefers a method in which the coccyx is palpated with the index finger of the nondominant hand, and then the finger slides cephalad until the sacral cornu and sacral hiatus are palpated. In children younger than age 3 years, both the sacral cornu and the sacral hiatus can be palpated simultaneously with one finger. This finger can now serve as a guide to correct placement of the needle into the sacrococcygeal ligament. Although some products have been designed specifically for pediatric regional anesthesia, a caudal block may be accomplished with a 20- or 22-G needle or intravenous catheter. After creation of a skin "nick," the caudal needle is engaged into the sacrococcygeal ligament at a 45° angle to the long axis of the sacrum with the needle bevel facing anteriorly. Once the needle is fully engaged, the angle is decreased and the needle is advanced. A "pop" is typically appreciated as the needle tip enters the caudal canal, and the needle should be advanced 1 to 2 mm further. If an intravenous catheter is used, the catheter should slide off the stylet without resistance. It is important not to advance a needle too far into the caudal space or to force a catheter off a stylet because dural puncture may occur.

Next aspirate for cerebrospinal fluid or blood, and if the result is negative, proceed with a test dose of local anesthetic. The test dose should contain 0.5 μg/kg body weight of epinephrine (0.1 mL/kg of a 1:200,000 epinephrine-containing solution, maximum 15 μg or 3 mL). A positive response to the test dose should involve a clinically significant increase in heart rate or blood pressure in less than 1 min. Desparmet and colleagues[66] reported that pretreatment with atropine is necessary in order to elicit tachycardia reliably if a positive response to a test dose were to occur in a patient anesthetized with halothane. There are no data published re-

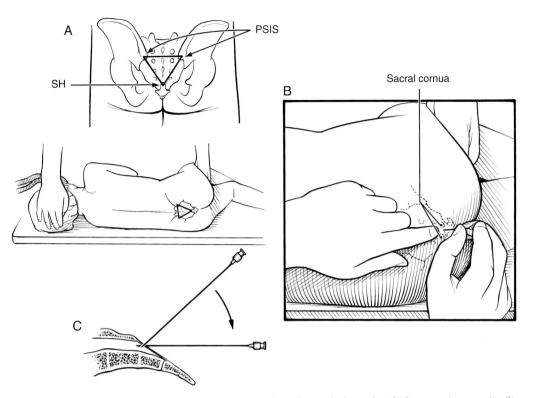

Figure 32–3 *A*, The sacral hiatus (SH) is located at the apex of an equilateral triangle formed with the posterior superior iliac spines (PSIS). *B*, Position of patient for caudal anesthesia. In the anesthetized patient, care should be taken not to flex the neck. This may cause airway obstruction in the patient without a tracheal tube or promote advancement of a tracheal tube into a bronchus. *C*, The angle of needle entry is decreased after engagement of the sacrococcygeal ligament.

garding test doses in children anesthetized with other anesthetics. Other investigators[67] have reported ST-segment changes on electrocardiogram, hypertension, and heart rate slowing as indications of an intravascular injection. The local anesthetic should flow without resistance into the caudal space. If it does not, the needle or catheter tip is either in subcutaneous tissue or in periosteum. The palmar aspect of the fingers can be used to palpate over the sacrum for subcutaneous injection. After the test dose, the remainder of the dose can be given incrementally in 2 to 3 min. The total volume of local anesthetic solution to be administered depends on the desired level of anesthesia. Although there are several formulas and charts available to calculate the volume of local anesthetic needed to achieve certain amounts of segmental spread,[68-73] the author prefers the simple estimate that 0.5 mL/kg results in an adequate sacral block for lower extremity and perineal procedures, and 1 mL/kg (maximum 25 mL) should be adequate for lower abdominal procedures. Care should be taken not to exceed the total recommended dose of local anesthetic.

A caudal catheter should be inserted if repeated dosing of local anesthetic is anticipated, if a high abdominal or thoracic procedure is to be performed, or if the use of regional analgesia is planned postoperatively (Fig. 32–4). The use of an adult-sized (i.e., 20 G) catheter is acceptable and standard in children and neonates. An 18-G intravenous catheter first must be inserted into the caudal space in order to thread the catheter.

Measure the distance externally from the sacral hiatus to the desired level for the catheter tip before placing the catheter. A catheter can be threaded from the caudal space to as high as C-6.[74] Several complications have occurred during placement of caudally inserted thoracic catheters, including intravascular placement,

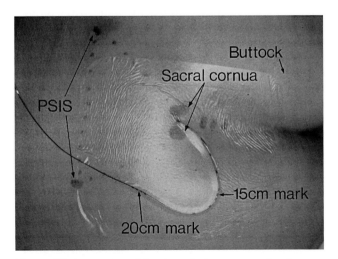

Figure 32–4 A 20-G caudal catheter is shown secured under a clear occlusive dressing with the 10-cm mark at the entry site in the sacral hiatus. This catheter can be used for repeated dosing of local anesthetics intraoperatively as well as for neuraxial analgesia postoperatively. PSIS, posterior superior iliac spines. (Courtesy of Elliot J. Krane, M.D. With permission.)

coiling, intrathecal placement, failure to thread to the desired level, and catheter migration into dural sleeves.[75–77]

When a caudal catheter is used for abdominal or thoracic operation, the site of local anesthetic delivery needs to be in close proximity to the desired spinal segments involved with the surgical procedure. If this is the case, an initial dose of 0.25 to 0.5 mL/kg of local anesthetic should provide adequate spread, and additional volume can be titrated on the basis of changes in vital signs during the procedure or by determining block level. Subsequent doses through the catheter should be approximately 50% of the original dose and should be given only if there is evidence of successful block with the original dose (i.e., predetermined dermatome distribution of anesthesia or the ability to maintain anesthesia with low inspired concentrations of volatile agents). The dosing interval for lidocaine with epinephrine is about 45 to 60 min and for bupivacaine with epinephrine, 90 min. Before each "top-up" dose, the epidural catheter should be aspirated to check for the presence of blood or cerebrospinal fluid, and a test dose should be administered. If there are no signs of intravascular injection, the remainder of the dose should be delivered in increments; dosing should be halted if it is clear the catheter has become intravascular.

Lumbar Epidural Anesthesia

The use of lumbar epidural anesthesia is much less frequent than caudal anesthesia in the author's practice. For children older than age 7 years having high abdominal or thoracic operation for which regional anesthesia is to be used, the author inserts a lumbar epidural in contrast to a caudal catheter. The technique used is similar to that for an adult. With sterile conditions, a Tuohy needle is inserted into the L3-4 or L4-5 interspace and the epidural space is located by using a loss of resistance technique with saline. An epidural catheter is inserted 3 cm beyond the needle tip; the needle is removed, and the catheter is secured with an occlusive dressing. Currently, there are 20-G, 5-cm needles that can be used with a 22-G catheter with stylet, although the author typically uses an 18-G needle with a 20-G catheter. The distance from the skin to the epidural space depends on the site of needle insertion and the age of the patient. Kosaka and associates[78] used the following formula:

$$\text{Distance (mm)} = 18 + \text{age in years} \times 1.3$$

The test dose and local anesthetic dose administered are the same as for lumbar or thoracic, caudally inserted epidural catheters (i.e., 0.25 to 0.5 mL/kg local anesthetic).

Thoracic Epidural Anesthesia

Ecoffey and colleagues[79] have described the use of thoracic epidural anesthesia in pediatric patients. In all cases, catheter placement occurred after induction of anesthesia. This is not a technique currently used in the author's department and would be recommended only for the anesthesiologist who has considerable experience with thoracic catheter insertion in adults and knowledge of the use of epidural anesthesia in children.

Neuraxial Analgesia

The first report of epidural administration of opioids for postoperative analgesia in children was by Jensen[80] in 1981. Since then, neuraxial analgesia has been used successfully in pediatric patients after lower extremity, perineal, abdominal, thoracic, and cardiac procedures (Table 32–3).[81–90] The most common methods of providing analgesia are single or repeated dosing of preservative-free morphine or continuous infusions of local anesthetics (with or without an added opioid). When preservative-free morphine is administered by intermittent bolus, catheter tip localization in proximity to spinal nerves supplying the surgical site is not as crucial because morphine diffuses rostrally within the cerebrospinal fluid to a greater extent than the more lipid-soluble opioids.[91]

If an epidural infusion of local anesthetic is to be used, an epidural catheter is placed by either the caudal or the lumbar approach and threaded to a level approximating the nerve roots supplying the affected dermatomes. Owing to the theoretic concern of causing spinal cord injury during placement of a thoracic epidural catheter in a heavily sedated or anesthetized child, the use of thoracic epidural catheters is not common and the published experience with thoracic epidural analgesia is limited.[82, 85, 92, 93]

More recently, it has become popular to add an opioid to a local anesthetic infusion in order to decrease the amount of local anesthetic required to provide analgesia and to decrease the risk of local anesthetic systemic toxicity. The author typically starts with 0.1% bupivacaine mixed with either 2 μg/mL of fentanyl or 10 μg/mL of preservative-free morphine. Recommended starting and maximum infusion rates for continuous epidural infusions of bupivacaine are shown in Tables 32–4 and 32–5. Neonates have a lower clearance of bupivacaine compared with older infants and children, and their infusion rate should not exceed 0.25 mg/kg per h. For older infants, toddlers, and children, the bupivacaine infusion rate should not exceed 0.5 mg/kg per h.[94] Higher infusion rates may increase the risk for seizure occurrence.[95, 96] An early sign of toxic responses in the central nervous system may be agitation, which is difficult to distinguish from inadequate analgesia or hunger in younger preverbal children. Patients with a preexisting seizure disorder may be at increased risk of local anesthetic–induced seizures, and their infusion rates should be decreased accordingly.[97, 98] Tobin and colleagues[98] have recommended using lidocaine infusions in place of bupivacaine because of the ease of measuring serum lidocaine concentration in most hospitals. Measurement of serial

Table 32–3 Epidural Administration of Morphine for Pediatric Neuraxial Analgesia

AUTHOR	PROCEDURES,* no.	AGE, yr	OPERATIONS†	ROUTE OF MORPHINE ADMINISTRATION	LOCAL ANESTHETIC OTHER THAN TEST DOSE	MORPHINE DOSE RANGE, mg/kg	REPEAT MORPHINE DOSES EPIDURALLY	DURATION OF ANALGESIA, MEAN ± SD (RANGE), h	EPISODES OF RESPIRATORY DEPRESSION
Jensen[80]	7	2–7	Hypospadias‡	Caudal	No	0.05	No	20 ± 9.9	None
Martin[81]	20	5.6 ± 0.69§	Circumcision	Caudal	Bupiv 0.5%	0.02	No	9.7 ± 1.4||	None
Shapiro et al[82]	5	3–11	Thoracotomy Laparotomy	Thoracic	No	0.5–2 mg¶	Yes	(4–25)	None
Glenski et al[83]	15	4–18	Cholecystectomy Thoracotomy	Lumbar	No	0.12 (0.07–0.16)	Yes	10.8 ± 4 (6.3–17.5)	None
Dalens et al[84]	14	2 days–7	Orthopedic	Lumbar	Lido 1% + bupiv 0.5%	0.05	No	17 ± 3.3	None
	27		Orthopedic	Lumbar	Etido 1% + bupiv 0.5%	0.05	No	20.6 ± 5.3	None
Attia et al[85]	20	2–15	Abdominal Urologic	Lumbar Thoracic	No	0.05	Yes	19.5 ± 8	
Krane et al[86]	8	1–16	Hypospadias Orthopedic	Caudal	No	0.1	No	9.9 (4.0– >24)	None
	7	2–12	Hypospadias Orthopedic	Caudal	No#	0.1	No	14.4 (4–23.6)	None
Rosen and Rosen[87]	16	2.0–12.0	Cardiac Abdominal Urologic Orthopedic	Caudal	No	0.075	No	6 (2–12)	None
Krane et al[88]	9	1.2–7	Abdominal Urologic Orthopedic	Caudal	No#	0.033	Yes	10.0 ± 3.3	None
	9	1.3–7.9	Abdominal Urologic Orthopedic	Caudal	No#	0.067	Yes	10.4 ± 4.2	None
	8	1.7–5.4	Abdominal Urologic Orthopedic	Caudal	No#	0.1	Yes	13.3 ± 4.7	1
Valley and Bailey[89]	130	1 day–16	Abdominal Thoracic Orthopedic	Caudal	Bupiv 0.25% (n = 12)	0.07	Yes (n = 14)	(4–24)	8**
Wolf et al[90]	15	1.2–6.7	Penile	Caudal	Bupiv 0.25%	0.05	No	(2– >24)	None

*In several of the reports, patients underwent repeated operations for which morphine was administered epidurally.
†All orthopedic operations involved the pelvis or lower extremities.
‡An additional six patients received 0.05 mg/kg of caudal morphine for circumcision. Duration of analgesia was not determined for this group.
§Mean ± standard error of mean.
||Six of the 20 patients did not require additional analgesics.
¶Morphine dose based on age not weight. Morphine dose/kg of body weight not specified.
#Lidocaine 1% was used to confirm correct catheter placement.
**Seven patients who had respiratory depression were <1 year old. Seven patients who had respiratory depression received opioids intravenously in addition to morphine epidurally.
Bupiv, bupivacaine; etido, etidocaine; lido, lidocaine.

Table 32–4 Continuous Epidural Infusions: Recommended Initial Infusion Rate of Bupivacaine

PATIENT WEIGHT, kg	BUPIVACAINE CONCENTRATION, %			
	0.0625 1/16	0.1 1/10	0.125 1/8	0.25 1/4
5	1*	1	1	NR
10	3	2	1	1
15	4	3	2	1
20	5	4	3	1
25	7	5	3	2
30	8	6	4	2
35	9	7	5	2
40	11	8	5	3
45	12	9	6	3
50	12	10	7	3
55	12	11	7	4
60	12	12	8	4
65	12	12	9	4
70	12	12	9	5

*All infusion rates are mL/h.
NR = not recommended.

lidocaine levels aids in avoiding local anesthetic accumulation to toxic levels.

The author considers several factors before deciding to proceed with regional analgesia either with intermittent epidural dosing of opioids or with continuous infusion of local anesthetic:

1. Desires of the patient and family.

2. Age of the patient (owing to lack of safety data, the epidural administration of opioids in a patient younger than age 1 year without a tracheal tube is not recommended).

3. The epidural catheter insertion site is determined primarily by the operative site and the age of the patient. A caudally placed catheter is typically used for all patients younger than age 6 years. For patients older than age 6 years, caudal catheters are used for lower extremity, perineal, genital, and lower abdominal pro-

Table 32–5 Continuous Epidural Infusions: Recommended Maximum Infusion Rate of Bupivacaine

PATIENT WEIGHT, kg	BUPIVACAINE CONCENTRATION, %			
	0.0625 1/16	0.1 1/10	0.125 1/8	0.25 1/4
5	2*	1.2	1	NR
10	8	5	4	2
15	12	7	6	3
20	16	10	8	4
25	20	12	10	5
30	24	15	12	6
35	24	17	14	7
40	24	20	16	8
45	24	22	18	9
50	24	24	20	10
55	24	24	22	11
60	24	24	24	12
65	24	24	24	13
70	24	24	24	14

*All infusion rates are mL/h.
NR, not recommended.

cedures and lumbar epidural catheters are used for upper abdominal and thoracic procedures. For caudally inserted thoracic epidural catheters, epidurography with water-soluble contrast material is recommended to confirm catheter tip placement.

4. If the catheter tip is not in close proximity to the involved spinal dermatome, a water-soluble opioid should be used. Currently, the only opioid for which there is a substantial amount of published data on the pediatric population is preservative-free morphine. For caudal catheters, an epidural dose of morphine of 0.03 to 0.05 mg/kg usually provides analgesia for up to 6 h and often longer.

5. Because of the risk of delayed respiratory depression, 12 h of in-hospital observation is required after an epidural dose of opioid.[99] Care is taken to ensure that an epidural dose of opioid would not interfere with intended hospital dismissal plans.

6. It is not necessary to admit patients receiving epidural analgesia to the Intensive Care Unit, but all patients must be cared for on a hospital ward where the nursing staff is familiar with the epidural use of opioids and local anesthetics. For patients receiving opioids epidurally, respiratory rate is measured and an assessment for excessive sedation is performed every hour for the first 24 h and every 4 h thereafter. Other vital signs are measured every 4 h. When in bed or unattended, all patients have continuous pulse oximetry. Pulse oximetry may be discontinued 12 h after the last epidural dose of opioid. Suction equipment, oxygen, face mask and reservoir bag, and naloxone are all kept at the bedside.

7. A member of the Acute Pain Service is always available for consultation and visits each patient daily. A physician member of the Department of Anesthesiology is always in the hospital and able to respond to an emergency.

8. Because there is up to a 46% incidence reported for urinary retention after epidural administration of morphine, the author discourages the use of this practice in patients without indwelling urinary bladder catheters.[84, 85] The need to perform intermittent catheterization on a child or adolescent for urinary retention is traumatic. If the need for bladder catheterization arises during epidural analgesia and is not responsive to medical management, an indwelling bladder catheter is inserted and is removed 6 h after the final epidural dose of opioids.

9. Supplemental oral or intravenous administration of opioids or sedatives is generally avoided. If these types of medications are to be administered, this occurs only by order of a physician member of the Acute Pain Service.

Peripheral Nerve Blocks

Peripheral nerve blocks and intravenous regional anesthesia are not as widely used for children as they are for adults. Even though there are reports of the use of intravenous regional anesthesia in children,[100–103] it is not used in the author's practice because of the concern for local anesthetic leak and tourniquet system failure.[104–106] The use of combinations of local anesthetic, opioid, and a nondepolarizing neuromuscular blocker for intravenous regional anesthesia has been examined in adults, with the goal of decreasing total local anesthetic dose.[107] Results of this type of research have not been extended to the pediatric population.

The common nerve blocks used in the pediatric population are the penile block for circumcision or plastic operations on the penis, ilioinguinal and iliohypogastric blocks for supplementary anesthesia for inguinal herniorrhaphy or orchiopexy, femoral nerve block for femur fracture reduction, femoral nerve block plus lateral femoral cutaneous nerve block for muscle biopsy or skin graft harvesting, and intercostal nerve block for post-thoracotomy analgesia. The techniques for performing these blocks in children are similar to those described for adults. Relationships between anatomic landmarks are similar, but in smaller children shorter distances between landmarks must be taken into account. The use of a peripheral nerve stimulator can aid in nerve location in the heavily sedated or anesthetized child. Disposable Teflon-coated block needles designed for use in small children are available.[108] When performing these blocks, avoid intravascular injection and do not exceed the recommended total local anesthetic dose.

Penile Nerve Block

Dorsal penile nerve blocks can be used alone or in conjunction with general anesthesia or deep sedation to provide anesthesia and analgesia for circumcision or operations on the distal portion of the penis. Sensation to the shaft and glans of the penis is via the paired dorsal penile nerves. These nerves are terminal branches of the pudendal nerves, which derive their fibers from the second through fourth sacral spinal nerves via the sacral plexus. The dorsal nerve of the penis lies inferior to the pubic bone just lateral to the symphysis pubis and enters the subpubic space. Scarpa's fascia is the anterior boundary of the subpubic space. The pubic bone and the perineal membrane form the posterior boundary. Portions of the fascia covering the corpora cavernosa as they form the penile crura determine the horizontal boundary. This fascia extends to the shaft of the penis, where it becomes Buck's fascia. The subpubic space is fat filled and divided in the midline by the fundiform (suspensory) ligament to form two noncommunicating compartments.[109] The dorsal nerve of the penis leaves the subpubic space and passes internal to Buck's fascia parallel to the long axis and on the dorsolateral surface of the corpora cavernosa. An artery is associated with each nerve within Buck's fascia. A single dorsal vein of the penis is midline also within the fascia, and several subcutaneous veins may be present external to the fascia (Figs. 32–5 and 32–6).

The dorsal nerve of the penis may be blocked at two locations: within the subpubic space and at the base of the penis. The child should be in the recumbent posi-

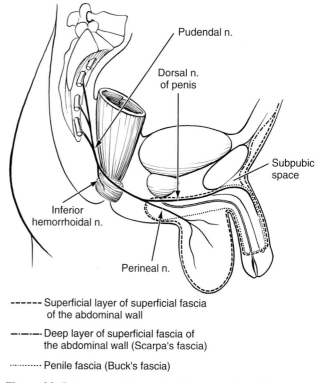

------ Superficial layer of superficial fascia of the abdominal wall

–·–·– Deep layer of superficial fascia of the abdominal wall (Scarpa's fascia)

·········· Penile fascia (Buck's fascia)

Figure 32–5 Anatomy of the pudendal nerve (n.) and its branches: fascia superficialis of the abdominal wall, Scarpa's fascia, subpubic space, superficial layer of the superficial fascia of the abdominal wall, penile fascia (Buck's fascia), pudendal nerve, inferior hemorrhoidal nerve, dorsal nerve of the penis, and peroneal nerve. (Redrawn from Dalens B, Vanneuville G, Dechelotte P: Penile block via the subpubic space in 100 children. Anesth Analg 1989; 69: 41-45.)

tion, and slight downward traction is applied to the penis. Use of a short-beveled needle permits greater appreciation of passage through fascial planes, which can be quite thin in young children. Dalens and co-workers[109] described a two-puncture technique to perform a subpubic block. The needle is inserted 0.5 cm (in infants) to 1 cm (in older children) lateral to the symphysis pubis and immediately below the inferior ramus of the pubic bone. Angle the needle posterocaudally and slightly medial. As the needle is advanced, an initial give will be appreciated as the needle traverses the fascia superficialis. Advance the needle another 5 mm, and Scarpa's fascia should be pierced. The needle tip now lies within the subpubic space. After a negative result of aspiration, inject 0.1 mL/kg body weight of 0.5% bupivacaine or 1% lidocaine (Fig. 32–6A).

Brown and Schulte-Steinberg[110] described a single-puncture technique (Fig. 32–6B). The needle is advanced to the symphysis pubis in the midline. Withdraw the needle slightly, reposition it with a slight lateral angle, and advance it off the edge of the symphysis. A give or pop should be appreciated within 5 mm as the advancing needle traverses Scarpa's fascia. Aspirate for blood, and if the result is negative, inject local anesthetic. Withdraw the needle and angle it lat-

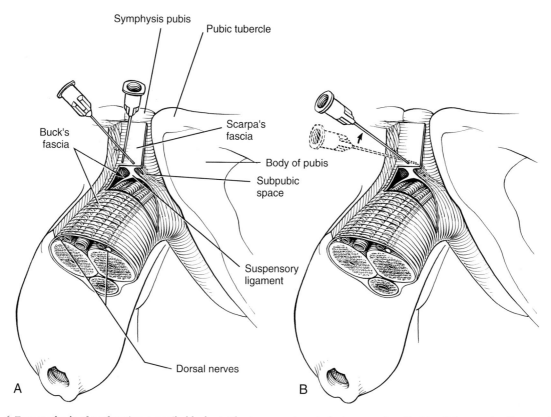

Figure 32–6 Two methods of performing a penile block. *A,* The two-puncture technique, as described by Dalens and colleagues.[109] *B,* The single-puncture technique, as described by Brown and Schulte-Steinberg.[110]

erally in the other direction for injection into the other subpubic compartment. Bacon[111] described a single-injection technique. For this to be successful, local anesthetic must either diffuse across the suspensory ligament or needle placement must be deep into the space and internal to Buck's fascia within the small triangular space containing the nerves (and arteries and vein).

Dorsal nerves of the penis can be blocked at the base of the penis by placing gentle traction on the penis and piercing the skin at approximately 20° to 25° from the parasagittal plane at the 2 o'clock and 10 o'clock positions. Buck's fascia should be pierced between 3 and 5 mm from the skin surface. Lidocaine 1% (0.4 mL) is used for each injection for neonatal circumcision, and 0.1 mL/kg of either 0.25% or 0.5% bupivacaine is used for older children.[112, 113] Broadman and colleagues[114] described using a subcutaneous ring of local anesthetic placed around the base of the penis. With their technique, no attempt is made to inject within Buck's fascia, and total dose of bupivacaine 0.25% is limited to less than 2 mg/kg, with a maximum of 5 mL (Fig. 32–7).

Complications reported from penile nerve blocks include accidental use of epinephrine instead of 1% lidocaine[115] and delayed penile ischemia possibly related to compression or injury of vascular beds.[116] Because the dorsal penile arteries are end arteries and they lie within close proximity to the penile nerves, epinephrine should not be used for this block. Also, when injecting into the base of the penis, deposition of exces-

sive volumes of local anesthetic may cause compression of the vascular structures within Buck's fascia.

Local anesthetic infiltration into the foreskin at the level of the corona has also been used to provide anesthesia for circumcision.[117] Several authors[118–120] have

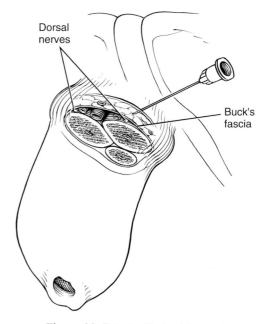

Figure 32–7 A ring block of the penis.

reported successful analgesia after circumcision with topical application of 2% lidocaine jelly or spray. To the author's knowledge, studies assessing systemic local anesthetic levels using these methods have not been published.

Ilioinguinal and Iliohypogastric Nerve Block

Ilioinguinal and iliohypogastric nerve blocks are useful for providing postoperative analgesia for inguinal herniorrhaphy or orchiopexy.[121–123] The blocks can be done in conjunction with a general anesthetic and can be performed either before or after the operation, depending in part on surgeon preference. These blocks are inadequate for operative anesthesia, especially because spermatic cord structures are often manipulated and receive their innervation from branches of T-10. If general anesthesia needs to be avoided for inguinal herniorrhaphy or orchiopexy, either a caudal or a spinal block is an alternative.

The iliohypogastric nerve has its origin from branches of T-12 and L-1. It initially is located along the inner surface of the quadratus lumborum muscle. Within the pelvis, the nerve follows a circular course determined by the shape of the iliac crest. Initially the nerve is located between the transverse abdominis muscle and the internal oblique muscle. Near the anterior superior iliac spine, the nerve pierces the internal oblique muscle and then lies between the external oblique and the internal oblique muscles. Cutaneous branches of the nerve provide sensation to the inguinal ligament and overlying area.

The ilioinguinal nerve originates from L-1 and follows a course similar to that of the iliohypogastric nerve. At the level of the anterior superior iliac spine, it lies between the transverse abdominis and the internal oblique muscles. Anteromedial to the anterior superior iliac spine, the nerve pierces the internal oblique muscle and then enters the scrotum to provide sensation to the superior portion of the scrotum and inner part of the thigh (Fig. 32–8).

With the patient in the supine position after sterile preparation of the skin, a short-beveled 25-G needle is inserted 1 cm medial and 1 cm superior to the anterior superior iliac spine. The needle is advanced in an inferolateral direction until it comes into contact with the iliac wing. Half of the local anesthetic dose is injected as the needle is withdrawn. This should provide effective block of the iliohypogastric nerve. With the same entry point, the needle is advanced in a posterior and inferior direction (toward the inguinal ligament) until a pop is appreciated as the needle pierces the external oblique fascia. The remainder of the local anesthetic dose is injected. This portion of the dose spreads between the external and internal oblique muscles and anesthetizes the ilioinguinal nerve as it emerges from the internal oblique muscle near this point (Fig. 32–8).

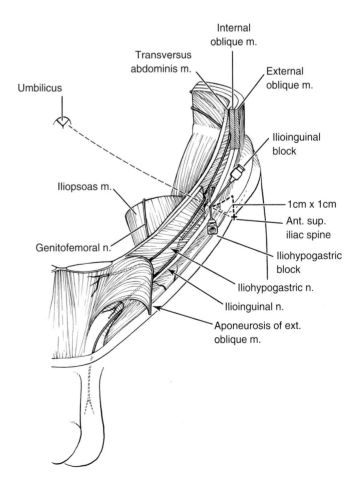

Figure 32–8 The iliohypogastric nerve block and the ilioinguinal nerve block. Ant., anterior; ext., external; m., muscle; n., nerve; sup., superior.

Typically, a unilateral block can be accomplished with 4 mL of local anesthetic solution. The concentration of local anesthetic should therefore reflect the total volume (and dose of local anesthetic) anticipated to be administered. Usually either 0.25% or 0.5% bupivacaine with or without epinephrine is used. The total bupivacaine dose should be less than 2 mg/kg (4 mg/kg if epinephrine-containing local anesthetic is used). Within this dose range, toxic plasma bupivacaine levels should not result.[15, 24]

If the block is to be performed at the completion of the operation, equivalent analgesia can be obtained by infiltration of local anesthetic through the lateral edge of the inguinal incision.[123]

Several studies[122, 123] have demonstrated that ilioinguinal and iliohypogastric nerve blocks are as effective as caudal epidural anesthesia for postoperative analgesia after herniorrhaphy or orchiopexy.

A side effect of this block was transient quadriceps femoris weakness and walking difficulty in several patients who had received 0.5% bupivacaine. This is presumably secondary to transient motor block of the femoral nerve and can be confirmed by documenting ipsilateral sensory loss over the anterior thigh, weakness in the quadriceps femoris, and decreased knee jerk.[124, 125] It is possible that this side effect is caused by passage of the local anesthetic to the femoral nerve via areolar tissue superficial to the external oblique aponeurosis.[126] Use of 0.25% bupivacaine may help minimize this side effect.

Femoral Nerve Block

The lateral femoral cutaneous, femoral and genitofemoral, and obturator nerves provide sensation to the lateral, anterior, and medial aspects of the thigh, respectively. Use of a femoral nerve block has been advocated as an excellent means of analgesia in the emergency setting in the evaluation and reduction of femoral midshaft fractures.[25, 127–129] Combined femoral nerve and lateral femoral cutaneous nerve block can be used for muscle biopsies as part of the evaluation of myopathy or susceptibility to malignant hyperthermia.[130] Block of all four nerves supplying the thigh would be necessary for procedures involving more extensive tissue dissection (e.g., removal of implants, femoral biopsy, repair of slipped capital femoral epiphysis).

All four nerves originate from the lumbar plexus (L-2 to L-4) and initially lie within the fascia iliaca compartment anterior to the quadratus lumborum and posterior to the iliopsoas muscles. The femoral nerve supplies sensory fibers to the anterior aspect of the thigh and the femoral midshaft and its periosteum and motor fibers to the quadriceps muscles. The nerve enters the groin posterior to the inguinal ligament and lateral and deep to the femoral vessels within the femoral triangle. The nerve divides into anterior and posterior bundles at or near the level of the inguinal ligament.[131]

To perform a femoral nerve block, have the patient lie supine. Palpate the femoral artery pulse at a level 1 cm inferior to the inguinal ligament. Keep one finger on the pulse and insert a 25-G needle immediately lateral to the artery to a depth deeper than the artery. Two pops can often be appreciated as the fascia lata and the fascia iliaca are pierced[132] (Fig. 32–9). After a negative result of aspiration, local anesthetic is injected in a radiating fashion around the nerve. Solicitation of paresthesia or use of a nerve stimulator may be of benefit in locating the nerve. Bupivacaine 0.25% to 0.5% can be used with or without epinephrine (maximum dose 2 mg/kg without epinephrine, 4 mg/kg with epinephrine). The maximum necessary dose is 10 mL. Onset of analgesia can be expected in less than 20 min, and duration of analgesia is usually about 6 h. Ronchi and colleagues[25] used 2 mg/kg of 0.5% bupivacaine without epinephrine on 14 children with femur fractures. Plasma bupivacaine levels were measured in nine of the children. The range of maximum plasma bupivacaine concentrations was 0.37 to 1.52 µg/mL. No patient exhibited any signs of local anesthetic systemic toxicity.

Winnie and associates[133] proposed a method of blocking the femoral, obturator, and lateral femoral cutaneous nerves with a single injection of local anesthetic (the 3-in-1 block). Use of this method in children has had varied degrees of success.[131, 134] Dalens and coworkers[131] advocated the use of the fascia iliaca compartment block for blocking all four nerves of the thigh.

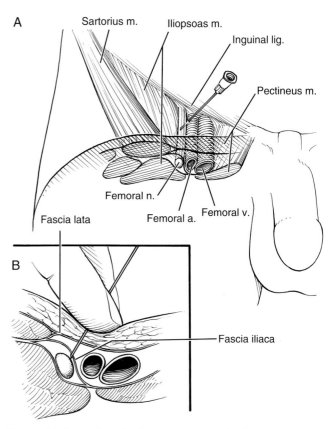

Figure 32–9 *A* and *B*, The femoral nerve (n.) lies between the fascia lata and the fascia iliaca, lateral to the femoral artery (a.) and vein (v.). lig., ligament; m., muscle.

With the patient in the supine position, a line from the anterior superior iliac spine to the pubic tubercle is drawn and divided into thirds. At a point 5 cm caudal from where the lateral one third meets the medial two thirds, a short-beveled needle is inserted posteriorly in a parasagittal plane. With a syringe attached to the needle and gentle constant pressure applied, a loss of resistance will be appreciated as the needle first pierces the fascia lata and subsequently the fascia iliaca. At this point, local anesthetic is injected while pressure is applied caudally to promote rostral spread of local anesthetic. A larger volume of local anesthetic is required for this block (0.5 to 0.7 mL/kg). Comparing the fascia iliaca compartment block with the 3-in-1 block, Dalens and associates[131] found a higher incidence of motor block with the 3-in-1 block and an equal extent of complete sensory anesthesia in the distribution of the femoral nerve. However, there was a significantly greater extent of sensory anesthesia of the lateral femoral cutaneous, obturator, and genito-femoral nerves with the fascia iliaca compartment block.

The lateral femoral cutaneous nerve supplies sensory fibers to the lateral aspect of the thigh. It can be blocked by depositing a wall of local anesthetic in its position near the inguinal ligament. With the patient in the supine position, a short-beveled needle is inserted 1 cm medial and 1 cm inferior to the anterior superior iliac spine (2.5 cm medial and 2.5 cm inferior to the anterior superior iliac spine in adult-sized patients). The needle is advanced until the fascia lata is pierced, and the local anesthetic is injected as the needle is withdrawn. The needle is reinserted in a slightly more medial direction, and the process is repeated with local anesthetic injection in a fanwise manner both deep and superficial to the fascia lata. A total local anesthetic volume of 0.1 to 0.2 mL/kg of either 0.25% bupivacaine or 1% lidocaine should be sufficient.

Intercostal Nerve Block

Each intercostal nerve originates from the dorsal ramus of its corresponding thoracic spinal nerve. The relationship between the intercostal nerve and the muscles of the intercostal space[135] is shown in Figure 32–10. The nerve is accompanied by an intercostal artery and vein and lies in the intercostal groove on the inferior aspect of the rib. A lateral cutaneous nerve branches off at approximately the midaxillary line. This nerve supplies sensation to the anterolateral, lateral, and posterolateral portions of the thorax. In order to adequately block the intercostal nerve, local anesthetic must be deposited proximal to its division.

Intercostal nerve blocks are useful in children to provide analgesia during or after thoracotomy. The blocks can be accomplished percutaneously either before or after operation or under direct vision by the surgeon through the parietal pleura when the thorax and pleural cavity are open. When this block is performed in association with general anesthesia, the patient should be in the lateral position and the site to be

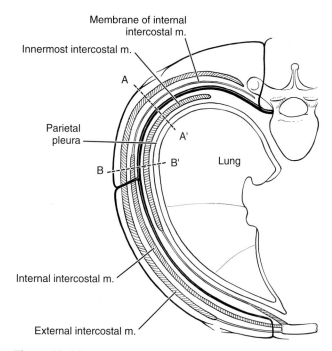

Figure 32–10 The initial course of the intercostal nerve is on the inner surface of the thorax external to the parietal pleura. In the region between the vertebral articulation and the angle of the rib, the nerve is external to the parietal pleura and the innermost intercostal muscle (m.) and internal to the external intercostal muscle and the membrane of the internal intercostal muscle (line A–A'). Distal to the angle of the rib, the nerve lies internal to the external intercostal muscle and the internal intercostal muscle and lies external to the innermost intercostal muscle and the parietal pleura (line B–B'). (Redrawn from Anderson JE: Grant's Atlas of Anatomy, 7th ed, Figure 1–13. Baltimore, Williams & Wilkins, 1978.)

blocked, nondependent. The upper arm is flexed and internally rotated to remove obstruction by the scapula. A procedure is followed similar to that described by Mulroy.[136] Injections are made at the angle of the rib just lateral to sacrospinalis musculature. The involved intercostal space and one or two spaces above and below should be blocked.

Locate and mark the angle of the ribs above the nerves to be blocked. A 22-G, short-beveled needle with an attached syringe filled with local anesthetic should be used. Apply gentle cephalad traction on the skin, and insert the needle over the angle of the rib. The needle is inserted perpendicular to the width of the rib and then angulated approximately 20° cephalad and advanced until it intercepts the lower edge of the rib as the skin is allowed to retract caudally. Anesthesiologists then rest their cephalad hand (right hand if the patient is in the right lateral decubitus position) on the thorax just cephalad to the intercostal space to be blocked and grasp the hub and shaft of the needle. All movements of the needle are accomplished with the hand resting on the thorax to allow for maximal steadiness and to avoid unintentional deep insertion. The needle is walked off the inferior edge of the rib and a loss of resistance is appreciated as the needle is advanced through the external and internal intercostal muscles. Care must be taken to keep the needle in a

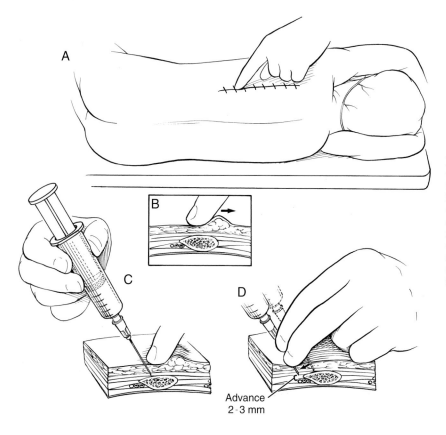

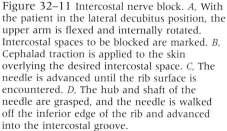

Figure 32–11 Intercostal nerve block. *A,* With the patient in the lateral decubitus position, the upper arm is flexed and internally rotated. Intercostal spaces to be blocked are marked. *B,* Cephalad traction is applied to the skin overlying the desired intercostal space. *C,* The needle is advanced until the rib surface is encountered. *D,* The hub and shaft of the needle are grasped, and the needle is walked off the inferior edge of the rib and advanced into the intercostal groove.

parallel orientation to its final 20° cephalad angle of insertion onto the rib. Entry into the intercostal groove should occur 1 to 2 mm deeper than the edge of the rib. The needle is now fixed in place by the index finger and thumb of the hand that has been guiding its position. Aspirate for the presence of air or blood. If the result of aspiration is negative, inject 1 to 4 mL of local anesthetic (Fig. 32–11). Because the goal of the procedure is prolonged analgesia, usually bupivacaine 0.25% or 0.5% with epinephrine 1:200,000 (5 μg/mL) is used. The dose needed to block each nerve depends on the size of the patient and is usually between 1 and 4 mL.

Local anesthetic absorption tends to be higher for intercostal nerve blocks than for other blocks.[12] Also, the time to peak concentration is shorter for children than for adults.[26, 27] Rothstein and colleagues[27] demonstrated whole blood bupivacaine levels greater than 2 μg/mL when 4 mg/kg of 0.5% bupivacaine with epinephrine 1:200,000 was used for intercostal blocks in children after thoracotomy. Peak blood concentrations occurred in less than 10 min in the majority of cases. For this reason, the author recommends decreasing the maximum allowable dose of bupivacaine with epinephrine to 3 mg/kg.

References

1. Williamson PS, Williamson ML: Physiologic stress reduction by a local anesthetic during newborn circumcision. Pediatrics 1983; 71: 36–40.
2. Stang HJ, Gunnar MR, Snellman L, et al: Local anesthesia for neonatal circumcision. Effects on distress and cortisol response. JAMA 1988; 259: 1507–1511.
3. Murat I, Walker J, Esteve C, et al: Effect of lumbar epidural anaesthesia on plasma cortisol levels in children. Can J Anaesth 1988; 35: 20–24.
4. Dick W: Is there a place for regional anesthesia in pediatrics?—No. Acta Anaesthesiol Belg 1988; 39: 185–189.
5. Dohi S, Naito H, Takahashi T: Age-related changes in blood pressure and duration of motor block in spinal anesthesia. Anesthesiology 1979; 50: 319–323.
6. Murat I, Delleur MM, Esteve C, et al: Continuous extradural anaesthesia in children. Clinical and haemodynamic implications. Br J Anaesth 1987; 59: 1441–1450.
7. Rudolph AM: Congenital Diseases of the Heart; Clinical-Physiologic Considerations in Diagnosis and Management. Chicago, Year Book Medical Publishers, 1974.
8. Finley JP, Hamilton R, MacKenzie MG: Heart rate response to tilting in newborns in quiet and active sleep. Biol Neonate 1984; 45: 1–10.
9. Waldman S, Krauss AN, Auld PA: Baroreceptors in preterm infants: their relationship to maturity and disease. Dev Med Child Neurol 1979; 21: 714–722.
10. Payen D, Ecoffey C, Carli P, et al: Pulsed Doppler ascending aortic, carotid, brachial, and femoral artery blood flows during caudal anesthesia in infants. Anesthesiology 1987; 67: 681–685.
11. Berkowitz S, Greene BA: Spinal anesthesia in children: report based on 350 patients under 13 years of age. Anesthesiology 1951; 12: 376–387.
12. Tucker GT: Pharmacokinetics of local anaesthetics. Br J Anaesth 1986; 58: 717–731.
13. Morselli PL, Franco-Morselli R, Bossi L: Clinical pharmacokinetics in newborns and infants. Age-related differences and therapeutic implications. Clin Pharmacokinet 1980; 5: 485–527.
14. Bokesch PM, Castaneda AR, Ziemer G, et al: The influence of a right-to-left cardiac shunt on lidocaine pharmacokinetics. Anesthesiology 1987; 67: 739–744.
15. Stow PJ, Scott A, Phillips A, et al: Plasma bupivacaine concentrations during caudal analgesia and ilioinguinal-iliohypogastric nerve block in children. Anaesthesia 1988; 43: 650–653.

16. Ecoffey C, Desparmet J, Maury M, et al: Bupivacaine in children: pharmacokinetics following caudal anesthesia. Anesthesiology 1985; 63: 447–448.

17. Mazoit JX, Denson DD, Samii K: Pharmacokinetics of bupivacaine following caudal anesthesia in infants. Anesthesiology 1988; 68: 387–391.

18. Takasaki M: Blood concentrations of lidocaine, mepivacaine and bupivacaine during caudal analgesia in children. Acta Anaesthesiol Scand 1984; 28: 211–214.

19. Yaster M, Aronoff D, Kornhauser DM, et al: The pharmacokinetics of lidocaine during caudal anesthesia in children. (Abstract.) Anesthesiology 1985; 63(Suppl): a465.

20. Ecoffey C, Desparmet J, Berdeaux A, et al: Pharmacokinetics of lignocaine in children following caudal anaesthesia. Br J Anaesth 1984; 56: 1399–1402.

21. Campbell RJ, Ilett KF, Dusci L: Plasma bupivacaine concentrations after axillary block in children. Anaesth Intensive Care 1986; 14: 343–346.

22. Maxwell LG, Yaster M, Wetzel RC, et al: Penile nerve block for newborn circumcision. Obstet Gynecol 1987; 70: 415–419.

23. Sfez M, Le Mapihan Y, Mazoit X, et al: Local anesthetic serum concentrations after penile nerve block in children. Anesth Analg 1990; 71: 423–426.

24. Epstein RH, Larijani GE, Wolfson PJ, et al: Plasma bupivacaine concentrations following ilioinguinal-iliohypogastric nerve blockade in children. Anesthesiology 1988; 69: 773–776.

25. Ronchi L, Rosenbaum D, Athouel A, et al: Femoral nerve blockade in children using bupivacaine. Anesthesiology 1989; 70: 622–624.

26. Bricker SRW, Telford RJ, Booker PD: Pharmacokinetics of bupivacaine following intraoperative intercostal nerve block in neonates and in infants aged less than 6 months. Anesthesiology 1989; 70: 942–947.

27. Rothstein P, Arthur GR, Feldman HS, et al: Bupivacaine for intercostal nerve blocks in children: blood concentrations and pharmacokinetics. Anesth Analg 1986; 65: 625–632.

28. Shand DG: Alpha 1-acid glycoprotein and plasma lidocaine binding. Clin Pharmacokinet 1984; 9(Suppl 1): 27–31.

29. Tucker GT, Mather LE: Clinical pharmacokinetics of local anaesthetics. Clin Pharmacokinet 1979; 4: 241–278.

30. Zsigmond EK, Downs JR: Plasma cholinesterase activity in newborns and infants. Can Anaesth Soc J 1971; 18: 278–285.

31. Henderson K, Sethna NF, Berde CB: Continuous caudal anesthesia for inguinal hernia repair in former preterm infants. J Clin Anesth 1993; 5: 129–133.

32. Ross JD: Deficient activity of DPNH-dependent methemoglobin diaphorase in cord blood erythrocytes. Blood 1963; 21: 51–62.

33. Ross JD, Desforges JF: Reduction of methemoglobin by erythrocytes from cord blood: further evidence of deficient enzyme activity in the newborn period. Pediatrics 1959; 23: 718–726.

34. Bunn HF: Human hemoglobins: normal and abnormal; methemoglobinemia. In Nathan DG, Oski FA (eds): Hematology of Infancy and Childhood, 4th ed, pp 698–731. Philadelphia, WB Saunders Co, 1993.

35. Duncan PG, Kobrinsky N: Prilocaine-induced methemoglobinemia in a newborn infant. Anesthesiology 1983; 59: 75–76.

36. Gregory GA: Out-patient anesthesia. In Miller RD (ed): Anesthesia, pp 1323–1333. New York, Churchill Livingstone, 1981.

37. Gregory GA, Steward DJ: Life-threatening perioperative apnea in the ex-"premie." (Editorial.) Anesthesiology 1983; 59: 495–498.

38. Steward DJ: Preterm infants are more prone to complications following minor surgery than are term infants. Anesthesiology 1982; 56: 304–306.

39. Liu LM, Coté CJ, Goudsouzian NG, et al: Life-threatening apnea in infants recovering from anesthesia. Anesthesiology 1983; 59: 506–510.

40. Welborn LG, Ramirez N, Oh TH, et al: Postanesthetic apnea and periodic breathing in infants. Anesthesiology 1986; 65: 658–661.

41. Kurth CD, Spitzer AR, Broennle AM, et al: Postoperative apnea in preterm infants. Anesthesiology 1987; 66: 483–488.

42. Welborn LG, Rice LJ, Hannallah RS, et al: Postoperative apnea in former preterm infants: prospective comparison of spinal and general anesthesia. Anesthesiology 1990; 72: 838–842.

43. Gray HT: A study of spinal anaesthesia in children and infants from a series of 200 cases. Lancet 1909; Sept 25: 913; 991.

44. Robson CH: Anesthesia in children. Am J Surg 1936; 34: 468–473.

45. Melman E, Penuelas JA, Marrufo J: Regional anesthesia in children. Anesth Analg 1975; 54: 387–390.

46. Blaise GA, Roy WL: Spinal anaesthesia for minor paediatric surgery. Can Anaesth Soc J 1986; 33: 227–230.

47. Gouvela MA: Raquianestesia para pacientes pediátricos: experiência pessoal em 50 casos. Rev Bras Anestesiol 1970; 20: 501–511.

48. Blaise G, Roy WL: Spinal anesthesia in children. (Letter to the editor.) Anesth Analg 1984; 63: 1140–1141.

49. Abajian JC, Mellish RW, Browne AF, et al: Spinal anesthesia for surgery in the high-risk infant. Anesth Analg 1984; 63: 359–362.

50. Mahe V, Ecoffey C: Spinal anesthesia with isobaric bupivacaine in infants. Anesthesiology 1988; 68: 601–603.

51. Gleason CA, Martin RJ, Anderson JV, et al: Optimal position for a spinal tap in preterm infants. Pediatrics 1983; 71: 31–35.

52. Weisman LE, Merenstein GB, Steenbarger JR: The effect of lumbar puncture position in sick neonates. Am J Dis Child 1983; 137: 1077–1079.

53. Choremis C, Economos D, Papadatos C, et al: Intraspinal epidermoid tumours (cholesteatomas) in patients treated for tuberculous meningitis. Lancet 1956; 2: 437–439.

54. Manno NJ, Uihlein A, Kernohan JW: Intraspinal epidermoids. J Neurosurg 1962; 19: 754–765.

55. Batnitzky S, Keucher TR, Mealey J Jr, et al: Iatrogenic intraspinal epidermoid tumors. JAMA 1977; 237: 148–150.

56. Wright TE, Orr RJ, Haberkern CM, et al: Complications during spinal anesthesia in infants: high spinal blockade. Anesthesiology 1990; 73: 1290–1292.

57. McGown RG: Caudal analgesia in children. Five hundred cases for procedures below the diaphragm. Anaesthesia 1982; 37: 806–818.

58. Broadman LM, Hannallah RS, Norden JM, et al: "Kiddie caudals": experience with 1154 consecutive cases without complications. (Abstract.) Anesth Analg 1987; 66(Suppl): s18.

59. Dalens B, Hasnaoui A: Caudal anesthesia in pediatric surgery: success rate and adverse effects in 750 consecutive patients. Anesth Analg 1989; 68: 83–89.

60. Fortuna A: Caudal analgesia: a simple and safe technique in paediatric surgery. Br J Anaesth 1967; 39: 165–170.

61. Desparmet JF: Total spinal anesthesia after caudal anesthesia in an infant. Anesth Analg 1990; 70: 665–667.

62. Matsumiya N, Dohi S, Takahashi H, et al: Cardiovascular collapse in an infant after caudal anesthesia with a lidocaine-epinephrine solution. Anesth Analg 1986; 65: 1074–1076.

63. Ved SA, Pinosky M, Nocodemus H: Ventricular tachycardia and brief cardiovascular collapse in two infants after caudal anesthesia using a bupivacaine-epinephrine solution. Anesthesiology 1993; 79: 1121–1123.

64. Spear RM, Deshpande JK, Maxwell LG: Caudal anesthesia in the awake, high-risk infant. Anesthesiology 1988; 69: 407–409.

65. Gunter JB, Watcha MF, Forestner JE, et al: Caudal epidural anesthesia in conscious premature and high-risk infants. J Pediatr Surg 1991; 26: 9–14.

66. Desparmet J, Mateo J, Ecoffey C, et al: Efficacy of an epidural test dose in children anesthetized with halothane. Anesthesiology 1990; 72: 249–251.

67. Freid EB, Bailey AG, Valley RD: Electrocardiographic and hemodynamic changes associated with unintentional intravascular injection of bupivacaine with epinephrine in infants. Anesthesiology 1993; 79: 394–398.

68. Armitage EN: Regional anaesthesia in pediatrics. Clin Anesthesiol 1985; 3: 553–568.

69. Bromage PR: Ageing and epidural dose requirements: segmental spread and predictability of epidural analgesia in youth and extreme age. Br J Anaesth 1969; 41: 1016–1022.

70. Schulte-Steinberg O, Rahlfs VW: Spread of extradural analgesia following caudal injection in children. A statistical study. Br J Anaesth 1977; 49: 1027–1034.

71. Takasaki M, Dohi S, Kawabata Y, et al: Dosage of lidocaine for caudal anesthesia in infants and children. Anesthesiology 1977; 47: 527–529.

72. Satoyoshi M, Kamiyama Y: Caudal anaesthesia for upper abdominal surgery in infants and children: a simple calculation of the volume of local anaesthetic. Acta Anaesthesiol Scand 1984; 28: 57–60.

73. Busoni P, Andreuccetti T: The spread of caudal analgesia in children: a mathematical model. Anaesth Intensive Care 1986; 14: 140–144.

74. Bösenberg AT, Bland BA, Schulte-Steinberg O, et al: Thoracic epidural anesthesia via caudal route in infants. Anesthesiology 1988; 69: 265–269.

75. Gunter JB, Eng C: Thoracic epidural anesthesia via the caudal approach in children. Anesthesiology 1992; 76: 935–938.

76. van Niekerk J, Bax-Vermeire BM, Geurts JW, et al: Epidurography in premature infants. Anaesthesia 1990; 45: 722–725.

77. Rasch DK, Webster DE, Pollard TG, et al: Lumbar and thoracic epidural analgesia via the caudal approach for postoperative pain relief in infants and children. Can J Anaesth 1990; 37: 359–362.

78. Kosaka Y, Sato K, Kawaguchi R: Distance from the skin to the epidural space in children. Masui 1974; 23: 874–875.

79. Ecoffey C, Dubousset AM, Samii K: Lumbar and thoracic epidural anesthesia for urologic and upper abdominal surgery in infants and children. Anesthesiology 1986; 65: 87–90.

80. Jensen BH: Caudal block for post-operative pain relief in children after genital operations. A comparison between bupivacaine and morphine. Acta Anaesthesiol Scand 1981; 25: 373–375.

81. Martin LV: Postoperative analgesia after circumcision in children. Br J Anaesth 1982; 54: 1263–1266.

82. Shapiro LA, Jedeikin RJ, Shalev D, et al: Epidural morphine analgesia in children. Anesthesiology 1984; 61: 210–212.

83. Glenski JA, Warner MA, Dawson B, et al: Postoperative use of epidurally administered morphine in children and adolescents. Mayo Clin Proc 1984; 59: 530–533.

84. Dalens B, Tanguy A, Haberer JP: Lumbar epidural anesthesia for operative and postoperative pain relief in infants and young children. Anesth Analg 1986; 65: 1069–1073.

85. Attia J, Ecoffey C, Sandouk P, et al: Epidural morphine in children: pharmacokinetics and CO_2 sensitivity. Anesthesiology 1986; 65: 590–594.

86. Krane EJ, Jacobson LE, Lynn AM, et al: Caudal morphine for postoperative analgesia in children: a comparison with caudal bupivacaine and intravenous morphine. Anesth Analg 1987; 66: 647–653.

87. Rosen KR, Rosen DA: Caudal epidural morphine for control of pain following open heart surgery in children. Anesthesiology 1989; 70: 418–421.

88. Krane EJ, Tyler DC, Jacobson LE: The dose response of caudal morphine in children. Anesthesiology 1989; 71: 48–52.

89. Valley RD, Bailey AG: Caudal morphine for postoperative analgesia in infants and children: a report of 138 cases. Anesth Analg 1991; 72: 120–124.

90. Wolf AR, Hughes D, Hobbs AJ, et al: Combined morphine-bupivacaine caudals for reconstructive penile surgery in children: systemic absorption of morphine and postoperative analgesia. Anaesth Intensive Care 1991; 19: 17–21.

91. Bromage PR, Camporesi EM, Durant PA, et al: Rostral spread of epidural morphine. Anesthesiology 1982; 56: 431–436.

92. Meignier M, Souron R, Le Neel JC: Postoperative dorsal epidural analgesia in the child with respiratory disabilities. Anesthesiology 1983; 59: 473–475.

93. Tobias JD, Lowe S, O'Dell N, et al: Thoracic epidural anaesthesia in infants and children. Can J Anaesth 1993; 40: 879–882.

94. Mevorach DL, Perkins FM, Isaacson SA: Bupivacaine toxicity secondary to continuous caudal epidural infusion in children. (Letter to the editor.) Anesth Analg 1993; 77: 1305–1306.

95. McCloskey JJ, Haun SE, Deshpande JK: Bupivacaine toxicity secondary to continuous caudal epidural infusion in children. Anesth Analg 1992; 75: 287–290.

96. Berde CB: Convulsions associated with pediatric regional anesthesia. (Editorial.) Anesth Analg 1992; 75: 164–166.

97. Agarwal R, Gutlove DP, Lockhart CH: Seizures occurring in pediatric patients receiving continuous infusion of bupivacaine. Anesth Analg 1992; 75: 284–286.

98. Tobin JR, Kost-Byerly S, Greenberg RS, et al: Continuous lidocaine epidural analgesia in children. (Abstract.) Anesthesiology 1993; 79(Suppl): a1131.

99. Krane EJ: Delayed respiratory depression in a child after caudal epidural morphine. Anesth Analg 1988; 67: 79–82.

100. Carrel ED, Eyring EJ: Intravenous regional anesthesia for childhood fractures. J Trauma 1971; 11: 301–305.

101. FitzGerald B: Intravenous regional anaesthesia in children. Br J Anaesth 1976; 48: 485–486.

102. Barnes CL, Blasier RD, Dodge BM: Intravenous regional anesthesia: a safe and cost-effective outpatient anesthetic for upper extremity fracture treatment in children. J Pediatr Orthop 1991; 11: 717–720.

103. Juliano PJ, Mazur JM, Cummings RJ, et al: Low-dose lidocaine intravenous regional anesthesia for forearm fractures in children. J Pediatr Orthop 1992; 12: 633–635.

104. Rosenberg PH, Kalso EA, Tuominen MK, et al: Acute bupivacaine toxicity as a result of venous leakage under the tourniquet cuff during a Bier block. Anesthesiology 1983; 58: 95–98.

105. Heath ML: Bupivicaine toxicity and Bier blocks. (Letter to the editor.) Anesthesiology 1983; 59: 481.

106. Grice SC, Morell RC, Balestrieri FJ, et al: Intravenous regional anesthesia: evaluation and prevention of leakage under the tourniquet. Anesthesiology 1986; 65: 316–320.

107. Abdulla WY, Fadhil NM: A new approach to intravenous regional anesthesia. Anesth Analg 1992; 75: 597–601.

108. Sethna NF, Berde CB: Pediatric regional anesthesia equipment. Int Anesthesiol Clin 1992; 30: 163–176.

109. Dalens B, Vanneuville G, Dechelotte P: Penile block via the subpubic space in 100 children. Anesth Analg 1989; 69: 41–45.

110. Brown TCK, Schulte-Steinberg O: Neural blockade for pediatric surgery. In Cousins MJ, Bridenbaugh PO (eds): Neural Blockade in Clinical Anesthesia and Management of Pain, 2nd ed, pp 669–692. Philadelphia, JB Lippincott, 1988.

111. Bacon AK: An alternative block for post circumcision analgesia. Anaesth Intensive Care 1977; 5: 63–64.

112. Soliman MG, Tremblay NA: Nerve block of the penis for postoperative pain relief in children. Anesth Analg 1978; 57: 495–498.

113. Kirya C, Werthmann MW Jr: Neonatal circumcision and penile dorsal nerve block—a painless procedure. J Pediatr 1978; 92: 998–1000.

114. Broadman LM, Hannallah RS, Belman AB, et al: Post-circumcision analgesia—a prospective evaluation of subcutaneous ring block of the penis. Anesthesiology 1987; 67: 399–402.

115. Berens R, Pontus SP Jr: A complication associated with dorsal penile nerve block. Reg Anesth 1990; 15: 309–310.

116. Sara CA, Lowry CJ: A complication of circumcision and dorsal nerve block of the penis. Anaesth Intensive Care 1984; 13: 79–85.

117. Masciello AL: Anesthesia for neonatal circumcision: local anesthesia is better than dorsal penile nerve block. Obstet Gynecol 1990; 75: 834–838.

118. Tree-Trakarn T, Pirayavaraporn S: Postoperative pain relief for circumcision in children: comparison among morphine, nerve block, and topical analgesia. Anesthesiology 1985; 62: 519–522.

119. Tree-Trakarn T, Pirayavaraporn S, Lertakyamanee J: Topical analgesia for relief of post-circumcision pain. Anesthesiology 1987; 67: 395–399.

120. Andersen KH: A new method of analgesia for relief of circumcision pain. Anaesthesia 1989; 44: 118–120.

121. Langer JC, Shandling B, Rosenberg M: Intraoperative bupivacaine during outpatient hernia repair in children: a randomized double blind trial. J Pediatr Surg 1987; 22: 267–270.

122. Markham SJ, Tomlinson J, Hain WR: Ilioinguinal nerve block in children. A comparison with caudal block for intra and postoperative analgesia. Anaesthesia 1986; 41: 1098–1103.

123. Hannallah RS, Broadman LM, Belman AB, et al: Comparison of caudal and ilioinguinal/iliohypogastric nerve blocks for control of post-orchiopexy pain in pediatric ambulatory surgery. Anesthesiology 1987; 66: 832–834.

124. Shandling B, Steward DJ: Regional analgesia for postoperative pain in pediatric outpatient surgery. J Pediatr Surg 1980; 15: 477–480.

125. Roy-Shapira A, Amoury RA, Ashcraft KW, et al: Transient quadriceps paresis following local inguinal block for postoperative pain control. J Pediatr Surg 1985; 20: 554–555.

126. Chan TY, Davidson T: Femoral nerve block after intra-operative subcutaneous bupivacaine injection. (Letter to the editor.) Anaesthesia 1990; 45: 163–164.

127. Berry FR: Analgesia in patients with fractured shaft of femur. Anaesthesia 1977; 32: 576–577.

128. Grossbard GD, Love BR: Femoral nerve block: a simple and safe method of instant analgesia for femoral shaft fractures in children. Aust N Z J Surg 1979; 49: 592–594.

129. Tondare AS, Nadkarni AV: Femoral nerve block for fractured shaft of femur. Can Anaesth Soc J 1982; 29: 270–271.

130. Berkowitz A, Rosenberg H: Femoral block with mepivacaine for muscle biopsy in malignant hyperthermia patients. Anesthesiology 1985; 62: 651–652.

131. Dalens B, Vanneuville G, Tanguy A: Comparison of the fascia iliaca compartment block with the 3-in-1 block in children. Anesth Analg 1989; 69: 705–713.

132. Khoo ST, Brown TC: Femoral nerve block—the anatomical basis for a single injection technique. Anaesth Intensive Care 1983; 11: 40–42.

133. Winnie AP, Ramamurthy S, Durrani Z: The inguinal paravascular technic of lumbar plexus anesthesia: the "3-in-1 block." Anesth Analg 1973; 52: 989–996.

134. Rosen KR, Broadman LM: Anaesthesia for diagnostic muscle biopsy in an infant with Pompe's disease. Can Anaesth Soc J 1986; 33: 790–794.

135. Gardner E, Gray DJ, O'Rahilly R: Thoracic wall and mediastinum. In Gardner E, Gray DJ, O'Rahilly R (eds): Anatomy: A Regional Study of Human Structure, 4th ed, pp 266–279. Philadelphia, WB Saunders Co, 1975.

136. Mulroy MF: Regional Anesthesia: An Illustrated Procedural Guide, pp 121–130. Boston, Little, Brown, 1989.

CHAPTER 33

Outpatients

Michael F. Mulroy, M.D.

The advantages of avoiding general anesthesia have been recognized since the advent of outpatient surgery. The usual side effects of general anesthetic techniques—nausea, emesis, and postoperative pain and sedation—delay dismissal from an outpatient unit and may necessitate overnight admission. The techniques of spinal, epidural, and peripheral nerve block anesthesia are advantageous in outpatient surgery units for decreasing the intensity and number of side effects and speeding dismissal.

Advantages of Regional Anesthesia

Avoiding Emesis

Reviews of ambulatory surgery experience consistently identify nausea and vomiting as the most frequent anesthesia-related cause of delay in dismissal[1, 2] and unplanned admission, with rates of 0.5% to 2%.[3] It is also a primary source of patient dissatisfaction in ambulatory surgery recovery.[4] Nausea is most frequently associated with general anesthesia and occurs in 20% to 30% of patients.[5] Opioid use may be associated with an incidence of vomiting as high as 40%.[6, 7] Although this can be decreased by the use of antiemetics, these drugs can prolong recovery by producing somnolence and also lead to other delayed side effects, such as dysphoria after dismissal.[8] The intravenous agent propofol is associated with less nausea and vomiting than other general anesthetic agents, but the incidence is still as high as 23%.[9] Desflurane also does not lessen nausea compared with other inhalation anesthetics, with an incidence of emesis of 40%.[7, 9] The incidence of emesis is lower after regional techniques, especially if excessive opioid premedication is avoided.

Relieving Pain

Postoperative pain is usually the second major cause of unplanned admission after outpatient surgery. Long-acting local anesthetics, such as bupivacaine or ropivacaine, used for upper or lower extremity blocks can produce 4 to 24 h of analgesia, which allows the patient to travel home in comfort.[10] This period of analgesia provides a more positive experience and decreases the use of opioid analgesics given orally, which are also associated with nausea that delays dismissal. Infiltration of the wound after hernia repair[11] or other major abdominal surgery can decrease postoperative pain and reliance on opioids. The approach is extremely effective in pediatric patients. This technique is underused and deserves more consideration by the anesthesiologist and surgeon in the outpatient setting.

Decreasing Nursing Care

With fewer side effects than from the use of general anesthesia (especially emesis and pain) and with a higher degree of mental alertness at admission, the regional anesthesia patient represents a decreased nursing burden in the postanesthesia care unit. Patients with upper extremity or retrobulbar blocks usually bypass the first-stage recovery areas and are transferred directly to the step-down units in most institutions.

Shortening Time to Dismissal

If side effects are minimized, recovery time can be decreased. More rapid dismissal has been demonstrated after arthroscopic procedures when leg block or epidural anesthesia is compared with general anesthesia.

Patel and colleagues[12] showed that peripheral nerve block of the leg with either of the two techniques was superior to general anesthesia in providing rapid dismissal after arthroscopy. Allen and coworkers[13] showed that patients receiving axillary blocks were dismissed 1 h sooner than similar patients undergoing the same operation with propofol–nitrous oxide general anesthesia administered by mask. The patients who had brachial blocks required no supplemental analgesics and less nursing care. Interscalene brachial plexus block has also been shown to produce shorter times to dismissal than isoflurane general anesthesia when used for shoulder arthroscopy in outpatients.[14]

The more rapid return of alertness after regional anesthesia, if heavy sedation is avoided, is intuitively comprehensible. Peripheral nerve blocks allow for almost immediate dismissal from the ambulatory unit. Spinal or epidural block may delay dismissal until motor function has returned in the lower extremity. Nevertheless, several studies of epidural anesthesia have shown dismissal times of 2 h after chloroprocaine or 3 h after lidocaine block,[15] which compare favorably to the 120- to 200-min delays needed with isoflurane or desflurane[7] or even the 120 min required to achieve "street fitness" after propofol.[16] These newer general anesthetic agents produce more rapid recovery than the previous outpatient general anesthetics, but the return of full mental alertness is still delayed, often because of the necessity for analgesic or antiemetic drugs in the recovery period.[17]

Head and Neck Procedures

Types of Operations

The two major categories of outpatient head and neck procedures suitable for regional techniques are cataract extraction and facial plastic surgery. The former represents a large number of outpatient procedures in most centers and is an ideal application for regional anesthesia. For plastic surgery, local infiltration is the most common anesthetic, although this is usually performed by the surgeon rather than an anesthesiologist.

Regional Techniques

For eye surgery, a retrobulbar block is usually performed. Peribulbar block is a frequent alternative but has a higher need for supplemental injections and requires more time for onset. Both are acceptable, and both have a low rate of complications.[18] In most institutions, the block is performed by the ophthalmologist, but anesthesiologists are involved in many centers. Performance of the block by the anesthesiologist can facilitate operating room turnover by having the block performed in a separate location while the ophthalmologist finishes the dressing and paperwork on the previous lightly sedated patient in the operating room. Although some sedation and analgesia are usually

required for the performance of the facial nerve block or the retrobulbar injection itself, further sedation is rarely needed intraoperatively, and these patients usually are ready to move to the recovery area in a wheelchair.

Choice of Drugs

For eye anesthesia, bupivacaine is the most commonly used drug because of its long duration and excellent akinesia of the extraocular muscles. Epinephrine is usually added to prolong duration, and hyaluronidase is added to facilitate the spread of anesthesia. For the facial nerve block, a shorter-acting drug such as lidocaine or mepivacaine allows early return of sensory function. The more proximal injections of the facial nerve (near the ear) often produce a facial droop that is disconcerting to the patient and family, and early resolution is desirable.

For subcutaneous infiltration for plastic surgery, lidocaine or bupivacaine is effective. Lower concentrations are needed for skin anesthesia than for peripheral nerve blocks, and the lower drug dose also decreases the potential for absorption of toxic amounts of drug from this vascular region.

Upper Extremity Procedures

The ideal demonstration of alertness, postoperative analgesia, and rapid dismissal occurs with the use of regional anesthesia for upper extremity surgery. Allen and colleagues[13] showed that patients receiving axillary blocks can leave the postanesthesia care unit 1 h sooner than similar patients undergoing the same operation with propofol–nitrous oxide general anesthesia administered by mask. The patients who had arm blocks required no supplemental analgesics and less nursing care. Brown and associates[14] also showed that interscalene block provides more rapid recovery than isoflurane general anesthesia for shoulder arthroscopy. The Mayo Clinic experience[10] showed that regional anesthesia provided excellent anesthesia, with rapid recovery and a high degree of patient satisfaction.

Types of Operations

Arm surgery is frequently performed in an outpatient setting. Common operations include procedures on the hand, forearm, and shoulder. In the hand itself, carpal tunnel release, excision of ganglions and neuromas, and minor fracture repairs as well as tendon repairs and plastic surgery procedures are performed. These require anesthesia of the three major nerves of the hand: radial, median, and ulnar. Procedures on the forearm frequently include insertion of arteriovenous fistulas and grafts in renal failure patients, in addition to orthopedic procedures on tendons and bone. These procedures require additional anesthesia of the musculocutaneous, medial brachial cutaneous, and medial antebrachial cutaneous nerves. Diagnostic arthroscopy of the shoulder is frequently performed in the outpatient setting, as are minor procedures such as acromioplasty. This requires anesthesia of the brachial plexus and the lower cervical roots, which provides sensory anesthesia to the dorsum of the shoulder.

Selection of Anesthesia

For the anesthesiologist, the simplest and most reliable anesthesia for the lower arm is the intravenous regional technique, which is usually ascribed to August Bier (Fig. 33–1). It is suitable for most superficial surgical procedures on extremities that take less than 90 min to perform; the limiting factor is tourniquet time.

The major risk of this technique is the unintentional or premature release of the tourniquet or inadequate tourniquet pressure, with resulting excessive blood levels of the local anesthetic drug. Close monitoring is essential, and two-stage release of the tourniquet is required if tourniquet time is less than 40 min. It is recommended that the tourniquet pressure be at least

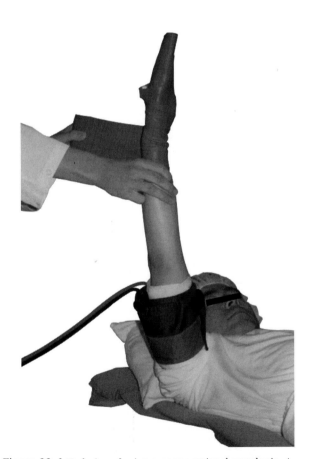

Figure 33–1 Technique for intravenous regional anesthesia. A small intravenous catheter is placed in the hand, and the tourniquet is applied at the top of the upper arm. A single tourniquet may be used for shorter operations and may provide more reliable compression of the venous system than the double-tourniquet system shown. Exsanguination of the arm is attained by elevation of the arm and wrapping it with the von Esmarch elastic bandage. The tourniquet is then inflated and the local anesthetic is injected.

100 mm Hg above the patient's normal systolic pressure if leakage of the local anesthetic drug under the tourniquet into the systemic circulation is to be prevented. The use of a wide blood pressure cuff and slow injection of the local anesthetic in a peripheral vein after full exsanguination of the arm decreases the potential for leakage of local anesthetic under the cuff.[19] This technique is unsuitable when a tourniquet is contraindicated, as in amputations or vascular access procedures. This technique does not provide any residual analgesia but does give full return of arm function before dismissal.

If more profound anesthesia of the upper extremity is required, regional block of the brachial plexus is favored. The plexus can be anesthetized in the interscalene groove, as it crosses the first rib, or in the axilla. Each technique has its advantages and proponents. The supraclavicular approach is avoided by some in treating outpatients because of the small incidence of pneumothorax. Nevertheless, it provides the best anesthesia for all four nerves of the hand and forearm. An interscalene block is less likely to produce pneumothorax and is extremely useful for shoulder procedures, including arthroscopy, acromioplasty, and rotator cuff repair.[14] The axillary approach provides anesthesia to the forearm, as long as care is taken to block the musculocutaneous nerve by infiltration. This approach anesthetizes all three nerves that cross the wrist and is excellent for hand surgery. The main problem of brachial plexus block for outpatient surgery is that it may take 15 to 20 min to produce surgical levels of anesthesia. A major advantage is that these blocks can provide prolonged analgesia for the dismissal home, but the corollary is that the extremity must be padded carefully and the patient cautioned to protect it as long as the numbness persists.

Choice of Drugs

Virtually any of the local anesthetics can be used for peripheral nerve blocks. Lidocaine in a 1.5% concentration is adequate. Many patients appreciate the slightly longer duration of postoperative analgesia that is provided by mepivacaine in a 1.25% to 1.5% concentration. The duration of both agents can be prolonged by the addition of epinephrine. The longest duration can be provided by the use of bupivacaine in 0.375% to 0.5% concentrations. This can provide as much as 12 to 24 h of analgesia in the upper extremity.

Although analgesia is often desirable, the patient also suffers from the persistent numbness that is associated with it. This can be annoying to some patients, who may express a concern about the eventual return of sensation in their arms. It also represents a slight increase in risk, because patients can injure an anesthetized extremity by direct trauma or by resting the extremity in a position that produces pressure on skin or superficial nerves. For this reason, many clinicians use the intermediate-duration anesthetic mepivacaine as a compromise in providing postoperative analgesia, with a reasonable return of function within 6 to 8 h after the performance of the block.

The addition of opioids to local anesthetic solutions for peripheral nerve blocks has been attempted but does not appear to provide any additional prolongation of analgesia.

Lower Abdominal Procedures

Indications

Abdominal surgery with regional anesthesia is usually limited to superficial operations or to minimally invasive procedures, such as laparoscopic surgery. The most common example is gynecologic procedures, which range from diagnostic investigation to removal of ovarian cysts or more extensive fertility evaluations. Even cholecystectomy is being performed with this technique on an outpatient basis. The other major category of abdominal wall surgery is hernia repair. This most commonly is performed in the inguinal area, but it can also involve femoral hernias or herniations of other areas of the abdominal wall musculature. Pediatric procedures such as hernia repair and urogenital surgery are strong indications for regional techniques in providing postoperative analgesia.

Choice of Techniques

Unilateral and bilateral intercostal nerve blocks are ideally suited for surgical procedures on the abdomen and chest wall. This procedure does involve a small risk of pneumothorax but does not limit ambulation or function and does not create the sympathetic block seen with central (peridural or spinal) blocks. Early ambulation and dismissal make this a particularly effective choice for outpatients. Intercostal block is technically more difficult and does require some time for adequate onset of anesthesia.

Spinal and epidural anesthesia are the simplest and most reliable of the regional techniques. The dense, reliable anesthesia provided must be balanced against the longer times to dismissal and greater physiologic changes with these blocks. Nevertheless, they are useful in outpatients.

A major limitation of spinal anesthesia has been the incidence of post-dural puncture headache. This approaches 5% to 10% among inpatients, but it can be decreased to less than 1% by the use of a 25- or 27-G rounded-bevel (Whitacre, Sprotte) spinal needle and by restricting the technique to older patients.[20] Needles smaller than 25 to 27 G increase the technical difficulty of the procedure and do not appear to offer further advantages. In patients older than 40 years of age, the incidence of post-dural puncture headache appears to be less than 1%, but it approaches 2% for patients younger than 40 years of age. In one half of these patients, headaches develop that are severe enough to require treatment with an epidural blood patch. Ambulation by itself does not appear to increase the risk of headache.[21-23] If a headache does occur, treatment with an epidural blood patch on an outpatient basis is effective in remedying this complication without the need for a hospital admission.[24]

In younger patients, epidural anesthesia is a suitable alternative. It does not completely eliminate the potential for post-dural puncture headache, because unintentional dural punctures occur. Caudal and lumbar epidural anesthesia are more difficult technically and slightly less reliable than subarachnoid block, but they have been used successfully for perineal, lower extremity orthopedic, and gynecologic procedures.[25] Epidural anesthesia is also effective for lithotripsy operations, providing alertness and rapid dismissal.[26] Another application of epidural anesthesia is in the repair of inguinal or femoral hernias.[11] If the operation is predictably short, a single-injection technique is sufficient. Epidural anesthesia allows the additional advantage of inserting a catheter to provide reinjection of additional anesthetic.

Unlike peripheral nerve blocks, the goal of neuraxial blocks in the outpatient is to use short-acting drugs to allow early ambulation. This removes the advantage of postoperative analgesia provided by the local anesthetic in extremity blocks. The surgeon may delay the onset of postoperative pain by supplementing the short-acting epidural anesthetic with wound infiltration by a long-acting local anesthetic drug such as 0.25% bupivacaine or ropivacaine. For groin surgery, this technique is preferable to reliance on a "hernia block" that may involve femoral nerve anesthesia, which may be prolonged and limit ambulation. Patients who have adequate surgical anesthesia with a combination of epidural and local infiltration may be dismissed comfortably to their homes before postoperative pain is perceived.[11]

Choice of Drugs

Lidocaine is the current standard drug for outpatient subarachnoid anesthesia. The 1.5% or 2% solution can be used alone as an isobaric preparation for lower abdominal procedures. Lidocaine is also available in a premixed hyperbaric solution of 5% local anesthetic with 7.5% dextrose. Hyperbaric solutions generally spread farther (usually at least to the T-4 level) with the patient in the supine position, but isobaric solutions remain at a lower level (Fig. 33–2). Duration of anesthesia is a function of the total milligrams in the dose and the extent of spread. The same dose provides longer anesthesia as an isobaric solution (limited spread) than as a hyperbaric solution (Table 33–1).[27]

The duration of lidocaine spinal anesthesia varies but is somewhat prolonged by the addition of epinephrine. Epinephrine appears to prolong the average duration (at the knee) from 90 to 120 min.[28] For abdominal surgery, the duration is shorter, and epinephrine has less effect in prolonging anesthesia, although it may prolong resolution of the block.[29] Epinephrine does prolong the time to voiding.[30] The addition of 10 to 20 μg of fentanyl has the interesting property of pro-

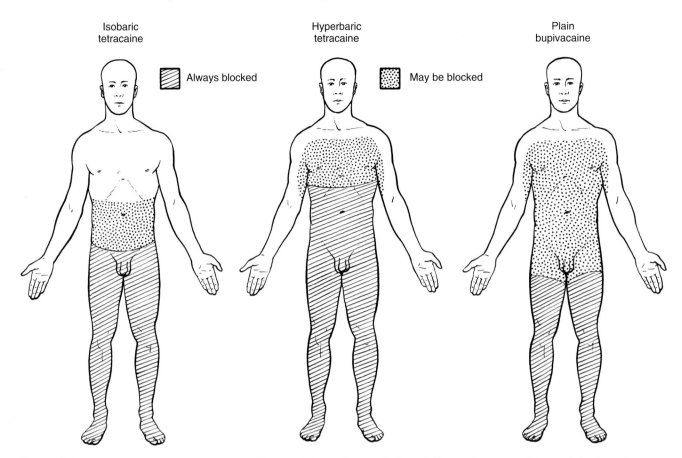

Isobaric tetracaine   Hyperbaric tetracaine   Plain bupivacaine

Always blocked   May be blocked

Figure 33–2 Extent of spinal anesthesia. The probable spread of anesthesia with three different solutions, each injected slowly at the interspace between L-3 and L-4, in the classic lateral midline position. (Modified from Wildsmith JAW, Rocco AG: Current concepts in spinal anesthesia. Reg Anesth 1985; 10: 119–124.)

longing lower abdominal anesthesia as much as epinephrine but not prolonging the time to voiding or recovery.[31]

The safety of lidocaine has been questioned. Although it has been used for many years for subarachnoid anesthesia, Lambert and colleagues[32] showed that the commercial 5% solution is toxic to amphibian nerves in an in vitro setting when applied directly to the nerve. Even diluted solutions (approximately 2%) appear to produce irreversible block.[33] This laboratory finding does not appear to correlate with the absence of clinical toxicity in standard practice, presumably be-

cause the lidocaine is diluted immediately after injection by the large volume of cerebrospinal fluid and because nerves are not exposed to toxic concentrations directly.

There has been concern about a clinical syndrome of persistent back and lower leg pain of 24- to 48-h duration after lidocaine spinal anesthesia that is referred to as "transient radicular irritation."[34] This appears to occur more frequently after lidocaine than after other local anesthetic drugs, and it may affect as many as 15% of patients, regardless of the concentration of lidocaine used.[35] This side effect is irritating but tran-

Table 33–1 Duration of Spinal Anesthesia With 50 mg of Lidocaine

		DURATION, min				
LIDOCAINE SOLUTION	**HEIGHT**	**Two-Segment Regression**	**T-12 Surgical Anesthesia**	**Motor Block**	**L-1 Regression**	**S-2 Regression**
5% plain	T-4	50	49	106	75	144
5% dextrose	T-3	65	61		109	150
5% epinephrine	T-4	56	45	108	96	156
5% fentanyl	T-3	70	75	89	125	157
1.5% dextrose	T-3	39	29		73	99
1.5% plain	T-6	56	20		104	130

Data from Chiu AA, Liu S, Carpenter RL, et al: The effects of epinephrine on lidocaine spinal anesthesia: a cross-over study. Anesth Analg 1995; 80: 735–739; Liu SL, Chiu AA, Carpenter RL, et al: Fentanyl prolongs lidocaine spinal anesthesia without prolonging recovery. Anesth Analg 1995; 80: 730–734.

sient, and it needs to be considered in the decision to use lidocaine, just as the potential for transient sore throat and muscle pain is considered in the decision to intubate an outpatient.

Procaine lasts approximately 30 min less than lidocaine for spinal anesthesia. It is commercially available in a 10% solution, but it should be diluted to a maximum concentration of 5%. It can be used as an isobaric solution when diluted with an equal volume of cerebrospinal fluid or a hypobaric solution when diluted with sterile water. Mixing with 10% glucose produces a hyperbaric solution. The dose requirement is usually 30% to 50% greater than for lidocaine. For a short-duration anesthetic, its onset of action is surprisingly slow.

Rarely, the use of bupivacaine or tetracaine without epinephrine for spinal anesthesia may be appropriate for an early morning procedure that is anticipated to last for 2 to 3 h. However, the longer duration and greater need for urinary catheterization with these drugs make them generally unsuitable for outpatient use.

For epidural anesthesia in the outpatient setting, chloroprocaine is an excellent choice because of its rapid onset and short duration. The duration of anesthesia is generally 45 to 60 min, and the block resolves in 2 to 3 h after injection. Previous problems of neurotoxicity have been remedied by the removal of 0.2% sodium bisulfite as a preservative, but the current formulation of 2-chloroprocaine with ethylenediaminetetraacetic acid as a preservative has been associated with reports of severe back pain after the use of large volumes in healthy young outpatients. This problem appears to be most frequently associated with volumes of greater than 30 mL, and the use of smaller volumes is associated with no greater incidence of back pain than with lidocaine.[36] It appears prudent to limit 2-chloroprocaine to procedures requiring 60 min or less time or for use as an additional medication after a lidocaine epidural block, when only a slightly longer period of analgesia is required.

The intermediate-acting amino-amide anesthetics lidocaine and mepivacaine appear to be safe and reliable in the usual clinical epidural doses and do not unduly prolong recovery. For initiating epidural anesthesia, 2% lidocaine or 1.5% mepivacaine is useful. The duration of block is somewhat longer with mepivacaine (Fig. 33-3). They can be used for single-injection techniques of 90 min or less. If uncertainty about duration exists, a continuous technique with either of these is still preferable to the injection of a longer-acting drug. If longer anesthesia is needed, a reinjection with 1.5% lidocaine usually gives an additional hour or more, and 2% chloroprocaine is ideal if the procedure is going to extend only an additional 30 or 45 min.

Bupivacaine and etidocaine have little use in outpatient epidural anesthesia because of their long duration of action.

Perineal Procedures

Types of Operations

Perirectal surgery is frequently performed on an outpatient basis. This includes repairs of fistula in ano and pilonidal cysts. Resections of Bartholin cysts of the vagina and other minor plastic procedures are commonly done on an outpatient basis. Some centers allow outpatients to undergo vaginal hysterectomy.

Choice of Techniques

These procedures require primarily sacral anesthesia. The use of a caudal injection in the peridural space is ideal. Caudal anesthesia, like epidural anesthesia, requires a longer time for diffusion of the anesthetic through the dural membrane, and it has a longer time to onset than spinal anesthesia. Caudal anesthesia is technically more difficult and often impractical in the presence of a pilonidal cyst (usually at the site of the intended injection) or with widespread infection in the perirectal area.

An excellent alternative is a spinal anesthetic, which can be tailored to produce primarily sacral anesthesia. A simple modification is to use a saddle block. This involves the use of a hyperbaric solution injected with the patient in the sitting position (Fig. 33-4). If that position is maintained for a minimum of 5 min, most of the anesthetic (provided that a small dose is used)

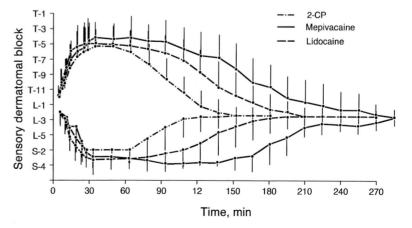

Figure 33-3 Duration of epidural anesthesia. Sensory dermatomal block level (with standard deviations) versus time after injection of 20 mL of 3% 2-chloroprocaine (2-CP), 1.5% lidocaine, or 1.5% mepivacaine with 1:200,000 epinephrine at the interspace between L-2 and L-3. The average total durations were 133, 182, and 247 min, respectively. (From Kopacz D, Mulroy MS: Chloroprocaine and lidocaine decrease hospital stay and admission rate after outpatient epidural anesthesia. Reg Anesth 1990; 15: 19–25.)

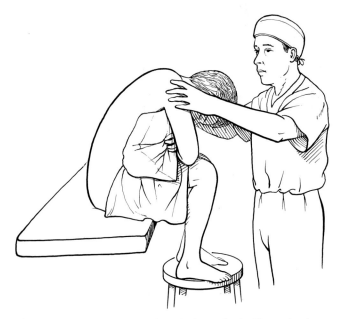

Figure 33–4 Sitting position for spinal anesthesia. The patient's legs are allowed to hang over the edge of the bed, and the feet are supported on a stool to encourage flexion of the lower spine. The shoulders are hunched forward, and the patient is encouraged to grasp firmly onto a pillow held over the abdomen. If sedation is given, an assistant should help the patient to maintain the position and should monitor the vital signs. This position is optimal for identifying the midline in obese patients or those with unusual spinal anatomy.

affects the sacral roots. This technique is ideal for patients who will be in the lithotomy position. Many of the perineal procedures are performed with the patient in the prone jackknife position. In this situation, the injection of a hypobaric spinal solution when the patient is on the operating room table is an excellent alternative (Fig. 33–5). This injection provides immediate onset of anesthesia, with no need to reposition the patient after the injection of the anesthetic. Spinal anesthetics have a rapid onset of anesthesia that allows the operation to proceed virtually as soon as the skin preparation is complete.

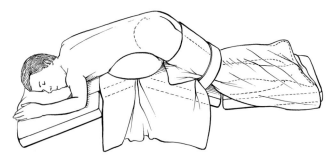

Figure 33–5 Jackknife position. Hypobaric spinal anesthesia can be administered with the patient positioned on a flexed operating table, as used for rectal procedures. The flexion point of the table should be directly under the hip joint, and the use of a pillow under the hips helps accentuate the flexion needed to identify the lumbar spinous processes. Aspiration of the spinal needle is often necessary to confirm dural puncture, because the lower cerebrospinal fluid pressure in this position does not necessarily generate a spontaneous flow of fluid.

Choice of Drugs

These operations usually are short, and the use of chloroprocaine or lidocaine for caudal block is usually sufficient. For subarachnoid saddle block, hyperbaric lidocaine is ideal. The commercial 5% solution is already hyperbaric because of the glucose it contains. The 2% solution can be made hyperbaric by the addition of glucose. For hypobaric injection, the 2% solution can be diluted with sterile water. Two milliliters of lidocaine (40 mg) with an equal volume of water produces excellent perianal anesthesia lasting an hour or more. This block does not "fix" solidly in the sacral region, and the level of anesthesia may rise by several dermatomes after the patient is returned to the supine position. These patients should have their sympathetic block assessed before the head of the bed is elevated in the recovery unit.

Lower Extremity Procedures

Types of Operations

Orthopedic procedures on the lower extremity account for a large proportion of procedures in most outpatient units. The most common are arthroscopic procedures on the knee. This approach can include simple diagnostic evaluation or a more extensive removal of a meniscus or even an anterior cruciate ligament repair. Other common lower extremity procedures are ankle and foot operations. Repairs of minor bunion defects and hammer toes are excellent candidates for outpatient surgery. Many other extensive bone deformities are treated on an outpatient basis with excellent success.

Choice of Techniques

In the leg, intravenous regional block is also possible but requires a larger volume of local anesthetic. It is ideal because of the rapid onset and high reliability, but it does not provide postoperative analgesia and does carry a slightly greater risk of systemic toxicity (because of the larger volume) than intravenous regional block of the arm.

For denser anesthesia, any combination of sciatic, femoral, lateral femoral cutaneous, and obturator nerve blocks is possible for lengthy and involved procedures. These blocks are particularly appropriate anesthesia for fractures and dislocations of the ankle or distal leg, especially for arthroscopic procedures. Unfortunately, femoral nerve block interferes with ambulation by disrupting quadriceps muscle function. A lateral femoral cutaneous nerve block frequently is the technique of choice for obtaining analgesia for taking skin for minor skin grafts. All of these peripheral nerve blocks require a longer time for onset of sufficient anesthesia than intravenous regional or spinal blocks.

An excellent alternative is block of the sciatic nerve at the knee in the popliteal fossa.[37] By including block of the distal femoral (saphenous) nerve near the tibial head, total anesthesia of the lower leg below the knee can be attained without loss of control of the extremity, although the patient requires crutches and generous padding of the foot to allow safe dismissal.

Use of the ankle block for an operation on the foot, reviewed and described by McCutcheon[38] and Schurman,[39] is especially valuable for procedures on the sole of the foot, as for cuts, foreign bodies, and plantar warts, because this is a sensitive area but tough and difficult to infiltrate locally. It also provides anesthesia for extensive foot surgery, such as bunionectomies. A midcalf tourniquet, if properly applied, is well tolerated by most patients for at least 30 min; this is helpful for most procedures on the foot.

Neuraxial blocks with spinal or epidural anesthesia are an excellent alternative for lower extremity operation. Epidural block is usually sufficient for knee surgery, and it allows the flexibility of extending the duration indefinitely for diagnostic arthroscopies. This advantage comes at the price of a slightly slower onset than spinal anesthesia. Epidural blocks also provide a segmental distribution of anesthesia that is slower in onset in the lower lumbar and sacral roots and may not be ideal for foot or ankle procedures. For procedures of predictable duration, spinal block is ideal. The rapid onset of profound anesthesia in the lumbar and sacral distribution provides immediate surgical anesthesia.

Choice of Drugs

As with the upper extremity blocks, bupivacaine in 0.375% to 0.5% concentrations provides the longest duration of analgesia, often lasting 18 to 24 h in the lower extremity. This prolonged analgesia comes at the price of prolonged sensory and motor block and a slightly increased risk of injury to the numbed extremity. As in the upper extremity, the use of mepivacaine or lidocaine appears to be a reasonable compromise. In the lower extremity, the use of a shorter-duration drug is even more appropriate, because even minimal motor block can significantly interfere with ambulation, especially if a block is performed at the level of the groin rather than at the knee or the ankle. For intravenous regional anesthesia, 0.5% lidocaine without additives appears to be the most efficacious solution. A quantity of 50 mL is appropriate for the upper extremity, but 100 mL are usually required for intravenous regional anesthesia of the lower extremity.

For epidural and spinal anesthesia, the considerations mentioned for lower abdominal surgery apply. For an epidural block, slightly higher doses may be required to produce sacral spread, with a resultant higher thoracic spread. Spinal anesthesia may require less drug. Lidocaine in a 50-mg dose is often sufficient (Table 33–2).

General Considerations for Outpatient Anesthesia

Modifications of Premedication

Most outpatients are more nervous than they admit, and the attitude of the medical personnel is of enor-

Table 33–2 Anesthetic Doses for Spinal Anesthesia

ANESTHETIC	DOSE, mg	
	Lower Extremity	Abdominal Area
Procaine	50–75	75–100
Lidocaine	40–50	60–75
Bupivacaine	4–6	6–8

mous psychologic importance in relieving this anxiety. Some patients benefit from a pharmacologic sedative; however, this may lead to lack of cooperation, and the result is a patient who requires prolonged supervision and may be unfit to go home. Although rapport, gentleness, and skill in performing the block frequently can make premedication unnecessary, preoperative sedation for regional anesthesia may be appropriate.

Midazolam (1 to 2 mg) may be given orally, intramuscularly, or (most frequently) intravenously. The amnestic effect of the benzodiazepines is an excellent asset to regional anesthesia, often eliminating the recall of sometimes unpleasant needle insertions or paresthesias. The sedative-amnestic effect can limit its usefulness if the patient becomes confused and can no longer cooperate with a block technique. Heavy sedation can also prolong time to dismissal, and moderate doses of midazolam are recommended, usually not to exceed 5 mg in a healthy adult.[40] It is important to avoid the temptation to titrate this drug to objective signs of sedation, such as slurred speech or somnolence. The sedative and amnestic effects are present at levels associated with apparent full consciousness,[41] and the use of higher doses merely prolongs recovery. The duration of midazolam sedation is generally 30 min, but higher doses and their use for "conscious sedation" delay dismissal. The availability of flumazenil is not a justification for excessive doses.

For uncomfortable procedures, which probably include all needle insertions, sedation and amnesia are not enough. Analgesia should be provided. The short-acting opioid fentanyl, in 50- to 100-μg doses, is ideal for outpatient use because it attenuates patient discomfort associated with the performance of the blocks or eliciting of a paresthesia, but it does not abolish patient cooperation. Excessive doses must be avoided because of the risk of respiratory depression and the potential for increased nausea and vomiting.[40] The short-acting analgesics alfentanil and remifentanil may be appealing, but their duration is too brief to be useful for the performance of most blocks.

If further sedation is needed intraoperatively, small quantities of these drugs may be titrated to effect. An alternative is the intravenous administration of propofol in doses of 25 to 50 μg/kg per min. At this infusion rate, sedation is provided with minimal hangover and delay of recovery. Methohexital is another alternative that involves lower cost but may require longer recovery and produce an unwanted excitement or "antianalgesic" phase.[42]

Table 33–3 Bicarbonate Doses for Local Anesthetic Solutions

ANESTHETIC	BICARBONATE, mEq
Chloroprocaine	1 per 30 mL of local anesthetic
Lidocaine	1 per 10 mL of local anesthetic
Bupivacaine	0.1 per 10 mL of local anesthetic

Time Considerations

The major hesitation about using regional techniques in the outpatient setting is the additional time required to perform the blocks. Several options can decrease the delay in initiating regional techniques. The foremost is to perform the block in an area separate from the operating room, as in an induction room or a corner of the postanesthesia care unit, where the technique may be performed while the nursing and housekeeping staff are preparing the operating room. This usually allows the additional 10 to 15 min needed for adequate onset of local anesthetics used with most procedures. If the blocks are performed in the operating room, the surgeons must be advised that there will be an inevitable delay, and they must not be allowed to start the surgical procedure until adequate anesthesia is achieved. In this situation, the addition of sodium bicarbonate to local anesthetic solution can often decrease time to onset of adequate anesthesia by 3 to 5 min (Table 33–3).[43–45]

The choice of regional techniques that have rapid onset, such as intravenous regional and spinal anesthesia, is an excellent decision in this situation. Additional personnel can allow the anesthesiologist to start a block earlier, and if there are enough staff members to allow an assistant to take a patient to the recovery room while a block is initiated on the next patient, turnover time is greatly decreased. Another alternative is to transfer the care of the patient to an operating room nurse toward the end of the procedure if minimal intraoperative sedation has been given. This works well with retrobulbar and upper extremity blocks, when the patient is stable and alert as the dressing is being applied.

Another major consideration is the education of the surgeon regarding the advantages of regional techniques. Allen and coworkers[13] showed that it did take 18 min longer to perform axillary blocks than to perform general anesthesia with propofol for hand surgery patients. Nevertheless, with the use of an induction room, they did not delay the turnover of the surgical suite and were able to show significant advantages in postoperative recovery. When surgeons and administrators become aware of these advantages, they will support the occasional short delays necessitated by the performance of regional techniques.

Dismissal Criteria

Before dismissal, patients should recover sufficiently from anesthesia to approach their preoperative physical and mental status. This does not imply full recovery, particularly if a peripheral block technique has been used, because the block is likely to continue to be effective. If the patients are properly instructed, they can usually be sent home during this period. The risk of a delayed systemic toxic reaction after 30 min decreases rapidly and is remote after 1 h. Careful instruction must be given to avoid injury, and the patients must be provided with an appropriate sling or protection for the numb extremity or anesthetized area. If a sympathetic block remains, elevation of the vasodilated extremity is especially useful.

Those who have received epidural or spinal block must have full recovery of motor function before dismissal. If all sensory anesthesia has regressed, particularly with a full return of perineal sensation, then sympathetic block and orthostatic hypotension should not be a problem on ambulation.[46] Urinary retention is not a frequent problem, but it can occur after neuraxial blocks, especially in older men and in operations with groin or perineal incisions. The frequency of retention is related to the duration of the local anesthetic agent,[11, 47] and short-duration drugs should be chosen preferentially for neuraxial blocks. The addition of epinephrine increases the potential for urinary retention.[30] With drugs such as lidocaine, the incidence of retention has even been reported as lower than with general anesthesia.[48] Although many outpatient units require voiding before dismissal, this is often awkward and stressful for the young outpatient. The bladder can be assessed by physical examination or ultrasound, and simple catheter drainage can be performed if distension is detected. After this (or if no distension is present), most patients can be dismissed to their homes with instructions to return to the emergency department if problems develop later.

In addition to resolution of the block, patients must also meet standard criteria for mental alertness, analgesia, and ability to tolerate oral fluids (Table 33–4). Because most of the patients who have had regional block anesthesia have had minimal premedication or sedation, they spend a shorter time in the postoperative recovery unit than those who have had general anesthesia. Studies[49] conducted in an ambulatory surgery unit comparing the recovery time and complications after general anesthesia and epidural anesthesia when used for outpatient laparoscopies demonstrated a significant advantage for epidural anesthesia.

The requirements of adequate analgesia and absence of nausea are not usually problems when regional

Table 33–4 Outpatient Surgery Dismissal Criteria

CRITERION	COMMENT
Be alert	Better with regional techniques, provided heavy sedation avoided
Ambulate	More rapid with regional anesthesia for the extremities
Analgesic	Ideal with peripheral nerve blocks
Eat	Earlier with regional
Void	Rare problem

techniques have been used. When the effects of the regional block wear off, the patient may need an analgesic, which should be prescribed as part of the postoperative care. An effective analgesic for operations on extremities is provided by elevation and immobilization. Oral administration of opioid analgesics is often associated with the onset of nausea in the postanesthesia care unit and should be avoided if possible. The use of alternative analgesics, such as nonsteroidal anti-inflammatory drugs like ketorolac, has been shown to decrease opioid requirements without producing nausea or respiratory depression. Ketorolac has been effective in decreasing opioid requirements in the outpatient setting, and it may be sufficient by itself to provide analgesia for minor surgical procedures. It is particularly effective in orthopedic and urologic procedures, although contraindicated in the presence of significant coagulopathy or renal disease. Other nonsteroidal anti-inflammatory preparations given orally are equally effective (if oral therapy is tolerated) and are usually less expensive.

Nausea is a frequent side effect of orally administered opioid analgesics. Antihistamines such as diphenhydramine or major tranquilizers such as droperidol may be effective treatments, but they may also produce somnolence and delay dismissal. Droperidol has been associated with postoperative dysphoria.[8] Metoclopramide may be a more desirable first-line antiemetic. Serotonin antagonists such as ondansetron are considerably more expensive, but they may be cost effective in the clinical setting of severe nausea or persistent emesis.

The use of local infiltration with local anesthetics is another excellent alternative. A field block or local infiltration of the wound at the termination of the operation can be accomplished with a long-acting local anesthetic drug, which allows a prolonged period of postoperative analgesia while the patient is recovering. This is especially effective in pediatric patients. Instillation of bupivacaine into knee joints after arthroscopy also decreases opioid requirements.[50] The use of morphine in joints may be helpful in situations in which inflammation is present,[51] but the reports of its effectiveness remain inconclusive.[52]

In most institutions in which procedures are being performed on outpatients, the patients are provided with a form that warns of possible sequelae, a brief instruction sheet on postoperative care, appointments with the responsible physician, and advice about food or drink. The form emphasizes the need for patients to be accompanied by a responsible adult to and from the surgical center and at home for the first 24 h. Other relevant information can also be given at the same time, including warnings about possible complications and the availability of a 24-h telephone contact. For patients receiving spinal blocks, a description of the possibility of post-dural puncture headache should be provided and a follow-up at 48 or 72 h should be considered because of the potential for late onset of this complication.

Summary

Regional techniques offer significant advantages to outpatients, especially in providing a high degree of alertness and analgesia at the time of dismissal. The decreased incidence of nausea and emesis also speeds dismissal and increases patient satisfaction, and the nursing care in the postanesthesia care unit is generally decreased. These advantages require some modifications in the choice of techniques, drugs, and sedation. The common complaint of surgical delay in a rapid-turnover outpatient unit can be decreased by these appropriate choices.

Regional techniques deserve wider application in outpatient surgery, and the following concepts can ease the integration of regional anesthesia into your outpatient practice. First, for all outpatients, the anesthesiologist should avoid long-acting or heavy doses of sedation. They negate all of the advantages of rapid recovery and decreased emesis that regional anesthesia otherwise provides. Second, for epidural and subarachnoid blocks, the shortest-acting local anesthetic should be used to provide rapid dismissal. The surgeon should be encouraged to supplement with infiltration of the wound using long-acting local anesthetics to provide postoperative analgesia. Third, surgeons will always be unhappy about the additional time required to perform regional techniques. This can be circumvented by identifying for them the advantages of rapid dismissal and lower rate of side effects, as well as the choice of rapid-onset techniques (spinal, intravenous regional) and rapid-acting drugs. The addition of bicarbonate to the local anesthetic usually speeds onset by 3 to 5 min. Ideally, the blocks are performed in an area other than the operating room to minimize the delay in case turnover.

References

1. Meridy HW: Criteria for selection of ambulatory surgical patients and guidelines for anesthetic management: a retrospective study of 1553 cases. Anesth Analg 1982; 61: 921–926.
2. White PF, Shafer A: Nausea and vomiting: causes and prophylaxis. Semin Anesth 1987; 6: 300–308.
3. Gold BS, Kitz DS, Lecky JH, et al: Unanticipated admission to the hospital following ambulatory surgery. JAMA 1989; 262: 3008–3010.
4. Orkin F: What do patients want? Preferences for immediate postoperative recovery. (Abstract.) Anesth Analg 1992; 74: S225.
5. Watcha MF, White PF: Postoperative nausea and vomiting. Its etiology, treatment, and prevention. Anesthesiology 1992; 77: 162–184.
6. Campbell WI: Analgesic side effects and minor surgery: which analgesic for minor and day-case surgery? Br J Anaesth 1990; 64: 617–620.
7. Ghouri AF, Bodner M, White PF: Recovery profile after desflurane-nitrous oxide versus isoflurane-nitrous oxide in outpatients. Anesthesiology 1991; 74: 419–424.
8. Melnick B, Sawyer R, Karambelkar D, et al: Delayed side effects of droperidol after ambulatory general anesthesia. Anesth Analg 1989; 69: 748–751.
9. Van Hemelrijck J, Smith I, White PF: Use of desflurane for outpatient anesthesia. A comparison with propofol and nitrous oxide. Anesthesiology 1991; 75: 197–203.
10. Davis WJ, Lennon RL, Wedel DJ: Brachial plexus anesthesia for outpatient surgical procedures on an upper extremity. Mayo Clin Proc 1991; 66: 470–473.
11. Ryan JA Jr, Adye BA, Jolly PC, et al: Outpatient inguinal herniorrhaphy with both regional and local anesthesia. Am J Surg 1984; 148: 313–316.
12. Patel NJ, Flashburg MH, Paskin S, et al: A regional anesthetic

technique compared to general anesthesia for outpatient knee arthroscopy. Anesth Analg 1986; 65: 185–187.

13. Allen HW, Mulroy MF, Fundis K, et al: Regional versus propofol general anesthesia for outpatient hand surgery. (Abstract.) Anesthesiology 1993; 79: A1.

14. Brown AR, Weiss R, Greenberg C, et al: Interscalene block for shoulder arthroscopy: comparison with general anesthesia. Arthroscopy 1993; 9: 295–300.

15. Neal JM, Deck JJ, Lewis MA, et al: A double-blind comparison of epidural 2-chloroprocaine vs. lidocaine for outpatient knee arthroscopy. (Abstract.) Anesthesiology 1993; 79: A12.

16. Doze VA, Westphal LM, White PF: Comparison of propofol with methohexital for outpatient anesthesia. Anesth Analg 1986; 65: 1189–1195.

17. White PF: Studies of desflurane in outpatient anesthesia. Anesth Analg 1992; 75: S47–S54.

18. Wong DH: Regional anaesthesia for intraocular surgery. Can J Anaesth 1993; 40: 635–657.

19. Grice SC, Morell RC, Balestrieri FJ, et al: Intravenous regional anesthesia: evaluation and prevention of leakage under the tourniquet. Anesthesiology 1986; 65: 316–320.

20. Buettner J, Wresch KP, Klose R: Postdural puncture headache: comparison of 25-gauge Whitacre and Quincke needles. Reg Anesth 1993; 18: 166–169.

21. Carbaat PA, van Crevel H: Lumbar puncture headache: controlled study on the preventive effect of 24 hours' bed rest. Lancet 1981; 2: 1133–1135.

22. Thornberry EA, Thomas TA: Posture and post-spinal headache. A controlled trial in 80 obstetric patients. Br J Anaesth 1988; 60: 195–197.

23. Jones RJ: The role of recumbency in the prevention and treatment of postspinal headache. Anesth Analg 1974; 53: 788–796.

24. Mulroy MF: Spinal headaches: management and avoidance. In Brown DL (ed): Problems in Anesthesia. Regional Anesthesia at the Virginia Mason Medical Center: A Clinical Perspective, vol 1, pp 602–611. Philadelphia, JB Lippincott, 1987.

25. Bridenbaugh LD, Soderstrom RM: Lumbar epidural block anesthesia for outpatient laparoscopy. J Reprod Med 1979; 23: 85–86.

26. Kopacz D, Mulroy MS: Chloroprocaine and lidocaine decrease hospital stay and admission rate after outpatient epidural anesthesia. Reg Anesth 1990; 15: 19–25.

27. Liu S, Pollock JE, Mulroy MF, et al: Comparison of 5%, 1.5% with dextrose, and 1.5% dextrose free lidocaine solutions for spinal anesthesia in human volunteers. Anesth Analg 1995; 81: 697–702.

28. Moore DC, Chadwick HS, Ready LB: Epinephrine prolongs lidocaine spinal: pain in the operative site the most accurate method of determining local anesthetic duration. Anesthesiology 1987; 67: 416–418.

29. Chambers WA, Littlewood DG, Logan MR, et al: Effect of added epinephrine on spinal anesthesia with lidocaine. Anesth Analg 1981; 60: 417–420.

30. Chiu AA, Liu S, Carpenter RL, et al: The effects of epinephrine on lidocaine spinal anesthesia: a cross-over study. Anesth Analg 1995; 80: 735–739.

31. Liu SL, Chiu AA, Carpenter RL, et al: Fentanyl prolongs lidocaine spinal anesthesia without prolonging recovery. Anesth Analg 1995; 80: 730–734.

32. Lambert LA, Lambert DH, Strichartz GR: Irreversible conduction block in isolated nerve by high concentrations of local anesthetics. Anesthesiology 1994; 80: 1082–1093.

33. Bainton CR, Strichartz GR: Concentration dependence of lidocaine-induced irreversible conduction loss in frog nerve. Anesthesiology 1994; 81: 657–667.

34. Schneider M, Ettlin T, Kaufmann M, et al: Transient neurologic toxicity after hyperbaric subarachnoid anesthesia with 5% lidocaine. Anesth Analg 1993; 76: 1154–1157.

35. Pollock JE, Mulroy MF, Stephenson C: Spinal anesthetics and the incidence of transient radicular irritation. (Abstract.) Anesthesiology 1994; 81: A1029.

36. Stevens RA, Urmey WF, Urquhart BL, et al: Back pain after epidural anesthesia with chloroprocaine. Anesthesiology 1993; 78: 492–497.

37. Rorie DK, Byer DE, Nelson DO, et al: Assessment of block of the sciatic nerve in the popliteal fossa. Anesth Analg 1980; 59: 371–376.

38. McCutcheon R: Regional anaesthesia for the foot. Can Anaesth Soc J 1965; 12: 465–474.

39. Schurman DJ: Ankle-block anesthesia for foot surgery. Anesthesiology 1976; 44: 348–352.

40. Shafer A, White PF, Urquhart ML, et al: Outpatient premedication: use of midazolam and opioid analgesics. Anesthesiology 1989; 71: 495–501.

41. Philip BK: Hazards of amnesia after midazolam in ambulatory surgical patients. (Letter to the editor.) Anesth Analg 1987; 66: 97–98.

42. White PF: Continuous infusions of thiopental, methohexital or etomidate as adjuvants to nitrous oxide for outpatient anesthesia. (Abstract.) Anesth Analg 1984; 63: 282.

43. DiFazio CA, Carron H, Grosslight KR, et al: Comparison of pH-adjusted lidocaine solutions for epidural anesthesia. Anesth Analg 1986; 65: 760–764.

44. Hilgier M: Alkalinization of bupivacaine for brachial plexus block. Reg Anesth 1985; 10: 59–61.

45. McMorland GH, Douglas MJ, Jeffery WK, et al: Effect of pH-adjustment of bupivacaine on onset and duration of epidural analgesia in parturients. Can Anaesth Soc J 1986; 33: 537–541.

46. Pflug AE, Aasheim GM, Foster C: Sequence of return of neurological function and criteria for safe ambulation following subarachnoid block (spinal anaesthetic). Can Anaesth Soc J 1978; 25: 133–139.

47. Bridenbaugh LD: Catheterization after long- and short-acting local anesthetics for continuous caudal block for vaginal delivery. Anesthesiology 1977; 46: 357–359.

48. Petros JG, Rimm EB, Robillard RJ, et al: Factors influencing postoperative urinary retention in patients undergoing elective inguinal herniorrhaphy. Am J Surg 1991; 161: 431–433.

49. Mulroy M, Bridenbaugh LD: Regional anesthetic techniques for outpatient surgery. Int Anesthesiol Clin 1982; 20: 71–80.

50. Smith I, Van Hemelrijck J, White PF, et al: Effects of local anesthesia on recovery after outpatient arthroscopy. Anesth Analg 1991; 73: 536–539.

51. Khoury GF, Chen AC, Garland DE, et al: Intraarticular morphine, bupivacaine, and morphine/bupivacaine for pain control after knee videoarthroscopy. Anesthesiology 1992; 77: 263–266.

52. Heard SO, Edwards WT, Ferrari D, et al: Analgesic effect of intraarticular bupivacaine or morphine after arthroscopic knee surgery: a randomized, prospective, double-blind study. Anesth Analg 1992; 74: 822–826.

CHAPTER 34

Analgesia During Labor and Delivery

Robert D. Vincent, Jr., M.D., David H. Chestnut, M.D.

"Then the Lord God said to the woman, 'Why have you done this?' The woman said, 'The serpent deceived me and I ate.' . . . To the woman He said: 'I will make great your distress in childbearing; in pain shall you bring forth children.' "
—Genesis 3:13, 16

The primary focus of this chapter is the application of regional anesthetic techniques to provide analgesia during labor and delivery. We emphasize the uses and controversies of neuraxial (i.e., epidural, spinal) blocks and review the provision of intrapartum analgesia for women with preeclampsia or obesity. We also discuss alternative techniques for treating the pain of parturition.

Pain During Parturition

There is little doubt that childbirth rates among the most intense measurable sources of pain. For example, Melzack[1] reported that the severity of labor pain ex-

ceeded that of most pain syndromes treated in a population of pain clinic patients (Fig. 34–1). Without analgesia, at least two thirds of women characterize their pain intensity as distressing, horrible, or excruciating during the late first stage of labor.[2]

Pain during labor is multifactorial in origin and varies in intensity and in location as labor progresses in a given patient. Dilation of the cervix and lower uterine segment and contraction of the body of the uterus are responsible for much of the pain during early labor.[3] These noxious impulses are transmitted through the 11th and 12th spinal nerves, resulting in pain over the lower abdominal wall, lower back, and upper sacrum (Figs. 34–2 and 34–3). As the intensity of uterine contractions increases, pain may spread cephalad to the 10th thoracic dermatome and caudad to the first and second lumbar dermatomes (Fig. 34–4).

The pain during this late first stage of labor is a composite of at least three different kinds of pain, which may be expressed in different degrees by each patient.[4] First, almost all laboring women experience lower abdominal pain during uterine contractions. This

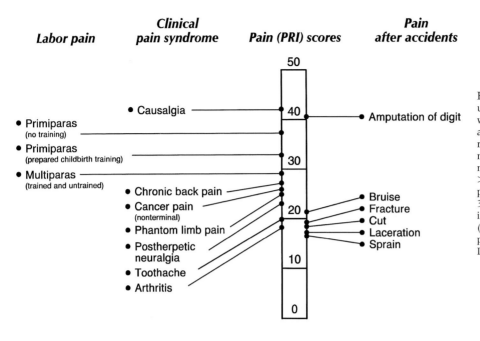

Figure 34–1 Comparison of pain scores using the McGill Pain Questionnaire, with responses from women during labor and from a population of emergency room patients. Scoring: 2 to 11, very mild pain; 12 to 21, mild pain; 22 to 31, moderate pain; 32 to 41, severe pain; >41, intolerable pain. Among primiparas, 30% had moderate pain, 38% had severe pain, and 23% had intolerable pain. PRI, pain rating index. (Modified from Melzack R: The myth of painless childbirth [The John J. Bonica Lecture]. Pain 1984; 19: 321–337.)

pain is usually intermittent and is often described as sharp, cramping, and pulling (Table 34–1). Second, nearly three fourths of laboring women also complain of intermittent back pain during contractions.[4, 5] Adjectives commonly used to describe intermittent back pain include gnawing, hot, and dull. Third, among women with intermittent back pain during contractions, almost one half also experience continuous back pain between contractions.[5] This pain is separate and qualitatively distinct from the intermittent back pain occurring only during contractions. It is especially dis-

tressing because it does not allow the patient to have an interlude in which to summon her internal resources for the next uterine contraction.[5] Possible sources of the continuous back pain of labor include traction and pressure on the adnexa uteri and parietal peritoneum and the structures they envelop; pressure and stretch on the bladder, urethra, or rectum; pressure on one or more roots of the lumbosacral plexus; and reflex skeletal muscle spasm.[3]

During the second stage of labor, the pain of parturition is a product of distension of the vagina, vulva, and perineum (Fig. 34–5). These stimuli are transmitted through the second, third, and fourth sacral nerves and result in pain over the perineal area.

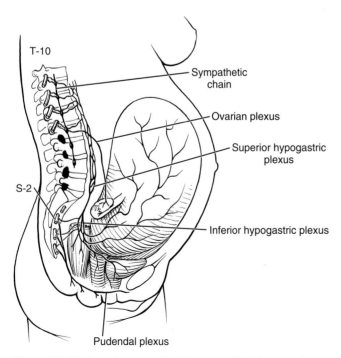

Figure 34–2 Pain pathways during labor. (Modified from Bonica JJ: Principles and Practice of Obstetric Analgesia and Anesthesia, vol 1, p 110. Philadelphia, FA Davis, 1967.)

Table 34–1 Sensory Terms Selected by Laboring Women to Describe Each Source of Labor Pain and Percentages of Women Who Chose Them

SENSORY TERM	LABORING WOMEN, %		
	Front Contractions	Back Contractions	Back Continuous
Sharp	41		
Gnawing		37	
Cramping	48		
Pressing			40
Pulling	43		40
Hot		37	33
Stinging			40
Dull		42	
Aching			33
Heavy			40
Taut	59	42	33

All patients experienced lower abdominal pain during contractions. Seventy-four percent also experienced low-back pain during labor. In 44% of these women, continuous back pain was rated more severe than was contraction back pain.

Table includes only percentages for descriptors selected by at least 33% of patients.

Data from Melzack R, Schaffelberg D: Low-back pain during labor. Am J Obstet Gynecol 1987; 156: 901–905.

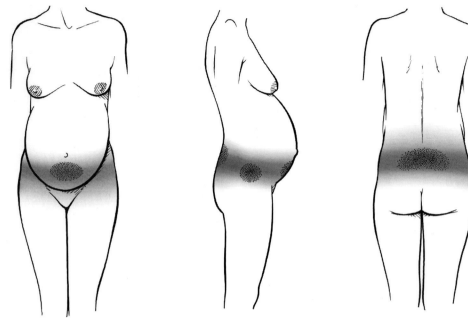

Figure 34–3 Area of reference of pain during the first stage of labor. The density of stippling and shading indicates the intensity of pain. (Modified from Bonica JJ: Principles and Practice of Obstetric Analgesia and Anesthesia, vol 1, p 108. Philadelphia, FA Davis, 1967.)

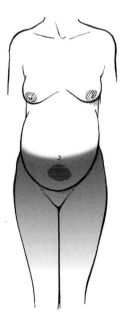
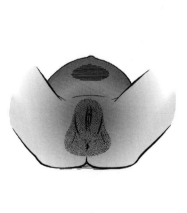
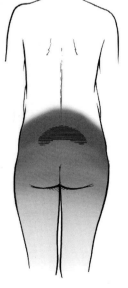

Figure 34–4 Area of reference of pain during the late first stage and early second stage of labor. The density of stippling and shading indicates the intensity of pain. (Modified from Bonica JJ: Principles and Practice of Obstetric Analgesia and Anesthesia, vol 1, p 109. Philadelphia, FA Davis, 1967.)

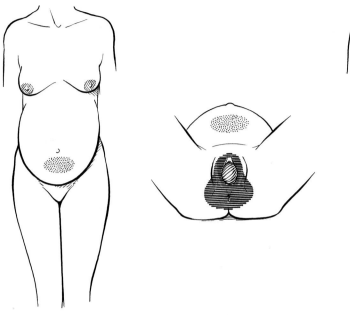

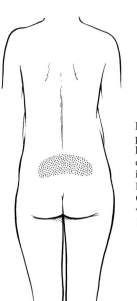

Figure 34–5 Area of reference of pain during the late second stage of labor and actual delivery. The density of stippling and shading indicates the intensity of pain. (Modified from Bonica JJ: Principles and Practice of Obstetric Analgesia and Anesthesia, vol 1, p 109. Philadelphia, FA Davis, 1967.)

Although the previous description may be typical for the average laboring patient, there are variations in the intensity and location of pain from one patient to another. Melzack and colleagues[6] recorded the intensity and spatial distribution of pain in six women at two or more different times during the first stage of labor. Some women experienced widespread pain over the abdomen, back, and perineum, but others had pain in limited, discrete areas (Fig. 34–6). Several variables may help to predict which parturients are more likely to experience severe pain during childbirth. Nulliparity, lower socioeconomic status, younger maternal age, history of low-back pain during menstruation, increased maternal or fetal weight, and intravenous administration of oxytocin are all associated with increased pain during labor and delivery.[2, 4, 6] Labor pain was reduced in women who attended prepared childbirth classes and in those who performed aerobic-conditioning exercises during pregnancy.[6–8]

Neuraxial Anesthesia Techniques

Epidural Analgesia

Epidural injection of a dilute solution of local anesthetic, with or without an opioid, is the most effective method of providing analgesia during labor and delivery. It is the standard with which all new analgesic modalities should be compared. Much of the clinical

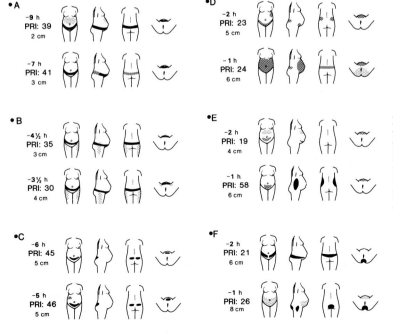

Figure 34–6 A to F, Spatial distribution of pain in six women at various times before delivery, with pain rating index (PRI) scores and the amount of cervical dilation. Pain intensity: dots, mild; cross-hatching, moderate; and solid areas, severe. (Reprinted from Melzack R, Kinch RA, Dobkin P, et al: Severity of labour pain: influence of physical as well as psychologic variables. Can Med Assoc J 1984; 130: 579–584.)

research in obstetric anesthesia has been directed at fine tuning rather than replacing continuous epidural techniques. No other form of analgesia is available that combines the reliability, safety, and flexibility of continuous epidural analgesia during childbirth.

Preliminary Considerations

Other than uncontrolled maternal hemorrhage, significant coagulopathy, and patient refusal, there are few absolute contraindications to epidural analgesia during labor. There are hypothetical risks to extensive sympathetic block in women with primary pulmonary hypertension and specific cardiac diseases (e.g., Eisenmenger syndrome, aortic stenosis). It is unclear whether segmental lower thoracic epidural analgesia during labor exposes these women to unnecessary risk. A difficult airway or obesity should not discourage the anesthesiologist from initiating epidural analgesia during labor, and a nonreassuring fetal heart rate pattern is not a contraindication to epidural analgesia. In these circumstances, the anesthesiologist should proceed expeditiously, although with caution, after consultation with the obstetrician. Prior placement of a functioning epidural catheter may prove useful if urgent forceps or cesarean delivery is required because of fetal distress.

We do not insist on any screening laboratory tests before instituting an epidural block in healthy parturients during labor. Instead, specific tests (e.g., platelet count, fibrinogen, prothrombin time, partial thromboplastin time) are indicated only if the clinical history or physical examination reveals abnormalities, such as placental abruption, immunologic thrombocytopenic purpura, preeclampsia, bruising, and bleeding from venipuncture sites. There is no evidence that a carefully administered epidural anesthetic is associated with increased maternal or fetal risk in a parturient with normovolemic anemia, and we do not routinely check the maternal venous hemoglobin concentration before proceeding with epidural analgesia.

After the anesthesiologist has evaluated the patient and she consents to receive epidural analgesia, two criteria must be met before initiating the block.[9] First, an obstetrician or other qualified individual must have examined the patient. Second, a physician with hospital privileges in obstetrics must have evaluated the progress of labor and the status of the mother and fetus. This physician must be readily available to manage any obstetric complications that may arise during the epidural block.

Test Dose and Induction of Epidural Analgesia

Most fetuses tolerate small decreases in maternal blood pressure, which often coincide with the induction of epidural analgesia. This may occur in part because an epidural block decreases maternal catecholamine concentrations during labor.[10]

More severe hypotension results in a significant decrease in uterine blood flow, which could jeopardize a fetus with marginal reserve.[11] Intravenous hydration with a non–dextrose-containing electrolyte solution should precede the induction of epidural analgesia in most circumstances. Collins and coworkers[12] observed that prehydration with 1 L of Hartmann's (lactated Ringer's) solution 10 to 15 min before epidural block decreased the incidence of maternal hypotension from 28% to 2% and the occurrence of abnormal fetal heart rate tracings from 34% to 12%. We usually administer at least 500 mL of lactated Ringer's solution just before injecting a local anesthetic epidurally. Possible exceptions to this practice are circumstances in which there is an urgent need to prevent unwanted premature maternal expulsive efforts, such as frank breech presentation in a woman who presents in advanced labor with planned vaginal delivery. In this situation, the anesthesiologist should be prepared to treat decreases in maternal blood pressure aggressively with intravenously administered ephedrine.

The anesthesiologist should always consider the initial dose of local anesthetic administered through an epidural needle or catheter to be a test for detection of occult subarachnoid or intravenous placement. Testing of an epidural catheter in a laboring patient is confounded by pain-induced fluctuations in maternal heart rate during uterine contractions and the potential deleterious effect of intravenously administered catecholamines on uterine blood flow.[13–15] Although 10 to 15 μg of epinephrine given intravenously provide a sensitive marker for detecting intravenous injection, the α-adrenergic effects of epinephrine may cause a transient decrease in uterine blood flow.[15] Fortunately, most healthy fetuses with ample reserve easily tolerate a transient, modest reduction in uterine blood flow.[16, 17] However, Leighton and colleagues[13] observed that the fetuses of two laboring women given 15 μg of epinephrine intravenously developed evidence of distress that lasted 10 to 12 min. An alternative method of detecting intravascular injection (e.g., air, local anesthetic only) may be considered in the rare situations in which even a small decrease in blood flow could produce devastating consequences.[18, 19]

At the University of Iowa Hospitals and Clinics, we typically inject an epidural test dose of 3 mL of 1.5% lidocaine with epinephrine (5 μg/mL) after gentle aspiration of the catheter. This method allows us to test for intravenous and subarachnoid administration with a single injection. An abrupt increase in maternal heart rate signals the possibility of intravascular catheter placement. A marked increase in blood pressure may also indicate intravenous injection, because a few patients respond to intravenous injection of epinephrine by developing hypertension and bradycardia.[13, 17]

The sensitivity and specificity of the test dose may be improved by delaying injection until immediately after a uterine contraction and by observing the patient for symptoms indicative of intravascular administration (e.g., palpitations, lightheadedness, dizziness). Rapid onset of a sacral block (i.e., S-2 sensory block within 2 min) should alert the physician to the possibility of unintentional intrathecal injection (Fig. 34–7).[20]

Some anesthesiologists prefer to induce epidural analgesia through the needle and to give subsequent doses through the epidural catheter. Under these con-

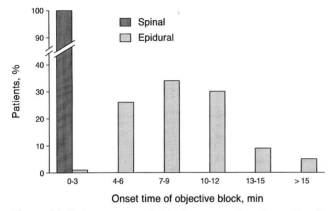

Figure 34–7 Time to onset of objective sensory loss after epidural and spinal administration of 30 to 45 mg of hyperbaric lidocaine solution. After subarachnoid injection, objective sensory block developed in all patients by 2 min; the mean time to sensory block at S-2 was 1.45 min. In contrast, only one patient demonstrated objective sensory loss after epidural injection within 4 min. This patient had sensory loss at the L-2 dermatome 3 min after injection. (Data from Abraham RA, Harris AP, Maxwell LG, et al: The efficacy of 1.5% lidocaine with 7.5% dextrose and epinephrine as an epidural test dose for obstetrics. Anesthesiology 1986; 64: 116–119.)

ditions, a test dose should be given through the catheter even if the result of an earlier test dose given through the needle was negative.

The dose of local anesthetic necessary to establish effective analgesia for labor depends on the intensity and location of the patient's pain. These factors depend on the variables discussed earlier, the amount of cervical dilation, and the position of the fetal head at the time epidural analgesia is requested. Typically, 25 to 30 mg of bupivacaine produce effective analgesia during the first stage of labor.[21–23] The volume of the epidural injectant also appears to play a significant role in producing satisfactory anesthesia. For example, 12 mL of 0.25% bupivacaine produced analgesia superior to that resulting from 6 mL of 0.5% bupivacaine.[21] Smaller quantities of bupivacaine may be required to achieve analgesia if several milliliters of 1.5% lidocaine were given earlier as a test dose. We usually inject an initial bolus of 5 mL of 0.25% bupivacaine 3 to 5 min after a negative response to a test dose. If pain relief is inadequate after several minutes, additional aliquots (not exceeding 5 mL each) of 0.25% bupivacaine are titrated to achieve satisfactory analgesia. We prefer to remain at the patient's bedside until the hemodynamic changes and the cephalad spread of anesthetic level have stabilized after each epidural bolus of local anesthetic.

Maintenance of Epidural Analgesia During Labor

Continuous infusions of local anesthetic solutions, with or without opioids, have largely replaced intermittent epidural bolus injection techniques for maintenance of epidural analgesia during labor. Others[23–28] have reported that 0.125% bupivacaine (10–14 mL/h) provides effective labor analgesia without causing a high incidence of profound motor block. In addition to

facilitating the efforts of the anesthesiologist, who must manage epidural analgesia in several women simultaneously, this technique minimizes fluctuations in sensory and motor block associated with intermittent top-up injections of local anesthetic. If the epidural catheter migrates into a vein, the risk of local anesthetic systemic toxicity from continuous intravenous infusion of analgesic doses of bupivacaine is minimal.

Patient-controlled epidural analgesia (PCEA) is an alternative to conventional epidural infusion techniques for maintenance of labor analgesia. Some investigators[29, 30] have reported that patient-controlled dosing decreased the hourly bupivacaine consumption without impairing the quality of analgesia. A typical regimen includes 3- to 4-mL boluses of 0.125% bupivacaine triggered by a patient-activated demand button, with intervening lockout periods of 10 to 20 min. One modification to pure PCEA is to include the use of a continuous background infusion of bupivacaine at about 4 to 6 mL/h; however, there are no data to show that this improves the overall quality of analgesia.[23]

A potential benefit of PCEA is the decreased necessity for the anesthesiologist to administer periodic supplemental boluses of local anesthetic, which are often necessary with conventional continuous-infusion techniques. Viscomi and Eisenach[31] reported that the incidence of supplemental injections was halved by the use of PCEA compared with continuous-infusion administration (36% versus 71%). PCEA may prove useful in busy obstetric units or in circumstances in which personnel is limited. Another advantage of PCEA is that it avoids unnecessary analgesia in women who prefer to preserve some sensation of their uterine contractions.[29] It is difficult to recommend PCEA for universal use, because the benefits are modest, it requires an expensive device, and it introduces another source of failure (pump malfunction due to overpressure occurred in almost one fourth of patients in one study).[30]

The American Society of Anesthesiologists recommended[9] that the parturient's vital signs and the fetal heart rate be monitored and documented by a qualified individual during induction and maintenance of epidural analgesia. We determine the blood pressure at 2- to 3-min intervals during induction of epidural analgesia, and subsequently, we monitor the maternal vital signs at 15-min intervals. We monitor the fetal heart rate continuously during induction and maintenance of analgesia. We also assess and record the sensory

Table 34–2 Bromage Motor Block Scale

BROMAGE CRITERION	DEGREE OF MOTOR BLOCK	SCORE, %
Free movement of legs and feet	None	0
Just able to flex the knees with free movement of the feet	Partial	33
Unable to flex the knees but with free movement of the feet	Almost complete	66
Unable to move legs or feet	Complete	100

Data from Bromage PR: A comparison of the hydrochloride and carbon dioxide salts of lidocaine and prilocaine in epidural analgesia. Acta Anaesthesiol Scand Suppl 1965; 16: 55–69.

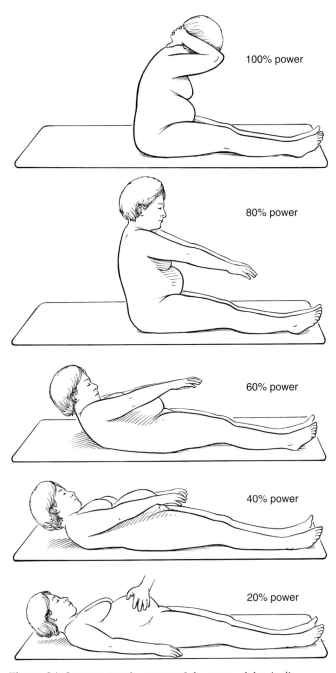

100% power

80% power

60% power

40% power

20% power

Figure 34–8 Measuring the power of the rectus abdominalis muscles (RAM). For the RAM test, the parturient is asked to come slowly to a sitting position when lying perfectly supine on the bed. (Redrawn from Van Zundert A, Vaes L, Soetens M, et al: Measuring motor blockade during lumbar epidural analgesia for vaginal delivery. Obstet Anesth Dig 1984; 4: 31–34.)

level of anesthesia intermittently; we are perplexed that there seems to be a reluctance on the part of some anesthesiologists to do this. We often use the Bromage scale to quantitate the degree of motor block present after a prolonged infusion of local anesthetic (Table 34–2).[32] Alternatively, some anesthesiologists think a test of the rectus abdominal muscles is a more appropriate test of motor function during labor (Fig. 34–8).[33]

Parturients must be instructed to avoid the supine position throughout labor to minimize the occurrence

of aortocaval compression. Anesthesiologists and obstetricians should not be reassured by the presence of normal brachial artery blood pressure measurements in supine parturients, because these may overestimate uterine artery perfusion pressures.[34] We encourage patients to alternate the left and right lateral positions throughout labor, because this practice may help decrease the occurrence of unilateral analgesia.[21] After the successful induction of epidural analgesia, we gradually elevate the head of the patient's bed as labor progresses. This may allow preferential caudal spread of the local anesthetic solution, thereby improving the quality of analgesia during the second stage.[35, 36]

Occasionally, a unilateral anesthetic or unblocked segment develops despite positional efforts to improve analgesia in an unanesthetized site. Fortunately, these are usually successfully remedied by additional boluses of local anesthetic with the patient placed in the proper position (i.e., painful side dependent).[37] If this is unsuccessful, withdrawing the epidural catheter 1 or 2 cm often improves the distribution of anesthetic within the epidural space. The rationale underlying this maneuver comes from radiographic data demonstrating that catheters advanced about 5 cm into the epidural space lie at a more favorable position and yield superior analgesia than those advanced much farther into the space.[35] A preliminary study[38] found that catheter withdrawal was successful in improving analgesia in two thirds of one-sided blocks. We withdraw a marginally functioning epidural catheter 1 to 2 cm if we are reasonably sure that all ports still remain in the epidural space. If analgesia remains unilateral after a bolus is administered through a repositioned catheter, we recommend replacement of the catheter.

Epidurally Administered Opioids During Labor

Epidurally administered opioids alone are not as effective as epidurally administered local anesthetics for providing analgesia during labor.[39–42] For example, Hughes and associates[41] found that 5 mg of morphine applied epidurally was almost always inadequate for relieving pain during labor. Although better results were achieved by increasing the dose to 7.5 mg, analgesia remained inferior to that produced by bupivacaine given epidurally (Fig. 34–9). Others[39, 41] found that neonatal arterial base excess values and early neurobehavioral scores were each lower after epidural morphine than after epidural bupivacaine. Lipid-soluble opioids alone also provide unreliable epidural analgesia during labor. For instance, fentanyl 100 μg and sufentanil 10 μg given epidurally were each found to be ineffective in treating labor pain.[40, 43]

Despite the inadequacy of opioids alone as epidural analgesics during labor, there are proven benefits and little maternal or fetal risk to the practice of administering lipid-soluble opioids epidurally in conjunction with local anesthetics during labor. Opioids hasten the onset of analgesia, prolong the duration, and increase the intensity of analgesia when added to epidural local anesthetics (Fig. 34–10).[44–49] A practical advantage of adding opioids to epidural local anesthetics is that they

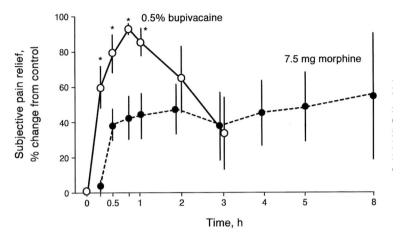

Figure 34–9 Subjective pain relief calculated from the Visual Linear Analog Scale (mean ± standard error of mean) contrasting morphine 7.5 mg given epidurally, with 0.5% bupivacaine given epidurally over time. The asterisk indicates a significant difference ($P < .01$). (Data from Hughes SC, Rosen MA, Shnider SM, et al: Maternal and neonatal effects of epidural morphine for labor and delivery. Anesth Analg 1984; 63: 319–324.)

decrease the number of supplemental bolus injections required to treat inadequate analgesia.[44] Opioids decrease local anesthetic requirements during labor, which decreases the incidence of profound motor block.[43, 46, 50–52] Because intense motor block is associated with a greater number of instrumented deliveries, it has tempted some to speculate that epidurally applied local anesthetic-opioid mixtures would be an ideal epidural anesthetic from the perspective of maximizing the percentage of spontaneous deliveries.

Two studies found that the epidural administration of an opioid in conjunction with bupivacaine increased the probability of a spontaneous vaginal delivery compared with epidural injection of bupivacaine alone.[51, 53] In a large multicenter study, Vertommen and colleagues[51] reported that there were fewer forceps deliveries in women given bupivacaine-sufentanil mixtures epidurally compared with those given only bupivacaine epidurally (Table 34–3). Unfortunately, most studies have not been able to substantiate the ability of epidural opioids to decrease the incidence of instrumented deliveries.[23, 44–47, 52] Nevertheless, the potential to achieve excellent analgesia with less motor block had led many anesthesiologists to routinely include an opioid with an epidural infusion of local anesthetic during

labor. A participants' survey at the 1993 Annual Meeting of The Society for Obstetric Anesthesia and Perinatology revealed that 73% of respondents routinely administer local anesthetic-opioid infusions during labor.[54]

An opioid should be added to a local anesthetic infusion during labor with the intention of decreasing the total dose of local anesthetic. For example, 0.0625% bupivacaine with 2 μg/mL of fentanyl produces analgesia similar to that provided by 0.125% bupivacaine alone.[52] Epidural administration of a lipid-soluble opioid is often effective for the treatment of any breakthrough pain that may develop despite the presence of a T-10 level of analgesia. For instance, Reynolds and O'Sullivan[48] observed that an epidurally administered bolus consisting of 100 μg of fentanyl and 10 mg of bupivacaine was consistently more effective than a bolus of 25 mg of bupivacaine for diminishing perineal pain during advanced labor.

Pruritus, nausea, and sedation are all greater after epidural administration of morphine than after epidural administration of bupivacaine. Pruritus seems to be the main side effect observed after epidural administration of fentanyl or sufentanil, although it is rarely severe and seldom requires treatment. Butorphanol and meperidine have each been used as a supplement to epidural administration of bupivacaine with some success.[46, 47] However, these opioids offer no real overall advantage for epidural use compared with fentanyl and sufentanil. For example, pruritus is less common after epidural administration of butorphanol, but somnolence is more prevalent.

Table 34–3 Incidence of Instrumental Delivery for Epidural Bupivacaine-Sufentanil and Epidural Bupivacaine Groups

| PARITY | INSTRUMENTAL DELIVERY, % | |
	Bupivacaine-Sufentanil ($n = 324$)	Bupivacaine (Control) ($n = 304$)
Nulliparous	34*	45
Parous	12*	22
Total	24*	36

Women in the bupivacaine-sufentanil group were given 10 mL of 0.125% bupivacaine with epinephrine 1:800,000 and sufentanil 10 μg for the initial three epidural injectons. Sufentanil was not administered with the fourth and subsequent injections. Women in the bupivacaine (control) group were given epidural injections of 10 mL of 0.125% bupivacaine with epinephrine 1:800,000 on each request for analgesia.

*$P < 0.01$ versus bupivacaine (control) group.

Data from Vertommen JD, Vandermeulen E, Van Aken H, et al.: The effects of the addition of sufentanil to 0.125% bupivacaine on the quality of analgesia during labor and on the incidence of instrumental deliveries. Anesthesiology 1991; 74: 809–819.

Epidural Analgesia for Delivery

If analgesia is maintained throughout the second stage of labor, it is mandatory to anesthetize the S-2 through S-4 nerve roots. Women who progress into the second stage of labor soon after induction of epidural analgesia seldom have adequate sacral blocks and often require additional boluses of local anesthetic at delivery, especially if episiotomy incision or the application of forceps is intended.[55] In these circumstances, epidural administration of 2% or 3% 2-chloroprocaine

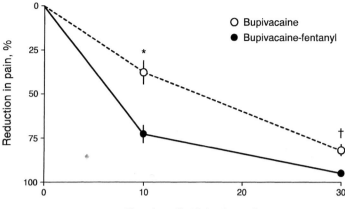

Figure 34–10 Percentage reduction in visual analog pain scores 10 and 30 min after the first epidural injection of 4 mL of 0.3% bupivacaine with or without 80 μg of fentanyl. *$P <$ .001, †$P <$ .01. (Data from Justins DM, Francis D, Houlton PG, et al: A controlled trial of extradural fentanyl in labour. Br J Anaesth 1982; 54: 409–414.)

usually achieves sensory sacral anesthesia in about 10 min. However, women who have received prolonged infusions of local anesthetic during labor often have adequate sacral anesthesia and may not require additional local anesthetic at delivery.

Controversies in Epidural Anesthesia

Does Epidural Analgesia Decrease the Efficacy of Uterine Contractions and Increase the Probability of Cesarean Section for Dystocia?

Even the occasional obstetric anesthesiologist is aware that there is disagreement regarding the influence of epidural analgesia on the effectiveness of uterine contractions. For instance, Willdeck-Lund and coworkers[56] observed that epidural injection of bupivacaine, with or without epinephrine, was followed by a transient decrease in the intensity, although not the frequency, of uterine contractions measured by an intrauterine pressure catheter (Fig. 34–11). Thorp and colleagues[57] observed that the rate of cervical dilation during the first stage of labor was slower in women randomized to receive bupivacaine epidurally than in those given meperidine intravenously (Fig. 34–12). However, Craft and associates[58] found that uterine contractility was attenuated only when local anesthetic solutions containing epinephrine were injected into the epidural space.

Behrens and colleagues[59] reported that, in a small nonrandomized study, epidural administration of bupivacaine without epinephrine decreased uterine activity and maternal plasma concentrations of oxytocin and a metabolite of prostaglandin $F_{2\alpha}$ 60 min after injection (Fig. 34–13). They hypothesized that epidural analgesia inhibited the reflex release of oxytocin, which subsequently blocked prostaglandin $F_{2\alpha}$ release, leading to the attenuation in uterine contractility. In a preliminary study, Cheek and coworkers[60] found that a 1-L bolus of fluids given intravenously (but not epidural injection of a local anesthetic) resulted in diminished uterine activity for about 20 min. Their data suggested that dilution of circulating factors (e.g., oxytocin, prostaglandins) by acute hydration may be responsible for the transient decrease in uterine activity some have observed after initiating epidural analgesia. This hypothesis is supported by the findings of Willdeck-Lund and colleagues,[56] who observed that "the [uterine] activity had already declined . . . during the

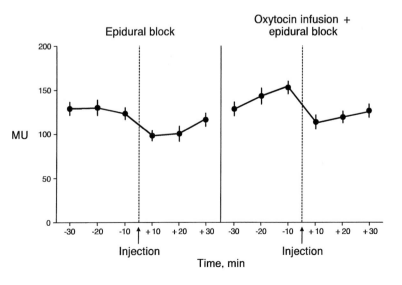

Figure 34–11 Uterine activity (Montevideo units [MU]), given as the mean ± standard error of mean, before and after epidural injection of local anesthetic. Notice that uterine activity was decreasing immediately before epidural injection. This may represent an effect of intravenous hydration rather than the epidural block. (Data from Willdeck-Lund G, Lindmark G, Nilsson BA: Effect of segmental epidural analgesia upon the uterine activity with special reference to the use of different local anaesthetic agents. Acta Anaesth Scand 1979; 23: 519–528.)

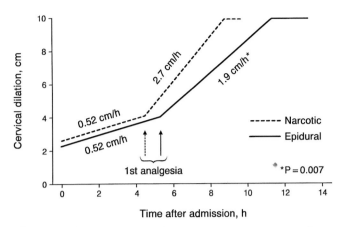

Figure 34–12 Progression of labor for the group given meperidine parenterally and the group given bupivacaine epidurally. The rate of cervical dilation after the first request for analgesia was significantly slower in the epidural group. Nine women in the epidural group were receiving oxytocin at the time of the initial analgesic treatment, compared with only three in the meperidine group. (Data from Thorp JA, Hu DH, Albin RM, et al: The effect of intrapartum epidural analgesia on nulliparous labor: a randomized, controlled, prospective trial. Am J Obstet Gynecol 1993; 169: 851–858.)

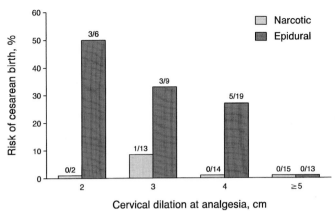

Figure 34–14 Risk of cesarean section versus cervical dilation at first request for analgesia. Early epidural placement increased the probability of cesarean section. There were no cesarean births performed in the group having epidural placement at ≥5 cm cervical dilation. (Data from Thorp JA, Hu DH, Albin RM, et al: The effect of intrapartum epidural analgesia on nulliparous labor: a randomized, controlled, prospective trial. Am J Obstet Gynecol 1993; 169: 851–858.)

preliminary preparations for the block . . . ." These investigators attributed the decrease in uterine activity just before epidural injection to an "increased endogenous release of catecholamines in response to the stress of the procedure." We interpret their data to suggest that acute intravenous hydration was in part responsible for the transient decrease in uterine contractility observed in this and other similar investigations.

Earlier studies[61–63] found that women given epidural analgesia were more likely to be delivered by cesarean section than women given medication systemically or no analgesia. Many physicians dismissed the negative outcomes of these retrospective reviews on the basis that patients who progress rapidly through labor often have less pain and are not as likely to request regional analgesia. However, a prospective study[57] reported that women randomized to receive epidural block were more than 10 times as likely (25% versus 2.2%) to

require cesarean delivery than those in a control group given only intravenous analgesia with meperidine. They observed that the increased incidence of cesarean deliveries occurred only among women given epidural analgesia in early labor. Eleven (32%) of 34 parturients given epidural block before the cervix was dilated 5 cm ultimately had cesarean delivery, compared with 0 of 13 in whom epidural analgesia was delayed until the cervix was dilated at least 5 cm (Fig. 34–14).

These results are not supported by other studies and the experience of many anesthesiologists and obstetricians. For example, Philipsen and Jensen[64] randomized 111 term parturients to receive either bupivacaine (0.375%) epidurally or meperidine intramuscularly for analgesia during labor. The time from analgesic administration until full cervical dilation was similar in the two groups, suggesting that the rate of cervical dilation was unaffected by type of analgesia. The cesarean section rate did not differ significantly between the two groups (Table 34–4). Regrettably, these investigators

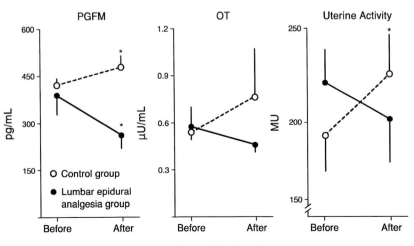

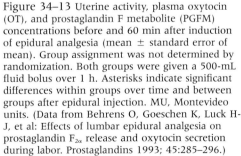

Figure 34–13 Uterine activity, plasma oxytocin (OT), and prostaglandin F metabolite (PGFM) concentrations before and 60 min after induction of epidural analgesia (mean ± standard error of mean). Group assignment was not determined by randomization. Both groups were given a 500-mL fluid bolus over 1 h. Asterisks indicate significant differences within groups over time and between groups after epidural injection. MU, Montevideo units. (Data from Behrens O, Goeschen K, Luck H-J, et al: Effects of lumbar epidural analgesia on prostaglandin $F_{2\alpha}$ release and oxytocin secretion during labor. Prostaglandins 1993; 45:285–296.)

Table 34–4 Progress of Labor and Mode of Delivery for Epidural Block Versus Meperidine Given Parenterally in Women of Mixed Parity

VARIABLE	BUPIVACAINE EPIDURALLY (n = 57)	MEPERIDINE PARENTERALLY (n = 54)	P
Progress of Labor, min			
Time from injection of analgesic to full cervical dilation	197	180	NS
Duration of second stage	47	37	NS (P = 0.106)
Total duration of labor	805	657	NS (P = 0.088)
Method of Delivery, no. (%)			
Spontaneous	33 (58)	34 (63)	NS
Vacuum extraction	13 (23)	14 (26)	NS
Forceps	1 (2)	0	NS
Cesarean section	10 (17)	6 (11)	NS

Bupivacaine was not administered epidurally after the cervix had dilated beyond 8 cm.

Median values are listed for progress of labor.

There were nine cesarean sections for cephalopelvic disproportion in the epidural group compared with three in the meperidine group (P = 0.153, NS)

Data from Philipsen T, Jensen N-H: Epidural block or parenteral pethidine as analgesic in labour; a randomized study concerning progress in labour and instrumental deliveries. Eur J Obstet Gynecol Reprod Biol 1989; 30: 27–33.

enrolled too few patients to state with confidence that epidural anesthesia did not cause a modest increase in the incidence of cesarean section, but their results stand in opposition to the dramatic increase in the cesarean section rate in the epidural group in the study by Thorp and associates.[57]

Perhaps most illuminating are data from institutions where the use of epidural analgesia increased abruptly over a short period. These studies[65, 66] uniformly refute the contribution of epidural analgesia to what some have called the epidemic of cesarean sections. For example, Larson[65] reported that the cesarean section rate decreased from 28% to 23% in the 12 months after a labor epidural service was instituted (Table 34–5). The increased number of women attempting vaginal birth after cesarean delivery was probably responsible for the lower rate after the availability of epidural analgesia.

Table 34–5 Effect of Initiating a Labor Epidural Service on the Rate of Cesarean and Forceps Deliveries

VARIABLE	JUNE 1989 TO MAY 1990 (NO LABOR EPIDURAL ANALGESIA SERVICE)	JULY 1990 TO JUNE 1991 (IN-HOUSE EPIDURAL ANALGESIA SERVICE)
Labor epidural rate, %	0	31.6
Cesarean section rate, %	27.6	22.9*
Forceps rate, %	8.4	9.2
Vaginal births after cesarean section, no.	65	113

*P < 0.001 between time periods.

The increased number of women electing to attempt vaginal births after cesarean section after epidural analgesia became available was likely responsible for the decrease in cesarean section rate in the latter time period.

Data from Larson DD: The effect of initiating an obstetric anesthesiology service on rate of cesarean section and rate of forceps delivery. Presented at the Annual Meeting of the Society for Obstetric Anesthesiology and Perinatology, Charleston, SC, May 8, 1992.

We think a carefully performed epidural block is unlikely to increase a parturient's likelihood of requiring a cesarean delivery. Women who request epidural analgesia may have anatomic differences (e.g., smaller pelvic dimensions) or less effective uterine contractions (or both) than women who are given opioids parenterally or no analgesia during labor.[67] Ideally, evaluations of epidural or intrathecal analgesia on the progress of labor should be limited to prospective randomized studies in well-defined patient populations (e.g., nulliparous women not receiving oxytocin). However, the quality of patient care and perhaps the clinical relevance of withholding an effective form of pain control (i.e., epidural analgesia) from women in severe pain must be questioned when no comparable alternative exists.

When Is the Best Time to Begin Epidural Analgesia During Labor?

Some physicians prefer to delay administration of epidural analgesia during labor because of concern that premature initiation of epidural block may interfere with labor.[3, 68] For example, Bonica[3] recommended delaying induction of epidural anesthesia until the cervix was dilated to at least 5 cm in nulliparous women and 4 cm in parous women, whether or not the parturient was receiving oxytocin intravenously. Data from Thorp and colleagues,[57] implicating early induction of epidural block as a causative factor in increasing the likelihood of a cesarean section, strongly argue against inducing epidural analgesia before the cervix has dilated to at least 5 cm in nulliparous women.

We[69] completed two separate studies that demonstrated no adverse consequences from inducing epidural analgesia during early labor. In the first study, we randomized 149 nulliparous women in active labor who were receiving an infusion of oxytocin to receive early (<5 cm cervical dilation) or late (≥5 cm cervical dilation) induction of epidural analgesia. Women in the late group were initially given nalbuphine intravenously for analgesia but were eligible to receive epidural analgesia 1 h after a second dose of nalbuphine or when the cervix had dilated to at least 5 cm. In the second study,[70] we used an identical protocol but restricted our analysis to 334 women in spontaneous labor (i.e., not receiving oxytocin) at the time of randomization. In both studies, early administration of epidural analgesia did not adversely affect any measure of obstetric outcome (Tables 34–6 and 34–7). Fetal arterial pH at delivery was slightly higher in the early epidural groups in both studies. Not surprisingly, we observed marked differences in analgesia after the initial treatment, which persisted for approximately 3 h after randomization (Fig. 34–15). These results have encouraged us to offer epidural analgesia regardless of cervical dilation, if a diagnosis of active labor has been established and the patient is uncomfortable, and at the point that she no longer wants to ambulate. However, one study[71] suggested that it is safe for patients in early labor to ambulate for brief periods (i.e., ≤ 5

Table 34–6 Early Versus Late Induction of Epidural Analgesia and Progress of Labor, Position of the Vertex at Delivery, and Mode of Delivery

VARIABLE	EARLY (*n* = 172)	LATE (*n* = 162)	P
Progress of Labor			
Cervix at randomization, cm*	4 (0.5)	4 (0.5)	NS
Cervix at time of epidural test dose, cm*	4 (0.5)	5 (0.25)	<0.0001
Time from randomization to full cervical dilation, min†	329 ± 197	359 ± 214	NS
Required oxytocin after randomization, %	31	38	NS
Duration of second stage, min†	85 ± 65	88 ± 62	NS
Position of Vertex at Delivery			
Occiput anterior, %	87	88	NS
Occiput posterior or transverse, %	13	12	NS
Mode of Delivery			
Spontaneous vaginal, %	53	49	NS
Instrumental vaginal, %	37	43	NS
Cesarean section, %	10	8	NS

Patients in the early group received bupivacaine epidurally at the first request for pain relief after randomization. Patients in the late group were given bupivacaine epidurally only after the cervix had dilated to at least 5 cm or 1 h after a second intravenous dose of nalbuphine.

*Median (quartile deviation).
†Mean ± standard deviation.

Data from Chestnut DH, McGrath JM, Vincent RD Jr, et al.: Does early administration of epidural analgesia affect obstetric outcome in nulliparous women who are in spontaneous labor? Anesthesiology 1994; 80: 1201–1208.

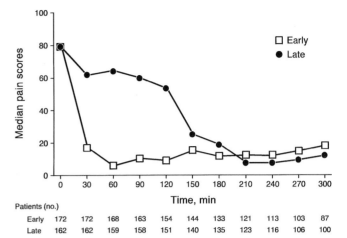

Figure 34–15 Median pain scores over time in women given early (<5 cm) or late (≥5 cm) epidural analgesia. Patients in the early group had significantly lower pain scores at all measurements between 30 and 150 min. (Data from Chestnut DH, McGrath JM, Vincent RD Jr, et al: Does early administration of epidural analgesia affect obstetric outcome in nulliparous women who are in spontaneous labor? Anesthesiology 1994; 80: 1201–1208.)

Table 34–7. Early Versus Late Induction of Epidural Analgesia and Neonatal Condition

VARIABLE	EARLY (*n* = 172)	LATE (*n* = 162)	P
Naloxone administered to infant, no. (%)	0	5 (3)	<0.05
Umbilical artery blood			
pH	7.25 ± 0.07	7.23 ± 0.07	<0.05
PCO_2, mm Hg	46 ± 9	48 ± 9	NS
PO_2, mm Hg	20 ± 6	20 ± 6	NS
Umbilical venous blood			
pH	7.33 ± 0.06	7.31 ± 0.07	<0.01
PCO_2, mm Hg	37 ± 6	39 ± 8	<0.05
PO_2, mm Hg	29 ± 6	28 ± 6	NS

All values mean ± standard deviation unless noted otherwise.

Lower fetal umbilical arterial and venous pH measurements in the late group were probably secondary to slightly higher maternal PCO_2 secondary to increased intravenous nalbuphine administration.

Data from Chestnut DH, McGrath JM, Vincent RD Jr, et al.: Does early administration of epidural analgesia affect obstetric outcome in nulliparous women who are in spontaneous labor? Anesthesiology 1994; 80: 1201–1208.

min) with assistance after epidural administration of an opioid, with or without a dilute solution of local anesthetic. The investigators concluded that a parturient must have no evidence of orthostatic hypotension and that she be able to perform a partial knee bend while standing before being allowed to ambulate during neuraxial analgesia.

Does Epidural Analgesia Increase the Incidence of Fetal Malposition, Prolong the Second Stage of Labor, and Increase the Probability of Forceps Delivery?

In 1977, Hoult and coworkers[72] reported that the incidence of malposition of the fetal head was greatly increased (21% versus 6%) when epidural analgesia was given during labor. They hypothesized that epidural anesthesia decreased pelvic floor muscle tone, which interfered with the normal anterior rotation of the fetal occiput during fetal descent. Thorp and colleagues[57, 63] also reported an association between epidural analgesia and a higher incidence of persistent occiput posterior or transverse positions. Jouppila and associates[73] were not able to corroborate an increased incidence of fetal head malpositions in women given segmental (T-10 to T-12) epidural analgesia initiated early in labor (average cervical dilation = 3 cm). They attributed the low rate of occurrence (6%) of malpositions in the epidural group to preservation of pelvic muscle tone secondary to the low doses of local anesthetic used. There is no proven relationship between the severity of pelvic floor muscle relaxation and abnormal fetal head position at delivery. Nevertheless, because motor block offers no advantage during labor, it seems prudent to select epidural or spinal techniques that minimize the severity of sacral muscle paralysis.

Analgesic management of the second stage of labor is sometimes problematic. Continuing an epidural infusion of local anesthetic during the second stage of labor results in superior analgesia at the cost of prolonging the second stage of labor and increasing the probability of an instrumental delivery (Fig. 34–16, Table 34–8).[74, 75] Several mechanisms may be responsible for the delay. First, epidural analgesia–induced sensory block of the sacral dermatomes may obliterate the

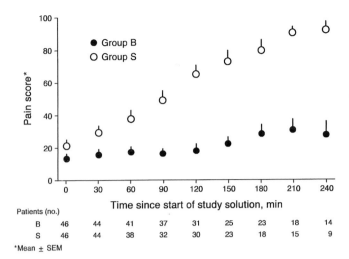

Patients (no.)

B	46	44	41	37	31	25	23	18	14
S	46	44	38	32	30	23	18	15	9

*Mean ± SEM

Figure 34–16 Pain scores for bupivacaine (B) given epidurally and isotonic saline (S) given epidurally during the second stage of labor. When the cervix was ≥8 cm dilated, the continuous epidural infusion of 0.125% bupivacaine was replaced with a coded study solution of 0.125% bupivacaine or isotonic saline. The mean pain scores were significantly lower in the bupivacaine group at each 30-min measurement after starting the study solution. (Data from Chestnut DH, Vandewalker GE, Owen CL, et al: The influence of continuous epidural bupivacaine analgesia on the second stage of labor and method of delivery in nulliparous women. Anesthesiology 1987; 66: 774–780.)

parturient's bearing-down reflex. Second, motor block of the lower abdominal muscles may decrease the patient's ability to generate optimal expulsive efforts. Third, epidural analgesia may attenuate a predelivery surge in maternal oxytocin secretion, which may diminish the intensity of uterine contractions during the second stage of labor. In a small, nonrandomized study,

Goodfellow and colleagues[76] observed no change in maternal plasma oxytocin concentrations during the second stage of labor in women given epidural analgesia. In contrast, maternal plasma oxytocin concentrations increased significantly in women given alternative forms of analgesia during labor.

A second stage of labor exceeding 2 h is not necessarily associated with a greater incidence of fetal acidosis or adverse long-term sequelae if the fetus is closely monitored (Table 34–9).[77, 78] The American College of Obstetricians and Gynecologists now considers the second stage to be prolonged only after it has exceeded 3 h in nulliparous women given epidural analgesia.[79] We routinely continue the epidural infusion into the second stage of labor. If the fetal vertex descends appropriately (i.e., ≥ 1 cm/h) and the maternal expulsive efforts are judged to be adequate, we do not discontinue the infusion before delivery.

Spinal Analgesia

One decade ago, several groups of investigators first tried to produce labor analgesia with intrathecally administered morphine alone.[80, 81] Their expectations that morphine given spinally would result in acceptable labor analgesia without local anesthetic-induced sympathetic and motor block were largely unmet, because the pain relief was often slow in onset, inconsistent in quality (especially for the second stage), and accompanied by a high incidence of troubling side effects. For instance, Abboud and coworkers[81] reported that adequate pain relief was usually not evident until at least 45 min after spinal administration of 0.5 to 1 mg of morphine (Fig. 34–17). They also observed a high frequency of pruritus, nausea, urinary retention, and sedation persisting for some time after delivery (Table 34–10). Perhaps most troubling was the respiratory depression (7 breaths/min) that developed in one woman 14 h after injection of morphine intrathecally. Even a low risk of respiratory depression is difficult to accept in healthy postpartum women who would otherwise not require intensive respiratory monitoring.

The discovery that lipid-soluble opioids (i.e., fentanyl, sufentanil) given intrathecally produce rapid-

Table 34–8. Bupivacaine Given Epidurally Versus Placebo Administration and the Second Stage of Labor

VARIABLE	BUPIVACAINE (n = 46)	ISOTONIC SALINE (CONTROL) (n = 46)	P
Duration of second stage, min	124 ± 70	94 ± 54	<0.05
Motor block at delivery*			
None, %	52	89	<0.005
Partial, %	39	9	
Almost complete, %	9	2	
Complete, %	0	0	
Mode of delivery			
Cesarean section, %	13	13	NS
Vaginal, %	87	87	NS
Spontaneous, %	41	63	<0.05
Low forceps, %	26	15	
Midvacuum followed by low forceps, %	13	0	
Midforceps, %	7	9	

After cervical dilation reached 8 cm, women were given either 0.125% bupivacaine or isotonic saline epidurally until delivery.
*Bromage classification used for quantification of motor block.
Data from Chestnut DH, Vandewalker GE, Owen CL, et al.: The influence of continuous epidural bupivacaine analgesia on the second stage of labor and method of delivery in nulliparous women. Anesthesiology 1987; 66: 774–780.

Table 34–9. Neonatal Outcome According to the Duration of the Second Stage of Labor

OUTCOME	NEONATES, %	
	0 to 120 min	>120 min
Birth weight > 4,000 g	10	16
One-min Apgar score < 7	10	22*
Five-min Apgar score < 7	1.5	0
Umbilical artery pH < 7.20	5.1	3.3
Umbilical cord base excess < −6	31	25
Intensive care nursery admission	1.7	2

*P < 0.05 between groups.
A prolonged second stage did not impose an increased hazard to the fetus, provided there was close fetal monitoring.
Data from Moon JM, Smith CV, Rayburn WF: Perinatal outcome after a prolonged second stage of labor. J Reprod Med 1990; 35: 229–231.

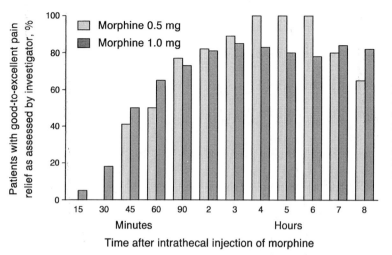

Figure 34–17 Percentage of patients having good to excellent pain relief after intrathecal injection of 0.5 mg or 1.0 mg of morphine. At least 45 min were required for most women to experience pain relief after injection. Maximal pain relief did not occur until 90 to 120 min after administration. (Data from Abboud TK, Shnider SM, Dailey PA, et al: Intrathecal administration of hyperbaric morphine for the relief of pain in labour. Br J Anaesth 1984; 56: 1351–1359.)

onset, excellent first-stage analgesia has rejuvenated interest in spinal analgesia during labor. For example, sufentanil (10 μg) produces analgesia in less than 10 min, with a duration of about 2 h.[82, 83] Analgesia after intrathecal administration of fentanyl (25 μg) is less effective than after sufentanil (10 μg), but this may be because the two doses are not equianalgesic.[82] Systemic potency ratios between opioids may not be applicable to subarachnoid administration, because they reflect the ability of the drugs to cross the dural membrane and gain receptor access.[84] Limitations to the use of lipid-soluble opioids for labor analgesia include their relatively brief duration of action and their inability to produce adequate pain relief during the second stage. These objections could be overcome by using a spinal microcatheter to give repeat bolus doses of an opioid during the first stage and then a single small dose of hyperbaric local anesthetic for sacral analgesia before delivery.[85] Unfortunately, the regulatory concern regarding the safety of spinal microcatheters makes it unlikely that such a technique will be available to most anesthesiologists in the immediate future.[86]

In some patients (e.g., women with aortic stenosis or Eisenmenger syndrome) in whom maintenance of

sympathetic tone is an important goal, the anesthesiologist may wish to use an intrathecal technique to administer opioids despite the uncertain quality of second-stage analgesia and the high incidence of maternal side effects. Leighton and colleagues[87] demonstrated that it is possible to combine a lipid-soluble opioid (25 μg of fentanyl) with a small dose of morphine (0.25 mg), given spinally for the purpose of achieving rapid onset of analgesia with an extended duration of action (Fig. 34–18). Nevertheless, 40% of their patients still required epidural injection of a local anesthetic to control pain before delivery. One enhancement of this technique would be to request the obstetrician to perform a pudendal block during the late first stage or early second stage of labor to decrease the intensity of sacral pain.[88] If there is not an anesthesiologist available to treat the rare life-threatening complications that may arise during the course of epidural analgesia, the relative safety of spinal administration of small doses

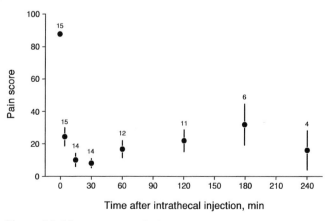

Figure 34–18 Mean ± standard error of mean of pain scores during labor after intrathecal injection of 25 μg of fentanyl and 0.25 mg of morphine. Six of the 15 patients required epidural injection of bupivacaine to produce adequate analgesia (140 ± 51 min after intrathecal injection of opioids). The number of patients still laboring with intrathecal opioid analgesia is shown above each data point. (Data from Leighton BL, DeSimone CA, Norris MC, et al: Intrathecal narcotics for labor revisited: the combination of fentanyl and morphine intrathecally provides rapid onset of profound, prolonged analgesia. Anesth Analg 1989; 69: 122–125.)

Table 34–10. Percentage of Patients Who Had Adverse Side Effects After Intrathecal Injection of Morphine (0.5 mg and 1.0 mg)

	PATIENTS, %		
SIDE EFFECT	0.5 mg (*n* = 12)	1.0 mg (*n* = 18)	Combined Data (*n* = 30)
Pruritus	58	94	80
Nausea or vomiting	50	56	53
Urinary retention	42	44	43
Drowsiness or dizziness	33	50	43
Respiratory depression	0	6	3
Headache	0	5	3

Pruritus began 3 to 5 h after intrathecal injection of morphine and lasted up to 30 h.

Modified from Abboud TK, Shnider SM, Dailey PA, et al: Intrathecal administration of hyperbaric morphine for the relief of pain in labour. Br J Anaesth 1984; 56: 1351–1359.

of lipid-soluble opioids increases their attractiveness as an analgesic modality during labor.

Local anesthetics are rarely injected intrathecally to produce labor analgesia. Although intrathecal injections of local anesthetics produce analgesia rapidly, they produce more motor block than epidural injections of local anesthetics.[89] Problems with continuous spinal delivery systems limit the use of intrathecal local anesthetics to a single dose. The use of spinal local anesthetics during labor is usually restricted to providing anesthesia during instrumental delivery. Intrathecal injection of hyperbaric lidocaine (25 mg) provides adequate sacral anesthesia for outlet or low-forceps delivery.[3] Alternatively, a slightly larger dose (e.g., 40 mg of lidocaine) may be given to provide satisfactory anesthesia (T-10) for a midforceps delivery.[3]

Combined Epidural and Spinal Analgesia

The remarkable ability of intrathecally applied lipid-soluble opioids to produce rapid onset of pain relief during the first stage of labor is one feature that cannot be equaled by epidural techniques. Some anesthesiologists facilitate the onset of analgesia by injecting a single dose of fentanyl or sufentanil intrathecally immediately after identification of the epidural space and before placing the epidural catheter (Fig. 34–19).[90, 91] An ideal situation for such a method may be when a parturient writhing in severe pain requests labor analgesia before the anesthesiologist has had an opportunity to give an adequate crystalloid preload intravenously. A single spinal injection of fentanyl or sufentanil decreases the number of painful contractions until effective analgesia is achieved. Thereafter, if analgesia is acceptable, local anesthetics injected through the catheter may be delayed until pain returns, usually in about 2 h. It is possible, but unproved, that such a technique decreases the adverse effects ascribed to local anesthetic-induced motor block.

Lumbar Sympathetic Block

Bilateral lumbar sympathetic block is seldom used for labor analgesia, because it lacks many of the advantages of and has at least as many disadvantages as continuous epidural analgesia.[92] The lumbar sympathetic block is technically more difficult to perform and requires needle sticks that are more painful than an epidural block. It does not provide sacral analgesia for the second stage of labor. Results of an earlier study suggested that this procedure may actually accelerate the first stage of labor or convert an abnormal uterine contraction pattern into a normal one.[93] Because this study did not include a control group, it is impossible to distinguish the effects of the block from the increase in uterine activity that naturally occurs over time. In either case, we see no justification for the routine use of this technique for the purpose of improving the efficacy of uterine contractions.

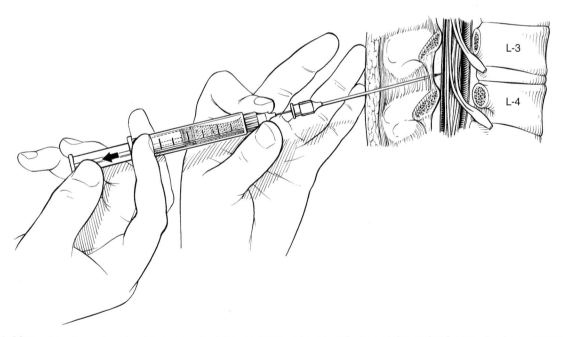

Figure 34–19 Combined spinal epidural technique for labor analgesia. After identification of the epidural space, dural puncture is performed with an atraumatic spinal needle (e.g., 120-mm or 150-mm 24-G Sprotte) placed through the lumen of an 88-mm epidural needle. Injection of 25 μg of fentanyl or 10 μg of sufentanil produces noticeable analgesia within 5 min. When the sensation of pain returns, the epidural catheter is then injected to produce analgesia. In some cases (e.g., when the depth of the epidural space is greater than 1 cm and a 120-mm spinal needle is used), it is necessary to abandon the technique or slowly advance both needles in tandem to obtain return of cerebrospinal fluid. Although unproved, the latter approach appears to carry the risk of dural puncture with a large-gauge epidural needle. An alternative method is to perform intrathecal injection of opioid as a separate procedure before attempting epidural catheter placement.

Transcutaneous Electrical Nerve Stimulation and Intracutaneous Nerve Stimulation

Some physicians[94, 95] have used transcutaneous electrical nerve stimulation over the lower lumbar area in the hope of creating a presynaptic inhibition of uterine and cervical afferent pain fibers. In an earlier study,[95] transcutaneous electrical nerve stimulation significantly decreased low-back pain during the first stage of labor, but the overall analgesic benefit appeared to be modest. Some investigators[95] have commented that the analgesic effect of transcutaneous electrical nerve stimulation is comparable to that of meperidine given intravenously. One positive attribute of transcutaneous electrical nerve stimulation is that it causes absolutely no fetal or maternal morbidity. However, a major drawback of transcutaneous electrical nerve stimulation is that it often creates electrical interference with the fetal heart rate waveform when used concurrently with an internal fetal scalp electrode.

Several studies have shown promising results from intradermal injections of sterile water for the treatment of severe back pain during the first stage of labor. Lytzen and associates[96] and Trolle and colleagues[97] reported that injections of sterile water intradermally along the sacral border produced analgesia in about 2 min that lasted up to 3 h. Hypothetically, intradermal injection of sterile water causes local irritation that decreases the perception of uterine visceral pain. The effect was apparently not placebo-mediated, because intradermal injection of saline did not produce a similar analgesic effect (Table 34–11). Intradermal injections of sterile water or other substances cannot provide complete analgesia during childbirth, but these results suggest that this technique deserves further investigation as a possible complement to neuraxial or intravenous analgesic methods.

Blocks Performed by Obstetricians

Obstetricians may perform paracervical blocks for labor analgesia if neuraxial techniques are contraindi-

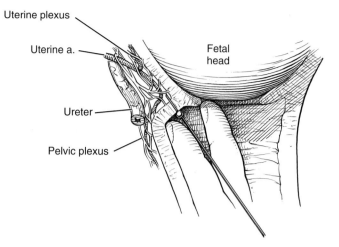

Figure 34–20 Technique for paracervical block. Between 5 and 6 mL of local anesthetic (e.g., 1% lidocaine) are injected into the mucosa of the cervix at the 4 and 8 o'clock positions or the 3 and 9 o'clock positions. a., artery. (Redrawn from Bonica JJ: Principles and Practice of Obstetric Analgesia and Anesthesia, vol 1, p 515. Philadelphia, FA Davis, 1967.)

cated or not available. Interruption of neural pathways in the uterovaginal plexus produces first-stage analgesia by blocking the pain of uterine contractions (Fig. 34–20).[3, 92] Analgesia develops rapidly after a paracervical block but tends to wear off precipitously within 60 to 90 min of injection. The block may need to be repeated as soon as the parturient begins to sense discomfort.

The greatest concern limiting the use of paracervical block is the high incidence of fetal heart rate changes reported after using the technique.[98, 99] Shnider and coworkers[98] observed fetal bradycardia and tachycardia after paracervical injection of local anesthetic in 24% and 4% of cases, respectively. Possible causes of paracervical anesthesia-induced fetal bradycardia include reflex bradycardia secondary to manipulation of the fetal head, uterus, or uterine blood vessels[100]; local anesthetic-induced central nervous system or myocardial depression or both[101, 102]; increased uterine tone or activity leading to decreased uteroplacental perfusion[103, 104]; and local anesthetic-induced uterine artery vasoconstriction.[103, 105–107] Most observers now favor decreased uteroplacental perfusion resulting from one of the last two mechanisms as the more probable explanation for decreased fetal heart rate after paracervical injection. Factors that may predispose to fetal heart rate changes after this technique include nulliparity, prematurity, and preexisting fetal compromise.[98] Others argue that the technique provides effective analgesia and adds little fetal risk if performed properly.[108, 109]

A pudendal nerve block may be used to produce perineal (S-2 through S-4) analgesia during the late first stage or early second stage of labor (Fig. 34–21).[3, 92] The pudendal nerve block is a useful anesthetic supplement if paracervical analgesia, intrathecally administered opioids, or systemically administered opioids have been given to produce analgesia during the first stage of labor.[88]

Table 34–11. Mean Pain Scores Before and After Intradermal Blocks With Sterile Water or Saline Solution

TIME OF ASSESSMENT	MEAN PAIN SCORE		
	Sterile Water (n = 141)	Saline Solution (n = 131)	P
Immediately before block	83	81	NS
After block			
1 h	29.5	76	<0.001
2 h	53.5	82	<0.001

The posterior superior iliac spines were palpated and marked. Two additional marks were made 2 cm inferior and 1 cm medial to the initial marks. Injection of 0.1 mL of sterile water at these points produced a small white papule surrounded with an erythematous halo. Typically, the parturient experienced a sharp burning sensation during injection, which subsided in about 30 s.

Data from Trolle B, Moller M, Kronborg H, et al: The effect of sterile water blocks on low back labor pain. Am J Obstet Gynecol 1991; 164: 1277–1281.

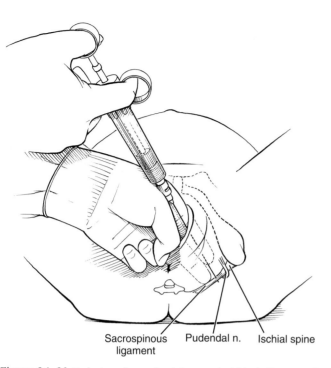

Figure 34–21 Technique for pudendal nerve (n.) block. Between 5 and 10 mL of local anesthetic (e.g., 1% lidocaine) are injected just below each ischial spine. (Redrawn from Bonica JJ: Principles and Practice of Obstetric Analgesia and Anesthesia, vol 1, p 493. Philadelphia, FA Davis, 1967.)

Obstetric Analgesia in the Parturient With Complications

Preeclampsia

Many consider preeclampsia to be a strong indication for continuous epidural analgesia during labor. A greater incidence of uteroplacental insufficiency in preeclamptic women translates into a higher probability of emergency cesarean delivery for fetal distress. Early induction of epidural analgesia may enable the physician to obtain a surgical level of analgesia promptly when fetal deterioration mandates immediate operative delivery. Avoidance of general anesthesia may be especially important in preeclamptic women because increased facial, pharyngeal, and laryngeal edema may exaggerate the difficulty of endotracheal intubation.[110, 111] Epidural anesthesia for cesarean section avoids the hypertensive response accompanying laryngoscopy and tracheal intubation.[112, 113] Severe hypotension is less likely after induction of epidural anesthesia than after induction of spinal anesthesia, because the onset of sympathetic block is slower after epidural injection of a local anesthetic. Evidence also indicates that epidural analgesia may have a favorable effect on uteroplacental perfusion in preeclamptic parturients.[114, 115] Epidural analgesia-induced peripheral vasodilation and reductions in maternal catecholamine concentrations may diminish the incidence of extreme hypertension that may otherwise require aggressive antihypertensive therapy.

Because of concern that neuraxial blocks may place preeclamptic women with quantitative and qualitative platelet deficits at an increased risk of spinal cord compression from an expanding intraspinal hematoma, many anesthesiologists usually avoid performing neuraxial anesthesia in preeclamptic patients if a recent platelet count is severely depressed. The finding that some preeclamptic women have abnormal platelet function despite an acceptable number of platelets has prompted some anesthesiologists to recommend tests of platelet function (e.g., bleeding time) before proceeding with epidural or spinal blocks. Ramanathan and colleagues[116] observed abnormal bleeding times (> 10 min) in almost 70% of women with platelet counts between 100,000/μL and 150,000/μL (Fig. 34–22). Initially, these data appeared to support the views of those who recommended routinely performing bleeding function tests in all preeclamptic women as an additional measure to help detect women who might be at a high risk for intraspinal hematoma after neuraxial analgesia. Others argue that the bleeding time test is of little value in predicting which patients are at a greater risk of clinically significant bleeding.[117] Lao and associates[118] reported that an intraspinal (subdural) hematoma developed in one preeclamptic woman after attempted epidural anesthesia despite a reassuring bleeding time (3 min) and platelet count (425,000/μL). This case makes reliance on any laboratory criterion in this setting questionable.

At the University of Iowa Hospitals and Clinics, we have not arbitrarily selected a minimum platelet count as a criterion for administering an epidural block to toxemic women. The decision to proceed with epidural analgesia in an individual preeclamptic patient should balance the rare, but catastrophic, risk of paraplegia with the specific benefits to that particular patient, such as pain relief, increased uteroplacental blood flow, and avoidance of general anesthesia in the presence of

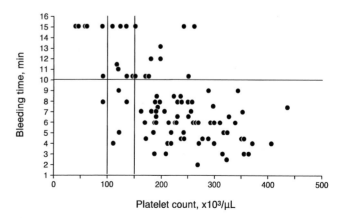

Figure 34–22 Platelet counts and corresponding bleeding times in women with preeclampsia. Overall, 7.5% of preeclamptic women had thrombocytopenia (<100,000 cells/μL), and 24.5% had prolonged bleeding times (>10 min). Nine of the 13 women with platelet counts between 100,000/μL and 150,000/μL had prolonged bleeding times. (Data from Ramanathan J, Sibai BM, Vu T, et al: Correlation between bleeding times and platelet counts in women with preeclampsia undergoing cesarean section. Anesthesiology 1989; 71: 188–191.)

profound upper airway edema. We think the best and perhaps only use of the bleeding time test is to justify the use of a neuraxial anesthetic in a woman without clinical evidence of coagulopathy but who has a low or rapidly decreasing platelet count.

Obesity

The morbidly obese parturient is especially challenging to the obstetric anesthesiologist. Identification of the epidural space is more difficult, and catheter malfunction is more likely. Hood and Dewan[119] reported that the initial catheter (thought to be in the epidural space) failed in 42% of morbidly obese women (> 300 lb), compared with only 6% of average-sized women. This is especially worrisome, because 62% of their obese population eventually underwent cesarean delivery. Because an obese gravida is more likely to require operative delivery and because tracheal intubation is a more risky endeavor in this population, it is reassuring to have a reliable epidural catheter in place throughout labor. In some situations, it may be appropriate to have a candid discussion with an obese parturient soon after admission about the impact of body habitus on anesthetic risk and the ability of an epidural block to circumvent some of those risks.

The anesthesiologist must be extraordinarily cautious when securing an epidural catheter in an obese parturient. Because deflexion may withdraw the catheter from the epidural space as much as 2.5 cm in obese patients, we do not tape the epidural catheter to the skin until the patient has deflexed her lumbar spine.[120]

Alternative Methods of Providing Analgesia During Labor

Psychoprophylactic Methods

The psychoprophylactic methods of Lamaze, Leboyer, Harris, and Bradley incorporate psychologic and physical preparation for childbirth.[121, 122] Typically, these methods include patient education in obstetric physiology, with instruction in relaxation techniques and breathing exercises. Participation by the husband or a close friend is encouraged during the preparation classes and during labor and delivery. Although participation in these classes may relieve some of the apprehension related to the birthing process, expectant mothers should not receive an unrealistic expectation of the analgesic benefits of psychotherapeutic maneuvers. Under the best circumstances, the perception of pain is decreased no more than 30%.[7] The mother may experience feelings of failure and guilt if labor eventually becomes painful.[123] Patients who attend prepared childbirth training classes should be informed that psychoprophylactic methods do not exclude the use of regional or systemic analgesia during labor.

Parenteral Methods

Meperidine is the opioid most frequently used systemically for labor analgesia. Typically, 25 to 50 mg of meperidine is given intravenously about every 2 to 4 h.[124] Unfortunately, meperidine given intravenously (and all other opioids) is usually ineffective in eliminating the pain of parturition when it is administered in doses consistent with maternal and fetal safety.[125] This is especially true in patients experiencing severe, incapacitating labor pain. Some data suggest that a shorter-acting opioid (e.g., fentanyl) may be a better selection than meperidine for minimizing the incidence of maternal side effects and fetal morbidity. Rayburn and colleagues[126] reported that analgesia was similar but that the incidence of nausea, vomiting, and sedation was less in women given fentanyl (50 to 100 μg) intravenously hourly than in a similar group given meperidine (25 to 50 mg) intravenously periodically during labor (Table 34–12). Fewer infants of the fentanyl-treated mothers required naloxone than those of the meperidine-treated mothers.

These data prompt us to question whether the investigational opioid remifentanil, which has much shorter duration of action than fentanyl, will prove to be a useful analgesic during labor. This will depend on whether doses necessary to achieve adequate analgesia result in a high incidence of maternal obtundation between contractions and whether transplacental transfer results in neonatal depression.

The most appropriate use of opioids given systemically may be when more effective (e.g., epidural, intrathecal) techniques are not available or when labor is expected to be brief and without severe pain.

Small boluses of ketamine (e.g., 0.2 to 0.4 mg/kg) given intravenously may be used if rapid, brief analgesia is desired. Akamatsu and coworkers[127] gave women

Table 34–12. Comparison of Fentanyl Given Intravenously and Meperidine Given Intravenously for Analgesia During Labor

VARIABLE	FENTANYL (*n* = 49)	MEPERIDINE (*n* = 56)	*P*
Pain score (0 to 10 scale)			
4 to 7 cm cervical dilation	5.9 ± 0.4	6.1 ± 0.3	NS
8 to 10 cm cervical dilation	8.9 ± 0.5	9.0 ± 0.5	NS
Need for antiemetic therapy, %	0	11	<0.05
Prolonged sedation, %	0	20	<0.05
Decreased fetal heart rate variability, %	49	52	NS
Abnormal fetal heart rate pattern, %	4	7	NS

Patients were randomized to receive either fentanyl 50 to 100 μg intravenously hourly or meperidine 25 to 50 mg intravenously every 2 to 3 h. There were fewer side effects in the group given fentanyl intravenously. Note the poor quality of analgesia with both opioids (especially during late labor), even though nearly half of each group was composed of multiparous women.

Modified from Rayburn WF, Smith CV, Parriott JE, et al.: Randomized comparison of meperidine and fentanyl during labor. Obstet Gynecol 1989; 74: 604–606. Reprinted with permission of The American College of Obstetricians and Gynecologists.

ketamine (12.5 to 25 mg repeated as needed, but ≤ 100 mg) intravenously for relief of pain during vaginal delivery. Of 80 women, 78 denied having pain, but all lacked recall of the delivery. Although the presence of a dream state always accompanied analgesia, they found that only one patient remarked that the experience was unpleasant. Because most women prefer to recall the events of delivery, this technique is rarely used.

Inhalational Techniques

Nitrous oxide and low concentrations of the potent inhalational agents have been administered for analgesia during labor and delivery.[128–131] Overall, these agents decrease but do not abolish the pain of uterine contractions. Nitrous oxide is the inhalation anesthetic most often used to produce analgesia during childbirth. Because of its relatively rapid onset, some prefer to give nitrous oxide intermittently during uterine contractions with the hope that unacceptable sedation will not occur during periods of minimal stimulation. Nitrous oxide administration must be begun some time in advance of each uterine contraction to achieve reasonable analgesia. Waud and Waud[132] recommended that the patient should initiate inhalation of nitrous oxide 45 s before the anticipated onset of each uterine contraction, because about 60 s is required to achieve a maximal effect. An alternative approach designed to eliminate the guesswork associated with predicting the beginning of each contraction is to administer lower concentrations (e.g., 30%) of nitrous oxide between contractions and increase the concentration to 50% at the onset of each contraction. The latter method requires the presence of an anesthesiologist and an anesthesia machine.

Some anesthesiologists advocate the use of subanesthetic concentrations of the potent inhalation anesthetics rather than nitrous oxide to produce analgesia during vaginal delivery.[133–135] The advantage of the potent inhalation agents over nitrous oxide is that they allow administration of almost 100% oxygen with the anesthetic. Abboud and colleagues[133] observed similar analgesia during the second stage of labor by using 40% nitrous oxide or 0.5% enflurane. However, fetal umbilical venous oxygen saturation tended to be higher in women who inhaled enflurane in oxygen.

Concerns about maintaining a reasonable level of consciousness mandate close supervision of women receiving any inhalational anesthetic during labor. Antacid prophylaxis should precede each administration in case excessive somnolence leads to pulmonary aspiration of gastric contents. The anesthesiologist should always begin with a low concentration (e.g., 40% nitrous oxide, 0.25% enflurane) and increase the concentration slowly, provided the patient remains responsive and cooperative. If the patient becomes stuporous or agitated, the anesthetic should be discontinued immediately, and 100% oxygen should be given. Inhalation of nitrous oxide or a subanesthetic concentration of a potent inhalation agent should be restricted to

brief periods of administration (e.g., late during the second stage of labor).

Economic Issues

As insurance companies and health maintenance organizations search for ways to control expenditures, costs for labor analgesia services are beginning to come under scrutiny. Some third-party payers have denied reimbursement for epidural analgesia administered for the sole purpose of providing intrapartum analgesia (i.e., without "medical indication"). For this reason, the American College of Obstetricians and Gynecologists and the American Society of Anesthesiologists have emphasized that "maternal request is sufficient justification for pain relief during labor."[136] They point out that "there is no other circumstance where it is considered acceptable for a person to experience severe pain, amenable to safe intervention, while under a physician's care."[136]

Maintaining a labor epidural service often represents an inefficient use of an anesthesiologist's time, especially if no more than one block is administered concurrently. We welcome the introduction of a new analgesic technique that is effective, safe, and inexpensive to deliver, but pending the discovery of such a new method, neuraxial blocks remain the technique of choice for women who experience severe pain during childbirth.

Summary

Childbirth rates among the most intense measurable sources of pain. The intensity and distribution of the pain may vary greatly among patients and even in a given patient as labor progresses. Continuous administration of epidural local anesthetic solutions, with or without opioids, is the most effective, flexible, and proven method of providing analgesia during labor and delivery.

Among the several advantages of adding a lipid-soluble opioid to an epidural local anesthetic infusion during labor, perhaps the greatest benefit is a decreased dose of local anesthetic, achieving excellent analgesia while decreasing the severity of a motor block.

There is controversy regarding the influence of epidural block on the efficacy of uterine contractions. Intravenous hydration and epinephrine-containing local anesthetic solutions may be contributors to the decrease in uterine contractility reported by some investigators. The possibility that epidural analgesia may transiently decrease uterine activity must be balanced against the benefits of pain relief.

It is not clear that epidural analgesia results in an increased incidence of fetal head malposition. However, women with fetal head malposition are more likely to request intrapartum analgesia.

Morphine alone given intrathecally produces analgesia that is slow in onset, with a high incidence of side effects. Small subarachnoid doses of fentanyl or sufentanil produce immediate onset of analgesia (although it is relatively brief) during the first stage of labor with relatively few adverse effects.

The physician should consider early administration of epidural analgesia in preeclamptic women. This practice may enable the anesthesiologist to achieve a surgical level of anesthesia rapidly if fetal deterioration occurs. As an added advantage, epidural analgesia may have a beneficial effect on uteroplacental perfusion in preeclamptic women.

REFERENCES

1. Melzack R: The myth of painless childbirth. (John J. Bonica lecture.) Pain 1984; 19: 321–337.
2. Brown ST, Campbell D, Kurtz A: Characteristics of labor pain at two stages of cervical dilation. Pain 1989; 38: 289–295.
3. Bonica JJ: Principles and Practice of Obstetric Analgesia and Anesthesia, vol 2. Philadelphia, FA Davis, 1969.
4. Melzack R, Belanger E: Labour pain: correlations with menstrual pain and acute low-back pain before and during pregnancy. Pain 1989; 36: 225–229.
5. Melzack R, Schaffelberg D: Low-back pain during labor. Am J Obstet Gynecol 1987; 156: 901–905.
6. Melzack R, Kinch R, Dobkin P, et al: Severity of labour pain: influence of physical as well as psychologic variables. Can Med Assoc J 1984; 130: 579–584.
7. Melzack R, Taenzer P, Feldman P, et al: Labour is still painful after prepared childbirth training. Can Med Assoc J 1981; 125: 357–363.
8. Varrassi G, Bazzano C, Edwards WT: Effects of physical activity on maternal plasma beta-endorphin levels and perception of labor pain. Am J Obstet Gynecol 1989; 160: 707–712.
9. American Society of Anesthesiologists: Guidelines for Regional Anesthesia in Obstetrics. Chicago, American Society of Anesthesiologists, 1988.
10. Shnider SM, Abboud TK, Artal R, et al: Maternal catecholamines decrease during labor after lumbar epidural anesthesia. Am J Obstet Gynecol 1983; 147: 13–15.
11. Greiss FC Jr, Crandell DL: Therapy for hypotension induced by spinal anesthesia during pregnancy: observations on gravid ewes. JAMA 1965; 191: 793–796.
12. Collins KM, Bevan DR, Beard RW: Fluid loading to reduce abnormalities of fetal heart rate and maternal hypotension during epidural analgesia in labour. Br Med J 1978; 2: 1460–1461.
13. Leighton BL, Norris MC, Sosis M, et al: Limitations of epinephrine as a marker of intravascular injection in laboring women. Anesthesiology 1987; 66: 688–691.
14. Norris MC, Grieco WM, Arkoosh VA: Maternal and fetal effects of isoproterenol in the gravid ewe. Presented at the Annual Meeting of the Society for Obstetric Anesthesiology and Perinatology, Palm Springs, CA, May 6, 1993.
15. Hood DD, Dewan DM, James FM III: Maternal and fetal effects of epinephrine in gravid ewes. Anesthesiology 1986; 64: 610–613.
16. Colonna-Romano P, Lingaraju N, Godfrey SD, et al: Epidural test dose and intravascular injection in obstetrics: sensitivity, specificity, and lowest effective dose. Anesth Analg 1992; 75: 372–376.
17. Gieraerts R, Van Zundert A, De Wolf A, et al: Ten ml bupivacaine 0.125% with 12.5 micrograms epinephrine is a reliable epidural test dose to detect inadvertent intravascular injection in obstetric patients. A double-blind study. Acta Anaesthesiol Scand 1992; 36: 656–659.
18. Leighton BL, Gross JB: Air: an effective indicator of intravenously located epidural catheters. Anesthesiology 1989; 71: 848–851.
19. Roetman KJ, Eisenach JC: Evaluation of lidocaine as an intravenous test dose for epidural anesthesia. (Abstract.) Anesthesiology 1988; 69: A669.
20. Abraham RA, Harris AP, Maxwell LG, et al: The efficacy of 1.5% lidocaine with 7.5% dextrose and epinephrine as an epidural test dose for obstetrics. Anesthesiology 1986; 64: 116–119.
21. Rolbin SH, Cole AF, Hew EM, et al: Effect of lateral position and volume on the spread of epidural anaesthesia in the parturient. Can Anaesth Soc J 1981; 28: 431–435.
22. Bleyaert A, Soetens M, Vaes L, et al: Bupivacaine, 0.125 per cent, in obstetric epidural analgesia: experience in three thousand cases. Anesthesiology 1979; 51: 435–438.
23. Lysak SZ, Eisenach JC, Dobson CE II: Patient-controlled epidural analgesia during labor: a comparison of three solutions with a continuous infusion control. Anesthesiology 1990; 72: 44–49.
24. Eddleston JM, Maresh M, Horsman EL, et al: Comparison of the maternal and fetal effects associated with intermittent or continuous infusion of extradural analgesia. Br J Anaesth 1992; 69: 154–158.
25. Bogod DG, Rosen M, Rees GA: Extradural infusion of 0.125% bupivacaine at 10 ml h^{-1} to women during labour. Br J Anaesth 1987; 59: 325–330.
26. Li DF, Rees GA, Rosen M: Continuous extradural infusion of 0.0625% or 0.125% bupivacaine for pain relief in primigravid labour. Br J Anaesth 1985; 57: 264–270.
27. Evans KR, Carrie LE: Continuous epidural infusion of bupivacaine in labour: a simple method. Anaesthesia 1979; 34: 310–315.
28. Abboud TK, Afrasiabi A, Sarkis F, et al: Continuous infusion epidural analgesia in parturients receiving bupivacaine, chloroprocaine, or lidocaine—maternal, fetal, and neonatal effects. Anesth Analg 1984; 63: 421–428.
29. Gambling DR, Yu P, Cole C, et al: A comparative study of patient controlled epidural analgesia (PCEA) and continuous infusion epidural analgesia (CIEA) during labour. Can J Anaesth 1988; 35: 249–254.
30. Ferrante FM, Lu L, Jamison SB, et al: Patient-controlled epidural analgesia: demand dosing. Anesth Analg 1991; 73: 547–552.
31. Viscomi C, Eisenach JC: Patient-controlled epidural analgesia during labor. Obstet Gynecol 1991; 77: 348–351.
32. Bromage PR: A comparison of the hydrochloride and carbon dioxide salts of lidocaine and prilocaine in epidural analgesia. Acta Anaesthesiol Scand Suppl 1965; 16: 55–69.
33. Van Zundert A, Vaes L, Soetens M, et al: Measuring motor blockade during lumbar epidural analgesia for vaginal delivery. Obstet Anesth Dig 1984; 4: 31–34.
34. Bieniarz J, Branda LA, Maqueda E, et al: Aortocaval compression by the uterus in late pregnancy. 3. Unreliability of the sphygmomanometric method in estimating urine artery pressure. Am J Obstet Gynecol 1968; 102: 1106–1115.
35. Matouskova A, Hanson B, Rosmark U: Continuous mini-infusion of bupivacaine into the epidural space during labor. Part I: Radiographic visualization of the epidural catheters. Acta Obstet Gynecol Scand Suppl 1979; 83: 15–29.
36. Matouskova A, Dottori O, Forssman L, et al: An improved method of epidural analgesia with reduced instrumental delivery rate. Acta Obstet Gynecol Scand 1975; 54: 231–235.
37. Ducrow M: The occurrence of unblocked segments during continuous lumbar epidural analgesia for pain relief in labour. Br J Anaesth 1971; 43: 1172–1174.
38. Stein A: Epidural catheters gone astray: Can they be saved? Presented at the Annual Meeting of the Society for Obstetric Anesthesiology and Perinatology, Charleston, SC, May 7, 1992.
39. Writer WD, James FM III, Wheeler AS: Double-blind comparison of morphine and bupivacaine for continuous epidural analgesia in labor. Anesthesiology 1981; 54: 215–219.
40. Cohen SE, Tan S, Albright GA, et al: Epidural fentanyl/bupivacaine mixtures for obstetric analgesia. Anesthesiology 1987; 67: 403–407.
41. Hughes SC, Rosen MA, Shnider SM, et al: Maternal and neonatal effects of epidural morphine for labor and delivery. Anesth Analg 1984; 63: 319–324.
42. Husemeyer RP, O'Connor MC, Davenport HT: Failure of epidural morphine to relieve pain in labour. Anaesthesia 1980; 35: 161–163.

43. Camann WR, Denney RA, Holby ED, et al: A comparison of intrathecal, epidural, and intravenous sufentanil for labor analgesia. Anesthesiology 1992; 77: 884–887.

44. Phillips G: Continuous infusion epidural analgesia in labor: the effect of adding sufentanil to 0.125% bupivacaine. Anesth Analg 1988; 67: 462–465.

45. Celleno D, Capogna G: Epidural fentanyl plus bupivacaine 0.125 per cent for labour: analgesic effects. Can J Anaesth 1988; 35: 375–378.

46. Hunt CO, Naulty JS, Malinow AM, et al: Epidural butorphanol-bupivacaine for analgesia during labor and delivery. Anesth Analg 1989; 68: 323–327.

47. Edwards ND, Hartley M, Clyburn P, et al: Epidural pethidine and bupivacaine in labour. Anaesthesia 1992; 47: 435–437.

48. Reynolds F, O'Sullivan G: Epidural fentanyl and perineal pain in labour. Anaesthesia 1989; 44: 341–344.

49. Justins DM, Francis D, Houlton PG, et al: A controlled trial of extradural fentanyl in labour. Br J Anaesth 1982; 54: 409–414.

50. Sinatra RS, Goldstein R, Sevarino FB: The clinical effectiveness of epidural bupivacaine, bupivacaine with lidocaine, and bupivacaine with fentanyl for labor analgesia. J Clin Anesth 1991; 3: 219–224.

51. Vertommen JD, Vandermeulen E, Van Aken H, et al: The effects of the addition of sufentanil to 0.125% bupivacaine on the quality of analgesia during labor and on the incidence of instrumental deliveries. Anesthesiology 1991; 74: 809–814.

52. Chestnut DH, Owen CL, Bates JN, et al: Continuous infusion epidural analgesia during labor: a randomized, double-blind comparison of 0.0625% bupivacaine/0.0002% fentanyl versus 0.125% bupivacaine. Anesthesiology 1988; 68: 754–759.

53. Murphy JD, Henderson K, Bowden MI, et al: Bupivacaine versus bupivacaine plus fentanyl for epidural analgesia: effect on maternal satisfaction. Br Med J 1991; 302: 564–567.

54. Society for Obstetric Anesthesia and Perinatology: Program Abstracts and Membership Directory, p 132. Chicago, Society for Obstetric Anesthesia and Perinatology, 1993.

55. Yarnell RW, Ewing DA, Tierney E, et al: Sacralization of epidural block with repeated doses of 0.25% bupivacaine during labor. Reg Anesth 1990; 15: 275–279.

56. Willdeck-Lund G, Lindmark G, Nilsson BA: Effect of segmental epidural analgesia upon the uterine activity with special reference to the use of different local anaesthetic agents. Acta Anaesthesiol Scand 1979; 23: 519–528.

57. Thorp JA, Hu DH, Albin RM, et al: The effect of intrapartum epidural analgesia on nulliparous labor: a randomized, controlled, prospective trial. Am J Obstet Gynecol 1993; 169: 851–858.

58. Craft JB Jr, Epstein BS, Coakley CS: Effect of lidocaine with epinephrine versus lidocaine (plain) on induced labor. Anesth Analg 1972; 51: 243–246.

59. Behrens O, Goeschen K, Luck HJ, et al: Effects of lumbar epidural analgesia on prostaglandin F2 alpha release and oxytocin secretion during labor. Prostaglandins 1993; 45: 285–296.

60. Cheek TG, Samuels P, Tobin M, et al: Rapid intravenous saline infusion decreases uterine activity in labor: epidural analgesia does not. (Abstract.) Anesthesiology 1989; 71: A884.

61. Diro M, Beydoun SN: Segmental epidural analgesia in labor: a matched control study. J Natl Med Assoc 1985; 77: 569–573.

62. Thorp JA, Parisi VM, Boylan PC, et al: The effect of continuous epidural analgesia on cesarean section for dystocia in nulliparous women. Am J Obstet Gynecol 1989; 161: 670–675.

63. Thorp JA, Eckert LO, Ang MS, et al: Epidural analgesia and cesarean section for dystocia: risk factors in nulliparas. Am J Perinatol 1991; 8: 402–410.

64. Philipsen T, Jensen NH: Epidural block or parenteral pethidine as analgesic in labour; a randomized study concerning progress in labour and instrumental deliveries. Eur J Obstet Gynecol Reprod Biol 1989; 30: 27–33.

65. Larson DD: The effect of initiating an obstetric anesthesiology service on rate of cesarean section and rate of forceps delivery. Presented at the Annual Meeting of the Society for Obstetric Anesthesiology and Perinatology, Charleston, SC, May 8, 1992.

66. Mancuso JJ: Epidural analgesia in an army medical center: impact on cesarean and instrumental vaginal deliveries. Presented at the Annual Meeting of the Society for Obstetric Anesthesiology and Perinatology, Palm Springs, CA, May 6, 1993.

67. Floberg J, Belfrage P, Ohlsen H: Influence of the pelvic outlet capacity on fetal head presentation at delivery. Acta Obstet Gynecol Scand 1987; 66: 127–130.

68. Read MD, Hunt LP, Anderson JM, et al: Epidural block and the progress and outcome of labour. J Obstet Gynaecol 1983; 4: 35–39.

69. Chestnut DH, McGrath JM, Vincent RD Jr, et al: Does early administration of epidural analgesia affect obstetric outcome in nulliparous women who are in spontaneous labor? Anesthesiology 1994; 80: 1201–1208.

70. Chestnut DH, Vincent RD Jr, McGrath JM, et al: Does early administration of epidural analgesia affect obstetric outcome in nulliparous women who are receiving intravenous oxytocin? Anesthesiology 1994; 80: 1193–1200.

71. Breen TW, Shapiro T, Glass B, et al: Epidural anesthesia for labor in an ambulatory patient. Anesth Analg 1993; 77: 919–924.

72. Hoult IJ, MacLennan AH, Carrie LE: Lumbar epidural analgesia in labour: relation to fetal malposition and instrumental delivery. Br Med J 1977; 1: 14–16.

73. Jouppila R, Jouppila P, Karinen JM, et al: Segmental epidural analgesia in labour: related to the progress of labour, fetal malposition and instrumental delivery. Acta Obstet Gynecol Scand 1979; 58: 135–139.

74. Chestnut DH, Laszewski LJ, Pollack KL, et al: Continuous epidural infusion of 0.0625% bupivacaine–0.0002% fentanyl during the second stage of labor. Anesthesiology 1990; 72: 613–618.

75. Chestnut DH, Vandewalker GE, Owen CL, et al: The influence of continuous epidural bupivacaine analgesia on the second stage of labor and method of delivery in nulliparous women. Anesthesiology 1987; 66: 774–780.

76. Goodfellow CF, Hull MG, Swaab DF, et al: Oxytocin deficiency at delivery with epidural analgesia. Br J Obstet Gynaecol 1983; 90: 214–219.

77. Moon JM, Smith CV, Rayburn WF: Perinatal outcome after a prolonged second stage of labor. J Reprod Med 1990; 35: 229–231.

78. Reynolds JL, Yudkin PL: Changes in the management of labour: 1. Length and management of the second stage. Can Med Assoc J 1987; 136: 1041–1045.

79. American College of Obstetricians and Gynecologists: Dystocia. In ACOG Technical Bulletin, no. 112. Washington, DC, American College of Obstetricians and Gynecologists, December 1989.

80. Baraka A, Noueihid R, Hajj S: Intrathecal injection of morphine for obstetric analgesia. Anesthesiology 1981; 54: 136–140.

81. Abboud TK, Shnider SM, Dailey PA, et al: Intrathecal administration of hyperbaric morphine for the relief of pain in labour. Br J Anaesth 1984; 56: 1351–1360.

82. Leicht CH, Evans DE, Durkan WJ, et al: Sufentanil vs fentanyl intrathecally for labor analgesia. (Abstract.) Anesth Analg 1991; 72: S159.

83. Grieco WM, Norris MC, Leighton BL, et al: Intrathecal sufentanil labor analgesia: the effects of adding morphine or epinephrine. Anesth Analg 1993; 77: 1149–1154.

84. McQuay HJ, Sullivan AF, Smallman K, et al: Intrathecal opioids, potency and lipophilicity. Pain 1989; 36: 111–115.

85. Zakowski MI, Goldstein MJ, Ramanathan S, et al: Intrathecal fentanyl for labor analgesia. (Abstract.) Anesthesiology 1991; 75: A840.

86. Benson JS: FDA Safety Alert: Cauda Equina Syndrome Associated With Use of Small-Bore Catheters in Continuous Spinal Anesthesia. Rockville, MD, Food and Drug Administration, May 29, 1992.

87. Leighton BL, DeSimone CA, Norris MC, et al: Intrathecal narcotics for labor revisited: the combination of fentanyl and morphine intrathecally provides rapid onset of profound, prolonged analgesia. Anesth Analg 1989; 69: 122–125.

88. Pollack KL, Chestnut DH, Wenstrom KD: Anesthetic management of a parturient with Eisenmenger's syndrome. Anesth Analg 1990; 70: 212–215.

89. McHale S, Mitchell V, Howsam S, et al: Continuous subarachnoid infusion of 0.125% bupivacaine for analgesia during labour. Br J Anaesth 1992; 69: 634–636.

90. Abouleish E, Rawal N, Shaw J, et al: Intrathecal morphine 0.2 mg versus epidural bupivacaine 0.125% or their combination: effects on parturients. Anesthesiology 1991; 74: 711–716.

91. Cohen SE, Cherry CM, Holbrook RH Jr, et al: Intrathecal sufentanil for labor analgesia—sensory changes, side effects, and fetal heart rate changes. Anesth Analg 1993; 77: 1155–1160.

92. Shnider SM, Levinson G, Ralston DH: Regional anesthesia for labor and delivery. In Shnider SM, Levinson G (eds): Anesthesia for Obstetrics, 3rd ed, pp 135–155. Baltimore, Williams & Wilkins, 1993.

93. Hunter CA Jr: Uterine motility studies during labor: observations on bilateral sympathetic nerve block in the normal and abnormal first stage of labor. Am J Obstet Gynecol 1963; 85: 681–685.

94. Augustinsson LE, Bohlin P, Bundsen P, et al: Pain relief during delivery by transcutaneous electrical nerve stimulation. Pain 1977; 4: 59–65.

95. Bundsen P, Peterson LE, Selstam U: Pain relief in labor by transcutaneous electrical nerve stimulation. A prospective matched study. Acta Obstet Gynecol Scand 1981; 60: 459–468.

96. Lytzen T, Cederberg L, Moller-Nielsen J: Relief of low back pain in labor by using intracutaneous nerve stimulation (INS) with sterile water papules. Acta Obstet Gynecol Scand 1989; 68: 341–343.

97. Trolle B, Moller M, Kronborg H, et al: The effect of sterile water blocks on low back labor pain. Am J Obstet Gynecol 1991; 164: 1277–1281.

98. Shnider SM, Asling JH, Holl JW, et al: Paracervical block anesthesia in obstetrics. I. Fetal complications and neonatal morbidity. Am J Obstet Gynecol 1970; 107: 619–625.

99. Goins JR: Experience with mepivacaine paracervical block in an obstetric private practice. Am J Obstet Gynecol 1992; 167: 342–344.

100. Rogers RE: Fetal bradycardia associated with paracervical block anesthesia in labor. Am J Obstet Gynecol 1970; 106: 913–916.

101. Asling JH, Shnider SM, Margolis AJ, et al: Paracervical block anesthesia in obstetrics. II. Etiology of fetal bradycardia following paracervical block anesthesia. Am J Obstet Gynecol 1970; 107: 626–634.

102. Shnider SM, Asling JH, Margolis AJ, et al: High fetal blood levels of mepivacaine and fetal bradycardia. (Letter to the editor.) N Engl J Med 1968; 279: 947–948.

103. Fishburne JI Jr, Greiss FC Jr, Hopkinson R, et al: Responses of the gravid uterine vasculature to arterial levels of local anesthetic agents. Am J Obstet Gynecol 1979; 133: 753–757.

104. Morishima HO, Covino BG, Yeh MN, et al: Bradycardia in the fetal baboon following paracervical block anesthesia. Am J Obstet Gynecol 1981; 140: 775–780.

105. Noren H, Lindblom B, Kallfelt B: Effects of bupivacaine and calcium antagonists on the rat uterine artery. Acta Anaesthesiol Scand 1991; 35: 77–80.

106. Noren H, Lindblom B, Kallfelt B: Effects of bupivacaine and calcium antagonists on human uterine arteries in pregnant and non-pregnant women. Acta Anaesthesiol Scand 1991; 35: 488–491.

107. Gibbs CP, Noel SC: Response of arterial segments from gravid human uterus to multiple concentrations of lignocaine. Br J Anaesth 1977; 49: 409–412.

108. Day TW: Community use of paracervical block in labor. J Fam Pract 1989; 28: 545–550.

109. Carlsson BM, Johansson M, Westin B: Fetal heart rate pattern before and after paracervical anesthesia. A prospective study. Acta Obstet Gynecol Scand 1987; 66: 391–395.

110. Seager SJ, Macdonald R: Laryngeal oedema and pre-eclampsia. Anaesthesia 1980; 35: 360–362.

111. Keeri-Szanto M: Laryngeal oedema complicating obstetric anaesthesia. (Letter to the editor.) Anaesthesia 1978; 33: 272.

112. Hodgkinson R, Husain FJ, Hayashi RH: Systemic and pulmonary blood pressure during caesarean section in parturients with gestational hypertension. Can Anaesth Soc J 1980; 27: 389–394.

113. Gutsche BB, Cheek TG: Anesthetic considerations in pre-eclampsia-eclampsia. In Shnider SM, Levinson G (eds): Anesthesia for Obstetrics, 3rd ed, pp 305–336. Baltimore, Williams & Wilkins, 1993.

114. Ramos-Santos E, Devoe LD, Wakefield ML, et al: The effects of epidural anesthesia on the Doppler velocimetry of umbilical and uterine arteries in normal and hypertensive patients during active term labor. Obstet Gynecol 1991; 77: 20–26.

115. Jouppila P, Jouppila R, Hollmen A, et al: Lumbar epidural analgesia to improve intervillous blood flow during labor in severe preeclampsia. Obstet Gynecol 1982; 59: 158–161.

116. Ramanathan J, Sibai BM, Vu T, et al: Correlation between bleeding times and platelet counts in women with preeclampsia undergoing cesarean section. Anesthesiology 1989; 71: 188–191.

117. Lind SE: The bleeding time does not predict surgical bleeding. Blood 1991; 77: 2547–2552.

118. Lao TT, Halpern SH, MacDonald D, et al: Spinal subdural haematoma in a parturient after attempted epidural anaesthesia. Can J Anaesth 1993; 40: 340–345.

119. Hood DD, Dewan DM: Anesthetic and obstetric outcome in morbidly obese parturients. Anesthesiology 1993; 79: 1210–1218.

120. Webster SG: Migration of epidural catheters. (Letter to the editor.) Anaesthesia 1986; 41: 654.

121. Beischer NA, Mackay EV, Purcal NK: Care of the Pregnant Woman and Her Baby, 2nd ed, pp 111–120. Sydney, WB Saunders/Baillière Tindall, 1989.

122. Russell KP, Niebyl JR: Eastman's Expectant Motherhood, 8th ed, pp 137–153. Boston, Little, Brown & Co, 1989.

123. Guzman Sanchez A, Segura Ortega L, Panduro Baron JG: Psychological reaction due to failure using the Lamaze method. Int J Gynaecol Obstet 1985; 23: 343–346.

124. American College of Obstetricians and Gynecologists: Obstetric anesthesia and analgesia. In ACOG Technical Bulletin, no. 112. Washington, DC, American College of Obstetricians and Gynecologists, 1988.

125. Rayburn W, Leuschen MP, Earl R, et al: Intravenous meperidine during labor: a randomized comparison between nursing- and patient-controlled administration. Obstet Gynecol 1989; 74: 702–706.

126. Rayburn WF, Smith CV, Parriott JE, et al: Randomized comparison of meperidine and fentanyl during labor. Obstet Gynecol 1989; 74: 604–606.

127. Akamatsu TJ, Bonica JJ, Rehmet R, et al: Experiences with the use of ketamine for parturition. I. Primary anesthetic for vaginal delivery. Anesth Analg 1974; 53: 284–287.

128. Jones PL, Rosen M, Mushin WW, et al: Methoxyflurane and nitrous oxide as obstetric analgesics. I. A comparison by continuous administration. Br Med J 1969; 3: 255–259.

129. Rosen M, Mushin WW, Jones PL, et al: Field trial of methoxyflurane, nitrous oxide, and trichloroethylene as obstetric analgesics. Br Med J 1969; 3: 263–267.

130. Holdcroft A, Morgan M: An assessment of the analgesic effect in labour of pethidine and 50 per cent nitrous oxide in oxygen (Entonox). J Obstet Gynaecol Br Commonw 1974; 81: 603–607.

131. Anonymous. Clinical trials of different concentrations of oxygen and nitrous oxide for obstetric analgesia. Report to the Medical Research Council of the Committee on Nitrous Oxide and Oxygen Analgesia in Midwifery. Br Med J 1970; 1: 709–713.

132. Waud BE, Waud DR: Calculated kinetics of distribution of nitrous oxide and methoxyflurane during intermittent administration in obstetrics. Anesthesiology 1970; 32: 306–316.

133. Abboud TK, Shnider SM, Wright RG, et al: Enflurane analgesia in obstetrics. Anesth Analg 1981; 60: 133–137.

134. McLeod DD, Ramayya GP, Tunstall ME: Self-administered isoflurane in labour. A comparative study with Entonox. Anaesthesia 1985; 40: 424–426.

135. Wee MY, Hasan MA, Thomas TA: Isoflurane in labour. Anaesthesia 1993; 48: 369–372.

136. Pain relief during labor. In Joint Statement of the American College of Obstetricians and Gynecologists and the American Society of Anesthesiologists, 1992.

CHAPTER 35
Cesarean Section Anesthesia

M. Joanne Douglas, M.D., F.R.C.P.C.

During the 1970s, the rate at which cesarean sections were performed increased dramatically in most countries. The only country to show a decrease in its rate since that time is Sweden.[1] The rate for 1979 to 1981 in the United States was 16.9 per 100 hospital births, increasing to 23.6 per 100 hospital births in 1989 to 1990.[2] The most common reasons for cesarean section are elective, repeat cesarean section; dystocia (cephalopelvic disproportion, failure to progress in labor); abnormal presentation, such as breech or transverse lie; fetal distress; and problems such as abnormal placentation (placenta previa) or uterine abnormalities.

Efforts to decrease the cesarean section rate have focused on challenging the dictum "once a cesarean always a cesarean."[3-5] As trial of labor after cesarean section becomes a more common practice, it is reasonable to anticipate a decline in the cesarean section rate.

Physiologic Changes in Pregnancy and Their Impact on Anesthesia

The anesthetic choice, drug requirement, and variation in technique are affected by the physiologic changes in pregnancy (Table 35–1). Although some of these changes have greater implications for general anesthesia, an inadequate block and complications arising during regional anesthesia may result in a need for rapid induction of general anesthesia.

Oxygen consumption increases steadily throughout gestation.[6] A concomitant decrease in functional residual capacity and residual volume[6] makes the parturient prone to desaturation during apnea,[7] which is worsened by obesity[8] and the supine position. It is essential to preoxygenate the patient before induction of general anesthesia, which can be accomplished by 3 min of breathing 100% oxygen or four vital capacity breaths of 100% oxygen.[9]

Hyperventilation begins early in pregnancy, with an increase of 50% in minute ventilation by term.[6] This increase is greater than would be expected from the increase in oxygen consumption, body weight, or basal metabolic rate and may predispose the parturient to dyspnea during regional anesthesia. Interstitial lung water may be increased at term,[10] which increases the risk of hypoxemia, pulmonary edema, and aspiration pneumonitis after pulmonary aspiration. Supplemental oxygen by nasal prongs or face mask during regional anesthesia benefits the mother and the fetus.[11, 12]

Of greater significance are changes to the maternal airway. Fat deposition is altered during pregnancy, with additional fat in the area of the neck and breasts, potentially increasing the difficulty of positioning for intubation. The nasopharyngeal congestion results in an airway that may be narrowed and mucosa that may be more friable. The airway must be assessed before induction of general anesthesia, even if this was done previously, because it may change during labor.[13]

Reflux of gastric contents into the esophagus depends on the relationships among gastric pressure, lower esophageal sphincter tone, esophageal pressure, and upper esophageal sphincter tone.[14] Gastric pressure is increased during pregnancy as a result of pressure from the enlarging uterus. There is a high incidence of gastroesophageal reflux in late pregnancy.[15] Gastric emptying is normal in late pregnancy[16, 17] but may be delayed by labor,[18] especially if opioids have been administered.[19] This applies to parenteral and epidural opioids.[20, 21] Because of the high incidence of gastroesophageal reflux, all parturients must be con-

Table 35–1 Physiologic Changes in Pregnancy and Their Anesthetic Implications

PHYSIOLOGIC CHANGE	MATERNAL IMPLICATION	ANESTHETIC IMPLICATION
↑ Oxygen consumption	Prone to desaturation	Preoxygenation for GA
↓ FRC, ↓ RV	Dyspnea	Induction GA more rapid
Hyperventilation		Supplemental O₂ for regional anesthesia
↑ Vascularity of nasopharynx	NP congestion	Difficult intubation
	Laryngeal edema with preeclampsia	
↑ Fat in breasts and neck		
↑ Cardiac output	CHF cardiac patient	↑ Induction GA
↓ Vascular resistance	Prone to ↓ BP	↓ BP with regional
↑ Vasomotor response		↑ Intravenous fluid bolus
↑ Aortocaval compression	↓ BP when supine	LUD
	↑ Vascularity of epidural space	More difficult to resuscitate
		↑ Risk venous cannulation
↑ Sensitivity of nervous tissue		↓ MAC
		↓ LA dose
↑ Gastric pressure	"Heartburn"	↑ Risk pulmonary aspiration
↓ LES tone		
↓ Gastric emptying		↑ Risk maternal mortality

BP, blood pressure; CHF, congestive heart failure; FRC, functional residual capacity; GA, general anesthesia; LA, local anesthetic; LES, lower esophageal sphincter; LUD, left uterine displacement; MAC, minimum alveolar concentration; NP, nasopharyngeal; RV, residual volume.

sidered at risk for pulmonary aspiration of gastric contents and appropriate precautions must be taken.

Cardiac output increases steadily throughout gestation, plateauing at about 26 to 30 weeks.[6] In the uncomplicated pregnancy, this is of little significance, but in the parturient with cardiac disease, congestive heart failure may develop. The combination of decreased functional residual capacity and residual volume and increased minute ventilation and cardiac output results in a more rapid uptake of volatile anesthetics and a more rapid induction of anesthesia.

In normal pregnancy, blood pressure decreases during the second trimester as a result of a decrease in systemic and pulmonary vascular resistance. This decrease in vascular resistance, combined with a greater maternal dependence on vasomotor response[22] to maintain blood pressure, results in a more profound response to sympathectomy during regional anesthesia. This underlines the rationale for administration of a fluid bolus before regional anesthesia.

In a pregnant patient, the uterus causes aortocaval compression, which may result in maternal hypotension if the parturient is placed supine[23] (Fig. 35–1). During cesarean section, it is important to displace the uterus by rotating the operating room table to the left or placing a wedge under the right hip.[24, 25] It has also been suggested that the lateral (tightly curled) position for insertion of an epidural catheter may cause aortocaval compression.[26]

Compression of the vena cava accentuates venous engorgement in the epidural space, decreasing its capacity for local anesthetic and increasing the risk of venous cannulation during epidural catheter insertion.

Pregnancy increases the sensitivity of nervous tissue to the effects of local and general anesthetics.[27–29] As a result, there is a decreased anesthetic requirement (lower minimum alveolar concentration) during general anesthesia and an increased risk of local anesthetic systemic toxicity.[30]

To offset the risk of hemorrhage at birth, there is an increase in factors V, VIII, and X and in fibrinogen, with a concomitant decrease in fibrinolytic factors.

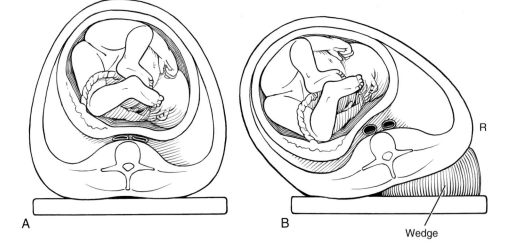

Figure 35–1 Importance of left uterine displacement in the supine position. *A,* The undisplaced uterus is compressing the aorta and inferior vena cava. *B,* The uterus is displaced to the left, with no compression of the aorta and inferior vena cava. R, right.

This, combined with stasis from the pregnant uterus compressing pelvic veins, increases the risk of thromboembolic disease. Parturients who are at risk for thromboembolism are those with a history of thromboembolic disease; a deficiency of protein S, C, or antithrombin III; or lupus anticoagulant antibodies. Prophylactic, subcutaneous injection of heparin is frequently ordered for these patients to prevent thromboembolic disease. The dose of heparin is designed to maintain the activated partial thromboplastin time within the normal range. Heparin is generally considered a contraindication to regional anesthesia, but many anesthesiologists feel comfortable offering it to these patients, providing there is no evidence of bleeding or bruising.

A decrease in the albumin level and changes in hepatic metabolism and renal function alter protein binding, metabolism, and clearance of certain drugs.[6] The decreased albumin level affects the binding of acidic drugs (e.g., salicylates, anticonvulsants, benzodiazepines), necessitating an adjustment of dosage during gestation. Hepatic enzyme induction by progesterone speeds elimination of some drugs, and increases in renal plasma flow and glomerular filtration rate increase the clearance of drugs such as pancuronium. A decrease in plasma cholinesterase lengthens recovery times from succinylcholine and 2-chloroprocaine, mainly in the postpartum period.[31]

Certain pregnancy-related conditions also affect anesthesia. Preeclampsia-induced laryngeal edema may interfere with intubation,[32, 33] but a shift of the P_{50} value to the left with preeclampsia decreases the release of oxygen to the tissues.[34]

Placental Transfer of Anesthetic Agents and Fetal and Neonatal Effects

Although the placenta serves as an interface between the mother and her fetus, most drugs administered to the mother reach the fetus. Lipid solubility is the main determinant of placental transfer, but the concentration of drug at the placental site determines the degree of fetal exposure.[35]

Measurement of plasma drug concentration in the mother and newborn by sampling the umbilical artery, umbilical vein, and maternal vein provides an estimate of fetal drug exposure. Measurement of uteroplacental blood flow and of fetal umbilical and aortic blood flow velocity with Doppler ultrasonography has been used to determine the effects of anesthetic techniques (Table 35–2).

Neonatal Apgar scores and acid-base status provide an indirect measure of drug effect. Testing of newborns for subtle drug effects has focused on the neonates' muscle tone and their response to certain stimuli. These neurobehavioral scoring systems are the Brazelton Neonatal Behavioral Assessment Scale, Scanlon Early Neonatal Neurobehavioral Scale, and the Neurologic and Adaptive Capacity Score of Amiel-Tison. The last test is the easiest to perform and more

Table 35–2 Effects of Regional Anesthesia for Cesarean Section on Uteroplacental and Fetal Circulations

ANESTHETIC	BLOOD FLOW	EFFECT	REFERENCE
Epidural	Uteroplacental	None	Alahuhta et al[36]
			Long et al[37]
		Impaired	Baumann et al[38]
	Fetal	None	Alahuhta et al[36]
			Lindblad et al[39]
	Uterine and umbilical	None	Marx et al[40]
			Morrow et al[41]
			Veille et al[42]
		Beneficial	Giles et al[43]
Spinal	Umbilical artery	None	Fairlie et al[44]
	Placental	None	Jouppila et al[45]

closely examines motor tone, a factor more likely affected by anesthetic agents.[46]

Local anesthetics are weak bases, and their placental transfer is enhanced by fetal hypoxia and acidosis. Bupivacaine, the most highly protein bound of the local anesthetics, has limited placental transfer, but it can still be detected in the newborn urine for 36 h after delivery (Fig. 35–2).[46] Lidocaine is less protein bound than bupivacaine, making more drug available for transfer. 2-Chloroprocaine is rapidly metabolized by plasma cholinesterase, limiting its placental transfer and neonatal effects. Neurobehavioral studies of the newborns after epidural anesthesia with these local anesthetics find subtle effects that are probably of no clinical significance.[46] Ropivacaine, a new amide local anesthetic, is under review for use in obstetric anesthesia. It produces less motor block and probably has fewer cardiac effects than bupivacaine during a systemic toxic reaction.[47]

Anesthetic induction agents such as thiopental, ketamine, propofol, diazepam, and midazolam readily cross the placenta and can be detected within minutes in the umbilical venous blood.[35] Thiopental is still considered

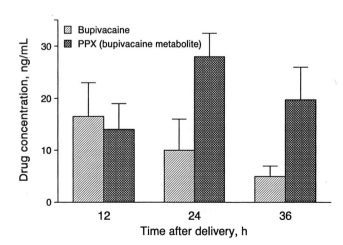

Figure 35–2 Neonatal excretion of bupivacaine and 2,6-piperolylxylidine (PPX) for 36 h after spinal anesthesia for delivery (mean ± SEM). (Redrawn from Kuhnert BR, Zuspan KJ, Kuhnert PM, et al: Bupivacaine disposition in mother, fetus and neonate after spinal anesthesia for cesarean section. Anesth Analg 1987; 66: 407–412.)

the standard induction agent for cesarean section, because the other agents fail to demonstrate any advantage in neonatal outcome. The benzodiazepines (diazepam, midazolam) reduce neonatal performance, as indicated by muscle tone and temperature regulation.

Nitrous oxide is used to supplement the volatile anesthetic agents during general anesthesia. It crosses the placenta rapidly,[35] and its effects on the neonate are related to the duration of intrapartum exposure. Volatile anesthetic agents also cross the placenta easily and may decrease neonatal performance. Neonates born after general anesthesia have a higher incidence of lower Apgar scores than those born after regional anesthesia.[48] Induction to delivery time appears to be an important variable for general anesthesia, and uterine incision to delivery time is important for regional anesthesia.[49]

The neuromuscular blocking agents are highly ionized and do not readily cross the placenta.[35]

Most anesthetic agents are transmitted to the infant through breast milk but appear to have little influence on the neonate. An exception to this is meperidine, which administered in repeated doses has caused significant neurobehavioral depression.[50]

Maternal Complications During Anesthesia for Cesarean Section

Maternal Mortality

The major cause of anesthesia-related maternal mortality is difficult intubation, with or without pulmonary aspiration of gastric contents. The Confidential Enquiry Into Maternal Deaths in the United Kingdom for 1988 to 1990[51] listed 5 maternal deaths directly related to anesthesia and an additional 10 in which anesthesia was a contributory factor (Tables 35–3 and 35–4). Of these 15, 9 were linked to anesthesia for cesarean section (3 of the 5 direct deaths). Respiratory complications (difficulty with intubation, pulmonary aspiration, and adult respiratory distress syndrome) were the major causes of anesthetic-related maternal death (Table 35–3).[52]

In the United States, a survey of anesthesia-related maternal mortality for 1979 to 1990 found 150 deaths.[53] Sixty-eight percent occurred during or shortly after cesarean delivery, and of these deaths, 48% were associated with general anesthesia (aspiration of gastric contents, anoxia due to induction or intubation problems, unspecified cardiac arrest approximately at the time of delivery). Twenty-two percent were related to regional anesthesia (Table 35–5) and resulted from local anesthetic systemic toxicity or high spinal or epidural block. Some of these deaths would have included those attributed to bupivacaine cardiotoxicity. Several common risk factors lead to complications or anesthetic-related deaths, most of which are avoidable (Table 35–6).

Hemorrhage

Hemorrhage is a major risk factor for maternal mortality. Although the parturient is considered to be in a hypercoagulable state, several factors may increase the risk of hemorrhage (Table 35–7).

If the placenta is located over a previous uterine incision, it may be abnormally adherent to the uterine wall (placenta accreta)[54] (Fig. 35–3). In attempting to remove the placenta, severe hemorrhage may occur. The major risk factor for placenta accreta is placenta previa, especially when it is combined with previous cesarean section; the risk increases with each cesarean section. Previous uterine surgery and a history of retained placenta are other risk factors. The anesthesiologist should be prepared to manage massive hemorrhage. Hysterectomy may be required to control the bleeding.[55]

Table 35–3 Causes of Maternal Death Directly Resulting From Anesthesia for Cesarean Section in the United Kingdom

CAUSE	1985–1987	1988–1990
Difficult or failed intubation	5	1
With pulmonary aspiration	0	0
With anoxic cardiac arrest	5	1
Pulmonary aspiration	1	2
Cardiovascular collapse (epidural in patient with aortic insufficiency)	1*	0
Total	7	3

*Regional anesthesia.

Data from Report on Confidential Enquiries Into Maternal Deaths in the United Kingdom 1985–1987 and 1988–1990. London, Her Majesty's Stationery Office, 1991 and 1994.

Table 35–4 Causes of Maternal Mortality in Which Anesthesia for Cesarean Section Contributed in the United Kingdom, 1985–1990

CAUSE	1985–1987	1988–1990
Hemorrhage	2	2
Bronchopneumonia (?aspiration)	0	1
ARDS (?aspiration)	0	2
Failure of postoperative care	4	1
Primary pulmonary hypertension	2	0
Valvular heart disease	1	0
Ischemic heart disease	1	0
Drug related (salbutamol)	1	0
Pheochromocytoma	1	0
Total	12	6

ARDS, adult respiratory distress syndrome.

Data from Report on Confidential Enquiries Into Maternal Deaths in the United Kingdom 1985–1987 and 1988–1990. London, Her Majesty's Stationery Office, 1991 and 1994.

Table 35–5 Risk Factors for Maternal Mortality Associated With Regional Anesthesia

Aspiration
High block
Mismanagement of hypotension
Local anesthetic systemic toxicity

Table 35–6 Risk Factors for Anesthetic-Related Maternal Mortality

Inexperienced anesthesiologist
Lack of adequately trained and experienced help
Failure of communication between obstetrician and anesthesiologist
Inadequate precautions to prevent gastric regurgitation
Substandard postoperative care: inadequate reversal, sedation
Associated factor: inappropriate management of hemorrhage

Data from Report on Confidential Enquiries Into Maternal Deaths in the United Kingdom 1985–1987. London, Her Majesty's Stationery Office, 1991.

The other major cause of massive blood loss during cesarean section is uterine hypotonia or atony. Sometimes, only a small segment of the uterus remains uncontracted, despite the administration of oxytocin. If oxytocin, ergonovine, or both do not cause uterine contraction, prostaglandin $F_{2\alpha}$ may be used. This agent has potent cardiovascular and bronchopulmonary effects and may produce bronchospasm, hypertension, hypotension, and fever.[56–59] Cardiovascular collapse has occurred after an unintentional administration of an overdose.[60]

Debate exists between anesthesiologists and obstetricians about the role of volatile anesthetic agents in uterine hypotonia and blood loss. Several retrospective studies[61, 62] suggested that there is greater blood loss when general anesthesia is used. The possible risk of increased blood loss during general anesthesia with volatile anesthetic agents has to be balanced against the risk of patient awareness of intraoperative events during general anesthesia when these agents are not used.

Certain pregnancy-related conditions, such as prolonged fetal death in utero, amniotic fluid embolism, and abruptio placenta, increase the risk of disseminated intravascular coagulopathy and hemorrhage. Preeclampsia is also associated with coagulation abnormalities. One of the most common is a decrease in the number of platelets. In one study,[63] 55% of patients with hemolysis, elevated liver enzymes, and low platelets (HELLP syndrome) required blood transfusion.

Patients at risk for hemorrhage should have a minimum of two large-bore intravenous catheters and four units of blood crossmatched and readily available. Hys-

Table 35–7 Risk Factors for Hemorrhage at Cesarean Section*

GENERAL FACTORS	SPECIFIC FACTORS
Placenta	Previa, especially anterior
	Accreta
	Abruptio
Uterine hypotonia	Overdistended uterus: large baby, hydramnios, multiple gestation
	History retained placenta
	Prolonged labor
	Chorioamnionitis
Coagulation abnormality	Congenital, DIC, HELLP

*There is debate about the use of general anesthesia.
DIC, disseminated intravascular coagulopathy; HELLP, hemolysis, elevated liver enzymes, low platelets.

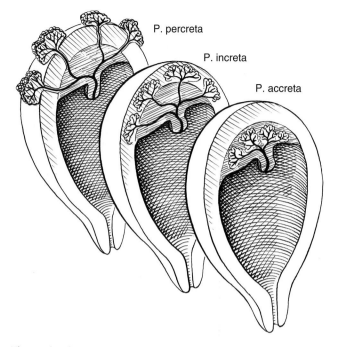

Figure 35–3 Classification of placenta (P.) accreta based on degree of penetration of myometrium. (Redrawn from Kamani AAS, Gambling DR, Christilaw J, et al: Anaesthetic management of patients with placenta accreta. Can J Anaesth 1987; 34; 613–617.)

terectomy may be required to control ongoing blood loss.[55]

Many patients at risk for hemorrhage are donating their own blood (autologous donation) to decrease the risk for viral transmission from donor blood. Risks from this procedure appear to be minimal.[64]

Precordial Doppler Events

In 1987, Malinow and coworkers[65] reported that there was a change in the precordial Doppler signal in approximately 50% of patients during cesarean section while regional anesthesia was being administered. This change occurred at the time of hysterotomy and correlated with complaints of chest pain. They attributed these changes to venous air embolism. These findings have been confirmed, as have the decrease in oxygen saturation and ST segment depression on the electrocardiogram.[66, 67] Although more common during regional anesthesia, these changes also occur during general anesthesia.[66–68] Echocardiography confirms that these embolic events are air emboli.[66] Clinically, these events are usually insignificant, but there are case reports of massive air embolism during cesarean section.[69]

Electrocardiographic Changes

Palmer and colleagues[70] also examined patient complaints of dyspnea and chest pain during regional anesthesia. They correlated these symptoms with electrocardiographic changes that suggested myocardial ischemia. Zakowski and coworkers[71] studied the 12-lead electrocardiogram and plasma levels of myocardial-specific creatine kinase in patients with ST segment abnormalities and concluded that these abnormalities were not caused by myocardial ischemia and were not clinically significant. Spectral analysis of heart rate variability[72] suggested that ST segment depression results from diminished cardiac sympathetic tone.

Amniotic Fluid Embolism

Amniotic fluid embolism is more commonly associated with labor than with cesarean section and has a high incidence of maternal mortality. Quance[73] reported a case of amniotic fluid embolism that occurred 1 min after delivery during cesarean section and was detected by a decrease in oxygen saturation. The patient had no complaints, but an arterial blood gas monitor showed hypoxemia (Pao_2 of 49 mm Hg). After transfer to the intensive care unit, she felt unwell, and cardiac arrest occurred. Sudden cardiovascular collapse and disseminated intravascular coagulopathy are the hallmarks of amniotic fluid embolism, which may occur during cesarean section.

If amniotic fluid embolism is suspected, pulmonary and radial artery catheters should be inserted to monitor hemodynamic changes. Two large-bore intravenous cannulas should also be inserted. Management is aimed at cardiopulmonary resuscitation and specific therapy to support left ventricular function and correct the coagulopathy.

Cardiac Arrest

Cardiac arrest in healthy parturients during cesarean section has been caused by pulmonary embolism or local anesthetic systemic toxicity and has occurred in patients with known or unrecognized cardiac disease such as valvular stenosis, cardiomyopathy, or primary pulmonary hypertension. After reports of cardiac arrest with unintentional intravenous injection of large doses of bupivacaine, attention focused on resuscitation of the parturient. Kasten and Martin[74] found that it was difficult to resuscitate dogs from bupivacaine-induced cardiac arrest when there was partial vena caval occlusion. Because aortocaval compression interferes with venous return to the heart, it is important to displace the uterus to the left during cardiopulmonary resuscitation of the parturient (see Fig. 35–1).[75] If this maneuver is unsuccessful, the fetus should be delivered immediately to facilitate resuscitation.[76]

Unexplained cardiac arrest has occurred during spinal anesthesia in healthy nonpregnant patients approximately 30 min after induction of anesthesia.[77] Most of these patients were reportedly stable before the arrest. The mechanism may be parasympathetic-sympathetic imbalance in the presence of blockade of cardioaccelerator fibers by the spinal anesthetic. Another report described a similar case in a parturient.[78]

Table 35–8 Preoperative Preparation

Assessment	
Mother	Airway; cardiovascular stability
Fetus	Fetal heart rate; position of fetus
Placenta	Location
Neutralize gastric contents	Nonparticulate antacid in all cases; ranitidine or metoclopramide for GA
Position	Left uterine displacement; arrange pillows for intubating position
Assistance	Ensure adequate, trained assistance for cricoid pressure for GA or for positioning for regional anesthesia
Oxygen	Preoxygenation before GA; supplemental O_2 during regional anesthesia
Monitors	NIBP, pulse oximetry, and ECG; end-tidal CO_2 and peripheral nerve stimulator for GA
Intravenous access	At least one large-bore intravenous catheter, minimum size 18-G; if hemorrhage is anticipated, two large-bore catheters

ECG, electrocardiogram; GA, general anesthesia; NIBP, noninvasive blood pressure.

Preoperative Preparation

The pregnancy-related changes necessitate a thorough evaluation of the parturient before selecting an anesthetic technique (Table 35–8).

Maternal Assessment

Even though a regional technique is chosen, it may be necessary to rapidly induce general anesthesia to protect the airway, to augment an inadequate or incomplete block, or because of unanticipated lengthy surgery. Assessment of the airway is therefore mandatory and includes evaluation of mouth opening, teeth (missing, loose, caps), mandibular size and shape, visibility of the pharyngeal structures, mental-hyoid distance, head and neck extension and flexion, and structures which may impact on the airway such as the breasts[79–81] (Table 35–9). The anesthesiologist must have a plan for managing an unexpected difficult or failed intubation (failed intubation drill), because it is not always possible to predict a difficult airway.[79, 82, 83]

Because all parturients are considered at risk for gastroesophageal reflux, it is necessary to ascertain the time of their last food and fluid intake. It may be possible to postpone the operation until ranitidine and

Table 35–9 Risk Factors for Difficult Intubation

Difficulty with visualization of oropharyngeal structures (Mallampati class IV 11.3 times the risk of class I)
Short neck
Obesity
Maxillary incisors: missing, single, protruding all increase risk
Receding mandible

Data from Rocke DA, Murray WB, Rout CC, et al: Relative risk analysis of factors associated with difficult intubation in obstetric anesthesia. Anesthesiology 1992; 77: 67–73.

metoclopramide are effective in raising gastric pH and decreasing gastric volume. The anesthesiologist must ensure that a nonparticulate antacid is administered immediately before induction of regional or general anesthesia.

In addition to a normal preanesthetic evaluation, the anesthesiologist must know if the patient has been on any medications antepartum or intrapartum. Treatment with low-dose aspirin (60 mg) is used to promote fetal growth, to prevent preeclampsia, and for management of antibody-related problems (lupus anticoagulant, anticardiolipin antibodies).[84] Aspirin may also be used in combination with low-dose, prophylactic heparin in patients considered at risk for thromboembolism. Regional anesthesia should not be denied to parturients receiving low-dose aspirin and heparin if there is no clinical evidence of bleeding or bruising.[85, 86] A normal activated partial thromboplastin time measured 3 h after the last dose of heparin is reassuring. In patients with lupus anticoagulant, the activated partial thromboplastin time may be artificially prolonged, but they are not at risk of bleeding.[87]

Other medications of importance to the anesthesiologist are magnesium sulfate, which is used in the management of preeclampsia and preterm labor; calcium channel antagonists (nifedipine) for preterm labor and hypertension; and β-adrenergic agonists (ritodrine, terbutaline) for preterm labor. The anesthetic implications of these medications are listed in Table 35–10.

Fetal Assessment

Fetal assessment is important before induction of anesthesia for cesarean section. If the cesarean is for breech position, this decision should be reevaluated, because the fetus may have changed position to a vertex since the last assessment. The fetal heart rate should also be checked, because in utero fetal death has occurred before cesarean section. If identified preoperatively, legal action can be avoided, and an operative delivery may be circumvented.

Many cesarean sections are performed for fetal distress that occurs during labor. Because the fetal heart rate often recovers during transfer from the labor room to the operating room, the fetal heart should be checked before induction of anesthesia. A normal fetal heart rate may alter the decision for operative birth or allow the patient to have a choice of anesthetic technique.

Assessing the Risk of Hemorrhage

Placental location should be assessed, especially if it is previa in a patient having a repeat cesarean section. Other risk factors should be specifically sought (see Table 35–7).

Maternal Monitoring

Standard monitors for anesthesia for cesarean section include pulse oximetry, blood pressure (noninvasive automatic form preferred), and electrocardiogram. For general anesthesia, a peripheral nerve stimulator and an end-tidal CO_2 monitor are essential. Invasive arterial blood pressure monitoring is useful in parturients with significant cardiac disease (mitral stenosis, aortic stenosis) or severe preeclampsia or who have a high risk of hemorrhage because of placenta previa or placenta accreta. Pulmonary artery catheter monitoring guides fluid management and changing hemodynamics in parturients with a fixed cardiac output, such as those with aortic stenosis or mitral stenosis.

Regional Anesthesia

Regional anesthesia is preferred to general anesthesia, because the awake parturient can maintain her airway, avoid the risks of pulmonary aspiration, and participate in the birth experience (Table 35–11). Regional techniques include epidural, spinal, combined spinal-epidural, and local anesthetic infiltration.

Measurement of Doppler ultrasound velocity is a noninvasive method of assessing the effects of anes-

Table 35–10 Medications Prescribed by Obstetricians and Their Anesthetic Implications

DRUG	CLINICAL USE	ANESTHETIC IMPLICATION
Magnesium sulfate	Tocolysis, preeclampsia	1. Sedation 2. Potentiation of NM block 3. Attenuation of CV response hemorrhage 4. ↓ BP with regional anesthesia (?) 5. Risk of pulmonary edema 6. ↓ Response to oxytocin
Calcium channel antagonists	Antihypertensive, tocolysis	1. CV depression during therapy or during anesthesia with volatile anesthetics 2. ↓ Response to oxytocin (?)
β-Sympathomimetics	Tocolysis	1. Risk of pulmonary edema 2. Tachyarrhythmias
Prostaglandin $F_{2\alpha}$	↑ Uterine tone	1. Pulmonary hypertension 2. Bronchospasm
Nitroglycerin	Antihypertensive, tocolysis	↓ BP if inappropriate fluid resuscitation

CV, cardiovascular; NM, neuromuscular.

Table 35–11 Comparison of Regional Anesthesia and General Anesthesia

VARIABLE	GENERAL ANESTHESIA	REGIONAL ANESTHESIA
Onset time	Rapid	Fast with spinal; slower with epidural
Cardiovascular	↑ BP, HR with intubation	More risk of lowered BP
Maternal participation	None	Awake mother
Postoperative analgesia	Parenteral narcotics	Spinal opioids
Duration of anesthesia	Unlimited	May be limited
Maternal mortality	Greater risk	Less risk

BP, blood pressure; HR, heart rate.

thetic techniques on fetal aortic, umbilical, and maternal uterine artery blood flow velocity. Epidural and spinal anesthesia maintain fetoplacental circulation in the healthy mother, providing there is no hypotension.[36–45, 88] The choice of vasopressor and local anesthetic also has no influence.[41, 89–91]

Complications of Regional Anesthesia for Cesarean Section

Hypotension

Hypotension commonly occurs during spinal and epidural anesthesia. The speed of onset is commonly thought to be more rapid with spinal anesthesia[92] than with incremental epidural injection of the local anesthetic, but not all agree.[93] Hypotension is less common in laboring parturients. Measures used to prevent and to treat hypotension include left uterine displacement, intravenous volume preloading, and judicious use of vasopressors.

Intravenous administration of fluids (20 mL/kg) before initiating the block decreases the severity of hypotension, making it more amenable to treatment with further fluids and vasopressors.[94, 95] In the presence of fetal distress, the physician does not have to wait until the entire volume has been administered before initiating regional anesthesia.[96]

There is no advantage to the use of colloid rather than crystalloid for volume preloading. Rapid infusion of a dextrose-containing solution before delivery of the fetus may result in neonatal hypoglycemia.[97] A non–glucose-containing crystalloid fluid such as isotonic saline or lactated Ringer's should be used.

Neuraxial block should be induced slowly in patients who have been treated with β-adrenergic agonists (ritodrine, terbutaline) and in patients with preeclampsia because these patients are at risk of pulmonary edema developing with excess fluids.

Ephedrine is the most commonly used vasopressor in obstetrics, because it maintains uterine perfusion while increasing blood pressure.[98–100] Until recently, phenylephrine, a pure α-adrenergic receptor agonist, was thought to decrease uteroplacental blood flow. However, small doses (50 to 100 μg) of phenylephrine do not have detrimental effects on the healthy fetus.[101, 102]

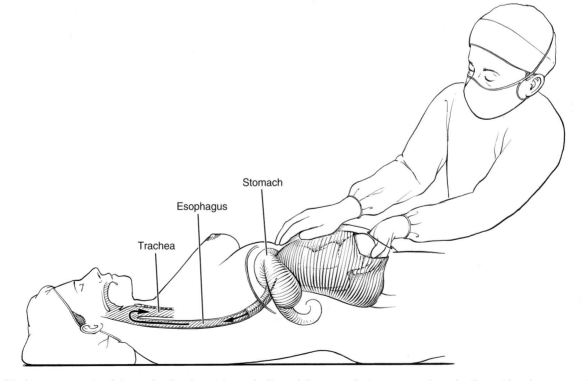

Figure 35–4 Pressure on the abdomen by the obstetrician to facilitate delivery results in gastroesophageal reflux with pulmonary aspiration of gastric contents.

Table 35–12 Comparison of Spinal and Epidural Anesthesia

SPINAL	EPIDURAL
More rapid onset, denser block	Titratable
Single-shot technique; duration limited by drug used	Flexible duration
Less shivering	Perhaps a lower incidence of hypotension
Less systemic absorption	May produce local anesthetic systemic toxicity
Less placental transfer	Greater placental transfer

Prevention of hypotension may be more important than the vasopressor selected. Prophylactic ephedrine infusions (50 mg in 500 mL of crystalloid) may be beneficial during spinal anesthesia.[103] Ephedrine crosses the placenta, increasing fetal heart rate and beat-to-beat variability[104] and causing changes in the spectral electroencephalogram in neonates.[105]

Pulmonary Aspiration

Pulmonary aspiration of gastric contents usually is associated with general anesthesia. However, aspiration has occurred during regional anesthesia after vomiting in a parturient with a high block and in one who was overly sedated (Fig. 35–4).

Spinal Anesthesia

Spinal anesthesia is used more frequently than epidural anesthesia because of its rapid onset, profound anesthesia and motor block, fixed end point in identifying the space, use of a smaller needle, lower dose of local anesthetic,[106] and less risk of incomplete or inadequate blocks (Table 35–12). Spinal anesthesia is largely a single-injection technique and therefore limited in its duration by the drug used. Hypotension may be more profound and rapid in onset (Table 35–13). With the use of smaller-gauge, pencil-point spinal needles, the overall risk of severe post–dural puncture headache (PDPH) is probably similar to that after unintentional dural puncture during attempted epidural anesthesia.[107]

Continuous spinal anesthesia techniques were greeted with enthusiasm as a means of combining the benefits of a spinal anesthetic with the ability to titrate the dose and control the degree of hypotension and the extent of block. Because of regulatory sanctions on the use of microcatheters, this technique has largely been abandoned, but in certain situations, it is still useful. Unintentional dural puncture, occurring during attempted insertion of an epidural catheter, can be converted to a continuous spinal anesthesia technique by inserting the epidural catheter through the needle into the subarachnoid space and using incremental injection. This is advantageous when the epidural space is difficult to identify, as in an obese parturient.[108]

Height, weight, and body mass index do not affect the spread of intrathecal bupivacaine in the term parturient (Fig. 35–5).[109] Adequate anesthesia is more likely to occur if spinal anesthesia is induced in the right lateral than in the left lateral position.[110, 111] A block between T-4 and T-1 increases patient comfort.

Bupivacaine is commonly used owing to its longer duration of action. Hyperbaric and isobaric bupivacaine (10 to 15 mg) produce excellent anesthesia.[112] Increasing the dose of intrathecally administered bupivacaine decreases the incidence of visceral pain.[113]

Epinephrine (0.2 mg) improves the quality of analgesia from 0.75% hyperbaric bupivacaine, increases the degree of motor block, and prolongs the time to sensory and motor recovery.[114] Fentanyl (10 μg) added to the local anesthetic improves comfort during peritoneal traction.[115] Other opioids are added for postoperative pain relief.[116–118] Meperidine has been used successfully as a single agent for cesarean section.[119, 120]

Side effects of spinal anesthesia include inadequate

Table 35–13 A Suggested Method of Spinal Anesthesia Administration for Cesarean Section

1. Administer sodium citrate (30 mL) on admission to the operating room.
2. Administer a fluid bolus intravenously (isotonic saline or Ringer's lactate), 20 mL/kg body weight (1.5 to 2 L), preinduction.
3. Assess airway.
4. Induce spinal anesthesia in the sitting or right lateral position.
5. Use small-gauge, pencil-point needle (25-G Whitacre, 24-G Sprotte) to inject the interspace between L2 to L3 or L3 to L4.
6. Local anesthetic (10–15 mg of hyperbaric 0.75% bupivacaine, 75 mg isobaric 2% lidocaine); add 10 μg of fentanyl or 250 μg of morphine or both for analgesia intraoperatively or postoperatively or both.
7. Position the parturient with left uterine displacement.
8. Administer oxygen by face mask or nasal prongs.
9. Monitor blood pressure every minute until stable.
10. To treat hypotension, administer fluids and vasopressor intravenously (ephedrine by intermittent bolus or infusion or, if tachycardia, use 50–100 μg of phenylephrine).

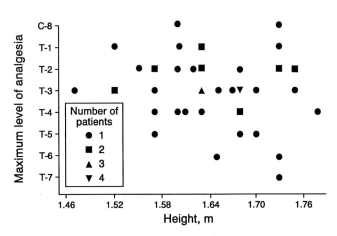

Figure 35–5 Relation between height and maximum cephalad spread of block after 12 mg hyperbaric bupivacaine in 47 term parturients. (Redrawn from Norris MC: Height, weight, and the spread of subarachnoid hyperbaric bupivacaine in the term parturient. Anesth Analg 1988; 67: 555–558.)

block (rare compared with epidural anesthesia), hypotension, nausea, shivering (less than with epidural block), total spinal block, and PDPH.[121] The incidence of PDPH is greater in pregnant patients than in other surgical patients. For this reason, spinal anesthesia was often avoided for cesarean section. The incidence of PDPH after use of the 24-G Sprotte or 25-G Whitacre needle has been acceptably low.[107] The incidence is higher with smaller-gauge Quincke needles, but the cost of the Quincke is less than that of the Sprotte and Whitacre needles. The cost of the needles has to be balanced against the risk of PDPH and the associated costs of a longer hospital stay and need for autologous epidural blood patch.

Another side effect is unexpectedly high block after induction of spinal anesthesia in parturients with inadequate epidural anesthesia.[122–125] Possible reasons include increased pressure on the subarachnoid space from the volume of fluid (local anesthetic) in the epidural space or transfer of additional local anesthetic from the epidural space into the subarachnoid space through the dural puncture.

Epidural Anesthesia

Epidural anesthesia is used less often in healthy parturients for elective cesarean section because of its slower onset of action, less reliable anesthesia, and poorer motor block. The slower onset of action is advantageous if hypotension is hazardous, as in patients with a fixed cardiac output or preeclampsia. Epidural anesthesia is used frequently for cesarean sections after labor, with extension of the block used for labor analgesia. When a functioning epidural catheter is in situ, rapid onset of anesthesia for cesarean section can be obtained by the use of a more rapid-acting local anesthetic, such as 3% 2-chloroprocaine. Adjustment of the pH of lidocaine and bupivacaine[126, 127] decreases the time to onset of block, as does addition of epinephrine.[128] Glosten and colleagues[129] reported that 24% of epidural blocks placed for labor were inadequate for cesarean delivery. Migration of the epidural catheter is one possible reason for this.[130, 131]

Side effects of epidural anesthesia for cesarean section include unintentional dural puncture; hypotension; unilateral, patchy, or inadequate blocks; intravenous injection of local anesthetic; local anesthetic systemic toxicity; shivering, which may make monitoring difficult; and a higher than expected block (unexpected spinal, subdural block).[132]

It is important to use an epidural test dose to detect intravenous or intrathecal catheter placement, followed by incremental injection of local anesthetic. There is considerable debate about the ideal test dose.[30] Whichever agent or technique is used, the best method of detecting inappropriate placement is to consider each incremental injection as a test dose.[133]

Combined Spinal-Epidural Anesthesia

In an effort to obtain the best qualities of spinal anesthesia (rapid onset, profound sensory and motor block) and those of epidural anesthesia (more controlled level, slower onset of hypotension, flexibility with respect to duration of operation), some anesthesiologists combine the two techniques.[134, 135]

Initially, the epidural space is identified with a standard Tuohy or Husted needle. Through this needle, a long, small-gauge pencil-point needle is inserted into the subarachnoid space. Local anesthetic, usually in a slightly lower dose than would be used for a single-shot spinal block, is injected through the spinal needle. That needle is withdrawn, the epidural catheter is inserted, the epidural needle is removed, and the catheter is taped in position. After positioning the patient and initial monitoring, the block height is assessed. If it is lower than required for the operation, additional local anesthetic is injected through the epidural catheter to raise the block to the desired height.

It may be difficult to determine the placement of the epidural catheter before its use. The position of the catheter could be intravenous, intrathecal, or outside the epidural space, or the catheter may have exited through an intervertebral foramen, resulting in an unsuccessful block (Fig. 35–6). This problem of a misplaced epidural catheter usually is identified early during a routine epidural block. Isobaric local anesthetic probably should be used for the subarachnoid block, because the patient may need to maintain the sitting or lateral position for a longer time while the epidural catheter is inserted and secured.

Analgesia After Cesarean Section

Epidural and intrathecal opioids are used for analgesia after cesarean section.[136, 137] Because the side effects

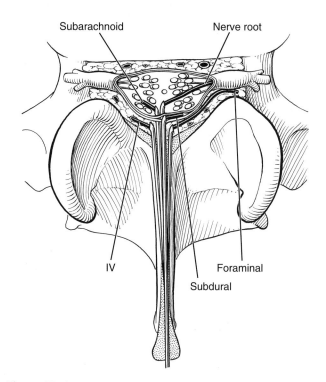

Figure 35–6 Locations of the epidural catheter that may lead to complications with the combined spinal-epidural technique. IV, intravenous.

of pruritus, nausea, vomiting, and respiratory depression are dose related, the doses of morphine used intrathecally and epidurally are 100 to 250 µg and 3 to 5 mg, respectively. Respiratory depression occurs with epidural and intrathecal injection of morphine and fentanyl[138, 139] but is equivalent to that seen after intramuscular injection of opioids.[140–143] Recurrence of herpes simplex labialis may be related to pruritus.[144]

Local Anesthetic Infiltration

Local anesthetic infiltration for cesarean section has been thoroughly described in the literature. Reports recount its use in two parturients: one with severe kyphoscoliosis and paraplegia for whom there were concerns about postoperative ventilatory management[145] and another in whom attempts at tracheal intubation and spinal anesthesia failed.[146] Although rarely required, it is another possible technique for selected patients.

General Anesthesia

General anesthesia is used if regional techniques are contraindicated or if a regional technique proves unsatisfactory intraoperatively (Table 35–14). Because anesthetic-related maternal morbidity and mortality occur more often with general anesthesia, emphasis should be placed on securing the airway rapidly. The anesthesiologist should try to neutralize acidic gastric contents by administering a nonparticulate antacid (0.3 M sodium citrate) immediately before induction. If the procedure is elective, administer ranitidine intravenously (50 mg) 30 min preoperatively to neutralize the pH[147] and metoclopramide (10 mg) intravenously 20 min preoperatively to promote gastric emptying.

When Mendelson[148] first described the classic syndrome of pulmonary pneumonitis after pulmonary aspiration, most general anesthesia was performed without tracheal intubation. Anesthesiologists subsequently changed their technique to include rapid-sequence induction with tracheal intubation using cricoid pressure.[149] When difficulty was encountered, many persisted in their efforts to intubate, forgetting the need for oxygenation. This resulted in a greater number of hypoxic deaths. Current techniques are designed to prevent these events.

Approximately 1 of 500 intubations in parturients fails.[79] Although airway assessment has improved our ability to predict the difficult airway, in one study,[80]

Table 35–14 Indications for General Anesthesia

Patient refusal of regional anesthesia
Severe fetal distress without a preexisting epidural catheter
Maternal hemodynamic instability (e.g., hemorrhage, fixed cardiac output)
Coagulopathy
Septicemia or sepsis at site of insertion
Inadequate regional anesthesia during operation

25% of difficult intubations were not predicted. There are several excellent reviews of this topic.[79, 80, 82] In the case of a potentially difficult airway, evaluation of the awake patient is indicated after the topical application of local anesthetic. Even if the larynx is seen easily, intubation of the awake patient is mandatory, with induction after the airway is secured. Paralysis shifts the larynx anteriorly,[150] making visualization more difficult in the paralyzed patient. Intubation using fiberoptics in the awake patient is another alternative.

Preoxygenation, achieved by breathing 100% oxygen for 3 min or four vital capacity breaths,[9] decreases the risk of desaturation during apnea. Rapid-sequence induction and intubation are performed with thiopental (4 mg/kg) or ketamine (1 mg/kg)[151] when the patient is hemodynamically unstable, followed by succinylcholine (1.5 mg/kg). If succinylcholine is contraindicated, intubation can be done in the awake patient, followed by induction with thiopental. Vecuronium (0.25 mg/kg) is an alternative to succinylcholine.[152]

Because thiopental causes a rapid reduction in upper esophageal sphincter pressure, cricoid pressure should be applied by a trained assistant as soon as induction is begun.[14] A pressure of 10 N (approximately 1 kg) can be tolerated without discomfort by patients. To prevent passive regurgitation, this should be increased to 30 N (3 kg) after unconsciousness occurs.[14] After intubation, the position of the tracheal tube is confirmed by the presence of end-tidal CO_2 and chest auscultation. Maternal hyperoxia has beneficial effects for the fetus.[153] An F_{IO_2} of 0.5 with nitrous oxide and 0.66 minimum alveolar concentration of a volatile agent, such as isoflurane, provides adequate oxygenation with a decreased incidence of awareness. Concerns about uterine hypotonia and increased bleeding during cesarean section with general anesthesia with volatile agents have to be balanced against the risks of maternal recall.[154]

Maintenance of anesthesia is achieved with muscle relaxants, opioids given intravenously, and an appropriate concentration of nitrous oxide and volatile agent. Emergence is another critical time for aspiration in the parturient. Extubation should occur when the parturient is fully awake and on her side (Table 35–15).

Specific Situations

Emergency Induction

There is an increased risk of maternal mortality with emergency cesarean section, because the reason for the cesarean section (hemorrhage, fetal distress) frequently dictates a need for general anesthesia. It is important to assess the risks to the mother and the fetus before induction of anesthesia.

In situations of acute, severe fetal distress, without a preexisting epidural catheter, general anesthesia is usually considered to be more rapid. However, the risk of a difficult airway outweighs the slightly longer time associated with induction of spinal anesthesia; the maternal risk of general anesthesia outweighs fetal risk

Table 35–15 A Suggested Method of General Anesthesia Administration for Cesarean Section

---

1. Establish intravenous access.
2. Neutralize gastric contents.
    Elective: Ranitidine 50 mg IV (30 min preop) or 150 mg PO (90 min preop)
    Sodium citrate 30 mL PO on admission to OR
    Emergency: Sodium citrate 30 mL PO on admission to OR
3. Assess the airway.
4. Position the patient with left uterine displacement. Pillows or towels are placed under the head or neck to optimize the position for intubation.
5. Attach monitors: ECG, NIBP, pulse oximeter, peripheral nerve stimulator, end-tidal CO_2.
6. Check anesthetic machine and its monitors.
7. Preoxygenate the patient using 100% oxygen for 3 min or four vital capacity breaths of 100% oxygen.
8. Rapid-sequence induction with cricoid pressure is achieved with thiopental (4 mg/kg), succinylcholine (1.5 mg/kg), and intubation with a small, cuffed tracheal tube.
9. Maintenance consists of N_2O/O_2 (50:50), isoflurane, enflurane, or halothane with a 0.66 minimum alveolar concentration.
10. IV opioids are given after delivery; neuromuscular blocker is titrated to response using a nerve stimulator.
11. Extubate when the patient is awake.

ECG, electrocardiogram; IV, intravenously; NIBP, noninvasive blood pressure; OR, operating room; PO, orally; preop, preoperatively.

from longer induction of regional technique. Marx and coworkers[155] showed that subarachnoid block for fetal distress resulted in similar umbilical blood gases but better 1-min Apgar scores than with general anesthesia.

Several techniques can decrease the risk to the parturient. Good communication between the obstetrician and the anesthesiologist allows early identification and assessment of the at-risk parturient. This enables the development of alternative strategies, such as epidural anesthesia during labor. It also allows the anesthesiologist to examine the airway and to explain the risks and benefits of the different techniques.

In these high-risk parturients, the anesthesiologist should ensure that the epidural catheter, inserted for labor, is working effectively before an emergency occurs. The block can then be extended rapidly to provide surgical anesthesia. In hemodynamically stable parturients without an epidural block, spinal anesthesia can be induced rapidly.

Morbid Obesity

Morbidly obese parturients have a higher incidence of cesarean section and other obstetric complications.[156] There frequently is difficulty with intubation for general anesthesia and with obtaining successful regional anesthesia.[157] Obese parturients are more likely to require repeat placement of the epidural catheter, with an initial failure rate of 42%. Dense upper thoracic epidural anesthesia combined with panniculus retraction may cause respiratory or cardiovascular problems.[158] Spinal anesthesia has been used successfully, although repeated attempts may be required. Difficulty with controlling the level of block and the possibility

of prolonged surgical time may make it a less desirable technique than epidural anesthesia. If an unintentional dural puncture occurs during insertion of the epidural catheter, consideration should be given to converting the technique to a continuous spinal block by threading the epidural catheter into the subarachnoid space. Local anesthetic can then be titrated to provide surgical anesthesia.[159]

Cesarean Delivery of the Preterm Infant

Cesarean delivery is frequently indicated for delivery of the preterm infant as a result of breech or transverse lie, fetal distress, intrauterine growth retardation, preeclampsia, and dystocia. Neonatal outcome is usually better after regional anesthesia.[160]

Cesarean section often occurs after failure to stop preterm labor with magnesium sulfate or the β-adrenergic receptor agonists, ritodrine or terbutaline. Ritodrine and terbutaline have profound cardiovascular effects that persist for 30 to 90 min after they are discontinued.[161] Reported complications during anesthesia in these patients include maternal hypotension, intraoperative pulmonary edema, sinus tachycardia, and ventricular arrhythmias. If possible, anesthesia should be deferred for a minimum of 30 min after discontinuation of these drugs. Administration of excess fluids may cause pulmonary edema because these patients frequently have a positive fluid balance.

General anesthesia is also not without risk. Halothane should be avoided because it sensitizes the myocardium to catecholamine-induced arrhythmias.[161] Hyperventilation should be avoided because it may potentiate the hypokalemia that occurs during treatment with β-adrenergic agents. It is not necessary to replace potassium, because it is only transferred intracellularly.

Magnesium sulfate therapy has anesthetic implications, because it increases sedation and neuromuscular block produced by nondepolarizing muscle relaxants.[161]

Cesarean delivery is often indicated in the preterm infant owing to an abnormal presentation (breech, transverse lie). After uterine incision, uterine contraction may interfere with delivery of the infant. Uterine relaxation permits extraction of the infant without extending the uterine incision. In the past, this was provided by deep halothane anesthesia, which requires general anesthesia with tracheal intubation. Nitroglycerin (100 µg) provides rapid, short-term uterine relaxation with minimal effects on the cardiovascular system, providing the patient is hemodynamically stable.[162]

Conclusions

Spinal anesthesia has many advantages for cesarean section and is the technique I prefer. It has a rapid onset and similar side effects to epidural anesthesia and, with the increasing use of spinal opioids, provides excellent postoperative pain relief. When I perform a spinal or epidural block, I ask the patient to assist me by telling me where she feels the pressure as the needle enters the interspinous space. If she states it is to one side, I alter the direction of the needle. This is an efficient method of identifying the midline, even in obese parturients and in those with scoliosis. Another simple technique that seems to limit the upper spread of spinal anesthesia is to flex the neck. Although some blocks reach T-1, they do not seem to migrate further cephalad.

I use several soft signs to determine the efficacy of an epidural block for operation, because many of my patients speak limited English. These soft signs include the temperature of their feet, motor power, and decrease in diastolic blood pressure. In patients with a preexisting epidural block from labor, temperature and pinprick sensation may be impaired when they arrive at the operating room. The use of these soft signs improves the chance of a successful surgical anesthetic.

Because of the reports of high blocks following spinal anesthesia after an inadequate epidural block, I try to determine whether the epidural anesthetic is working by using a maximum of 10 mL of local anesthetic. If I am not convinced that it is working efficiently, I induce spinal anesthesia early, not when the epidural space is filled with a large volume of local anesthetic.

With general anesthesia, preparation for intubation is key. The physician must be prepared before starting to anesthetically induce the patient. The pillows should be arranged so the head and neck are in the "sniffing" position. The operating room table is raised to a suitable height for the anesthesiologist, not for the surgeon. It can be raised or lowered after the trachea is intubated.

The assistant must know what to do. The anesthesiologist should take a few seconds to teach the assistant if there is any doubt. I recommend that the person applying cricoid pressure place one hand under the cervical spine while applying cricoid pressure with the other. This helps to maintain the "sniffing" position and seems to make intubation easier. It also keeps the assistant's attention focused on maintaining cricoid pressure. If intubation is impossible, oxygenate!

References

1. Notzon FC, Cnattingius S, Bergsjo P, et al: Cesarean section delivery in the 1980s: international comparison by indication. Am J Obstet Gynecol 1994; 170: 495–504.
2. Anonymous: Rates of cesarean delivery—United States, 1991. MMWR Morb Mortal Wkly Rep 1993; 42: 285–289.
3. Flamm BL, Goings JR, Liu Y, et al: Elective repeat cesarean delivery versus trial of labor: a prospective multicenter study. Obstet Gynecol 1994; 83: 927–932.
4. Iglesias S, Burn R, Saunders LD: Reducing the cesarean section rate in a rural community hospital. (Published erratum appears in Can Med Assoc J 1992; 146: 1701.) Can Med Assoc J 1991; 145: 1459–1464.
5. Cowan RK, Kinch RA, Ellis B, et al: Trial of labor following cesarean delivery. Obstet Gynecol 1994; 83: 933–936.
6. Cohen SE: Physiological alterations of pregnancy. Clin Anaesthesiol 1986; 4: 33–46.
7. Archer GW Jr, Marx GF: Arterial oxygen tension during apnoea in parturient women. Br J Anaesth 1974; 46: 358–360.
8. Jense HG, Dubin SA, Silverstein PI, et al: Effect of obesity on safe duration of apnea in anesthetized humans. Anesth Analg 1991; 72: 89–93.
9. Norris MC, Dewan DM: Preoxygenation for cesarean section: a comparison of two techniques. Anesthesiology 1985; 62: 827–829.
10. MacLennan FM, MacDonald AF, Campbell DM: Lung water during the puerperium. Anaesthesia 1987; 42: 141–147.
11. Ramanathan S, Gandhi S, Arismendy J, et al: Oxygen transfer from mother to fetus during cesarean section under epidural anesthesia. Anesth Analg 1982; 61: 576–581.
12. Crosby ET, Halpern SH: Supplemental maternal oxygen therapy during caesarean section under epidural anaesthesia: a comparison of nasal prongs and face mask. Can J Anaesth 1992; 39: 313–316.
13. Farcon EL, Kim MH, Marx GF: Changing Mallampati score during labour. Can J Anaesth 1994; 41: 50–51.
14. Vanner RG: Mechanisms of regurgitation and its prevention with cricoid pressure. Int J Obstet Anesth 1993; 2: 207–215.
15. Vanner RG, Goodman NW: Gastro-oesophageal reflux in pregnancy at term and after delivery. Anaesthesia 1989; 44: 808–811.
16. Sandhar BK, Elliott RH, Windram I, et al: Peripartum changes in gastric emptying. Anaesthesia 1992; 47: 196–198.
17. Macfie AG, Magides AD, Richmond MN, et al: Gastric emptying in pregnancy. Br J Anaesth 1991; 67: 54–57.
18. Carp H, Jayaram A, Stoll M: Ultrasound examination of the stomach contents of parturients. Anesth Analg 1992; 74: 683–687.
19. O'Sullivan GM, Sutton AJ, Thompson SA, et al: Noninvasive measurement of gastric emptying in obstetric patients. Anesth Analg 1987; 66: 505–511.
20. Geddes SM, Thorburn J, Logan RW: Gastric emptying following caesarean section and the effect of epidural fentanyl. Anaesthesia 1991; 46: 1016–1018.
21. Ewah B, Yau K, King M, et al: Effect of epidural opioids on gastric emptying in labour. Int J Obstet Anesth 1993; 2: 125–128.
22. Goodlin RC: Venous reactivity and pregnancy abnormalities. Acta Obstet Gynecol Scand 1986; 65: 345–348.
23. Marx GF: Aortocaval compression syndrome: its 50-year history. (Editorial.) Int J Obstet Anesth 1992; 1: 60–64.
24. Crawford JS, Burton M, Davies P: Time and lateral tilt at caesarean section. Br J Anaesth 1972; 44: 477–484.
25. Ellington C, Katz VL, Watson WJ, et al: The effect of lateral tilt on maternal and fetal hemodynamic variables. Obstet Gynecol 1991; 77: 201–203.
26. Andrews PJ, Ackerman WE III, Juneja MM: Aortocaval compression in the sitting and lateral decubitus positions during extradural catheter placement in the parturient. Can J Anaesth 1993; 40: 320–324.
27. Datta S, Lambert DH, Gregus J, et al: Differential sensitivities of mammalian nerve fibers during pregnancy. Anesth Analg 1983; 62: 1070–1072.
28. Butterworth JF IV, Walker FO, Lysak SZ: Pregnancy increases median nerve susceptibility to lidocaine. Anesthesiology 1990; 72: 962–965.
29. Palahniuk RJ, Shnider SM, Eger EI II: Pregnancy decreases the requirement for inhaled anesthetic agents. Anesthesiology 1974; 41: 82–83.
30. Santos AC, Pedersen H: Current controversies in obstetric anesthesia. Anesth Analg 1994; 78: 753–760.
31. Robson N, Robertson I, Whittaker M: Plasma cholinesterase changes during the puerperium. Anaesthesia 1986; 41: 243–249.
32. Hein HA: Cardiorespiratory arrest with laryngeal oedema in pregnancy-induced hypertension. Can Anaesth Soc J 1984; 31: 210–212.
33. Rocke DA, Scoones GP: Rapidly progressive laryngeal oedema associated with pregnancy-aggravated hypertension. Anaesthesia 1992; 47: 141–143.
34. Kambam JR, Handte RE, Brown WU, et al: Effect of normal and preeclamptic pregnancies on the oxyhemoglobin dissociation curve. Anesthesiology 1986; 65: 426–427.
35. Reynolds F: Placental transfer of drugs used by anaesthetists. Anaesth Rev 1989; 6: 151–183.

36. Alahuhta S, Räsänen J, Jouppila R, et al: Uteroplacental and fetal haemodynamics during extradural anaesthesia for caesarean section. Br J Anaesth 1991; 66: 319–323.

37. Long MG, Price M, Spencer JA: Uteroplacental perfusion after epidural analgesia for elective caesarean section. Br J Obstet Gynaecol 1988; 95: 1081–1082.

38. Baumann H, Alon E, Atanassoff P, et al: Effect of epidural anesthesia for cesarean delivery on maternal femoral arterial and venous, uteroplacental, and umbilical blood flow velocities and waveforms. Obstet Gynecol 1990; 75: 194–198.

39. Lindblad A, Bernow J, Vernersson E, et al: Effects of extradural anaesthesia on human fetal blood flow in utero. Comparison of three local anaesthetic solutions. Br J Anaesth 1987; 59: 1265–1272.

40. Marx GF, Patel S, Berman JA, et al: Umbilical blood flow velocity waveforms in different maternal positions and with epidural analgesia. Obstet Gynecol 1986; 68: 61–64.

41. Morrow RJ, Rolbin SH, Ritchie JW, et al: Epidural anaesthesia and blood flow velocity in mother and fetus. Can J Anaesth 1989; 36: 519–522.

42. Veille JC, Youngstrom P, Kanaan C, et al: Human umbilical artery flow velocity waveforms before and after regional anesthesia for cesarean section. Obstet Gynecol 1988; 72: 890–893.

43. Giles WB, Lah FX, Trudinger BJ: The effect of epidural anaesthesia for caesarean section on maternal uterine and fetal umbilical artery blood flow velocity waveforms. Br J Obstet Gynaecol 1987; 94: 55–59.

44. Fairlie FM, Kirkwood I, Lang GD, et al: Umbilical artery flow velocity waveforms during spinal anesthesia. Eur J Obstet Gynecol Reprod Biol 1991; 38: 3–7.

45. Jouppila P, Jouppila R, Barinoff T, et al: Placental blood flow during caesarean section performed under subarachnoid blockade. Br J Anaesth 1984; 56: 1379–1383.

46. Kuhnert BR, Linn PL, Kuhnert PM: Obstetric medication and neonatal behavior. Current controversies. Clin Perinatol 1985; 12: 423–440.

47. Scott DB, Lee A, Fagan D, et al: Acute toxicity of ropivacaine compared with that of bupivacaine. Anesth Analg 1989; 69: 563–569.

48. Ong BY, Cohen MM, Palahniuk RJ: Anesthesia for cesarean section—effects on neonates. Anesth Analg 1989; 68: 270–275.

49. Datta S, Ostheimer GW, Weiss JB, et al: Neonatal effect of prolonged anesthetic induction for cesarean section. Obstet Gynecol 1981; 58: 331–335.

50. Lee JJ, Rubin AP: Breast feeding and anaesthesia. Anaesthesia 1993; 48: 616–625.

51. Report on Confidential Enquiries Into Maternal Deaths in the United Kingdom 1985–87. London, Her Majesty's Stationery Office, 1991.

52. Report on Confidential Enquiries Into Maternal Deaths in the United Kingdom 1988–90. London, Her Majesty's Stationery Office, 1994.

53. Hawkins J, Koonin L, Palmer S, et al: Anesthesia-related maternal deaths in the United States: A twelve year review 1979–1990. (Abstract.) In Proceedings of the Annual Meeting of the Society for Obstetric Anesthesia and Perinatology, p 7, Palm Springs, 1993.

54. Kamani AA, Gambling DR, Christilaw J, et al: Anaesthetic management of patients with placenta accreta. Can J Anaesth 1987; 34: 613–617.

55. Chestnut DH, Dewan DM, Redick LF, et al: Anesthetic management for obstetric hysterectomy: a multi-institutional study. Anesthesiology 1989; 70: 607–610.

56. Hankins GD, Berryman GK, Scott RT Jr, et al: Maternal arterial desaturation with 15-methyl prostaglandin F_2 alpha for uterine atony. Obstet Gynecol 1988; 72: 367–370.

57. Reedy MB, McMillion JS, Engvall WR, et al: Inadvertent administration of prostaglandin E_1 instead of prostaglandin $F_{2\alpha}$ in a patient with uterine atony and hemorrhage. Obstet Gynecol 1992; 79: 890–894.

58. Secher NJ, Thayssen P, Arnsbo P, et al: Effect of prostaglandin E_2 and $F_{2\alpha}$ on the systemic and pulmonary circulation in pregnant anesthetized women. Acta Obstet Gynecol Scand 1982; 61: 213–218.

59. Phelan JP, Meguiar RV, Matey D, et al: Dramatic pyrexic and cardiovascular response to intravaginal prostaglandin E_2. Am J Obstet Gynecol 1978; 132: 28–32.

60. Douglas MJ, Farquharson DF, Ross PL, et al: Cardiovascular collapse following an overdose of prostaglandin $F_{2\alpha}$: a case report. Can J Anaesth 1989; 36: 466–469.

61. Combs CA, Murphy EL, Laros RK Jr: Factors associated with hemorrhage in cesarean deliveries. Obstet Gynecol 1991; 77: 77–82.

62. Naef RW III, Chauhan SP, Chevalier SP, et al: Prediction of hemorrhage at cesarean delivery. Obstet Gynecol 1994; 83: 923–926.

63. Sibai BM, Ramadan MK, Usta I, et al: Maternal morbidity and mortality in 442 pregnancies with hemolysis, elevated liver enzymes, and low platelets (HELLP syndrome). Am J Obstet Gynecol 1993; 169: 1000–1006.

64. McVay PA, Hoag RW, Hoag MS, et al: Safety and use of autologous blood donation during the third trimester of pregnancy (with discussion). Am J Obstet Gynecol 1989; 160: 1479–1488.

65. Malinow AM, Naulty JS, Hunt CO, et al: Precordial ultrasonic monitoring during cesarean delivery. Anesthesiology 1987; 66: 816–819.

66. Fong J, Gadalla F, Pierri MK, et al: Are Doppler-detected venous emboli during cesarean section air emboli? (Published erratum appears in Anesth Analg 1990; 71: 574.) Anesth Analg 1990; 71: 254–257.

67. Vartikar JV, Johnson MD, Datta S: Precordial Doppler monitoring and pulse oximetry during cesarean delivery: detection of venous air embolism. Reg Anesth 1989; 14: 145–148.

68. Matthews NC, Greer G: Embolism during caesarean section. Anaesthesia 1990; 45: 964–965.

69. Younker D, Rodriguez V, Kavanagh J: Massive air embolism during cesarean section. Anesthesiology 1986; 65: 77–79.

70. Palmer CM, Norris MC, Giudici MC, et al: Incidence of electrocardiographic changes during cesarean delivery under regional anesthesia. Anesth Analg 1990; 70: 36–43.

71. Zakowski MI, Ramanthan S, Baratta JB, et al: Electrocardiographic changes during cesarean section: a cause for concern? Anesth Analg 1993; 76: 162–167.

72. Eisenach JC, Tuttle R, Stein A: Is ST segment depression of the electrocardiogram during cesarean section merely due to cardiac sympathetic block? Anesth Analg 1994; 78: 287–292.

73. Quance D: Amniotic fluid embolism: Detection by pulse oximetry. Anesthesiology 1988; 68: 951–952.

74. Kasten GW, Martin ST: Resuscitation from bupivacaine-induced cardiovascular toxicity during partial inferior vena cava occlusion. Anesth Analg 1986; 65: 341–344.

75. Lindsay SL, Hanson GC: Cardiac arrest in near-term pregnancy. Anaesthesia 1987; 42: 1074–1077.

76. Marx GF: Cardiopulmonary resuscitation of late-pregnant women. (Letter to the editor.) Anesthesiology 1982; 56: 156.

77. Caplan RA, Ward RJ, Posner K, et al: Unexpected cardiac arrest during spinal anesthesia: a closed claims analysis of predisposing factors. Anesthesiology 1988; 68: 5–11.

78. Jewett JF: Committee on maternal welfare. Anesthetic death. N Engl J Med 1974; 291: 48–49.

79. Davies JM, Weeks S, Crone LA, et al: Difficult intubation in the parturient. Can J Anaesth 1989; 36: 668–674.

80. Wilson ME, Spiegelhalter D, Robertson JA, et al: Predicting difficult intubation. Br J Anaesth 1988; 61: 211–216.

81. Rocke DA, Murray WB, Rout CC, et al: Relative risk analysis of factors associated with difficult intubation in obstetric anesthesia. Anesthesiology 1992; 77: 67–73.

82. Benumof JL: Management of the difficult adult airway. With special emphasis on awake tracheal intubation. (Published erratum appears in Anesthesiology 1993; 78: 224.) Anesthesiology 1991; 75: 1087–1110.

83. Hewett E, Livingstone P: Management of failed endotracheal intubation at caesarean section. Anaesth Intensive Care 1990; 18: 330–335.

84. Sibai BM, Mirro R, Chesney CM, et al: Low-dose aspirin in pregnancy. Obstet Gynecol 1989; 74: 551–557.

85. Horlocker TT, Wedel DJ, Offord KP: Does preoperative antiplatelet therapy increase the risk of hemorrhagic complications associated with regional anesthesia? Anesth Analg 1990; 70: 631–634.

86. de Swiet M, Redman CW: Aspirin, extradural anaesthesia and the MRC Collaborative Low-Dose Aspirin Study in Pregnancy (CLASP). (Letter to the editor.) Br J Anaesth 1992; 69: 109–110.

87. Malinow AM, Rickford WJ, Mokriski BL, et al: Lupus anticoagulant. Implications for obstetric anaesthetists. Anaesthesia 1987; 42: 1291–1293.

88. Lindblad A, Bernow J, Marsal K: Fetal blood flow during intrathecal anaesthesia for elective caesarean section. Br J Anaesth 1988; 61: 376–381.

89. Wright PM, Iftikhar M, Fitzpatrick KT, et al: Vasopressor therapy for hypotension during epidural anesthesia for cesarean section: effects on maternal and fetal flow velocity ratios. Anesth Analg 1992; 75: 56–63.

90. Räsänen J, Alahuhta S, Kangas-Saarela T, et al: The effects of ephedrine and etilefrine on uterine and fetal blood flow and on fetal myocardial function during spinal anaesthesia for caesarean section. Int J Obstet Anesth 1991; 1: 3–8.

91. Alahuhta S, Räsänen J, Jouppila P, et al: Ephedrine and phenylephrine for avoiding maternal hypotension due to spinal anaesthesia for caesarean section. Int J Obstet Anesth 1992; 1: 129–134.

92. McCrae AF, Wildsmith JAW: Prevention and treatment of hypotension during central neural block. Br J Anaesth 1993; 70: 672–680.

93. Defalque RJ: Compared effects of spinal and extradural anesthesia upon blood pressure. Anesthesiology 1962; 23: 627–630.

94. Caritis SN, Abouleish E, Edelstone DI, et al: Fetal acid-base state following spinal or epidural anesthesia for cesarean section. Obstet Gynecol 1980; 56: 610–615.

95. Marx GF, Cosmi EV, Wollman SB: Biochemical status and clinical condition of mother and infant at cesarean section. Anesth Analg 1969; 48: 986–994.

96. Rout CC, Rocke DA, Levin J, et al: A reevaluation of the role of crystalloid preload in the prevention of hypotension associated with spinal anesthesia for elective cesarean section. Anesthesiology 1993; 79: 262–269.

97. Kenepp NB, Kumar S, Shelley WC, et al: Fetal and neonatal hazards of maternal hydration with 5% dextrose before caesarean section. Lancet 1982; 1: 1150–1152.

98. James FM III, Greiss FC Jr, Kemp RA: An evaluation of vasopressor therapy for maternal hypotension during spinal anesthesia. Anesthesiology 1970; 33: 25–34.

99. Ralston DH, Shnider SM, deLorimier AA: Effects of equipotent ephedrine, metaraminol, mephentermine, and methoxamine on uterine blood flow in the pregnant ewe. Anesthesiology 1974; 40: 354–370.

100. Tong C, Eisenach JC: The vascular mechanism of ephedrine's beneficial effect on uterine perfusion during pregnancy. Anesthesiology 1992; 76: 792–798.

101. Ramanathan S, Grant GJ: Vasopressor therapy for hypotension due to epidural anesthesia for cesarean section. Acta Anaesthesiol Scand 1988; 32: 559–565.

102. Moran DH, Perillo M, LaPorta RF, et al: Phenylephrine in the prevention of hypotension following spinal anesthesia for cesarean delivery. J Clin Anesth 1991; 3: 301–305.

103. Kang YG, Abouleish E, Caritis S: Prophylactic intravenous ephedrine infusion during spinal anesthesia for cesarean section. Anesth Analg 1982; 61: 839–842.

104. Hughes SC, Ward MG, Levinson G, et al: Placental transfer of ephedrine does not affect neonatal outcome. Anesthesiology 1985; 63: 217–219.

105. Kangas-Saarela T, Hollmen AI, Tolonen U, et al: Does ephedrine influence newborn neurobehavioural responses and spectral EEG when used to prevent maternal hypotension during caesarean section? Acta Anaesthesiol Scand 1990; 34: 8–16.

106. Kuhnert BR, Zuspan KJ, Kuhnert PM, et al: Bupivacaine disposition in mother, fetus, and neonate after spinal anesthesia for cesarean section. Anesth Analg 1987; 66: 407–412.

107. Campbell DC, Douglas MJ, Pavy TJG, et al: Comparison of the 25-gauge Whitacre with the 24-gauge Sprotte spinal needle for elective caesarean section: cost implications. Can J Anaesth 1993; 40: 1131–1135.

108. Norris MC, Leighton BL: Continuous spinal anesthesia after unintentional dural puncture in parturients. Reg Anesth 1990; 15: 285–287.

109. Norris MC: Height, weight, and the spread of subarachnoid hyperbaric bupivacaine in the term parturient. Anesth Analg 1988; 67: 555–558.

110. Sprague DH: Effects of position and uterine displacement on spinal anesthesia for cesarean section. Anesthesiology 1976; 44: 164–166.

111. Russell IF: Effect of posture during the induction of subarachnoid analgesia for caesarean section. Right v. left lateral. Br J Anaesth 1987; 59: 342–346.

112. Russell IF, Holmqvist ELO: Subarachnoid analgesia for caesarean section. A double-blind comparison of plain and hyperbaric 0.5% bupivacaine. Br J Anaesth 1987; 59: 347–353.

113. Pedersen H, Santos AC, Steinberg ES, et al: Incidence of visceral pain during cesarean section: the effect of varying doses of spinal bupivacaine. Anesth Analg 1989; 69: 46–49.

114. Abouleish EI: Epinephrine improves the quality of spinal hyperbaric bupivacaine for cesarean section. Anesth Analg 1987; 66: 395–400.

115. Ward ME, Kliffer AP, Gambling DR, et al: Effect of combining fentanyl with morphine/bupivacaine for elective C/S under spinal. (Abstract.) Anesthesiology 1993; 79(Suppl 3A): A1023.

116. Abouleish E, Rawal N, Fallon K, et al: Combined intrathecal morphine and bupivacaine for cesarean section. Anesth Analg 1988; 67: 370–374.

117. Abboud TK, Dror A, Mosaad P, et al: Mini-dose intrathecal morphine for the relief of post-cesarean section pain: safety, efficacy, and ventilatory responses to carbon dioxide. Anesth Analg 1988; 67: 137–143.

118. Abouleish E, Rawal N, Rashad MN: The addition of 0.2 mg subarachnoid morphine to hyperbaric bupivacaine for cesarean delivery: a prospective study of 856 cases. Reg Anesth 1991; 16: 137–140.

119. Camann WR, Bader AM: Spinal anesthesia for cesarean delivery with meperidine as the sole agent. Int J Obstet Anesth 1992; 1: 156–158.

120. Kafle SK: Intrathecal meperidine for elective caesarean section: a comparison with lidocaine. Can J Anaesth 1993; 40: 718–721.

121. Juhani TP, Hannele H: Complications during spinal anesthesia for cesarean delivery: a clinical report of one year's experience. Reg Anesth 1993; 18: 128–131.

122. Beck GN, Griffiths AG: Failed extradural anaesthesia for caesarean section. Complication of subsequent spinal block. Anaesthesia 1992; 47: 690–692.

123. Stone PA, Thorburn J, Lamb KSR: Complications of spinal anaesthesia following extradural block for caesarean section. Br J Anaesth 1989; 62: 335–337.

124. Mets B, Broccoli E, Brown AR: Is spinal anesthesia after failed epidural anesthesia contraindicated for cesarean section? Anesth Analg 1993; 77: 629–631.

125. Leach A, Smith GB: Subarachnoid spread of epidural local anaesthetic following dural puncture. Anaesthesia 1988; 43: 671–674.

126. McMorland GH, Douglas MJ, Axelson JE, et al: The effect of pH adjustment of bupivacaine on onset and duration of epidural anaesthesia for caesarean section. Can J Anaesth 1988; 35: 457–461.

127. DiFazio CA, Carron H, Grosslight KR, et al: Comparison of pH-adjusted lidocaine solutions for epidural anesthesia. Anesth Analg 1986; 65: 760–764.

128. Price ML, Reynolds F, Morgan BM: Extending epidural blockade for emergency caesarean section. Evaluation of 2% lignocaine with adrenaline. Int J Obstet Anesth 1991; 1: 13–18.

129. Glosten B, Chadwick HS, Ross BK, et al: Failed regional anesthesia for cesarean delivery. (Abstract.) In Proceedings of the Annual Meeting of the Society for Obstetric Anesthesia and Perinatology, p 13, Philadelphia, 1994.

130. Crosby ET: Epidural catheter migration during labour: an hypothesis for inadequate analgesia. Can J Anaesth 1990; 37: 789–793.

131. Bishton IM, Martin PH, Vernon JM, et al: Factors influencing epidural catheter migration. Anaesthesia 1992; 47: 610–612.

132. Morgan B: Unexpectedly extensive conduction blocks in obstetric epidural analgesia. Anaesthesia 1990; 45: 148–152.

133. Van Zundert A, Vaes L, Soetens M, et al: Every dose given in epidural analgesia for vaginal delivery can be a test dose. Anesthesiology 1987; 67: 436–440.

134. Rawal N, Schollin J, Wesstrom G: Epidural versus combined spinal epidural block for cesarean section. Acta Anaesthesiol Scand 1988; 32: 61–66.
135. Fan SZ, Susetio L, Wang YP, et al: Low dose of intrathecal hyperbaric bupivacaine combined with epidural lidocaine for cesarean section—a balance block technique. Anesth Analg 1994; 78: 474–477.
136. Kotelko DM, Dailey PA, Shnider SM, et al: Epidural morphine analgesia after cesarean delivery. Obstet Gynecol 1984; 63: 409–413.
137. Fuller JG, McMorland GH, Douglas MJ, et al: Epidural morphine for analgesia after caesarean section: a report of 4880 patients. Can J Anaesth 1990; 37: 636–640.
138. Brockway MS, Noble DW, Sharwood-Smith GH, et al: Profound respiratory depression after extradural fentanyl. Br J Anaesth 1990; 64: 243–245.
139. Palmer CM: Early respiratory depression following intrathecal fentanyl-morphine combination. Anesthesiology 1991; 74: 1153–1155.
140. Brose WG, Cohen SE: Oxyhemoglobin saturation following cesarean section in patients receiving epidural morphine, PCA, or IM meperidine analgesia. Anesthesiology 1989; 70: 948–953.
141. Daley MD, Sandler AN, Turner KE, et al: A comparison of epidural and intramuscular morphine in patients following cesarean section. Anesthesiology 1990; 72: 289–294.
142. Eisenach JC, Grice SC, Dewan DM: Patient-controlled analgesia following cesarean section: a comparison with epidural and intramuscular narcotics. Anesthesiology 1988; 68: 444–448.
143. Harrison DM, Sinatra R, Morgese L, et al: Epidural narcotic and patient-controlled analgesia for post-cesarean section pain relief. Anesthesiology 1988; 68: 454–457.
144. Crone LA, Conly JM, Clark KM, et al: Recurrent herpes simplex virus labialis and the use of epidural morphine in obstetric patients. Anesth Analg 1988; 67: 318–323.
145. Ranney B, Stanage WF: Advantages of local anesthesia for cesarean section. Obstet Gynecol 1975; 45: 163–167.
146. Cooper MG, Feeney EM, Joseph M, et al: Local anaesthetic infiltration for caesarean section. Anaesth Intensive Care 1989; 17: 198–201.
147. Rout CC, Rocke DA, Gouws E: Intravenous ranitidine reduces the risk of acid aspiration of gastric contents at emergency cesarean section. (Published erratum appears in Anesth Analg 1993; 76: 1180.) Anesth Analg 1993; 76: 156–161.
148. Mendelson CL: The aspiration of stomach contents into the lungs during obstetric anesthesia. Am J Obstet Gynecol 1946; 52: 191–204.
149. Sellick BA: Cricoid pressure to control regurgitation of stomach contents during induction of anaesthesia. Lancet 1961; 2: 404–406.
150. Sivarajan M, Fink BR: The position and the state of the larynx during general anesthesia and muscle paralysis. Anesthesiology 1990; 72: 439–442.
151. Holdcroft A, Morgan M: Intravenous induction agents for caesarean section. Anaesthesia 1989; 44: 719–720.
152. Lennon RL, Olson RA, Gronert GA: Atracurium or vecuronium for rapid sequence endotracheal intubation. Anesthesiology 1986; 64: 510–513.
153. Marx GF, Mateo CV: Effects of different oxygen concentrations during general anesthesia for elective caesarean section. Can Anaesth Soc J 1971; 18: 587–593.
154. Baraka A, Louis F, Noueihid R, et al: Awareness following different techniques of general anaesthesia for caesarean section. Br J Anaesth 1989; 62: 645–648.
155. Marx GF, Luykx WM, Cohen S: Fetal-neonatal status following caesarean section for fetal distress. Br J Anaesth 1984; 56: 1009–1013.
156. Perlow JH, Morgan MA: Massive maternal obesity and perioperative cesarean morbidity. Am J Obstet Gynecol 1994; 170: 560–565.
157. Hood DD, Dewan DM: Anesthetic and obstetric outcome in morbidly obese parturients. Anesthesiology 1993; 79: 1210–1218.
158. Hodgkinson R, Husain FJ: Caesarean section associated with gross obesity. Br J Anaesth 1980; 52: 919–923.
159. Milligan KR, Carp H: Continuous spinal anaesthesia for caesarean section in the morbidly obese. Int J Obstet Anesth 1992; 1: 111–113.
160. Rolbin SH, Cohen MM, Levinton CM, et al: The premature infant: anesthesia for cesarean delivery. Anesth Analg 1994; 78: 912–917.
161. Douglas MJ, Ward ME: Current pharmacology and the obstetric anesthesiologist. Int Anesth Clin 1994; 32(2): 1–10.
162. Mayer DC, Weeks SK: Antepartum uterine relaxation with nitroglycerin at caesarean delivery. Can J Anaesth 1992; 39: 166–169.

CHAPTER 36

Postdelivery Analgesia

David M. Ransom, M.D., Craig H. Leicht, M.D., M.P.H.

Historical Perspective

Throughout the ages, methods have been sought to relieve the discomfort associated with childbirth. As early as 2600 BC, the Chinese, Greeks, Egyptians, and others used various pain-relieving modalities to ease suffering during childbirth.[1] Early accounts mention only efforts to decrease pain during childbirth and do not address the issue of pain relief in the postpartum period, despite anecdotal reports[2] that cesarean sections were performed during this time. At least two issues are responsible for this apparent insensitivity by early medical practitioners. First, before the late 1700s, most cesarean sections were performed only in an attempt to save the fetus after maternal death, a practice mandated at that time by the Catholic Church for baptismal purposes.[2] Second, until the Renaissance period, miracles and faith healing rather than scientific method were the prevailing therapies, with patients often failing to survive into the postdelivery period.[3] Early medical practitioners condemned the performance of cesarean deliveries because of suboptimal analgesia and the high incidence of death due to hemorrhage and sepsis.[2]

Early in the 19th century, the Prussian pharmacist Sertürner isolated the alkaloid morphine, identifying it as the opiate substance whose pain-relieving properties had been touted for centuries.[4] During the mid-19th century, chloroform, nitrous oxide, and ether were being put into clinical use for operative procedures. Concomitantly, cesarean sections were being performed with greater safety and minimal pain and were considered seriously as an option to vaginal delivery. Still, the focus of physicians was on pain control during childbirth and the perioperative period. It was not until the early 1900s, when George Crile advanced his anociassociation theory that postoperative pain control could exert a positive influence on the results of operation, that postdelivery analgesia was considered worthy of recognition.[4] Oral analgesics were commonplace after vaginal delivery during this time, with intramuscular administration of opioids providing the mainstay of therapy after operative deliveries. By 1952, a growing dissatisfaction with intramuscular administration of opioids was emerging, eventually prompting experimentation with other routes of opioid administration.[4]

In 1963, Roe[5] showed that opioids administered intravenously by intermittent bolus doses provided better pain relief than larger doses administered intramuscularly. Unfortunately, the duration of analgesia was brief, and increasing the dose produced unwanted side effects. This led to experimentation by several practitioners with continuous intravenous infusions, but the difficulty in identifying an ideal dose that afforded good analgesia without untoward effects or the need for intermittent bolus supplementation limited the utility of this technique.[6] With the advent of patient-controlled analgesia (PCA) in the late 1960s, intravenous analgesia became more effective, and advances in this modality have kept it at the forefront of postoperative analgesic options.

At roughly the same time that intravenous administration of opioids was undergoing scrutiny, a renewed interest in epidural analgesia had prompted several investigators to experiment with opioid administration by this route. Behar and colleagues[7] in 1979 were the first to administer opioids epidurally for postoperative pain relief, and at the same time Wang and coworkers[8] began using opioids intrathecally for pain relief in the outpatient setting. These two methods enjoy wide clinical acceptance today and represent the standard for postcesarean analgesia at this time. For pain after vaginal delivery, oral medications continue to be the most commonly prescribed analgesics, with the newer nonsteroidal agents assuming a prominent role.

Analgesia After Vaginal Delivery

Any discussion of postdelivery obstetric analgesia would be incomplete without a discussion of analgesic options for the parturient after vaginal delivery. Topical therapy such as cold stimuli from ice packs and cold sitz baths as well as topical anesthetics are often used initially for pain relief after vaginal delivery. However, episiotomy pain and uterine cramping are often insufficiently relieved with these interventional modalities during the immediate postpartum period. Because both of these pain entities are attributed in part to prostaglandin release, aspirin and the nonsteroidal anti-inflammatory drugs are useful in relieving this pain. Opioids relieve episiotomy pain by inhibiting the release of excitatory transmitters from the nociceptive pain receptors stimulated in response to tissue injury at the episiotomy site. The oral preparations of these agents have been extensively studied in this patient population and are indeed useful for control of mild to moderate pain.

Ibuprofen is the nonsteroidal anti-inflammatory drug we prefer because of its low cost and lack of effect on infants who are breast-fed.[9] Aspirin is an effective alternative but does require more frequent dosing. Potential adverse effects of ibuprofen and other nonsteroidal anti-inflammatory drugs include gastrointestinal irritation and platelet inhibition in susceptible patients. Because of the short duration of therapy with the nonsteroidal agents, the incidence of related problems has been minimal in this patient population.

Oral preparations of opioids containing codeine are often used in the postpartum patient, but in studies by Bloomfield and colleagues,[10, 11] the analgesic effect was indistinguishable from that of the nonsteroidal anti-inflammatory drugs. Because of this and the potential for nausea, vomiting, and central nervous system effects such as sedation and dizziness, many physicians prefer to limit the use of codeine-containing preparations for postdelivery analgesia.

Traditional Postcesarean Analgesia

As early as 1961, Keats and associates[12] described the inadequacies of traditional postoperative pain management techniques, such as nurse-administered intramuscular and intravenous analgesics. Graves and colleagues[13] attributed the undertreatment of pain by traditional methods to the cyclic nature of a patient's request for pain medication (Fig. 36–1). Each step in this cycle delays analgesia, and Graves and his colleagues estimated that 30 min passed between the time a patient requested medication and the time the injection was given. This regimen resulted in a pattern of high peak blood levels of analgesic accompanied by patient sedation immediately after injection, followed by subtherapeutic concentrations and renewed perception of pain on patient awakening, leading into the next cycle. Patient satisfaction with pain medication administered in this manner was low, particularly in

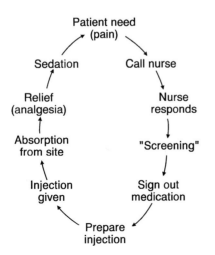

Figure 36–1 The cyclic character of conventional analgesic therapy. (Redrawn from Graves DA, Foster TS, Batenhorst RL, et al: Patient-controlled analgesia. Ann Intern Med 1983; 99: 360–366.)

women after cesarean delivery because of their intense desire but decreased ability to interact with their newborn.[14]

Patient-Controlled Analgesia

Sechzer[15] first described PCA using intermittent intravenous bolus doses of opioids in 1968. He demonstrated that consistent pain relief could be achieved with less medication when opioids were administered by nurses on request from the patient. Early acceptance of his technique was limited because this practice was labor intensive for nursing staff. After investigators perfected automated techniques of administration, intravenously administered PCA gained wide acceptance.

The ability of the patient to self-administer pain medication offers several advantages over traditional methods. Many patients hesitate to request pain medication from nursing personnel, feeling it is a sign of weakness or that they are bothering the nursing staff. The autonomy of PCA affords this subgroup of patients improved pain relief and contributes to their psychologic well-being by placing them in control of their pain management. Less sedation is experienced by patients who have PCA with opioids than with opioids given intramuscularly because the PCA route of administration eliminates the use of concomitantly administered sedatives with each dose and results in lower overall medication usage.[12, 16] This is of particular benefit in the parturient who is anxious to interact with her newborn. Pain relief with intravenous PCA has been reported[16, 17] to be more immediate and superior to intramuscular injections, although at least one group of investigators[14] has disputed this observation. Statistically significant decreases in the number of pulmonary complications occurring postoperatively in patients who had PCA compared with those receiving intramuscular analgesia were reported by Nayman.[18] This has been suggested by other researchers[17] as well, especially in subpopulations susceptible to pulmonary insults after surgical procedures, such as obese patients. Painful intramuscular injections are eliminated, promoting greater patient acceptance. Tamsen and coworkers[19] reported that 92% of patients using PCA considered the technique very effective, which is indicative of the high degree of patient satisfaction with this modality of pain relief.

Although side effects and complications are rare, they do exist. In 1970, Scott[20] described a case of generalized convulsions during PCA that was attributed to toxic blood levels of opioid. Frank respiratory depression was reported in two patients by Tamsen and colleagues[19] based on blood gas assessment. Both patients were also hypovolemic, and as fluid resuscitation was performed, their respiratory depression gradually disappeared, allowing both to continue PCA. Other side effects observed by Tamsen's group included drowsiness in 68% of patients, dry mouth in 43%, and nausea in 14%. Rayburn and associates[16] observed pruritus in 1 of 67 patients in a PCA group. The patient required drug therapy (hydroxyzine) but did not have to discon-

Table 36–1 Costs Attributable to Postcesarean Analgesia: Nursing Time Plus Pharmacy Charges

| | COST, $ | | | | |
INTERVENTIONS	EM (n = 128)	EM + F (n = 245)	SM (n = 48)	IM (n = 165)	PCA (n = 98)
Side effects	30.74	28.20	26.59	15.99	1.53
Analgesia	28.06	33.59	20.32	74.61	129.25
Monitoring	45.00	45.00	45.00	7.85	7.85
Total	103.80	106.79	91.91	98.45	138.63*

*P = .05 versus all other groups (significant differences stated only for total costs).

EM, epidural morphine; EM + F, epidural morphine + fentanyl; IM, intramuscular analgesia; PCA, patient-controlled analgesia; SM, subarachnoid morphine; n, number of patients.

From Cohen SE, Suback LL, Brose WG, et al: Analgesia after cesarean delivery: patient evaluations and costs of five opioid techniques. Reg Anesth 1991; 16: 141–149.

tinue the infusion. The cost of therapy with PCA is only slightly more than that of the other currently available analgesic modalities[21] (Table 36–1).

Relatively little information exists regarding the optimal analgesic agent for use in PCA, but drugs such as meperidine and fentanyl seem to be favored over drugs such as buprenorphine, morphine, and methadone.[13, 22, 23] The pharmacokinetics and pharmacodynamics of the agent chosen for PCA administration must be considered, and agents that result in a peak analgesic effect within minutes coupled with minimal sedation are preferred.[13]

Neuraxial Analgesia

Neuraxial analgesia typically encompasses epidural and intrathecal administration of analgesics to provide postdelivery pain relief. The use of these modalities is logical because many women have analgesics administered epidurally or intrathecally for labor or operative analgesia.

Epidural Analgesia

The excellent analgesia afforded by the epidural route is well substantiated in the literature.[24–28] Since 1979, when Behar and colleagues[7] first administered morphine epidurally for postoperative pain relief, clinicians have used this route for delivering postoperative analgesia. Although some centers may use epidural analgesia for postoperative pain control in patients delivering vaginally, the most widespread use is in patients who have undergone cesarean delivery.

Historically, opioids have been the agents of choice for postdelivery epidural analgesia. Opioids administered epidurally exert a combined effect on the spinal opioid receptors identified by Yaksh and Rudy[29] and on supraspinal and presynaptic opioid receptors, producing excellent analgesia at lower doses than opioids administered intramuscularly or intravenously. The lower dose requirement produces fewer side effects, resulting in no muscle weakness or loss of motor performance and minimal sensory impairment other than the relief of pain.

Opioids can be administered epidurally in various

ways. A single epidural dose of opioid is typically administered after completion of cesarean delivery just before removal of the epidural catheter. Morphine is the drug most often used in this way, with a dose typically ranging from 2 to 7.5 mg. Although the lower dose has been used successfully by some, Rosen and colleagues,[26] in reviewing the literature, found most investigators reported ineffective analgesia for operative procedures on the abdomen with a dose of 2 mg. When doses of 5 and 7.5 mg were administered, they found no reported difference in time of onset, peak analgesia, or duration of analgesia between the two doses. This is an important finding, because the incidence and severity of side effects appear to be dose dependent. Patients generally report a slow onset of pain relief with morphine, but they ultimately enjoy between 24 and 30 h of pain relief after a single epidural dose of morphine without supplementation by oral medications (Table 36–2). This duration of action is somewhat longer than that reported for morphine administered epidurally after other surgical procedures,[30, 31] and it may result from a subconscious suppression of pain recognition by the parturient who is preoccupied with her newborn or secondary to the physiologic changes that accompany pregnancy.

Postcesarean analgesia can also involve the combination of opioids with other known analgesic agents. The addition of local anesthetic, as reported by Hanson and coworkers,[32] improves the onset of action of morphine, but in their hands it did not improve the side-effect profile of this opioid. Moore and colleagues[33] described the use of low-dose morphine (2.5 mg) administered epidurally in conjunction with 60 mg of ketorolac

Table 36–2 Epidural Administration of Morphine After Cesarean Section: Analgesia in 1000 Patients

OUTCOME	MEASUREMENT
Good to excellent pain relief, %	85
Duration of analgesia (mean ± SEM), h	23 ± 0.4
Patients requesting no further analgesics, %	16
Patients requesting only oral analgesics, %	44

SEM, standard error of the mean.

Data from Leicht CH, Hughes SC, Dailey PA, et al: Epidural morphine sulfate for analgesia after cesarean section: a prospective report of 1000 patients. (Abstract.) Anesthesiology 1986; 65: A366.

given intravenously at the conclusion of cesarean delivery, followed by 30 mg of ketorolac administered every 6 h thereafter for 24 h. Patient satisfaction with pain control is markedly increased by this combination therapy, and side effects have been decreased considerably, although recommendations are to limit the combined use to mothers not planning to breast-feed their infants. Similarly, other investigators have used intramuscular or intravenous administration of diclofenac[34] or ketoprofen[35] in combination with morphine and have observed an opioid-sparing effect with these agents as well. Because of the action of these nonsteroidal anti-inflammatory medications, an additional benefit may be predicted if they are used preemptively in the delivery situation. Their use in this manner is not recommended, however, because of concerns about premature ductus arteriosus closure in the fetus.

Huntoon and associates[36] found epidurally administered clonidine to be somewhat efficacious for postdelivery analgesia after continuous epidurally administered bupivacaine for cesarean delivery. However, they concluded that clonidine may offer few advantages over traditional opioid therapy, may increase the incidence of side effects—especially hypotension,[37] and may be less effective after 2-chloroprocaine has been administered for analgesia during the cesarean procedure.

Other opioids have been advocated for use as a single bolus before epidural catheter removal, but the results have been somewhat disappointing. Fentanyl has a rapid onset of action, but the duration of pain relief is short, usually lasting only 2 to 4 h. Meperidine, sufentanil, and methadone also do not provide a satisfactory duration of action when administered as a single bolus before epidural catheter removal.[31, 38] In the past, we have used the 5-mg dose of morphine through the epidural route when used alone as a single bolus because it offers adequate pain relief in relation to side effects and has a satisfactory duration of action. However, we more commonly use 2.5 mg of morphine given epidurally in conjunction with intravenous or intramuscular administration of ketorolac, similar to the method suggested by Moore and colleagues.[33] This appears to provide the best ratio of pain relief to side effects for pain management in our patient population.

Continuous epidural infusions of fentanyl in doses ranging from 50 to 100 μg/h have gained popularity during the past few years. However, the literature is somewhat divided in terms of the clinical utility of this route of administration, because it may offer no benefit over continuous intravenous administration[39] and may result in the patient receiving more opioid than required.[40] Several investigators[41–45] have experimented with continuous opioid administration by means of epidural PCA. This method combines the superior analgesia of epidural administration of opioids with the improved analgesia resulting from patient participation.[14] Various opioids, including morphine, hydromorphone, meperidine, and fentanyl, have been administered in this manner. The greatest patient satisfaction appears to be with agents of intermediate lipophilicity such as meperidine and hydromorphone. The highly

lipophilic agents such as fentanyl are rapidly absorbed systemically, resulting in concentrations similar to, and therefore of no benefit over, intravenous PCA. The low lipophilic agents such as morphine have a prolonged time to onset and increased incidence of side effects.[42] Overall, PCA administered epidurally is associated with earlier return of bowel sounds, earlier resumption of solid diet, and earlier hospital dismissal than PCA administered intravenously.[41] Pruritus and nausea, however, prevent a more widespread use of this route of administration.

Side effects most commonly reported after epidural administration of opioids are similar to those seen with other routes of opioid administration and include respiratory depression, pruritus, nausea, and urinary retention. The most serious is delayed respiratory depression. Opioids are potent analgesic drugs, and respiratory depression is a potential concern with their use, regardless of the route of administration. In the parturient, however, the incidence after epidural administration may be somewhat less than in the general population owing to the increased respiratory drive that occurs during pregnancy. Leicht and coworkers[46] demonstrated that the incidence of clinical respiratory depression in the parturient after 5 mg of epidurally administered morphine sulfate may be as low as 0.1% to 0.2% (Table 36–3). Factors that may increase the potential for respiratory depression include the spinal level at which the opioid is administered and also supplemental parenteral opioid administration. The latter factor is of particular concern to the anesthesiologist because the postoperative care for the parturient is often rendered in a location away from surgical and labor and delivery suites where the anesthesiologist, of necessity, is stationed. It is therefore important to have a mechanism in place such as standard written orders or a protocol that allows for the management of the parturient's pain in locations where an anesthesiologist may not be physically present but is immediately available.

When delayed respiratory depression does occur, it is most often reported within 8 to 12 h of bolus opioid administration (Fig. 36–2). Morphine seems to be the agent most likely to result in respiratory depression, particularly of a delayed nature, because of its low lipid solubility. This characteristic allows for accumulation of morphine in the cerebrospinal fluid, enhancing the

Table 36–3 Epidural Administration of Morphine After Cesarean Section: Side Effects in 1000 Patients

SIDE EFFECT	PATIENTS, %
Pruritus	
Severe	4
Moderate	23
Requiring treatment	29
Nausea and vomiting	20
Respiratory depression	0.4
Potentially life threatening	0.1

Data from Leicht CH, Hughes SC, Dailey PA, et al: Epidural morphine sulfate for analgesia after cesarean section: a prospective report of 1000 patients. (Abstract.) Anesthesiology 1986; 65: A366.

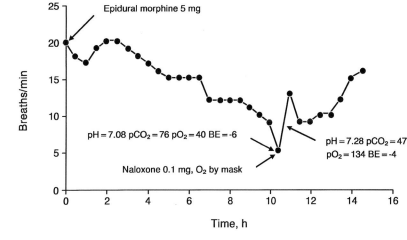

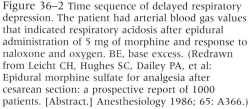

Figure 36–2 Time sequence of delayed respiratory depression. The patient had arterial blood gas values that indicated respiratory acidosis after epidural administration of 5 mg of morphine and response to naloxone and oxygen. BE, base excess. (Redrawn from Leicht CH, Hughes SC, Dailey PA, et al: Epidural morphine sulfate for analgesia after cesarean section: a prospective report of 1000 patients. [Abstract.] Anesthesiology 1986; 65: A366.)

potential for rostral spread.[47] Respiratory depression, immediate or delayed, is an ongoing concern with the use of continuous opioid infusions. Although opioids, including those administered epidurally, have the potential to cause respiratory depression, this should not preclude their use in a setting where appropriate patient monitoring is maintained.

The incidence of nausea and vomiting is somewhat variable with opioids given epidurally but appears to be greatest in patients receiving morphine epidurally instead of more lipid-soluble agents. The incidence varies between 15% and 30% of the obstetric population. Commonly used antiemetics such as droperidol, metoclopramide, and even transdermal scopolamine may be effective in relieving this symptom.[48]

Pruritus, although usually minor, may occur in as many as 80% of patients receiving opioids epidurally.[25] One third of patients experiencing pruritus ultimately request treatment for this side effect.[46, 49] Intravenously administered opioid antagonists such as naloxone have been somewhat effective in relieving this symptom and, contrary to popular belief, do not always reverse the analgesic effect of the opioid.[50] If an antagonist is administered within the first 30 min after fentanyl administration, however, a decreased analgesic effect may result.[51] Diphenhydramine has also been used successfully for controlling pruritus in parturients receiving postoperative analgesics. A novel treatment option for pruritus secondary to epidural administration of morphine is the use of subhypnotic doses of propofol. Borgeat and colleagues[52] successfully treated morphine-induced pruritus in approximately 85% of patients by giving 10 mg of propofol intravenously. The side effects were minimal in their patient population.

Urinary retention has also been reported after epidural administration of opioids for postdelivery analgesia. Although poorly understood, the mechanism is thought to result from the opioid's effect on sacral spinal nerves, which inhibits the micturition reflex.[48] Chadwick and Ross[48] reported less than a 5% incidence of urinary retention after epidural administration of opioids for postdelivery pain management. In general, this is not a significant problem in the obstetric population, because it is the practice of many obstetricians to

leave an indwelling urinary catheter in place for 24 h after a cesarean delivery.

Intrathecal Analgesia

Local anesthetics administered intrathecally for obstetric care may last into the postdelivery period, but they are not the best choice for pain control after the surgical procedure has been completed because of the accompanying motor block. Similar to epidural administration of morphine, intrathecal administration of opioids provides an analgesic effect as a result of a direct action on spinal opioid receptors in the substantia gelatinosa of the dorsal horn of the spinal cord. This pain-relieving effect is selective in that sensory, motor, and sympathetic function remain essentially intact after administration of analgesic doses. Maintenance of vascular tone resulting from little or no sympathetic effect without a motor block facilitates early patient mobility.

Intrathecal administration of morphine has been used for postoperative analgesia for many years. A single dose of morphine can be administered intrathecally at the time a regional technique is performed. Analgesic duration is roughly 24 h after administration. Initial acceptance of this technique was low because of the high incidence of side effects. However, as practitioners learned that lower doses of morphine given intrathecally provided adequate analgesia while dramatically decreasing side effects, the use of this technique increased significantly.[53] Brookshire and colleagues,[54] experimenting with the opioid antagonist naloxone, found that intravenous administration of this agent after intrathecal administration of 1 mg of morphine decreased the incidence of side effects without affecting the analgesic properties. Routine use of naloxone to counter side effects is unnecessary when a lower dose of morphine is selected for intrathecal administration.

The potentially harmful effects of morphine given intrathecally are dose related, depending on the rate of absorption and on movement within the cerebrospinal fluid. Most practitioners use 0.1 to 0.5 mg of morphine for postoperative analgesia, and the incidence of side effects is much lower than it once was. More lipophilic opioids such as fentanyl have been administered intrathecally and offer the advantage of more rapid absorption and therefore quicker effect. Their duration of action is much shorter, however, and limits their use in patients receiving a single intrathecal injection at the start of a surgical procedure. We use low-dose morphine given intrathecally in conjunction with ketorolac given intravenously or intramuscularly, similar to what Moore and associates[33] described with morphine given epidurally. This combination provides excellent analgesia in the postoperative period and decreases the incidence of side effects caused by morphine. However, because of prescribing changes instituted by the manufacturer of ketorolac, we limit the use of this combination to those patients who will not be breast-feeding their newborns.

The side effects of opioids given intrathecally are similar to those described during epidural analgesia. As with opioids given epidurally, the greatest concern is for delayed respiratory depression. Postoperative monitoring of these patients is essential for the duration of the analgesic effect. Although many monitoring devices have been evaluated, we use close nursing observation in the postoperative setting for a minimum of 24 h as our mainstay for monitoring parturients after opioids are given intrathecally. For higher-risk patients, pulse oximetry may be added to monitor respiratory status more closely.

Administration of intrathecal analgesia through an indwelling catheter has increased in popularity for obstetric patients. Because of a concern over the safety of leaving an indwelling catheter in the intrathecal space for extended periods, most anesthesiologists using this technique remove the catheter after delivery is complete. Bevacqua and colleagues[55] evaluated the presence of intrathecal catheters in the postdelivery setting as a cause of infections. Their work indicates that intrathecal catheter usage may be an option provided the catheter is not left in place longer than 96 h. Because of the significance of a central nervous system infection, particularly in the postdelivery setting, we rarely leave intrathecal catheters in place after the surgical procedure is completed. We do, however, inject low-dose morphine intrathecally before removal of the catheter.

Summary

During the past few years, many innovations have occurred in the field of obstetric anesthesia. Postcesarean analgesia is one area that has benefited particularly from the new techniques. The use of intermittent intravenous and intramuscular bolus administration of opioids has been replaced primarily by the superior analgesia afforded by PCA, epidural analgesia, and intrathecal analgesia. These techniques continue to be refined, resulting in more effective pain management, earlier resumption of normal activities, and earlier hospital dismissal.[21, 56] With the increased emphasis by the federal government and third-party payers on medical cost control, it is important to appreciate that the use of these newer methods of pain control is not apparently associated with increased costs in most cases.[21] A new standard for postcesarean pain management has been achieved with the advent of these new techniques that maintains the anesthesiologist in a position of leadership in this vital area of pain management.

References

1. Lull CB, Hingson RA: Control of Pain in Childbirth, 2nd ed, pp 121–130. Philadelphia, JB Lippincott, 1945.
2. Phelan JP, Clark SL (eds): Cesarean Delivery, chap 1. New York, Elsevier Publishing, 1988.
3. Madigan SR, Raj PP: History and current status of pain management. In Raj PP: Practical Management of Pain, 2nd ed, pp 3–15. St. Louis, Mosby Year Book, 1992.
4. Raj PP: The problem of postoperative pain—an epidemiologic perspective. In Ferrante FM, VadeBoncouer TR (eds): Postoperative Pain Management, pp 1–16. New York, Churchill Livingstone, 1993.
5. Roe BB: Are postoperative narcotics necessary? Arch Surg 1963; 87: 912–915.
6. Parker RK: Postoperative analgesia: Systemic techniques. In Chestnut DH (ed): Obstetric Anesthesia: Principles & Practice, pp 501–512. St. Louis, Mosby–Year Book, 1994.
7. Behar M, Magora F, Olshwang D, et al: Epidural morphine in treatment of pain. Lancet 1979; 1: 527–529.
8. Wang JK, Nauss LA, Thomas JE: Pain relief by intrathecally applied morphine in man. Anesthesiology 1979; 50: 149–151.
9. Windle ML, Booker LA, Rayburn WF: Postpartum pain after vaginal delivery: a review of comparative analgesic trials. J Reprod Med 1989; 34: 891–895.
10. Bloomfield SS, Barden TP, Mitchell J: Naproxen, aspirin, and codeine in postpartum uterine pain. Clin Pharmacol Ther 1977; 21: 414–421.
11. Bloomfield SS, Mitchell J, Cissell G, et al: Flurbiprofen, aspirin, codeine, and placebo for postpartum uterine pain. Am J Med 1986; 80: 65–70.
12. Keats AS, Telford J, Kurosu Y: "Potentiation" of meperidine by promethazine. Anesthesiology 1961; 22: 34–41.
13. Graves DA, Foster TS, Batenhorst RL, et al: Patient-controlled analgesia. Ann Intern Med 1983; 99: 360–366.
14. Harrison DM, Sinatra R, Morgese L, et al: Epidural narcotic and patient-controlled analgesia for post-cesarean section pain relief. Anesthesiology 1988; 68: 454–457.
15. Sechzer PH: Objective measurement of pain. Anesthesiology 1968; 29: 209–210.
16. Rayburn WF, Geranis BJ, Ramadei CA, et al: Patient-controlled analgesia for post-cesarean section pain. Obstet Gynecol 1988; 72: 136–139.
17. White PF: Use of patient-controlled analgesia for management of acute pain. JAMA 1988; 259: 243–247.
18. Nayman J: Measurement and control of postoperative pain. Ann R Coll Surg Engl 1979; 61: 419–426.
19. Tamsen A, Hartvig P, Fagerlund C, et al: Patient-controlled analgesic therapy: clinical experience. Acta Anaesthesiol Scand Suppl 1982; 74: 157–160.
20. Scott JS: Obstetric analgesia: A consideration of labor pain and a patient-controlled technique for its relief with meperidine. Am J Obstet Gynecol 1970; 106: 959–978.
21. Cohen SE, Subak LL, Brose WG, et al: Analgesia after cesarean delivery: patient evaluations and costs of five opioid techniques. Reg Anesth 1991; 16: 141–149.
22. Gibbs JM, Johnson HD, Davis FM: Patient administration of I.V. buprenorphine for postoperative pain relief using the "Cardiff" demand analgesia apparatus. Br J Anaesth 1982; 54: 279–284.
23. Dahlstrom B, Tamsen A, Paalzow L, et al: Patient-controlled analgesic therapy, Part IV: Pharmacokinetics and analgesic plasma concentrations of morphine. Clin Pharmacokinet 1982; 7: 266–279.
24. Farabow WS, Roberson VO, Maxey J, et al: A twenty-year retrospective analysis of the efficacy of epidural analgesia-anes-

thesia when administered and/or managed by obstetricians. Am J Obstet Gynecol 1993; 169: 270–278.

25. Westmore MD: Epidural opioids in obstetrics—a review. Anaesth Intensive Care 1990; 18: 292–300.

26. Rosen MA, Hughes SC, Shnider SM, et al: Epidural morphine for the relief of postoperative pain after cesarean delivery. Anesth Analg 1983; 62: 666–672.

27. Kotelko DM, Dailey PA, Shnider SM, et al: Epidural morphine analgesia after cesarean delivery. Obstet Gynecol 1984; 63: 409–413.

28. Fuller JG, McMorland GH, Douglas MJ, et al: Epidural morphine for analgesia after caesarean section: a report of 4880 patients. Can J Anaesth 1990; 37: 636–640.

29. Yaksh TL, Rudy TA: Analgesia mediated by a direct spinal action of narcotics. Science 1976; 192: 1357–1358.

30. Rutter DV, Skewes DG, Morgan M: Extradural opioids for post-operative analgesia: a double-blind comparison of pethidine, fentanyl and morphine. Br J Anaesth 1981; 53: 915–920.

31. Torda TA, Pybus DA: Comparison of four narcotic analgesics for extradural analgesia. Br J Anaesth 1982; 54: 291–295.

32. Hanson AL, Hanson B, Matousek M: Epidural anesthesia for cesarean section: the effect of morphine-bupivacaine administered epidurally for intra- and postoperative pain relief. Acta Obstet Gynecol Scand 1984; 63: 135–140.

33. Moore CH, Fragneto RY, Pan PH, et al: Combination low-dose epidural morphine and parenteral ketorolac tromethamine for postcesarean pain relief. (Abstract 49.) Proceedings of the Twenty-Sixth Annual Meeting of the Society for Obstetric Anesthesia and Perinatology (SOAP), Philadelphia, May 1994.

34. Sun HL, Wu CC, Lin MS, et al: Combination of low-dose epidural morphine and intramuscular diclofenac sodium in postcesarean analgesia. Anesth Analg 1992; 75: 64–68.

35. Rorarius MG, Suominen P, Baer GA, et al: Diclofenac and ketoprofen for pain treatment after elective caesarean section. Br J Anaesth 1993; 70: 293–297.

36. Huntoon M, Eisenach JC, Boese P: Epidural clonidine after cesarean section: appropriate dose and effect of prior local anesthetic. Anesthesiology 1992; 76: 187–193.

37. Mogensen T, Eliasen K, Ejlersen E, et al: Epidural clonidine enhances postoperative analgesia from a combined low-dose epidural bupivacaine and morphine regimen. Anesth Analg 1992; 75: 607–610.

38. Dottrens M, Rifat K, Morel DR: Comparison of extradural administration of sufentanil, morphine and sufentanil-morphine combination after caesarean section. Br J Anaesth 1992; 69: 9–12.

39. Ellis DJ, Millar WL, Reisner LS: A randomized double-blind comparison of epidural versus intravenous fentanyl infusion for analgesia after cesarean section. Anesthesiology 1990; 72: 981–986.

40. Parker RK, White PF: Epidural patient-controlled analgesia: an alternative to intravenous patient-controlled analgesia for pain relief after cesarean delivery. Anesth Analg 1992; 75: 245–251.

41. Marlowe S, Engstrom R, White PF: Epidural patient-controlled analgesia (PCA): an alternative to continuous epidural infusions. Pain 1989; 37: 97–101.

42. Yarnell RW, Polis T, Reid GN, et al: Patient-controlled analgesia with epidural meperidine after elective cesarean section. Reg Anesth 1992; 17: 329–333.

43. Yu PY, Gambling DR: A comparative study of patient-controlled epidural fentanyl and single dose epidural morphine for post-caesarean analgesia. Can J Anaesth 1993; 40: 416–420.

44. Parker RK, Sawaki Y, White PF: Epidural patient-controlled analgesia: influence of bupivacaine and hydromorphone basal infusion on pain control after cesarean delivery. Anesth Analg 1992; 75: 740–746.

45. Cohen S, Amar D, Pantuck CB, et al: Epidural patient-controlled analgesia after cesarean section: buprenorphine–0.015% bupivacaine with epinephrine versus fentanyl–0.015% bupivacaine with and without epinephrine. Anesth Analg 1992; 74: 226–230.

46. Leicht CH, Hughes SC, Dailey PA, et al: Epidural morphine sulfate for analgesia after cesarean section: a prospective report of 1000 patients. (Abstract.) Anesthesiology 1986; 65:A366.

47. Cousins MJ, Mather LE: Intrathecal and epidural administration of opioids. Anesthesiology 1984; 61: 276–310.

48. Chadwick HS, Ross BK: Analgesia for post-cesarean delivery pain. Anesthiol Clin North Am 1989; 7: 133–153.

49. Rah KH, Baxter RW, Perera F, et al: Epidural morphine analgesia after cesarean delivery. Anesth Rev 1987; 3: 8–16.

50. Dailey PA, Brookshire GL, Shnider SM, et al: The effects of naloxone associated with the intrathecal use of morphine in labor. Anesth Analg 1985; 64: 658–666.

51. Brownridge P, Frewin DB: A comparative study of techniques of postoperative analgesia following caesarean section and lower abdominal surgery. Anaesth Intensive Care 1985; 13: 123–130.

52. Borgeat A, Wilder-Smith OH, Saiah M, et al: Subhypnotic doses of propofol relieve pruritus induced by epidural and intrathecal morphine. Anesthesiology 1992; 76: 510–512.

53. Nordberg G, Hedner T, Mellstrand T, et al: Pharmacokinetic aspects of intrathecal morphine analgesia. Anesthesiology 1984; 60: 448–454.

54. Brookshire GL, Shnider SM, Abboud TK, et al: Effects of naloxone on the mother and neonate after intrathecal morphine for labor analgesia. (Abstract.) Anesthesiology 1983; 59:A417.

55. Bevacqua BK, Slucky AV, Cleary WF: Is postoperative intrathecal catheter use associated with central nervous system infection? Anesthesiology 1994; 80: 1234–1240.

56. Stenkamp SJ, Easterling TR, Chadwick HS: Effect of epidural and intrathecal morphine on the length of hospital stay after cesarean section. Anesth Analg 1989; 68: 66–69.

CHAPTER 37

Anesthesiology-Based Acute Pain Services: A Contemporary View

L. Brian Ready, M.D., F.R.C.P.C.,
Narinder Rawal, M.D., Ph.D.

The role of anesthesiologists as members of interdisciplinary teams that evaluate and treat chronic and cancer pain has been established for more than 40 years, but it was not until 1988 that an anesthesiology-based acute pain service was popularized.[1] In this chapter, the origins and short history of acute pain services are discussed. The current worldwide status of acute pain services is reviewed; the section on Europe was prepared by Dr. Narinder Rawal, and the section on other countries was prepared by Dr. L. Brian Ready. We define the common features of all or most acute pain services from among our widely differing organizational features and methods to provide care.

Origins and History of Anesthesiology-Based Acute Pain Services

In the late 1970s and early 1980s, several analgesic techniques were introduced into clinical practice. Most important among these were epidural and intrathecal administration of opioid analgesia and patient-controlled analgesia (PCA). Anesthesiologists in many parts of the world were quick to recognize the importance and value of these techniques and asserted leadership in scientifically investigating them and making them available to patients. The usual historic treatment of postoperative pain (i.e., intramuscular administration of opioids prescribed as needed) was frequently ineffective, but postoperative pain relief was important and possible.

Much of the early improvement in postoperative analgesia was provided by dedicated, individual anesthesiologists, and although this was admirable, many surgical patients continued to receive inadequate pain relief. Only when anesthesiologists undertook collaboration, especially with nurses, surgeons, and pharmacists, did programs begin to evolve that were designed to meet the analgesic needs of surgical patients throughout entire institutions. This was the birth of the concept of acute pain services.

Several anesthesiology departments in the United States had independently developed acute pain services by the mid-1980s; initial reports[1-3] of their success appeared in 1988. Numerous reports about acute pain services have continued to appear, including many from other parts of the world.[4-35] Although the initial reports centered on adult surgical patients, it was not long before pediatric anesthesiologists recognized the potential benefits of an organized approach to providing comfort for their patients. Subsequently, several pediatric acute pain services were described.[36-38]

Current Status of Acute Pain Services

The solution to many problems of postoperative pain management lies not so much in the development of new techniques as in development of an organization to exploit existing expertise. This is one of the main conclusions of interdisciplinary expert committee reports by the National Health and Medical Research Council of Australia,[39] the Royal College of Surgeons of England and the College of Anaesthetists,[40] the U.S. Department of Health and Human Services,[41] and the International Association for the Study of Pain.[42] These committees also published guidelines that recommend actions such as using pain assessment tools, frequent pain assessment and evaluation of treatment efficacy, and bedside pain documentation systems. One of the most important recommendations was for an effective organization of postoperative pain service using a team approach.

The need for a collaborative, interdisciplinary approach to improve the quality of postoperative pain relief is becoming apparent, and this type of postoperative pain management will continue to gain importance, comparable to that of the multidisciplinary pain clinic for treatment of chronic pain. Less clear is the type of organization necessary for this collaborative approach. In the United States, there has been some controversy about the role of the anesthesiologist in acute pain services. According to one school of thought, the ultimate responsibility for pain management belongs to the surgeon who caused pain through surgery; the anesthesiologist is a consultant pain expert available to the surgeon. To quote Bridenbaugh, "It is not the function of the anesthesiologist to run around the hospital filling up epidural catheters with various analgesic mixtures or setting infusion pumps. Far better that this time be used in teaching or performing regional nerve blocks appropriate for acute pain relief."[43] The proponents of the other and more popular school of thought have no doubt that anesthesiologists are uniquely qualified to assume the responsibility for developing, organizing, and sustaining acute pain services.[1, 44]

Anesthesiology-based comprehensive acute pain services are being established in the United States.[1, 45] Experience from Europe has shown that it is possible to have well-functioning acute pain services without having to follow either school of thought. In the United States, 24-h acute pain services provide good-quality analgesia by using PCA and epidural techniques for increasing numbers of surgical patients. Most major institutions in the United States have acute pain services. Such comprehensive pain-management teams usually consist of staff anesthesiologists, resident anesthesiologists, specially trained nurses, and pharmacists; sometimes, physiotherapists are also included. Patients under the care of acute pain services are visited and assessed regularly by one or more members of the team. A pain fellow or anesthesiology resident is on call for the acute pain service.[1, 25, 45] However, it is estimated that less than 30% of the total United States surgical population (about 23 million operations per year) have access to organized acute pain services (Carr D, Raj P, Stanton-Hicks M: personal communication). Although pain management is often very satisfactory, the economic costs of such services are high (average cost, $200 to $300/patient), and the benefits are not available to all surgical patients because of reimbursement regulations.

Different methods have been used to gather the information on acute pain services, including a review of published manuscripts and several original surveys conducted to identify current availability and characteristics of acute pain services. In the section on European countries, the surveys were comprehensive, coordinated, and consistent from one country to another in their design. The information from other countries comes from the available literature or from recently conducted surveys that varied considerably with regard to their design and degree of complexity. This makes detailed comparisons among non-European countries inappropriate.

Europe

Few European hospitals have organized acute pain services. The United States model is not transferable to most European hospitals because of state-controlled health services and cost issues.[46] Except for the work of a few enthusiasts,[21, 34, 47–51] the situation in Europe is generally unsatisfactory.[34, 46–48] Models for acute pain services have been proposed in Germany,[49] the United Kingdom,[6, 34, 47] Switzerland,[50, 51] and Sweden.[21] However, these models are from individual institutions, and their impact on pain management on a countrywide basis is unclear.

Since publication of the report[40] by a joint working party of the Royal College of Surgeons of England and the College of Anaesthetists in 1990, there has been considerable interest in improving postoperative pain relief in the United Kingdom. This has centered on development of high-dependency units and acute pain teams and expansion in the use of techniques such as PCA.[34, 52, 53] It has been estimated that less than 30% of British hospitals have a high-dependency unit. If complex analgesia techniques such as epidural analgesia, PCA, and regional blocks are restricted to high-dependency units, there would be little improvement in the quality of pain relief for most patients undergoing surgery.[34] A few nurse-based acute pain services have been successfully implemented in the United Kingdom.[1, 45] The lack of organized acute pain services at most institutions mainly results from administrative difficulties and financial restrictions (Table 37–1). Even when resources are available, it may be difficult to introduce new analgesia techniques on surgical wards because of practical constraints, communication problems, and nursing policies. In a new hospital in the United Kingdom (Telford), a senior and junior anesthesiologist were available for 24-h acute pain services. This acute pain service was successful in increasing the use of continuous intravenous administration of opioid therapy and PCA. However, more than 50% of patients

Table 37–1 17-Nation European Survey on Acute Pain Management

REASONS FOR NOT USING POSTOPERATIVE ANALGESIC TECHNIQUE OF CHOICE	HOSPITALS, %	
	Mean	Range
Administrative problems*	24	10–60
Economic reasons†	32	20–66

*Lack of qualified nurses or reluctant surgeons.
†Lack of personnel for teaching or lack of equipment.

continued to receive intermittent intramuscular administration of opioids, and it was not possible to introduce epidural technique on the wards because of nursing regulations in the United Kingdom that do not allow nurses to administer drugs into epidural catheters or to reprogram PCA pumps. The procedure of recharging syringes in syringe pumps may be acceptable to some nurses, but it is considered an extended role by others.[6]

In Germany, there are an estimated 20 to 25 acute pain services. These are run mostly by anesthesiologists-in-training and special pain nurses. In 1993, the German Societies of Surgeons and Anesthesiologists proposed the implementation of multidisciplinary acute pain services. The role of anesthesiologists on surgical wards was also defined (Maier C: personal communication, 1994). In Kiel, Germany, an anesthesiologist-in-training from the recovery unit is responsible for the acute pain service. All patients receiving regional blocks or PCA are visited daily on surgical wards. Other patients are treated on the basis of standard protocols. This acute pain service has been functioning satisfactorily since 1985.[49]

In France, acute pain services (i.e., formal administrative organization of postoperative pain evaluation and treatment) have been developed in a limited number of institutions. Most of these are university hospitals, but some private institutions also have acute pain services. In these institutions, the organization of acute pain services depends on the personal involvement of one or two staff anesthesiologists. There are no national guidelines in France, but occasionally, institutional guidelines have been established for treatment and monitoring of postoperative pain (Bonnet F: personal communication, 1994).

Nurse-based acute pain services are available in a few Italian hospitals. A designated anesthesiologist has overall responsibility, but the anesthesiologist does not work full-time with the acute pain service (Bertini L, Tagariello V: personal communication, 1994). In exceptional cases, acute pain services are run by a full-time senior anesthesiologist or nurse. Such acute pain services are found in Switzerland,[50] Belgium, and the United Kingdom.[6, 47]

There seems to be an awakening of interest in establishing acute pain services in European hospitals. This was one of the conclusions of a 17-nation European survey[53a] that included Austria, Belgium, Denmark, Finland, France, Germany, Greece, Iceland, Ireland, Italy, Netherlands, Norway, Portugal, Spain, Sweden, Switzerland, and the United Kingdom. In this survey, 5 to 10 experts from each country (depending on the country's population) were asked to answer questions about hospital policy regarding acute pain. An established expert on pain was designated as a country coordinator for each country. This country coordinator provided the names of other national pain experts. The country coordinators were requested to provide the names of experts from hospitals that would be representative for that country in terms of geography and teaching or nonteaching institutions.

A 67-page questionnaire consisting of more than 200 questions was mailed to participating pain experts. All of these experts were senior anesthesiologists. The questions were related to the following aspects of acute pain and its management:

1. Total number of operations, preoperative evaluations, and postoperative analgesia techniques
   2. PCA technique
   3. Regional analgesia techniques
   4. Preemptive analgesia
   5. Obstetric analgesia
   6. Trauma and burn pain
   7. Pediatric pain
   8. Pain management in outpatient surgery
   9. Acutely painful medical conditions
   10. Organization of postoperative pain services
   11. Economic costs and regulations
   12. Education

The questionnaire response rate was quite high (62%). Of the 105 hospitals surveyed, only 37% (range, 10% to 80%) had some kind of acute pain service. The availability of special units (intermediate ward, step-down unit) for patients requiring prolonged pain relief by techniques such as epidural analgesia and PCA varied considerably (Fig. 37–1). Similarly, the number of postanesthesia care unit beds as a proportion of total hospital beds ranged from 0.19% (Italy) to 5.79% (Norway) (Fig. 37–2). These factors can be expected to influence European postoperative analgesia routines.

Most European anesthesiologists were dissatisfied with pain management on surgical wards; the situation was considered satisfactory in postanesthesia care units (Table 37–2). A range of 20% to 67% of anesthesiologists from 10 of 17 countries surveyed reported economic reasons for their inability to provide analgesic treatment of choice (Table 37–3). These results are similar to those of a survey in the United Kingdom by Semple and Jackson[52] and a survey in Canada by Zimmermann and Stewart.[53] The 17-nation European survey also showed that anesthesiologists had responsibility for acute pain services in 50% of hospitals, an advisory role in 42% of hospitals, and no role at all in 8% of hospitals. Few anesthesiologists in Austria and Spain thought they had any significant role in pain management on surgical wards. Organized acute pain services were reported from some hospitals in Belgium, Germany, Ireland, Netherlands, Sweden, Switzerland, and the United Kingdom. In the remaining hospitals, anesthesiologists were available for consultation as part of a regular anesthesia service. Centers that did have acute pain services were usually run by anesthesiologists-in-training, and senior anesthesiologists were available for consultation and block procedures if necessary. Nurse-based, anesthesiologist-supervised acute pain services have been developed at some centers in France, Norway, Sweden, Switzerland, and the United Kingdom. In both models, the anesthesiologist on call has responsibility for acute pain services after regular working hours.

About 60% of hospitals surveyed had pain centers for management of chronic pain and cancer pain. In

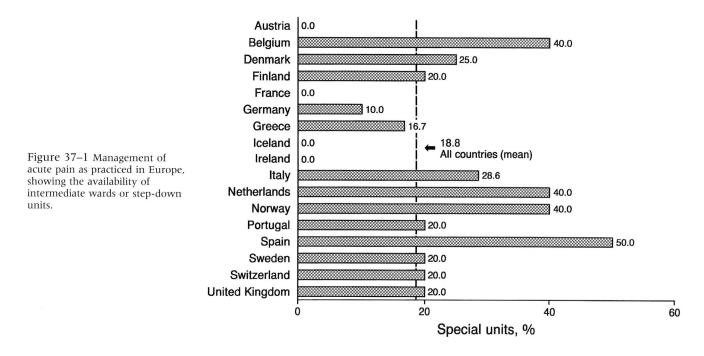

Figure 37–1 Management of acute pain as practiced in Europe, showing the availability of intermediate wards or step-down units.

some hospitals, specialists from these pain centers are consulted for acute pain problems. None of the participating hospitals had anesthesiology-based comprehensive acute pain services, as in the United States.

Anesthesiologists in most European hospitals routinely visit surgical wards to evaluate patients preoperatively and to provide postoperative analgesia when requested by the surgeon. The idea of anesthesiologists working outside the operating suite is not as revolutionary as it is in the United States.[3] However, in Europe and in the United States, the patients who benefit from the expertise of anesthesiologists are those who are selected by the surgeons. The number of referred

patients varies, but they almost always constitute a small percentage of the total surgical population.[1, 6, 34]

Simpler and less expensive models have to be developed if the aim is to improve the quality of postoperative analgesia for every patient. The organization should also include patients who undergo outpatient surgery. In countries with state-financed health services and budgetary restraints, the anesthesiology-based comprehensive, multidisciplinary postoperative pain control teams appear unrealistic for many institutions. This was evident from the results of the European survey in that none of the respondents had an acute pain service at their hospital. Most surgical pa-

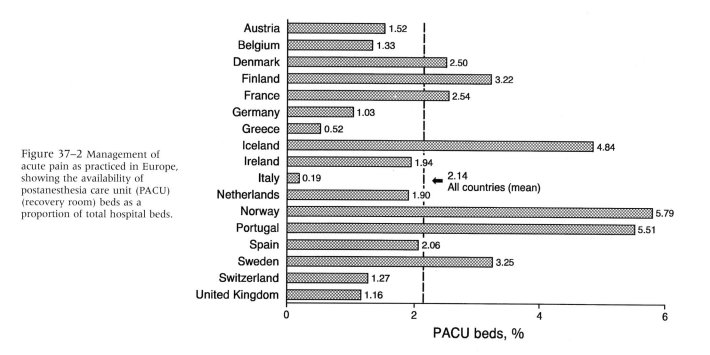

Figure 37–2 Management of acute pain as practiced in Europe, showing the availability of postanesthesia care unit (PACU) (recovery room) beds as a proportion of total hospital beds.

Table 37–2 17-Nation European Survey on Acute Pain Management

ARE YOU SATISFIED WITH THE CURRENT SITUATION REGARDING POSTOPERATIVE ANALGESIA AT YOUR HOSPITAL?	ANESTHESIOLOGISTS, %			
	PACU		Surgical Ward	
	Mean	*Range*	*Mean*	*Range*
Satisfied/very satisfied	68	50–100	42	20–80
Dissatisfied/very dissatisfied	7*	10–33	55†	40–80
No response	25	10–100	3	0–20

*Belgium, France, Germany, and Spain.
†Every country.
PACU, postanesthesia care unit.

tients are American Society of Anesthesiologists physical status class I or II, and most surgical procedures are such that early restoration of respiratory function or early ambulation is not a major problem. Such patients can often be managed adequately by appropriate use of peripherally acting analgesics such as nonsteroidal anti-inflammatory drugs, centrally acting systemic opioids, or both. Even in hospitals in the United States with well-functioning acute pain services, epidural and PCA techniques are used for only 10% to 25% of all patients undergoing surgery[1,6,34,52] (Carr D, Raj P, Stanton-Hicks M: personal communication, 1995).

Other Countries

United States

Because no published source of information could be found that quantified anesthesiology-based acute pain services in the United States, a simple survey was undertaken in April 1994 to address the issue. Initially, a list was obtained of all hospitals in the country with 30 or more beds. Institutions with fewer than 100 beds were eliminated, leaving 2254 institutions. After stratifying them geographically to ensure responses from all parts of the country, a sample of 500 was randomly selected. A questionnaire was mailed to the

Table 37–3 Management of Acute Pain in Europe: Inability to Provide Treatment of Choice Because of Economic Reasons

COUNTRY	ANESTHESIOLOGISTS, %*
Belgium	40
Finland	20
Greece	40
Ireland	40
Netherlands	33
Norway	20
Portugal	20
Sweden	40
Switzerland	20
United Kingdom	67

*Percentage of anesthesiologists who believe it is common or very common.
Data from 17-nation European survey on management of acute pain.

Table 37–4 Results of the Survey on Anesthesiology-Based Acute Pain Services in Institutions in the United States

VARIABLE	RESPONSES	
	No.	%
Responses received	324	65
Institutions with an anesthesiology-based acute pain service	236	73
Institutions offering patient-controlled analgesia	310	96

director of the Department of Anesthesiology at each institution. It contained the following questions:

1. Is there an anesthesiology-based acute pain service in your hospital?
2. Is PCA used in your hospital?
3. What group or groups of physicians manage PCA—anesthesiologists, surgeons, oncologists, other (specify)?
4. What is the ZIP code of your hospital? (This question was included to help confirm widespread geographic representation).

The large proportion of respondents in the United States indicating the existence of an anesthesiology-based acute pain service at their institutions was a surprise (Table 37–4). Because all institutions were randomly selected and their responses were anonymous, it is not known what proportion of these were academic centers. Based on ZIP codes, it was confirmed that the pattern was widespread throughout the country, although it is likely that the types and levels of services provided varied considerably (Table 37–5)[54].

Canada

In this chapter, information on acute pain services in Canada comes entirely from a survey of university-

Table 37–5 Therapist Groups Managing Patient-Controlled Analgesia (PCA) in United States Institutions

THERAPIST GROUP	INSTITUTIONS INDICATING PARTICIPATION OF THE GROUP IN PCA MANAGEMENT	
	No.	%
Anesthesiologists	221	68
Anesthesiologists exclusively	65	20
Anesthesiologists and surgeons exclusively	56	17
Surgeons exclusively	49	15
Registered nurses*	21	7
Internists (including oncologists)	14	4
Obstetricians	10	3
Family medicine	6	2
Certified registered nurse anesthetists*	2	0.6
Pharmacy*	2	0.6

*In these groups, physicians provided the necessary signature on the PCA orders but had little or no other participation in patient care.

Modified from Ready LB: How many acute pain services are there in the United States, and who is managing patient-controlled analgesia? (Letter to the editor.) Anesthesiology 1995; 82: 322.

affiliated teaching hospitals conducted in December 1991 and subsequently published in 1993.[35] The aims of the survey were to determine the prevalence, structure, and function of acute pain services and to determine the use and management of PCA and epidural administration of opioid analgesia at teaching hospitals in Canada.

Fifty-six questionnaires were mailed, and 47 (84%) responses were received. Twenty-five (53%) hospitals operated an acute pain service. Of the 22 hospitals without an organized acute pain service, 17 (36% of all respondents) were attempting to start one. Problems encountered most commonly in the process were financial (e.g., cost of equipment), difficulty freeing anesthesiology staff from the operating room, and perception by the nursing and surgical staff that the improvement of postoperative analgesia was not a priority. Most services were multidisciplinary, with 60% having a nurse and 29% having a pharmacist. Acute pain services were found in 33% of hospitals with fewer than 200 active surgical beds and 67% of larger hospitals.

Regardless of the presence of an acute pain service, PCA was used in 32 (68%) hospitals and opioid analgesia given epidurally was used in 41 (87%), but only 15 (32%) provided opioid analgesia epidurally on general wards.

Complications were observed with PCA and epidural administration of opioid analgesia. From the data, the estimated incidence of severe respiratory depression was 0.03% with PCA and 0.13% with opioid analgesia given epidurally. No deaths were reported with either technique at the time of the survey.

It was concluded from this survey that there is great interest in postoperative pain management in university-affiliated teaching hospitals in Canada. Little is known about interest or activity within other institutions. If trends in Canada are similar to those in the United States, it would be expected that many private hospitals also have developed acute pain services.

Australia

Acute pain services have been described in Australia,[17] but until recently, little was known about the prevalence of such facilities. A survey conducted in 1991 sheds considerable light on the topic. The Australia Wide Survey of Acute Pain Management Facilities was sponsored by the special interest group of the Faculty of Anaesthetists, Royal Australian Colleges of Surgeons. The survey was conducted in 1991 by Dr. Roger Goucke, Consultant Anaesthetist, Pain Management Clinic, Sir Charles Gairdner Hospital, The Queen Elizabeth II Medical Centre, Nedlands, Western Australia.

One hundred seventy-seven questionnaires were mailed to all metropolitan teaching hospitals, major private and government nonteaching hospitals, and a range of larger country hospitals; all were expected to have acute surgical services. It became apparent that some of the institutions on the original list (e.g., psychiatric institutions, hospice centers) did not have sur-

gical facilities. That group was removed for purposes of the survey, leaving 150 that consisted primarily of university centers and major subregional centers. From these, 111 replies were received—a response rate of 74%. Of these, 79 (71%) were metropolitan and 32 (29%) were nonmetropolitan. Seventy-three (66%) were classified as teaching hospitals.

Of the 111 hospitals surveyed, 37 (33%) had a formal acute pain service. Only three (3%) were nonteaching hospitals with no acute pain service. Thirty-one hospitals indicated they would like such a resource or had plans to develop one (Table 37-6). Twenty-five of the nonteaching hospitals provided similar responses.

The acute pain management techniques available in the responding institutions were as follows. In hospitals with acute pain services, patient care was provided by specialist anesthetists, anesthetic registrars, and dedicated nurses; wide variations were reported in availability and time dedicated to acute pain management by the members of each group. Dedicated nurses played a role in 24 (65%) acute pain services with nondedicated positions. Secretarial support was available in 31 of the 37 acute pain services. It is likely that the considerable interest in developing acute pain services that was demonstrated in 1991 resulted in additional facilities in the country.

New Zealand

A survey of medical institutions in New Zealand was undertaken and completed in May 1994. The survey was conducted by Dr. Alan Merry, Department of Anaesthesia and Mary-Ann Judge, Clinical Nurse Specialist, Green Lane Hospital, Green Lane West, Auckland 3, New Zealand.

Eighty-three hospitals received a telephone call, a survey by mail, or both. Responses were obtained from 62 (75%) of the hospitals: 38 designated as primarily public and 24 as private. The private hospitals all had fewer than 150 beds. The public hospitals were subdivided into two categories: 150 or more beds and fewer than 150 beds. There were 12 (19%) hospitals, all larger public institutions, with formal acute pain services and an additional 28 (45%) institutions with

Table 37-6 1991 Acute Pain Service Survey Results of Australian Hospitals

	RESPONSES			
	Teaching Hospitals (n = 73)		Nonteaching Hospitals (n = 38)	
ANALGESIC TECHNIQUE	No.	%	No.	%
Intravenous infusions of opioid	71	97	37	97
Patient-controlled analgesia	65	89	21	55
Epidurally administered opioids	70	96	34	89
Epidurally administered local anesthetic and opioids	69	95	33	87
Perioperative NSAIDS (n = 82)	52	71	26	68

NSAIDs, nonsteroidal anti-inflammatory drugs.

Table 37–7 Distribution of Acute Pain Services in New Zealand Hospitals, Circa 1994

ACUTE PAIN SERVICE	HOSPITALS, NO.		
	Private < 150 Beds (n = 24)	Public ≤ 150 Beds (n = 16)	Public ≥ 150 Beds (n = 22)
Formal	0	0	12
Informal	8	11	9
None	16	5	1

informal acute pain services. Details of the distribution of acute pain services are shown in Table 37–7.

Many anesthesiologists in New Zealand offer modern postoperative pain-relieving methods to their patients. Table 37–8 shows the availability of some of these methods. In most private hospitals, a close doctor-patient relationship is maintained. Consultant anesthesiologists and surgeons work together as teams to provide postoperative care. This approach, even in a small hospital, frequently results in close supervision of analgesic management. PCA and epidural routes of administration of opioid analgesia are used quite widely in these hospitals, even in the absence of a formal acute pain service. The issue of who makes the decision about postoperative use of PCA and epidural administration of opioid analgesia in New Zealand hospitals is addressed in Table 37–9. An apparent trend revealed in this table is of more shared decision making (i.e.,

Table 37–8 Treatment Modalities for Acute Pain Available in New Zealand Hospitals, Circa 1994

TREATMENT MODALITY	ACUTE PAIN SERVICE		
	None (n = 22)	Informal (n = 28)	Formal (n = 12)
Patient-controlled analgesia			
Total	19	24	12
Used on wards	19	24	12
Used in high-dependency unit	2	7	5
Bolus mode only	12	14	6
Bolus plus infusion modes only	1	4	0
Either mode	6	6	6
Intravenous infusion of opioids			
Total	14	23	6
Used on wards	13	21	4
Used in high-dependency unit	5	10	5
Epidural analgesia: boluses			
Total	8	11	1
Used on wards	7	7	1
Used in high-dependency unit	2	3	1
Epidural analgesia: infusions			
Total	12	23	12
Used on wards	11	16	9
Used in high-dependency unit	4	11	6
Infusions of local anesthetic into plexus			
Total	2	7	9
Used on wards	2	6	8
Used in high-dependency unit	0	3	3
NSAIDs as part of routine care	4	24	11

NSAIDs, nonsteroidal anti-inflammatory drugs.

Table 37–9 Decision Making Regarding Patient-Controlled Analgesia and Epidural Analgesia in New Zealand, Circa 1994

DECISION MAKER	ACUTE PAIN SERVICE		
	None (n = 22)	Informal (n = 28)	Formal (n = 12)
Patient-controlled analgesia			
Anesthesiologists only	12	10	2
Surgeons only	1	0	0
Anesthesiologists in combination with others	6	14	10
NA	3	4	0
Epidural analgesia			
Anesthesiologists only	15	21	2
Surgeons only	1	0	0
Anesthesiologists in combination with others	2	4	10
NA	4	3	0

NA, not applicable; the modality is not used.

presumably more collaboration) among various hospital personnel when the institution has an acute pain service.

Miscellaneous Countries

Reports have described organized approaches to postoperative pain management in several other countries. Although it is not possible to determine whether the practices described were isolated or widespread in those countries, the publications at least indicate some degree of interest. Examples of countries with some documented acute pain service experience include Columbia,[4] Malaysia,[55] and South Africa.[29]

Development of a Low-Cost Model

Despite differences in health care systems around the world, three common problems stand out. First, most surgical patients do not have access to acute pain services. Second, even in the hospitals that have acute pain services, most patients are not under the care of acute pain services and therefore receive traditional and often inadequate pain treatments. Third, quality assurance recommendations, such as frequent assessment and documentation of pain intensity and treatment efficacy, have not been implemented.

In most situations, the initial improvement can be gained without significant expense by improving education of all involved with management of postoperative pain; in the long-term, adequate funding has to be provided for the safe introduction of newer techniques such as epidural administration of opioids or local anesthetics (or both) and PCA on surgical wards.[46] Optimal application of pain control techniques depends on cooperation among the members of the health care team. Any pain management organization has to be modified to fit the individual institution, depending on its size, the nursing practices, and the volume and complexity of surgical procedures.[1]

At Örebro Medical Center Hospital in Sweden, a nurse-based anesthesiologist-supervised acute pain service was introduced in February 1991. This low-cost system is based on the concept that postoperative pain relief can be improved by provision of in-service training for medical and nursing staff, regular recording of pain intensity and treatment efficacy, optimal use of systemically administered opioids (including use of PCA) and peripherally acting analgesics, and the use of epidural technique and regional blocks in appropriate patients.

At the time of preoperative evaluation, patients are informed about pain assessment by the Visual Analog Scale (VAS) and about pain management techniques that are available and the rationale underlying their use. This is reinforced by informational brochures and wall posters that inform the patients about the importance of effective postoperative pain relief, frequent assessment of pain intensity by VAS, analgesia options such as intramuscularly administered opioids, PCA, epidural technique, regional blocks, routine use of acetaminophen suppositories every 6 h, and the importance of requesting pain medication before pain becomes severe. Patients who require specialized postoperative care and monitoring (PCA, epidural blocks, and regional blocks) are identified at this time. Patients are also informed that every effort will be made to keep their VAS score at or below 3 on the 10-grade scale.

Regardless of age, all patients receive acetaminophen rectally every 6 h. This is started before surgery or on the operating room table immediately after operation.

Patients who have undergone an operation (during general or regional anesthesia) are asked to grade their pain severity on the VAS. This is done every 3 h and the score is recorded on a specially reserved place on the vital sign chart. The idea is to emphasize that routine scoring of pain is as important as recording of temperature, heart rate, and blood pressure (Fig. 37–3A). To evaluate the effect of prescribed treatment, pain intensity is also scored before and about 45 min after treatment (see Fig. 37–3B). Pain intensity is recorded more frequently (every hour) in the following circumstances: patients in an intensive care unit, patients in a postanesthesia care unit, patients undergoing outpatient surgery, and patients receiving PCA or opioids epidurally.

Appropriate protocols, pain management guidelines, standard orders, and monitoring routines have been developed in cooperation with surgeons for each surgical section. Specially trained acute pain nurses make daily rounds of all surgery departments. Their duties are described in Table 37–10. In this organization, the treatment of individual patients is based on standard orders and protocols developed jointly by the section anesthesiologist, surgeon, and ward nurse. This gives nurses the flexibility to administer the analgesics when necessary. In Sweden, nurses, including ward nurses, are allowed to inject drugs intravenously and through epidural catheters.

The duties of the section anesthesiologist consist of providing anesthesia services and acute pain services (see Table 37–10). The section anesthesiologist selects

Table 37–10 Organization of Acute Pain Services at Örebro Medical Center Hospital, Sweden

HEALTH CARE MEMBER*	RESPONSIBILITIES
Acute pain anesthesiologist	Responsible for coordinating hospitalwide and acute pain services in-service teaching for medical and nursing staff
Section anesthesiologist	Responsible for postoperative pain management on own surgical ward
"Pain representative" ward surgeon	Formally responsible for pain management on own surgical ward
"Pain representative" day nurse	Responsible for implementation of pain management guidelines and monitoring routines on the wards
"Pain representative" night nurse	
Acute pain nurse (nurse anesthetist)	Daily rounds of all surgical wards Check VAS score recording on charts Help with technical problems (PCA, epidural block) Refer problem patients to section pain anesthesiologist

*The health care members ("pain representatives") meet four times each year with the leadership of the acute pain anesthesiologist.
PCA, patient-controlled analgesia; VAS, Visual Analog Scale.

the patients for special pain therapies such as PCA, epidural block, and peripheral nerve block. During regular working hours, this anesthesiologist is available for consultation or any emergency, and later, the anesthesiologist on call has the same function.

Nurse and physician education are crucial for successful implementation of any pain management program. At Örebro Medical Center Hospital, the educational program consists of an overview of relevant anatomy, physiology, pharmacology, goals of therapy, and risks. Clear instructions are also provided regarding dose of analgesia, treatment of inadequate analgesia, patient monitoring, and potential complications and their management. Nurse responsibility and physician accountability are also defined. To facilitate implementation of pain management guidelines and monitoring routines on the ward, two ward nurses from each surgical department (day nurse and night nurse) are also included (see Table 37–10). There is a clear understanding between surgeons and anesthesiologists regarding responsibility to avoid the problems of conflicting orders. To decrease the risk of errors and to standardize clinical care hospitalwide, printed protocols and standard orders have been developed jointly to permit the use of opioids by intramuscular route (Table 37–11), intravenous PCA (Table 37–12), and epidural route (Table 37–13) on surgical wards.

At Örebro Medical Center Hospital during the last 15 years, major abdominal and thoracic surgery were routinely performed during a combination of epidural and general anesthesia. Major knee and hip surgery were routinely performed during combined spinal-epidural block. For all such patients, postoperative analgesia is provided by epidural administration of local anesthetics or opioids (or both). Preoperatively, all epidural catheters are placed in the operating room holding area. PCA is initiated in the postanesthesia care unit most of the time and continued on the wards.

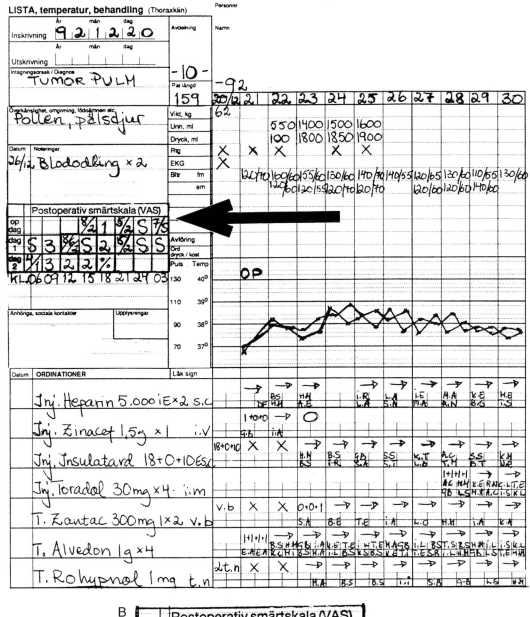

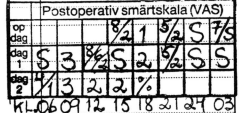

Figure 37–3 *A*, A typical bedside vital sign chart in Sweden. To emphasize the importance of regular pain scoring, a stamp (arrow) for recording Visual Analog Scale (VAS) score every 3 h is placed in a space close to the space for recording temperature, pulse, and blood pressure. This facilitates the discussion of postoperative pain on surgical rounds. Pain intensity above 3 on the 10-grade VAS is treated promptly. A glance at the chart provides information about adequacy of analgesia and about sleep during the entire treatment period. Easy identification of patients in whom pain is poorly controlled permits prompt revision of management plans. *B*, A close-up of the VAS recording stamp. VAS is recorded every 3 h; it is also recorded before and about 45 min after treatment. If VAS score is above 3 despite treatment, a second dose of analgesic (50% of first dose) is given. For example, on day 1 after an operation at 12 noon, pain intensity decreased from 8 to 6 after the first injection. An anesthesiologist or acute pain nurse is contacted if analgesia is still inadequate after a second injection. The dose and route of analgesic administration are recorded in the nurse's report. For patients receiving patient-controlled analgesia and opioids given spinally, respiratory rate, sedation level, and VAS score are monitored every hour and documented separately. Appropriate modifications are made for outpatient surgical patients. */*, patient received pain therapy (e.g., 8/2 = VAS score 8 before treatment and 2 after treatment); S, patient asleep; ●/●, termination of VAS scoring (when three consecutive measurements show VAS score at or below 3 without any treatment); op dag, operation day; dag 1, day 1 (after operation); dag 2, day 2; KL, time (clock time).

Table 37–11 Standard Orders for Morphine Given Intramuscularly on Surgical Wards

Record pain intensity (on bedside flow sheet) every 3 h; VAS recording may be terminated only when VAS score is 3 or below without treatment on three consecutive measurements

Unless contraindicated (e.g., liver disease), give every adult patient 1 g acetaminophen rectally (suppository) 4 times/day as base analgesic medication until VAS recording is terminated; for children, 15 to 20 mg/kg rectally

In addition, give morphine 7.5 to 10 mg when VAS score is above 3 (decrease dose by 25% to 50% in elderly and very sick patients); recheck and record VAS score about 45 min after morphine injection; if VAS score is still above 3, give additional morphine (50% of initial dose)

Contact acute pain nurse or section anesthesiologist if VAS score is still above 3 after second dose; after working hours, contact the anesthesiologist on call

VAS, Visual Analog Scale.

The acute pain anesthesiologist and acute pain nurse coordinate pain management routines among the surgical sections and the acute pain anesthesiologist chairs quarterly "pain representative" meetings of section anesthesiologists, surgeons, and day and night ward nurses (see Table 37–10). The usual topics for discussion at these meetings are practical pain problems, protocol modifications, suggestions for improvement of services, and introduction of new techniques.

With the organization described, the only additional cost is that of the acute pain nurse. A second acute pain nurse has recently joined the acute pain service for night and weekend coverage. At Örebro Medical Center Hospital, about 18,000 to 20,000 surgical procedures are performed annually, and all of these patients can be expected to benefit from this organization. The cost of two acute pain nurses is about $60,000 in United States dollars, or less than $4.00 per patient. In

Table 37–12 Standard Orders for Patient-Controlled Analgesia (PCA) on Surgical Wards

Unless contraindicated (e.g., liver disease), give 1 g acetaminophen 4 times/day rectally (suppository) as base analgesic medication until VAS recording is terminated; for children, 15 to 20 mg/kg rectally

Drug: morphine (1 mg/mL)

Loading dose: titrated to clinical effect (VAS score 3 or below) in postanesthesia care unit

Bolus dose: 1 to 1.5 mg (depending on type of operation, ASA status)*

Lock-out interval: 6 min

Monitoring: respiratory rate, level of sedation† (on 4-grade scale), and pain intensity (VAS) every hour

If respiratory rate <10/min or sedation level 4, give 0.4 mg of naloxone intravenously and contact the anesthesiologist on call

Even after termination of PCA therapy, the departmental routine of VAS recording every 3 h must be continued until VAS score is 3 or below without treatment on three consecutive measurements

For inadequate analgesia or problems related to PCA, contact acute pain nurse or section anesthesiologist; after working hours, contact the anesthesiologist on call

*Dose adjustments made by acute pain nurse after consultation with section anesthesiologist.

†Sedation scale: 1, fully awake; 2, mild sedation; 3, sedate but arousable; 4, deep sedation, not responding.

ASA, American Society of Anesthesiologists; VAS, Visual Analog Scale.

Table 37–13 Standard Orders for Morphine Given Epidurally on Surgical Wards

Unless contraindicated (e.g., liver disease), give 1 g acetaminophen 4 times/day rectally (suppository) as base analgesic medication until VAS recording is terminated; for children, 15 to 20 mg/kg rectally

Drug: morphine (0.4 mg/mL)

Dose: 4 mg when VAS score is at or above 3; reduce dose (2 mg) for elderly and high-risk patients*

Monitoring: after every injection, respiratory rate and sedation level† (on 4-grade scale) every 30 min for 2 h followed by every hour for 10 h‡

Urinary retention: if patient has not passed urine within 6 h postoperatively, in-and-out catheterization of bladder

If respiratory rate <10/min or sedation level 4, give 0.4 mg of naloxone intravenously and contact the anesthesiologist on call

Maintain intravenous access for at least 12 h after last dose of morphine given epidurally

Even after termination of epidural administration of morphine therapy, the departmental routine of VAS recording every 3 h must be continued until VAS score is 3 or below without treatment on three consecutive measurements

For inadequate analgesia or problems with epidural administration of morphine, contact acute pain nurse or section anesthesiologist; after working hours, contact the anesthesiologist on call

*Patient selection and dose adjustments made by acute pain nurse after consultation with section anesthesiologist.

†Sedation scale: 1, fully awake; 2, mild sedation; 3, sedated but arousable; 4, deep sedation, not responding.

‡This monitoring routine is now approved by the Swedish Society of Anesthesiology and Intensive Care.

the fee-for-service system, which is still within the state-financed health services, this cost is included in the cost for anesthesia services for which the anesthesia department is reimbursed from the budgets of different surgical specialties. Despite major economic restraints, the surgeons have agreed to bear the added costs of acute pain nurses. The acute pain services were introduced gradually on a departmental basis. The implementation of the services for the entire hospital took about 18 months.

The routine use of the VAS on surgical wards has demonstrated for surgeons and ward nurses that even repeated intramuscular injections of opioids may be unable to maintain VAS scores that are considered acceptable (VAS score ≤3) for the department. This is particularly true in patients with severe pain, such as those undergoing upper abdominal, thoracic, or knee surgery. This has resulted in increased requests for and better acceptance of techniques such as PCA and epidural analgesia on the surgical wards. The development of a structured program with readily available assistance is appreciated by nurses and surgeons on the ward. Since the introduction of this organization, no major complications have occurred. Although all anesthesiologists are involved with the postoperative pain management of their patients, the section anesthesiologists (see Table 37–10) are responsible for developing protocols and standard orders for their section. This system is professionally more stimulating; the anesthesiologists provide the continuity of patient care because they are routinely involved in preoperative assessment, intraoperative management, and postoperative follow-up.

Nurse-based pain services have been reported[34, 47] in some centers in the United Kingdom. Gould and colleagues[47] reported considerable improvement in postoperative analgesia after sequential introduction of such services, regular pain assessment, and frequent use of intramuscular analgesia. Similarly, Wheatley and coworkers[34] demonstrated improved pain scores in 660 patients receiving PCA or epidural therapy; pain scores were assessed at 1- to 4-h intervals in addition to the 24-h VAS score. A major difference in the Swedish model is the hospitalwide implementation of recording pain intensity on the vital sign chart every 3 h (hourly for PCA or epidural analgesia) and routine recording of treatment efficacy, making pain "visible." This model benefits every patient who undergoes surgery, including those treated on an ambulatory basis. After study visits, more than 30 Swedish hospitals are in various stages of introducing routine VAS score recording and other aspects of this model. More than 100 anesthesiologists or nurses outside Sweden have also shown interest by requests for patient information brochures, protocols, and study visits.

This implementation is a first step in an ongoing quality assurance (performance improvement) program. The next step is to introduce routine pain scoring during movement, not just at rest. Although questionnaire surveys and random checks have been done, a systematic audit of the outcome of the acute pain service is necessary. The greatly increased "pain awareness" may facilitate the introduction of new ideas and modalities for improved pain relief. This model is primarily for postoperative pain management, but frequent pain recording and documentation of treatment efficacy in this manner and as a component of quality assurance can be used in other specialties that have patients with acute or chronic pain.

At Örebro Medical Center Hospital, pain intensity (VAS) is recorded every 3 h in the Emergency Department and the Department of Infectious Diseases. In the Department of Oncology and the Department of Gynecological Oncology, pain intensity is checked and recorded once or twice daily. The model can also be modified to fit local institutional conditions in other countries. In some institutions, modifications would be necessary to accommodate special regulations such as handling of narcotic drugs and epidural and intrathecal injections of drugs by nurses.

Principles Common to Acute Pain Services

The concept of interested and skilled pain therapists collaborating to provide improved postoperative analgesia within hospitals appears to be universally applicable. The approaches to providing this improvement depend on factors such as availability and interest of anesthesiologists, surgical populations and practice in different countries, varied nursing practices and levels of interest, beliefs of different societies with regard to postoperative pain, medical resources, reimbursement practices, and levels of support by government or private health care agencies. Despite tremendous differences, many countries now embrace the provision of coordinated postoperative analgesia that acute pain services can provide. Although the structure and methods vary, we think several basic principles apply wherever acute pain services are used:

1. Belief in the importance of postoperative pain relief and the improvement in function that accompanies it

2. Recognition of the large degree of variability among surgical patients with regard to the amount of pain experienced and the amount of analgesic medication needed to adequately control it

3. Belief in the need to provide comprehensive education to hospital personnel regarding postoperative pain

4. Belief that regular pain assessment and documentation are essential to the process of improving postoperative pain

5. Belief in the importance of collaborative efforts, especially among anesthesiologists, nurses, surgeons, and pharmacists

6. Recognition of the importance of regular medical evaluation and availability of experts at all times

7. Recognition of the value of institutional protocols for ordering and administering analgesic therapy

8. Recognition that the side effects associated with analgesic methods are common and can interfere with optimal pain relief

9. Recognition of the need for a process for tracking the quality and safety of the postoperative analgesia that is provided

As the availability of acute pain services worldwide continues to grow, the improved pain relief they make possible can be of immeasurable benefit to countless future patients.

References

1. Ready LB, Oden R, Chadwick HS, et al: Development of an anesthesiology-based postoperative pain management service. Anesthesiology 1988; 68: 100–106.
2. Ramsey DH: Perioperative pain: Establishing an analgesia service. In Brown DL (ed): Problems in Anesthesia: Perioperative Analgesia, pp 321–326. Philadelphia, JB Lippincott, 1988.
3. Saidman LJ: The anesthesiologist outside the operating room: a new and exciting opportunity. (Editorial.) Anesthesiology 1988; 68: 1–2.
4. Bejarano P, Duque C, Griego J, et al: "Naughty goblins" during the establishment of a PCA program. (Abstract.) In Proceedings of the 7th World Congress on Pain, Paris, p 392. Seattle, IASP Publications, 1993.
5. Breivik H, Högström H, Curatoto M, et al: Developing a hospitalwide postoperative pain service. (Abstract.) Acta Anaesthesiol Scand Suppl 1993; 100: 223.
6. Cartwright PD, Helfinger RG, Howell JJ, et al: Introducing an acute pain service. Anaesthesia 1991; 46: 188–191.
7. Chien BB, Burke RG, Hunter DJ: An extensive experience with postoperative pain relief using postoperative fentanyl infusion. Arch Surg 1991; 126: 692–695.
8. Cross DA, Hunt JB: Feasibility of epidural morphine for postoperative analgesia in a small community hospital. Anesth Analg 1991; 72: 765–768.
9. Domsky M, Kwartowitz J: Efficacy of subarachnoid morphine in a community hospital. Reg Anesth 1992; 17: 279–282.
10. Gould TH, Crosby DL, Harmer M, et al: Policy for controlling

pain after surgery: effect of sequential changes in management. Br Med J 1992; 305: 1187–1193.

11. Hart L, Macintyre PE, Winefield H, et al: Re-evaluation of patient, medical and nursing staff attitudes to postoperative opioid analgesia after the establishment of an acute pain service: stage 2 of a longitudinal study. (Abstract.) In Proceedings of the 7th World Congress on Pain, Paris, p 397. Seattle, IASP Publications, 1993.

12. Hoopman P: Nursing considerations for acute pain management. In Ferrante FM, VadeBoncouer TR (eds): Postoperative Pain Management, pp 605–612. New York, Churchill Livingstone, 1993.

13. Judge M, Merry AF: The assessment of the impact of the introduction of an acute pain management service. (Abstract.) In Proceedings of the 7th World Congress on Pain, Paris, p 398. Seattle, IASP Publications, 1993.

14. Kinnear SB, Macintyre PE, Hart L, et al: Pain relief for cholecystectomy patients before and after the start of an acute pain service: stage 2 of a longitudinal study. (Abstract.) In Proceedings of the 7th World Congress on Pain, Paris, p 397. Seattle, IASP Publications, 1993.

15. Lauder GR, Sutton D: The acute pain service and GP referral practices. (Letter to the editor.) Anaesthesia 1993; 48: 454.

16. Le Sage EM: Financial aspects of acute pain management. In Ferrante FM, VadeBoncouer TR (eds): Postoperative Pain Management, pp 599–604. New York, Churchill Livingstone, 1993.

17. Macintyre PE, Runciman WB, Webb RK: An acute pain service in an Australian teaching hospital: the first year. Med J Aust 1990; 153: 417–421.

18. McKenna M, Murphy DF: The role of the nurse in the acute pain service. (Abstract.) In Proceedings of the 7th World Congress on Pain, Paris, p 398. Seattle, IASP Publications, 1993.

19. Pasero CL, Hubbard L: Development of an acute pain service monitoring and evaluation system. Qual Rev Bull 1991; 17: 396–401.

20. Rawal N: Postoperative Smärta Och Dess Behandling. Örebro, Kabi Pharmacia, 1991.

21. Rawal N, Berggren L: Organization of acute pain services: a low-cost model. Pain 1994; 57: 117–123.

22. Ready LB: The acute pain service. Acta Anaesthesiol Belg 1992; 43: 21–27.

23. Ready LB: Acute pain service unit. Acta Anaesthesiol Scand Suppl 1993; 100: 137–140.

24. Ready LB: Postoperative pain treatment on wards–USA experience. Acta Anaesthesiol Scand Suppl 1993; 100: 1–5.

25. Ready LB, Wild LM: Organization of an acute pain service: training and manpower. Anesthesiol Clin North Am 1989; 7: 229–239.

26. Salomäki TE, Laitinen JO, Nuutinen LS: Postoperative pain management on wards—Finnish experience. Acta Anaesthesiol Scand Suppl 1993; 100: 9–11.

27. Schug SA, Haridas RP: Development and organizational structure of an acute pain service in a major teaching hospital. Aust NZ J Surg 1993; 63: 8–13.

28. Schug SA, Torrie JJ: Safety assessment of postoperative pain management by an acute pain service. Pain 1993; 55: 387–391.

29. Shipton EA, Beeton AG, Minkowitz HS: Introducing a patient-controlled analgesia-based acute pain relief service into southern Africa—the first 10 months. S Afr Med J 1993; 83: 501–505.

30. Smith G: Pain after surgery. (Editorial.) Br J Anaesth 1991; 67: 233–234.

31. VadeBoncouer TR, Ferrante FM: Management of a postoperative pain service at a teaching hospital. In Ferrante FM, VadeBoncouer TR (eds): Postoperative Pain Management, pp 625–639. New York, Churchill Livingstone, 1993.

32. Watt JW, Wiles JR: Does an acute pain service require a high

dependency unit? (Letter to the editor.) Anaesthesia 1991; 46: 789–790.

33. Wenrich J: Acute pain service in a community hospital. J Post Anesth Nurs 1991; 6: 324–330.

34. Wheatley RG, Madej TH, Jackson IJ, et al: The first year's experience of an acute pain service. Br J Anaesth 1991; 67: 353–359.

35. Zimmermann DL, Stewart J: Postoperative pain management and acute pain service activity in Canada. Can J Anaesth 1993; 40: 568–575.

36. Berde C, Sethna NF, Masek B, et al: Pediatric pain clinics: recommendations for their development. Pediatrician 1989; 16: 94–102.

37. Berde CB: A pediatric pain service. Am Soc Anesthiol Refresh Course Lect 1989; 134: 1–7.

38. Shapiro BS, Cohen DE, Covelman KW, et al: Experience of an interdisciplinary pediatric pain service. Pediatrics 1991; 88: 1226–1232.

39. National Health and Medical Research Council (Australia): Management of Severe Pain. Canberra, Australia, 1988.

40. Royal College of Surgeons of England and the College of Anaesthetists: Report of the Working Party on Pain After Surgery, September 1990.

41. U.S. Department of Health and Human Services: Acute Pain Management: Clinical Practice Guideline. AHCPR Publication No. 92–0032, USA, 1992.

42. Ready LB, Edwards WT, and the International Association for the Study of Pain (Task Force on Acute Pain): Management of Acute Pain: a Practical Guide. Seattle, IASP Publications, 1992.

43. Bridenbaugh DL: Acute pain therapy: whose responsibility? Reg Anesth 1990; 15: 223–231.

44. Moore DC: The 1990 John J. Bonica lecture: the role of the anesthesiologist in managing postoperative pain. Reg Anesth 1990; 15: 223–231.

45. Brown DL, Carpenter RL: Perioperative analgesia: a review of risks and benefits. J Cardiothorac Anesth 1990; 4: 368–383.

46. Harmer M: Postoperative pain relief—time to take our heads out of the sand? (Editorial.) Anaesthesia 1991; 46: 167–168.

47. Gould TH, Crosby DL, Harmer M, et al: Policy for controlling pain after surgery: effect of sequential changes in management. Br Med J 1992; 305: 1187–1193.

48. Black AM: Taking pains to take away pain. (Editorial.) Br Med J 1991; 302: 1165–1166.

49. Maier C, Kibbel K, Mercker S, et al: Postoperative Schmerztherapie auf Allgemeinen Krankenpflegestationen. Analyse der achtjährigen Tätigkeit eines Anästhesiologischen Akutschmerzdienstes. Anaesthesist 1994; 43: 385–397.

50. Breivik H: Recommendations for foundation of a hospital-wide postoperative pain service: a European view. Pain Digest 1993; 3: 27–30.

51. Alon E, Biro P, Himmelscher S: Zur Lage der Schmerzbehandlung durch Anästhesiologen in der Deutschschweiz. Eur J Pain 1993; 14: 91–96.

52. Semple P, Jackson IJ: Postoperative pain control: a survey of current practice. Anaesthesia 1991; 46: 1074–1076.

53. Zimmermann DL, Stewart J: Postoperative pain management and acute pain service activity in Canada. Can J Anaesth 1993; 40: 568–575.

53a. Rawal N: Epidural and intrathecal opioids for postoperative pain management in Europe—a 17-nation survey. (Abstract.) Reg Anesth 1995; 20: A45.

54. Ready LB: How many acute pain services are there in the United States, and who is managing patient-controlled analgesia? (Letter to the editor.) Anesthesiology 1995; 82: 322.

55. Delilkan AE, Vijayan R: Experience with an acute pain service in a developing country. (Abstract.) In Proceedings of the 7th World Congress on Pain, Paris, p 395. Seattle, IASP Publications, 1993.

CHAPTER 38

Analgesic Techniques

Timothy R. Lubenow, M.D.

The expanding awareness of the epidemiology and pathophysiology of pain has led to an ever-increasing number of methods to manage postoperative pain. This chapter reviews the physiology and modulation of nociception. After this conceptual review of pain processing, various analgesic techniques suitable for managing postoperative pain are described. Neuraxial techniques are described in detail because they represent a common modality for pain management and have been the most extensively studied. Peripheral nerve blocks that have applications for postoperative pain are highlighted, as are some nonpharmacologic therapies.

Physiology of Nociception

Somatosensory Receptors and Peripheral Afferent Fibers

Nociception describes the process of detection, transduction, and transmission of noxious stimuli. Stimuli are generated from thermal, mechanical, or chemical tissue damage and activate nociceptors, which are free nerve endings. Nociceptors can be further classified into exteroceptors, which receive stimuli from the skin surface, and interoceptors, which are located in the walls of viscera or deep body structures. In addition to nociceptors, the skin is richly innervated by specialized somatosensory receptors that interpret other forms of stimulation (Table 38–1). Each sensory unit includes an end-organ receptor with its accompanying axon, dorsal root ganglion, and axon terminals in the spinal cord.[1] In contrast to these special somatosensory receptors, nociceptors exhibit high response thresholds and persistent discharge to suprathreshold stimuli without rapid adaptation and are associated with the smaller receptive fields and small afferent nerve fiber endings.[2] Nerve fibers were initially described according to the

presence or absence of myelination and the type of covering. Nerve fibers may be covered with neurilemma or myelin or both. The speed of conduction is determined by the presence or absence of myelination as well as the fiber size. Small, unmyelinated afferent fibers transmit at a slower speed than larger, myelinated afferent fibers.[1] Erlanger and Gasser[3] described the first functional classification of peripheral nerve fibers. Nerve fibers were categorized into three groups (A, B, and C), depending on size, degree of myelination, rapidity of conduction, and distribution of fibers. Refinement of this classification has resulted in the functional subdivision of the class A fibers into the subtypes of α, β, γ, and δ.[4]

Class A Fibers

These neurons, composed of large myelinated axons, exhibit a low threshold for activation, conduct impulses at a fast speed of 5 to 100 m/s, and measure 1 to 20 μm in diameter. Class A-δ fibers mediate pain sensation, whereas class A-α fibers transmit motor and proprioceptive impulses. Class A-β and A-γ fibers are responsible for cutaneous touch and pressure and regulation of muscle spindle reflexes, respectively.

Class B Fibers

These neurons constitute the medium-sized myelinated fibers with intermediate conduction velocity ranging from 3 to 14 m/s and have a diameter less than 3 μm. They have a higher threshold—that is, a lower excitability—than class A fibers but have a lower threshold than class C fibers. Postganglionic sympathetic as well as visceral afferents belong to this group.

Class C Fibers

Class C fibers are unmyelinated or thinly myelinated and have the slowest conduction velocities—in the

644

Table 38–1 Somatosensory and Nociceptive Receptors and the Corresponding Sensations

RECEPTOR	SENSATION PERCEIVED
Golgi-Mazzoni ending	Pressure
Pacinian corpuscle	Pressure
Ruffini ending	Heat
Krause end bulb	Cold
Free nerve ending (nociceptor)	Pain
Meissner corpuscle	Touch
Merkel disk	Touch
Nerve fibers on hair follicles	Touch

From Lubenow TR, McCarthy RJ, Ivankovich AD: Management of acute postoperative pain. In Barash PG, Cullen BF, Stoelting RK (eds): Clinical Anesthesia, 2nd ed, pp 1547–1577. Philadelphia, JB Lippincott, 1992.

range of 0.5 to 2 m/s. This class of nerve fibers is composed of preganglionic autonomic fibers and pain fibers. Approximately 50% to 80% of C fibers modulate nociceptive stimuli. An additional classification of afferent muscle nerve fibers used by neurophysiologists divides the large myelinated fibers into three functional groups (IA, IB, and II), placing the thinly myelinated (III) and unmyelinated fibers (IV) into separate groups. The muscle afferents of Erlanger and Gasser's class A-α fibers are subdivided into two groups: IA and IB. Fibers from the annulospiral endings of the muscle spindles are group IA, whereas the group IB fibers emanate from the Golgi tendon organs. Group II consists of the tactile and proprioceptor fibers of classes A-β and A-γ, respectively, whereas the primary nociceptive nerve fibers of classes A-δ and C are equivalent to groups III and IV, respectively.

Spinal Cord and Brain Pathways

The process of nociception is initiated with activation of a nociceptor. This nociceptive receptor transmits the afferent impulse along the peripheral afferent neuron, which is referred to as the first-order neuron. This has its cell body located in the dorsal root ganglion and sends axonal projections into the dorsal horn and other areas of the spinal cord. At this point in the dorsal horn, a synapse occurs with a second-order afferent neuron, which can be categorized depending on the afferent input it receives as a nociceptive-specific or a wide dynamic range neuron (Fig. 38–1). Nociceptive-specific neurons transmit afferent impulses only from nociceptive afferent fibers, whereas A-β, A-δ, and C fibers communicate with wide dynamic range neurons. In the dorsal horn, the first-order neurons also communicate with the cell bodies of the sympathetic nervous system as well as ventral motor nuclei either directly or through internuncial neuron connections.[5] The cell body of the second-order neuron lies in the dorsal horn, and axonal projections of this neuron cross to the contralateral side of the cord. From here, the second-order afferent neuron ascends within the lateral spinothalamic tract to synapse in the thalamus. Along the way, this neuron divides and sends small axonal branches that synapse in the midline structures

of the brain stem in the region of the reticular formation, nucleus raphe magnus, and periaqueductal gray. In the thalamus, the second-order neuron synapses with a third-order afferent neuron, which then sends axonal connections into the sensory cortex. Thus, the afferent processing of a pain stimulus follows an intricate, multistep pathway to the cerebral cortex.

Modulation of Nociception

Nociceptors, with their accompanying afferent sensory neural pathways, detect noxious stimuli and transmit this information when appropriately stimulated. Modification of this stimulation occurs at several levels in the pathway before perception of the signal at the cerebral cortex. This modulation can occur in the periphery or at any point where synaptic transmission occurs.

Peripheral Modulation

Peripheral modulation occurs by either the liberation or the elimination of certain algetic substances in the

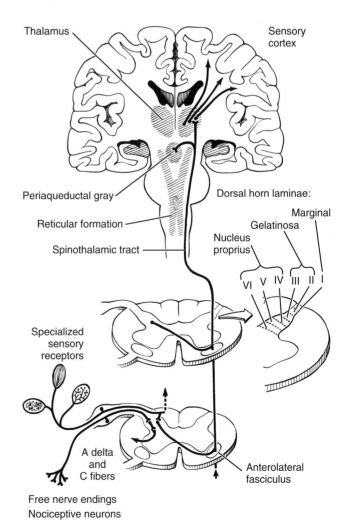

Figure 38–1 Afferent sensory pathways for pain transmission.

vicinity of the nociceptor. Algetic mediators—such as lactic acid, serotonin, bradykinin, potassium and hydrogen ions, histamine, and the prostaglandins—sensitize and excite nociceptors and act as mediators of inflammation. This effect occurs either directly or indirectly because of alterations in the peripheral microcirculation. Aspirin and nonsteroidal anti-inflammatory drugs exert an analgesic effect by inhibiting prostaglandin synthesis and decreasing prostaglandin E_1– and E_2–mediated sensitization of nociceptors within the periphery.

Spinal Modulation

Modulation within the spinal cord results from the action of neurotransmitter substances in the dorsal horn or from spinal reflexes that convey efferent impulses back to the peripheral nociceptive field. The excitatory amino acids L-glutamate and aspartate in particular and several neuropeptides, including vasoactive intestinal peptide, cholecystokinin, gastrin-releasing peptide, angiotensin II, and calcitonin gene–related peptide, are found in the central terminals of the first-order afferent neurons and have been shown to modulate transmission of nociceptive afferent signals.[6] Substance P, which is found in the synaptic vesicles of unmyelinated C fibers, is a neurotransmitter that enhances or transmits pain stimuli.[*, 8] Inhibitory substances involved in the regulation of afferent impulses in the dorsal horn include the enkephalins, norepinephrine, and serotonin. Somatostatin, a neuropeptide found in cells that do not contain substance P, may represent another inhibitory neuropeptide involved in afferent modulation.[8, 9]

Afferent modulating mechanisms at the spinal level may also involve spinal reflexes in which afferent signals evoke direct somatic or sympathetic efferent impulses (or both). These impulses discharge in the vicinity of the efferent nociceptive synapses. For example, skeletal muscle spasm in an injured area is part of the somatic efferent reflex that is induced as a result of nociceptive afferent signal processing. Increased skeletal muscle tone initiates more nociceptive signals in the positive feedback loop from the muscles in the surgical field. In addition, spinal reflexes may involve the discharge of efferent sympathetic signals evoked by the nociceptive impulse (Fig. 38–2). These efferent sympathetic signals emanate from cell bodies located in the intermediolateral cell column of the spinal cord. The cell bodies receive internuncial projections from the dorsal horn. The sympathetic reflex produces smooth muscle spasm, vasoconstriction, and liberation of norepinephrine in the vicinity of the wound, which exacerbates pain. This further changes the microcirculation and induces change within the local chemical milieu. The release of norepinephrine has been shown to produce and augment pain after injury.[10]

Brain Stem

Descending inhibitory tracts in the brain stem have cell bodies that originate in the region of the periaque-

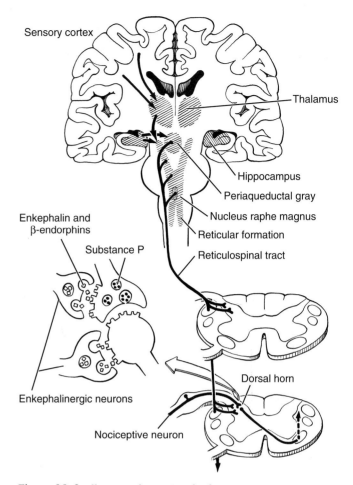

Figure 38–2 Efferent pathways involved in nociceptive modulation.

ductal gray, nucleus raphe magnus, and reticular formation. From these midline brain stem structures, the inhibitory tracts descend in the dorsal lateral fasciculus of the spinal cord and synapse in the dorsal horn at each spinal cord level. Neurotransmitters are released that act either presynaptically on the first-order afferent neuron or postsynaptically on the second-order afferent neuron of the spinothalamic tract. Alternatively, they may act on the internuncial neuron pool. Internuncial neurons can also be inhibitory in nature and can regulate synaptic transmission between primary and secondary afferent neurons in the dorsal horn. At least two groups of these descending inhibitory nerve tracts have been identified as participants.

One group of fibers involves the opioid system and contains the neurotransmitters β-endorphin and enkephalin as well as other neuropeptides. Several studies have demonstrated that analgesia may be produced during electrical stimulation of the periaqueductal gray and that this effect is blocked by naloxone.[11–13] These opioid projections from the nucleus raphe magnus and reticular formation interface presynaptically with the first-order afferent neurons. Neurotransmitters released from these projections then hyperpolarize class A-δ and C fibers, which serves to negate or shunt the depolarizing current that approaches the terminal end plate, thereby diminishing the release of the neurotransmitters such as substance P (Fig. 38–2). In addition to the presynaptic modulation, studies have shown that exogenously applied opioids will inhibit L-glutamate–evoked discharge of dorsal horn neurons, suggesting that opioids exert a direct postsynaptic effect as well.[14, 15] In summary, opioids modulate transmission of afferent impulses in the dorsal horn region presynaptically at the level of the first-order afferent neuron. The neurotransmitter that is released from the descending inhibitory pathways hyperpolarizes the afferent terminals to block neurotransmitter release. Evidence also suggests that opioids exert a direct inhibitory effect on the postsynaptic membrane potential as well.

Besides the descending opioid inhibitory pathway, an α-adrenergic pathway has been identified that also originates from locations in the periaqueductal gray and reticular formation. Stimulation of this pathway inhibits synaptic transmission in the dorsal horn similar to the inhibition produced by the opioid system. Electrostimulation of these pathways and intracerebral injections of α_2 agonists can inhibit spinal nociceptive reflexes. This effect can be antagonized by the intrathecal administration of α_2-adrenergic antagonists.[16, 17] Further evidence of this α_2-adrenergic pathway stems from the observation that intrathecal administration of α_2-adrenergic agonists produces analgesia. This implies that the α_2 adrenoreceptor is responsible for this antinociceptive effect.[18, 19] The α_2-adrenergic fibers descend in the dorsolateral fasciculus in a manner similar to that of the opioid fibers and synapse in the substantia gelatinosa region of the dorsal horn. Norepinephrine as well as serotonin is released from these nerve terminals and produces hypopolarization of the first-order neurons, internuncial neurons, and wide dynamic range neurons. In addition, there are some α_2-adrenoreceptor projections into the ventral gray matter of the motor nuclei.

At the cellular level, the opioid and α_2 receptors share a similar mechanism of action. Opioid and α_2-adrenergic receptors belong to a family of membrane-bound receptors that are coupled to a G protein (Fig. 38–3).[20, 21] The G protein is a membrane-bound protein consisting of multiple subunits situated along the cytosolic aspect of the membrane. Normally, the G protein is inactive when aligned and not interacting with the α_2 or opioid receptor. When bound by an agonist, the G protein undergoes a conformational change that results in the cleaving of the α_1 subunit. The α_1 subunit is then activated by hydrolysis of a high-energy phosphate bond. The activated α_1 subunit then diffuses along the inner aspect of the cell where it exerts its intracellular effect. With regard to pain transmission, the activated α_1 subunit binds to the inner aspect of the potassium ion channel, leaving the channel in its open position. With the potassium channel locked into the open position, the potassium ions flow down their concentration gradient, resulting in hypopolarization of the neuron. This hypopolarization makes the resting membrane potential more negative and results in a decreased quantity of neurotransmitter release from presynaptic terminals as well as a decreased sensitivity

Nociceptive Nerve Membrane

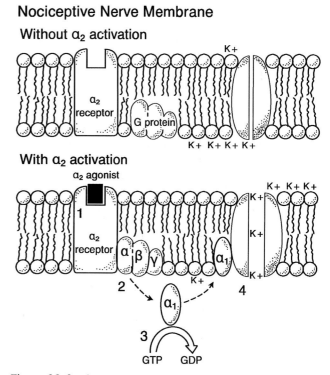

Figure 38–3 Schematic representation of G protein–linked receptor, which participates in either α-adrenergic or opioidergic modulation. (Adapted from Maze M, Tranquilli W: Anesthesiology 1991; 74: 581; in Lubenow TR, McCarthy RJ, Ivankovich AD: Management of acute postoperative pain. In Barash PG, Cullen BF, Stoelting RK [eds]: Clinical Anesthesia, 2nd ed, pp 1547–1577. Philadelphia, JB Lippincott, 1992.)

of the postsynaptic membrane. Hypopolarization of the nerve may also be modulated somewhat by inhibition of calcium movement.[21-23]

Higher Central Nervous System

The cerebral cortex has several interconnections that communicate with the reticular formation, periaqueductal gray, and other structures in the brain and brain stem. A basic review of the dimensions of perceptual psychology is required to understand the role of higher cortical function. Perception is the phenomenon by which noxious stimuli reach consciousness. Input from the cortex is necessary to provide interpretation and to give meaning to the stimuli. Perception can then be divided into two categories: cognition and attention. Cognitive functions are those abilities to recognize, discriminate, memorize, or judge afferent information that stems from external stimuli. Therefore, cognitive modulation of pain involves the patient's ability to relate a painful experience to another event. For example, pain experienced in a pleasant environment elicits less pain response than pain experienced in a setting of depression. The other area of perception is attention. Attention operates on the premise that only a fixed amount of afferent stimulation can reach cortical centers. If a patient in pain concentrates on separate and unrelated images, it is possible to decrease the effect of a painful sensation. This is achieved because the patient is focused on something else. The positive impact on pain from biofeedback or hypnosis also operates on this principle.

Neuraxial Analgesia

The technique of spinal analgesia was described initially by Bier and Toeffler in 1898 and that of sacral analgesia, by Sicard and Cathelin in 1901. A major advance in the application of neuraxial analgesia was made in 1949 with the description by Cleland[24] of the use of an epidural catheter for continuous postoperative analgesia. Analgesia in this setting was maintained for 1 to 5 days postoperatively by the administration of intermittent boluses of a local anesthetic. Effective analgesia was achieved, although this was at a cost of a significant sympathetic block for which all patients required at least a single dose of a vasopressor. Additional shortcomings of this technique were fluctuating levels of analgesia that occurred as the effect of the local anesthetic bolus wore off and the medical staff required to reinject patients every several hours.

Because of the shortcomings of the intermittent-dosing technique, the continuous infusion of local anesthetics into the neuraxis was subsequently recommended as an alternative to the intermittent-bolus technique. The continuous infusion of local anesthetics simplified maintenance of analgesia, but the use of local anesthetics in concentrations sufficient to produce pain relief usually resulted in sensory and sometimes motor block. These effects are unwanted in the postoperative period because sensory block and motor block prohibit ambulation, an important factor in postoperative convalescence.

Although it has been recognized that injection of local anesthetics into the spinal canal could provide effective analgesia, it was the demonstration that opioids could produce intense spinal analgesia that has been responsible for the explosive growth of the practice of neuraxial analgesia. The increased interest in this route of administration has been a direct result of the shortcomings of intramuscular and intravenous therapies. By interrupting or modulating pain transmissions at the level of communication between the first- and second-order neurons, a method is provided for effective analgesia without the associated central nervous system depression and cyclic nature of pain associated with other parenteral routes of administration.

Intrathecal

The intrathecal delivery of opioids has the advantage of providing prolonged postoperative analgesia after a single injection. This is a practical approach to postoperative pain management, especially in conjunction with a subarachnoid local anesthetic block for surgical anesthesia. The onset and duration of analgesia depend on the particular opioid used and are related to the relative hydrophilicity or lipophilicity of the opioid.

The onset of analgesic effect after the administration of a lipophilic opioid is faster than that of a hydrophilic compound, whereas the duration of effect is longer with a more hydrophilic medication. Morphine, for example, has been shown to produce a peak analgesic effect in 20 to 60 min that lasts for approximately 2 to 12 h with doses ranging from 0.25 mg to 4 mg.[25, 26] In routine clinical practice, 0.25 to 1 mg of morphine can be expected to provide effective analgesia. Doses in the range of 0.25 to 0.5 mg generally maintain analgesic efficacy while minimizing the potential for respiratory depression.[25] Doses of 0.5 mg to 1 mg warrant closer observation for respiratory depression. Lipophilic opioids such as sufentanil have an onset of action within minutes but a much shorter duration of action, ranging from 2 to 4 h.

Intermittent intrathecal injections share many of the problems of other intermittent-injection techniques: lack of titratability and extensive time and personnel requirements for monitoring and reinjection. In addition, there are data that demonstrate that the intrathecal route of administration is associated with a higher incidence of side effects compared with the epidural route and has a greater risk of respiratory depression owing to the greater rostral spread of the drug. Extensive clinical experience with continuous epidural infusions suggests they may be preferable to intrathecal techniques. The practical aspects of maintaining a catheter in the intrathecal space for a prolonged time and reports of cauda equina syndrome after continuous spinal anesthesia may be additional reasons to use the continuous epidural infusion technique.[27]

Epidural

When planning epidural analgesia, one must consider whether continuous-infusion techniques, intermittent-bolus regimens, or a patient-assisted (also referred to as patient-controlled) modality should be used. To fully appreciate the differences among the various regimens, it is helpful to review the evolution of each technique. Conceptually, postoperative epidural analgesia is not new but rather evolved from the early use of local anesthetics by anesthesiologists skilled in regional anesthesia. In 1949,[24] the first description was published of postoperative analgesia by the intermittent-bolus administration of a local anesthetic for 1 to 5 days postoperatively. Although patients achieved effective analgesia, a significant sympathetic block accompanied the pain relief, and all patients required one or more doses of a vasopressor in the postoperative period. As with other intermittent-dosing regimens, this technique was also associated with fluctuating levels of pain relief as the effect of the bolus began to regress. A final problem inherent with the intermittent-dosing regimen is the labor intensiveness, which requires anesthesia personnel to reassess and redose the patient every several hours. In a busy pain service, this extensive time commitment would be prohibitive and could potentially compromise patient care. Because of these shortcomings, the continuous epidural infusion of local anesthetics was subsequently examined as an alternative to the intermittent-bolus administration.

The continuous infusion of dilute local anesthetic solutions simplified maintenance and improved postsurgical analgesic uniformity. However, concentrations sufficient to provide pain relief generally resulted in motor block. Motor block is undesirable in the postoperative period because the ability to ambulate, a key factor in postoperative convalescence, is compromised.

The discovery of spinal opioid receptors in the mid- and late 1970s focused interest on neuraxial administration of opioids and away from local anesthetics as the agents of choice for epidural analgesia. The early practice of epidural administration of opioids for analgesia paralleled the early use of local anesthetics in that bolus techniques were initially used. Early reports[28, 29] described intermittent epidural doses of morphine (up to 15 mg/day) for postsurgical analgesia. Although this technique provided excellent pain relief, it soon became apparent that the incidence and severity of side effects associated with these large doses limited its widespread clinical application. In an effort to mitigate the frequency and severity of opioid-induced side effects, El-Baz and coworkers[30] describe the continuous epidural infusion of morphine. In this particular study, patients were randomized to receive epidural injections of either bupivacaine 0.5% or morphine 5 mg or a continuous infusion of morphine 100 μg/h. Results from this study demonstrated that the continuous infusion of morphine provided equivalent analgesia and fewer side effects compared with the other treatment regimens.

The observation that a low-dose continuous epidural infusion provides analgesic intensity similar to much larger bolus doses[31–33] is not surprising if one examines the pharmacokinetics of epidurally administered morphine.[29, 34] Whether delivered epidurally or intravenously, 10 mg of morphine produces peak serum levels and decay curves that are nearly identical.[28, 29, 34] Although the period of pain relief resulting from the intravenous administration is short lived, epidurally administered morphine provides 12 h or more of analgesia. This finding indicates that a major proportion of an epidural bolus of a hydrophilic substance is absorbed via the systemic circulation. A relatively small amount of drug diffuses into the cerebrospinal fluid, and only a small fraction of drug diffuses into the spinal cord and binds to opioid receptors. A corollary to these observations indicates that the degree to which morphine spreads rostrally by bulk flow of cerebrospinal fluid, and therefore the incidence and severity of associated effects, is highly dose-dependent.[29, 34]

In an effort to achieve analgesic synergy from the desirable properties of epidural administration of local anesthetics and of opioids, several investigators[31, 32, 35–39] have described the concurrent use of morphine-bupivacaine or fentanyl-bupivacaine epidural infusions for postoperative pain relief. These combinations appear to provide pain relief of greater magnitude than that obtained with either drug alone while decreasing the incidence and severity of side effects. The theoretic basis for this combination therapy relates to the differ-

ent locations of action of the medications. Opioids produce analgesia by binding to opioid receptors in the substantia gelatinosa of the cord, whereas local anesthetics provide analgesia by blocking pain transmission at the nerve roots and dorsal root ganglion.

Choice of Opioid for Epidural Administration

The primary differences among opioids used for analgesia relate to their onset of action, duration of action, and propensity to produce side effects. Morphine, the first opioid to be used for epidural administration, has been the most extensively studied and remains a popular analgesic. Morphine solutions given epidurally provide prolonged duration of pain relief and greater dermatomal spread of analgesic compared with more hydrophilic opioids. These characteristics are well suited for either intermittent-bolus dosing or continuous epidural infusion. The major drawbacks of morphine given epidurally include a delayed onset of analgesia (60 min), a prolonged time to peak effect (90 to 120 min), and a relatively high incidence of associated side effects compared with the more lipophilic opioids. The major clinical advantage of the lipophilic opioids is the extremely rapid onset of analgesia they provide.[34, 39, 40] Unfortunately, the duration is quite limited (generally 2 to 4 h), thus mandating continuous infusion to provide practical postsurgical analgesia. Again, an additional advantage of the continuous infusion is the ability to coadminister a dilute bupivacaine solution.

Patient-Assisted Epidural Analgesia

The newest refinement in the application of epidural management of pain has been the description of patient-assisted epidural analgesia—also often referred to as patient-controlled epidural analgesia. Patient-assisted epidural analgesia represents a hybrid of the conventional continuous epidural infusion coupled with patient-activated epidural boluses to provide supplemental pain relief. Initially, the clinical approach to patient-controlled epidural administration of opioids for analgesia used an on-demand fixed dose or a minimal continuous infusion rate with superimposed demand doses.[39] With patient-controlled epidural analgesia, the intermittent dose provides most of the analgesia. In the more recently described patient-assisted epidural analgesia, the continuous infusion delivers the major analgesic dose while the patient-activated boluses are intended to provide supplemental analgesia for transient increases in analgesic requirements. The development of new infusion technologies has allowed combined modes of analgesic delivery to become safe, practical, and readily available.

Initiation and Maintenance of Therapy

Continuous epidural infusions of opioids or opioid-bupivacaine mixtures result in fewer fluctuations in concentration of drug in cerebrospinal fluid. However, one disadvantage of this technique is that it takes several hours to infuse enough medication epidurally to provide adequate analgesia. This delay in the onset of analgesia may be overcome by administering a small (5- to 10-mL) loading bolus of solution epidurally before beginning the infusion. Alternatively and preferably, the epidural infusion should be started intraoperatively to allow adequate spinal penetration and opioid receptor binding. This practice allows one to provide preemptive analgesia in order to provide antinociception before the surgical stimulus. This practice serves to optimize pain relief and smooths emergence from surgical anesthesia. To achieve this end, it is recommended that epidural catheters be placed preoperatively before the induction of anesthesia.

Preoperative placement of the epidural catheter allows the anesthesiologist to administer a test dose of local anesthetic while the patient is still awake and also allows the start of an infusion intraoperatively. The epidural catheter may be inserted by the anesthesiologist providing the surgical anesthesia or by another anesthesiologist. Several epidural solutions may be used (Table 38–2). Experience has shown that approximately 3 to 4 h is required to infuse enough medication into the epidural space to provide adequate analgesia on awakening. If the procedure is expected to be of short duration (e.g., 1 to 2 h), a 5- to 10-mL bolus of the infusion mixture may be given to hasten the onset of analgesia. Alternatively, patients may be given an epidural bolus of 0.5% bupivacaine combined with fentanyl (50 to 100 μg), sufentanil (30 μg), or morphine (1 to 5 mg). After operation, the epidural infusion is generally maintained at the same rate of infusion that was started intraoperatively. This may be titrated upward, or preferably the patient may be placed on a patient-assisted administration mode that allows the patient to self-administer additional medication.

Importance of Epidural Catheter Location

After epidural injection, morphine will be partitioned preferentially into cerebrospinal fluid, which then allows it to spread rostrally in the cerebrospinal fluid and saturate the entire length of the spinal cord.[34] Because of this property, morphine given epidurally may be infused at a low lumbar level and still provide analgesia for surgical procedures performed on the upper spinal segments such as the upper abdomen and thorax. Fentanyl, a more lipophilic opioid, is theorized to provide a segmental effect. This segmental effect is most likely due to the lipophilic binding to lipid structures in the spinal canal such as epidural fat and the lipid portion of the spinal cord. This segmental analgesia suggests one should place the epidural catheter to cover the expected dermatomes included in the surgical field. Suggested spinal segments that need to be blocked for various surgical procedures are as follows:

Thoracic	T-2 to T-12
Upper abdominal	T-4 to L-1
Renal	T-6 to L-1
Hip	T-12 to L-3
Lower abdominal and gynecologic	T-10 to L-5

Alternatively, one may use a simple rule of thumb that this author uses when deciding where to place the epidural catheter. Identify the superior aspect of the surgical incision, whether it is at the anterior abdominal wall or the lateral midaxillary line, and draw an imaginary straight line across to the midline posterior portion of the back. The catheter can then be inserted at that level or one spinal level below that. In general, it has been this author's observation that many anesthesiologists tend to place the epidural catheter too low when they expect to use fentanyl epidurally as the analgesic medication. One may still elect to place lumbar catheters for upper abdominal or thoracic operations and use fentanyl epidurally; however, the opioid dose requirements for lipophilic agents may be quite high when administered via these lumbar catheters. When given at higher infusion rates (e.g., 100 μg/h or greater), it is likely that the serum levels from epidural administration of fentanyl may approach the serum

Table 38–2 Epidural Administration of Opioids or Opioid-Bupivacaine Solutions

	INTERMITTENT INJECTION		
DRUG	**Dose**	**Onset, min**	**Duration, h**
Meperidine	25–100 mg	5–10	6
Morphine	0.5–5 mg	30–60	8–24
Hydromorphone	1 mg	13	12
Fentanyl	50–100 μg	4–10	4–6
Sufentanil	10–60 μg	7	2–4

	CONTINUOUS INFUSION		PATIENT-ASSISTED EPIDURAL*	
	Range, mL/h	**Continuous-Rate, mL/h**	**Patient-Assisted Bolus, mL**	**Interval, min**
Meperidine† (0.1%–0.25%)—Bupivacaine‡ (0.1%)[41]	2–10	5	1	12
Morphine 0.01%—Bupivacaine‡ 0.1%	3–6	3	1	20
Fentanyl§ 0.001%—Bupivacaine‡ 0.1%	4–10	5	1	12

*With patient-assisted epidural analgesia, the maximal hourly rate of continuous basal infusion and patient-assisted bolus should not exceed the maximum continuous infusion range for that agent.

†Meperidine concentrations may vary from 0.1% to 0.25% while patient is monitored for optimal analgesic effect (maximal meperidine dose, 25 mg/h).

‡Bupivacaine concentrations may vary from 0.06% to 0.125% while patient is monitored for optimal analgesic effect.

§Fentanyl concentration may vary downward to 0.0002% (5 μg/mL), particularly in elderly patients.

levels of parenterally administered fentanyl.[40] This latter concept is highlighted by the data from Guinard et al,[42] who showed that in patients recovering from thoracotomy, analgesia side effects were lowest and pulmonary function better maintained when thoracic epidural administration of fentanyl was used compared with lumbar epidural or intravenous administration of fentanyl. Nevertheless, these investigators questioned whether the benefits outweighed reluctance by many to administer fentanyl epidurally via the thoracic route.

Management of Inadequate Analgesia

Despite the optimal pain relief that epidural analgesia provides in the majority of patients, there are scenarios when patients experience inadequate pain relief. In these situations, it is recommended that a member of the acute pain service assess the patient and attempt to identify the cause of inadequate analgesia. To this end, it is recommended that an algorithm using a test dose of a local anesthetic be initiated to define more precisely the reason for inadequate analgesia. If a patient continues to have persistent pain despite a bolus of the epidural infusion medication, the anesthesiologist may administer a test dose of a 2% lidocaine solution with 1:200,000 epinephrine to confirm epidural catheter placement. The test dose generally yields one of three results. If a bilateral sensory block occurs in a few segmental dermatomes, correct catheter placement is confirmed. In this case, insufficient volume or dose of epidural infusion was the likely cause of inadequate pain relief and is resolved by increasing the rate of infusion. If a unilateral sensory block is obtained, the epidural catheter tip is most likely placed too far into the epidural space, with the tip located within an intervertebral foramen laterally. The catheter is then withdrawn 1 to 2 cm and the test dose is repeated. In the third scenario, no sensory block indicates that the epidural catheter is no longer in the epidural space. The catheter is removed and the patient may have another epidural catheter placed or alternatively may be switched to another mode of analgesic therapy. Despite this maneuver, if patients continue to have moderate or severe pain, small amounts of morphine (2 mg) given intravenously every 2 to 4 h are tolerated well without undue risk of respiratory depression. Alternatively, intravenous or intramuscular administration of ketorolac works well in this situation.

Patient Safety Considerations

Although the goal of epidural analgesia is improved pain relief, patient safety is the paramount consideration. Serious complications that may occur with epidural analgesia involve unintentional intrathecal administration of drug, infection-related problems, epidural hematoma, and respiratory depression. In order to decrease the incidence of these potential complications, several guidelines are useful:

1. The use of appropriate concentrations of local anesthetics (for example, 0.1% bupivacaine) allows ready diagnosis of subarachnoid catheter migration, which is identified by increasing levels of sensory block.

2. Daily examination of catheter insertion sites and monitoring of temperature curves and periodic evaluation for signs of meningeal irritation allow early detection of infection. If findings consistent with infection are present, it is prudent to remove the catheter and continue observation for infectious complications. In the experience at the author's institution of more than 10,000 cases of epidural analgesia, no cases of epidural abscess have been encountered. There has been a small number of subcutaneous infections that have resolved quickly with conservative therapy.

3. The placement of epidural catheters in patients who have received anticoagulants is controversial because of the risk of epidural hematoma formation. Data from the author's institution as well as the observations of others indicate that if epidural catheters are placed at least 1 h before heparinization, the incidence of clinically significant epidural hemorrhage is extremely low. Likewise, epidural catheters may be inserted safely in patients who will receive warfarin postoperatively as long as coagulation status is normal at the time of catheter insertion.

4. Respiratory monitoring to detect the occurrence of respiratory depression is a controversial issue that varies from institution to institution. It is often the primary reason that some institutions limit the use of epidural administration of opioids to patients in an intensive care or postanesthesia care unit. This practice limits the number of patients who can benefit from epidural analgesia. There is ample evidence from the author's institution as well as others that patients can safely receive opioids epidurally in the hospital ward setting provided that the anesthesiology team is responsible for all adjustments of analgesic and sedative medications. In addition, patients should have their respiratory rate and level of sedation observed once an hour. Apnea or electrocardiographic monitors can be used to supplement nursing observation but should not replace direct patient contact.

Caudal

In the adult population, caudal nerve blocks play a minor role in acute, postoperative pain management. The reason for this is that it is generally more difficult to perform caudal blocks in adults compared with lumbar epidural blocks. Continuous caudal analgesia has a limited utility because of the difficulty of inserting the catheter, but with this caveat, it may have a role in select individuals, such as those who have had extensive lumbar or thoracic spine surgery. In these situations where continuous caudal analgesia is used, the standard solutions for lumbar epidural analgesia may be given.

Peripheral Regional Block

The peripheral injection of local anesthetics to block nociception can be a useful component in acute, postoperative pain management. Peripheral nerve blocks are relatively simple to perform and have a historical record of effectiveness. The disadvantage is that they may provide pain relief of relatively brief duration. However, the pain relief afforded by regional nerve blocks may be superior to that achieved with systemic narcotics. Local anesthetics produce antinociception by blocking nerve transmission by inhibiting sodium channels. Local anesthetics diffuse across the nerve membrane in their uncharged form. Once inside the cell, the local anesthetic becomes charged once again and then binds to the inner aspect of sodium channels, preventing the influx of sodium ions necessary for depolarization. This leaves the membrane in its normal polarized condition, and an action potential cannot be generated.

Local Infiltration

The local infiltration of anesthetics in the vicinity of the surgical incision is a simple technique for providing postoperative analgesia for the initial several hours after minor operations. Care should be taken to aspirate before injection to avoid unintentional intravascular injection. However, even when blood has not been aspirated, it is still possible for local anesthetics to be delivered intravascularly. In addition to the hazards of intravascular local injection, another concern is to not exceed recommended dosing guidelines because of local anesthetic systemic toxicity. A unique role of local infiltration is the intra-articular injection of local anesthetics after arthroscopic procedures. This technique improves postoperative comfort and facilitates recuperation.[43, 44] Bupivacaine is the most commonly used local anesthetic (up to 100 mg). One report[45] also described intra-articular injection of morphine in small doses (e.g., 1 mg), which also provides effective pain relief. This observation has led to the speculation that there are opioid receptors peripherally.

Intercostal

Intercostal nerve blocks are helpful in providing analgesia for thoracic and upper abdominal operations. When performing an intercostal nerve block for extensive thoracic incisions, it is important to identify the sensory dermatomes affected by the surgical incision so that each dermatome can be blocked. Dermatomes that include the thoracostomy drainage tubes must also be blocked. With long midline abdominal incisions, a large volume of local anesthetic is needed for optimal pain relief. Careful consideration should be given to maximum dosage guidelines. Provision of adequate analgesia for these types of incisions requires multiple bilateral intercostal blocks. In many practices, postoperative pain management for abdominal or thoracic operation is more easily done with continuous epidural infusions. An additional disadvantage of intercostal blocks is the potential for pneumothorax with attendant respiratory compromise. Bupivacaine or bupivacaine with epinephrine is recommended for postsurgical pain relief. Adequate analgesia for surgical incision usually requires injection of local anesthetics into a minimum of two or three intercostal segments.

An alternative to the injection of local anesthetic on the intercostal nerve is cryoanalgesia, which involves the application of a cryoprobe along an intercostal nerve. This produces local freezing of a segment of the intercostal nerve, impairing neuronal transmission. This technique has been reported to produce reversible nerve disruption while preserving intraneural connective tissue. For optimal results, the cryoprobe needs to be applied on the intercostal nerve from within the chest by piercing the parietal pleura, and two levels below and above the incision need to be blocked. Nerve function after cryoanalgesia begins to recover within 2 to 3 weeks; complete recovery occurs within 1 to 3 months. Advantages of this technique are said to include a minimal incidence of neuritis or neuroma formation; however, this is controversial. Because of the extended period of postoperative analgesia, this technique may be advantageous when the postoperative analgesic requirement is expected to last for a prolonged time, such as for the individual with significant chest trauma or significant limitation of respiratory function.[46]

Intrapleural

Intrapleural regional analgesia involves the percutaneous placement of a catheter within the chest between the visceral and parietal pleura.[47] The procedure is generally performed with the patient in the lateral decubitus position. An intercostal space between the fifth and tenth ribs is chosen, and a 17-G Tuohy needle is inserted at the posterior axillary line. The needle is then walked over the superior aspect of the rib. A saline-lubricated glass syringe filled with 3 to 4 mL of air is attached to the needle, and the syringe needle is advanced as a unit with the needle bevel directed in a cephalad direction. Once the pleural space is entered, the negative intrapleural pressure draws the syringe plunger inward in a manner analogous to the hanging-drop technique for epidural site identification. An epidural catheter is then advanced 6 cm within the intrapleural space in a rapid fashion to prevent the development of a clinically significant pneumothorax. For patients on mechanical ventilation, positive pressure ventilation should be interrupted while the needle and catheter are being inserted in order to prevent injury to the lung. When patients are breathing spontaneously, the needle and catheter procedure should be performed during breath holding after end exhalation. To achieve a more extensive block, two catheters may need to be placed in the intrapleural space.[48] The intrapleural analgesia resulting from the intermittent injection of local anesthetics is useful for postoperative pain relief after upper abdominal operations such as an open cholecystectomy via a subcostal incision.[49] Effective postoperative pain relief requires intermittent intrapleural injections every 6 h with 20 mL of 0.25% to 0.5% bupivacaine. In closed chest procedures, a continuous infusion of bupivacaine may also be used. This avoids the fluctuating levels of analgesia that occur with any intermittent-bolus technique.

Intrapleural analgesia after thoracotomy has been examined by several authors[49, 50] and has been found to be less effective for post-thoracotomy pain than for other procedures in which the pleura is intact and there are no thoracostomy drainage tubes to divert the local anesthetic. Certain intercostal incisions such as those required for anterior thoracotomies require that pleural drainage tubes be clamped for a short time after each intermittent local anesthetic injection to allow the local anesthetic sufficient time to cross the parietal pleura and provide effective analgesia.[51] This intermittent clamping of the pleural drainage tubes may not be tolerated in patients with a moderate or large air leak from the pulmonary parenchyma after thoracotomy. The risk of pneumothorax and the problems of fluctuating levels of analgesia are limitations of this technique; pulmonary parenchymal damage has been reported[52] after this technique.

Ilioinguinal

Ilioinguinal nerve blocks are useful for pain management after inguinal or femoral herniorrhaphy, appendectomy, or procedures involving the scrotum. This technique is performed after palpation of the anterior superior iliac spine. A position two fingerbreadths medial and two fingerbreadths superior is identified, and an imaginary line from the anterior superior iliac spine to the umbilicus is drawn. The intersection of these points is the location of needle advancement. Generally, a 22-G, 8.75-cm needle is advanced posteriorly in the parasagittal plane in most adults. The needle is advanced slowly and bounced every several millimeters until a paresthesia is elicited. This indicates needle contact with the fascia immediately superficial to the external oblique muscle along which the ilioinguinal nerve is located. Once the needle is in this position, 10 to 15 mL of local anesthetic is injected. The needle is then withdrawn several millimeters and redirected laterally until the tip reaches the medial edge of the anterior superior iliac spine. An additional 10 to 15 mL of local anesthetic solution is then injected. Complications of this nerve block include hemorrhage and hematoma at the injection site. Occasionally, numbness in the distribution of the lateral femoral cutaneous nerve can also occur.

Penile

A penile nerve block provides effective analgesia after circumcision or orchiopexy. Bupivacaine 0.25% to 0.5% may be used. Two techniques are described for performing this block. One technique involves injecting half of the volume of local anesthetic at the 10 o'clock position at the base of the penis, with the remainder at the 2 o'clock position. An alternative technique involves infiltrating local anesthetic at the base of the subcutaneous tissue 360° around the base of the penis. Epinephrine-containing local anesthetics should not be used because of the risk of vasoconstriction and ischemic necrosis of the skin.

Brachial Plexus

Continuous postoperative brachial plexus analgesia has been described[53–56] with catheters placed via the interscalene, axillary, supraclavicular, or infraclavicular approach. A catheter-over-needle technique using an 18-G, 5-cm, Teflon-coated intravenous catheter placed over a 22-G needle is one method.[56] A nerve stimulator may be used to elicit paresthesias and identify contact with the neurovascular bundle. Another method for catheter placement uses a Seldinger technique. With this technique, the needle is placed with the aid of a nerve stimulator, after which a guidewire is passed through the needle. Sterile alligator clips connected to the nerve stimulator can then be placed on the guidewire after the needle is removed to confirm that the guidewire is still in contact with the brachial plexus. A 20-G catheter can be placed over the guidewire, which is then removed. For rapid sequential confirmation of correct catheter placement, the guidewire can be reinserted in the catheter and a nerve stimulator can be used to determine if paresthesias can still be elicited. Technical difficulty with this technique occurs in patients who have a significant amount of subcutaneous tissue through which the catheter needs to be advanced over the guidewire.

Postoperative brachial plexus analgesia has been described with bupivacaine 0.125% to 0.25% at rates ranging from 6 to 10 mL/h. When infusion rates are maintained in this range, it is unlikely that serum levels will reach toxic levels. It has been the author's experience that serum levels always remain far below toxic levels when these dosing parameters are used. This regimen does not preclude any commonly used dosages and volumes of any local anesthetic currently recommended for surgical anesthesia. The major disadvantage of this technique is postoperative catheter migration.

Opioid Analgesic Delivery Systems

The parenteral administration of opioids remains the primary route for the treatment of moderate to severe postoperative pain. Advances in microprocessor technology and newer applications of opioids have played a role in refining methods of delivery and decreasing side effects of parenterally administered opioids.

Intramuscular

The intramuscular administration of analgesics produces a rapid onset and time to peak effect. It is also a simple route of administration because no special infusion devices are required. However, pain at the injection site, patient apprehensiveness, potential for delayed respiratory depression, and wide variability in serum drug concentrations limit the use of this route. Absorption from intramuscular sites depends on the lipophilicity of the opioid as well as the blood flow to the area of the injection. After intramuscular injections of morphine or meperidine, plasma concentrations may vary as much as threefold to fivefold and time to peak concentration may vary from 4 to 108 min among patients.[56, 57] In addition, there is variability in the minimal analgesic plasma concentration for patients.[58]

Small changes in opioid concentrations (10% to 20% for a patient) may represent a spectrum of effects from inadequate analgesia to complete pain relief.[59] The relationship between plasma concentration and effect over time is depicted in Figure 38–4. Plasma concentration after intramuscular administration establishes a cyclic pattern of sedation, analgesia, and, finally, inadequate analgesia. When morphine is administered by this route on a 3- to 4-h basis, plasma concentrations exceed or meet analgesia requirements for only approximately 30% of the dosing interval because of the delay in absorption and the narrow therapeutic window.[57] This situation is exacerbated by the dynamic nature of pain. Newer methods of delivery, such as patient-controlled analgesia, circumvent these problems of intramuscular administration and provide more effective analgesia with fewer side effects by maintaining tighter control of plasma levels.

Although many opioids can be administered by the intramuscular route, only one nonsteroidal anti-inflammatory drug, ketorolac, is currently available for intramuscular injection. Ketorolac is a potent analgesic with limited anti-inflammatory properties and only moderate effects on platelet function. Many clinical trials have demonstrated the efficacy of this medication.

Intravenous

The intermittent intravenous injection of opioids is feasible in situations in which close continuous monitoring of the patient is available. With an intravenous bolus dose, the time delay for analgesic effect and the variability in plasma concentration seen with intramuscular administration are minimized. However, rapid redistribution of the drug shortens the duration of action and, in general, all of the limitations of intramuscular administration are present with intravenous administration. Continuous intravenous infusions offer the advantage of maintaining nearly consistent plasma drug concentrations. However, this does not take into account the dynamic nature of pain and the fluctuations in dosing requirements that occur with time.

Patient-Controlled Analgesia

Patient-controlled analgesia involves the self-administration of opioid medication via a patient-activated infusion device. By combining advantages of continuous infusion with the flexibility of interposed, small bolus injections as analgesic requirements vary, patient-controlled analgesia appears to be the answer for many patients' analgesic needs. This method has evolved from improved drug delivery systems coupled with advances in computer technology. The earliest patient-controlled analgesia devices permitted patients to titrate analgesic needs by delivering only small boluses intermittently. Technologic advances have allowed more sophisticated dosing schedules. Limits can be placed on the number of activations per unit time, with the patient given a minimum time interval that needs to elapse between patient activations (lock-out interval). Refinements of this delivery system permit concurrent administration of a background continuous infusion and patient-activated boluses. These new devices allow the system to record a profile of drug administration, including number and time of bolus deliveries, number of activations that did not result in bolus drug delivery, and total amounts of the agent administered. Patient-controlled analgesia has been shown to provide superior analgesia compared with traditional, on-demand intramuscular injections. Most patients tend to determine a pain level at which they feel comfortable and taper their dosages with time as they convalesce.[60] Patients' acceptance of patient-controlled analgesia is high, because they feel they have significant control over their therapy. One limitation of patient-controlled analgesia therapy is the selection of agents currently available for use in patient-controlled analgesia devices (Table 38–3).

Other Modalities

Transcutaneous Electrical Nerve Stimulation

Transcutaneous electrical nerve stimulation is a simple, noninvasive technique that uses electrical stimula-

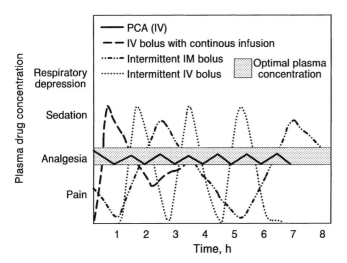

Figure 38–4 Relationship between pharmacologic effect over time at a specific plasma drug concentration and method of administration. IM, intramuscular; IV, intravenous; PCA, patient-controlled analgesia. (From Tuman KJ, McCarthy RJ, Ivankovich AD: Pain control in the postoperative cardiac surgery patient. Hosp Formulary 1988; 23: 580.)

Table 38–3 Patient-Controlled Analgesia: Bolus Doses, Lock-Out Intervals, and Continuous Infusion Rates for Various Parenteral Analgesics

DRUG	BOLUS DOSE, mg	LOCK-OUT INTERVAL, min	CONTINUOUS INFUSION, mg/h
Agonists			
Fentanyl citrate	0.015–0.05	3–10	0.02–0.1
Hydromorphone hydrochloride	0.10–0.5	5–15	0.2–0.5
Meperidine hydrochloride	5–15	5–15	5–40
Methadone hydrochloride	0.50–3.0	10–20	—
Morphine sulfate	0.50–3.0	5–20	1–10
Oxymorphone hydrochloride	0.20–0.8	5–15	0.1–1
Sufentanil citrate	0.003–0.015	3–10	0.004–0.03
Agonist-Antagonists			
Buprenorphine hydrochloride	0.03–0.2	10–20	—
Nalbupine hydrochloride	1–5	5–15	1–8
Pentazocine hydrochloride	5–30	5–15	6–40

From Lubenow TR, McCarthy RJ, Ivankovich AD: Management of acute postoperative pain. In Barash PG, Cullen BF, Stoelting RK (eds): Clinical Anesthesia, 2nd ed, pp 1547–1577. Philadelphia, JB Lippincott, 1992.

tion of the skin to provide pain relief. Transcutaneous electrical nerve stimulation initially was prescribed for the relief of chronic pain, but its use has been extended to include control of postoperative pain. Two or four electrodes are placed on the skin adjacent to the incision. These electrodes are then connected to a battery-operated pulse generator capable of varying stimulation mode, frequency, and amplitude. The mechanism by which pain relief is produced is thought to involve the release of endogenous enkephalins at the spinal cord level by the electrical stimulation of afferent cutaneous nerve fibers. This endogenous enkephalin release has an inhibitory effect on the dorsal horn and augments the descending inhibitory pathway. Partial reversal of the analgesia by naloxone supports this theory.[61] The degree of pain relief exhibited by patients varies from satisfactory to negligible in many instances. The advent of more effective techniques (e.g., patient-controlled analgesia and epidural analgesia) has made the use of transcutaneous electrical nerve stimulation for postoperative pain infrequent.

Psychologic Interventions

The use of a wide variety of analgesic techniques involving nerve blocks, neuraxial administration of opioids, or sophisticated intravenous infusions has produced dramatic changes in the management of pain during the past decade. However, it is at times necessary to augment these newer sophisticated techniques with various psychologic interventions. Psychotherapy is used widely in the treatment of chronic pain, and these cognitive and behavioral strategies have a role in the management of acute pain for certain patients. This cognitive approach to the treatment of pain uses interventions such as distraction or imagery that attempt to focus attention away from the painful event and toward more pleasant scenarios. In addition, communication with and education of the patients regarding their surroundings, treatment plans for their disease, natural history of the disease, and the hospital environment often decrease fear and anxiety about unknown events or situations in the perioperative period. This approach is often overlooked when dealing with patients who are unfamiliar with the hospital environment. Other psychologic interventions that may also be useful are relaxation techniques such as deep-breathing exercises or muscle-relaxation training, which have also been shown to decrease anxiety and muscle tension.[62, 63]

Summary

The recent interest in postoperative pain management has fostered the growth and development of a new subspecialty in anesthesiology directed at optimizing relief of postoperative pain. This growth has allowed anesthesiologists to extend their clinical practice in order to develop and refine new avenues. This chapter reviews the physiology and modulation of nociception, and a wide variety of analgesic techniques are compared and contrasted.

References

1. Bonica JJ: The anatomical basis of pain. In Bonica JJ (ed): The Management of Pain, pp 27–61. Philadelphia, Lea & Febiger, 1972.
2. Chapman CR, Bonica JJ: Acute pain. In Current Concepts, pp 4–16. Kalamazoo, The Upjohn Company, 1983.
3. Erlanger J, Gasser HS: Compound nature of action current of nerves as disclosed by cathode ray oscillograph. Am J Physiol 1924; 70: 624–666.
4. de Jong RH (ed): Physiology and Pharmacology of Local Anesthesia, pp 97–102. Springfield, Charles C Thomas, 1970.
5. Kerr FWL: The structured basis of pain: circuitry and pathways. In Ng LKY, Bonica JJ (eds): Pain, Discomfort and Humanitarian Care: Proceedings of the National Conference Held at the National Institutes of Health, Bethesda, Maryland, February 15–16, 1979, pp 49–60. New York, Elsevier, 1980.
6. Snyder SH: Peptide neurotransmitters with possible involvement in pain perception. In Bonica JJ (ed): Pain, pp 233–244. New York, Raven Press, 1980.
7. Henry JL: Effects of substance P on functionally identified units in cat spinal cord. Brain Res 1976; 114: 439–451.

8. Jessel TM, Mudge AW, Leeman SE, et al: Release of substance P and somatostatin in vivo from primary afferent terminals in mammalian spinal cord. Neuro Sci Abstr 1979; 5: 611.

9. Randic M, Miletic V: Depressant actions of methionine-enkephalin and somatostatin in cat dorsal horn neurones activated by noxious stimuli. Brain Res 1978; 152: 196–202.

10. Nathan PW: Involvement of the sympathetic nervous system in pain. In Kosterlitz HW, Terenius LY (eds): Dahlem Workshop on Pain and Society, Berlin, 1979, pp 311–324. Weinheim, Germany, Verlag Chemie, 1980.

11. Richardson DE, Akil H: Pain reduction by electrical brain stimulation in man. Part 1: Acute administration in periaqueductal and periventricular sites. J Neurosurg 1977; 47: 178–183.

12. Adams JE: Naloxone reversal of analgesia produced by brain stimulation in the human. Pain 1976; 2: 161–166.

13. Hosobuchi Y, Adams JE, Linchitz R: Pain relief by electrical stimulation of the central gray matter in humans and its reversal by naloxone. Science 1977; 197: 183–186.

14. Zieglgansberger W, Bayerl H: The mechanism of inhibition of neuronal activity by opiates in the spinal cord of cat. Brain Res 1976; 115: 111–128.

15. Zieglgansberger W, Tulloch IF: The effects of methionine- and leucine-enkephalin on spinal neurones of the cat. Brain Res 1979; 167: 53–64.

16. Camarata PJ, Yaksh TL: Characterization of the spinal adrenergic receptors mediating the spinal effects produced by the microinjection of morphine into the periaqueductal gray. Brain Res 1985; 336: 133–142.

17. Yaksh TL: Direct evidence that spinal serotonin and noradrenaline terminals mediate the spinal antinociceptive effects of morphine in the periaqueductal gray. Brain Res 1979; 160: 180–185.

18. Kuraishi Y, Harada Y, Takagi H: Noradrenaline regulation of pain-transmission in the spinal cord mediated by alpha-adrenoceptors. Brain Res 1979; 174: 333–336.

19. Reddy SV, Maderdrut JL, Yaksh TL: Spinal cord pharmacology of adrenergic agonist-mediated antinociception. J Pharmacol Exp Ther 1980; 213: 525–533.

20. North RA, Williams JT, Surprenant A, et al: Mu and delta receptors belong to a family of receptors that are coupled to potassium channels. Proc Natl Acad Sci U S A 1987; 84: 5487–5491.

21. Maze M, Tranquilli W: Alpha-2 adrenoceptor agonists: defining the role in clinical anesthesia. Anesthesiology 1991; 74: 581–605.

22. Sabbe MB, Yaksh TL: Pharmacology of spinal opioids. J Pain Symptom Manage 1990; 5: 191–203.

23. North RA, Yoshimura M: The actions of noradrenaline on neurones of the rat substantia gelatinosa in vitro. J Physiol (Lond) 1984; 349: 43–55.

24. Cleland JGP: Continuous peridural and caudal analgesia in surgery and early ambulation. Northwest Med 1949; 48: 26–34.

25. Abboud TK, Dror A, Mosaad P, et al: Mini-dose intrathecal morphine for the relief of post-cesarean section pain: safety, efficacy, and ventilatory responses to carbon dioxide. Anesth Analg 1988; 67: 137–143.

26. Aun C, Thomas D, St John-Jones L, et al: Intrathecal morphine in cardiac surgery. Eur J Anaesthesiol 1985; 2: 419–426.

27. Rigler ML, Drasner K, Krejcie TC, et al: Cauda equina syndrome after continuous spinal anesthesia. Anesth Analg 1991; 72: 275–281.

28. Bromage PR, Camporesi E, Chestnut D: Epidural narcotics for postoperative analgesia. Anesth Analg 1980; 59: 473–480.

29. Cousins MJ, Mather LE: Intrathecal and epidural administration of opioids. Anesthesiology 1984; 61: 276–310.

30. El-Baz NM, Faber LP, Jensik RJ: Continuous epidural infusion of morphine for treatment of pain after thoracic surgery: a new technique. Anesth Analg 1984; 63: 757–764.

31. Fischer RL, Lubenow TR, Liceaga A, et al: Comparison of continuous epidural infusion of fentanyl-bupivacaine and morphine-bupivacaine in management of postoperative pain. Anesth Analg 1988; 67: 559–563.

32. Hjortso NC, Lund C, Mogensen T, et al: Epidural morphine improves pain relief and maintains sensory analgesia during continuous epidural bupivacaine after abdominal surgery. Anesth Analg 1986; 65: 1033–1036.

33. Lubenow TR, Fischer RL, Besser TP, et al: Comparison of continuous epidural infusions of sufentanil-bupivacaine with morphine-bupivacaine. (Abstract.) Anesthesiology 1988; 69(Suppl): A397.

34. Bromage PR, Camporesi EM, Durant PA, et al: Nonrespiratory side effects of epidural morphine. Anesth Analg 1982; 61: 490–495.

35. Akerman B, Arwestrom E, Post C: Local anesthetics potentiate spinal morphine antinociception. Anesth Analg 1988; 67: 943–948.

36. Chestnut DH, Owen CL, Bates JN, et al: Continuous infusion epidural analgesia during labor: a randomized, double-blind comparison of 0.0625% bupivacaine/0.0002% fentanyl versus 0.125% bupivacaine. Anesthesiology 1988; 68: 754–759.

37. Cullen ML, Staren ED, el-Ganzouri A, et al: Continuous epidural infusion for analgesia after major abdominal operations: a randomized, prospective, double-blind study. Surgery 1985; 98: 718–728.

38. Logas WG, el-Baz N, el-Ganzouri A, et al: Continuous thoracic epidural analgesia for postoperative pain relief following thoracotomy: a randomized prospective study. Anesthesiology 1987; 67: 787–791.

39. Lubenow T, Durrani Z, Ivankovich A: Evaluation of continuous epidural fentanyl/butorphanol infusion for postoperative pain. (Abstract.) Anesthesiology 1990; 73(Suppl): A800.

40. Loper KA, Ready LB, Downey M, et al: Epidural and intravenous fentanyl infusions are clinically equivalent after knee surgery. Anesth Analg 1990; 70: 72–75.

41. Ferrante FM, VadeBoncouer TR: Epidural analgesia with combinations of local anesthetics and opioids. In Ferrante FM, VadeBoncouer TR (eds): Postoperative Pain Management, pp 305–333. New York, Churchill Livingstone, 1993.

42. Guinard JP, Mavrocordatos P, Chiolero R, et al: A randomized comparison of intravenous versus lumbar and thoracic epidural fentanyl for analgesia after thoracotomy. Anesthesiology 1992; 77: 1108–1115.

43. Benson H: The Relaxation Response. New York, William Morrow, 1975.

44. Hilgard ER: Hypnosis and pain. In Sternbach RA (ed): The Psychology of Pain, 2nd ed, pp 197–221. New York, Raven Press, 1986.

45. Boden BP, Fassler S, Cooper S, et al: Analgesic effect of intraarticular morphine, bupivacaine, and morphine/bupivacaine after arthroscopic knee surgery. Arthroscopy 1994; 10: 104–107.

46. Payne R, Foley KM: Advances in the management of cancer pain. Cancer Treat Rep 1984; 68: 173–183.

47. Coombs DW, Fratkin JD, Meier FA, et al: Neuropathologic lesions and CSF morphine concentrations during chronic continuous intraspinal morphine infusion. A clinical and post-mortem study. Pain 1985; 22: 337–351.

48. Coombs DW, Saunders RL, Gaylor M, et al: Epidural narcotic infusion reservoir: implantation technique and efficacy. Anesthesiology 1982; 56: 469–473.

49. Woods WA, Cohen SE: High-dose epidural morphine in a terminally ill patient. Anesthesiology 1982; 56: 311–312.

50. Greenberg HS, Taren J, Ensminger WD, et al: Benefit from and tolerance to continuous intrathecal infusion of morphine for intractable cancer pain. J Neurosurg 1982; 57: 360–364.

51. Coombs DW, Saunders RL, Lachance D, et al: Intrathecal morphine tolerance: use of intrathecal clonidine, DADLE, and intraventricular morphine. Anesthesiology 1985; 62: 358–363.

52. Murphy DF: Interpleural analgesia. Br J Anaesth 1993; 71: 426–434.

53. Miser AW, Davis DM, Hughes CS, et al: Continuous subcutaneous infusion of morphine in children with cancer. Am J Dis Child 1983; 137: 383–385.

54. Wang JK, Nauss LA, Thomas JE: Pain relief by intrathecally applied morphine in man. Anesthesiology 1979; 50: 149–151.

55. Coombs DW, Saunders RL, Gaylor MS, et al: Relief of continuous chronic pain by intraspinal narcotics infusion via an implanted reservoir. JAMA 1983; 250: 2336–2339.

56. Rigg JR, Browne RA, Davis C, et al: Variation in the disposition of morphine after i.m. administration in surgical patients. Br J Anaesth 1978; 50: 1125–1130.

57. Austin KL, Stapleton JV, Mather LE: Multiple intramuscular

injections: a major source of variability in analgesic response to meperidine. Pain 1980; 8: 47–62.

58. Dilke TF, Burry HC, Grahame R: Extradural corticosteroid injection in management of lumbar nerve root compression. Br Med J 1973; 2: 635–637.

59. Breivik H, Hesia PE, Molnar I, et al: Treatment of chronic low back pain and sciatica: comparison of caudal epidural injections of bupivacaine and methylprednisolone with bupivacaine followed by saline. Adv Pain Res Ther 1976; 1: 927–932.

60. Abram SE, Hopwood MB: What factors contribute to outcome with lumbar epidural steroids. In Bond MR, Charlton JE, Woolf CJ (eds): Proceedings of the VIth World Congress on Pain, pp 495–500. Amsterdam, Elsevier, 1991.

61. Chapman CR, Benedetti C: Analgesia following transcutaneous electrical stimulation and its partial reversal by a narcotic antagonist. Life Sci 1977; 21: 1645–1648.

62. Messahel FM, Tomlin PJ: Narcotic withdrawal syndrome after intrathecal administration of morphine. Br Med J 1981; 283: 471–472.

63. Hogan Q, Haddox JD, Abram S, et al: Epidural opiates and local anesthetics for the management of cancer pain. Pain 1991; 46: 271–279.

CHAPTER 39

Outcome After Epidural Anesthesia and Analgesia

Oscar A. de Leon-Casasola, M.D.

The first report on the use of opioids administered epidurally for the treatment of pain by Behar et al[1] opened a new field for clinical and basic research in anesthesiology. Currently, postoperative pain is being treated with parenteral administration of opioids delivered via intermittent bolus injections or patient-controlled analgesia, epidural administration of opioids delivered via intermittent bolus injections or continuous infusion, or in combinations with local anesthetics as a continuous infusion. Early studies[2, 3] showed that although patient satisfaction was higher with intravenous administration of patient-controlled analgesia, the quality of analgesia was superior when epidural administration of morphine was used. However, studies[4–8] using the lipid-soluble opioid fentanyl have shown that not only the quality of analgesia but also the incidence of side effects and the plasma levels may be comparable for the intravenous and the epidural routes (irrespective of the site of catheter insertion). Thus, continued use of postoperative, epidural analgesic techniques may be subject to physicians' ability to prove that the recovery of patients may be improved by perioperative epidural techniques.

The benefits associated with improved postoperative patient outcome are related to improved postoperative pulmonary, cardiovascular, gastrointestinal, immunologic, and coagulation function. Moreover, economic incentives resulting from less intensive care and overall hospitalization costs also play an important role in the choice of perioperative analgesic techniques.

The Pulmonary System

Postoperative Physiologic Changes

Decrease in pulmonary expiratory flows and volumes commonly occurs after operation. The changes are more striking in patients undergoing upper abdominal and thoracic procedures owing to the decrease in diaphragmatic function,[9, 10] increase in upper abdominal and intercostal muscle resting tone,[11, 12] and release of algetic substances. Reflex inhibition of phrenic nerve function appears to be responsible for the diaphragmatic dysfunction seen after upper abdominal and thoracic procedures.[10, 13, 14] Neither epidural nor parenteral administration of opioids results in a significant improvement in postoperative diaphragmatic dysfunction. Conversely, it appears that thoracic epidural anesthesia and analgesia with local anesthetics may block the inhibitory phrenic nerve reflexes, thus improving postoperative diaphragmatic function.[9, 10] Patients undergoing lower abdominal procedures are at a lower risk for pulmonary complications because they do not experience these physiologic aberrations.

Mechanical ventilation and inhalation anesthetics also appear to have an influence on postoperative pulmonary dysfunction.[15] Other risk factors include severe pain,[16] degree of preexisting lung disease,[17] length of surgical incisions,[18] obesity,[19] and advanced age.[20]

The most important postoperative physiologic aberration in pulmonary function is the decrease in functional residual capacity, which may be minimized in patients undergoing upper abdominal and thoracic procedures by improvements in dynamic pain control.

Dynamic pain control is defined as a target level of analgesia titrated to allow patients deep inspiration, coughing, and movement. The importance of this concept has been underscored by Bell,[21] who studied the influence of both resting and dynamic pain control on postoperative pulmonary function after abdominal aortic operation. If pain appeared during movement (dynamic pain), the rate of infusions was increased until analgesia was achieved. No differences in forced expiratory volume in 1 s and inspiratory force were found in patients allocated to either the epidural or the intravenous administration of patient-controlled analgesia treatment groups when only resting pain control was achieved. However, when their pulmonary function was tested once dynamic pain control was achieved, the epidural group demonstrated significantly improved pulmonary function (forced expiratory volume in 1 s = 61% ± 7 versus 30% ± 6 and inspiratory force = 38 cm H_2O ± 5 versus 25 cm H_2O ± 6, $P < .05$ epidural versus patient-controlled analgesia). Although this study is retrospective, these findings may partially explain the differences found in pulmonary function after upper abdominal or thoracic procedures in patients receiving epidural or parenteral administration of opioid therapy. Ideally, this study should be repeated in a prospective masked (double-blind) manner.

Postoperative Lung Function

In 1961, Simpson and collaborators[22] were the first to demonstrate that the use of epidural analgesia with local anesthetics was associated with a decrease in the incidence of postoperative pulmonary complications. Ten years later, Spence and Smith[23] demonstrated the superiority of epidural block over morphine given intramuscularly in restoring the forced expiratory volume in 1 s/forced vital capacity ratio toward normal after upper abdominal operation in healthy adults.

The demonstration of opioid receptors in the spinal cord[24] and the concept of selective spinal analgesia[1, 25] renewed the interest in studying the effects of spinal-mediated analgesia and postoperative pulmonary complications. Several prospective randomized studies have demonstrated that compared with opioids given parenterally or intercostal blocks, epidural analgesia decreased the incidence of pulmonary complications in patients who underwent upper abdominal[16, 19, 26–33] or thoracic surgical procedures.[34–36] In these studies, improvement in expiratory flows and ability to cough was associated with a lower incidence of postoperative pneumonia and respiratory failure, as judged by the incidence of tracheal reintubation and the need for mechanical ventilation. The author's group[37] has also demonstrated that patients receiving epidural anesthesia and analgesia with bupivacaine and morphine required less mechanical ventilation time and experienced a shorter stay in the intensive care unit. These studies support the concept that analgesia associated with dynamic pain control results in improved pulmonary outcome.

A meta-analysis of all randomized controlled trials examining the influence of analgesia on postoperative pulmonary function has been published.[38] The investigators included trials that assessed the effects of epidural administration of opioids or local anesthetics, local nerve blocks, and intravenous infusions of opioids on postoperative forced expiratory volume in 1 s, forced vital capacity, vital capacity, peak expiratory flow, arterial oxygenation, and incidence of atelectasis. Four or more studies must have been available in each

category to warrant inclusion in the analysis. Opioids given epidurally were associated with a significant improvement in pulmonary expiratory flows and arterial oxygenation, a decreased incidence of atelectasis, but no significant improvement in forced expiratory volume in 1 s compared with conventional therapy (opioids given intramuscularly as needed). Epidural administration of local anesthetics was associated with a significant decrease in postoperative pulmonary complications and improvement in arterial oxygenation compared with conventional therapy. Local nerve blocks produced a significant improvement in forced vital capacity, forced expiratory volume in 1 s, and peak expiratory flow but no significant decrease in the incidence of atelectasis compared with conventional therapy. Intravenous infusion of opioids significantly improved vital capacity but not arterial oxygenation compared with conventional therapy. Thus, all four therapies improved selected measures of pulmonary function. However, although this gives us information on the improvement of selected measures of pulmonary function, no outcome information can be derived because of the limitations in the studies.

Problems With the Design of Current Studies

Several variables determine the final pulmonary outcome of patients undergoing upper abdominal or thoracic procedures. Neuraxial administration of opioids or local anesthetics or both may partially restore lung volumes to the preoperative levels and improve pulmonary outcome; however, other factors also play an important role. Cigarette smoking, preoperative mucus hypersecretion, impairment of tracheobronchial secretion clearance, and degree of preoperative bronchospasm are well-recognized preoperative predictors of poor pulmonary outcome.[39] Moreover, smokers have a higher closing capacity (increasing the risk of atelectasis), and patients report increase in sputum volume and difficulty with expectoration 1 to 2 days after they stop smoking (frequent occurrence in the perioperative period).[39] Thus, studies addressing the influence of anesthetic-analgesic techniques on pulmonary outcome must consider the weighted value of these variables when evaluating final outcome.

Other important information that should be included in this type of study is what the goal of therapy was and how the analgesics were titrated to achieve the predetermined level of analgesia. A study conducted by Jayr and collaborators[40] illustrates common shortcomings in the clinical design of studies that compare epidural with parenteral analgesia and their effects on postoperative lung function. These investigators randomized patients to a continuous infusion of morphine given parenterally or a continuous infusion of morphine and bupivacaine given epidurally. Evaluation of their materials and methods revealed the following:

1. The epidurally administered doses of morphine were well below the expected mean utilization during the first 72 h postoperatively (0.25 versus 0.6 mg/h)

by patients undergoing the type of procedures reported in the study.

2. It was not established whether the researchers achieved dynamic pain control. The reported pain scores were evaluated only once in the morning. Thus, it is conceivable that after patients ambulated and became active, their dynamic pain scores increased, thereby restricting their ability to cough and mobilize secretions.

3. The use of breakthrough doses was not quantified. Because small fixed doses of morphine given epidurally were used, it is conceivable that patients required high doses of the breakthrough medication (acetaminophen), converting this to a comparison between morphine given parenterally and acetaminophen given intravenously.

4. The spirometry measurements were done early in the morning. Readings performed at peak of activity would show depressed effort-dependent forced expiratory volume in 1 s and forced vital capacity measurements if there were intergroup differences in the quality of dynamic pain control.

5. The number of patients who underwent either upper or lower abdominal operations in each group and the type of incisions used were not mentioned, even though it was reported that upper abdominal procedures were performed via midline or bicostal (chevron) incisions. Because bicostal incisions transect the rectus abdominis muscle, the degree of postoperative pulmonary dysfunction would be greater in this group of patients and is vital information for conclusions on the final outcome. Thus, when analyzing the literature for pulmonary outcome, it is important to consider all these variables that may significantly affect the final results.

Finally, pulmonary function testing via spirometry has been used to compare groups of patients receiving either epidural or parenteral analgesia. The purpose of pulmonary function testing is to identify those patients who are at risk of postoperative respiratory complications. However, no study has documented a correlation between an increase in lung volumes (as determined by spirometry) and a decrease in the incidence of atelectasis, pneumonias, cor pulmonale, or acute respiratory failure. From the physiology of postoperative pulmonary dysfunction, it appears that a postoperative analgesic technique that results in fewer pulmonary complications would also result in a significant increase in functional residual capacity. In an elegant study, Wahba and collaborators[41] investigated the effects of epidural analgesia on functional residual capacity. Postoperatively, patients had a mean 22% decrease in functional residual capacity while experiencing pain. After epidural administration of lidocaine, a 27% increase in functional residual capacity was reported. These results suggest that restoration of functional residual capacity in the postoperative period may be the mechanism by which epidural analgesia decreases postoperative pulmonary morbidity and shortens the duration that mechanical ventilation is needed in patients undergoing upper abdominal and thoracic procedures.

In summary, well-controlled studies have documented a significant improvement in postoperative pulmonary function when epidural analgesia was compared with opioids given parenterally. This may be the result of the level of pain control produced by the epidural techniques, which result in full dynamic pain control. Studies have searched for markers that quantify the improvement in pulmonary function in order to correlate them with improved outcome. Lung volumes as measured via spirometry partially achieve these goals. However, measuring the changes in functional residual capacity in combination with other lung volumes would be a more physiologically complete evaluation.

The Cardiovascular System

Postoperative Physiologic Changes

Studies[42-48] evaluating patients for perioperative myocardial infarction have determined that myocardial ischemia occurs most frequently in the first 36 to 48 h after operation. Mangano et al[42] found that myocardial infarction, unstable angina, and sudden death occurred 36 to 48 h after the onset of perioperative myocardial infarction. Several studies[48-51] have shown that most perioperative myocardial infarctions occur in the first 3 days after operation. Thus, if ischemia prophylaxis is to be effective, it can be theorized that therapy must continue for at least 72 h after the completion of the operation.

The incidence of postoperative myocardial ischemia may be closely related to the activation of the neuroendocrine response. As an example, plasma norepinephrine and renin levels are higher during episodes of silent ischemia.[52] In healthy humans, the coronary vessels dilate in response to nitric oxide and prostacyclin produced by the coronary endothelium in response to norepinephrine. When coronary atherosclerosis is present, the release of nitric oxide results in paradoxic coronary vasoconstriction.[53] Moreover, postoperative hypercoagulability is frequently experienced by patients with atherosclerotic disease.[54, 55] Thus, this vaso-occlusive phenomenon acting synergistically with a high degree of adrenergic tone may be responsible for the high incidence of postoperative myocardial ischemia and adverse outcome seen in surgical patients with coronary artery disease.

Cardiac Function

Postoperative epidural analgesia with bupivacaine and morphine may be associated with a better outcome in patients with coronary artery disease.[27, 56] Epidurally administered morphine attenuates the postoperative sympathetic nervous system activation that results in hypertension and tachycardia.[57] Local anesthetics administered in the thoracic epidural space may potentiate the cardioprotective effects of epidural morphine by (1) producing a cardiac sympathetic block resulting in vasodilatation of epicardial vessels previously exhibiting 100% physiologic stenosis[58]; (2) improving left ventricular function during ischemia[59]; and (3) depressing adrenergic neurotransmission in the coronary blood vessels, leading to inhibition of smooth muscle contraction.[60] Bupivacaine seems to have a greater effect than lidocaine.[60]

Decreases in myocardial oxygen supply appear to be the mechanism by which perioperative sympathetic system activation results in increased cardiac morbidity (via nitric oxide activation). Several studies[61–64] suggested that increases in myocardial oxygen demand correlate poorly with perioperative myocardial ischemia. These findings are in accord with results from basic research.

Selective sympathetic block of the heart (T-1 to T-5) achieved with local anesthetics delivered via a thoracic epidural catheter resulted in a decrease in myocardial oxygen demand and, to a certain extent, oxygen supply as well.[65–67] Hemodynamic changes associated with thoracic epidural block include a decrease in cardiac output, heart rate, and blood pressure.[68, 69] Although total coronary blood flow remains unchanged,[58, 70] blood flow to ischemic regions of the myocardium increases[58, 70, 71] via inhibition of sympathetically mediated coronary vasoconstriction that occurs distal to the coronary stenotic area,[58, 72] and regional distribution of myocardial blood flow improves by augmentation of endocardial blood flow.[70, 71] These effects are a direct result of the sympathetic block and the resulting local changes in the dynamics of the coronary vessels, because plasma levels of local anesthetics achieved after a thoracic epidural block will not produce the aforementioned coronary blood flow changes.[71]

Thus, the use of thoracic epidural block in patients with significant coronary artery disease (>70% obstruction) results in beneficial matching of the myocardial oxygen supply/demand ratio. Animal studies evaluating the effects of thoracic epidural block after controlled acute coronary occlusion have shown that (1) the regional metabolic changes produced by ischemia are allayed[73]; (2) the magnitude of ischemia may be lessened as interpreted from the decrease in the degree of ST-segment changes[73, 74]; and (3) the size of the infarcted area is decreased as well as the incidence of ventricular arrhythmias associated with the ischemic event.[73, 75]

Clinical studies support the findings in these animal studies. In patients with acute myocardial ischemia unresponsive to β-blockers, calcium channel antagonists, and nitrates, thoracic epidural block has been proved to be an effective treatment.[68, 76–78] Relief of ischemia in these patients probably occurred because of an increase in myocardial oxygen delivery (via coronary vasodilation) and a decrease in myocardial oxygen demand produced by a decrease in heart rate and left ventricular end-diastolic pressure. Patients in these studies experienced improvement in their hemodynamic profile (increase in cardiac index and decrease in heart rate and left ventricular end-diastolic pressure) with no hemodynamically significant hypotension or bradycardia. Consequently, thoracic epidural block may not only optimize the indices of myocardial oxygen

supply and demand but also be superior to combinations of β-blockers, calcium channel antagonists, and nitrates given intravenously during the acute episodes of myocardial ischemia.

In contrast, lumbar epidural block appears to lack the cardioprotective effects of thoracic epidural block. This may be the result of the limited cardiac sympathetic block associated with lumbar epidural anesthesia. In order to produce a T-1 to T-4 sympathetic block, the sensory block should be at least at the T-3 level. Consequently, hypotension may occur as a result of the extensive peripheral sympathetic block. Because blood flow distal to significant coronary lesions is pressure-dependent (in the absence of universal coronary vasodilation), oxygen delivery could be compromised because the reduction in oxygen demand is not proportional.[69, 79] There are no conclusive data demonstrating that the use of lumbar epidural block in patients with coronary artery disease has a negative impact on cardiac outcome.

Most of the studies evaluating the effects of lumbar epidural block on cardiac function analyzed the changes in wall motion abnormalities that occurred after the block was established.[69, 79, 80] Indeed, it is now recognized that not all regional wall motion abnormalities are necessarily indicative of acute myocardial ischemia.[64, 81] Preload and afterload changes may produce these abnormalities,[81, 82] explaining the results reported by Saada and coworkers[69, 79] and Baron et al.[80] However, a study[82] in a swine model of severe coronary artery stenosis demonstrated that the use of combined lumbar epidural-general anesthesia resulted in a moderate decrease in regional myocardial function as a result of a severe reduction in blood flow distal to the area of coronary stenosis.

These findings suggest that extensive epidural sensory block (C-7 to T-1 upper sensory level) may be associated with myocardial ischemia and should be avoided in patients with known coronary artery disease. Moreover, in supine humans, lumbar epidural block extending to the midthoracic region leads to a reflex vasoconstriction in the upper extremity and chest.[83] This may evoke a redistribution of blood at the expense of cardiac filling and further compromise coronary flow. Conversely, lumbar epidural block limited to the low thoracic regions may in fact improve myocardial performance.[80] Thus, it appears that lumbar epidural block is not associated with increased cardiac morbidity as long as coronary perfusion pressure is maintained.

Outcome Studies

Few studies have evaluated the efficacy of epidural anesthesia and analgesia on cardiac outcome. Studies[61–63] on intraoperative myocardial ischemia revealed that only 10% to 30% of these episodes are associated with intraoperative hemodynamic disturbances. Thus, it is not surprising that studies evaluating different anesthetic techniques found no difference in overall cardiac outcome.[63, 84, 85] Baron et al[85] demonstrated that in patients undergoing abdominal aortic reconstructions, intraoperative thoracic epidural anesthesia in combination with light general anesthesia was not associated with a decreased incidence of cardiovascular complications compared with general anesthesia. The incidence of postoperative myocardial infarction, congestive heart failure, and postoperative myocardial ischemia was similar in both groups. These results further support the notion that postoperative myocardial ischemia is the single most important predictor of postoperative cardiac outcome[42] and that well-performed intraoperative anesthetic technique has limited influence on postoperative cardiac outcome. Thus, if cardiac outcome is to be improved, postoperative techniques that aim to control postoperative myocardial ischemia should be implemented.

In the past several years, four studies[55, 86-88] evaluating the influence of postoperative epidural analgesia on myocardial ischemia have been published.

Beattie et al[55] evaluated, in a prospective fashion, 55 patients at risk for coronary artery disease. Patients were allocated to either epidural anesthesia–postoperative epidurally administered morphine therapy or general anesthesia–intermittent postoperative intravenously administered morphine therapy in a nonrandomized fashion. Most of the patients underwent vascular procedures. Overall, 18 patients experienced postoperative myocardial ischemia (33%): 5 (17%) in the epidural group versus 13 (50%) in the parenteral group ($P = .01$). The number of myocardial ischemic episodes was also greater in the parenteral group (25 versus 12, $P < .01$). Five patients had major morbid events (defined as new myocardial infarction, congestive heart failure, or arrhythmias requiring intensive care therapy): three (10%) in the epidural group versus two (8%) in the parenteral group.

The author and his collaborators[86] evaluated the influence of thoracic epidural anesthesia and analgesia on cardiac outcome after upper abdominal procedures for cancer. A total of 198 patients were evaluated in a nonrandomized fashion. Patients in the epidural group had a lower incidence of postoperative tachycardia (15 versus 58, $P = .00001$), hypertension (15 versus 49, $P = .0001$), and myocardial ischemia (5 versus 15, $P = .04$) than similar patients in the parenteral group. The difference in the incidence of myocardial infarction (0 versus 3, $P = .09$) was not statistically significant between the two groups, although a larger sample size might have allowed a difference to be documented.

Patient allocation in this study was not randomized. However, the two groups were similar with regard to demographics, preoperative cardiac risk, antianginal medications, American Society of Anesthesiologists class status, and type of operation. Moreover, the incidence of intraoperative myocardial ischemia, hemodynamic aberrations, and operating time was comparable, thus allowing for valid comparisons.

A large number of patients need to be studied to find differences in the final outcome between these types of treatment groups. If a therapy is to decrease the incidence of complications by one third (30% to 20% in the case of myocardial infarctions after postoperative ischemic episodes), approximately 3000 patients would

be required to demonstrate that aggressive therapy is useful (power of 0.80 for a 33% decrease in complications).[87] However, no study evaluating postoperative myocardial ischemia and infarctions has documented a single myocardial infarction occurring without previous myocardial ischemia. Thus, despite the lack of evidence in final cardiac outcome, it appears that the initial goal of therapy in patients with significant coronary artery disease should be to decrease the incidence of postoperative myocardial ischemia.

In contrast to these two reports, Weitz and collaborators[88] reported preliminary results of a study on postoperative myocardial ischemia in patients at risk for coronary artery disease. Patients receiving morphine by epidural or intravenous administration of patient-controlled analgesia for postoperative analgesia had the same incidence of postoperative myocardial ischemia. The same group has also documented that intense intravenous analgesia after coronary artery bypass graft operation was associated with a lower incidence of postoperative myocardial ischemia (but no infarctions) in this high-risk population. Moreover, the severity of the ischemic events was lower in the sufentanil-treated group. Thus, it appears that quality analgesia is associated with a lower incidence of postoperative myocardial events. However, it appears that combinations of local anesthetics and opioids provide optimal protection in the high-risk groups.

Christopherson et al[89] randomized 150 patients undergoing lower extremity revascularization procedures to receive general or epidural anesthesia. Postoperative analgesia was provided with morphine via patient-controlled analgesia for the general anesthesia group and fentanyl only via patient-controlled analgesia for the epidural group. However, the length of postoperative epidural analgesia was limited to 24 h, with morphine administered intramuscularly as needed thereafter. The incidence of postoperative myocardial ischemia and negative cardiac outcomes was similar in the two groups. These contrasting findings may result from study design and the natural history of postoperative myocardial ischemia and infarctions. Consequently, no definitive conclusions concerning the influence of postoperative epidural analgesia on postoperative cardiac outcome can be drawn from these data because the authors limited the duration of epidural analgesia to the first 24 h postoperatively.

In summary, few studies have evaluated the effects of postoperative epidural analgesia on cardiac outcome. Basic research data as well as pilot studies suggest that combinations of local anesthetics and opioids may be ideal to decrease the incidence of postoperative myocardial ischemia and possibly to improve postoperative cardiac outcome. A multicenter large-scale study will be needed to document that a decrease in postoperative myocardial ischemia results in a decrease in the incidence of postoperative negative myocardial events.

The Coagulation System

Postoperative Physiologic Changes

Surgical stress is associated with hypercoagulability as a result of an increase in the concentration of factor

VIII,[90, 91] von Willebrand factor,[91] and fibrinogen[92] and inhibition of fibrinolysis.[56, 92] It appears that facilitation of clotting is associated closely with many components of the neuroendocrine response to the surgical trauma. It is well known that corticosteroids and epinephrine may influence the coagulation state as well as the fibrinolytic activity.[93–95] Endogenous or exogenously induced high plasma levels of corticosteroids result in an increased concentration of factor VIII.[96] Likewise, the increase in factor VIII activity depends partially on the activation of β-adrenergic receptors.[94, 97]

Vasopressin has been linked to the rapid response exhibited by endothelial proteins involved in fibrinolysis.[98] Fibrinogen's synthesis is increased by the liver in response to stress.[99] Moreover, the increase in fibrinogen concentration may be mediated by several cytokines, particularly interleukin-2 and tumor necrosis factor.[100] Thus, there is a clear relationship between the neuroendocrine response elicited by the surgical injury and the postoperative hypercoagulable state.[101]

Postoperative Hypercoagulability

If we accept the premise that there is a direct cause-and-effect relationship between perioperative stress response and coagulation (i.e., the stress response to the surgical stimulus leads to hypercoagulability and inhibition of fibrinolysis), then we may find a perioperative technique that abolishes or diminishes the stress response to operation results in a decreased incidence of postoperative thrombosis. Epidural anesthesia for lower abdominal and lower extremity surgical procedures has been demonstrated to prevent this perioperative neuroendocrine activation[102–109] in contrast to general anesthesia with high-dose opioids.[110] Several authors have described the potential antithrombotic effect of local anesthetics by inhibition of platelet aggregation.[111–113] Moreover, epidural anesthesia limits the postoperative increase of factor VIII and von Willebrand factor.[90] This is an important effect because von Willebrand factor is an essential glycoprotein for the attachment of platelets to the injured vascular wall.[90, 114] Antithrombin III returns to preoperative concentrations more rapidly in patients receiving local anesthetics epidurally.[115] Thus, it is conceivable that epidural anesthesia is more effective than general anesthesia in preventing the shift in coagulative and fibrinolytic processes in the postoperative period.

More recently, two studies[27, 56] have elucidated other mechanisms associated with the decrease in postoperative clot formation. Tuman et al[27] used thromboelastography to make qualitative measurements of postoperative coagulation in patients who underwent vascular surgical procedures. They found that epidural block attenuated the hypercoagulable state experienced by patients who underwent vascular surgical procedures. Rosenfeld and associates[56] measured perioperative fibrinogen, plasminogen activator inhibitor–1, and D-dimer levels in patients who underwent peripheral vascular procedures during general or epidural anesthesia. Multiple logistic regression analysis indicated that gen-

eral anesthesia and plasminogen activator inhibitor–1 levels predicted postoperative arterial thrombotic complications. These findings suggest that impaired postoperative fibrinolysis may be the cause of thrombotic phenomena in the postoperative period. Plasminogen activator inhibitor–1 is a rapid and specific inhibitor of both tissue and urokinase-type plasminogen activators, possibly representing the primary regulator of plasminogen activation in vivo. Alterations in levels of plasminogen activator inhibitor–1 may lead to thrombosis or excessive bleeding.[116, 117] Plasminogen activator inhibitor–1 is a stress response marker and increases postoperatively in patients receiving general anesthesia.[118, 119] It is possible that this increase of plasminogen activator inhibitor–1 after operation during general anesthesia is the cause of the greater incidence of thrombosis experienced by this group of patients.

Outcome Studies

Tuman and associates[27] and Christopherson and colleagues[89] demonstrated that patients receiving epidural block for peripheral vascular reconstruction experienced a lower incidence of postoperative graft clotting. In the study by Tuman et al,[27] the incidence of graft failure was significantly lower in the epidural group (8/40 versus 1/40, $P = .013$). In the study by Christopherson et al,[89] similar findings were reported (11/51 versus 2/49, $P < .01$).

Several studies have evaluated the influence of neuraxial block on the incidence of postoperative deep vein thrombosis and pulmonary embolism after orthopedic procedures. Patients undergoing joint replacement of the lower extremities constitute an at-risk study population. The incidence of deep vein thrombosis after total knee arthroplasty has been reported to be as high as 88% in the untreated patients.

Modig et al[120] reported that epidural anesthesia followed by epidural analgesia with bupivacaine was superior to general anesthesia and postoperative parenteral analgesia. The incidence of deep vein thrombosis (20% versus 73%, $P < .01$) and pulmonary embolism (13% versus 47%, $P < .01$) was lower in patients receiving the epidural technique for total hip arthroplasty. A subsequent study[121] from the same group reported similar findings of femoropopliteal (13% versus 67%, $P < .01$) and calf and thigh (40% versus 77%, $P < .01$) thrombosis and incidence of pulmonary embolism (10% versus 33%, $P < .01$) in 60 patients who were randomized to receive either epidural or general anesthesia, respectively. More recently, Wille-Jorgensen et al[122] compared 33 patients receiving epidural anesthesia with 65 patients who received general anesthesia for total hip arthroplasty. They also reported a significantly lower incidence of deep vein thrombosis and pulmonary embolism in patients who received epidural anesthesia (9% versus 31% and 1% versus 9%, respectively; $P < .01$ for both comparisons). Davis and collaborators[123] reported similar findings for postoperative deep vein thrombosis when they compared spinal with general anesthesia (13% versus 27%, $P < .01$) in 140 patients undergoing total hip replacement.

In patients undergoing total knee arthroplasty, Sharrock et al[124] found that the incidence of deep vein thrombosis was lower in patients receiving epidural anesthesia than general anesthesia (48% versus 64%, $P < .01$, $N = 491$).

However, in the literature on coagulation outcome after orthopedic procedures, mechanical ventilation seems to worsen stasis by decreasing venous return and has been implicated as a cause of deep vein thrombosis.[125] This concept is supported by Donadoni et al,[115] who found a lower incidence of deep vein thrombosis after epidural anesthesia compared with either general anesthesia or combined epidural-general anesthesia for total hip replacement (25% versus 45% versus 38%, respectively).

In summary, epidural anesthesia with or without postoperative epidural analgesia appears to directly affect postoperative outcome in patients undergoing orthopedic procedures and vascular procedures on the abdominal and lower extremity vessels. Proposed mechanisms include increased arterial inflow and changes in venous capacitance and in the rate of venous flow produced by the sympathetic block. Altered coagulation and improved fibrinolysis also appear to play a significant role.

Most of the studies addressing postoperative outcome appear to stress the need for postoperative epidural analgesia in order to improve outcome. However, the coagulation system is the only system positively affected by the use of intraoperative neuraxial block without the use of postoperative neuraxial analgesia.

The Gastrointestinal System

Postoperative Physiologic Changes

Postoperative gastrointestinal paralysis (ileus) is an important and common problem after intra-abdominal surgical procedures. The surgical trauma activates, via spinal afferents, inhibitory nonadrenergic, noncholinergic vagal efferents and sympathetic efferents that inhibit excitatory vagal efferents.[126, 127] The resultant inhibition in gastrointestinal motility is most persistent in the stomach (1 to 2 days) and the colon (2 to 3 days), whereas the activity of the small bowel returns to normal a few hours after operation.

Postoperative Ileus

Postoperative neuraxial analgesia with 0.25% bupivacaine alone has been shown to decrease gastrointestinal transit time from 150 hours to 35 hours in patients who underwent colon resection.[126] Moreover, studies[128, 129] in volunteers have shown that gastric emptying and oral-to-cecal transit time are not affected by thoracic analgesia with bupivacaine given epidurally.

Conversely, the parenteral administration of opioids for pain control has been associated with a significant increase in gastrointestinal transit time compared with epidurally administered local anesthetics.[126, 127, 130–134] Moreover, opioids given epidurally inhibit motility in both the proximal and distal colon.[135, 136] This may be due to the inability of the epidurally administered opioid to block somatic and sympathetic nerve transmission.[137] This leaves intact the inhibitory reflexes that mediate postoperative ileus. The delay in the postoperative return of gastrointestinal function associated with morphine given parenterally is related to the production of clusters of short, nonmigrating, phasic spike bursts in the myoelectric plexus of the colon.[130] This results in an uncoordinated action potential that does not generate peristalsis within the colon. This phenomenon is not encountered after the epidural administration of morphine.[130] Nevertheless, the benefit of epidural administration of opioids may be marginal compared with local anesthetics alone.

In conclusion, the use of epidural analgesia with only bupivacaine prevents the inhibition of gastrointestinal motility caused by surgical trauma. Negative effects on propulsive gastrointestinal motility result from both epidural and parenteral administration of opioids, but epidural administration is associated with less delay in the return of gastrointestinal function than parenteral administration is.

Outcome Studies

Postoperative ileus is a clinically important problem. It delays the administration of enteral feeding, potentially resulting in morbidity or prolonged hospitalization or both. For example, early enteral feeding has been associated with attenuation of the neuroendocrine response to the stress of operation, improvement in wound healing, and reduction in postoperative septic complications.[138–140] The humane and financial implications of decreasing the incidence of postoperative sepsis are obvious. Moreover, the cost of prolonged postoperative ileus has been estimated to be $750 million annually.[141]

Most available data support the use of epidural techniques for pain control when postoperative gastrointestinal recovery is optimized.[126, 127, 130–134] However, two studies found that bupivacaine given epidurally was not effective in preventing ileus in the postoperative period.[142, 143] In these two studies, epidural local anesthetics were administered for only 24 h. Analgesia was subsequently provided with opioids, explaining the contrasting results.

Few studies have evaluated combinations of local anesthetics and opioids. Theoretically, the synergistic effects between the two drugs would allow lower doses of opioids to be used and result in less inhibition of gastrointestinal function. In patients undergoing radical hysterectomies, the author and his colleagues[144] demonstrated that those who received epidural analgesia required fewer days of nasogastric tube therapy (4 versus 8 days, $P = .0001$), tolerated solid food sooner (6 versus 11 days, $P < .0001$), and had a shorter hospitalization period (10 versus 14 days, P = .0001) compared with a patient-controlled analgesia group.

In summary, the majority of studies support the concept that postoperative epidural administration of local anesthetics results in a decrease in the duration of postoperative ileus. Epidurally administered opioids also appear to provide more rapid recovery than parenterally administered opioids. In order to experience significant benefits, it appears that epidural postoperative analgesia has to be administered for at least 72 h.

The Immunologic System

Postoperative Physiologic Changes

In the past several years, a considerable amount of clinical research has focused on techniques that improve global cardiovascular and pulmonary function in the perioperative period. This is justified because sudden deterioration in the function of either organ system results in severe morbidity and mortality. With the improvement in the prevention and management of cardiopulmonary complications, other sources of postoperative morbidity have been studied. This is the case for postoperative infections, sepsis, and multiple organ failure.

The usual immunologic response to surgical trauma includes a rapid deterioration of immunocompetence that peaks on the third postoperative day and a slow return to normal immunocompetence during the next 1 to 3 weeks. This recovery may take longer in patients exposed to extensive surgical procedures or with preexisting medical conditions. Mediators of the immunodepression in the perioperative period include (1) the neuroendocrine stress response (e.g., cortisol), (2) drugs administered in the perioperative period such as opioids given intravenously[145] and anesthetics given by inhalation,[146] and (3) local tissue inflammatory products released during tissue manipulation.

Postoperative Immune Function

Tubaro and collaborators[147] demonstrated that the parenteral administration of morphine in animals was associated with an increased susceptibility to infection. Clinicians have also hypothesized that the immunodepression seen in opioid-addicted patients may be related, in part, to their opioid use. Yeager and Colacchio[148] have shown in a murine model that administration of morphine (15 mg/kg subcutaneously every 6 h for 24 h) resulted in a measurable decline of natural killer cell cytotoxicity (cellular immunity test that evaluates lymphocyte toxicity against tumor cells, virus, and some bacteria). This decline in cytotoxicity was not observed when ketorolac was used at analgesic doses. Moreover, when human volunteers were exposed to oral and intravenous administration of morphine for 30 to 60 h, antibody-dependent cellular cytotoxicity and natural killer cell cytotoxicity were depressed.[149] These findings support results in animal studies show-

ing that natural killer cell cytotoxicity is also inhibited when morphine is administered parenterally without the stimulus of operation.[150] Thus, morphine inhibition of lymphocyte activity is mediated by an opioid-dependent mechanism in the lymphocyte.[150]

In contrast, the use of epidural anesthesia and analgesia may play a significant role in preserving perioperative cellular immunity. In one study, patients who received epidural anesthesia and analgesia appeared to have a more rapid return of natural killer cell cytotoxic function than patients who received general anesthesia and ketorolac (3 versus 7 to 10 days). Ketorolac was included in the perioperative care of patients who received general anesthesia to inhibit eicosanoids, especially prostaglandin E_2, which are thought to have immunosuppressive effects after major trauma or operation (Yeager MP: Personal communication). Tonnesen and Wahlgreen[151] and Ryhanen et al[152] also demonstrated that the use of epidural anesthesia and analgesia in patients undergoing hysterectomies and epidural anesthesia in patients undergoing elective cesarean deliveries was also associated with preservation of postoperative natural killer cell cytotoxic function compared with patients who received general anesthesia. A decrease in natural killer cell cytotoxicity has been shown experimentally to result in accelerated tumor growth and an increase in the number of metastases.[153-155]

In the past two decades, other immunologic defects have also been described in patients recovering from operation and trauma. Quantitative and qualitative postoperative lymphocytic dysfunction has been clearly documented in humans.[156-158]

Outcome Studies

Although there is no conclusive evidence that parenteral administration of opioids is associated with an increased susceptibility to infection, outcome results suggest that avoidance of postoperative parenteral administration of opioids may help decrease the incidence of postoperative immune suppression and infection.[26, 27] In the study by Yeager et al,[26] patients receiving epidural anesthesia and analgesia had a lower incidence of infections (2/28 versus 10/25, P = .07). Similar results were reported by Tuman et al.[27] Patients receiving epidural anesthesia and analgesia also had a significantly lower incidence of infections (2/40 versus 8/40, P = .04).

In summary, opioids given parenterally and the neuroendocrine response to surgical procedures lead to perioperative immunodepression. Initial studies have documented that there is a decrease in the rate of postoperative infections experienced by patients undergoing operation with neuraxial techniques and epidural analgesia.

Patient Recovery

Both the scrutiny of institutional performance improvement programs and incentives to dismiss patients earlier from the hospital have shifted attention to finding new ways of improving surgical outcome that result in a decrease in the length of intensive care unit and hospital stays.

Fewer cardiorespiratory complications, faster convalescence, and earlier ambulation and oral intake can result in lower hospital costs. The influence of postoperative pain control in improving clinical outcome is being studied extensively. However, the evidence remains controversial because some studies are retrospective and end points for quality of pain control are not well defined. Drugs used, drug concentrations, and mode of administration also differ among studies. Furthermore, some studies emanate from European centers where incentive for early dismissal may not be as critical as in the United States.

In most studies, sample sizes were relatively small and, although statistical significance was demonstrated, erroneous conclusions may result from a type I (alpha) error. Likewise, generalization may be a problem and readers must evaluate whether the patient population studied, the anesthetic technique, and the feasibility of using epidural anesthesia-analgesia have any clinical relevance in their practice.

Studies[8, 32, 159-163] documenting a decrease in hospitalization time related to a lower incidence of complications have invariably included postoperative epidural analgesia in their anesthetic plan. The decreased hospitalization time in these studies[19, 26, 27, 37, 70] was related mainly to an improvement in cardiorespiratory function that resulted in a decreased incidence of complications. These benefits resulted in lower hospitalization costs and physician charges despite similar hospitalization times for both groups in some of the studies.[27, 28, 162]

In 1974, Pflug and collaborators[159] studied the effects of postoperative epidural analgesia on pulmonary complications after cholecystectomy and hip surgery performed during general anesthesia. They documented a decreased hospitalization (47% decrease, $P < .05$) compared with the group of patients who received opioids parenterally.

Miller and coworkers[32] also reported a briefer hospitalization in patients who received postoperative epidural analgesia with opioids when evaluating the effects of postoperative epidural analgesia with opioids on respiratory function.

Another study by Jacobs[160] suggested that availability of an acute pain service saved more than $200,000 annually as a result of hospital beds not being occupied by the 47 patients dismissed early with improved acute pain control.

More recently, Bellamy and coworkers[162] reported earlier dismissal from the hospital after anterior cruciate ligament repair when epidural anesthesia and analgesia with morphine was compared with morphine given intravenously by patient-controlled analgesia. Walmsly et al[163] corroborated these results in patients undergoing nephrectomies.

The author and associates[37] also reported a briefer intensive care unit and hospitalization stay in high-risk cancer patients receiving intraoperative epidural-general anesthesia and postoperative analgesia with

bupivacaine and morphine. Overall patient comparisons and comparisons according to the site of operation were made. Patients undergoing thoracic and upper and lower abdominal procedures experienced significantly less time on ventilators and briefer intensive care unit and hospital stays than comparable patients receiving general anesthesia followed by intravenously administered patient-controlled analgesia. On the basis of their per diem hospital reimbursement, their estimated 1-year treatment costs were decreased by half from $11,274,672 (general-routine analgesia group) to $6,548,247.

Other studies[164] have documented shorter hospital stays but no decrease in overall hospital cost. Potential explanations include differences in laboratory tests used in the perioperative period and physicians' practice regarding dismissal (early morning versus early afternoon). Thus, future studies evaluating overall cost must find a way to control these variables to adequately compare treatment regimens.

Conclusion

Epidural anesthesia along with postoperative epidural analgesia not only provides excellent pain control but also improves respiratory function and cardiac stability and is associated with a lower incidence of thromboembolic events, briefer period of postoperative ileus and immunodepression, and overall faster recovery that leads to shorter intensive care unit and hospital stays. High-risk patients with decreased organ reserve undergoing extensive surgical procedures may benefit from this therapy by experiencing less stressful intraoperative and postoperative periods.

References

1. Behar M, Magora F, Olshwang D, et al: Epidural morphine in treatment of pain. Lancet 1979; 1: 527–529.
2. Harrison DM, Sinatra R, Morgese L, et al: Epidural narcotic and patient-controlled analgesia for post-cesarean section pain relief. Anesthesiology 1988; 68: 454–457.
3. Eisenach JC, Grice SC, Dewan DM: Patient-controlled analgesia following cesarean section: a comparison with epidural and intramuscular narcotics. Anesthesiology 1988; 68: 444–448.
4. Ellis DJ, Millar WL, Reisner LS: A randomized double-blind comparison of epidural versus intravenous fentanyl infusion for analgesia after cesarean section. Anesthesiology 1990; 72: 981–986.
5. Loper KA, Ready LB, Downey M, et al: Epidural and intravenous fentanyl infusions are clinically equivalent after knee surgery. Anesth Analg 1990; 70: 72–75.
6. Glass PS, Estok P, Ginsberg B, et al: Use of patient-controlled analgesia to compare the efficacy of epidural to intravenous fentanyl administration. Anesth Analg 1992; 74: 345–351.
7. Sandler AN, Stringer D, Panos L, et al: A randomized, double-blind comparison of lumbar epidural and intravenous fentanyl infusions for postthoracotomy pain relief. Analgesic, pharmacokinetic, and respiratory effects. Anesthesiology 1992; 77: 626–634.
8. Guinard JP, Mavrocordatos P, Chiolero R, et al: A randomized comparison of intravenous versus lumbar and thoracic epidural fentanyl for analgesia after thoracotomy. Anesthesiology 1992; 77: 1108–1115.
9. Manikian B, Cantineau JP, Bertrand M, et al: Improvement of

diaphragmatic function by a thoracic extradural block after upper abdominal surgery. Anesthesiology 1988; 68: 379–386.

10. Pansard JL, Mankikian B, Bertrand M, et al: Effects of thoracic extradural block on diaphragmatic electrical activity and contractility after upper abdominal surgery. Anesthesiology 1993; 78: 63–71.

11. Craig DB: Postoperative recovery of pulmonary function. Anesth Analg 1981; 60: 46–52.

12. Duggan J, Drummond GB: Activity of lower intercostal and abdominal muscle after upper abdominal surgery. Anesth Analg 1987; 66: 852–855.

13. Ford GT, Whitelaw WA, Rosenal TW, et al: Diaphragmatic function after upper abdominal surgery in humans. Am Rev Respir Dis 1987; 127: 431–435.

14. Simonneau G, Vivien A, Sartene R, et al: Diaphragm dysfunction induced by upper abdominal surgery. Role of postoperative pain. Am Rev Respir Dis 1983; 128: 899–903.

15. Nunn JF: Effects of anaesthesia on respiration. Br J Anaesth 1990; 65: 54–62.

16. Cuschieri RJ, Morran CG, Howie JC, et al: Postoperative pain and pulmonary complications: comparison of three analgesic regimens. Br J Surg 1985; 72: 495–498.

17. Garibaldi RA, Britt MR, Coleman ML, et al: Risk factors for postoperative pneumonia. Am J Med 1981; 70: 677–680.

18. Rademaker BM, Ringers J, Odoom JA, et al: Pulmonary function and stress response after laparoscopic cholecystectomy: comparison with subcostal incision and influence of thoracic epidural analgesia. Anesth Analg 1992; 75: 381–385.

19. Rawal N, Sjostrand U, Christoffersson E, et al: Comparison of intramuscular and epidural morphine for postoperative analgesia in the grossly obese: influence on postoperative ambulation and pulmonary function. Anesth Analg 1984; 63: 583–592.

20. Wahba WM: Influence of aging on lung function—clinical significance of changes from age twenty. Anesth Analg 1983; 62: 764–776.

21. Bell SD: The correlation between pulmonary function and resting and dynamic pain scores in post aortic surgery patients. (Abstract.) Anesth Analg 1991; 72(Suppl): S18.

22. Simpson BR, Parkhouse J, Marshall R, et al: Extradural analgesia and the prevention of postoperative respiratory complications. Br J Anaesth 1961; 33: 628–641.

23. Spence AA, Smith G: Postoperative analgesia and lung function: a comparison of morphine with extradural block. Br J Anaesth 1971; 43: 144–148.

24. Lamotte C, Pert CB, Snyder SH: Opiate receptor binding in primate spinal cord: distribution and changes after dorsal root section. Brain Res 1976; 112: 407–412.

25. Cousins MJ, Mather LE, Glynn CJ, et al: Selective spinal analgesia. (Letter to the editor.) Lancet 1979; 1: 1141–1142.

26. Yeager MP, Glass DD, Neff RK, et al: Epidural anesthesia and analgesia in high-risk surgical patients. Anesthesiology 1987; 66: 729–736.

27. Tuman KJ, McCarthy RJ, March RJ, et al: Effects of epidural anesthesia and analgesia on coagulation and outcome after major vascular surgery. Anesth Analg 1991; 73: 696–704.

28. Bromage PR, Camporesi E, Chestnut D: Epidural narcotics for postoperative analgesia. Anesth Analg 1980; 59: 473–480.

29. Hendolin H, Lahtinen J, Lansimies E, et al: The effect of thoracic epidural analgesia on respiratory function after cholecystectomy. Acta Anaesthesiol Scand 1987; 31: 645–651.

30. Rawal N, Sjostrand UH, Dahlstrom B, et al: Epidural morphine for postoperative pain relief: a comparative study with intramuscular narcotic and intercostal nerve block. Anesth Analg 1982; 61: 93–98.

31. Rybro L, Schurizek BA, Petersen TK, et al: Postoperative analgesia and lung function: a comparison of intramuscular with epidural morphine. Acta Anaesthesiol Scand 1982; 26: 514–518.

32. Miller L, Gertel M, Fox GS, et al: Comparison of effect of narcotic and epidural analgesia on postoperative respiratory function. Am J Surg 1976; 131: 291–294.

33. Cullen ML, Staren ED, el-Ganzouri A, et al: Continuous epidural infusion for analgesia after major abdominal operations: a randomized, prospective, double-blind study. Surgery 1985; 98: 718–728.

34. Buckley DN, Macintosh J, Beattie WS, et al: Epidural analgesia prevents loss of lung volume. (Abstract.) Anesthesiology 1990; 73(Suppl): A764.

35. Hasenbos M, van Egmond J, Gielen M, et al: Post-operative analgesia by high thoracic epidural versus intramuscular nicomorphine after thoracotomy. Part III. The effects of pre- and post-operative analgesia on morbidity. Acta Anaesthesiol Scand 1987; 31: 608–615.

36. Shulman M, Sandler AN, Bradley JW, et al: Postthoracotomy pain and pulmonary function following epidural and systemic morphine. Anesthesiology 1984; 61: 569–575.

37. de Leon-Casasola OA, Parker BM, Lema MJ, et al: Epidural analgesia versus intravenous patient-controlled analgesia. Differences in the postoperative course of cancer patients. Reg Anesth 1994; 19: 307–315.

38. Chalmers TC, Ballantyne JC, Carr DR, et al: Comparative effects of analgesic therapies upon postoperative pulmonary function: meta-analysis. (Abstract #358.) 7th World Congress of Pain, p 136, 1993.

39. Pearce AC, Jones RM: Smoking and anesthesia: preoperative abstinence and perioperative morbidity. Anesthesiology 1984; 61: 576–584.

40. Jayr C, Thomas H, Rey A, et al: Postoperative pulmonary complications. Epidural analgesia using bupivacaine and opioids versus parenteral opioids. Anesthesiology 1993; 78: 666–676.

41. Wahba WM, Don HF, Craig DB: Post-operative epidural analgesia: effects on lung volumes. Can Anaesth Soc J 1975; 22: 519–527.

42. Mangano DT, Browner WS, Hollenberg M, et al: Association of perioperative myocardial ischemia with cardiac morbidity and mortality in men undergoing noncardiac surgery. N Engl J Med 1990; 323: 1781–1788.

43. Mangano DT, Siliciano D, Hollenberg M, et al: Postoperative myocardial ischemia. Therapeutic trials using intensive analgesia following surgery. Anesthesiology 1992; 76: 342–353.

44. McCann RL, Clements FM: Silent myocardial ischemia in patients undergoing peripheral vascular surgery: incidence and association with perioperative cardiac morbidity and mortality. J Vasc Surg 1989; 9: 583–587.

45. Ouyang P, Gerstenblith G, Furman WR, et al: Frequency and significance of early postoperative silent myocardial ischemia in patients having peripheral vascular surgery. Am J Cardiol 1989; 64: 1113–1116.

46. Pasternack PF, Grossi EA, Baumann FG, et al: The value of silent myocardial ischemia monitoring in the prediction of perioperative myocardial infarction in patients undergoing peripheral vascular surgery. J Vasc Surg 1989; 10: 617–625.

47. Raby KE, Barry J, Creager MA, et al: Detection and significance of intraoperative and postoperative myocardial ischemia in peripheral vascular surgery. JAMA 1992; 268: 222–227.

48. Becker RC, Underwood DA: Myocardial infarction in patients undergoing noncardiac surgery. Cleve Clin J Med 1987; 54: 25–28.

49. Plumlee JE, Boettner RB: Myocardial infarction during and following anesthesia and operation. South Med J 1972; 65: 886–889.

50. Rao TL, Jacobs KH, El-Etr AA: Reinfarction following anesthesia in patients with myocardial infarction. Anesthesiology 1983; 59: 499–505.

51. Tarhan S, Moffitt EA, Taylor WF, et al: Myocardial infarction after general anesthesia. JAMA 1972; 220: 1451–1454.

52. Lee DD, Kimura S, DeQuattro V: Noradrenergic activity and silent ischaemia in hypertensive patients with stable angina: effect of metoprolol. Lancet 1989; 1: 403–406.

53. Vanhoutte PM, Shimokawa H: Endothelium-derived relaxing factor and coronary vasospasm. Circulation 1989; 80: 1–9.

54. McDaniel MD, Pearce WH, Yao JS, et al: Sequential changes in coagulation and platelet function following femorotibial bypass. J Vasc Surg 1984; 1: 261–268.

55. Beattie WS, Buckley DN, Forrest JB: Epidural morphine reduces the risk of postoperative myocardial ischaemia in patients with cardiac risk factors. Can J Anaesth 1993; 40: 532–541.

56. Rosenfeld BA, Beattie C, Christopherson R, et al: The effects of different anesthetic regimens on fibrinolysis and the development of postoperative arterial thrombosis. Anesthesiology 1993; 79: 435–443.

57. Breslow MJ, Jordan DA, Christopherson R, et al: Epidural morphine decreases postoperative hypertension by attenuating sympathetic nervous system hyperactivity. JAMA 1989; 261: 3577–3581.

58. Blomberg S, Emanuelsson H, Kvist H, et al: Effects of thoracic epidural anesthesia on coronary arteries and arterioles in patients with coronary artery disease. Anesthesiology 1990; 73: 840–847.

59. Kock M, Blomberg S, Emanuelsson H, et al: Thoracic epidural anesthesia improves global and regional left ventricular function during stress-induced myocardial ischemia in patients with coronary artery disease. Anesth Analg 1990; 71: 625–630.

60. Szocik JF, Gardner CA, Webb RC: Inhibitory effects of bupivacaine and lidocaine on adrenergic neuroeffector junctions in rat tail artery. Anesthesiology 1993; 78: 911–917.

61. Mangano DT, Hollenberg M, Fegert G, et al: Perioperative myocardial ischemia in patients undergoing noncardiac surgery—I: incidence and severity during the 4 day perioperative period. J Am Coll Cardiol 1991; 17: 843–850.

62. Hollenberg M, Mangano DT, Browner WS, et al: Predictors of postoperative myocardial ischemia in patients undergoing noncardiac surgery. JAMA 1992; 268: 205–209.

63. Slogoff S, Keats AS: Randomized trial of primary anesthetic agents on outcome of coronary artery bypass operations. Anesthesiology 1989; 70: 179–188.

64. Leung JM, O'Kelly BF, Mangano DT: Relationship of regional wall motion abnormalities to hemodynamic indices of myocardial oxygen supply and demand in patients undergoing CABG surgery. Anesthesiology 1990; 73: 802–814.

65. Hasenbos M, Liem TH, Kerkkamp H, et al: The influence of high thoracic epidural analgesia on the cardiovascular system. Acta Anaesthesiol Belg 1988; 39: 49–54.

66. Reiz S, Nath S, Rais O: Effects of thoracic epidural block and prenalterol on coronary vascular resistance and myocardial metabolism in patients with coronary artery disease. Acta Anaesthesiol Scand 1980; 24: 11–16.

67. Reiz S, Haggmark S, Rydvall A, et al: Beta-blockers and thoracic epidural analgesia. Cardioprotective and synergistic effects. Acta Anaesthesiol Scand Suppl 1982; 76: 54–61.

68. Blomberg S, Emanuelsson H, Ricksten SE: Thoracic epidural anesthesia and central hemodynamics in patients with unstable angina pectoris. Anesth Analg 1989; 69: 558–562.

69. Saada M, Catoire P, Bonnet F, et al: Effect of thoracic epidural analgesia combined with general anesthesia on segmental wall motion assessed by transesophageal echocardiography. Anesth Analg 1992; 75: 329–335.

70. Reiz S, Balfors E, Sorenson MB, et al: Coronary hemodynamic effects of general anesthesia and surgery. Modification by epidural analgesia in patients with ischemic heart disease. Reg Anesth 1982; 7(Suppl): 8–18.

71. Davis RF, DeBoer LW, Maroko PR: Thoracic epidural anesthesia reduces myocardial infarct size after coronary artery occlusion in dogs. Anesth Analg 1986; 65: 711–717.

72. Heusch G, Deussen A, Thamer V: Cardiac sympathetic nerve activity and progressive vasoconstriction distal to coronary stenoses: feed-back aggravation of myocardial ischemia. J Auton Nerv Syst 1985; 13: 311–326.

73. Tsuchida H, Omote T, Miyamoto M, et al: Effects of thoracic epidural anesthesia on myocardial pH and metabolism during ischemia. Acta Anaesthesiol Scand 1991; 35: 508–512.

74. Vik-Mo H, Ottesen S, Renck H: Cardiac effects of thoracic epidural analgesia before and during acute coronary artery occlusion in open-chest dogs. Scand J Clin Lab Invest 1978; 38: 737–746.

75. Blomberg S, Ricksten SE: Thoracic epidural anaesthesia decreases the incidence of ventricular arrhythmias during acute myocardial ischaemia in the anaesthetized rat. Acta Anaesthesiol Scand 1988; 32: 173–178.

76. Tevelenok IuA: Peridural anesthesia in the acute period of myocardial infarct. (Russian.) Anesteziol Reanimatol 1977; 3: 36–39.

77. Toft P, Jorgensen A: Continuous thoracic epidural analgesia for the control of pain in myocardial infarction. Intensive Care Med 1987; 13: 388–389.

78. Blomberg S, Curelaru I, Emanuelsson H, et al: Thoracic epidural anaesthesia in patients with unstable angina pectoris. Eur Heart J 1989; 10: 437–444.

79. Saada M, Duval AM, Bonnet F, et al: Abnormalities in myocardial segmental wall motion during lumbar epidural anesthesia. Anesthesiology 1989; 71: 26–32.

80. Baron JF, Coriat P, Mundler O, et al: Left ventricular global and regional function during lumbar epidural anesthesia in patients with and without angina pectoris. Anesthesiology 1987; 66: 621–627.

81. Vandenberg BF, Kerber RE: Transesophageal echocardiography and intraoperative monitoring of left ventricular function. (Editorial.) Anesthesiology 1990; 73: 799–801.

82. Mergner GW, Stolte AL, Frame WB, et al: Combined epidural analgesia and general anesthesia induce ischemia distal to a severe coronary artery stenosis in swine. Anesth Analg 1994; 78: 37–45.

83. Arndt JO, Hock A, Stanton-Hicks M, et al: Peridural anesthesia and the distribution of blood in supine humans. Anesthesiology 1985; 63: 616–623.

84. Tuman KJ, McCarthy RJ, Spiess BD, et al: Does choice of anesthetic agent significantly affect outcome after coronary artery surgery? Anesthesiology 1989; 70: 189–198.

85. Baron JF, Bertrand M, Barre E, et al: Combined epidural and general anesthesia versus general anesthesia for abdominal aortic surgery. Anesthesiology 1991; 75: 611–618.

86. de Leon-Casasola OA, Karabella D, Lema MJ, et al: Postoperative myocardial ischemia: epidural versus intravenous PCA analgesia: a pilot project. Reg Anesth 1995; 20: 105–112.

87. de Leon-Casasola OA, Lema MJ: Intensive analgesia reduces postoperative myocardial ischemia? I. (Letter to the editor.) Anesthesiology 1992; 77: 404–405.

88. Weitz S, Drasner K, Cohen N, et al: PCA vs epidural morphine: comparison of perioperative myocardial ischemia. Reg Anesth 1993; 18: 2S–4S.

89. Christopherson R, Beattie C, Frank SM, et al: Perioperative morbidity in patients randomized to epidural or general anesthesia for lower extremity vascular surgery. Anesthesiology 1993; 79: 422–434.

90. Bredbacka S, Blomback M, Hagnevik K, et al: Pre- and postoperative changes in coagulation and fibrinolytic variables during abdominal hysterectomy under epidural or general anaesthesia. Acta Anaesthesiol Scand 1986; 30: 204–210.

91. Kuitunen A, Hynynen M, Salmenpera M, et al: Anaesthesia affects plasma concentrations of vasopressin, von Willebrand factor and coagulation factor VIII in cardiac surgical patients. Br J Anaesth 1993; 70: 173–180.

92. Freyburger G, Janvier G, Dief S, et al: Fibrinolytic and hemorrheologic alterations during and after elective aortic graft surgery: implications for postoperative management. Anesth Analg 1993; 76: 504–512

93. Isacson S: Effect of prednisolone on the coagulation and fibrinolytic systems. Scand J Haematol 1970; 7: 212–216.

94. Gader AMA, Clarkson AR, Cash JD: The plasminogen activator and coagulation factor VIII responses to adrenalin, noradrenaline, isoprenaline and salbutamol in man. Thromb Res 1973; 2: 9–16.

95. Britton BJ, Hawkey C, Wood WG, et al: Stress—a significant factor in venous thrombosis? Br J Surg 1974; 61: 814–820.

96. Sjoberg HE, Blomback M, Granberg PO: Thromboembolic complications, heparin treatment in increase in coagulation factors in Cushing's syndrome. Acta Med Scand 1976; 199:95–98.

97. Cash JD, Woodfield DG, Allan AG: Adrenergic mechanisms in the systemic plasminogen active response to adrenaline in man. Br J Haematol 1970; 18: 487–494.

98. Grant PJ, Tate GM, Davies JA, et al: Intra-operative activation of coagulation—a stimulus to thrombosis mediated by vasopressin? Thromb Haemost 1986; 55: 104–107.

99. Fey GH, Fuller GM: Regulation of acute phase gene expression by inflammatory mediators. Mol Biol Med 1974; 3: 323–328.

100. Lane A, Graham L, Cook M, et al: Cytokine production by cholesterol-loaded human peripheral monocyte-macrophages: the effect on fibrinogen mRNA levels in a hepatoma cell-line (HepG2). Biochim Biophys Acta 1991; 1097: 161–165.

101. Esmon CT, Taylor FB Jr, Snow TR: Inflammation and coagulation: linked processes potentially regulated through a common

pathway mediated by protein C. Thromb Haemost 1991; 66: 160–165.

102. Vedrinne C, Vedrinne JM, Guiraud M, et al: Nitrogen-sparing effect of epidural administration of local anesthetics in colon surgery. Anesth Analg 1989; 69: 354–359.

103. Tsuji H, Shirasaka C, Asoh T, et al: Effects of epidural administration of local anaesthetics or morphine on postoperative nitrogen loss and catabolic hormones. Br J Surg 1987; 74: 421–425.

104. Rutberg H, Hakanson E, Anderberg B, et al: Effects of the extradural administration of morphine, or bupivacaine, on the endocrine response to upper abdominal surgery. Br J Anaesth 1984; 56: 233–238.

105. Kehlet H: Epidural analgesia and the endocrine-metabolic response to surgery. Update and perspectives. Acta Anaesthesiol Scand 1984; 28: 125–127.

106. Kehlet H: The modifying effect of general and regional anesthesia on the endocrine-metabolic response to surgery. Reg Anesth 1982; 7(Suppl): S38–S48.

107. Kehlet H: Influence of epidural analgesia on the endocrine-metabolic response to surgery. Acta Anaesthesiol Scand Suppl 1978; 70: 39–42.

108. Engquist A, Brandt MR, Fernandes A, et al: The blocking effect of epidural analgesia on the adrenocortical and hyperglycemic responses to surgery. Acta Anaesthesiol Scand 1977; 21: 330–335.

109. Lush D, Thorpe JN, Richardson DJ, et al: The effect of epidural analgesia on the adrenocortical response to surgery. Br J Anaesth 1972; 44: 1169–1172.

110. Philbin DM, Rosow CE, Schneider RC, et al: Fentanyl and sufentanil anesthesia revisited: how much is enough? Anesthesiology 1990; 73: 5–11.

111. Borg T, Modig J: Potential anti-thrombotic effects of local anaesthetics due to their inhibition of platelet aggregation. Acta Anaesthesiol Scand 1985; 29: 739–742.

112. Henny CP, Odoom JA, ten Cate H, et al: Effects of extradural bupivacaine on the haemostatic system. Br J Anaesth 1986; 58: 301–305.

113. Feinstein MG, Fiekers J, Fraser C: An analysis of the mechanism of local anesthetic inhibition of platelet aggregation and secretion. J Pharmacol Exp Ther 1976; 197: 215–228.

114. Sixma JJ, de Groot PG: von Willebrand factor and the blood vessel wall. Mayo Clin Proc 1991; 66: 628–633.

115. Donadoni R, Baele G, Devulder J, et al: Coagulation and fibrinolytic parameters in patients undergoing total hip replacement: influence of the anaesthesia technique. Acta Anaesthesiol Scand 1989; 33: 588–592.

116. Schleef RR, Higgins DL, Pillemer E, et al: Bleeding diathesis due to decreased functional activity of type 1 plasminogen activator inhibitor. J Clin Invest 1989; 83: 1747–1752.

117. Haggroth L, Mattsson C, Felding P, et al: Plasminogen activator inhibitors in plasma and platelets from patients with recurrent venous thrombosis and pregnant women. Thromb Res 1986; 42: 585–594.

118. Aillaud MF, Juhan-Vague I, Alessi MC, et al: Increased PA-inhibitor levels in the postoperative period—no cause-effect relation with increased cortisol. Thromb Haemost 1985; 54: 466–468.

119. Kluft C, Verheijen JH, Jie AF, et al: The postoperative fibrinolytic shutdown: a rapidly reverting acute phase pattern for the fast-acting inhibitor of tissue-type plasminogen activator after trauma. Scand J Clin Lab Invest 1985; 45: 605–610.

120. Modig J, Hjelmstedt A, Sahlstedt B, et al: Comparative influences of epidural and general anaesthesia on deep venous thrombosis and pulmonary embolism after total hip replacement. Acta Chir Scand 1981; 147: 125–130.

121. Modig J, Borg T, Karlstrom G, et al: Thromboembolism after total hip replacement: role of epidural and general anesthesia. Anesth Analg 1983; 62: 174–180.

122. Wille-Jorgensen P, Christenson SW, Bjerg-Nielsen A, et al: Prevention of thromboembolism following elective hip surgery. The value of regional anesthesia and graded compression stockings. Clin Orthop 1989; 247: 163–167.

123. Davis FM, Quince M, Laurenson VG: Deep vein thrombosis and anaesthetic technique in emergency hip surgery. Br Med J 1980; 281: 1528–1529.

124. Sharrock NE, Haas SB, Hargett MJ, et al: Effects of epidural anesthesia on the incidence of deep-vein thrombosis after total knee arthroplasty. J Bone Joint Surg Am 1991; 73: 502–506.

125. Takkunen O, Takkunen H: Peak airway pressure as pointer to risk of postoperative deep venous thrombosis. (Letter to the editor.) Lancet 1982; 1: 1066.

126. Ahn H, Bronge A, Johansson K, et al: Effect of continuous postoperative epidural analgesia on intestinal motility. Br J Surg 1988; 75: 1176–1178.

127. Glise H, Abrahamsson H: Reflex inhibition of gastric motility pathophysiological aspects. Scand J Gastroenterol Suppl 1984; 89: 77–82.

128. Thoren T, Wattwil M: Effects on gastric emptying of thoracic epidural analgesia with morphine or bupivacaine. Anesth Analg 1988; 67: 687–694.

129. Thoren T, Wattwil M, Jarnerot G, et al: Epidural and spinal anesthesia do not influence gastric emptying and small intestinal transit in volunteers. Reg Anesth 1989; 14: 35–42.

130. Frantzides CT, Cowles V, Salaymeh B, et al: Morphine effects on human colonic myoelectric activity in the postoperative period. Am J Surg 1992; 163: 144–148.

131. England DW, Davis IJ, Timmins AE, et al: Gastric emptying: a study to compare the effects of intrathecal morphine and i.m. papaveretum analgesia. Br J Anaesth 1987; 59: 1403–1407.

132. Scheinin B, Asantila R, Orko R: The effect of bupivacaine and morphine on pain and bowel function after colonic surgery. Acta Anaesthesiol Scand 1987; 31: 161–164.

133. Thoren T, Sundberg A, Wattwil M, et al: Effects of epidural bupivacaine and epidural morphine on bowel function and pain after hysterectomy. Acta Anaesthesiol Scand 1989; 33: 181–185.

134. Thorn SE, Wattwil M, Naslund I: Postoperative epidural morphine, but not epidural bupivacaine, delays gastric emptying on the first day after cholecystectomy. Reg Anesth 1992; 17: 91–94.

135. Porreca F, Mosberg HI, Hurst R, et al: Roles of mu, delta and kappa opioid receptors in spinal and supraspinal mediation of gastrointestinal transit effects and hot-plate analgesia in the mouse. J Pharmacol Exp Ther 1984; 230: 341–348.

136. Bardon T, Ruckebusch Y: Comparative effects of opiate agonists on proximal and distal colonic motility in dogs. Eur J Pharmacol 1985; 110: 329–334.

137. Lund C, Selmar P, Hansen OB, et al: Effect of extradural morphine on somatosensory evoked potentials to dermatomal stimulation. Br J Anaesth 1987; 59: 1408–1411.

138. Saito H, Trocki O, Alexander JW, et al: The effect of route of nutrient administration on the nutritional state, catabolic hormone secretion, and gut mucosal integrity after burn injury. J Parenter Enteral Nutr 1987; 11: 1–7.

139. Moore FA, Feliciano DV, Andrassy RJ, et al: Early enteral feeding, compared with parenteral, reduces postoperative septic complications. The results of a meta-analysis. Ann Surg 1992; 216: 172–183.

140. Shou J, Lappin J, Minnard EA, et al: Total parenteral nutrition, bacterial translocation, and host immune function. Am J Surg 1994; 167: 145–150.

141. Moss G, Regal ME, Lichtig L: Reducing postoperative pain, narcotics, and length of hospitalization. Surgery 1986; 99: 206–210.

142. Hjortso NC, Neumann P, Frosig F, et al: A controlled study on the effect of epidural analgesia with local anaesthetics and morphine on morbidity after abdominal surgery. Acta Anaesthesiol Scand 1985; 29: 790–796.

143. Wallin G, Cassuto J, Hogstrom S, et al: Failure of epidural anesthesia to prevent postoperative paralytic ileus. Anesthesiology 1986; 65: 292–297.

144. de Leon-Casasola OA, Karabela D, Lema MJ: The effects of epidural bupivacaine-morphine and intravenous PCA morphine on bowel function and pain after radical hysterectomies. J Clin Anesth. (In press.)

145. Stevenson GW, Hall SC, Rudnick S, et al: The effect of anesthetic agents on the human immune response. Anesthesiology 1990; 72: 542–552.

146. Markovic SN, Knight PR, Murasko DM: Inhibition of interferon stimulation of natural killer cell activity in mice anesthetized

with halothane or isoflurane. Anesthesiology 1993; 78: 700–706.

147. Tubaro E, Borelli G, Croce C, et al: Effect of morphine on resistance to infection. J Infect Dis 1983; 148: 656–666.

148. Yeager MP, Colacchio TA: Effect of morphine on growth of metastatic colon cancer in vivo. Arch Surg 1991; 126: 454–456.

149. Yeager MP, Yu CT, Campbell AS, et al: Effect of morphine and beta-endorphin on human Fc receptor–dependent and natural killer cell functions. Clin Immunol Immunopathol 1992; 62: 336–343.

150. Bayer BM, Daussin S, Hernandez M, et al: Morphine inhibition of lymphocyte activity is mediated by an opioid dependent mechanism. Neuropharmacology 1990; 29: 369–374.

151. Tonnesen E, Wahlgreen C: Influence of extradural and general anaesthesia on natural killer cell activity and lymphocyte subpopulations in patients undergoing hysterectomy. Br J Anaesth 1988; 60: 500–507.

152. Ryhanen P, Jouppila R, Lanning M, et al: Natural killer cell activity after elective cesarean section under general and epidural anesthesia in healthy parturients and their newborns. Gynecol Obstet Invest 1985; 19: 139–142.

153. Ben-Eliyahu S, Yirmiya R, Liebeskind JC, et al: Stress increases metastatic spread of a mammary tumor in rats: evidence for mediation by the immune system. Brain Behav Immun 1991; 5: 193–205.

154. Herberman RB, Ortaldo JR: Natural killer cells: their roles in defenses against disease. Science 1981; 214: 24–30.

155. Poste G, Fidler IJ: The pathogenesis of cancer metastasis. Nature 1980; 283: 139–146.

156. Moore TC, Spruck CH, Leduc LE: Depression of lymphocyte traffic in sheep by anaesthesia and associated changes in efferent-lymph PGE2 and antibody levels. Immunology 1988; 63: 139–143.

157. Slade MS, Simmons RL, Yunis E, et al: Immunodepression after major surgery in normal patients. Surgery 1975; 78: 363–372.

158. Uchida A, Kolb R, Micksche M: Generation of suppressor cells for natural killer activity in cancer patients after surgery. J Natl Cancer Inst 1982; 68: 735–741.

159. Pflug AE, Murphy TM, Butler SH, et al: The effects of postoperative peridural analgesia on pulmonary therapy and pulmonary complications. Anesthesiology 1974; 41: 8–17.

160. Jacobs DF: Cost-effectiveness of specialized psychological programs for reducing hospital stays and outpatient visits. J Clin Psychol 1987; 43: 729–735.

161. Kehlet H: Anesthetic technique and surgical convalescence. Acta Chir Scand Suppl 1989; 550: 182–188.

162. Bellamy CD, McDonnell FJ, Colclough GW: Postoperative epidural pain management results in shorter hospital stay than IV PCA morphine: a comparison in anterior cruciate ligament repair. (Abstract.) Anesthesiology 1989; 71(Suppl): A686.

163. Walmsly PHN, Colclough GW, Mazloomdoost M, et al: Epidural PCA/infusion for post-nephrectomy pain: shorter hospitalization. (Abstract.) Anesth Analg 1989; 71(Suppl): A684.

164. Baysinger CL, Harkins TL, Horger EO, et al: Intrathecal morphine sulfate versus intravenous patient controlled analgesia following cesarean section: a comparison of hospital costs and duration of stay. (Abstract.) Anesth Analg 1994; 78: S22.

Chronic Pain

CHAPTER 40

Pharmacology of Pain Control

Stephen E. Abram, M.D.

In 1979, the initial report[1] of use of intrathecally applied morphine in humans consisted of eight case reports of patients with cancer pain treated with a single spinal injection of morphine (0.5 to 1.0 mg), which produced complete pain relief for 12 to 24 h. These patients reported no side effects or complications and demonstrated normal neurologic function. It appeared from these preliminary reports that neuraxial opioid administration would relieve intractable pain for many patients and that the answer to the problem of unmanageable pain depended only on development of satisfactory long-term infusion techniques.[2] Although such delivery systems have come into widespread use, the overall success of long-term neuraxial opioid administration has not been as high as anticipated.

Evidence that neuraxial administration of opioids was not without problems came soon after the publication of these first reports, when Ventafridda and colleagues[3] demonstrated the development of tolerance in eight patients with cancer pain who were receiving daily intrathecal injections of morphine. There is no question that certain patients who experience inadequate analgesia or intolerable side effects (or both) from systemic administration of opioids have an excellent response to spinal or epidural administration of the same drugs. In some series, satisfactory analgesia has been reported with morphine alone in 75% to 85% of patients.[4, 5] However, there are many patients who fail to experience adequate analgesia or who quickly lose the analgesic effect from neuraxial application of opioids.

The inability to manage certain intractable pain problems with systemic or spinal administration of μ-opioid receptor agonists has led to a search for agents that affect other types of opioid receptors or nonopioid receptors or that have effects that are not receptor mediated. Local anesthetic agents have been shown in animal models[6] to exert superadditive analgesic effects when combined with spinally administered opioids. Although some patients who receive neuraxial administration of opioids experience intolerable motor or sensory block with the addition of local anesthetic doses adequate to relieve pain, others experience satisfactory analgesia at minimal concentrations of local anesthetic.[7]

Some research has been done on the ability of non–μ-opioid receptor agonists to provide analgesia under conditions of μ-opioid resistance or tolerance. Agents that act at the δ receptor appear, from animal[8] and human[9] studies, to have some promise.

A wide variety of nonopioid receptor agonists have analgesic properties when administered spinally. Adrenergic agents, particularly those that exert substantial α_2 activity, are analgesic in several animal models.[10, 11] This is one of the few classes of nonopioid receptor agonists that have been used for chronic administration in humans.[12] Other receptor agonists that have analgesic properties include γ-aminobutyric acid (GABA)$_A$ and GABA$_B$ agonists, cholinergic agents, somatostatin, and adenosine agonists. Some of these agents appear to have synergistic effects when combined with opioids, and others may exert some protection against development of tolerance to opioids.[11]

There are several classes of drugs under development that have little or no direct analgesic effect but can influence the development of hyperalgesia by blocking the ability of noxious stimuli to increase the sensitivity and responsiveness of central nervous system neurons that are activated by painful stimuli. *N*-methyl D-aspartate (NMDA) receptors in the dorsal horn are ordinarily unresponsive to excitatory amino acids released from primary afferent terminals. However, after repetitive noxious stimulation, these receptors are enabled, and their activation leads to a series of intracellular events that magnify and prolong the neural responses to subsequent sensory stimuli.[13] Agents that block the NMDA receptor or that block the production of other mediators of the hyperalgesic state are capable of decreasing the sensitization of dorsal horn neurons by noxious stimulation.[13–16] It is not clear whether drugs that inhibit spinal sensitization will be useful clinically. They may prove effective when used before a noxious stimulus (such as preoperatively) but may be ineffective in influencing pain perception after hyperalgesia has become established, as in treating chronic pain and cancer pain.

Much information is available about the peripheral events that lead to alterations of nociceptor sensitivity or to peripheral neural activity associated with nerve injury. It is often important to address the peripheral changes initiating a painful condition as well as the central changes that occur secondarily when seeking solutions to intractable pain problems. Several classes of drugs, including nonsteroidal anti-inflammatory drugs (NSAIDs), steroids, axoplasmic-transport blockers, sodium channel blockers, and under certain circumstances, opioids, can modify peripheral nerve activity associated with the activation of nociceptors or injury to afferent nerves.

It is frustrating that the explosion of research on the pharmacology of analgesic agents has resulted in few new clinical agents or techniques. However, such research has greatly advanced our understanding of the physiology of sensory processing, and various new pharmacologic interventions are forthcoming.

Central Nervous System Modulation of Sensory Input

Excitatory Amino Acids

Excitatory amino acids such as glutamate and aspartate are the principal nociceptive neurotransmitters involved in the activation of dorsal horn cells by primary afferent terminals. It was demonstrated as early as 1959 that glutamate was capable of exciting certain spinal cord neurons.[17] Glutamate later was localized, along with substance P, in nerve terminals in the superficial dorsal horn,[18] and the spinal cord release of glutamate has been shown to increase in response to noxious stimulation.[19]

There are several discrete types of excitatory amino acid receptors in the dorsal horn. The AMPA receptor, so named because of its selective responsiveness to the excitatory amino acid, α-amino-3-hydroxy-5-methyl-4-isoxazopropionic acid, responds unconditionally to glutamate, producing a rapid, short-lived depolarization. AMPA receptor depolarization is initiated and terminated within a time frame lasting tens of milliseconds.[13] Activation of the NMDA receptor produces potentials lasting seconds or longer. The NMDA receptor is ordinarily unresponsive to a brief stimulus or to the initial release of glutamate. At physiologic Mg^{2+}

concentrations and a normal resting potential of -70 mV, dorsal horn neurons are unresponsive to NMDA. This voltage-dependent block can be overcome by prior depolarization of other receptors such as the AMPA receptor or the NK-1 neurokinin receptor, which responds to substance P.[13] The brief response to a short-lived stimulus is converted to a prolonged response, one likely to be perceived as pain, after repetitive stimulation. The phenomenon of "windup," the progressive increase in response to repetitive, brief C-fiber intensity stimulation, appears to be NMDA receptor mediated and can be blocked by pretreatment with NMDA receptor antagonists.[20] Several research models have been developed in which C-fiber sensitization of dorsal horn neurons is induced. This sensitization is consistently blocked by NMDA antagonists.[21–24]

NMDA antagonists appear to be effective at inhibiting the sensitization phenomenon when given before the noxious stimulus but have little or no analgesic effect when administered after the stimulus, even when given within several minutes. One model of spinal sensitization is the formalin test, a paradigm commonly used in rodents. A small amount of dilute formalin is injected subcutaneously in the hindfoot, which results in a brief (3–5 min) period of flinching or licking the paw. This subsides for about 10 min but recommences about 20 min after injection and lasts another 30 to 40 min. It is the period of resumed pain behavior (phase 2) that is the result of NMDA receptor–mediated spinal sensitization. The pretreatment of animals with intrathecal administration of MK801, a highly selective NMDA antagonist, has little effect on the initial (phase 1) flinching but markedly attenuates phase 2 activity.[21] However, if the drug is given several minutes after the formalin injection, it has no effect (Fig. 40–1).

Of the several classes of NMDA receptor antagonists, the most familiar are the noncompetitive antagonists, which act at a site within the ion-conducting channel gated by the NMDA receptor.[25] Many of the drugs in this class belong to the group of phencyclidine-like drugs, such as ketamine and MK801. The only NMDA antagonist in widespread use in humans is ketamine, which probably has a small number of actions that are unrelated to its excitatory amino acid–antagonizing properties. Ketamine has undergone several trials in which it was administered epidurally for postoperative pain in subdissociative doses.[26, 27] The results were mixed, with some studies confirming its analgesic properties in this setting and others failing to show substantial benefit.

It is in the field of chronic pain management, particularly the treatment of hyperalgesic states such as nerve injury and reflex sympathetic dystrophy, that these agents may have promise. One case report[28] attested to the analgesic effect of an NMDA antagonist on chronic pain. The NMDA antagonist 3-(2-carboxypiperazin-4-yl)propyl-1-phosphonic acid (CPP) was administered intrathecally to a patient with neuropathic pain. The drug did little for the constant pain or allodynia, but it markedly suppressed the increasing spreading pain induced by mechanical stimulation.

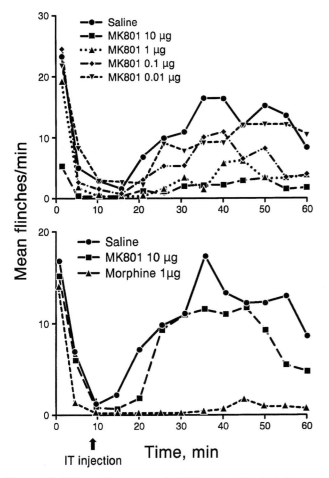

Figure 40–1 Time-effect curves of MK801 given 15 min before injection of formalin into the right hindpaw show the number of flinches per minute observed after formalin. Each line represents the group mean of four to six animals. Time-effect curves for morphine (1 μg) and MK801 (10 μg) given 9 min after formalin injection. IT, intrathecal. (From Yamamoto T, Yaksh TL: Comparison of the antinociceptive effects of pre- and posttreatment with intrathecal morphine and MK801, an NMDA antagonist, on the formalin test in the rat. Anesthesiology 1992; 77: 757–763.)

Ketamine-like psychotomimetic effects developed several hours after administration.

In addition to the short-term sensitization of dorsal horn cells by excitatory amino acids, there is evidence for prolonged increases in responsiveness of spinal cord neurons to sensory inputs. Changes in dorsal horn neural function known as synaptic plasticity may last hours to days. A similar phenomenon known as long-term potentiation is seen in the hippocampus and is associated with learning and memory function.[29] As with the spinal cord phenomenon of augmented transmission of nociceptive transmission (allodynia, hyperalgesia), long-term potentiation in the hippocampus is NMDA receptor mediated.[30] There is considerable evidence that intense or prolonged release of excitatory amino acids can lead to damage or loss of neurons within the central nervous system and that such neurotoxicity is mediated at least in part by the NMDA receptor.[31] After some types of peripheral nerve lesions in animals, the appearance of small, dark neurons in the substantia gelatinosa has been reported coincidentally with the development of thermal hyperalgesia.[13] There is speculation that these cells represent degenerating inhibitory interneurons damaged by the large amounts of glutamate released by C-fiber barrages from the injured nerve segment.[13]

Neuropeptides

Several neuropeptides are released in the dorsal horn in response to noxious stimulation. These include substance P, neurokinin A, somatostatin, calcitonin gene-related peptide, and galanin.[14] The principal receptor affected by substance P is the NK-1 receptor. Located postsynaptically, activation of this receptor decreases K^+ efflux, increasing excitability of the neuron; opioids and adrenergic agonists enhance K^+ efflux. The duration of substance P activity is relatively short because of rapid enzymatic degradation. Neurokinin A, which also affects the NK-1 receptor, resists enzymatic destruction[32] and may potentiate NMDA receptor activity for hours after injury or inflammation. The intrathecal injection of NK-1 receptor antagonists has blocked the hyperalgesia associated with subcutaneous formalin injection[33] or sciatic nerve ligation.[34]

Intracellular Mechanisms

One of the intracellular mechanisms implicated in the development of hyperalgesia is the stimulation of prostaglandin synthesis in the central nervous system. Ferreira[35] demonstrated that intracerebroventricular administration of NSAIDs inhibited carrageenan-evoked hyperalgesia in the rat hindpaw. Yaksh[36] reported that intrathecal administration of acetylsalicylic acid in rats inhibited the pain behavior evoked by intraperitoneal injection of an irritant at doses that were ineffective systemically. Another study[37] demonstrated that many NSAIDs, when administered intrathecally in rats, inhibit the behavioral response to subcutaneous formalin injection of the hindpaw. Systemic administration of the same drugs required about 100 times higher doses to achieve the same effect[37] (Table 40–1).

It is postulated that high-threshold (nociceptive) afferent activation produces Ca^{2+} influx in dorsal horn cells by membrane depolarization and NMDA receptor activation. Ca^{2+} influx then results in the activation of phospholipase A_2 and increased production of intracellular arachidonic acid and the products of the prostaglandin cascade. The resultant spinal cord accumulation of prostaglandins augments the hyperalgesic state through mechanisms not yet identified. Intrathecally administered prostaglandins are capable of inducing a hyperalgesic state,[36] and hyperalgesia induced by intrathecal administration of NMDA is inhibited by intrathecal administration of NSAIDs.[16] Unlike the situation with NMDA antagonists, there is an appreciable effect even when the drug is given after the injection of formalin (Fig. 40–2).[37] After appropriate neurotoxi-

Table 40–1 Inhibitory Effects of Intrathecally and Intraperitoneally Administered Nonsteroidal Anti-inflammatory Drugs on the 2a Phase (10–39 min) of the Formalin Test, Presented as Percent of Control Response*

DRUG	IT ID_{50}† 95% CI, nmol	IP ID_{50}† 95% CI, μmol	IT POTENCY RATIO‡ vs. ASA	IP POTENCY RATIO vs. ASA	POTENCY RATIO,§ IP vs. IT
Acetylsalicylic acid	27.0 (18–41)	8.0 (5.4–11.8)	1.0	1.0	182 (175–188)
Indomethacin	1.9 (1.2–4.0)	2.6 (1.3–5.3)	14	3.0	807 (759–857)
Flurbiprofen	2.1 (1.0–4.3)	3.1 (2.3–4.1)	13	2.5	930 (902–959)
Ketorolac	5.2 (3.2–8.3)	3.0 (2.4–3.8)	5.2	2.6	216 (209–223)
Zomepirac	5.9 (3.9–8.9)	5.5 (2.1–14)	4.5	1.4	307 (234–400)
S(+)ibuprofen	15.7 (6.7–36)		1.7		
Ibuprofen (racemic)	18.9 (9.3–38)		1.4		
Acetaminophen	257 (163–405)	6.0 (0.8–44)	0.1	1.3	23 (22–24)
R(−)ibuprofen	>270		>0.1		

*ID_{50} values and 95% CI calculated from regression lines shown in Figures 2 and 6 in reference 37.
†The ID_{50} value represents the total dose resulting in 50% inhibition of the formalin control response.
‡Potency ratio showing the relative potency compared with the potency of ASA (i.e., indomethacin is 14 times more potent than ASA in inhibiting the formalin response after IT administration).
§Relative potency with 95% CI of dose (total doses)-response regression lines from IT vs. IP administration.
ASA, acetylsalicylic acid; CI, confidence interval; IP, intraperitoneal; IT, intrathecal.
From Malmberg AB, Yaksh TL: Antinociceptive actions of spinal nonsteroidal anti-inflammatory agents on the formalin test in the rat. J Pharmacol Exp Ther 1992; 263: 136–146.

cology studies of intrathecal administration of NSAIDs, human applications may prove to be of value, particularly in conditions that are contingent on spinal sensitization.

It seems logical that spinal administration of corticosteroids or other agents that block prostaglandin production through inhibition of phospholipase A_2 would be capable of blocking spinal sensitization in a manner similar to that of NSAIDs. Such effects may help explain the beneficial effects of epidural steroid injections in patients with radiculopathy. However, spinally administered steroids[38] and other phospholipase A_2 inhibitors[39] produced little or no suppression of the sensitization-dependent response (phase 2) on the formalin test in rats.

A series of events involving several intracellular chemical messengers is triggered by the action of excitatory amino acids and neuropeptides on NMDA and other excitatory amino acid (e.g., metabotropic) receptors. The activation of intracellular phospholipase C stimulates the formation of inositol triphosphate and diacylglycerol, substances that have been implicated in the development of nociceptor-induced plasticity. Inositol triphosphate stimulates the release of intracellular Ca^{2+} stores, and diacylglycerol leads to increased production of protein kinase C. Increases in intracellular Ca^{2+} and protein kinase C are thought to enhance NMDA receptor excitation and to increase the expression of proto-oncogenes such as *FOS* and *JUN*, which act as third messengers that control transcription of genes that encode various neuropeptides capable of modulating responses to noxious stimuli.[14] Agents that inhibit production of phospholipase C (e.g., neomycin) or protein kinase C (e.g., H-7) decrease the delayed hyperalgesic response to subcutaneous formalin injection in rats.[39]

Another mechanism by which responsiveness to noxious stimulation is enhanced involves the production of intracellular nitric oxide. It has been proposed that the activation of the NMDA receptor leads to an influx of Ca^{2+}, which activates the enzyme nitric oxide synthase through a calcium-calmodulin mechanism.

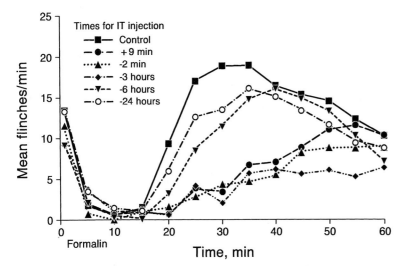

Figure 40–2 Time-effect curve with ketorolac (27 nmol) administered intrathecally (IT) 2 min or 3, 6, and 24 h before and 9 min after formalin ($n = 20$ for controls, 4 to 6 for treated animals). Notice the persistence of effect even when the drug is given after the noxious stimulus. (From Malmberg AB, Yaksh TL: Antinociceptive actions of spinal nonsteroidal anti-inflammatory agents on the formalin test in the rat. J Pharmacol Exp Ther 1992; 263: 136–146.)

Nitric oxide is produced by the action of the enzyme on L-arginine. Nitric oxide, which is rapidly diffusible inside and outside the cell, activates guanylate cyclase to increase production of cyclic guanosine monophosphate (cGMP). Within the target cell, this leads to production of protein kinases (enhanced NMDA responsiveness, altered gene expression), and in the primary afferent terminal, there is enhanced release of excitatory amino acids and peptides such as substance P and calcitonin gene-related peptide. Nitric oxide may also decrease function of inhibitory interneurons in the vicinity of the affected neurons.[15] A composite of the intracellular events initiated by the release of excitatory

amino acids and substance P from nociceptive primary afferent terminals is shown in Figure 40–3.

If the preceding theory is valid, drugs that block the activity of nitric oxide synthase should decrease nociceptor-driven spinal sensitization. Malmberg and Yaksh[40] demonstrated that NG-nitro-L-arginine methyl ester (L-NAME), an arginine analogue that acts as a nitric oxide synthase inhibitor, was effective in blocking the development of phase 2 of the formalin test in rats. Intrathecal injection of L-NAME 10 or 30 min before the subcutaneous injection of formalin dramatically decreased the delayed (phase 2) flinching. When given 9 min after the formalin injection, the L-NAME still

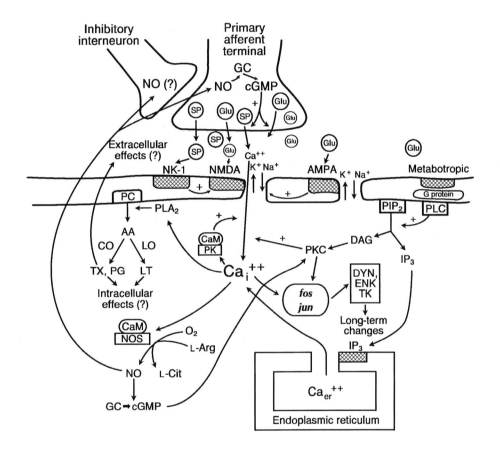

Figure 40–3 Sequences of events leading to sensitization of dorsal horn neurons after injury and intense nociceptive stimulation. Intense activation of a primary afferent neuron stimulates release of glutamate (Glu) and substance P (SP). The N-methyl-D-aspartate (NMDA) receptor, at physiologic Mg^{2+} levels, is initially unresponsive to Glu, but after depolarization of the α-amino-3-hydroxy-5-methyl-4-isoxazoproprionic acid (AMPA) receptor by Glu or the neurokinin (NK-1) receptor by SP, it becomes responsive to Glu, allowing Ca^{2+} influx. The action of Glu on the metabotropic receptor stimulates G-protein–mediated activation of phospholipase C (PLC), which catalyzes hydrolysis of phosphatidylinositol 4,5-bisphosphate (PIP_2) to produce inositol triphosphate (IP_3) and diacylglycerol (DAG). DAG stimulates production of protein kinase C (PKC), which is activated in the presence of high levels of intracellular Ca^{2+} (Ca_i^{2+}). IP_3 stimulates release of intracellular Ca^{2+} from intracellular stores within the endoplasmic reticulum (Ca_{er}^{2+}). Increased PKC induces a sustained increase in membrane permeability and, in conjunction with increased intracellular Ca^{2+}, leads to increased expression of proto-oncogenes such as *fos* and *jun*. The proteins produced by these proto-oncogenes encode a number of neuropeptides such as enkephalins (ENK), dynorphin (DYN), and tachykinins (TK). Increased Ca_i^{2+} also leads to activation of calcium-calmodulin–dependent protein kinase (CaM PK), which produces a brief increase in membrane permeability, and to activation of phospholipase A_2 (PLA_2) and to activation of nitric oxide synthase (NOS) through a calcium-calmodulin mechanism. PLA_2 catalyzes the conversion of phosphatidylcholine (PC) to arachidonic acid (AA), which is acted on by cyclooxygenase (CO) to produce prostaglandins (PG) and thromboxanes (TX) and by lipoxygenase (LO) to produce leukotrienes (LT). NOS catalyzes the production of nitric oxide (NO) and L-citrulline (L-Cit) from L-arginine (L-Arg). NO activates soluble guanylate cyclase (GC), which increases the intracellular content of cyclic guanosine monophosphate (cGMP) and leads to increased production of protein kinases, such as PKC, and alterations in gene expression. NO diffuses out of the cell to the primary afferent terminal, where, through a GC and cGMP mechanism, it increases the release of glutamate. It is speculated that NO may interfere with release of inhibitory neurotransmitters from inhibitory neurons.

produced some phase 2 suppression, although it was not as pronounced as when given before the noxious stimulus (Fig. 40–4).

Inhibitory Neurotransmitters

Several classes of drugs are capable of suppressing activation of dorsal horn neurons by noxious stimuli. At least six general classes of receptors can modify processing of nociceptive information and diminish behavioral responses to stimuli that ordinarily produce pain.

Opioid Receptors

Spinally administered opioids produce significant dose-dependent analgesia by action on the dorsal horn of the spinal cord. The analgesic effect of opioids in the dorsal horn appears to depend on two distinct mechanisms: presynaptic inhibition of the release of neurotransmitters from small primary afferents[41, 42] and hyperpolarization of postsynaptic neurons produced by opening of K^+ channels.[41]

The first mechanism, blockade of neurotransmitter release, should effectively protect dorsal horn neurons from the sensitizing effects of excitatory amino acids such as glutamate in much the same way that regional anesthesia exerts a preemptive effect. Yamamoto and Yaksh[21] demonstrated that spinally administered morphine produced profound analgesia on the first and second phases of the formalin test in rats, suggesting that opioid analgesia is effective despite spinal sensitization. However, Woolf and Wall[43] demonstrated that much larger doses of morphine were required to suppress the activity of dorsal horn cells when given after, rather than before, the noxious stimulus. Spinal injection of opioids, administered before subcutaneous injection of formalin and reversed with opioid antagonists several minutes after the noxious stimulus, also suppresses pain-related behavior[44] and dorsal horn

neural activity[45] associated with the second or sensitization-dependent phase of the formalin test. However, systemically administered opioids do not appear to block spinal sensitization when used in a similar paradigm.[46]

It seems likely that opioids are much more capable of blocking release of neurotransmitters from dorsal horn afferents and protecting dorsal horn neurons from sensitization when given spinally. From the experimental data regarding the timing of spinal administration of opioids, the neuraxial administration of opioids could be expected to provide better postoperative analgesia when initiated preoperatively as opposed to postoperatively, but few studies have investigated this effect.[47]

The analgesic action of systemically administered opioids is more complex and is not as well understood. It appears likely that systemically administered opioids, even in doses that produce profound analgesia, may not exert substantial spinal effects.[48] Several lines of evidence support such a statement. First, spinal cord opioid concentrations measured after modest doses given intrathecally are about 10-fold higher than those measured after high doses given systemically.[48, 49] Second, the analgesic effect of morphine given systemically is substantially decreased after high spinal transection in animals, but the analgesic effect of spinal morphine is preserved,[50] indicating that opioids given systemically exert their effects principally at supraspinal sites. Third, some evidence indicates that systemically or supraspinally administered opioids may not produce inhibition of C-fiber–evoked activity in spinal cord neurons.

Although it has been widely accepted that supraspinal effects of opioids are mediated by descending inhibitory pathways,[51–53] a few studies have failed to demonstrate spinal inhibition from injections of morphine into the periaqueductal gray,[54] intracerebroventricular morphine,[55] or systemically administered morphine.[56] This remains a controversial issue. Even if systemically administered morphine produces much of its analgesia through a descending inhibitory action on spinal cord

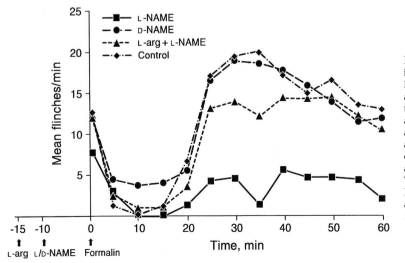

Figure 40–4 Time-effect curve for intrathecal injection of NG-nitro-L-arginine methyl ester (L-NAME; 370 nmol), D-NAME (3.7 mmol), and L-arginine (L-arg; 4.7 mmol) + L-NAME (370 nmol) on the formalin test in rats. L- and D-NAME were administered 10 min before formalin injection, and L-arginine was injected 5 min before L-NAME. The data are presented as the mean (four to eight rats per line) of the number of flinches per minute versus the time after formalin injection. (From Malmberg AB, Yaksh TL: Spinal nitric oxide synthesis inhibition blocks NMDA-induced thermal hyperalgesia and produces antinociception in the formalin test in rats. Pain 1993; 54: 291–300.)

neurons, such effects may be qualitatively different from the effects of spinally administered opioids.

Even though the initial reports[1, 2] of the efficacy of intrathecal and epidural administration of morphine for the treatment of intractable pain were highly encouraging, the reality is that many cancer patients, particularly those who have become resistant to systemically administered opioids, have less than optimal responses to neuraxial injection of opioids. In many institutions, patients tend to be referred for epidural injections late in the course of their illness, when metastases are widespread, nociceptive inputs are high, and tolerance is a substantial problem. Such was the case in a study by Hogan and coworkers,[7] who found that 10 of 16 patients, selected from a total of 1205 cancer admissions, required local infusions of anesthetic along with epidurally applied morphine to achieve satisfactory analgesia. Du Pen and colleagues[57] found that only 68 (18%) of 375 patients failed to achieve satisfactory analgesia with neuraxial administration of opioids alone. Sixty-one of those 68 patients experienced satisfactory analgesia with the addition of local anesthetic drugs. In other studies,[4, 5] satisfactory analgesia has been reported with morphine alone in 75% to 85% of patients. It is likely that the patients in such reports were selected earlier in the course of their disease, although this is difficult to assess from the information provided.

Most experience with chronic administration of opioids has been with morphine. Its long duration and its position as the only opioid that is approved by the Food and Drug Administration for spinal and epidural administration in the United States make it the obvious choice. However, other agents may be advantageous in certain situations. The most obvious drawback to morphine for chronic administration is the occasional dramatic tolerance that develops, particularly among cancer patients. In some patients, this may be true pharmacologic tolerance: escalation of the dose required to produce a previously obtained effect or reduction of effect from continued administration of a given dose.[58] This phenomenon is related to loss of agonist effect on a receptor after chronic exposure and probably represents a reduction in the agonist-receptor interaction (decrease in number of effective receptors or a decrease in receptor affinity) or a change in receptor-effector coupling.[58]

When pharmacologic tolerance occurs, more potent opioids may be advantageous. A more potent drug is capable of producing a maximal effect at a lower level of receptor occupation than a less potent drug. Suppose, for example, that to achieve a certain degree of analgesia morphine must occupy 50% of available opioid receptors, but sufentanil produces the same effect when only 10% of receptors are occupied. After a period of chronic administration, 60% of the receptors become unresponsive. There is no way that morphine can interact with enough receptors to produce the same effect, but sufentanil can still occupy 10% of the original receptor population and can retain its maximal effect. Stevens and Yaksh[58] showed a much smaller shift in dose-response curves with highly potent drugs such as sufentanil than with lower potency drugs such as morphine during chronic intrathecal administration in rats.

The use of more potent drugs may be a reasonable choice for patients in whom troublesome tolerance to morphine has developed, but there is almost no clinical data available to prove or disprove this hypothesis. We have instituted epidural infusions of sufentanil in a few patients who had become unresponsive to epidural infusions of morphine and found no improvement in analgesia. It is not clear, however, whether these patients were pharmacologically tolerant or epidural scarring and fibrosis had developed. The latter is the more likely explanation in at least one of those patients.

Boersma and associates[59] reported a series of 15 patients who received epidural infusions of sufentanil at doses ranging from 150 to 500 μg per day for cancer pain. Most patients required little or no additional narcotics. Unfortunately, the report presents no data on previous requirements for systemically administered opioids or on the rate of escalation of sufentanil doses. The investigators do point out that sufentanil, as with other lipid-soluble drugs, exerts its spinal effects over a narrow segmental range, such that the pain associated with distant metastases is poorly controlled. Morphine, a much more polar molecule, resides in the cerebrospinal fluid for long periods and migrates throughout the neuraxis.

Another potential drawback to the use of the potent, short-acting, lipid-soluble drugs is the possibility that they do not reach the spinal cord in high concentrations when administered epidurally. There is now considerable evidence from studies of epidural administration of opioids for postoperative analgesia that the analgesic effect of epidural infusions of fentanyl and alfentanil is mainly the result of systemic uptake of the drugs and that epidural infusions are no more effective than intravenous infusions.[60-63] However, de Leon-Casasola and Lema[64] found that epidural infusions of sufentanil combined with bupivacaine were clearly more effective than epidural infusions of morphine and bupivacaine for postoperative pain among patients chronically on high doses of opioids given systemically. They reported better analgesic scores and lower relative opioid doses after switching from morphine to sufentanil.

Another reason for the development of a decreased response to opioids is that the amount of noxious stimulation is increased. This is a common reason for increases in dose requirements among terminal cancer patients. Yaksh[65] demonstrated that higher doses of opioids were required in rats to suppress responses to noxious heat when a more intense stimulus was applied (60° C, 52° C, and 48° C) in the hot plate test. However, the shift in dose-response curve is much greater for morphine than for sufentanil. This phenomenon is probably another reflection of the receptor-occupation requirements of more potent compared with less potent drugs. For an intense stimulus, the receptor-occupation requirement may be more than a less potent drug can achieve, but a highly potent drug may have enough receptor "reserve" to achieve acceptable analgesia with a modest increase in dose. There is little clinical data available to test this hypothesis.

An alternative to the idea of shifting to more potent μ-receptor agonists in patients tolerant to conventional opioids is the use of drugs that act on other types of opioid receptors. The selective κ agonists that have been used in laboratory investigations are not available clinically, and the clinically available opioids that possess κ-agonist properties also have some degree of μ-receptor antagonism, making them unsuitable for use in opioid-tolerant patients, because they may precipitate acute withdrawal.

It has been postulated that δ-opioid receptor agonists may be of some benefit for patients tolerant to μ-receptor agonists. Animals rendered tolerant to μ agonists show no diminution in the analgesic effect of [D-Ala²-D-Leu⁵]enkephalin (DADL), a moderately selective δ-receptor agonist.[8] DADL has been used neuraxially in only one clinical series,[9] which compared intrathecal administration of DADL and morphine in 10 patients who were tolerant to systemic μ opioids. DADL was more effective than morphine in six patients, equally effective in one, and less effective in three patients. Side effects, mainly somnolence, were comparable for the two agents.

Enkephalinase inhibitors prolong the activity of endogenously released opiate peptides, producing dose-dependent but submaximal analgesia similar in quality to that produced by exogenous opioids.[66] Because endogenous peptides, such as met-enkephalin, have some δ-receptor agonist effect, administration of such agents may prove useful in μ-receptor agonist-tolerant individuals.

Alpha₂-Adrenergic Agonists

Agents such as clonidine and 2-(2,6-diethylphenyl-amino)-2-imidazoline (ST-91), injected intrathecally in rats, have been shown to have analgesic effects in the hot plate and the tail flick paradigms.[10] In primate studies, clonidine and ST-91 were capable of producing dose-dependent, long-lasting elevation of the pain threshold to electric shock, and this effect was antagonized by phentolamine.[11] Coadministration of inactive doses of morphine and ST-91 produced near-maximal analgesia, which, unlike morphine alone, failed to show any degree of tolerance over a 21-day period. Animal studies suggested that spinal administration of α₂-adrenergic agents may be able to restore effective analgesia for morphine-tolerant patients.

In 1989, Eisenach and colleagues[12] looked systematically at the short-term analgesic effects of epidural injection of clonidine in nine cancer pain patients. Patients were given three escalating doses on consecutive days. One group received 100 to 300 mg of clonidine, the second group received 400 to 600 mg, and the third group received 700 to 900 mg. Pain was otherwise treated with patient-controlled analgesia with morphine. Visual Analog Score and morphine requirements during patient-controlled analgesia were followed for 6 h after each injection, along with data on

hemodynamic changes and side effects. There was some degree of analgesia in all patients. The reductions in Visual Analog Scores were dose related, as were decreases in heart rate and blood pressure and the incidence of somnolence. Seven patients were maintained on clonidine plus morphine infusions at home for as long as 5 months. Most of these patients were pleased with the degree of analgesia it provided, and some reported less nausea and sedation. There was minimal escalation of clonidine or morphine during the combined infusions. This study appears to confirm clonidine's potential advantage over opioids alone in providing ongoing analgesia without appreciable loss of effect over time.

Coombs and coworkers[67] reported the use of continuous intrathecal infusion of clonidine in a patient whose pain was poorly controlled with high doses of morphine given intrathecally and methadone given orally. Pain was well controlled, and opioid requirements decreased dramatically for about 2 weeks. However, orthostatic hypotension was a troublesome problem. In the ensuing days, the patient's response to the clonidine diminished. It is not clear whether this represented tolerance to the drug or escalating nociceptive input from the tumor. DADL provided no additional analgesic effect in this patient. Other studies[68, 69] reported that clonidine provides comparable short-term analgesia in chronic pain, but there is little additional data on long-term efficacy and tolerance in these studies.

Later studies indicate that neuraxial injection of α₂-adrenergic agonists may not have as much advantage over opioids as originally speculated. Takano and Yaksh[70] demonstrated that tolerance to clonidine, dexmedetomidine, and ST-91 occurred over a 5- to 7-day period of continuous intrathecal administration. One study of the use of epidural injection of clonidine for postoperative pain demonstrated some respiratory depression and the usual side effects of sedation, hypotension, and bradycardia.[71] Several postoperative studies have failed to show a better response to neuraxial administration of clonidine than to systemic administration.[72]

GABA-Receptor Agonists

Baclofen, a GABA_B-receptor agonist, when delivered intrathecally, had analgesic effects similar to those of clonidine and ST-91 in the primate shock-titration model.[11] Some tolerance developed during repeated daily injections but not to the extent seen with morphine. Like clonidine, baclofen provided effective analgesia in morphine-tolerant animals. Unlike morphine and the adrenergic agonists, baclofen produced a dose-dependent motor block in the lower limbs. It was this property that provided the impetus for baclofen's introduction into clinical practice.

There has been considerable demonstration of the efficacy of continuous intrathecal infusion of baclofen, administered by implantable, programmable electronic infusion pumps, in controlling spasticity.[73] Most patients selected have had multiple sclerosis or spinal cord injury. The technique has been effective in patients poorly responsive to oral baclofen or other antispasmodics. Although there is usually some dose escalation over time, most patients do not become tolerant to the point of loss of drug effect. Few data are available on the analgesic, as opposed to the antispasmodic, effect of intrathecal baclofen in humans.

Benzodiazepines, which act at a site on $GABA_A$ receptors to augment the effect of GABA in increasing chloride conductance,[74] have analgesic effects when injected intrathecally in animals.[75] Because agents that act directly on $GABA_A$ receptors (e.g., muscimol) do not produce analgesia at doses that do not block motor function,[76] it is not clear how the benzodiazepines do so. There has been one study of the use of intrathecal injection of midazolam in chronic pain. Serrao and colleagues[77] compared the effect of 2 mg midazolam given intrathecally with that of methylprednisolone given epidurally in patients with chronic back pain. There was similar improvement in analgesia scores for both groups over 2 months, but more patients in the midazolam group were able to decrease their use of analgesic medication. It is not clear whether there was any real long-term improvement in either group.

Cholinergic Agonists

Cholinergic receptors have been identified in the dorsal horn of the spinal cord, and intrathecal administration of muscarinic cholinergic agonists produces atropine-reversible antinociception.[78] The intrathecal administration of neostigmine augments the analgesic effect of intrathecal administration of morphine[79] and clonidine,[80] and isobolographic analysis has shown that the addition of intrathecal injection of neostigmine produces synergistic analgesic effects when combined with intrathecal injection of morphine or clonidine in rats.[81] Spinally administered neostigmine produces an increase in blood pressure[82] and can offset the hypotension associated with the intrathecal administration of clonidine in sheep.[83]

Somatostatin-Receptor Agonists

Somatostatin is another substance that has been reported to produce analgesia when injected intraspinally. In one report,[84] intrathecal infusion of somatostatin provided satisfactory analgesia in two patients with cancer pain. Both patients had experienced good analgesia with low doses (2 to 3 mg/day) of morphine given epidurally, and these trials did not represent the worst-case scenario. Another report[85] described effective postoperative analgesia during continuous epidural infusion of somatostatin. The investigators of these reports offered little explanation of the mechanism of analgesia, other than to speculate, on the basis of a lack of reversal of analgesia by naloxone in two of their patients, that it was not opiate receptor mediated. It seems unlikely that further human investigation of this substance will continue because toxic effects have been observed in the spinal cord in rats and cats after intrathecal administration,[86] and analgesia is observed only at concentrations that are in or near the neurotoxic range.[87] In addition to its potential for neurotoxicity, somatostatin has the added disadvantage of being a peptide with chemical instability and rapid enzymatic degradation.

A stable analogue of somatostatin, octreotide, produced analgesia for periods of up to 3 months with intrathecal administration in cancer patients.[88] Analgesia was seen in a small number of patients who were unresponsive to systemic or spinal administration of opioids.

Adenosine Agonists

Intrathecal administration of adenosine and its analogues produces analgesia in several experimental paradigms,[89–91] and the blockade of endogenous adenosine by spinal application of theophylline results in hyperalgesia.[92] Spinally administered morphine may at least partially act through an adenosine-mediated mechanism.[90, 91] Two classes of adenosine receptors (A_1 and A_2) have been identified, and agonists of both receptor subtypes have been identified as being analgesic.[89, 93]

Peripheral Mechanisms of Pain Modulation

Physiology of Nociceptive Afferents

Several classes of nociceptors, receptors that respond exclusively to intense, potentially tissue-injuring stimuli, exist in somatic tissues. There is considerable controversy regarding the existence of true nociceptors in visceral structures, and many researchers argue that visceral pain results from the high-frequency discharge of visceral afferents that ordinarily subserve other functions.[94, 95]

Cutaneous nociceptors, which are most accessible to the researcher, have been best characterized. They are classified according to their fiber type (Aδ or C) and to their response characteristics. A listing of the more commonly reported types of nociceptors is seen in Table 40–2. In addition to these commonly reported receptor types,[96] there are reports of C fibers that respond only to intense thermal or mechanical stimulation and of thinly myelinated polymodal fibers that respond in a manner similar to C-polymodal nociceptors.

Table 40–2 Cutaneous Nociceptors

TYPE OF NOCICEPTOR	FIBER TYPE	STIMULUS
High-threshold mechanoreceptor	Aδ	Mechanical*
C-polymodal nociceptor	C	Mechanical, heat, chemical
C-mechano-heat nociceptor	C	Mechanical, heat
A-mechano-heat nociceptor	Aδ	Mechanical, heat

*Response to noxious heat after high-temperature sensitization.

The C and Aδ fibers that appear to have nociceptive function have been found in muscle, tendons, and fascia. These muscle nociceptors have a range of response characteristics; some respond to stretch, some to strong contraction and ischemia, and some to chemicals such as bradykinin.[97] Joints are richly innervated with C and Aδ fibers, many of which appear to be responsive to noxious stimuli.[98] Responsiveness of joint nociceptors is greatly enhanced during inflammation.[99]

Sensitization of nociceptors in peripheral tissues has been recognized for many years to be a mechanism for the development of hyperalgesia. Several substances that are released during tissue injury, such as bradykinin, histamine, and 5-hydroxytryptamine, are capable of lowering response thresholds of nociceptors.[100] Several eicosanoids also are important in sensitization of nociceptors. They are formed by the action of phospholipase A_2 on cell membrane phospholipids, producing arachidonic acid. Arachidonic acid is acted on by cyclooxygenase to produce cyclic endoperoxides, the precursors of prostaglandins, prostacyclin, and thromboxanes. At least two of the prostaglandins (E_2 and $F_{2\alpha}$) are capable of increasing nociceptor sensitivity, and prostacyclin potentiates the edema induced by bradykinin and histamine.[100]

Arachidonic acid is acted on by lipoxygenase to produce several intermediates that are converted to leukotrienes. These substances do not appear to be important in the mediation of pain and hyperalgesia but have been implicated in the development of a sensitized state that depends on the presence of polymorphonuclear leukocytes.[96]

Corticosteroids exert at least a portion of their anti-inflammatory effect by inhibiting phospholipase A_2, decreasing production of prostaglandins and leukotrienes. Until recently, the analgesic effect of NSAIDs was thought to be entirely peripheral, mediated primarily through inhibition of cyclooxygenase and the subsequent decrease in tissue prostaglandins. We now know that prostaglandins may have substantial sensory modulating effects in the brain and spinal cord. We have assumed that opioids produce their analgesic effects through central nervous system mechanisms, and such views are supported by the lack of behavioral or electrophysiologic effects of opioids when injected into uninjured tissues or perineurally.[101] However, there is evidence that opioids can alter peripheral nociceptor function in injured or inflamed tissues. Evidence comes from the observation (which is not seen in all studies) that small intra-articular doses of morphine can provide analgesia after arthroscopic knee surgery.[102, 103] One mechanism that has been proposed for the analgesic effect of opioids in inflamed tissues is blockade of release of substance P from nociceptor nerve endings in the periphery.[104]

Pathophysiology of Pain After Nerve Injury

Several mechanisms are involved in the generation of chronic pain after peripheral nerve injuries. Injured nerve segments are capable of initiating spontaneous nerve activity,[105, 106] and there is evidence that dorsal root ganglia proximal to injured nerves participate in abnormal impulse generation.[105] Spontaneous generation of ectopic impulses from experimentally created neuromas is augmented by sympathetic stimulation or by local instillation of norepinephrine,[107, 108] and injection of epinephrine around painful neuromas in human patients causes an intense increase in pain.[109] A sympathetically mediated increase in ectopic impulse generation is one of many possible mechanisms to explain the therapeutic response to sympathetic block or sympatholytic drugs in patients with neuropathic pain. Devor[110] proposed that after nerve injury sodium and calcium channel proteins and adrenergic receptor proteins are transported axoplasmically to the injured segment and that adrenergic receptor stimulation enhances the spontaneous depolarization mediated by the new ion channels. Evidence for the role of axoplasmic transport in the development of spontaneous ectopic activity is provided by a study showing that axoplasmic transport blockers such as colchicine, applied to the nerve at the time of injury, decreased subsequent spontaneous activity[111] and abolished the thermal hyperalgesia that develops after chronic nerve constriction.[112]

Drugs that block sodium channels, such as local anesthetics, appear to decrease spontaneous activity arising from injured nerve segments and from adjacent dorsal root ganglia. Devor and associates[105] demonstrated decreased spontaneous activity originating from neuromas after intravascular (carotid artery) injection of 0.5 mg of lidocaine in rats and complete cessation of ectopic activity originating from dorsal root ganglia with the same dose. Tanelian and MacIver,[106] using an in vitro corneal nerve injury model, demonstrated suppression of spontaneous discharge from Aδ and C fibers with lidocaine concentrations of 2 to 15 μg/mL. In a study by Abram and Yaksh,[113] intravenous administration of lidocaine was shown to ameliorate the hyperalgesia to noxious thermal stimulation after sciatic nerve ligation injury in rats. The effect was significant at doses that produced 1 μg/mL blood levels and lasted at least 3 hours in all animals and more than 24 hours in some (Fig. 40–5). This same study demonstrated that lidocaine given intravenously was capable of partially blocking the hyperalgesic response to formalin injection, but it did so only at blood levels greater than 6 μg/mL. Lidocaine did not block spinal hypersensitivity if it was administered after the formalin injection.[113] The investigators concluded that the antihyperalgesic effect of lidocaine in nerve injury was most likely the result of action on the peripheral nerve and not related to central nervous system effects.[113]

Systemic administration of local anesthetics can diminish the severity of neuropathic pain[114–116] and decrease the intensity and extent of associated allodynia[116] at doses that do not produce symptoms of systemic toxicity. Although lidocaine is not an ideal therapeutic agent for long-term therapy because of the need for parenteral administration and the potential accumulation of a toxic metabolite, monoethylglycine xylidide,[117] it has been used chronically as a subcutaneous infusion,[117] and some patients experience days to

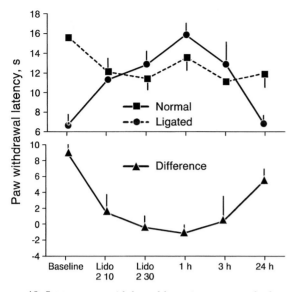

Figure 40–5 Mean paw withdrawal latencies (s ± standard error of the mean) for normal and ligated (nerve injured) limbs 10 and 30 min after bolus injection of 3 mL 2 mg/mL lidocaine (*Lido* 2 10, *Lido* 2 30) and 1, 3, and 24 h after the infusion was discontinued. (From Abram SE, Yaksh TL: Systemic lidocaine blocks nerve injury-induced hyperalgesia and nociceptor-driven spinal sensitization in the rat. Anesthesiology 1994; 80: 383–391.)

weeks of pain reduction after a single administration.[115] Orally effective sodium channel blocking agents, such as mexiletine, have suppressed ectopic discharge from neuromas in animals[118] and may be efficacious for some patients with neuropathic pain that is temporarily responsive to lidocaine.[119]

Ectopic neural discharge originating in neuromas can be decreased by topical application of corticosteroids at the time of nerve injury.[120] Steroids have also produced prolonged suppression of ongoing discharge from neuromas that are already active.[120] This phenomenon may explain much of the beneficial effect of the epidural injection of corticosteroids in patients with nerve root pathologic conditions associated with lumbar or cervical disk disease and the occasional benefit from local infiltration of injured nerves with local anesthetic plus corticosteroids.

References

1. Wang JK, Nauss LA, Thomas JE: Pain relief by intrathecally applied morphine in man. Anesthesiology 1979; 50: 149–151.
2. Behar M, Magora F, Olshwang D, et al: Epidural morphine in treatment of pain. Lancet 1979; 1: 527–529.
3. Ventafridda V, Figliuzzi M, Tamburini M, et al: Clinical observation on analgesia elicited by intrathecal morphine in cancer patients. Adv Pain Res Ther 1979; 3: 559–565.
4. Shetter AG, Hadley MN, Wilkinson E: Administration of intraspinal morphine sulfate for the treatment of intractable cancer pain. Neurosurgery 1986; 18: 740–747.
5. Penn RD, Paice JA: Chronic intrathecal morphine for intractable pain. J Neurosurg 1987; 67: 182–186.
6. Penning JP, Yaksh TL: Interaction of intrathecal morphine with bupivacaine and lidocaine in the rat. Anesthesiology 1992; 77: 1186–2000.
7. Hogan Q, Haddox JD, Abram S, et al: Epidural opiates and local anesthetics for the management of cancer pain. Pain 1991; 46: 271–279.
8. Yaksh TL: In vivo studies on spinal opiate receptor systems mediating antinociception. I. Mu and delta receptor profiles in the primate. J Pharmacol Exp Ther 1983; 226: 303–316.
9. Moulin DE, Max MB, Kaiko RF, et al: The analgesic efficacy of intrathecal D-Ala²-D-Leu⁵-enkephalin in cancer patients with chronic pain. Pain 1985; 23: 213–221.
10. Yaksh TL: Pharmacology of spinal adrenergic systems which modulate spinal nociceptive processing. Pharmacol Biochem Behav 1985; 22: 845–858.
11. Yaksh TL, Reddy SV: Studies in the primate on the analgetic effects associated with intrathecal actions of opiates, alpha-adrenergic agonists and baclofen. Anesthesiology 1981; 54: 451–467.
12. Eisenach JC, Rauck RL, Buzzanell C, et al: Epidural clonidine analgesia for intractable cancer pain: phase I. Anesthesiology 1989; 71: 647–652.
13. Wilcox GL: Excitatory neurotransmitters and pain. In Bond MR, Charlton JE, Woolf CJ (eds): Proceedings of the VIth World Congress on Pain, pp 97–117. Amsterdam, Elsevier, 1991.
14. Coderre TJ, Katz J, Vaccarino AL, et al: Contribution of central neuroplasticity to pathological pain: review of clinical and experimental evidence. Pain 1993; 52: 259–285.
15. Meller ST, Gebhart GF: Nitric oxide (NO) and nociceptive processing in the spinal cord. Pain 1993; 52: 127–136.
16. Malmberg AB, Yaksh TL: Hyperalgesia mediated by spinal glutamate or substance P receptor blocked by spinal cyclooxygenase inhibition. Science 1992; 257: 1276–1279.
17. Curtis DR, Phillis JW, Watkins JC: Chemical excitation of spinal neurones. Nature 1959; 183: 611–612.
18. Battaglia G, Rustioni A: Coexistence of glutamate and substance P in dorsal root ganglion neurons of the rat and monkey. J Comp Neurol 1988; 277: 302–312.
19. Skilling SR, Smullin DH, Beitz AJ, et al: Extracellular amino acid concentrations in the dorsal spinal cord of freely moving rats following veratridine and nociceptive stimulation. J Neurochem 1988; 51: 127–132.
20. Mendell LM: Physiological properties of unmyelinated fiber projection to the spinal cord. Exp Neurol 1966; 16: 316–332.
21. Yamamoto T, Yaksh TL: Comparison of the antinociceptive effects of pre- and posttreatment with intrathecal morphine and MK801, an NMDA antagonist, on the formalin test in the rat. Anesthesiology 1992; 77: 757–763.
22. Yamamoto T, Yaksh TL: Spinal pharmacology of thermal hyperesthesia induced by constriction injury of sciatic nerve. Excitatory amino acid antagonists. Pain 1992; 49: 121–128.
23. Yaksh TL: Behavioral and autonomic correlates of the tactile evoked allodynia produced by spinal glycine inhibition: effects of modulatory receptor systems and excitatory amino acid antagonists. Pain 1989; 37: 111–123.
24. Seltzer Z, Cohn S, Ginzburg R, et al: Modulation of neuropathic pain behavior in rats by spinal disinhibition and NMDA receptor blockade of injury discharge. Pain 1991; 45: 69–75.
25. Lodge D, Johnson KM: Noncompetitive excitatory amino acid receptor antagonists. Trends Pharmacol Sci 1990; 11: 81–86.
26. Islas JA, Astorga J, Laredo M: Epidural ketamine for control of postoperative pain. Anesth Analg 1985; 64: 1161–1162.
27. Ravat F, Dorne R, Baechle JP, et al: Epidural ketamine or morphine for postoperative analgesia. Anesthesiology 1987; 66: 819–822.
28. Kristensen JD, Svensson B, Gordh T Jr: The NMDA-receptor antagonist CPP abolishes neurogenic 'wind-up pain' after intrathecal administration in humans. Pain 1992; 51: 249–253.
29. Bliss TV, Collingridge GL: A synaptic model of memory: long-term potentiation in the hippocampus. Nature 1993; 361: 31–39.
30. Collingridge GL, Herron CE, Lester RA: Frequency-dependent N-methyl-D-aspartate receptor-mediated synaptic transmission in rat hippocampus. J Physiol (Lond) 1988; 399: 301–312.
31. Meldrum B, Garthwaite J: Excitatory amino acid neurotoxicity and neurodegenerative disease. Trends Pharmacol Sci 1990; 11: 379–387.
32. Hope PJ, Schaible H-G, Jarrott B, et al: Release and persistence of immunoreactive neurokinin A in the spinal cord is associated with chemical arthritis. (Abstract.) Pain 1990; 5: S230.

33. Yamamoto T, Yaksh TL: Stereospecific effects of a nonpeptidic NK1 selective antagonist, CP-96,345: antinociception in the absence of motor dysfunction. Life Sci 1991; 49: 1955–1963.

34. Yamamoto T, Yaksh TL: Effects of intrathecal capsaicin and an NK-1 antagonist, CP,96-345, on the thermal hyperalgesia observed following unilateral constriction of the sciatic nerve in the rat. Pain 1992; 51: 329–334.

35. Ferreira SH: Prostaglandins: peripheral and central analgesia. Adv Pain Res Ther 1983; 5: 627–634.

36. Yaksh TL: Central and peripheral mechanisms for the antialgesic action of acetylsalicylic acid. In Barnett HJM, Hirsh J, Mustard JF (eds): Acetylsalicylic Acid: New Uses for an Old Drug, pp 137–151. New York, Raven Press, 1982.

37. Malmberg AB, Yaksh TL: Antinociceptive actions of spinal nonsteroidal anti-inflammatory agents on the formalin test in the rat. J Pharmacol Exp Ther 1992; 263: 136–146.

38. Abram SE, Marsala M, Yaksh TL: Analgesic and neurotoxic effects of intrathecal corticosteroids in rats. Anesthesiology 1994; 81: 1198–1205.

39. Coderre TJ: Contribution of protein kinase C to central sensitization and persistent pain following tissue injury. Neurosci Lett 1992; 140: 181–184.

40. Malmberg AB, Yaksh TL: Spinal nitric oxide synthesis inhibition blocks NMDA-induced thermal hyperalgesia and produces antinociception in the formalin test in rats. Pain 1993; 54: 291–300.

41. Dickenson AH: Mechanisms of the analgesic actions of opiates and opioids. Br Med Bull 1991; 47: 690–702.

42. Chang HM, Berde CB, Holz GG IV, et al: Sufentanil, morphine, met-enkephalin, and kappa-agonist (U-50,488H) inhibit substance P release from primary sensory neurons: a model for presynaptic spinal opioid actions. Anesthesiology 1989; 70: 672–677.

43. Woolf CJ, Wall PD: Morphine-sensitive and morphine-insensitive actions of C-fibre input on the rat spinal cord. Neurosci Lett 1986; 64: 221–225.

44. Abram SE, Yaksh TL: Morphine, but not inhalation anesthesia, blocks post-injury facilitation. The role of preemptive suppression of afferent transmission. Anesthesiology 1993; 78: 713–721.

45. Dickenson AH, Sullivan AF: Subcutaneous formalin-induced activity of dorsal horn neurones in the rat: differential response to an intrathecal opiate administered pre or post formalin. Pain 1987; 30: 349–360.

46. Abram SE, Olson EE: Systemic opioids do not suppress spinal sensitization after subcutaneous formalin in rats. Anesthesiology 1994; 80: 1114–1119.

47. Katz J, Kavanagh BP, Sandler AN, et al: Preemptive analgesia. Clinical evidence of neuroplasticity contributing to postoperative pain. Anesthesiology 1992; 77: 439–446.

48. Gustafsson LL, Post C, Edvardsen B, et al: Distribution of morphine and meperidine after intrathecal administration in rat and mouse. Anesthesiology 1985; 63: 483–489.

49. Bolander H, Kourtopoulos H, Lundberg S, et al: Morphine concentrations in serum, brain and cerebrospinal fluid in the rat after intravenous administration of a single dose. J Pharm Pharmacol 1983; 35: 656–659.

50. Advokat C, Burton P: Antinociceptive effect of systemic and intrathecal morphine in spinally transected rats. Eur J Pharmacol 1987; 139: 335–343.

51. Fields HL, Basbaum AI: Brainstem control of spinal pain-transmission neurons. Annu Rev Physiol 1978; 40: 217–248.

52. Barton C, Basbaum AI, Fields HL: Dissociation of supraspinal and spinal actions of morphine: a quantitative evaluation. Brain Res 1980; 188: 487–498.

53. Jones SL, Gebhart GF: Inhibition of spinal nociceptive transmission from the midbrain, pons and medulla in the rat: activation of descending inhibition by morphine, glutamate and electrical stimulation. Brain Res 1988; 460: 281–296.

54. Dickenson AH, Le Bars D: Lack of evidence for increased descending inhibition on the dorsal horn of the rat following periaqueductal grey morphine microinjections. Br J Pharmacol 1987; 92: 271–280.

55. Bouhassira D, Villanueva L, Le Bars D: Intracerebroventricular morphine decreases descending inhibitions acting on lumbar dorsal horn neuronal activities related to pain in the rat. J Pharmacol Exp Ther 1988; 247: 332–342.

56. Duggan AW, Griersmith BT, North RA: Morphine and supraspinal inhibition of spinal neurones: evidence that morphine decreases tonic descending inhibition in the anaesthetized cat. Br J Pharmacol 1980; 69: 461–466.

57. Du Pen SL, Kharasch ED, Williams A, et al: Chronic epidural bupivacaine-opioid infusion in intractable cancer pain. Pain 1992; 49: 293–300.

58. Stevens CW, Yaksh TL: Potency of infused spinal antinociceptive agents is inversely related to magnitude of tolerance after continuous infusion. J Pharmacol Exp Ther 1989; 250: 1–8.

59. Boersma FP, Noorduin H, Vanden Bussche G: Epidural sufentanil for cancer pain control in outpatients. Reg Anesth 1989; 14: 293–297.

60. Loper KA, Ready LB, Downey M, et al: Epidural and intravenous fentanyl infusions are clinically equivalent after knee surgery. Anesth Analg 1990; 70: 72–75.

61. Guinard JP, Mavrocordatos P, Chiolero R, et al: A randomized comparison of intravenous versus lumbar and thoracic epidural fentanyl for analgesia after thoracotomy. Anesthesiology 1992; 77: 1108–1115.

62. Glass PS, Estok P, Ginsberg B, et al: Use of patient-controlled analgesia to compare the efficacy of epidural to intravenous fentanyl administration. Anesth Analg 1992; 74: 345–351.

63. Camu F, Debucquoy F: Alfentanil infusion for postoperative pain: a comparison of epidural and intravenous routes. Anesthesiology 1991; 75: 171–178.

64. de Leon-Casasola OA, Lema MJ: Epidural bupivacaine/sufentanil therapy for postoperative pain control in patients tolerant to opioid and unresponsive to epidural bupivacaine/morphine. Anesthesiology 1994; 80: 303–309.

65. Yaksh TL: The analgesic pharmacology of spinally administered mu opioid agonists. Eur J Pain 1990; 11: 66–71.

66. Oshita S, Yaksh TL, Chipkin R: The antinociceptive effects of intrathecally administered SCH32615, an enkephalinase inhibitor in the rat. Brain Res 1990; 515: 143–148.

67. Coombs DW, Saunders RL, Lachance D, et al: Intrathecal morphine tolerance: use of intrathecal clonidine, DADLE, and intraventricular morphine. Anesthesiology 1985; 62: 358–363.

68. Glynn C, Dawson D, Sanders R: A double-blind comparison between epidural morphine and epidural clonidine in patients with chronic non-cancer pain. Pain 1988; 34: 123–128.

69. Germain H, Neron A, Lomssy A: Analgesic effect of epidural clonidine. In Dubner R, Gebhart GF, Bond MR (eds): Proceedings of the Vth World Congress on Pain, pp 472–476. Amsterdam, Elsevier, 1988.

70. Takano Y, Yaksh TL: Chronic spinal infusion of dexmedetomidine, ST-91 and clonidine: spinal alpha 2 adrenoceptor subtypes and intrinsic activity. J Pharmacol Exp Ther 1993; 264: 327–335.

71. Narchi P, Benhamou D, Hamza J, et al: Ventilatory effects of epidural clonidine during the first 3 hours after caesarean section. Acta Anaesthesiol Scand 1992; 36: 791–795.

72. De Kock M, Crochet B, Morimont C, et al: Intravenous or epidural clonidine for intra- and postoperative analgesia. Anesthesiology 1993; 79: 525–531.

73. Penn RD, Savoy SM, Corcos D, et al: Intrathecal baclofen for severe spinal spasticity. N Engl J Med 1989; 320: 1517–1521.

74. Nishi S, Minota S, Karczmar AG: Primary afferent neurones: the ionic mechanism of GABA-mediated depolarization. Neuropharmacology 1974; 13: 215–219.

75. Goodchild CS, Serrao JM: Intrathecal midazolam in the rat: evidence for spinally-mediated analgesia. Br J Anaesth 1987; 59: 1563–1570.

76. Sawynok J: GABAergic mechanisms of analgesia: an update. Pharmacol Biochem Behav 1987; 26: 463–474.

77. Serrao JM, Marks RL, Morley SJ, et al: Intrathecal midazolam for the treatment of chronic mechanical low back pain: a controlled comparison with epidural steroid in a pilot study. Pain 1992; 48: 5–12.

78. Yaksh TL, Dirksen R, Harty GJ: Antinociceptive effects of intrathecally injected cholinomimetic drugs in the rat and cat. Eur J Pharmacol 1985; 117: 81–88.

79. Dirksen R, Nijhuis GM: The relevance of cholinergic transmission at the spinal level to opiate effectiveness. Eur J Pharmacol 1983; 91: 215–221.

80. Gordh T Jr, Jansson I, Hartvig P, et al: Interactions between noradrenergic and cholinergic mechanisms involved in spinal nociceptive processing. Acta Anaesthesiol Scand 1989; 33: 39–47.

81. Abram SE, Winne RP: Intrathecal acetyl cholinesterase inhibitors produce analgesia that is synergistic with morphine and clonidine in rats. Anesth Analg 1995; 81: 501–507.

82. Takahashi H, Buccafusco JJ: The sympathoexcitatory response following selective activation of a spinal cholinergic system in anesthetized rats. J Auton Nerv Syst 1991; 34: 59–67.

83. Williams JS, Tong C, Eisenach JC: Neostigmine counteracts spinal clonidine-induced hypotension in sheep. Anesthesiology 1993; 78: 301–307.

84. Meynadier J, Chrubasik J, Dubar M, et al: Intrathecal somatostatin in terminally ill patients. A report of two cases. Pain 1985; 23: 9–12.

85. Chrubasik J, Meynadier J, Scherpereel P, et al: The effect of epidural somatostatin on postoperative pain. Anesth Analg 1985; 64: 1085–1088.

86. Gaumann DM, Yaksh TL, Post C, et al: Intrathecal somatostatin in cat and mouse studies on pain, motor behavior, and histopathology. Anesth Analg 1989; 68: 623–632.

87. Mollenholt P, Post C, Rawal N, et al: Antinociceptive and neurotoxic' actions of somatostatin in rat spinal cord after intrathecal administration. Pain 1988; 32: 95–105.

88. Penn RD, Paice JA, Kroin JS: Octreotide: a potent new nonopiate analgesic for intrathecal infusion. Pain 1992; 49: 13–19.

89. Sawynok J, Sweeney MI, White TD: Classification of adenosine receptors mediating antinociception in the rat spinal cord. Br J Pharmacol 1986; 88: 923–930.

90. DeLander GE, Hopkins CJ: Spinal adenosine modulates descending antinociceptive pathways stimulated by morphine. J Pharmacol Exp Ther 1986; 239: 88–93.

91. Sweeney MI, White TD, Sawynok J: Involvement of adenosine in the spinal antinociceptive effects of morphine and noradrenaline. J Pharmacol Exp Ther 1987; 243: 657–665.

92. Jurna I: Cyclic nucleotides and aminophylline produce different effects on nociceptive motor and sensory responses in the rat spinal cord. Naunyn Schmiedebergs Arch Pharmacol 1984; 327: 23–30.

93. Yaksh TL, Sosnowski M, Sabbe M, et al: Spinal modulation of pain input. Adv Pain Res Ther 1989; 11: 291–310.

94. Malliani A: Cardiovascular sympathetic afferent fibers. Rev Physiol Biochem Pharmacol 1982; 94: 11–17.

95. Perl ER: Is pain a specific sensation? J Psychiatr Res 1971; 8: 273–287.

96. Raja SN, Meyer RA, Campbell JN: Peripheral mechanisms of somatic pain. Anesthesiology 1988; 68: 571–590.

97. Lynn B: The detection of injury and tissue damage. In Wall PD, Melzack R (eds): Textbook of Pain, pp 19–33. New York, Churchill Livingstone, 1984.

98. Burgess PR, Clark FJ: Characteristics of knee joint receptors in the cat. J Physiol (Lond) 1969; 203: 317–335.

99. Ferreira SH, Nakamura M: I—Prostaglandin hyperalgesia, a cAMP/Ca^{2+} dependent process. Prostaglandins 1979; 18: 179–190.

100. Terenius L: Biochemical mediators in pain. Triangle 1981; 20: 19–26.

101. Hargreaves KM, Loris JL: The peripheral analgesic effects of opioids. Am Pain Soc J 1993; 2: 51–59.

102. Stein C, Comisel K, Haimerl E, et al: Analgesic effect of intraarticular morphine after arthroscopic knee surgery. N Engl J Med 1991; 325: 1123–1126.

103. Raja S, Dickstein R, Johnson C: Intra-articular bupivacaine and morphine: comparison of analgesia following arthroscopic knee surgery. (Abstract.) Am Pain Soc J 1991; 10: 137.

104. Yaksh TL: Substance P release from knee joint afferent terminals: modulation by opioids. Brain Res 1988; 458: 319–324.

105. Devor M, Wall PD, Catalan N: Systemic lidocaine silences ectopic neuroma and DRG discharge without blocking nerve conduction. Pain 1992; 48: 261–268.

106. Tanelian DL, MacIver MB: Analgesic concentrations of lidocaine suppress tonic A-delta and C fiber discharges produced by acute injury. Anesthesiology 1991; 74: 934–936.

107. Blumberg H, Janig W: Discharge pattern of afferent fibers from a neuroma. Pain 1984; 20: 335–353.

108. Devor M, Janig W: Activation of myelinated afferents ending in a neuroma by stimulation of the sympathetic supply in the rat. Neurosci Lett 1981; 24: 43–47.

109. Chabal C, Jacobson L, Russell LC, et al: Pain response to perineuromal injection of normal saline, epinephrine, and lidocaine in humans. Pain 1992; 49: 9–12.

110. Devor M: Nerve pathophysiology and mechanisms of pain in causalgia. J Auton Nerv Syst 1983; 7: 371–384.

111. Devor M, Govrin-Lippmann R: Axoplasmic transport block reduces ectopic impulse generation in injured peripheral nerves. Pain 1983; 16: 73–85.

112. Yamamoto T, Yaksh TL: Effects of colchicine applied to the peripheral nerve on the thermal hyperalgesia evoked with chronic nerve constriction. Pain 1993; 55: 227–233.

113. Abram SE, Yaksh TL: Systemic lidocaine blocks nerve injury-induced hyperalgesia and nociceptor-driven spinal sensitization in the rat. Anesthesiology 1994; 80: 383–391.

114. Bach FW, Jensen TS, Kastrup J, et al: The effect of intravenous lidocaine on nociceptive processing in diabetic neuropathy. Pain 1990; 40: 29–34.

115. Boas RA, Covino BG, Shahnarian A: Analgesic responses to i.v. lignocaine. Br J Anaesth 1982; 54: 501–505.

116. Marchettini P, Lacerenza M, Marangoni C, et al: Lidocaine test in neuralgia. Pain 1992; 48: 377–382.

117. Brose WG, Cousins MJ: Subcutaneous lidocaine for treatment of neuropathic cancer pain. Pain 1991; 45: 145–148.

118. Chabal C, Russell LC, Burchiel KJ: The effect of intravenous lidocaine, tocainide, and mexiletine on spontaneously active fibers originating in rat sciatic neuromas. Pain 1989; 38: 333–338.

119. Dejgard A, Petersen P, Kastrup J: Mexiletine for treatment of chronic painful diabetic neuropathy. Lancet 1988; 1: 9–11.

120. Devor M, Govrin-Lippmann R, Raber P: Corticosteroids suppress ectopic neural discharge originating in experimental neuromas. Pain 1985; 22: 127–137.

CHAPTER 41

Benign Pain

John M. De Sio, M.D., Carol A. Warfield, M.D.,
Cynthia Kahn, M.D.

The knowledge of anatomy and pain physiology and skill in techniques of regional blocks used for surgical procedures are directly applicable to the understanding and management of chronic pain. As the role of the anesthesiologist has expanded beyond the operating suite to include the pain management center, so have the opportunities to apply these special skills and knowledge in new and beneficial ways. The use of regional techniques as part of a multimodal interdisciplinary approach to the diagnosis and treatment of chronic benign pain syndromes is discussed in this chapter.

Sympathetically Maintained Pain

Sympathetically maintained pain is one of several terms that have been used to describe a syndrome frequently observed in pain clinic patients. Initially referred to as causalgia,[1] other terms such as posttrau-matic pain syndrome, Sudeck's atrophy, algodystrophy, sympathetically maintained pain, sympathalgia, reflex sympathetic dystrophy, and traumatic vasospasm were developed to describe more accurately the hyperhidrosis, edema, temperature change, and atrophy of skin appendages that commonly occur in these patients. The lack of a single descriptive term reflects the diversity of the classic features of the syndrome. More commonly, patients have hyperalgesia and allodynia with pain of a burning quality.

Several hypotheses have been proposed to explain the pathophysiology of sympathetically maintained pain. Sudeck[2, 3] postulated that the syndrome was caused by an exaggerated inflammatory response to an injury. Roberts[4] proposed that sympathetically maintained pain resulted from tonic activity in myelinated mechanoreceptor afferent fibers. He speculated that this activity was induced by sympathetic efferent actions on sensory receptors. A peripheral nervous system abnormality involving α_1-adrenoreceptors has also

Table 41–1 Phases of Sympathetically Maintained Pain

PHASE (mo)	PAIN	OBJECTIVE FINDINGS
Acute (0–3)	Persistent, localized, worsened by movement, emotional disturbances, or visual or auditory stimuli; burning, aching pain with hyperpathia, hyperalgesia, and allodynia	Increased skin blood flow and temperature, hyperhidrosis, edema, increased hair growth, dependent rubor
Dystrophic (3–12)	Spreads proximally or distally, not dermatomal; hyperpathia more evident	Edema spreads proximally and becomes brawny; skin is cool, pale, cyanotic, and dry; muscle atrophy, decreased hair growth, cracked brittle nails, increased joint thickness with decreased range of motion, osteoporosis
Atrophic (>12)	Pain may involve other body parts, usually intractable	Progressive atrophy of skin, muscle, bone, and joints; pale, cyanotic skin with decreased temperature; irreversible trophic changes; smooth, glossy skin, stiff fixed joints, wasted muscles, contractures

been described[5] to explain the spontaneous pain observed in patients with sympathetically maintained pain. Although the complete pathophysiology of sympathetically maintained pain is unknown, it is widely accepted that changes occur at the spinal cord level that induce the continuous cycle of pain and the persistent signs of sympathetic hyperactivity of this painful syndrome.

Evaluation of a patient with suspected sympathetically maintained pain may be difficult. Depending on the duration of pain, the presenting symptoms can range from slight edema with an increase in skin temperature over the painful area to a completely contracted extremity with severe muscle wasting and intractable pain. Classically, sympathetically maintained pain has been divided into three phases (Table 41–1).

Traditionally, the diagnosis of sympathetically maintained pain is made empirically by using the presenting clinical features and the observed response to sympathetic blocks. In an attempt to hone the diagnostic criteria for sympathetically maintained pain, Veldman and colleagues[6] initiated a prospective study of 829 patients who presented with various features of sympathetically maintained pain. They concluded that patients should present with four of five signs or symptoms of unexplained diffuse pain, a difference in skin color or temperature relative to the other limb, and diffuse edema or limited range of motion before the diagnosis of sympathetically maintained pain is made. The occurrence of or increase in any of these signs or symptoms after use and the presence of signs or symptoms in an area larger than the area of primary injury are required for the diagnosis of this syndrome. Some of the testing modalities for these patients are listed in Table 41–2.

Block of efferent sympathetic fibers is a commonly used therapy in the treatment of sympathetically maintained pain. Temporary or permanent sympatholysis using local anesthetic or neurolytic agents, surgical sympathectomy, and orally or parenterally administered α-adrenergic blocking agents have been used to provide sympatholysis (Table 41–3).

Stellate Ganglion Block

Stellate ganglion blocks are most commonly indicated for the treatment of sympathetically maintained pain involving the head, neck, and upper extremities. The stellate ganglion is formed by the union of the

Table 41–2 Tests Used in Diagnosing Sympathetically Maintained Pain

Intravenous administration of phentolamine
Sympathetic block
Triple-phase bone scan (useful only in early, hyperemic phase)
Thermography
Sympathogalvanic skin response
Plethysmography
Xenon clearance test

Table 41–3 Therapeutic Modalities for Sympathetically Maintained Pain

BLOCK THERAPIES	SUPPLEMENTAL THERAPIES
Stellate ganglion block	α-Adrenergic blockers (phentolamine, prazosin)
Epidural or intrathecal block	Tricyclic antidepressants
Intravenous regional block (bretylium)	Physical therapy to decrease incidence of disuse atrophy
Lumbar sympathetic block	TENS therapy
Superior hypogastric plexus block	Spinal cord stimulation
Impar ganglion block	
Radiofrequency sympatholysis	
Surgical sympathectomy	

TENS, transcutaneous electrical nerve stimulation.

inferior cervical ganglion and the first thoracic ganglion (Fig. 41–1).

Usually, a paratracheal technique is used at a level slightly cephalad to the stellate ganglion to decrease the risk of a pneumothorax developing. With the patient in the supine position, a roll is placed between the scapulae to promote extension of the head. With the head rotated to the side opposite the block, the anesthesiologist's index and middle fingers are used to palpate the anterior tubercle of the transverse process of C-6 (Chassaignac's tubercle). This landmark is located medial to the carotid pulse and lateral to the trachea at the level of the cricoid cartilage. After a skin wheal is raised, a 22- to 25-G, 3-cm needle is advanced until it contacts the bony tubercle. The needle is then withdrawn 2 mm and secured at the skin. After a negative aspiration result, a test dose of 2 mL of local anesthetic is injected in 0.5-mL increments. After proper needle position is confirmed, a total of 10 to 15 mL of local anesthetic is injected in increments of 3 mL, with intermittent aspirations. Immediately after the injection, the patient assumes a sitting position to promote spread of the local anesthetic along the thoracic sympathetic

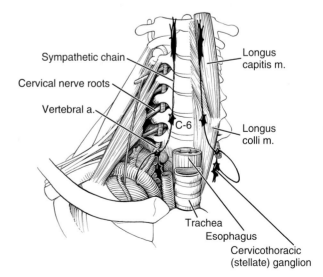

Figure 41–1 Stellate ganglion. Notice the proximity of the sympathetic trunk to the vertebral artery (a.) and the cervical nerve roots. m., muscle.

chain. An increase in arm temperature confirms the effectiveness of the sympathetic block.

Typical side effects include temporary hoarseness, feeling of a lump in the throat, and Horner's syndrome (i.e., miosis, ptosis, and enophthalmos). Complications include hematoma, pneumothorax, and brachial plexus or phrenic nerve block. Other complications include vertebral artery injection (less than 0.5 mL of 1% lidocaine can cause seizure) and epidural or intrathecal injection, which can result in a "high spinal."

Lumbar Sympathetic Block

A lumbar sympathetic block is often performed for the treatment of sympathetically maintained pain involving the pelvis or lower extremities. The lumbar sympathetic chain lies at the anterolateral aspect of the vertebral bodies, separated from the somatic nerves by the psoas muscle and its fascia (Fig. 41–2).

With the patient in the prone position, a pillow is placed beneath the abdomen to help attenuate the patient's lumbar lordosis. A skin wheal is raised 7 to 8 cm lateral to the spinous process of L-2, and a 20- to 22-G, 15-cm needle is advanced in a cephalomesiad direction until bone is contacted (in a three-needle technique, the procedure is performed at the L-2, L-3, and L-4 levels). The needle is then withdrawn and redirected until its tip lies at the anterolateral border of the vertebral body of L-2. After a negative result of aspiration for blood, a confirmatory test dose of 3 mL of 1% lidocaine with 1:200,000 epinephrine is injected. After a negative response to the test dose, a total of 15 to 30 mL of local anesthetic is injected incrementally. An increase in leg temperature confirms an effective sympathetic block. If the patient obtains significant or complete pain relief from the block, sympathetically maintained pain is thought to play a primary role in the patient's pain syndrome. Occasionally, the relief lasts only the duration of the local anesthetic. If this

occurs after repeated intermittent blocks, a catheter can be inserted percutaneously to provide prolonged interruption of the sympathetic nerves at this level.

Perforation of the aorta, vena cava, and kidney can occur during this procedure, as can somatic nerve root block at one or more levels. Hypotension can also occur but is more frequently observed when the block is performed bilaterally. Trauma to the nerve root, most often the L-1 root, can appear at presentation to be a genitofemoral neuralgia. An intrathecal, epidural, or intradiskal injection can occur, causing sensory and motor block, increased pain, and possibly infection.

Intravenous Regional Block

Hannington-Kiff[7] first described the successful use of intravenous regional injection of guanethidine for the treatment of causalgia. Ford and colleagues[8] looked at intravenous regional injection of bretylium (an adrenergic blocking agent with actions similar to guanethidine) for the treatment of sympathetically maintained pain. They observed that bretylium provided good to excellent pain relief that lasted up to 7 mo after treatment. They also found that bretylium was associated with fewer side effects (hypotension, diarrhea) compared with guanethidine (Fig. 41–3).

While the patient's electrocardiogram and blood pressure are continually monitored, two intravenous catheters are placed, one in any limb and the other in the distal part of the affected extremity. The painful extremity is then elevated for 2 min to promote venous drainage. A double pneumatic cuff is placed proximally and inflated to a minimum pressure of 100 mm Hg above the patient's systolic pressure. A solution containing 0.5% lidocaine (60 mL for the lower extremity and 40 mL for the upper extremity) with bretylium (2 mg/kg) is injected intravenously into the affected extremity. Pain scores are assessed every 10 min during

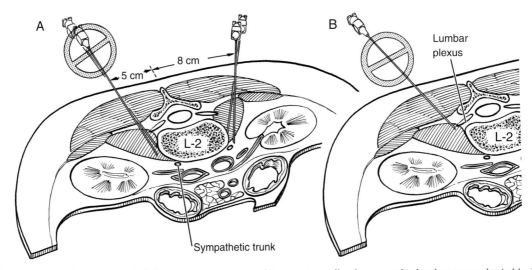

Figure 41–2 Cross-sectional anatomy at L-2 demonstrates correct and incorrect needle placement for lumbar sympathetic block. *A*, The needle enters the skin too close to the midline (5 cm) and cannot get past the lateral vertebral body to reach the sympathetic trunk. The final needle position is too lateral and within the psoas muscle. The opposite needle enters the skin 8 cm from the midline, a more favorable approach to slide past the vertebral body and achieve a satisfactory position in the area of the sympathetic trunk. *B*, The needle placement is too superficial, within the psoas muscle and near the lumbar plexus.

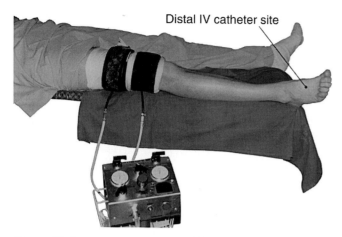
Distal IV catheter site

Figure 41–3 Intravenous (IV) regional bretylium block. The double pneumatic cuff is placed proximally after a distal intravenous catheter is placed in the affected extremity.

and up to 30 min after the block. The cuffs are deflated slowly 25 to 30 min after the injection.

Complications primarily result from early or unintentional release of pressure from the cuffs. A bolus of bretylium results in an initial hypertensive response, reflecting release of norepinephrine. These effects are short lived and are followed by a period of orthostatic hypotension as a result of the chemically induced sympathetic block. Gastrointestinal and central nervous system effects are minimal owing to the quaternary structure of bretylium. Systemic local anesthetic effects may also occur during premature cuff release.

Herpes Zoster

Herpes zoster results from reactivation of the varicella-zoster virus that lies dormant in the dorsal root ganglia of patients who have previously had chickenpox. The virus is most often reactivated in patients who experience a decline in immunity. The most common causes for the decrease in immunity are a severe infection, malignancy, and an iatrogenically introduced immunosuppressant. The chance of herpes zoster developing also increases with increasing age.

Acute Herpes Zoster

A patient with acute herpes zoster usually presents with pain localized to the dermatomal distribution of one or more affected posterior root ganglia. Eruptions along the dermatomes involved appear 4 to 5 d after the onset of pain and persist for 2 to 3 wk. Pain may be mild at first but can progress in severity and location. It usually is described as a sharp, shooting, burning pain that is made worse by any tactile stimulus. Overall, the acute phase of herpes zoster can last 3 to 4 wk, and in otherwise healthy individuals, it resolves without sequelae.

Postherpetic Neuralgia

Postherpetic neuralgia is a protracted syndrome of severe pain that develops after the resolution of an acute herpes zoster infection. Its occurrence in patients who have had herpes zoster is estimated to be between 7% and 55%,[9] with the chance of postherpetic neuralgia developing increasing with age; 50% of patients older than age 60 years with acute herpes zoster develop postherpetic neuralgia.

Typically, two types of pain occur simultaneously. A continuous, aching burning pain is associated with dysesthesia, and the patient becomes extremely sensitive to touch in the affected areas. Concomitantly, a feeling of tightness is accompanied by an itching sensation that also occurs along the dermatomes involved.[10]

Treatment

Sympathetic Block

Sympathetic block alone or in combination with a somatic nerve block early after the onset of pain or eruptions can provide prompt pain relief in patients with acute herpes zoster. Sympathetic blocks also appear to decrease the severity and duration of the eruptions and accelerate healing.[11] Blocks are performed each day for 5 to 7 d, depending on the response observed. If a positive response occurs, the blocks are repeated three times each week until the pain resolves.

A stellate ganglion block is indicated when herpes zoster involves an upper thoracic, cervical, or trigeminal nerve distribution. Although zoster does not often involve the lumbar or sacral roots, when it does, lumbar sympathetic blocks can be performed early in the disease process in an attempt to provide lasting pain relief. If these blocks are done within 5 to 7 d of the development of eruptions, they may decrease the incidence of postherpetic neuralgia by at least 30%.[11]

Somatic Nerve Block

Prolonged pain relief can be achieved after a somatic nerve block, which usually outlasts the duration of the local anesthetic used. These blocks are usually performed at the brachial plexus and intercostal, paravertebral, and sciatic nerves in patients with acute herpes zoster. The blocks appear to provide little benefit if done during the postherpetic phase of the disease.[12]

Epidural administration of local anesthetic has been successful in providing pain relief in patients with acute herpes zoster, in shortening the duration of the eruption, and in causing lesions to dry faster.[12] To treat patients with acute herpes zoster or postherpetic neuralgia, an epidural catheter is placed at the appropriate dermatomal level, and local anesthetic is injected daily for 3 to 5 d. The catheter is then removed, and the patient is assessed to determine the efficacy of the blocks. If some pain persists, two to three additional epidural injections can be done in conjunction with starting adjunctive therapies such as tricyclic antidepressants and nonsteroidal anti-inflammatory drugs (NSAIDs).

Intralesional Injection

Infiltration of local anesthetic and a locally acting steroid has been used for years to provide pain relief for patients with acute herpes zoster. Epstein[13] first reported the benefits of daily subcutaneous injections of 0.2% triamcinolone mixed with procaine for 5 to 13 d. More often, a combination of 1% lidocaine and 4 mg/mL of triamcinolone is administered into the subcutaneous tissue at the base of the vesicle in patients who fail to respond to a trial of sympathetic nerve blocks. These injections can be repeated daily during a 2-wk period or until a significant improvement is observed.

Other modalities available to treat acute herpes zoster include acyclovir given orally, topical application of a eutectic mixture of local anesthetics (EMLA cream), steroids given orally, and transcutaneous electrical nerve stimulation (TENS) therapy. Adjunctive therapies used in treating postherpetic neuralgia are topical application of capsaicin or NSAIDs and tricyclic antidepressants.

Myofascial Pain Syndrome

Myofascial pain syndrome is characterized by steady, aching muscle pain at multiple sites (usually more than three) and is often associated with nonrestorative sleep, morning stiffness, chronic fatigue, depression, decreased range of motion, and trigger points. A trigger point is a hyperirritable spot within a taut band of skeletal muscle or fascia. On compression of a trigger point, the patient experiences an increase in pain, often with spread to a larger area.[14] If untreated, the patient with myofascial pain syndrome may experience periods of exacerbation and remission of symptoms, with a gradual decline in physical capacity, loss of range of motion, and occasional sympathetic dysfunction. Other terms used to describe myofascial pain include fibromyalgia, fibrositis, muscular rheumatism, myalgia, myositis, myofibrositis, and myofascitis.

Myofascial pain can occur after acute, traumatic muscle injury or chronic muscle fatigue and overuse, or it may be associated with other chronic pain syndromes such as facet syndrome, failed laminectomy syndrome, and post-thoracotomy syndrome. The mechanism of onset is unclear, but one theory[15] proposes that injury to the muscle results in rupture of the sarcoplasmic reticulum and release of calcium, which causes sustained muscle contraction in the area of injury. The sustained contraction of the muscle fibers depletes adenosine triphosphate to a critical level, leading to ischemia and release of kinins, histamine, and prostaglandins. These chemical mediators lower the threshold for transmission of nociceptive impulses to the central nervous system, which results in increased muscle tension, sympathetic activity, and local ischemia. The patient experiences more muscle spasm and pain, and the cycle of pain, spasm, and more pain begins.

The first line of therapy is to inactivate trigger points by full stretching of the involved muscles. Travell and Simons[14] described a technique of using a vapocoolant spray before beginning muscle stretching and active range of motion exercises. The patient should perform the "spray and stretch" therapy three times each day, increasing the number of repetitions per session of the range of motion exercises and the number of sessions as tolerated.

Dry needling and injection of sterile water, saline, local anesthetic, and steroid have provided some benefit to patients with myofascial pain syndrome.[16] We prefer to inject the trigger point with local anesthetic, with or without the addition of steroid, to provide analgesia, relax the muscle, and increase blood flow to the area. The addition of steroid is advocated by some for its potent anti-inflammatory effect (Fig. 41-4).

The first step in the technique for injecting trigger points is to identify and mark them with a skin marker. The skin is cleaned with alcohol before injection. A sterile 22- or 25-G, 2.5- to 4-cm needle is attached to a syringe filled with 1% lidocaine or 0.25% bupivacaine. The physician calculates the toxic dose of local anesthetic and does not exceed that dose. A steroid such as triamcinolone (2 mg/mL) may be added to the local anesthetic. The patient may notice an increase in pain when the needle is inserted into the trigger point. The anesthesiologist injects 1 to 2 mL into each trigger point and assesses the degree of pain relief obtained. If the area is still painful, an additional 1 to 2 mL of local anesthetic is injected into the painful area. The physician then reassesses the myoneural block efficacy.

Once comfortable, the patient should begin a gentle physical therapy regimen. This may consist of ultra-

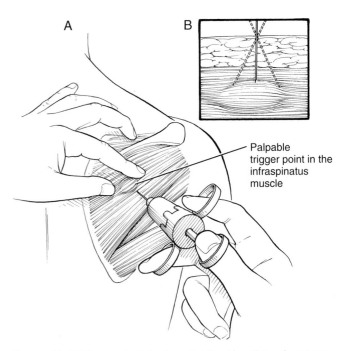

Palpable trigger point in the infraspinatus muscle

Figure 41-4 Trigger point injection. *A,* After identifying the trigger point and disinfecting the skin, a 25-G, 5-cm needle attached to a 10-mL syringe containing local anesthetic solution is advanced slowly toward the trigger point. As the needle approaches the trigger area, the patient experiences more local and referred pain and tenderness, and this experience is further aggravated during the injection of the local anesthetic solution. It is best to perform a fan-like injection by repeatedly withdrawing the needle and redirecting it as shown in the inset *(B).* (Modified from Bonica JJ [ed]: The Management of Pain. Philadelphia, Lea & Febiger, 1953.)

sound with electrical stimulation as tolerated for 15 min over the tender muscles, followed by heat application and limbering exercises. This regimen should be continued for the first 4 d after trigger point injection. The patient can then begin active stretching and strengthening exercises. NSAIDs, tricyclic antidepressants, and skeletal muscle relaxants may be used as supplemental therapy.

Complications after trigger point injections are rare. However, local anesthetic systemic toxicity is possible, as is pneumothorax when the trapezius muscle and other thoracic sites are treated.

Head and Neck Pain

Headache

Management of patients with intractable headaches is challenging. A thorough history should focus on the headache pattern, precipitating factors, associated sensory disturbances, and any coexisting symptoms. Details about the age at onset of the headaches as well as the quality, frequency, and duration of a typical headache can aid in making the correct diagnosis. A list should be made of over-the-counter and prescription medications the patient has taken and is currently using.

The physical examination should include vital signs, evaluation of the head and neck for trigger points, and palpation of bony prominences for point tenderness. A complete neurologic examination is conducted to look specifically for focal signs of neurologic disease. Funduscopic and otoscopic inspection should also be performed to eliminate the possibility of an underlying infectious or inflammatory cause of the headaches.

Although most types of headaches are treated with combinations of medications (Table 41–4), some causes of headache or head pain are amenable to nerve blocks.

Occipital Nerve Block

Occipital nerve block is indicated for the treatment of headaches resulting from occipital neuralgia. The occipital nerves are sensory branches of the C-2 and C-3 nerve roots. The headaches usually start in the occipital region but can radiate to other areas of the head and face (Fig. 41–5).

With the patient seated and the patient's neck flexed, the occiput is examined for a tender area along the nuchal ridge where the greater occipital nerve perforates the muscles of the neck midway between the mastoid process and the occipital protuberance. After a tender area is located, a 25-G, 3-cm needle is advanced until bone is contacted. After a negative aspiration result, 3 to 5 mL of 0.25% bupivacaine with 4 mg/mL of triamcinolone is injected. Pressure is then applied with a gauze pad to the injection site until the wheal resolves. Complications include infection and bleeding.

Most patients with occipital neuralgia obtain good, lasting pain relief from occipital nerve block. However, the block may have to be repeated before this occurs.

Sphenopalatine Ganglion Block

Indications for performing a sphenopalatine ganglion block include treating painful disorders of the head and facial regions.[17–20] A sphenopalatine ganglion block using 4% lidocaine has been as effective as cocaine in relieving pain from cluster headaches[21] (Fig. 41–6).

With the patient in the semireclined position, a cotton-tipped applicator soaked with 4% lidocaine is passed gently through the naris at an angle perpendicular to the coronal plane. The applicator is advanced until light contact is made with the nasopharynx posterior to the inferior turbinate. The procedure is then repeated through the naris at a more vertical angle so that contact is made behind the middle turbinate. Bilateral blocks are often used. Pledgets are left in place for 15 to 20 min, with the patient in the supine position.[22] Usually, the block is performed every other day for 1 wk and then three times each week for the next 2 wk in an attempt to provide lasting pain relief. The applicator is never forced, and a unilateral approach can be used if desired.

Adverse effects include bleeding, infection, local anesthetic systemic toxicity, and possibly a "high spinal" if the cribriform plate is entered by applying excessive pressure while inserting the applicator.

Facial Pain

Facial pain can be the result of many different conditions. In most cases, the cause can be readily determined (e.g., toothache, localized infection, or herpes zoster). However, with the complex anatomy of the face, the correct diagnosis can sometimes be difficult to make. It is important to obtain an accurate history of the facial pain, descriptors, intensity, and location, because this information may be sufficient to make the proper diagnosis. Aggravating factors such as chewing, talking, and swallowing should also be sought, because they may point to an underlying mechanical problem. Neurologic abnormalities should be assessed. The muscles of the face should be examined for trigger points

Table 41–4 Headache Syndromes and Common Medical Therapies

CHRONIC HEADACHE SYNDROMES	THERAPEUTIC OR PROPHYLACTIC AGENTS
Migraine	NSAIDs
Migraine with aura	Metoclopramide
Tension-type headache	β-Blockers
Cluster headache	Calcium channel antagonists
Chronic paroxysmal hemicrania	Serotonin antagonists (methysergide)
Posttraumatic headache	Serotonin agonists (sumatriptan)
Subacute headache (temporal arteritis, carotidynia, postendarterectomy headache)	Tricyclic antidepressants Ergotamine tartrate or caffeine Dihydroergotamine
Cranial neuralgias	Sodium valproate

NSAIDs, nonsteroidal anti-inflammatory drugs.

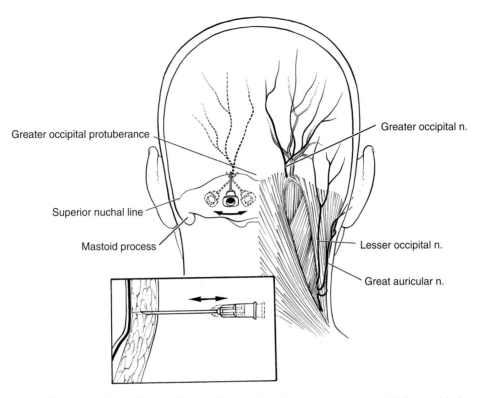

Figure 41–5 Greater occipital nerve (n.) block. The needle insertion site for performing a greater occipital nerve block is approximately midway between the mastoid process and the occipital protuberance on the affected side. *Inset,* After bone is contacted, the needle is slightly withdrawn before injection.

and evidence of nerve entrapment. Lesions on the skin should be documented, and evidence of hyperalgesia and allodynia should be sought, because hyperalgesia and allodynia may be early signs of a sympathetic or neuropathic origin of pain.

Gasserian Ganglion Block

Gasserian ganglion block (Fig. 41–7) is indicated for the diagnosis and treatment of trigeminal neuralgias. A 22-G, 10-cm needle is introduced, through an anterior

approach, 2.5 cm lateral to the corner of the mouth on the painful side and just medial to the masseter muscle. The needle is directed posteriorly and medially while the anesthesiologist keeps a finger in the patient's mouth to ensure the needle does not perforate the oral mucosa. The needle is advanced until it contacts the infratemporal fossa at the base of the skull. Next, the needle is walked off the bony surface until it slips into the foramen ovale. Many use fluoroscopic guidance for this procedure.

Once in the foramen, the needle is advanced 1 cm.

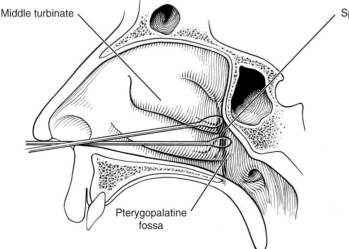

Figure 41–6 Sphenopalatine ganglion block. (Modified from Waldman SD: Evaluation and treatment of common headache and facial pain syndrome. In Raj PP: Practical Management of Pain, 2nd ed, pp 198–218. St. Louis, Mosby–Year Book, 1992.)

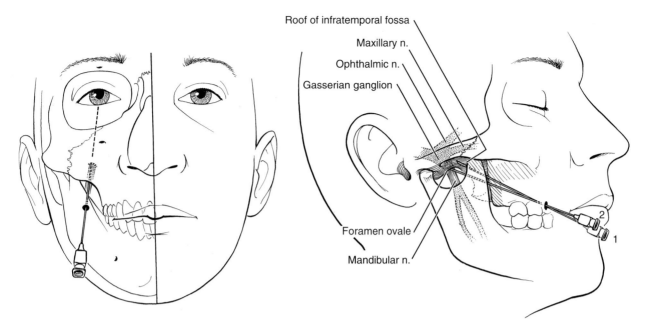

Roof of infratemporal fossa
Maxillary n.
Ophthalmic n.
Gasserian ganglion
Foramen ovale
Mandibular n.

Figure 41–7 Technique of gasserian ganglion block, showing the needle entry through foramen ovale into gasserian ganglion. The needle is withdrawn (1) and re-directed in a stepwise manner until foramen ovale is entered (2). If too medial, the needle may meet resistance from the pterygoid plate. If too posterior, the needle may penetrate a branch of the external carotid artery. n., nerve.

A paresthesia is usually elicited along one of the divisions of the trigeminal nerve. A paresthesia of the first or second division confirms needle placement in proximity to the gasserian ganglion. Aspiration is then attempted to exclude intravascular or intrathecal needle position.

After the proper position is confirmed, a diagnostic block is performed with 1% lidocaine administered in 0.25-mL increments until adequate pain relief is obtained. Some needle adjustment may be required. If the block is successful in providing pain relief, a neurolytic block with absolute alcohol can be performed after the same technique, although many refer these patients for thermocoagulation of the ganglion after the diagnosis is established.

If a neurolytic block is performed, an increase in pain usually occurs after the block and may last a few days. Bleeding and infection can also occur after a gasserian ganglion block. More serious complications may result from injection into the cerebrospinal fluid: unconsciousness and profound paralysis.

Blocks of the Divisions of the Trigeminal Nerve

Ophthalmic Nerve Block. The ophthalmic division of the trigeminal nerve is blocked by using the anterior approach to the foramen ovale. Once through the foramen, the needle is repositioned slightly until a paresthesia is obtained along the distribution of the ophthalmic nerve.

The branches of the ophthalmic nerve, the supraorbital nerve, and the supratrochlear nerve can be blocked to provide excellent analgesia of the forehead and scalp. The supraorbital nerve is located just superior to the orbit after the nerve exits the supraorbital foramen. A 25-G, 1.5-cm needle is used to contact the frontal bone at the junction of the medial and middle one third of the eyebrow on the painful side. After a negative aspiration result, 2 to 4 mL of 1% lidocaine is injected. An additional 2 mL of local anesthetic is deposited just medial to this area to block the supratrochlear nerve on the superomedial aspect of the orbit (Fig. 41–8).

Supraorbital and supratrochlear nerve blocks are associated with few adverse effects. Except for bleeding, infection, and a possible temporary increase in pain, the procedure is usually well tolerated.

Maxillary Nerve Block. This block is most commonly performed by using a lateral approach. With the patient in the supine position, a 22-G, 10-cm needle is inserted just inferior to the midpoint of the zygomatic arch. The needle is advanced medially through the coronoid notch of the mandible until it contacts the lateral pterygoid plate. It is walked anteriorly and cephalad to enter the pterygopalatine fossa, at which point a paresthesia of the maxillary nerve is usually obtained. After proper needle position is confirmed, 3 to 4 mL of 1% lidocaine is injected for diagnostic purposes. A hematoma occasionally occurs because of the vascularity in this region. Temporary blindness can also occur if the local anesthetic spreads proximally along the optic nerve.

Mandibular Nerve Block. The mandibular nerve is blocked by using an approach similar to that for the maxillary nerve. However, after the needle contacts the lateral pterygoid plate, it is walked posteriorly until a paresthesia of the mandibular nerve is obtained. After the proper needle position is confirmed and a negative result is obtained from aspiration, a diagnostic block is performed with 3 to 5 mL of 1% lidocaine. A hematoma may develop but is less likely to occur than after a maxillary nerve block. Temporary paralysis of the

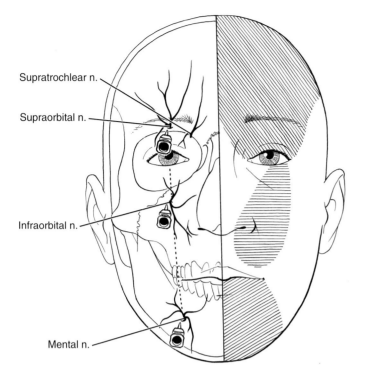

Supratrochlear n.

Supraorbital n.

Infraorbital n.

Mental n.

Figure 41–8 Technique of distal trigeminal nerve (n.) block. Notice the location of the foramen in the vertical plane through the corner of the mouth and pupil. Innervation by branches of these distal trigeminal nerves is shown on right side of face.

muscles of mastication can also occur, resulting in uncoordinated movements of the jaw.

Cervical or Radicular Strain

Nerve root irritation, myofascial dysfunction, arthritic conditions of the cervical spine, torticollis secondary to trauma or infection, and cancer in the head and neck region can cause neck pain. The therapies for each condition vary. When a history is taken from a patient with neck pain, it is important to determine the location of the pain and whether it radiates along a particular dermatome. The patient should be asked about associated signs and symptoms, such as headaches, limited range of motion in the neck, and sensory and motor deficits, that may coincide with the pain. Any initiating injuries that occurred at the onset of the pain should be discussed. The mechanism of the injury can reveal the underlying cause of pain; for example, whiplash or flexion-extension injuries are frequently associated with facet joint arthropathies.

Physical examination should include a complete neurologic assessment of the head, neck, and upper extremities. Any sensory or motor deficits as well as changes in skin color and temperature must be documented. If the pain began suddenly, radiographs should be made to eliminate the possibility of an underlying mechanical abnormality (e.g., fracture, dislocation, subluxation). Anteroposterior and lateral views should be made. A computed tomographic scan or magnetic resonance imaging of the cervical spine can be done to evaluate the intervertebral disks, nerve roots, facet joints, spinal cord, and thecal sac. If the evaluation fails to reveal any abnormalities, an electromyogram can be done to further clarify the continued complaint of neck pain. If the result is negative, a myofascial mechanism may be causative.

Cervical Epidural Injections of Steroids

Cervical epidural injections of steroids are primarily indicated for neck pain that occurs secondary to cervical disk disease. Pain from spinal stenosis causing foraminal narrowing or a preexisting arthritic condition may also be treatable with cervical epidural injections of steroids (Fig. 41–9).

With the patient in the sitting position, the patient's head is flexed to the chest. A 20-G, 5-cm winged needle or an 18-G, 10-cm Tuohy needle is placed at the appropriate (usually C-6 to C-7) interspace after the skin is anesthetized. The needle is advanced until it is firmly seated in the interspinous ligament. To use the "hanging drop" technique, the stylet of the needle is removed, and a drop of preservative-free saline is placed at the hub of the needle. The drop bulges outward owing to the firmness of the interspinous ligament. The wings of the needle should be held firmly between the fingertips, and the anesthesiologist's hands should be resting against the patient's shoulders. This allows a slow, smooth advance of the needle into the epidural space. When the epidural space is entered, the apparent negative pressure within the space causes the drop of saline at the hub of the needle to be drawn into the space. Alternatively, the "loss of resistance" technique to saline or air may be used. If no cerebrospinal fluid or blood is aspirated, 5 to 7 mL of saline or local anesthetic mixed with 50 mg of methylprednisolone or 80 mg of triamcinolone is injected. If partial improvement occurs, the patient may undergo another cervical epidural injection of steroid in 10 to 14 d. If

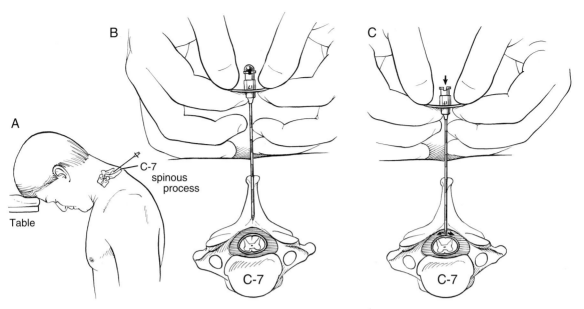

Figure 41–9 Cervical epidural steroid injection. *A,* While in the sitting position, the patient rests his forehead on the edge of a table to accentuate the cervical interspinous space. *B,* With both hands firmly resting on the back of the neck, the needle is slowly advanced until *(C)* the hanging drop is "sucked into" the needle and into the epidural space.

there is no improvement, the patient should consider other conservative therapy or surgical therapy.

Complications can occur, including a transient increase in neck pain and a spinal headache from dural puncture. Less often, epidural abscess,[23] hematoma,[24] and meningitis[25] have been reported.

Trigger Point Injections

Trigger point injections are indicated when a myofascial mechanism is suspected as the cause of neck pain.

Deep Cervical Plexus Block

The deep cervical plexus block is a useful anesthetic technique for surgical anesthesia and may be of some benefit in the diagnosis of vague neck discomfort[26] (Fig. 41–10).

With the patient placed in the supine position, the head is rotated opposite to the side to be blocked. The tip of the mastoid process and the transverse process of C-6 (Chassaignac's tubercle) are located, and a line is drawn connecting the landmarks. The transverse processes of C-2, C-3, and C-4 are located 1 cm posterior to this line and approximately 1.5 cm from each other. A 22-G, 5-cm needle is used to contact the transverse process of C-2 in a mesiocaudad direction. The needle is re-directed inferiorly until a paresthesia is obtained. After a negative aspiration result, 3 to 4 mL of 1% lidocaine is injected, and the procedure is repeated at the other two levels. A single-needle technique using a larger volume of local anesthetic places the needle at C-4.[27]

Because of the proximity of the vertebral artery to the cervical plexus, the possibility exists of an intra-arterial injection of local anesthetic, which can cause seizures. Other possible complications include epidural or intrathecal injection, phrenic nerve block, and a sympathetic block resulting in Horner's syndrome.

Chronic Abdominal and Pelvic Pain

The origin of chronic abdominal pain and chronic pelvic pain can be difficult to diagnose owing to the complex innervation of the abdominal and pelvic viscera. A complete history and physical examination are necessary to narrow the differential diagnosis of what otherwise can be a confusing and misleading picture.

Evaluation and Diagnosis

Pain of visceral origin is usually described as crampy, achy, or colicky. It may radiate to other intra-abdominal or intrathoracic structures or be felt as diffuse abdominal pain. Systemic symptoms such as nausea, vomiting, sweating, or diarrhea may accompany the pain. Pain from deep somatic structures is described as sharp, intense, and well localized and less commonly is referred to other areas such as deep pelvic structures or the back. Abdominal wall pain is usually caused by a local ongoing process such as a nerve entrapment or a myofascial pain syndrome. A patient with postsurgical scar pain presents with a demarcated area of tenderness along a previous surgical scar. Often, the pain can be acutely exacerbated by tapping the scar, which may indicate an underlying neuroma. Other factors that are helpful in determining the cause of abdominal or pelvic pain are the severity, location, and duration of the pain.

What factors make the pain worse and what can be done to obtain pain relief? The answers to these questions direct the clinician to the proper diagnosis and render the expense and occasional danger of much

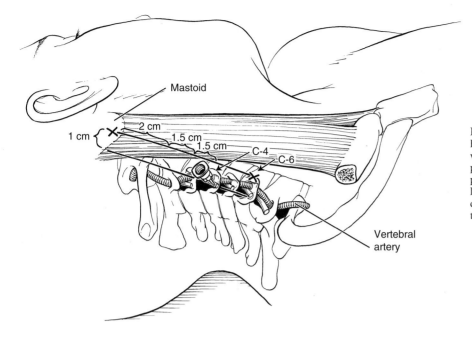

Figure 41–10 Cervical plexus block, highlighting the relationship between the vertebral artery and the deep cervical plexus. The needle insertion sites for performing this block typically lie along a line 1 cm below an imaginary line connecting the mastoid process with the transverse process of C-6.

investigation unnecessary in the patient with chronic, nonspecific abdominal or pelvic pain.

Rectus Entrapment Syndrome

Abdominal wall pain may be caused by rectus nerve entrapment syndrome or abdominal cutaneous nerve entrapment syndrome. Applegate[28] speculated that an area of point tenderness is produced by herniation of the neurovascular bundle through wide gaps in the rectus sheath. The pain is usually well localized at the exit site of the nerve from the muscle or occasionally may be widespread over the dermatome involved. The pain is described as achy, with intermittent periods of

severe, sharp pain of a burning quality. Lifting, turning, straining, or changes in position are frequently associated with increases in pain.[29] The feature that distinguishes nerve entrapment syndrome from pain of visceral origin is an immediate increase in tenderness that occurs with contraction of the abdominal musculature. Any of the intercostal nerves (T-7 to T-11) that traverse the rectus abdominis muscle may be involved in this syndrome (Fig. 41–11).

For diagnostic and therapeutic purposes, a 22-G, 3-cm needle is introduced into the point of maximal tenderness and 4 to 6 mL of 1% lidocaine and 4 mg/mL of triamcinolone are injected. Occasionally, pain relief can last for months, but the block usually must

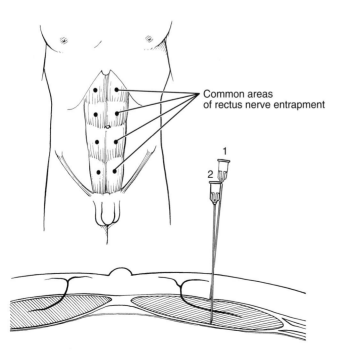

Figure 41–11 Rectus nerve entrapment block. Skin wheals are raised in the center of rectus segments. These are delineated by a vertical line through umbilicus and horizontal lines at the umbilical level and midway between the umbilicus and xiphisternum. A short-bevel needle contacts resistance of the anterior rectus sheath (1). The needle penetrates the rectus muscle and is halted by resistance of the posterior rectus sheath (2). The latter structure is absent below the line midway between the umbilicus and pubis. These two rectus injections are made last. (Modified from Thompson GE, Moore DC: Celiac plexus, intercostal, and minor peripheral blockade. In Cousins MJ, Bridenbaugh PO [eds]: Neural Blockade in Clinical Anesthesia and Management of Pain, 2nd ed, pp 503–530. Philadelphia, JB Lippincott, 1988.)

be repeated before lasting relief is achieved. Awareness of this condition and a proper evaluation of the abdominal wall are all that is needed to confirm or eliminate the presence of a cutaneous nerve entrapment syndrome.

Chronic Pancreatitis

Pain from chronic pancreatitis manifests as a constant, aching, sometimes burning sensation, often felt in the midepigastric area, that can radiate to the back. This condition generally occurs secondary to alcohol abuse but can also develop from a chronically obstructed pancreatic duct. It has been proposed that the pain results from either an increase in intraductal and intraparenchymal pancreatic pressure[30] or a neuritis of the sensory nerves that course through the inflamed pancreatic tissue.[31] Typically, the pain is made worse by eating, moving, or lying down and is improved by sitting or leaning forward. Some pain of varying intensity is always present. Acute attacks of pancreatitis can occur periodically and exacerbate the usual pain for days or weeks. When this occurs, a low thoracic epidural block with local anesthetic may provide adequate analgesia.[32]

Initial management includes an opioid and a nonopioid analgesic. Adjunctive medications such as tricyclic antidepressants, oral preparations of steroids, and enzyme therapy given orally[33] may also be helpful in providing pain relief. Endoscopic pancreatic stent placement may be successful in decompressing the ductal stenosis and providing pain relief.[34]

Although neurolytic celiac plexus blocks have been effective in relieving pain from pancreatic cancer,[35–37] results in patients with chronic pancreatitis have been disappointing. Because of the low long-term success rate and the risk of possible neurologic complications, neurolytic celiac plexus blocks are reserved, reluctantly, for patients with chronic pancreatitis who remain refractory to all other types of pain therapy.

Nerve Blocks

Celiac Plexus Blocks

The most common indication for a celiac plexus block is intractable pain secondary to pancreatic cancer or other upper gastrointestinal malignancy. Other painful conditions that may respond to a celiac plexus block include acute and chronic pancreatitis and some chronic benign abdominal pain syndromes[38] (Fig. 41–12).

Several approaches have been described for performing a celiac plexus block.[39–41] Typically, with the patient in the prone position, a 22-G, 15-cm needle is inserted approximately 7 to 8 cm lateral to the L-1 spinous process and immediately inferior to the 12th rib. The needle is advanced to contact the lateral aspect of the body of the L-1 vertebra; then the needle is withdrawn slightly and re-directed to graze the vertebral body. The needle is advanced to a point anterior to the anterior aspect of the L-1 vertebral body. The

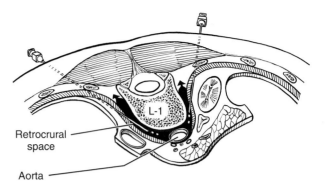

Figure 41–12 Celiac plexus block. The needle insertion site lies 7 to 8 cm lateral to the midline and immediately inferior to the 12th rib. After the needle contacts bone, it is repositioned to approximate the anterolateral aspect of the body of L-1.

procedure is repeated on the opposite side. With both needles in place and after a negative aspiration result is obtained, a test dose of 3 mL of 1% lidocaine is injected through each needle. After the test dose, a total of 15 to 25 mL of 1% lidocaine is injected on each side. If a positive diagnostic response occurs, the patient often returns the next day to undergo a neurolytic celiac plexus block. The neurolytic procedure is performed with 15 to 20 mL of 50% to 100% alcohol injected through each needle. Some practitioners are combining the diagnostic and neurolytic blocks in one procedure.

Diarrhea, hypotension, and occasionally a transient increase in pain can occur immediately after the block. Less frequently, kidney perforation, pneumothorax, retroperitoneal hematoma, and neurologic sequelae, such as neuralgia, paralysis of the lower extremities, and loss of sphincter control, can be seen. After an alcohol block, patients may develop phrenic irritation that manifests as hiccups and usually subsides within 48 h.

Superior Hypogastric Plexus Block

The superior hypogastric plexus is located in the retroperitoneal space within loose connective tissue. It lies anterior to the lower portion of the body of L-5 and the superior portion of S-1. A superior hypogastric plexus block is recommended for diagnostic and therapeutic purposes in patients with chronic pelvic pain and may be especially useful when pain is of neoplastic origin (Fig. 41–13).

With the patient in the prone position, a 22-G, 15-cm needle is introduced at a point 5 to 7 cm lateral to the spinous process of L-5. From a horizontal plane, the needle is oriented 30° caudad and 45° mesiad from the parasagittal plane. The needle is then advanced with fluoroscopic guidance until it approximates the anterolateral aspect of the L-5 vertebral body. The needle then is walked off the vertebral body in an inferior direction until it rests 1 cm past the anterior border of the lower one third of the L-5 vertebral body. After proper needle position is achieved, the contralateral needle is inserted in a similar fashion.[42] Injection of 3 to 5 mL of contrast medium should show spread con-

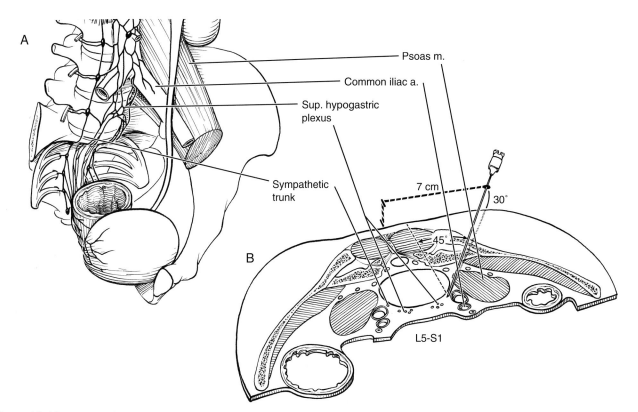

A

Psoas m.

Common iliac a.

Sup. hypogastric plexus

Sympathetic trunk

B

7 cm

30°

45°

L5-S1

Figure 41–13 *A,* Regional anatomy and needle placement for a superior (sup.) hypogastric plexus (SHP) block. *B,* Notice the proximity of the SHP to the iliac vessels. a., artery; m., muscle.

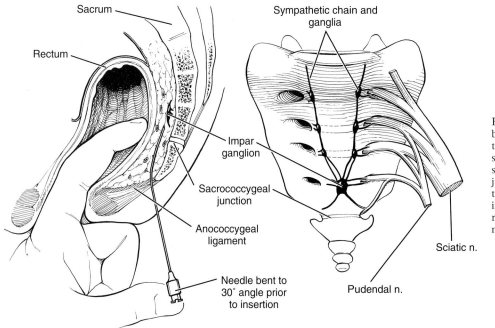

Sacrum

Rectum

Sympathetic chain and ganglia

Impar ganglion

Sacrococcygeal junction

Anococcygeal ligament

Sciatic n.

Needle bent to 30° angle prior to insertion

Pudendal n.

Figure 41–14 Impar ganglion block. The impar ganglion typically lies on the anterior surface of the sacrum, just superior to the sacrococcygeal junction. A 30° angle at the distal third of the needle before insertion and a finger in the rectum assist in obtaining proper needle position. n., nerve.

fined to the midline region on an anteroposterior view. A diagnostic block is performed with 10 mL of 1% lidocaine injected through each needle. If the patient reports a significant degree of pain relief, a neurolytic block is then performed with 10 mL of 10% phenol injected through each needle.

Possible sequelae from a superior hypogastric plexus block are retroperitoneal hematoma, infection, epidural or intrathecal injection, somatic nerve injury, renal or ureteral puncture, and impotence.

Impar Ganglion Block

The impar ganglion (i.e., Walther's ganglion) is formed by the direct convergence of the two sympathetic chains. It lies over the distal one third of the anterior border of the sacrum and extends inferiorly to the sacrococcygeal junction. Block of this ganglion is indicated for the relief of intractable perineal pain (Fig. 41–14).

With the patient in the lateral decubitus position, a skin wheal is raised in the midline at the superior aspect of the intergluteal crease over the anococcygeal ligament. A 22-G, 10-cm spinal needle previously bent to a 25° to 30° angle is introduced with its concavity oriented posteriorly. It is advanced until the tip is situated at the sacrococcygeal junction.[43] Next, 3 mL of contrast medium is injected, and the needle position in the retroperitoneal space is confirmed by fluoroscopy. A diagnostic block is performed with 10 mL of 1% lidocaine. If the patient experiences a significant amount of pain relief, a neurolytic injection is performed with 6 to 8 mL of 10% phenol.

Adverse outcomes can occur, including hematoma formation, infection secondary to needle perforation of the rectum, or an inability to properly position the needle because of tumor, resulting in an inadequate block.

Chest Pain

Chest pain is a common symptom in many acute disease states and some chronic benign conditions. The pain may have its origin in the thoracic wall or intrathoracic structures or be referred from areas below the diaphragm. An accurate history and thorough physical examination can narrow the list of possible causes. Details with respect to location, quality, duration, and frequency of pain should be obtained. Precipitating factors and associated symptoms can aid in distinguishing a visceral from a somatic origin of pain.[44] After the possibility of pain of cardiac origin has been eliminated, it is important to evaluate the patient systematically for other causes of chest pain. Between 10% and 30% of patients who present with typical anginal symptoms are later found to have normal coronary arteries and no other objective evidence of heart disease.[45–49] In this group of patients, the correct diagnosis may often rely on subtle physical findings and elimination of other, more easily diagnosed causes of chest pain.

Costochondritis

Costochondritis is one of the more common causes of chest pain, although it often goes undiagnosed. This syndrome is also referred to as the anterior chest wall syndrome, costosternal syndrome, and parasternal chondrodynia.[50] Pain and tenderness are commonly located over the anterior chest wall. The pain may radiate widely and subsequently be confused with intrathoracic or intra-abdominal disease. Palpation of the anterior chest wall is important in evaluating these patients. More than 90% of patients complain of exquisite point tenderness that is usually located over the upper costosternal junctions on the affected side. The pain may radiate to other areas of the chest wall or abdomen. There are no specific radiologic changes associated with costochondritis. In rare cases, calcium deposits are found in the costal cartilages.[51] Chest radiographs are important only to eliminate the possibility of any coexisting underlying disease.

Reassuring the patient that no cardiac disease is involved is the first step in treating this painful condition. NSAIDs usually provide lasting pain relief. However, if pain continues, injection of a local anesthetic and a locally acting steroid into the affected joint can provide analgesia. Generally, 3 to 5 mL of 1% lidocaine with 4 mg/mL of triamcinolone is injected into each painful joint. Pain relief is usually immediate and can last weeks to months.

Development of a pneumothorax is a possible complication of a costochondral injection. Hematoma formation, infection in the joint space, and a transient worsening of the pain are also possible.

Tietze's Syndrome

Tietze's syndrome is similar to costochondritis, with a few exceptions. First, a bulbous swelling is usually observed in the involved costal cartilage. This syndrome routinely affects only one level, generally the second or third costal cartilage in 80% of the patients.[52] Pain is described as moderate to severe and usually is well localized. There is a predilection for Tietze's syndrome to occur during the second and third decades of life, but it can occur in all age groups. Treatment is similar to that for costochondritis.

Intercostal Neuritis

The pain experienced from intercostal neuritis is described as a severe, sharp, shooting pain that, if untreated, can cause complete disability. There are several causes of intercostal neuritis; the most frequent are acute herpes zoster and postherpetic neuralgia. Postthoracotomy scars and metastatic tumors involving the chest wall can trap the intercostal nerves and cause this severely painful condition. Pain can radiate anteriorly and posteriorly along the dermatomal distribution of the nerve or nerves involved.

Intercostal neuritis may also be caused by painful rib

syndrome.[53] This syndrome consists of three features: pain in the lower chest or upper abdomen, a tender spot on the costal margin with reproduction of the pain by pressing on the tender spot, and instability of one or more ribs at the costosternal junction. This defect allows one rib to override the next, with subsequent compression of the intercostal nerve.

Treatment includes NSAIDs, TENS therapy, and possibly a series of intercostal nerve blocks. For refractory cases of painful rib syndrome, surgical stabilization of the rib cage is a consideration. For other causes of intercostal neuritis, intercostal nerve blocks are performed with 3 to 5 mL of 1% lidocaine and 4 mg/mL of triamcinolone at each involved level (Fig. 41–15). First, the inferior border of each rib corresponding to the affected intercostal nerves is located. Approximately 6 cm from the midline posteriorly (depending on body size), a 23-G, 3-cm needle is introduced and advanced to contact the rib with the anesthesiologist's nondominant hand securing the needle at the skin.

The needle is slowly walked off the inferior border of the rib and advanced 2 mm. After a negative aspiration result, the local anesthetic and steroid solution is injected. The procedure is repeated at each level involved. This therapy usually provides significant pain relief. However, if the relief is temporary, cryotherapy can be performed in an attempt to provide a longer duration of analgesia.

Development of a pneumothorax is a possible complication, but the incidence is less than 1%.[54] Other possible complications include infection, bleeding, local anesthetic systemic toxicity, and intravascular injection.

Intractable Chest Pain

Some patients experience typical anginal symptoms despite a failure to detect underlying cardiac disease during evaluation. These patients also appear to be

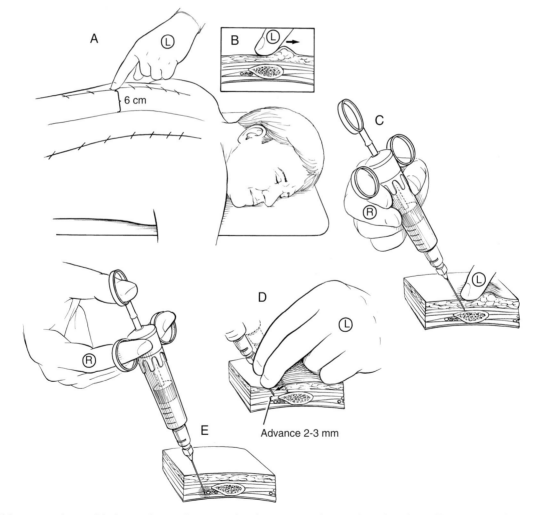

Figure 41–15 Intercostal nerve blocks. *A,* Skin markings are placed approximately 6 cm lateral to the midline, posteriorly over the ribs and corresponding to the affected intercostal nerves. *B,* Skin over the ribs is retracted superiorly to aid in correct needle placement. *C,* The needle is inserted to contact the rib while the skin remains retracted. *D,* As skin retraction is released, the needle is grasped proximally and slowly walked off the inferior edge of the rib. *E,* Once free of the inferior margin of the rib, the needle is advanced 2 to 3 mm, and after negative aspiration, the injection is performed. The left hand is removed to clarify needle position, but it should be in place to control advance of the needle once it is "walked off" the rib. L, left; R, right.

refractory to the usual antianginal therapies (e.g., nitroglycerin, calcium channel antagonists). Imipramine was found[55] to decrease the frequency of chest pain by approximately 50% at a dose of 50 mg nightly, presumably acting by a visceral analgesic effect in patients with normal coronary angiograms. Alternatively, patients with chronic chest pain secondary to severe inoperable cardiac disease may experience significant pain relief from nerve blocks, including thoracic epidural injections of local anesthetic or placement of an intrapleural catheter.[56] Chronic chest pain or referred sympathetic pain (shoulder-hand syndrome) may also be responsive to stellate ganglion blocks.[57] We have seen some patients with intractable chest pain of cardiac origin obtain various degrees of pain relief with low-dose opioid therapy. The clinical significance of this has yet to be determined.

Neuropathic Pain

Neuropathic pain may occur after injury to neural tissue due to systemic disease, infection, trauma, ischemia, deficiencies in metabolism or nutrition, genetic abnormalities, exposure to environmental toxins, or neurotoxic medications. Some common examples of neuropathic pain syndromes include diabetic neuropathy, acquired immunodeficiency syndrome (AIDS) neuropathy, postherpetic neuralgia, sympathetically maintained pain, carpal tunnel syndrome, nerve entrapment, phantom limb pain, alcoholic polyneuropathy, beriberi, Fabry's disease, thallium or mercury exposure, and neuropathy associated with isoniazid and cisplatin.

A patient may present with complaints of an intense burning pain, with episodes of lancinating pain. The patient may describe tingling, crawling, or electrical sensations in a localized area (dysesthesias). Nonpainful stimuli such as stroking the affected area may cause excruciating pain (allodynia), and normally painful stimuli may elicit an inordinate amount of pain (hyperalgesia). Changes in temperature and application of heat or cold to the affected area may exacerbate the pain.

Several possible mechanisms have been suggested to explain the origin of neuropathic pain.[58] After neural injury occurs, there is a loss of large, myelinated afferent fibers that inhibit transmission of painful stimuli to the dorsal horn cells. This deafferentation produces hyperactivity of the dorsal horn cells. In the periphery, at the site of neural injury, spontaneous ectopic neural impulses may occur as the nerve regenerates. The sympathetic nervous system becomes activated as the damaged C-fiber, primary nociceptive afferents regenerate. The C fibers release substance P and other neurotransmitters involved in producing local inflammation and hyperalgesia.[58]

The diagnosis of neuropathic pain is made by history and description of the patient's symptoms. A physical examination should document the presence of sensory or motor deficits (or both), which are often present in patients with neuropathic pain. The areas of hyperalgesia, allodynia, and dysesthesia should also be mapped. Decreases in the intensity of the pain or size of the affected area help to assess the efficacy of treatment.

Initial treatment of neuropathic pain usually consists of medications that decrease the spontaneous ectopic impulses generated by the damaged nerves.[59, 60] These include antidepressant medications (amitriptyline, nortriptyline, desipramine, doxepin, paroxetine), anticonvulsants (phenytoin, carbamazepine, clonazepam), and the antiarrhythmia drugs (lidocaine, mexiletine). Other medications that have been tried with varying success include baclofen and α-adrenergic blockers such as clonidine and terazosin. Topical medications such as capsaicin cream, which depletes substance P; topically applied lidocaine or EMLA cream, which provides local anesthesia; or clonidine patches, which decrease the cutaneous hypersensitivity in patients with a significant sympathetic component to their pain can be considered as adjunctive therapy. TENS has also been effective for some patients.[61]

To characterize the type of neuropathic pain more specifically and to aid in the selection of appropriate medications, many pain centers perform intravenous challenges with lidocaine, phenytoin, phentolamine, and fentanyl. The patients are fully monitored, and strict protocols are followed to minimize the possibility of placebo response and to assess patient response to the different medications. Lidocaine abolishes the ectopic impulses generated by damaged C-fiber afferent nociceptors. If the patient's pain is relieved by 2 to 5 mg/kg of lidocaine given intravenously, a trial of mexiletine given orally is considered.[62] Phenytoin (15 to 20 mg/kg) given intravenously also abolishes ectopic impulses generated by damaged nerves. If the patient responds to phenytoin given intravenously, phenytoin given orally can be prescribed.[63] The dose should be adjusted to maximize analgesic effect and minimize side effects. If intolerable side effects develop before pain relief is achieved, other anticonvulsants such as carbamazepine and clonazepam may be tried. Anticonvulsants are particularly effective in relieving the lancinating pain so often associated with neuropathy.

Phentolamine (35 to 40 mg infused in 30 min) given intravenously is an α-adrenergic antagonist that can be used to assess the degree of sympathetically maintained pain.[64] If the patient has more than a 50% reduction in pain after infusion, blockers such as clonidine or terazosin may be tried. A positive response to phentolamine challenge may indicate the potential benefit of sympathetic block with local anesthetic.[64] Sympathetic block has been especially effective in relieving burning pain associated with hyperesthesia, allodynia, and sensitivity to cold. Some patients have opioid-responsive pain. Although the use of opioids in chronic benign pain is controversial, some advocate a trial of fentanyl (up to 200 μg in 10 min) given intravenously. If the pain is sensitive to opioids, the patient should receive a long-acting agent such as morphine or methadone. This should be reserved only for patients who have failed to respond to all other therapies.[65]

Nerve blocks also play a role in the treatment of neuropathic pain. Peripheral nerve blocks or epidural blocks have been used as treatments for postherpetic neuralgia with some success. If the patient obtains better, longer-lasting relief after each block, the therapy should be continued until no further improvement occurs or the pain has resolved. Medications should be started early and combined to obtain maximum analgesic effect (e.g., use an anticonvulsant or antiarrhythmic plus an antidepressant in conjunction with nerve block therapy). Local anesthetic plus steroid injected into a painful scar or neuroma has resulted in prolonged relief from the burning component of neuropathic pain. Sympathetic blocks have provided relief to some patients with neuropathic pain due to thalamic syndrome, multiple sclerosis, or spinal cord trauma.

When all conservative treatment fails, dorsal root entry zone lesions[66] or placement of a dorsal column stimulator[67] can be considered. These procedures have helped some patients with phantom limb pain, postherpetic neuralgia, and peripheral neuropathies. Neuropathic pain can be extremely difficult to treat. The patient must participate actively in the treatment plan and understand that all of the pain may not be relieved, but that the pain symptoms can be controlled. The pain medicine specialist must coordinate an often complicated, multimodal treatment plan to achieve maximum analgesia with minimum side effects and overall improvement in the patient's ability to cope with the painful condition.

Low Back Pain

Chronic low back pain is one of the most common problems treated by pain management specialists. More than half of the population of the United States complain of low back pain at some point in their lives, with an annual incidence of 5%.[68] As many as 20% of workers are incapacitated by low back pain for more than 4 wk, with a cost to the U.S. economy of more than $15 billion annually.[69, 70]

In our institution, most patients first visit their primary physician for treatment of acute low back pain. They are treated with rest, NSAIDs, and possibly with a low-dose opioid analgesic for the first 4 to 6 wk after the onset of symptoms. If the pain is not relieved, if there is persistent radiculopathy, or if motor or sensory deficits have developed, they usually are referred to an orthopedist or a neurosurgeon for further evaluation. At this point, a computed tomographic scan or a magnetic resonance image may be obtained. If radiculitis is suspected, many surgeons request that the patient undergo evaluation by a pain specialist and treatment with steroids given epidurally before planning surgery.

Epidural injections of steroid are most effective in lumbosacral radiculopathy associated with disk herniation, bulging, or degeneration (i.e., patients with nerve root irritation). In one study,[71] 63% of patients who had the primary diagnosis of radicular pain, compared with 23% of patients with other primary diagnoses, responded to steroids given epidurally. The success rate is better for patients without prior operations, with

pain lasting less than 6 mo, and with no litigation or workers' compensation history.

Before initiation of any type of block therapy for low back pain, a complete history and physical examination should be performed, and available radiographic studies (lumbosacral spine films, computed tomography, magnetic resonance imaging) and electromyographic studies should be reviewed. It is important to eliminate fracture, tumor, and infection as possibilities and to document any preexisting neurologic deficits. A thorough back examination should include a full neurologic examination, with particular attention to reflexes, motor and sensory function, bowel and bladder control, and patient response to maneuvers such as straight-leg raising, spinal flexion, rotation, extension, palpation, and walking on heels or toes. If a patient complains of bowel or bladder incontinence or has saddle anesthesia on examination, the diagnosis of cauda equina syndrome should be made, and the patient should be referred to a surgeon immediately. If the patient is a candidate for epidural injection of steroid, documentation of symptoms and neurologic status before epidural injection of steroid provides a way to assess improvement after the injection.

Table 41–5 outlines some of the most common causes of low back pain that an anesthesiologist experienced in techniques of regional block may be asked to treat. Additional tests and diagnostic blocks that may help confirm a diagnosis are listed. Treatment plans consisting of blocks and supplemental therapies are also presented. The blocks described should be one component of a comprehensive approach to the diagnosis and treatment of low back pain.

Epidural Injections of Steroids

Epidural injections of steroids can be performed with the patient in the sitting or lateral decubitus position. It is recommended that the patient lie on the side most affected after the steroid has been injected. When drugs are injected into the epidural space, they are absorbed by the epidural fat, taken up by the epidural vessels, and diffuse through the dura mater and along adjacent nerve roots. The drug should be administered as close to the affected nerve roots as possible to maximize the amount of drug reaching the nerve root.

After entry into the epidural space has been achieved, steroid mixed with preservative-free saline or local anesthetic is injected. The use of saline or local anesthetic varies from center to center. There is no comprehensive study that substantiates a benefit of local anesthetic compared with saline. We routinely use 7 to 8 mL of preservative-free saline as the diluent for the steroid. Local anesthetic (1% lidocaine) occasionally is used for patients who have acute low back pain with severe, incapacitating symptoms. The local anesthetic is often helpful in transiently decreasing the pain and spasm.

The steroids used most often are methylprednisolone and triamcinolone. Methylprednisolone acetate suspension is an anti-inflammatory glucocorticoid that can

Table 41–5 Common Causes of Low Back Pain

DIAGNOSIS	FURTHER TESTS AND DIAGNOSTIC BLOCKS	TREATMENT
Herniated nucleus pulposus	CT, MRI, EMG	Bed rest (48 h), NSAIDs, PT, epidural steroids, surgery
Internal disk disruption	CT, diskography	NSAIDs, PT, back brace, epidural steroids
Spinal stenosis	CT, myelogram, MRI, EMG, selective nerve root block	NSAIDs, TENS, PT, epidural steroids, selective nerve root block, surgery
Spondylolisthesis	CT, EMG, selective nerve root block	NSAIDs, TENS, PT, epidural steroids, facet blocks, selective nerve root block, surgery
Facet syndrome	Facet injection	NSAIDs, PT, spinal manipulation, facet injection, radiofrequency facet denervation, dorsal rhizotomy
Failed back surgery syndrome	MRI, CT, EMG, diskography, selective nerve root block	NSAIDs, PT, multimodal conservative care if not a surgical candidate, dorsal column stimulation
Myofascial pain	Trigger point injection	NSAIDs, PT, trigger point injections
Piriformis syndrome	Trigger point injection	NSAIDs, PT and stretching, trigger point injections, surgical release of the piriformis muscle
Sacroiliac joint syndrome	Sacroiliac joint injection	NSAIDs, PT, sacroiliac joint injection, surgical fusion
Peripheral nerve entrapment	EMG, peripheral nerve block, selective nerve root block	Peripheral nerve block, neurolysis, surgical nerve release
Herpes zoster	EMG, selective nerve root block	Acyclovir, TENS, antidepressants, anticonvulsants, capsaicin, sympathetic block, selective nerve root block
Bone lesions	MRI, CT, bone scan, SMA-20, ESR, acid phosphatase, SPEP, lumbar puncture	Treat cause of bone lesions, NSAIDs and opioids as needed to control pain

CT, computed tomography; EMG, electromyography; ESR, erythrocyte sedimentation rate; MRI, magnetic resonance imaging; NSAIDs, nonsteroidal anti-inflammatory drugs; PT, physical therapy; SMA-20, sequential multiple analysis of 20 chemical constituents; SPEP, serum protein electrophoresis; TENS, transcutaneous electrical nerve stimulation.

be used for intramuscular, intralesional, intrasynovial, soft tissue, or epidural injection. It comes in concentrations of 40 mg/mL and 80 mg/mL and contains polyethylene glycol, myristyl-γ-picolinium chloride, and sodium chloride. Its pH is 3.5 to 7.0. A common dose for epidural injections of steroid is 40 to 80 mg. Triamcinolone diacetate suspension has glucocorticoid properties with virtually no mineralocorticoid activity. It comes in concentrations of 25 mg/mL and 40 mg/mL and contains polysorbate 80, polyethylene glycol, sodium chloride, and less than 0.9% benzyl alcohol. A common dose for epidural injections of steroid is 50 to 80 mg.

Although the diluents for the steroids are potentially neurotoxic at higher concentrations, animal studies have supported their relative safety, and no cases of direct neurotoxicity secondary to steroid in the epidural space have been documented. Aseptic meningitis, adhesive arachnoiditis, and conus medullaris syndrome have occurred after intrathecal injection of methylprednisolone. The use of epidural injections of morphine in conjunction with methylprednisolone is associated with significant risk of respiratory depression and other side effects of opioids, such as pruritus and nausea, without providing added benefit.[72]

Injections are performed at 2- to 4-wk intervals. This allows full assessment of the effect of the injections and the return of cortisol levels to normal between injections. The hypothalamic-pituitary-adrenal axis is suppressed, with decreased plasma cortisol levels for 3 to 5 wk after a typical epidural injection of steroid.[73] Our protocol calls for three injections within 6 mo. More frequent injections may result in prolonged adrenal suppression.[74]

Other complications and side effects seen (rarely) after epidural injections of steroid include spinal headache after unintentional dural puncture, iatrogenic Cushing syndrome, congestive heart failure secondary to fluid retention, changes in blood glucose levels, back pain at the site of injection or the exacerbation of the existing symptoms, facial flushing and rash, epidural abscess, meningitis, nerve root injury, durocutaneous fistula, and epidural hematoma.

Intra-articular and Medial Branch Block of the Facet Joint

Facet syndrome is used to describe patients with chronic, intractable back pain who have tenderness over the facet joints that is abolished after facet joint injection with local anesthetic (Fig. 41–16). To perform a facet joint injection, the patient should be prone, with the hips supported by pillows. The procedure should be done with fluoroscopic guidance. The table or fluoroscope should be manipulated to achieve the best view of the joint. This is often achieved when the fluoroscope beam is directed at a 30° to 45° angle to the sagittal plane. After the appropriate lumbar facet joint is clearly visualized and using sterile technique, the skin and deeper layers should be anesthetized with local anesthetic. A 22-G, 10-cm spinal needle is advanced into the joint by using fluoroscopic guidance. To confirm intra-articular placement, 0.5 mL of radio-contrast dye can be injected to visualize the S-shaped joint space before injection of 1.0 to 1.5 mL of local anesthetic (1% to 4% lidocaine or 0.25% to 0.5%

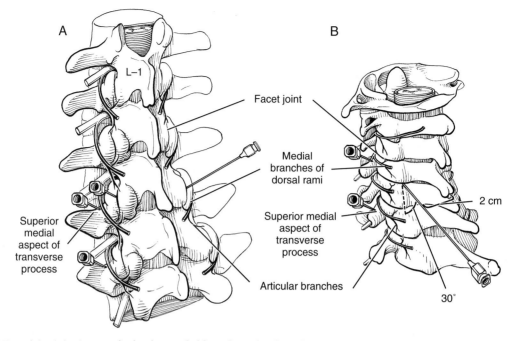

Figure 41–16 Facet joint injection. *A,* The lumbar medial branch sends a branch to the facet joint at the same level and to the facet joint directly below. Intra-articular needle placement is used for performing facet joint injection. *B,* A posterior oblique view of the cervical spine shows the courses of the third occipital nerve, the medial branches of the cervical dorsal rami, and their articular branches. The needles are drawn to indicate the target points for a third occipital nerve block and for C-5 and C-6 medial branch blocks. (*A,* Modified from Bogduk N: Back pain: zygapophysial blocks and epidural steroids. In Cousins MJ, Bridenbaugh PO [eds]: Neural Blockade in Clinical Anesthesia and Management of Pain, 2nd ed, pp 935–954. Philadelphia, JB Lippincott, 1988. *B,* Modified from Bogduk N, Marsland A: The cervical zygapophysial joints as a source of neck pain. Spine 1988; 13: 610–617.)

bupivacaine) with 10 to 20 mg of triamcinolone or methylprednisolone.

The medial branch of the posterior primary ramus provides sensory innervation to the lower pole of the facet joint at the level of exit from the intervertebral foramen and innervates the upper pole of the facet joint below. To block the innervation of one facet joint, two medial branches must be blocked: one medial branch as it arises from the nerve at the same level as the joint and the other medial branch as it descends from the posterior primary ramus of the nerve above.

To perform a medial branch block, the patient should be prone. After sterile preparation and draping, the skin and underlying tissues are anesthetized before introducing a 22-G spinal needle 5 cm lateral to the spinous process of the vertebra that provides an articular surface of the joint to be blocked. The needle should be directed obliquely with fluoroscopic guidance until it rests on the most medial aspect of the superior edge of the transverse process. Local anesthetic with steroid (1 to 2 mL) should be injected at each level. This approach may be particularly helpful in patients with severe arthritis or another joint abnormality that precludes easy access to the joint space.

Abolition of back pain after facet joint injection by either technique supports the diagnosis of lumbar facet syndrome. The block may provide prolonged pain relief. However, it is more likely that the patient will require additional facet joint blocks with local anesthetic and steroid, cryoanalgesia, or radiofrequency facet denervation to obtain any degree of sustained relief.[75, 76]

Complications after facet joint block are rare. Transient back pain may occur. Facet joint capsular rupture has been reported if more than 2 mL of injectant is used for intra-articular injections. Spinal anesthesia and an episode of chemical meningitis have occurred after unintentional dural puncture.

Lumbar and Transsacral Selective Nerve Root Blocks

A patient may have multilevel spinal abnormalities seen on radiographic studies but have only one or two specific nerve roots that are responsible for the pain. Identification of the source of the patient's pain allows the surgeon to confine the surgical treatment to the levels causing the pain. Selective nerve root blocks may be therapeutic, especially if steroid is deposited at the nerve root along with the local anesthetic. In some cases, an operation can be avoided altogether[77] (Fig. 41–17).

Selective lumbar somatic nerve root blocks of L-1 to L-5 are performed in the same manner as lumbar somatic nerve root blocks. The needle should be placed with fluoroscopic guidance. After the needle is confirmed to be in proper position, care should be taken to use only 1 to 2 mL of local anesthetic with 10 to 20 mg of triamcinolone in patients undergoing diagnostic

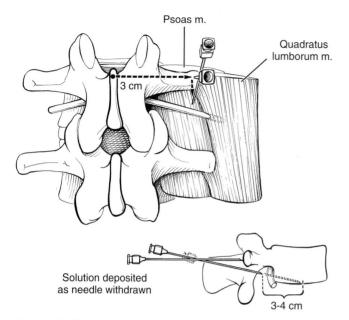

Figure 41–17 Lumbar nerve root block. The transverse process of L-2, spinal nerve at L-2, and spinous process of L-2 are shown. m., muscle. (Modified from Thompson GE, Moore DC: Celiac plexus, intercostal, and minor peripheral blockade. In Cousins MJ, Bridenbaugh PO [eds]: Neural Blockade in Clinical Anesthesia and Management of Pain, 2nd ed, pp 503–530. Philadelphia, JB Lippincott, 1988.)

or therapeutic blocks for low back pain (in contrast to the 5 to 7 mL placed at each level for surgical anesthesia). Greater volumes result in spread to other somatic nerve roots and confound the diagnostic results of the

block. The patient's response to each selective nerve root block should be carefully assessed by having the patient perform movements that had been painful.

Transsacral nerve root block can be helpful in the diagnosis and treatment of sacral nerve root lesions.[78] The sacrum is a wedge-shaped bone made of the five fused sacral vertebrae. Sacral nerve roots 1 through 4 exit through foramina within the sacral bone, and S-5 exits just caudad to the sacral cornua. Some perform selective transsacral blocks with fluoroscopy (Fig. 41–18); however, the sacral foramina are palpable in many patients.

The patient is placed in the prone position, with a pillow under the hips. After sterile preparation and draping, the skin and superficial tissues are anesthetized. A 22-G spinal needle should be inserted anteriorly in a parasagittal plane until it contacts periosteum. The needle should be adjusted with fluoroscopic guidance until it enters the posterior sacral foramen. If surface landmarks are used, the needle should be walked off the dorsum of the sacrum into the selected foramen. The needle is advanced until the tip is at the entrance of the anterior sacral foramen from which the nerve root exits. A lateral fluoroscopic view should confirm placement of the needle tip at the anterior border of the sacrum, within the anterior sacral foramen. Radiocontrast dye (1 mL) may also be injected to visualize the course of the nerve root.

Because the sacrum is wedge shaped, the distance between the anterior and posterior sacral foramina is approximately 2.5 cm at S-1, decreasing to 0.5 cm at S-4. These distances should be kept in mind if fluoroscopy is not used. If there is no paresthesia and no

Figure 41–18 Transsacral nerve root block. Although bony anatomic variability of the sacrum is common, it usually is most variable in the midline. The posterior sacral foramina generally lie on a line that passes from 2 to 3 cm medial to the posterior superior iliac spine (midway between S-1 and S-2) and 1 to 2 cm lateral to the sacral cornu. Depending on patient size, the S-2 and S-4 foramina can usually be found about 2 cm caudad from the line intersecting the posterior superior iliac spine and 1 to 2 cm cephalad to the sacral cornu, respectively. The S-3 foramen is equidistant between the two, and S-1 is equidistant above S-2. To perform this block, the patient is placed prone, with a pillow beneath the hips (as for caudal block). After first determining the depth by encountering the posterior bony plate of the sacrum, a needle is walked into the appropriate foramen and advanced an additional 1 to 2 cm to lie closer to the anterior primary ramus before injection of 4 to 8 mL of solution. m., muscle. (Modified from Bonica JJ, Buckley FP: Regional analgesia with local anesthetics. In Bonica JJ: The Management of Pain, 2nd ed, vol II, pp 1883–1966. Philadelphia, Lea & Febiger, 1990.)

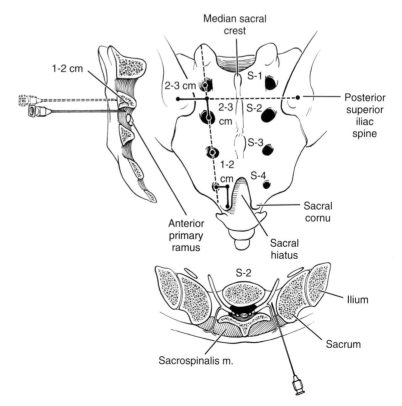

aspiration of blood or cerebrospinal fluid, 1 to 2 mL of local anesthetic with 20 mg of triamcinolone should be injected.

Reported complications after selective nerve root block include subarachnoid or epidural analgesia, intraneural injection, and sympathetic ganglion block. Some specialists think that complications can be minimized by fluoroscopy.

Sacroiliac Joint Injection

Although most pain in the sacroiliac region is referred, some low back, hip, or buttock pain may result from inflammation of the sacroiliac joint. Compression of the joint during physical examination and provocative maneuvers exacerbate the pain. Treatment consists of sacroiliac joint injection (Fig. 41–19) with local anesthetic and steroid, followed by physical therapy. NSAIDs also help to decrease chronic inflammation in the joint.[79] Rarely, the degeneration of the joint is so severe that the pain is not responsive to joint injections, oral medications, and physical therapy. A patient like this may require surgical joint fusion.

A sacroiliac joint injection can be performed with or without fluoroscopic guidance. If fluoroscopy is used, the patient is placed prone, with the opposite hip raised on a pillow. The patient should be positioned such that the anterior and posterior orifices of the lower one third of the joint are superimposed, maximizing visualization of the joint. This appears as a Y fluoroscopically.[80] After sterile preparation and draping and infiltration of the skin and underlying tissue with local anesthetic, a 22-G spinal needle is advanced vertically into the lower one third of the joint. Joint entry should be successful at a depth of 3 to 5 cm. If fluoroscopy is used, the entry to the joint should be confirmed with 1 to 2 mL of radiocontrast dye (e.g., Isovue-300 mixed with an equal amount of isotonic saline). If dye flow is not seen throughout the entire joint, another spinal needle is placed at one or two other points in the joint to maximize spread of local anesthetic and steroid. A total volume of 5 to 10 mL of 1% lidocaine or other dilute local anesthetic mixed with 20 to 40 mg triamcinolone can be injected. The patient's response after injection is assessed by provocative testing, and the patient is followed for the next 1 to 2 wk to determine whether a repeat block would be beneficial.

Blocks for Myofascial Pain in the Back

Some patients with no spinal or joint abnormality may complain of pain due to inflammation of the muscles and ligaments of the back. Trigger point injections to the large muscles of the back, in conjunction with physical therapy, often provide significant pain relief. Quadratus lumborum, piriformis, paraspinous muscle, and iliolumbar ligament injections have been helpful in treating patients with myofascial syndrome.

Pain in the Extremities

Extremity pain may be caused by compression, inflammation, ischemia, infection, systemic disease, exposure to toxic substances, or entrapment of nerves in the periphery and at the level of the nerve roots and

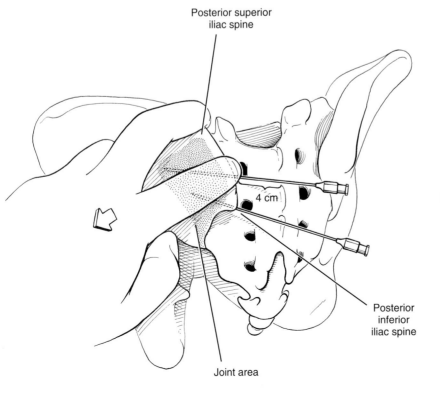

Posterior superior iliac spine

4 cm

Posterior inferior iliac spine

Joint area

Figure 41–19 Sacroiliac joint injection.

spinal cord. A history and physical examination can reveal the location and characteristics of the pain.

Common chronic pain syndromes in the upper extremities include carpal tunnel syndrome; arthritis; peripheral neuropathies due to nerve entrapment, diabetes, uremia, malnutrition, or toxins; reflex sympathetic dystrophy; myofascial pain; and phantom limb pain. Cervical disk or spine disease can produce radicular pain in the neck and upper extremities. Cardiac pain can also be referred to the arms, chest, and jaw.

Common chronic pain syndromes in the lower extremities include lumbosacral radiculopathy, arthritis, reflex sympathetic dystrophy, meralgia paresthetica, peripheral neuropathies, trochanteric bursitis, piriformis syndrome, and phantom limb pain.

Most extremity pain is managed with medications, surgical treatment, or both modalities. However, there are several instances in which the expertise of the anesthesiologist skilled in regional block may be beneficial. A cervical epidural injection of steroid may be performed if conservative therapy fails to eliminate the radicular symptoms associated with conditions such as cervical spondylosis, disk degeneration or herniation, and spinal stenosis.[81] In patients with carpal tunnel syndrome,[82] immobilization of the wrist with a splint and steroid injections beneath the carpal ligament are often helpful. For patients with painful scars or neuromas,[83] injection of local anesthetic with or without steroid to the painful areas, followed by deep massage, often provides relief for longer periods than the duration of action of the local anesthetic. Repeated injections can provide prolonged relief. Arthritis, painful neuritis due to infection (AIDS), or neuropathy secondary to systemic diseases (diabetes, multiple sclerosis, amyloidosis) usually responds best to medications. Other syndromes such as postherpetic neuralgia and reflex sympathetic dystrophy often respond to a combination of medications and block therapy.

Myofascial pain in the extremities may respond to a series of trigger point injections and physical therapy. Tenosynovitis resulting in a painful hand often responds to local injections of steroid.[84] Painful elbow is treated with deep heat, rest in the acute phase, and local anesthetic injections. Interscalene blocks of the brachial plexus followed by aggressive physical therapy can be performed as part of the treatment for frozen shoulder syndrome.[85] Intra-articular injections of local anesthetic and steroid also provide some relief. Postamputation phantom limb pain, Raynaud's syndrome, vasospasm, pain from arterial embolism, and acute herpes zoster can be treated with stellate ganglion block.

Patients with low back pain may complain of lower extremity pain as well. Compression of the lumbosacral nerve roots by an intervertebral disk, hypertrophy of the facet joints, or misalignment of the vertebrae due to spondylolysis or spondylolisthesis can produce radicular symptoms that respond to lumbar epidural injections of steroid, facet blocks, or selective nerve root blocks.

Occasionally, a patient presents with meralgia paresthetica.[86] The patient complains of a burning, tingling pain in the anterolateral thigh that is exacerbated by standing or walking and is sometimes relieved by flexion of the hip. Meralgia paresthetica is caused by entrapment of or trauma to the lateral femoral cutaneous nerve and is treated by perineural injection of a combination of local anesthetic and steroid. A series of injections may be necessary to obtain sustained relief (Fig. 41–20).

Trochanteric bursitis is one of the most frequent causes of hip pain.[87] The bursa lies between the greater trochanter and the fascia lata. When inflamed, the bursa causes pain that is localized to the area of the greater trochanter. Treatment consists of NSAIDs, rest from activities that exacerbate the pain, physical therapy, and intrabursal injection of local anesthetic and steroid to decrease pain and inflammation.

Piriformis syndrome (pseudosciatica) may be caused by spasm of the piriformis muscle.[88] The patient may complain of pain radiating from the sciatic notch down the leg in the distribution of the sciatic nerve. The patient may also complain of tenderness on palpation of the sciatic notch. Treatment consists of NSAIDs and injection of local anesthetic and steroid to the piriformis muscle (Fig. 41–21), followed by active physical therapy.

Postamputation phantom limb pain (experience of pain in the part of the limb that is no longer there) can be excruciating.[89] Sympathetic block before amputation, usually by placement of a lumbar epidural catheter and infusion of local anesthetic, may decrease the

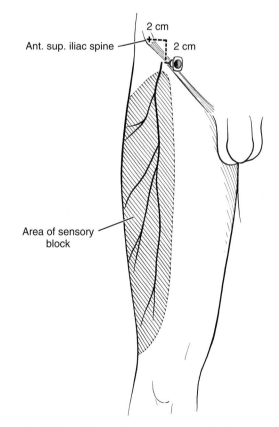

Figure 41–20 Lateral femoral cutaneous nerve block. Ant., anterior; sup., superior. (Modified from Bonica JJ [ed]: The Management of Pain. Philadelphia, Lea & Febiger, 1953.)

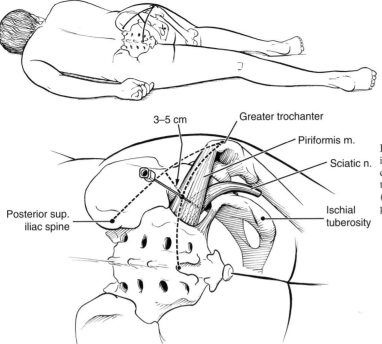

Figure 41–21 Piriformis muscle injection. The needle insertion site is 3 to 5 cm below the midpoint of a line connecting the posterior superior iliac spine and greater trochanter. m., muscle; n., nerve; sup., superior. (Modified from Brown DL: Atlas of Regional Anesthesia, p 84. Philadelphia, WB Saunders Co, 1992.)

incidence of phantom limb pain. If phantom limb pain does occur, sympatholysis using a lumbar sympathetic block or with a lumbar epidural injection of local anesthetic, antidepressant and anticonvulsant medications, psychologic support, TENS, and physical therapy may alleviate the symptoms.

A well-fitting prosthesis is crucial in preventing phantom limb pain and stump pain (pain that is located in the stump and does not extend beyond it).[90] Stump pain can be caused by neuromas or nerve entrapment in scar tissue. Injection with local anesthetic and steroid and deep massage of the scar may help. TENS and combinations of analgesics, anticonvulsants, and antidepressant medications can be used to treat intractable cases of stump pain.

References

1. Mitchell SW: Injuries of Nerves and Their Consequences. Philadelphia, JB Lippincott, 1872.
2. Sudeck P: Ueber die akute entzündliche Knochenatrophie. Arch Klin Chir 1900; 62: 147–156.
3. Sudeck P: Die sogen. Akute Knochenatrophie als Entzündungsvorgang. Chirurg 1942; 14: 449–458.
4. Roberts WJ: A hypothesis on the physiological basis for causalgia and related pains. Pain 1986; 24: 297–311.
5. Campbell JN, Meyer RA, Raja SN: Is nociceptor activation by alpha-1 adrenoreceptors the culprit in sympathetically maintained pain? Am Pain Soc J 1992; 1: 3–11.
6. Veldman PH, Reynen HM, Arntz IE, et al: Signs and symptoms of reflex sympathetic dystrophy: prospective study of 829 patients. Lancet 1993; 342: 1012–1016.
7. Hannington-Kiff JG: Intravenous regional sympathetic block with guanethidine. Lancet 1974; 1: 1019–1020.
8. Ford SR, Forrest WH Jr, Eltherington L: The treatment of reflex sympathetic dystrophy with intravenous regional bretylium. Anesthesiology 1988; 68: 137–140.
9. Katz J, Renck H: Handbook of Thoraco-Abdominal Nerve Block, p 181. Orlando, Grune & Stratton, 1987.
10. Reiestad F, McIlvaine WB, Barnes M, et al: Interpleural analgesia in the treatment of severe thoracic postherpetic neuralgia. Reg Anesth 1990; 15: 113–117.
11. Bonica JJ, Buckley FP: Regional analgesia with local anesthetics. In Bonica JJ (ed): The Management of Pain, 2nd ed, vol 2, pp 1883–1996. Philadelphia, Lea & Febiger, 1990.
12. Raj PP: Pain due to herpes zoster. In Raj PP: Practical Management of Pain, 2nd ed, pp 517–545. St. Louis, Mosby–Year Book, 1992.
13. Epstein E: Triamcinolone-procaine in the treatment of zoster and postzoster neuralgia. Calif Med 1971; 115: 6–10.
14. Travell JG, Simons DG: Myofascial Pain and Dysfunction: The Trigger Point Manual. Baltimore, Williams & Wilkins, 1983.
15. Brown BR Jr: Myofascial and musculoskeletal pain. Int Anesthesiol Clin 1983; 21: 139–151.
16. Frost FA, Jessen B, Siggaard-Andersen J: A controlled, double-blind comparison of mepivacaine injection versus saline injection for myofascial pain. Lancet 1980; 1: 499–500.
17. Ruskin AP: Sphenopalatine (nasal) ganglion: remote effects including "psychosomatic" symptoms, rage reaction, pain, and spasm. Arch Phys Med Rehabil 1979; 60: 353–359.
18. Ryan RE Jr, Facer GW: Sphenopalatine ganglion neuralgia and cluster headache: comparisons, contrasts, and treatment. Headache 1977; 17: 7–8.
19. Sparer W: Cessation of convulsive seizures following injection of alcohol into the sphenopalatine ganglia in three cases. Laryngoscope 1935; 45: 886–890.
20. Stewart D, Lambert V: Further observation on spheno-palatine ganglion. J Laryngol Otol 1934; 49: 319–322.
21. Kittrelle JP, Grouse DS, Seybold ME: Cluster headache. Local anesthetic abortive agents. Arch Neurol 1985; 42: 496–498.
22. Lebovits AH, Alfred H, Lefkowitz M: Sphenopalatine ganglion block: clinical use in the pain management clinic. Clin J Pain 1990; 6: 131–136.
23. Chan ST, Leung S: Spinal epidural abscess following steroid injection for sciatica. Case report. Spine 1989; 14: 106–108.
24. Williams KN, Jackowski A, Evans PJ: Epidural haematoma requiring surgical decompression following repeated cervical epidural steroid injections for chronic pain. Pain 1990; 42: 197–199.
25. Dougherty JH Jr, Fraser RA: Complications following intraspinal

injections of steroids. Report of two cases. J Neurosurg 1978; 48: 1023–1025.

26. Katz J: Somatic nerve blocks. In Raj PP: Practical Management of Pain, 2nd ed, pp 713–753. St. Louis, Mosby–Year Book, 1992.

27. Murphy TM: Somatic blockade. In Cousins MJ, Bridenbaugh PO (eds): Neural Blockade in Clinical Anesthesia and Management of Pain, pp 406–424. Philadelphia, JB Lippincott, 1980.

28. Applegate WV: Abdominal cutaneous nerve entrapment syndrome. Surgery 1972; 71: 118–124.

29. Doouss TW, Boas RA: The abdominal cutaneous nerve entrapment syndrome. N Z Med J 1975; 81: 473–475.

30. Okazaki K, Yamamoto Y, Kagiyama S, et al: Pressure of papillary sphincter zone and pancreatic main duct in patients with chronic pancreatitis in the early stage. Scand J Gastroenterol 1988; 23: 501–507.

31. Bockman DE, Buchler M, Malfertheiner P, et al: Analysis of nerves in chronic pancreatitis. Gastroenterology 1988; 94: 1459–1469.

32. Mulholland MW, Debas HT, Bonica JJ: Diseases of the liver, biliary system, and pancreas. In Bonica JJ: The Management of Pain, 2nd ed, vol 2, pp 1214–1231. Philadelphia, Lea & Febiger, 1990.

33. Ramo OJ, Puolakkainen PA, Seppala K, et al: Self-administration of enzyme substitution in the treatment of exocrine pancreatic insufficiency. Scand J Gastroenterol 1989; 24: 688–692.

34. Geenen JE, Rolny P: Endoscopic therapy of acute and chronic pancreatitis. Gastrointest Endosc 1991; 37: 377–382.

35. Owitz S, Koppolu S: Celiac plexus block: an overview. Mt Sinai J Med 1983; 50: 486–490.

36. Ischia S, Luzzani A, Ischia A, et al: A new approach to the neurolytic block of the coeliac plexus: the transaortic technique. Pain 1983; 16: 333–341.

37. Brown DL, Bulley CK, Quiel EL: Neurolytic celiac plexus block for pancreatic cancer pain. Anesth Analg 1987; 66: 869–873.

38. Hastings RH, McKay WR: Treatment of benign chronic abdominal pain with neurolytic celiac plexus block. Anesthesiology 1991; 75: 156–158.

39. Lieberman RP, Waldman SD: Celiac plexus neurolysis with the modified transaortic approach. Radiology 1990; 175: 274–276.

40. Ischia S, Ischia A, Polati E, et al: Three posterior percutaneous celiac plexus block techniques. A prospective, randomized study in 61 patients with pancreatic cancer pain. Anesthesiology 1992; 76: 534–540.

41. Fugere F, Lewis G: Coeliac plexus block for chronic pain syndromes. Can J Anaesth 1993; 40: 954–963.

42. Plancarte R, Amescua C, Patt RB, et al: Superior hypogastric plexus block for pelvic cancer pain. Anesthesiology 1990; 73: 236–239.

43. Plancarte R, Amescua C, Patt RB, et al: Presacral blockade of the ganglion of Walther (ganglion impar). (Abstract.) Anesthesiology 1990; 73: A751.

44. Cattau EL Jr: Noncardiac chest pain evaluation: clearing the air or more smoke? Am J Gastroenterol 1991; 86: 920–921.

45. Proudfit WL, Shirey EK, Sones FM Jr: Selective cine coronary arteriography. Correlation with clinical findings in 1,000 patients. Circulation 1966; 33: 901–910.

46. Kemp HG Jr, Vokonas PS, Cohn PF, et al: The anginal syndrome associated with normal coronary arteriograms. Report of a six year experience. Am J Med 1973; 54: 735–742.

47. Pasternak RC, Thibault GE, Savoia M, et al: Chest pain with angiographically insignificant coronary arterial obstruction. Clinical presentation and long-term follow-up. Am J Med 1980; 68: 813–817.

48. Dart AM, Davies HA, Dalal J, et al: 'Angina' and normal coronary arteriograms: a follow-up study. Eur Heart J 1980; 1: 97–100.

49. Papanicolaou MN, Califf RM, Hlatky MA, et al: Prognostic implications of angiographically normal and insignificantly narrowed coronary arteries. Am J Cardiol 1986; 58: 1181–1187.

50. Calabro JJ: Costochondritis. (Letter to the editor.) N Engl J Med 1977; 296: 946–947.

51. Wolf E, Stern S: Costosternal syndrome: its frequency and importance in the differential diagnosis of coronary heart disease. Arch Intern Med 1976; 136: 189–191.

52. Calabro JJ, Jeghers H, Miller KA, et al: Classification of anterior chest wall syndromes. (Letter to the editor.) JAMA 1980; 243: 1420–1421.

53. Scott EM, Scott BB: Painful rib syndrome—a review of 76 cases. Gut 1993; 34: 1006–1008.

54. Moore DC, Bush WH, Scurlock JE: Intercostal nerve block: a roentgenographic anatomic study of technique and absorption in humans. Anesth Analg 1980; 59: 815–825.

55. Cannon RO III, Quyyumi AA, Mincemoyer R, et al: Imipramine in patients with chest pain despite normal coronary angiograms. N Engl J Med 1994; 330: 1411–1417.

56. Bonica JJ: The Management of Pain, pp 1310–1361. Philadelphia, Lea & Febiger, 1953.

57. Hathaway BN, Hill GE, Ohmura A: Centrally induced sympathetic dystrophy of the upper extremity. Anesth Analg 1978; 57: 373–374.

58. Asbury AK, Fields HL: Pain due to peripheral nerve damage: an hypothesis. Neurology 1984; 34: 1587–1590.

59. Belgrade MJ, Lev BI: Diabetic neuropathy. Helping patients cope with their pain. Postgrad Med 1991; 90: 263–270.

60. Brooks PJ, Francisco GE: Drug therapy of diabetic neuropathy. Clin Podiatr Med Surg 1992; 9: 257–274.

61. Bates JA, Nathan PW: Transcutaneous electrical nerve stimulation for chronic pain. Anaesthesia 1980; 35: 817–822.

62. Ackerman WE III, Colclough GW, Juneja MM, et al: The management of oral mexiletine and intravenous lidocaine to treat chronic painful symmetrical distal diabetic neuropathy. J Ky Med Assoc 1991; 89: 500–501.

63. Swerdlow M: Anticonvulsant drugs and chronic pain. Clin Neuropharmacol 1984; 7: 51–82.

64. Arner S: Intravenous phentolamine test: diagnostic and prognostic use in reflex sympathetic dystrophy. Pain 1991; 46: 17–22.

65. Portenoy RK, Foley KM: Chronic use of opioid analgesics in non-malignant pain: report of 38 cases. Pain 1986; 25: 171–186.

66. Nashold BS Jr, Higgins AC, Blumenkopf B: Dorsal root entry zone lesions for pain relief. In Wilkins RH, Rangachary SS (eds): Neurosurgery, vol 3, pp 2433–2437. New York, McGraw-Hill, 1985.

67. Young RF: Evaluation of dorsal column stimulation in the treatment of chronic pain. Neurosurgery 1978; 3: 373–379.

68. Frymoyer JW: Back pain and sciatica. N Engl J Med 1988; 318: 291–300.

69. el-Khoury GY, Renfrew DL: Percutaneous procedures for the diagnosis and treatment of lower back pain: diskography, facet-joint injection, and epidural injection. AJR Am J Roentgenol 1991; 157: 685–691.

70. Haldeman S: North American Spine Society: failure of the pathology model to predict back pain. Spine 1990; 15: 718–724.

71. Benzon HT: Epidural steroid injections for low back pain and lumbosacral radiculopathy. Pain 1986; 24: 277–295.

72. Haddox JD: Lumbar and cervical epidural steroid therapy. Anesthesiol Clin North Am 1992; 10: 179–203.

73. Knight CL, Burnell JC: Systemic side-effects of extradural steroids. Anaesthesia 1980; 35: 593–594.

74. Jacobs S, Pullan PT, Potter JM, et al: Adrenal suppression following extradural steroids. Anaesthesia 1983; 38: 953–956.

75. Helbig T, Lee CK: The lumbar facet syndrome. Spine 1988; 13: 61–64.

76. Destouet JM, Gilula LA, Murphy WA, et al: Lumbar facet joint injection: indication, technique, clinical correlation, and preliminary results. Radiology 1982; 145: 321–325.

77. Dooley JF, McBroom RJ, Taguchi T, et al: Nerve root infiltration in the diagnosis of radicular pain. Spine 1988; 13: 79–83.

78. Clark AJ, Awad SA: Selective transsacral nerve root blocks. Reg Anesth 1990; 15: 125–129.

79. Mooney V: Understanding, examining for, and treating sacroiliac pain. J Musculoskel Med 1993; 10: 37–49.

80. Hendrix RW, Lin PJ, Kane WJ: Simplified aspiration or injection technique for the sacro-iliac joint. J Bone Joint Surg Am 1982; 64: 1249–1252.

81. Waldman SD: Complications of cervical epidural nerve blocks with steroids: a prospective study of 790 consecutive blocks. Reg Anesth 1989; 14: 149–151.

82. Seror P: Evaluation of the efficacy of infiltrative treatment in carpal tunnel syndrome. Electrophysiologic data and clinical applications. [French] Rev Rhum Mal Osteoartic 1989; 56: 307–312.

83. Chabal C, Jacobson L, Russell LC, et al: Pain response to perineuronal injection of normal saline, epinephrine, and lidocaine in humans. Pain 1992; 49: 9–12.
84. Witt J, Pess G, Gelberman RH: Treatment of de Quervain tenosynovitis. A prospective study of the results of injection of steroids and immobilization in a splint. J Bone Joint Surg Am 1991; 73: 219–222.
85. Bulgen DY, Binder AI, Hazleman BL, et al: Frozen shoulder: prospective clinical study with an evaluation of three treatment regimens. Ann Rheum Dis 1984; 43: 353–360.
86. Williams PH, Trzil KP: Management of meralgia paresthetica. J Neurosurg 1991; 74: 76–80.
87. Ege Rasmussen KJ, Fano N: Trochanteric bursitis. Treatment by corticosteroid injection. Scand J Rheumatol 1985; 14: 417–420.
88. Barton PM: Piriformis syndrome: a rational approach to management. Pain 1991; 47: 345–352.
89. Wesolowski JA, Lema MJ: Phantom limb pain. Reg Anesth 1993; 18: 121–127.
90. Davis RW: Phantom sensation, phantom pain, and stump pain. Arch Phys Med Rehabil 1993; 74: 79–91.

CHAPTER 42

Cancer Pain

Patricia Harrison, M.D., Mark J. Lema, M.D., Ph.D.

Next to incurability, the most feared complication of contracting cancer is intractable pain, and 50% to 70% of all cancer patients in the early stages of the disease experience significant pain. Between 60% and 90% of advanced-stage patients have pain as a main complaint.[1-7] When these rates are converted to the actual number of patients, about 1.2 million Americans experience pain related to their cancer each year.[2]

The most distressing statistic reveals that even today 40% of all cancer patients die in unrelieved pain. Studies by Cleeland and colleagues[8] using Eastern Cooperative Oncology Group physicians show that most cancer pain is undertreated by these specialists. Moreover, minority and elderly patients were at an even greater risk of experiencing unrelieved pain.

Barriers to Cancer Pain Control

In 1992, the American Cancer Society Advisory Group on Cancer Pain Relief concluded that three major barriers to effective cancer pain treatment exist and must be eliminated: physician barriers, patient barriers, and regulatory barriers.

Physician Barriers

Widespread misconceptions and knowledge deficits still exist among physicians and other health care professionals regarding the effective methods of treating cancer pain. Fundamental to the problem is the physician's and health professional's inability to quickly recognize and adequately assess pain in cancer patients. Studies by Grossman[9] demonstrated that physicians and nurses significantly underestimate the intensity of a patient's pain.

This knowledge deficit is being corrected by professional schools that are starting to educate their students about pain assessment and treatment. The American Society of Clinical Oncologists and the Society of Surgical Oncology have also implemented mandatory training programs in cancer pain assessment and treatment. The Agency for Health Care Policy and Research has published[10] and distributed cancer pain guidelines for use by all professionals.

Patient Barriers

Many patients are reluctant to report pain because they fear that the pain means the tumor has spread, they do not want to distract oncologists from finding a cure, and they worry about becoming addicted to the drugs used to alleviate pain. Moreover, family members often share the same feelings about opioid use and dependency.

These shocking facts indicate that widespread community programs educating patients and families about the myths and benefits of opioid analgesic therapy are essential for correcting this problem. Patients should be taught to evaluate their own pain intensity so they can take medications on a regular basis to prevent the onset of severe pain.

Regulatory Barriers

Most state laws make writing a prescription for opioids difficult for physicians by imposing many restrictions. The use of cumbersome triplicate forms, limited 15- to 30-day supplies, and laws that can lead to indictment of physicians for prescription abuse have largely deterred most primary care physicians from effectively titrating opioids to decrease pain. Instead, the patients are undermedicated or, if fortunate, referred to a pain clinic for pain relief.

The state governments must work in conjunction

with the medical societies to rewrite these laws so that cancer patients' suffering can be decreased by effective prescription-writing practices.

Pathophysiology of Cancer Pain

Causes of Cancer Pain

There are essentially five different causes of pain in cancer patients: acute cancer-related pain, chronic cancer-related pain, chronic pain unrelated to the cancer per se, pain in opioid-tolerant patients, and combinations of these causes seen in terminally ill patients (Table 42–1).

Several classic studies estimated the type of cancer pain seen in pain clinics.[3, 5, 11] Approximately 60% to 80% of all patients have tumor-related pain, 20% to 30% have treatment-related pain, and 10% to 15% have pain unrelated to the cancer. Twycross and Fairfield[5] found that about 80% of the cancer patients coming to their clinic had two or more anatomically distinct pain sites, and one third had four or more pain sites.

Classification of Cancer Pain

When cancer pain is classified, two components must be considered: pain duration and pain quality. Pain duration denotes the degree of chronicity. The three temporal conditions are acute pain, chronic pain, and incidental pain (joint pain, arthralgias) that occurs when moving. A pathophysiologic component is also described: somatic (nociceptive) pain, visceral pain, and neuropathic pain.

Somatic Pain

Somatic pain results from the activation of nociceptors in peripheral or deep tissues. The C and A-δ fibers transmit the pain sensation from the periphery to the dorsal horn and eventually cephalad through the spinothalamic tract to various parts of the midbrain and neocortex. The quality of this pain is described as a well-localized aching or gnawing pain. Bone pain and postsurgical pain are common causes of this condition.

Visceral Pain

When visceral structures are stretched, compressed, invaded, or distended, a poorly localized noxious pain is reported. Patients often describe the pain as deep, squeezing, crampy, and colic in nature. Referred pain, such as shoulder complaints when the diaphragm is invaded with liver tumor, and nausea and vomiting are common associated conditions. Pancreatic and colon carcinomas may produce this condition.

Neuropathic Pain

Direct injury to neural tissue from tumor infiltration or erosion or from cancer therapies can result in a noxious, intractable condition. Associated sensory, motor, and autonomic deficits can accompany the symptoms of burning, squeezing, and paroxysmal sharp pain. Examples of this pain include brachial and lumbar plexopathies and post-thoracotomy pain syndrome. A high incidence of patient suffering is associated with neuropathic pain.

Cancer Pain Syndromes

Although it is desirable for the clinician to classify pain according to its onset, duration, and nature, cancer pain often is experienced as several different types of pain. During the course of the disease, the pain may change as the result of tumor progression or regression after treatment. These changes may occur rapidly and illustrate the dynamic nature of cancer pain.

Acute Pain

Pain is often the presenting symptom of a patient with cancer. If it occurs early in the disease, patients may endure high levels of pain in the expectation that adequate anticancer therapy will relieve their symptoms. If it occurs late in the course, pain may signify disease recurrence, which is associated with significant anxiety, apprehension, and suffering. At this stage, acute pain may result from direct tumor involvement such as bony metastasis or may be visceral in nature.

Pain also is associated with diagnostic procedures such as blood sampling, lumbar puncture, bone marrow biopsy, angiography, and endoscopy. Many patients undergo surgery for tissue diagnosis or for removal of the tumor; such procedures can involve wideranging dissection and hence profound acute pain. Postoperative pain can occur later in the course of the disease as the result of surgery for tumor recurrence and may be complicated in patients in whom tolerance to opioids has developed. The different types of acute

Table 42–1 Types of Pain Experienced by Cancer Patients

Acute cancer-related pain
    Tumor spread
    Chemotherapy, radiotherapy, or surgery
    Debilitating effects of chronic illness
Chronic cancer-related pain
    Tumor destruction
    Cancer therapies
    Paraneoplastic pain
Pain unrelated to cancer
    Acute injury pain
    Disease-related pain
    Chronic pain not due to malignancy
Pain in opioid-tolerant cancer patients
    Current and previous drug addicts
    Patients taking opioids daily for several months
    Previous drug addict receiving methadone
Terminal illness pain
    Acute pain related to cachectic state
    Chronic pain
    Continuous acute pain associated with tumor progression

cancer pain syndromes are listed in Table 42–2, as described by Cherny and Portenoy.[12]

Anticancer therapy is frequently associated with painful sequelae such as skin burns, mucositis, pharyngitis, esophagitis, or proctitis after radiation therapy. Similarly, with drug chemotherapy, some patients experience mucositis, myalgias, gastrointestinal distension, or local irritation from tissue extravasation of the agent. Treatment-induced acute pain occasionally progresses to chronic pain. Usually, acute pain is self-limiting and is most effectively treated with opioid analgesics and nonsteroidal anti-inflammatory drugs (NSAIDs).

Chronic Pain Related to Cancer

The distinction between acute and chronic pain is often equivocal. If the acute cancer pain does not subside with initial therapy, patients experience pain of a more constant nature, the characteristics of which vary with the cause and the involved sites. An accurate diagnosis is essential to providing appropriate treatment. Chronic cancer pain syndromes, as described by Cherny and Portenoy,[12] are listed in Table 42–3.

Table 42–2 Acute Cancer Pain Syndromes

Diagnostic and therapeutic interventions
    Lumbar puncture headache
    Arterial or venous blood sampling
    Bone marrow biopsy
    Lumbar puncture
Postoperative
Therapeutic interventions
    Pleurodesis
    Tumor embolization
Analgesic techniques
    Injection pain
    Spinal opioid hyperalgesia syndrome
    Epidural injection pain
Anticancer therapies
Chemotherapy infusion techniques
    Intravenous infusion pain
        Venous spasm
        Chemical phlebitis
        Vesicant extravasation
        Anthracycline-associated flare reaction
    Hepatic artery infusion pain
    Intraperitoneal chemotherapy abdominal pain
Chemotherapy toxicity
    Mucositis
    Corticosteroid-induced perineal discomfort
    Painful peripheral neuropathy
    Diffuse bone pain from *trans*-retinoic acid or colony-stimulating factors
Hormonal therapy
    Luteinizing hormone–releasing factor tumor flare in prostate cancer
    Hormone-induced acute pain flare in breast cancer
Radiation therapy
    Incident pains
    Oropharyngeal mucositis
    Acute radiation enteritis and proctocolitis
Infection
    Acute herpetic neuralgia

Adapted from Cherny NI, Portenoy RK: The management of cancer pain. CA Cancer J Clin 1994; 44: 262–303.

Chronic pain related to cancer can be considered according to the following categories.

Tumor-Induced Pain

The nature and severity of pain caused by tumor growth depends on the structures that are involved. It may occur at the site of the primary tumor, occur at a site of metastasis, or be referred to a distant site (e.g., pain from a spinal tumor).

Somatic pain from invasion of bone is the most common cause of cancer pain.[5, 13] It is usually constant, with a gradual increase in intensity. The most common sites of metastasis are the spine, base of the skull, pelvis, and long bones, and multiple sites may exist. Metastases to vertebral bodies cause a dull and aching pain that, if located in the lumbar area, is exacerbated by lying or sitting and often relieved by standing. Associated radicular pain or other neurologic signs such as weakness or numbness often accompany the pain. In the sacral area, bowel and bladder dysfunction often occur. It is essential to make an accurate and early diagnosis to minimize permanent neurologic deficit.

Computed tomographic or magnetic resonance imaging studies are more accurate than bone scans or radiographs in demonstrating bone metastases that produce neurologic dysfunction. Tumor invasion of abdominal and pelvic organs manifests as visceral pain that is diffuse, poorly localized, and referred to dermatomes supplied by the corresponding spinal cord segments (e.g., midline thoracic back pain in pancreas cancer). Tumors often grow into a hollow viscus, causing obstruction, or may directly affect viscera such as liver, pancreas, spleen, and kidney, resulting in organ dysfunction. Pain therefore arises as a result of distension and stretching of the fascia or by direct tumor infiltration. Pain occurs frequently in pancreatic cancer but largely depends on the location of the tumor in that organ. In one series,[14] 72% of patients with tumors in the head of the pancreas had pain, compared with 87% of patients with tumors in the body or tail. However, pain in the latter group is more likely to occur late in the disease.

Tumor compression or infiltration of peripheral nerves frequently causes early pain[15] that is constant, burning and hyperpathic, hypoesthetic, or dysesthetic in the area of sensory loss. This syndrome, when associated with tumor infiltration of the brachial plexus, is called the Pancoast syndrome. Pain often arises initially in the shoulder and posterior arm in the distribution of C-8 to T-1 dermatomes. As it becomes progressively more severe, the pain extends to the medial part of the arm and hand. An associated Horner syndrome indicates the involvement of the sympathetic chain in the paravertebral space.[2] The features of causalgia with associated vasomotor changes occasionally develop.

In patients with urinary, colonic, or gynecologic malignancies, lumbosacral plexus involvement produces pain in the anterior thigh or groin if the upper plexus is involved (L-1 to L-3) or pain from the posterior part of the leg to the heel if the lower plexus is involved (L-5 to S-1).[15] Perianal sensory loss associated with

Table 42–3 Chronic Cancer Pain Syndromes

TUMOR-RELATED PAIN SYNDROMES	CANCER THERAPY–RELATED PAIN SYNDROMES
Bone pain	Postchemotherapy pain syndromes
Multifocal or generalized bone pain	Chronic painful peripheral neuropathy
Multiple bony metastases	Avascular necrosis of femoral or humeral head
Marrow expansion	Plexopathy associated with intra-arterial infusion
Vertebral syndromes	Chronic pain associated with hormonal therapy
Atlantoaxial destruction and odontoid fractures	Gynecomastia with hormonal therapy for prostate cancer
C-7 to T-11 syndrome	Chronic postsurgical pain syndromes
T-12 to L-1 syndrome	Postmastectomy pain syndrome
Sacral syndrome	Post–radical neck dissection pain
Back pain and epidural compression	Post-thoracotomy pain
Pain syndromes of the bony pelvis and hip	Postoperative frozen shoulder
Headache and facial pain	Phantom pain syndromes
Intracerebral tumor	Stump pain
Leptomeningeal metastases	Postsurgical pelvic floor myalgia
Base of skull metastases	Chronic postradiation pain syndromes
Painful cranial neuralgias	Plexopathies
Tumor involvement of the peripheral nervous system	Chronic radiation myelopathy
Tumor-related radiculopathy	Chronic radiation enteritis and proctitis
Postherpetic neuralgia	Burning perineum syndrome
Cervical plexopathy	Osteoradionecrosis
Brachial plexopathy	
Malignant lumbosacral plexopathy	
Tumor-related mononeuropathy	
Paraneoplastic painful peripheral neuropathy	
Pain syndromes of the viscera and miscellaneous tumor-related syndromes	
Hepatic distension syndrome	
Midline retroperitoneal syndrome	
Chronic intestinal obstruction	
Peritoneal carcinomatosis	
Malignant perineal pain	
Ureteric obstruction	
Paraneoplastic nociceptive pain syndrome	
Tumor-related gynecomastia	

Adapted from Cherny NI, Portenoy RK: The management of cancer pain. CA Cancer J Clin 1994; 44: 262–303.

dull, aching, midline pelvic pain indicates sacral plexus involvement.

Chemotherapy-Induced Pain

Several of the commonly used chemotherapy agents occasionally result in the development of chronic pain problems (see Table 42–3). The *Vinca* alkaloids in therapeutic doses can cause peripheral neuropathy.[16] This condition usually manifests as a dysesthesia of the hands and feet characterized by burning pain and is often associated with symmetric paresthesias.

Corticosteroid use is associated with a condition called steroid pseudorheumatism, which is seen on withdrawal of the medication[16]; the features include pain and tenderness in muscles and joints. Aseptic necrosis of bone, usually in the head of the femur or humerus, is also a side effect of chronic steroid use when pain precedes radiologic changes.

Mucositis occurs after certain chemotherapeutic agents, including cyclophosphamide, and after radiation therapy. The severity of this oral pain may make swallowing extremely difficult, and the patient requires parenteral fluid support and analgesics.

Radiation Therapy–Induced Pain

Irradiation, often used as a therapeutic modality for pain, can also be the primary therapeutic intervention for certain tumor types or as an adjuvant to surgery or chemotherapy. However, pain problems, which may be short term or delayed, occasionally arise after irradiation. Occasionally, they develop as chronic and intractable pain syndromes. Determinants of toxicity include the total dose (in Gray units) delivered, whether fractionation was used, prior irradiation and chemotherapy, concurrent infection, and the underlying tissue vascularization.[17]

The early problems result from painful mucosal thinning or ulceration and include oral mucositis, esophagitis, and perineal pain. Injury to the small intestine causes cramping and abdominal distension, with the possible later development of fistulae.[18] Myelopathy resulting from damage to the spinal cord may be transient, with the onset delayed up to 4 months after irradiation and perhaps regressing in 2 to 36 weeks. If progressive, the myelopathy begins 5 to 13 months after irradiation. Pain, an early symptom in 15% of patients,[13] is localized to the area of damage, referred with associated muscle weakness and painful dysesthesias,[16] or it rarely progresses to complete transverse myelopathy.

Fibrosis of a neural plexus may pose a difficult diagnostic problem, because it can mimic the presentation of a recurrent tumor. The most commonly involved nerves are those of the limbs and brachial plexus and, in these regions, pain is seen as early as 6 months or as delayed as 20 years after therapy. A previous history of radiation treatment with local skin changes, lymphedema of the limb, or evidence of radiation necrosis of bone without documented tumor recurrence aids in the diagnosis. Although rare, painful tumors can develop at the site of irradiation as late as 20 years after therapy. These are peripheral nerve tumors that produce burning, aching pain in the distribution of the involved nerve. When these tumors are surgically extirpated, a painful phantom syndrome usually develops.

Postsurgical Pain Syndromes

Pain After Thoracotomy. After thoracotomy, pain develops in the distribution of the intercostal nerves in a small number of patients as a result of partial or complete injury.[19] Pain most often develops 1 to 2 months after operation and is described as constant in the area of sensory loss, with occasional lancinating pain. This may be accompanied by dysesthesia at the scar and hyperesthesia in the surrounding area. Movement tends to exacerbate the pain, often resulting in a frozen shoulder because of decreased joint motion. Other sequelae include disuse atrophy of the arm or, rarely, reflex sympathetic dystrophy.

Pain After Mastectomy. Patients who have undergone radical mastectomy may have pain develop in the posterior part of the arm, axilla, and anterior chest wall as a result of damage to the intercostobrachial nerve.[19] Pain typically develops 1 to 2 months after the operation and is tight, constricting, and burning in nature. Patients tend to keep the arm in a flexed position close to the chest wall, because movement exacerbates the pain, and a frozen shoulder may develop from reduced joint motion.

Pain After Radical Neck Dissection. Pain can arise as a result of surgical intervention, including radical neck dissection. This pain is characterized as being constant, with dysesthesia and shock-like sensation as a result of interruption of the cervical plexus nerves.

Phantom Limb Pain. Phantom limb pain occurs in a significant number of patients after amputation of limbs and usually has a burning and cramping sensation in the area of the original limb. It can easily be differentiated from stump pain, which occurs at the site of the amputation, and can be elicited by palpation or percussion of the stump area.

Pain Unrelated to Cancer

Approximately 3% of the pain syndromes that occur in cancer patients have no relation to the underlying cancer or cancer treatment.[13] Most commonly, pain is caused by degenerative disk disease, arthritis, or migraine and has often been present before the diagnosis of cancer. In these patients, pain does not necessarily signify recurrent disease or metastases. However, a chronic illness behavior has already developed in many of these patients, and they require careful assessment and early psychologic intervention.

Cancer Pain and Opioid-Tolerant Patients

Opioid-tolerant pain patients are a challenging group for physicians. They may have used opioids illicitly in the past but are no longer using them. Many have a reluctance to take opioids for their cancer pain owing to a concern about the addiction potential and a fear of returning to a lifestyle that was so difficult to leave. These patients require support and an understanding of the necessity to treat the pain. The liberal use of adjuvant therapies, allowing decreased opioid doses, is also beneficial.

Some patients remain actively involved in illicit drug use, making it difficult to evaluate and treat them. The diagnosis of cancer and pain may lead them to increase their drug use in an attempt to manage their anxiety and depression. Their complaints are often misinterpreted as a request for more drugs, and they are best managed where pain and rehabilitation specialists can provide appropriate and adequate therapy. These patients may sell part of their prescriptions and seek additional pills.

Cancer pain that develops in patients who have been taking opioids for other medical conditions requires higher doses of opioids.[20] In these cases, the use of adjuvants and early intervention with block techniques or the use of more potent opioid-receptor agonists may avoid dose escalation without good pain control.[21]

Cancer Pain Therapy

This section is devoted to pharmacologic and invasive therapies. A patient with cancer pain requires a comprehensive assessment before an effective therapeutic approach can be devised. In most cases, pain can be adequately relieved by the administration of one of these therapies and by adopting a multidisciplinary approach to supportive care.

Oral and Parenteral Analgesia

Pharmacotherapy is the most widely used method of pain control. The three categories of analgesic medications that are commonly available are NSAIDs, opioid analgesics, and adjuvant agents. The analgesic ladder (Fig. 42–1) was originally developed by the Cancer Relief Program of the World Health Organization[22] and has become a widely accepted method of drug selection. The initial approach for patients with mild to moderate pain is to use an NSAID, with addition of an adjuvant agent if indicated. If this does not provide adequate relief or if the pain increases or is severe on presentation, an opioid should be instituted, with or without an NSAID or adjuvant drug.

Nonsteroidal Anti-inflammatory Drugs

The peripheral effects of an NSAID are thought to result from inhibition of the enzyme cyclooxygenase, decreasing tissue levels of prostaglandins, which are

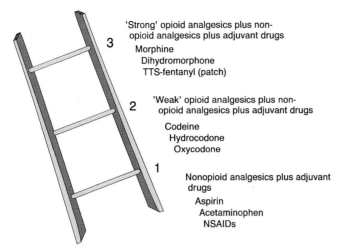

'Strong' opioid analgesics plus nonopioid analgesics plus adjuvant drugs

3 Morphine
Dihydromorphone
TTS-fentanyl (patch)

'Weak' opioid analgesics plus nonopioid analgesics plus adjuvant drugs

2 Codeine
Hydrocodone
Oxycodone

Nonopioid analgesics plus adjuvant
drugs

1 Aspirin
Acetaminophen
NSAIDs

Figure 42–1 Three-step ladder oral analgesic program for managing cancer pain. NSAIDs, nonsteroidal anti-inflammatory drugs; TTS, transdermal therapeutic system. (Modified, by permission, from Cancer Pain Relief and Palliative Care: Report of WHO Expert Committee. Geneva, World Health Organization, Technical Report Series, no. 804, 1990.)

the inflammatory mediators that sensitize peripheral nociceptors.[23] They have an anti-inflammatory action and a possible inhibitory effect on bone tumor growth by the inhibition of prostaglandin E_2 release. They may also have a centrally mediated analgesic effect.[24]

Acetaminophen has an analgesic effect by inhibiting nitric oxide synthetase, an action that is centrally and spinally mediated[25] and similar in efficacy to aspirin. It is often classified as an NSAID but has little peripheral anti-inflammatory action.

The NSAIDs possess a therapeutic ceiling dose above which further dose increments provide little analgesia. Toxicity, however, increases with increasing doses and includes nausea, gastritis, and platelet dysfunction. NSAIDs should therefore be used with caution in patients with peptic ulcer disease or a bleeding tendency.

The efficacy of NSAIDs in cancer pain can usually be evaluated after 1 week, when doses may be increased if a response has occurred. However, if there is no initial response, it is worthwhile switching to a different chemical formulation of NSAID. There may also be an advantage to using a nonacetylated salicylate if nausea develops, because these drugs appear to cause minimal gastrointestinal irritation and interference with platelet function. Table 42–4 lists the NSAIDs most frequently used in treating cancer pain.

Opioid Analgesics

Opioid analgesics are the mainstay of therapy for cancer pain. The objective when using these drugs is to control pain while minimizing distressing side effects. The success of this therapy depends on the expertise of the prescriber, who must have a knowledge of the nuances of pharmacologic features among opioids and experience in their use to make an appropriate selection for each patient.

Agonist-antagonist analgesic drugs are not very ef-

fective in the treatment of cancer pain because of their ceiling effect of analgesia, potential to precipitate withdrawal, and associated psychotropic side effects. The pure opioid agonists are used almost exclusively, and it is customary to prescribe for patients with moderate pain one of the weak opioids from the second rung of the analgesic ladder. These drugs include codeine, oxycodone, and hydrocodeine, and they are usually available in combination with acetaminophen or aspirin. Because of their nonopioid analgesic component, escalation of dosage is restricted to about 4 to 5 g of NSAID daily to prevent renal or hepatic dysfunction.

The availability of oxycodone alone, which is equipotent to morphine when given orally, also makes it a strong opioid. It is possible to titrate the dosage of oxycodone without restriction to treat more intense pain.

Patients who do not respond to weaker opioids are switched to a stronger opioid on the third rung of the ladder, most often morphine. This agent has been used extensively worldwide and has been endorsed by the World Health Organization.[22] It is also available in several formulations, therefore lending itself to administration by different routes, and as a sustained-release medication that can be administered orally two or three times daily. Because of the individual variations in response, it is worthwhile trying a different opioid, such as hydromorphone, levorphanol, or even oxycodone, if inadequate analgesia occurs with morphine. Table 42–5 provides a list of opioids used for treating cancer pain.

Meperidine is a frequently used opioid for acute pain, but it is generally not used for cancer pain. With long-term usage, the accumulation of the toxic metabolite normeperidine has been associated with central nervous system toxicity, including myoclonus, tremulousness, and seizures.[26]

When the physician selects a route for administration, factors such as gastrointestinal upset or obstruction, outpatient versus inpatient setting, and patient compliance should be addressed. The preferred and most economical route is the oral one, although some medications may be given rectally when doses by both routes are considered equivalent. Transdermal administration of fentanyl effectively bypasses the oral route. Other potential routes include subcutaneous, especially in a home or hospice setting, and intravenous, which is used frequently in hospitalized patients with severe pain who require rapid dose titration.

A widely accepted principle of effective management of cancer pain with opioids is dosage administration at fixed intervals on an around-the-clock basis; this provides sustained analgesia and avoids the peak and trough effects of medication given as needed. Additional opioids should also be available for breakthrough pain at all times during the course of treatment. Doses must be titrated to the patient's need, thereby avoiding side effects from overdosing or persistent pain from inadequate analgesia.

Adjuvant Therapy

Adjuvant medications are used in conjunction with oral or parenteral analgesics. They may have inherent

Table 42–4 Nonsteroidal Anti-Inflammatory Drugs

CLASS AND GENERIC NAME	APPROXIMATE HALF-LIFE, h	DOSING SCHEDULE	RECOMMENDED STARTING DOSE, mg/day	MAXIMUM RECOMMENDED DOSE, mg/day
p-Aminophenol derivatives				
Acetaminophen	2–4	q 4–6 h	2600	6000
Salicylates				
Acetylsalicylic acid	3–12	q 4–6 h	2600	6000
Choline magnesium trisalicylate	8–12	q 8–12 h	1500 × 1 then 500 q 12 h	4000
Salsalate	8–12	q 8–12 h	1500 × 1 then 500 q 12 h	4000
Diflunisal	8–12	q 12 h	1000 × 1 then 500 q 12 h	1500
Acetic acid derivatives				
Indomethacin	4–5	q 8–12 h	75	200
Sulindac	14	q 12 h	300	400
Tolmetin	1	q 6–8 h	600	2000
Ketorolac	4–7	q 4–6 h	120	240
Suprofen (ophth. 10 mg/mL)	2–4	q 6 h	600	600
Fenamates				
Mefenamic acid	2	q 6 h	1000	1000
Meclofenamate sodium	2–4	q 6–8 h	150	400
Proprionic acid derivatives				
Ibuprofen	3–4	q 4–8 h	1200	4200
Naproxen	13	q 12 h	500	1000
Fenoprofen	2–3	q 6 h	800	3200
Ketoprofen	2–3	q 6–8 h	150	300
Flurbiprofen	5–6	q 8–12 h	100	300
Diclofenac	2	q 6 h	75	200
Oxicam				
Piroxicam	45	q 24 h	20	40
Pyranocarboxylic acid				
Etodolac	7.3	q 4–6 h	800	1200
Naphthylalkanone				
Nabumetone	22–30	q 12–24 h	1000	2000

analgesic action, potentiate the effect of the opioid analgesics, or improve mood, sleep, nausea, anxiety, and somnolence.

The tricyclic antidepressants are known to have analgesic action, treat depression, improve sleep, and benefit patients with neuropathic pain, especially those with dysesthesias. The tertiary amines (e.g., amitriptyline, doxepin) are often the first line of therapy owing to their greater analgesic effect. If they cause excessive sedation, a secondary amine (e.g., desipramine, nortriptyline) can be used. Anticonvulsant drugs (e.g., carbamazepine, clonazepam, phenytoin) and the antispasmodic baclofen are helpful in patients with lancinating pain. Mexiletine, with action similar to a local anesthetic, is finding acceptance for use in neuropathic pain after success in the treatment of painful diabetic neuropathy.[27]

Corticosteroids are useful adjuvants; they have been shown to improve analgesia, mood, and appetite in the short term.[28] They are especially beneficial in patients with bone pain and in those with pain due to nerve trunk or spinal cord compression. Other medications that occasionally benefit patients are the benzodiazepines (anxiolytics) for patients in whom pain is accompanied by anxiety, haloperidol for the management of confusion, and phenothiazine for nausea and anxiety. A list of frequently used adjuvant drugs is provided in Table 42–6.

Table 42–5 Opioid Agonist Analgesic Drugs* for Treating Cancer Pain

DRUG	EQUIANALGESIC DOSE, mg		DURATION OF ACTION, h	COMMENT
	IM	Oral		
Morphine	10	30	3–4	
Oxycodone	15	30	2–4	
Codeine	130	200	2–4	
Hydromorphone	1.5	7.5	2–4	
Oxymorphone	1	10 (rectal)	3–4	No oral form
Levorphanol	2	4	4–8	Delayed toxicity (accumulation)
Methadone	10	20	4–8	Delayed toxicity (accumulation)

*Not recommended for cancer pain: propoxyphene, meperidine, partial opioid agonists, and opioid agonist-antagonists.
IM, intramuscular.

Table 42–6 Adjuvant Drugs

CLASS AND GENERIC NAME	DOSAGE RANGE, mg/day	COMMENTS
Antidepressants		
Amitriptyline	10–300	Burning or lancinating neuropathic pain; helpful in treating insomnia and depression
Imipramine	10–30	
Doxepin	30–300	
Desipramine	75–300	Start with lowest dose and titrate to effect
Nortriptyline	25–100	
Maprotiline	75–300	
Paroxetine	20–60	
Venlafaxine	75–225	
Anticonvulsants		
Carbamazepine	300–1600	Lancinating neuropathic pain; considered the first-line therapy
Phenytoin	300–400	
Clonazepam	2–8	
Valproate	375–3000	
Local anesthetics		
Mexiletine	300–900	Lancinating neuropathic pain refractory to other agents
Tocainide	600–1200	Safest agents compared with others in this table
Corticosteroids		
Cortisone	100–300	Neuropathic pain from nerve compression or inflammation or bone pain
Methylprednisone	10–30	
Dexamethasone	4–8	
Miscellaneous		
Baclofen	20–120	Antispasmodic, antineuropathic vasodilator for RSD pain; opioid potentiator, adrenergic agent, anxiolytic, major tranquilizer
Nifedipine	10–60	
Clonidine	0.1–0.3	
Benzodiazepines		
Phenothiazines		
Psychostimulants		
Dextroamphetamine	10–80	Enhance alertness
Methylphenidate	10–40	

RSD, reflex sympathetic dystrophy.

Transdermal Delivery

The transdermal therapeutic system with fentanyl has simplified the concept of continuous parenteral administration of opioid by a noninvasive method. This system has been beneficial in the treatment of cancer pain, with high patient preference.[29, 30] Fentanyl is the sole opioid available by this method because of its high lipid solubility. The transdermal therapeutic system with fentanyl contains a drug reservoir and rate-controlling membrane that allows fentanyl to diffuse slowly into the dermal layer, where it accumulates.

After initial application of the patch, serum levels gradually increase to peak concentration in 12 to 24 h, and effective analgesia occurs as early as 6 h.[31] The patches are marketed in 25-, 50-, 75-, and 100-μg/h dosages and are applied for 72 h. Because these dosages are additive, a patient requiring 150 μg/h of transdermal fentanyl may have two 75-μg/h patches or one 50- and one 100-μg/h patch applied. Some patients may experience 48 to 60 h of analgesia before requiring a new patch. Titration of dosage is slower than by conventional oral or parenteral routes, and breakthrough medication must be available. However, this system provides a convenient method of continuous opioid delivery, while bypassing the gastrointestinal tract.

Transdermal delivery is particularly advantageous in patients with head and neck tumors or esophageal cancer or in those with gastrointestinal involvement by tumor, vomiting, or obstruction.

Patient-Controlled Analgesia

Patient-controlled analgesia allows patients to treat their own pain by self-administering prescribed doses of opioids parenterally by using a small, sophisticated, programmable computerized pump. This technique has been widely used in the management of postoperative pain and was developed in response to the undertreatment of pain in hospitalized patients.[32] Intravenous or subcutaneous routes are used in the hospital or the home setting. The pump can be programmed to deliver a continuous infusion, in addition to which the patient can administer bolus injections at a preset dose and time interval. There appears to be no difference in the effects on respiratory function compared with other therapies.[21]

This mode of delivery is useful when the oral route is unavailable, the total dose required is excessive, benefit may be derived from providing increased patient control, and patient-controlled analgesia can provide immediate relief for breakthrough pain.[33] This method has an important application in the rapid relief and titration of dosage in patients with severe exacerbations of cancer pain and can be used in the home setting. However, with the increasing use of fentanyl patches, many patients are now able to achieve good pain control without patient-controlled analgesia, a more expensive technique in the home setting.

Neurosurgical Procedures

With the development of the multidisciplinary approach to pain management and with an increasing range of available pharmacologic agents, few patients require surgical intervention. The aim is to interrupt the nociceptive pathways in the peripheral nerves or at certain sites in the neuraxis.

The most commonly performed surgical procedure for cancer pain relief is anterolateral cordotomy, which targets the spinothalamic tract. This can be done by open technique, which has a significant morbidity; the complications include hemiparesis, urinary retention, and sexual impotence. Percutaneous cordotomy has largely replaced the open method and is usually performed during local anesthesia with fluoroscopic guidance. It is probably ineffective in neuropathic pain because of a central mechanism and has only limited use in visceral pain. Immediate complete pain relief is achieved in 60% to 80% of patients,[34] but this decreases to 40% to 50% at 6 to 12 months. Many patients in whom pain recurs also have paresthesias or dysesthesias develop.

Intraspinal Therapies

Intraspinal administration of opioids is frequently used in the treatment of pain, especially in patients whose pain is not controlled with oral medications. Opioids can be delivered by the spinal or epidural routes, and the advantages include profound analgesia, often at a much lower opioid dose without the motor, sensory, or sympathetic block associated with intraspinal local anesthetic administration.[35]

However, combinations of low-dose opioids given epidurally and a local anesthetic act synergistically to produce effective analgesia while decreasing the side effects. Opioids can be delivered by intermittent bolus injection or by continuous infusion. Morphine is the most commonly used opioid, although hydromorphone, fentanyl, sufentanil, and oxymorphone have also been successfully used.

Three systems used for chronic intraspinal opioid administration include percutaneous tunneled epidural or spinal catheters, tunneled catheters connected to subcutaneously implanted injection ports, and implanted infusion pump systems. Implantable pumps, although more convenient and less likely to cause infection, are more costly in the short term (life expectancy, 3 to 4 mo). Tolerance to chronic intraspinal administration of opioids occurs and is managed by increasing doses, changing to another opioid, or substi-

tuting local anesthetic for a short period. Other side effects include pruritus, urinary retention, somnolence, myoclonus, catheter infection, and rarely, respiratory depression.

Regional Blocks

Patients suffering from localized cancer pain, which manifests as peripheral neuralgia or visceral pain, are excellent candidates for regional block with neurolytic agents. These techniques are also appropriate in patients who are extremely ill or debilitated. Commonly used neurolytic substances are 3% to 12% phenol and 25% to 100% alcohol. These agents are thought to act by causing wallerian degeneration of the nerve fiber by means of protein denaturation and destruction of the myelin sheath.[36]

When peripheral neurolysis is indicated in the management of malignant pain, neural interruption is done proximal to the source of irritation. Because of the overlapping sensory receptive fields of peripheral nerves, blocks of neighboring segments are advised, especially in the case of intercostal nerves. A pretherapeutic diagnostic block with a local anesthetic is considered essential by many to evaluate the therapeutic effect and the impact of the resulting motor deficit. Accurate needle placement can avoid damage to adjacent structures and may be achieved easily with nerve stimulation devices or computed tomographic guidance. This is especially true for cranial and cervical nerve blocks. Transient postinjection neuritis may occur, and subsequent regeneration of peripheral nerves may be accompanied by neuritis or neuroma formation.

The sympathetic nervous system is largely responsible for visceral nociception. A diagnostic block of a sympathetic nerve plexus establishes the relative contribution of autonomic and visceral pain. It may also determine whether repeated blocks with a local anesthetic or a neurolytic agent will be beneficial.

Stellate Ganglion Block

The stellate ganglion lies anterior to the lateral process of the C-7 vertebra. Sympathetic nerve conduction to the ipsilateral head and upper extremity is interrupted by a block of this ganglion. Because of the proximity of other vital structures, many clinicians are reluctant to perform neurolytic blocks in this area. However, serial blocks with local anesthetic or neurolytic agents in dilute concentrations (3% to 6% phenol) after a diagnostic local anesthetic block have been recommended.[37] Potential complications include intravascular injection of the vertebral artery, phrenic and superior laryngeal nerve block, and rarely, intrathecal injection.[33]

Celiac Plexus Block

The celiac plexus lies on the anterolateral surface of the aorta at the T-12 to L-2 vertebral level. A block of this plexus affects visceral pain in many abdominal organs and has gained widespread acceptance for the treatment of pancreatic cancer pain. The incidence of pain relief has been reported[38] to be more than 84%, although occasionally repeat blocks are required. Possible complications include hypotension; intrathecal, epidural, or interpsoas injection; intravascular injection of the aorta or vena cava; puncture of the kidney, intestine, or lung; and paraplegia.

Hypogastric Plexus Block

The hypogastric plexus lies anterior to the body of the L-5 to S-1 vertebrae and controls sympathetic activity to the pelvis and lower limbs. A block of these nerves has been described for the treatment of pain associated with pelvic malignancy.[39, 40] Injury to sacral nerves, bladder or bowel perforation, intravascular injection, and urinary or fecal incontinence are potential complications.

Interpleural Analgesia

Another technique that deserves mention in the treatment of cancer pain is interpleural analgesia. This block has been successfully used for surgical anesthesia and in the management of some chronic states such as pancreatic pain[41] and post-thoracotomy pain syndrome.[42] It has also been used to alleviate acute exacerbations in various advanced cancer conditions.[43]

The mechanism of action of interpleural analgesia appears to be by somatic neural block, but an autonomic block has also been inferred.[41, 44] Diffusion of local anesthetic into the brachial plexus has resulted in the relief of upper extremity pain syndromes with the production of Horner's syndrome. The success of this block depends on the correct positioning of the patient such that the solution gravitates to the appropriate paravertebral area. Interpleural administration of phenol has also been used successfully in the long-term relief of cancer pain.[45]

Possible complications associated with this technique include tension pneumothorax, pleural infection, and local anesthetic systemic toxicity from rapid tissue absorption.

Diagnostic Considerations for Cancer Pain Management

Patient Assessment

The key to successful management of cancer pain involves a meticulous, thorough, and expeditious medical and psychologic assessment of cancer pain and the patient's response to it. Cherny and Portenoy[12] briefly outlined a step-wise assessment: data collection, provisional assessment, diagnostic investigations, development of a problem list, patient review of diagnoses, and institution of a multimodal therapeutic plan. Table 42–7 shows an abridged evaluation based on these six steps.

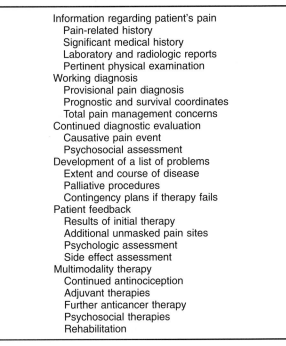

Table 42–7 Cancer Pain Assessment Steps

Information regarding patient's pain
  Pain-related history
  Significant medical history
  Laboratory and radiologic reports
  Pertinent physical examination
Working diagnosis
  Provisional pain diagnosis
  Prognostic and survival coordinates
  Total pain management concerns
Continued diagnostic evaluation
  Causative pain event
  Psychosocial assessment
Development of a list of problems
  Extent and course of disease
  Palliative procedures
  Contingency plans if therapy fails
Patient feedback
  Results of initial therapy
  Additional unmasked pain sites
  Psychologic assessment
  Side effect assessment
Multimodality therapy
  Continued antinociception
  Adjuvant therapies
  Further anticancer therapy
  Psychosocial therapies
  Rehabilitation

Practical Management Considerations

A few thoughts regarding the treatment of cancer pain patients may assist those starting cancer pain programs from repeating some early suboptimal situations.[21] The physician should determine if the prescribed therapy is compatible with the patient's home, social, and economic environments:

1. Is the patient capable of self-care?
2. Does the family support this daily care?
3. Is there a home care agency nearby that knows of this therapy and is willing to participate?
4. Are the local physicians agreeable to overseeing the primary physician's therapy?
5. Is there a 24-h hot line for pain patients having problems with the prescribed therapy?
6. Are the drugs, physical therapy, radiation therapy, or occupational therapy readily available in the patient's hometown?
7. New techniques should not be introduced for out-of-town patients.
8. New complaints of pain must be treated seriously, assuming a recurrence of disease until the possibility is eliminated.
9. The cost of therapy must be considered:
   a. Has a trial of oral or parenteral therapy been considered before invasive catheters or pumps?
   b. Were inexpensive NSAIDs used before expensive NSAIDs?
   c. Therapies requiring many return trips to the operating room should be avoided.
   d. Inclusion and exclusion criteria should be applied for the use of implantable pumps.

Conclusion

Regardless of the pain-control method selected, the most important aspect of medical care for the suffering cancer patient is reassurance that members of the pain team will work to alleviate the pain and that help will always be available for emergency intervention when acute exacerbations of chronic pain recur. Early and effective pain management and control of drug side effects greatly improve the quality of life remaining for these patients.

In the past, suffering patients asked to be put out of their misery, and the often helpless physician offered only words of comfort. Albert Schweitzer[46] called pain a ". . . more terrible lord of mankind than even death himself." Not treating patients' total pain—nociception, anger, depression, anxiety—is compelling them to select death over suffering. Physicians have the means to alleviate or eliminate approximately 95% of cancer pain for terminally ill patients. Moreover, medicine is not waiting for any scientific breakthroughs to adequately treat cancer pain. When relief from pain can be inserted into the death versus suffering option, we believe most people will choose a short-term trial of pain relief before death.

References

1. Johanson GA: Symptom character and prevalence during cancer patients' last days of life. Am J Hosp Palliat Care 1991; 8: 6–8, 18.
2. Bonica JJ, Ventafridda V, Twycross RG: Cancer pain. In Bonica JJ: The Management of Pain, 2nd ed, vol 1, pp 400–460. Philadelphia, Lea & Febiger, 1990.
3. Coyle N, Adelhardt J, Foley KM, et al: Character of terminal illness in the advanced cancer patient: pain and other symptoms during the last four weeks of life. J Pain Symptom Manage 1990; 5: 83–93.
4. Portenoy RK, Miransky J, Thaler HT, et al: Pain in ambulatory patients with lung or colon cancer. Prevalence, characteristics, and effect. Cancer 1992; 70: 1616–1624.
5. Twycross RG, Fairfield S: Pain in far-advanced cancer. Pain 1982; 14: 303–310.
6. Brescia FJ, Adler D, Gray G, et al: Hospitalized advanced cancer patients: a profile. J Pain Symptom Manage 1990; 5: 221–227.
7. Ventafridda V, Ripamonti C, De Conno F, et al: Symptom prevalence and control during cancer patients' last days of life. J Palliat Care 1990; 6: 7–11.
8. Cleeland CS, Gonin R, Hatfield AK, et al: Pain and its treatment in outpatients with metastatic cancer. N Engl J Med 1994; 330: 592–596.
9. Grossman SA: Is pain undertreated in cancer patients? Adv Oncol 1993; 9: 9–12.
10. Jacox A, Carr DB, Payne R, et al: Management of Cancer Pain. Clinical Practice Guideline No. 9. AHCPR Publication No. 94-0592. Rockville, MD, Agency for Health Care Policy and Research, U.S. Department of Health and Human Services, Public Health Service, March 1994.
11. Kanner RM, Foley KM: Patterns of narcotic drug use in a cancer pain clinic. Ann N Y Acad Sci 1981; 362: 161–172.
12. Cherny NI, Portenoy RK: The management of cancer pain. CA Cancer J Clin 1994; 44: 262–303.
13. Foley KM: Pain syndromes in patients with cancer. In Swerdlow M, Ventafridda V (eds): Cancer Pain, pp 45–54. Boston, MPT Press, 1987.
14. Buncher CR: Epidemiology of pancreatic cancer. In Moossa AR: Tumors of the Pancreas, pp 415–427. Baltimore, Williams & Wilkins, 1980.
15. Bonica JJ, Benedetti C: Management of cancer pain. In Moossa AR, Robson MC, Schimpff SC (eds): Comprehensive Textbook of Oncology, pp 443–477. Baltimore, Williams & Wilkins, 1986.
16. Payne R: Post chemotherapy and post radiation pain syndromes. In Foley KM (ed): Management of Cancer Pain. Syllabus of the Postgraduate Course of Memorial Sloan-Kettering Cancer Center, pp 73–93. New York, Memorial Sloan-Kettering Cancer Center, 1985.
17. Chapman CR: Pain related to cancer treatment. J Pain Symptom Manage 1988; 3: 188–193.
18. Palmer JJ: Radiation myelopathy. Brain 1972; 95: 109–122.
19. Kanner R: Postsurgical pain syndromes. In Foley KM (ed): Management of Cancer Pain. Syllabus of the Postgraduate Course of Memorial Sloan-Kettering Cancer Center, pp 65–72. New York, Memorial Sloan-Kettering Cancer Center, 1985.
20. de Leon-Casasola OA, Myers DP, Donaparthi S, et al: A comparison of postoperative epidural analgesia between patients with chronic cancer taking high doses of oral opioids versus opioid-naive patients. Anesth Analg 1993; 76: 302–307.
21. Lema MJ: Cancer pain management: an overview of current therapeutic regimens. Semin Anesth 1993; 12: 109–117.
22. World Health Organization: Cancer Pain Relief, pp 18–19. Geneva, Switzerland, World Health Organization, 1986.
23. Vane JR: Inhibition of prostaglandin synthesis as a mechanism of action for aspirin-like drugs. Nature New Biol 1971; 231: 232–235.
24. Willer JC, De Broucker T, Bussel B, et al: Central analgesic effect of ketoprofen in humans: electrophysiological evidence for a supraspinal mechanism in a double-blind and cross-over study. Pain 1989; 38: 1–7.
25. Piletta P, Porchet HC, Dayer P: Central analgesic effect of acetaminophen but not of aspirin. Clin Pharmacol Ther 1991; 49: 350–354.
26. Kaiko RF, Foley KM, Grabinski PY, et al: Central nervous system excitatory effects of meperidine in cancer patients. Ann Neurol 1983; 13: 180–185.
27. Dejgard A, Petersen P, Kastrup J: Mexiletine for treatment of chronic painful diabetic neuropathy. Lancet 1988; 1: 9–11.
28. Bruera E, Roca E, Cedaro L, et al: Action of oral methylprednisolone in terminal cancer patients: a prospective randomized double-blind study. Cancer Treat Rep 1985; 69: 751–754.
29. Miser AW, Narang PK, Dothage JA, et al: Transdermal fentanyl for pain control in patients with cancer. Pain 1989; 37: 15–21.
30. Maves TJ, Barcellos WA: Management of cancer pain with transdermal fentanyl: phase IV trial, University of Iowa. J Pain Symptom Manage 1992; 7(Suppl 3): S58–S62.
31. Plezia PM, Kramer TH, Linford J, et al: Transdermal fentanyl: pharmacokinetics and preliminary clinical evaluation. Pharmacotherapy 1989; 9: 2–9.
32. Burns JW, Hodsman NB, McLintock TT, et al: The influence of patient characteristics on the requirements for postoperative analgesia. A reassessment using patient-controlled analgesia. Anaesthesia 1989; 44: 2–6.
33. Ferrell BR, Nash CC, Warfield CC: The role of patient-controlled analgesia in the management of cancer pain. J Pain Symptom Manage 1992; 7: 149–154.
34. Lahuerta J, Lipton SA, Wells JCD: Percutaneous cervical cordotomy: results and complications in a recent series of 100 patients. Ann R Coll Surg Engl 1985; 67: 41–44.
35. Plummer JL, Cherry DA, Cousins MJ, et al: Long-term spinal administration of morphine in cancer and non-cancer pain: a retrospective study. Pain 1991; 44: 215–220.
36. Myers RR, Katz J: Neuropathology of neurolytic and semidestructive agents. In Cousins MJ, Bridenbaugh PO (eds): Neural Blockade in Clinical Anesthesia and Management of Pain, 2nd ed, pp 1031–1051. Philadelphia, JB Lippincott, 1988.
37. Löfström JB, Cousins MJ: Sympathetic neural blockade of upper and lower extremity. In Cousins MJ, Bridenbaugh PO (eds): Neural Blockade in Clinical Anesthesia and Management of Pain, 2nd ed, pp 461–500. Philadelphia, JB Lippincott, 1988.
38. Brown DL, Bulley CK, Quiel EL: Neurolytic celiac plexus block for pancreatic cancer pain. Anesth Analg 1987; 66: 869–873.
39. Jain S, Kestenbaum A, Shah N, et al: Hypogastric plexus block: a

new technique for treatment of perineal pain. (Abstract.) Anesth Analg 1990; 70: S175.

40. Plancarte R, Amescua C, Patt RB, et al: Superior hypogastric plexus block for pelvic cancer pain. Anesthesiology 1990; 73: 236–239.

41. Durrani Z, Winnie AP, Ikuta P: Interpleural catheter analgesia for pancreatic pain. Anesth Analg 1988; 67: 479–481.

42. Fineman SP: Long-term post-thoracotomy cancer pain management with interpleural bupivacaine. Anesth Analg 1989; 68: 694–697.

43. Myers DP, Lema MJ, de Leon-Casasola OA, et al: Interpleural analgesia for the treatment of severe cancer pain in terminally ill patients. J Pain Symptom Manage 1993; 8: 505–510.

44. Morrow JS, Squier RC: Sympathetic blockade with interpleural analgesia. (Abstract.) Anesthesiology 1989; 71: A662.

45. Lema MJ, Myers DP, De Leon-Casasola O, et al: Pleural phenol therapy for the treatment of chronic esophageal cancer pain. Reg Anesth 1992; 17: 166–170.

46. Schweitzer A: Cited in Familiar Medical Quotations. Boston, Little, Brown, 1968, p 356.

Index

Note: Page numbers in *italics* refer to illustrations; page numbers followed by (t) refer to tables.

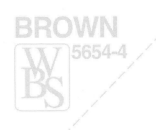

BROWN
5654-4

ISBN 0-7216-5654-4